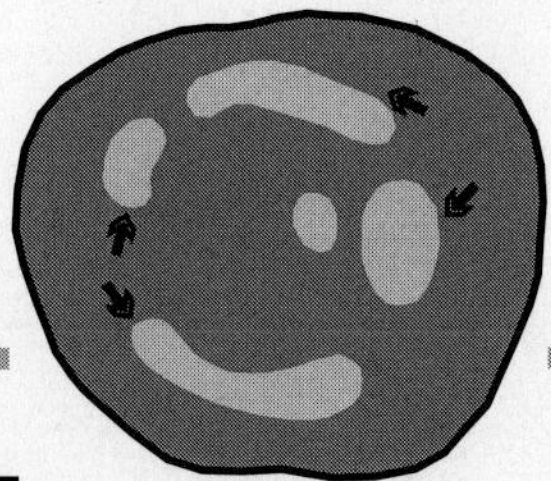

Neuro-Ophthalmology

Diagnosis and Management

GRANT T. LIU, M.D.
Associate Professor of Neurology and Ophthalmology

NICHOLAS J. VOLPE, M.D.
Associate Professor of Ophthalmology and Neurology

STEVEN L. GALETTA, M.D.
Van Meter Professor of Neurology and Ophthalmology

University of Pennsylvania School of Medicine
Hospital of the University of Pennsylvania
Scheie Eye Institute
Children's Hospital of Philadelphia
Philadelphia, Pennsylvania

W.B. SAUNDERS COMPANY
A Harcourt Health Sciences Company
Philadelphia London New York St Louis Sydney Toronto

W.B. SAUNDERS COMPANY
A Harcourt Health Sciences Company

The Curtis Center
Independence Square West
Philadelphia, Pennsylvania 19106

Library of Congress Cataloging-in-Publication Data

Liu, Grant T.

Neuro-ophthalmology / Grant T. Liu, Nicholas J. Volpe, Steven L. Galetta.—1st ed.

p. ; cm.

ISBN 0–7216–6533–0

1. Neuro-ophthalmology. I. Volpe, Nicholas J. II. Galetta, Steven L. III. Title.
[DNLM: 1. Eye Diseases. 2. Neurologic Manifestations. 3. Facial Nerve Diseases. 4.
Optic Nerve Diseases. 5. Visual Pathways—pathology. WW 460 L783n 2001]

RE725 .L58 2001
617.7′3—dc21 00-038805

Editor-in-Chief: Richard H. Lampert
Senior Editorial Assistant: Beth LoGiudice
Production Manager: Donna L. Morrissey

NEURO-OPHTHALMOLOGY
Diagnosis and Management ISBN 0–7216–6533–0

Printed in the United States of America

Last digit is the print number: 9 8 7 6 5 4 3 2 1

To Gerry, Francesca, and Genie

Foreword

It is a great joy to write in praise of the work of three talented physicians it was my privilege to teach. In this fascinating, scrupulously researched, and useful volume, they successfully summarize and organize for students and scholars the current wealth of knowledge in the field of neuro-ophthalmology. Their combined expertise in neurology and ophthalmology, and their professional training at many and diverse institutions, lend an unusually fresh perspective to the text. Special attention, for example, is paid here to the management of headaches, facial pain, and disorders of facial sensation, topics not often addressed in other texts. The anatomic approach to the afferent and efferent visual systems is given an especially clear presentation, and will be a valuable educational tool.

"Let the honor of your student," says the Talmud Torah, "be as dear to you as your own." I am proud of the small role I have played in the authors' education, and feel honored to be able to switch roles and learn from them.

Norman J. Schatz, M.D.
Key Biscayne, Florida

Preface

This book is designed for the students of neuro-ophthalmology: the practitioners, ophthalmology and neurology residents, and medical students dealing with patients with disturbances of the afferent visual pathways and efferent ocular motor systems. Although this book is not intended necessarily for the professors of neuro-ophthalmology, we hope that they will nevertheless approve of our efforts.

Our hope was to offer a book that could serve both as a guide for diagnosing and managing patients with neuro-ophthalmic problems and a one-volume textbook containing in-depth discussions of neuro-ophthalmic topics and disorders. With just three authors, our aim was to create a highly organized and uniform textbook, extensively illustrated and referenced, that would bridge the gap between neuro-ophthalmic handbooks containing tables, outlines, and flow-diagrams and neuro-ophthalmic encyclopedias.

How the Book Is Organized

The book is divided into four sections: history and examination, afferent disorders, efferent disorders, and headache. This initial grouping of the last three sections is symptom-based, and within each of those sections, the chapters then are divided neuroanatomically. Each chapter has roughly the same internal organization and starts with an introduction to the structures or disorders discussed, followed by a review of their neuroanatomy, symptoms, and signs. This is followed by a detailed discussion of the presentation, pathophysiology, diagnosis, neuroimaging and diagnostic studies, and management of the diseases which affect that structure.

Within the chapters, the liberal use of headings such as "neuro-ophthalmic manifestations" points the reader to exactly what he or she may want to know about a particular topic. The copious use of figures and tables aids the discussions, and the generous references direct those desiring to pursue a topic in greater depth. Repetition between chapters, sometimes unavoidable for the sake of completeness, was kept to a minimum by cross-referencing topics, figures, and tables. Because this is a book for clinicians, reviews of neuroanatomy and neurophysiology in most instances are based upon clinical and pathological observations in humans without extensive discussion of experimental literature involving nonhuman primates and other animals.

The first two chapters on history and examination were designed for students and residents unfamiliar with eliciting symptoms and signs in neuro-ophthalmic patients. The examination chapter also includes reviews of the neurological examination and the bedside neuro-ophthalmic evaluation of comatose patients. Often based on the history alone, the problem can be localized neuroanatomically and its etiology determined. The examination can then be used to support a suspected diagnosis and eliminate other causes.

The next section on afferent disorders discusses the diseases associated with structures responsible for transmitting and processing visual information coming from the eye. Here disorders of the retina, optic nerve, chiasm, and retrochiasmal structures, as well as disc swelling, higher cortical disorders, transient and functional visual loss, and hallucinations and illusions are discussed. Readers unfamiliar with these subjects or topical localization of visual field defects might first review Chapter 3, which contains an overview of afferent visual disorders and visual field testing.

The section on efferent disorders reviews conditions involving motor neuro-ophthalmic structures. Thus pupillary, eyelid, and facial nerve abnormalities, then eye movement and orbital disorders are discussed here. Eye movement disorders are covered in four chapters: Chapter 15 reviews causes of dysconjugate gaze including third, fourth, and sixth nerve palsies; Chapter 16 discusses abnormalities of conjugate gaze such as defective saccades and pursuit; Chapter 17 outlines conditions where the eyes move excessively as in nystagmus and nystagmoid movements; and Chapter 18 discusses eye movement and other abnormalities in orbital disorders.

Chapter 19: headache, facial pain, and disorders of facial sensation discusses topics such as migraine, cluster headache, trigeminal neuralgia, and trigeminal neuropathy.

Acknowledgments

In acknowledgment sections such as this, authors usually thank large lists of individuals who have helped them develop their careers and write their book. I am no different.

Firstly, I would also like to thank my parents for stressing and offering me an education. Martin Samuels, Dave Dawson, Michael Ronthal, Charles Barlow, Joseph Volpe, and Donald Bienfang at the Harvard Longwood Neurology Program were my teachers as a resident, and Michael Charness was the first there to encourage me to put pen to paper. I am indebted to my mentors in neuro-ophthalmology, Norman Schatz, Joel Glaser, J. Lawton Smith, and Simmons Lessell. I am fortunate to have learned from the who's who in neuro-ophthalmology.

My chairmen, Donald Silberberg, Robert Barchi, and Stuart Fine, created a clinical and academic atmosphere at the University of Pennsylvania where my practice and career could flourish. I have to thank my co-authors Steve and Nick for continuing my neuro-ophthalmic education. Steve is the best division chief that anybody could ask for, with his combination of vision, knowledge, clinical acumen, personality, guidance, and most importantly, tolerance. I have to thank the patients I have seen for allowing me to participate in their care and learn from them. My secretary Tracey Sears spent countless hours in the library retrieving hundreds of articles. I would also like to express my gratitude to Richard Lampert, our publisher at Saunders, for his advice and leeway despite missed deadlines, piecemeal chapters, and clinicians suffering from the pressures and time-demands of managed care medicine. I also have to acknowledge the help of numerous physicians who helped review chapters or sections of this book: Arthur Asburg, Shawn Bird, Elizabeth Engle, Kevin Judy, Susan Mandel, Donald Schotland, and Leslie Sutton. I would also like to thank our Biomedical Communications service for their help in preparing many of the figures.

Finally, I have to thank my children, Alessandra and Jonathan, for their patience while daddy spent hours on the computer at home writing portions of this book. However, I owe the most to my wife, Geraldine. She endured the last two years of medical school, internship, residency, fellowship, three moves along the east coast, and the promise of delayed gratification. I don't know why she puts up with a husband who attempts to juggle family, a clinical practice, an academic career, a book, and golf.

Now that "the book" is done, I am going to make that tee time with my wife, then take the kids out for ice cream.

Grant T. Liu, M.D.

My success and accomplishments would not have been possible without the support and sacrifices of many other people. My teachers and friends; Arthur Wolintz, M.D. for encouraging me, Joseph F. Rizzo, III, M.D. for lighting the fire, his neuro-ophthalmic imagination and true friendship, Simmons Lessell, M.D. my professional father and molder of clinicians, for teaching me by example, the art of neuro-ophthalmology and how to be a doctor and Stuart L. Fine, M.D. for his guidance, friendship and helping me to be the best I can be. My colleagues and comrades: Steven Galetta, M.D.; Grant Liu, M.D., Laura Balcer, M.D., and Mark Moster, M.D. from whom I continue to learn everyday. I would like to thank my colleagues at the Scheie Eye Institute and my students (past and future) who inspire me and allow me to function at the cutting edge. And finally, my family: my brothers Russell and Robert who are my best friends, my parents Nicholas and Lydia who priotized education in a nuturing environment, always give (gave) the best advice, always say (said) the right thing, my children Nicholas, Matthew, Lena, and Tessa for the joy they bring me every day, every moment as they bring things into perspective and most of all I acknowledge the love, support, companionship, sacrifice, and encouragement of my wife Francesca who makes everything I do possible.

Nicholas J. Volpe, M.D.

I would like to thank those individuals who have had a major impact in my life: My parents Louis and Winifred Galetta for their unending love. My coaches, Brother Pat Pennell, Frank McCartney, James Tuppeny, Irv Mondschein, and Bill Wagner for teaching me how to win and lose. My colleagues, Eric Raps, Robert I. Grossman, Lawrence Gray, Grant Liu, Nicholas Volpe, and Laura Balcer for their friendship and brilliance. My mentors Norman J. Schatz, Joel Glaser, J. Lawton-Smith, Donald Silberberg, Donald Gilden, and Arthur K. Asbury for teaching me with untiring enthusiasm. Finally, to my family, Genie, Kristin, Michael, and Matthew for their love and support and for making it all worthwhile.

Steven L. Galetta, M.D.

Contents

PART I

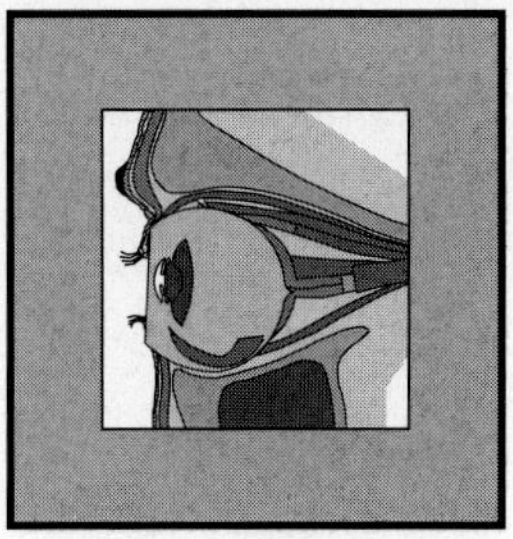

HISTORY AND EXAMINATION

CHAPTER 1

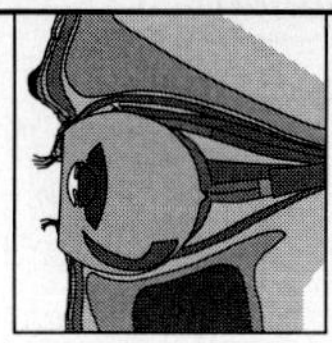

The Neuro-Ophthalmic History

As in any field of medicine, the neuro-ophthalmic history guides the physician's examination and differential diagnosis. From the beginning of the history taking, the physician should be attempting to categorize the patient's problem. Table 1–1, which mirrors the organization of this book, classifies neuro-ophthalmic disorders into three groups: afferent disorders, efferent disorders, and headache and abnormal facial sensations. It can be used as a guide in generating a differential diagnosis. Then, influenced by the patient's age, sex, underlying illnesses, and disease risk factors, the physician can narrow the list of potential diagnoses and shape the examination to confirm or eliminate each disorder.

Frequently, the correct neuro-ophthalmic disorder can be diagnosed based on the history alone. For instance, an otherwise healthy young woman with sudden vision loss in one eye with pain on eye movements probably has optic neuritis. An elderly man with hypertension, new binocular horizontal double vision worse at distance and in right gaze, and right periorbital pain most likely has a vasculopathic right sixth nerve palsy.

The various elements of the neuro-ophthalmic history (Table 1–2) will be reviewed in the context of neuro-ophthalmic disorders. Although important, topics such as physician demeanor, style, language use during history taking, the best environment for the interview, and the physician–patient relationship are beyond the scope of this chapter and are discussed eloquently in other textbooks.[1, 2]

CHIEF COMPLAINT

The patient's age should be ascertained first. Congenital neuro-ophthalmic problems are more likely to be seen in children, and degenerative and vascular disorders are seen predominantly in adults. Neoplasms occur at all ages, although the tumor types are age dependent. For instance, in children the most common causes of chiasmal compression are optic pathway tumors and craniopharyngiomas, while in adulthood, pituitary adenomas are the most likely culprit.

The patient's sex should be noted because of the predilection of some diseases for either men or women. For example, eye complications of breast cancer are obviously more prevalent in women, but optic neuritis, giant cell arteritis, and Duane's retraction syndrome are also more common in females.

Then the patient should be asked to summarize his or her complaint in one sentence. Simple statements such as "I can not see out of my left eye," "I have double vision," and "My left eyelid droops" are extremely helpful, and immediately allow the examiner to begin thinking about a differential diagnosis. However; when the complaint is a vague one such as "I haven't seen very well for 6 months," further historic investigation is necessary.

The chief complaint should be reduced to one sentence containing the patient's age, sex,

TABLE 1–1. Categorization of Neuro-ophthalmic Disorders

	Chapter
Visual loss and other disorders of the afferent visual pathway	
Visual loss: retinal disorders	4
Visual loss: optic neuropathies	5
Optic disc swelling: papilledema and other causes	6
Visual loss: chiasmal disorders	7
Visual loss: retrochiasmal disorders	8
Disorders of higher cortical visual function	9
Transient visual loss	10
Functional visual loss	11
Visual hallucinations and illusions	12
Efferent neuro-ophthalmic disorders	
Pupillary disorders	13
Eyelid and facial nerve disorders	14
Eye movement disorders: third, fourth, and sixth nerve palsies and other causes of diplopia and ocular misalignment	15
Eye movement disorders: gaze abnormalities	16
Eye movement disorders: nystagmus and nystagmoid eye movements	17
Orbital disease	18
Headache, facial pain, and disorders of facial sensation	19

These three major groups reflect the table of contents and organization of this book. During history taking, the examiner should attempt to categorize the patient's problem into one of these groups.

and complaint: "The patient is a 45-year-old woman with left facial pain," for example.

HISTORY OF PRESENT ILLNESS

The patient's chief complaint should be explored in further detail, including the temporal profile of events and any associated symptoms.

Detailing the Problem

Afferent Dysfunction. If the patient complains of visual loss, its pattern and degree should be explored to help localize the problem within the afferent visual pathway. The patient should be asked whether the right or left eye or both eyes are involved and whether the visual loss affects the nasal, temporal, superior, or inferior field of vision. Then the visual loss should be characterized according to its degree (complete blindness, grayness, or visual distortion, for example). Defects in color perception should be noted. Higher cortical visual dysfunction should be considered when the visual complaints are vague and unexplained by loss of clarity.

Efferent Dysfunction. The most common efferent neuro-ophthalmic complaint is double vision. Patients with diplopia should be asked whether their double vision is (1) binocular, (2) horizontal or vertical, and (3) worse in left-, right-, up-, or downgaze, or distance or near. Neurologic diplopia is almost always binocular, and the defective nerve or muscle can often be determined according to the direction in which the double vision is worse.

Blurred vision is a common complaint associated with refractive error, media opacity, and afferent dysfunction. However, the examiner should be aware that some patients complaining of blurred vision are actually found to have diplopia when questioned further.

Temporal Profile of Symptoms

The *chronicity, rapidity of onset,* and *pattern* of symptoms should be investigated.

Chronicity. When the symptoms first occurred should be established. This can be explored by asking, for instance, when the patient was last able to read small print. Some disorders, such as optic neuritis, usually resolve within several weeks or months. However, if visual loss has been present for several years, other diagnoses, such as a slowly growing meningioma, should be considered. Long-standing, and even intermittent, double vision implies a slowly expanding neoplasm or decompensated congenital strabismus.

Rapidity of Onset. A sudden onset of symptoms suggests a vascular process, such as a stroke. Inflammatory and infectious disorders may also present acutely. In contrast, symptoms associated with degenerative and com-

TABLE 1–2. The Neuro-ophthalmic History

Chief complaint
Age, sex, and major complaint
History of present illness
Detailing the problem
Temporal profile of symptoms
Associated symptoms
Past neurologic and ophthalmic history
Past medical and surgical history
Review of systems
Family history
Social history

pressive processes are usually more insidious, and the patient may not be able to date the exact beginning of the problem.

Pattern of Symptoms. The time course of symptoms can be extremely helpful. Progressive symptoms suggest compressive mass lesions, while those with acute onset that plateau or improve are more consistent with vascular or inflammatory processes. Episodic visual loss could be due to migraine, carotid disease, or seizures, for instance. Fluctuating ptosis or double vision that is particularly worse in the evening is highly suggestive of myasthenia gravis.

Associated Symptoms

The patient should be asked about neurologic or generalized symptoms that may not have been volunteered as related to the eye problem. For instance, headaches may be consistent with migraine, elevated intracranial pressure, and compressive mass lesions. Malaise, fevers, muscle aches, headaches, and jaw claudication indicate giant cell arteritis in an elderly patient with amaurosis fugax or frank visual loss. Pain is more typical of optic neuritis than ischemic optic neuropathy. Systemic weakness, dysphagia, and dyspnea suggest myasthenia gravis in a patient with ptosis or diplopia. On the other hand, in a patient with diplopia, dysarthria, and ataxia, a posterior fossa lesion is more likely.

PAST NEUROLOGIC AND OPHTHALMOLOGIC HISTORY

A history of any neurologic disease, such as migraines, strokes, transient ischemic attacks, head injury, or seizures, or prior neuroimaging should be investigated. Important questions regarding past ophthalmologic problems would include those concerning previous spectacle correction, cataracts, glaucoma, strabismus, amblyopia, eye patching, or surgery.

PAST MEDICAL AND SURGICAL HISTORY AND REVIEW OF SYSTEMS

Because many neuro-ophthalmic disorders are complications of underlying medical illnesses, careful exploration and documentation of the medical and surgical history and review of systems are paramount. Inquiry regarding the presence of hypertension, diabetes, coronary artery disease, arrhythmias, cardiac valvular disease, hypercholesterolemia, and peripheral vascular disease is extremely important, but any history of cancer, rheumatologic disorders, or infectious diseases may also be highly relevant.

SPECIAL CONSIDERATIONS IN CHILDREN

Diagnostic clues in children undergoing neuro-ophthalmic evaluation may be evident in the mother's pregnancy history, especially with regard to drug or alcohol exposure, viral illnesses, or change in fetal movements. Details of the birth, including length of gestation, birth weight, Apgar scores, and presence of perinatal difficulties, should be noted. A developmental history, with particular attention to milestones achieved in cognitive, motor, and language function, should be taken as well. Loss of milestones suggests a degenerative disorder, while developmental delay with slow achievement of milestones suggests a static encephalopathy due to hypoxemia, for instance.

FAMILY HISTORY

The history of any neurologic, ophthalmologic, or medical illnesses in related family members should be documented. In addition, many neuro-ophthalmic disorders, such as migraine, multiple sclerosis, and Leber's hereditary optic neuropathy, have a genetic predisposition, and so their presence in any relatives would strongly suggest their consideration.

SOCIAL HISTORY

Certain behaviors, such as illicit drug use, smoking, and alcohol consumption, may be important predisposing factors for neuro-ophthalmic disorders. For example, smoking is a risk factor for vascular disease, while alcohol may be associated with optic neuropathy.

Because occupational exposures also may be relevant, the examiner should inquire about the patient's job. Knowing the patient's occupation is also important in understanding how the patient's neuro-ophthalmic problem affects his or her everyday life. For instance, a dentist may be devastated by monocular visual loss and the subsequent inability to appreciate objects stereoscopically. On the other hand, an airline reservation agent, whose job likely does not require binocular vision, may not be affected as severely by a similar injury.

REFERENCES

1. Bates B: Interviewing and the health history. In: A Guide to Physical Examination, pp 1–27. Philadelphia, JB Lippincott, 1983.
2. DeGowin RL: The medical history. In: DeGowin & DeGowin's Bedside Diagnostic Examination, pp 14–35. New York, Macmillan Publishing Co, 1987.

CHAPTER 2

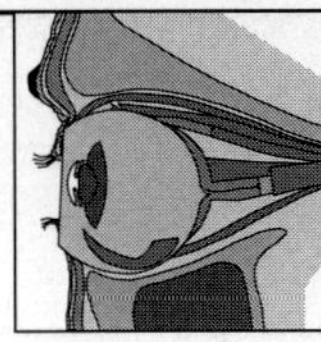

The Neuro-Ophthalmic Examination

The neuro-ophthalmic examination combines ophthalmic and neurologic techniques to assess the patient's vision, pupillary function, ocular motility, eyelids, orbits, funduscopic appearance, and neurologic status. In most cases, after obtaining the history, the examiner should have already formed an opinion regarding the possible localization and differential diagnosis. The examination then either supports or refutes these initial impressions; exam findings may also prompt consideration of other diagnoses.

In this chapter, the major elements of the neuro-ophthalmic examination (Table 2–1) will be reviewed, and in each section, processes that affect them will be mentioned briefly. The neuro-ophthalmic examination in comatose patients will also be reviewed. The reader should then refer to the appropriate chapters for more detailed differential diagnoses and discussions of the pathologic disorders.

AFFERENT VISUAL FUNCTION

Measurement of afferent visual function establishes many different aspects of how well the patient sees. Normal vision depends on an intact afferent visual pathway. Important functions to assess include visual acuity, color vision, and visual fields. The examiner must keep in mind that these are inherently subjective measurements and depend heavily on the patient's level of cooperation and effort.

Visual Acuity

Visual acuity is a measurement of the individual's capacity for visual discrimination of fine details of high contrast.[1] Best corrected visual acuity should be tested for each eye. Distance vision is assessed with a standard Snellen chart (Fig. 2–1A); and near vision, with a hand-held card (Fig. 2–1B). Ideally, best corrected vision should be assessed using current corrective lenses or manifest refraction. If these are unavailable, a pinhole will improve most mild to moderate refractive errors in cooperative patients. When acuity can not be corrected by a pinhole, nonrefractive causes of visual loss (see below) should be considered.

Acuity is most often recorded as *a fraction* (eg, 20/40), where the numerator refers to the distance (in feet) from which the patient sees the letters; and the denominator, the distance from which a patient with normal vision sees the same letters.[2] The normal eye can resolve a figure that subtends a visual angle of 5 minutes at a distance of 20 feet. At the distance at which a normal patient can see a line of letters on a Snellen eye chart, the widths of the lines on each letter subtend a visual angle of 1 minute, or one-fifth of the entire letter. 20/20−2 indicates the patient saw all the letters on the 20/20 line except two, while 20/20+2 means the patient was able to see the 20/20 letters plus two letters on the next (20/15) line. Visual acuity with the near card is often recorded using the standard Jaeger notation (J1, J3,

TABLE 2–1. Neuro-ophthalmic Examination

Afferent visual function
Visual acuity
Contrast sensitivity (optional)
Color perception
Confrontation visual fields
Amsler grid testing
Higher cortical visual function (optional)
Efferent system
Pupils
Size
Reactivity
Swinging flashlight test
Accommodation (optional)
Eyelids
Facial nerve function
Ocular motility
Inspection
Ductions
Vergences
Assessment of ocular misalignment
Slit-lamp examination/applanation tensions
Funduscopic examination
Directed neurologic examination
Mental status
Cranial nerves
Motor function
Cerebellar function
Sensation
Gait
Reflexes
Directed general examination

etc). Near acuities are not as accurate as those obtained at distance, especially when the card is not held at the requisite 14 inches. Most normal adults under age 40 have best corrected visual acuities of 20/20 or better in each eye.

If a patient is unable to read the largest Snellen letters (20/200 or 20/400), the acuity should be recorded by moving a 200-size letter toward the patient until it is seen (Fig. 2–2). That distance is recorded as the numerator. For example, an acuity of 4/200 means the patient was able to see the 200-size letter at 4 feet. Alternatively, the degree of vision can be recorded using the phrases "count fingers" (CF) (and at what distance), "detect hand motions" (HM), and "have light perception" (LP). An eye that is blind has "no light perception" (NLP).

In illiterate individuals or children unable to read letters, acuity can be tested with HOTV letters (Fig. 2–3), tumbling E's (Fig. 2–4), or Allen figures[3] (Fig. 2–5). In younger preverbal patients, assessment of fixing and following in most instances is sufficient. Caution should be applied when examining small infants, since visual fixation normally may be inconsistent or absent until 8 to 16 weeks of age.[4] When more precise documentation of visual acuities is required (for serial examinations, for instance), preferential looking tests (Teller acuities) may be used (Fig. 2–6).[5–8] These tests are based on the principle that a child would rather look at objects with a pattern stimulus (alternating black and white lines of specific widths) than at a homogeneous field. The smallest pattern that the child seems to prefer is an indicator of best visual acuity ("grating acuity"), which can be recorded in Snellen equivalents. Visual acuity in a newborn is roughly 20/400 to 20/600, improves to approximately 20/60 by 12 months of age, and then reaches the 20/20 level by 3 to 5 years of age.[9]

Ocular causes of reduced visual acuity include refractive error, amblyopia, macular lesion, or media opacity such as cataract, vitritis, or keratopathy. Neuro-ophthalmic processes that can decrease visual acuity are those that affect the optic nerve or chiasm. Disturbances that are posterior to the chiasm (retrochiasmal, ie, tract, optic radiations, and occipital lobe) affect visual acuity only if they are bilateral.[10]

Contrast Sensitivity

Contrast sensitivity testing with sine-wave or square-wave gratings may be a useful adjunct in the evaluation of visual acuity.[11] Conventional visual acuity measures spatial resolution at high contrast, while contrast sensitivity testing assesses spatial resolution when contrast varies. In one variation of the test, the patient is asked to identify in which direction the gratings, which span a spectrum of spatial and temporal frequencies and are arranged in increasing difficulty, are oriented. Another version, the Pelli–Robson test, is depicted in Figure 2–7. Contrast sensitivity testing should never replace acuity assessment, as its role seems limited to those situations where acuity is normal or near normal and further evaluation is desired.[12, 13] Optic neuropathies as well as media opacities and macular disease may reduce contrast sensitivity.

Color Perception

Color vision can be tested with standard pseudoisochromatic Ishihara or Hardy–Rand–

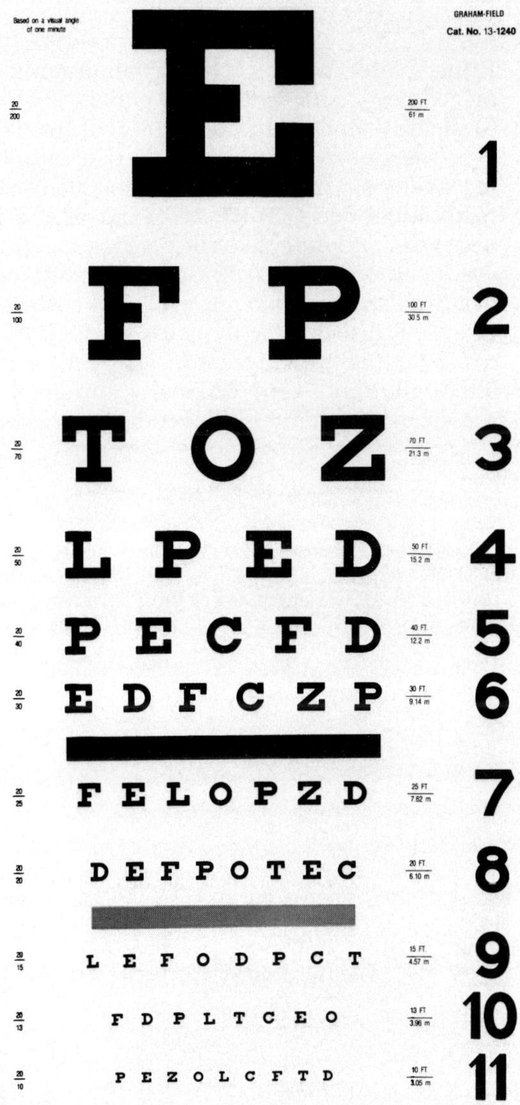

A

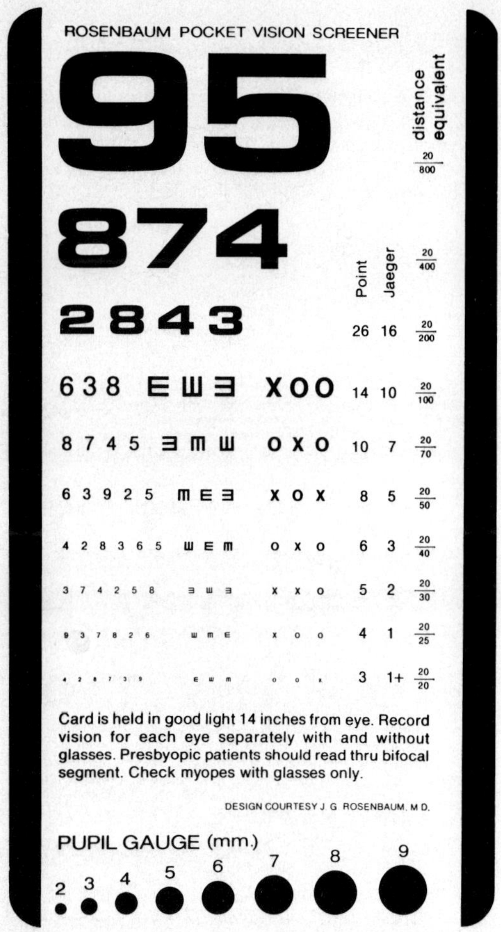

B

FIGURE 2–1. A. Snellen eye chart for testing visual acuity. The largest letter at the top is the 20/200 E, while the letters at the bottom represent the 20/10 line. **B.** Near card with pupil gauge. Note that near visual acuity is often recorded using the Jaeger notation, as in "Jaeger 2" or "J2" to indicate 20/30 near acuity.

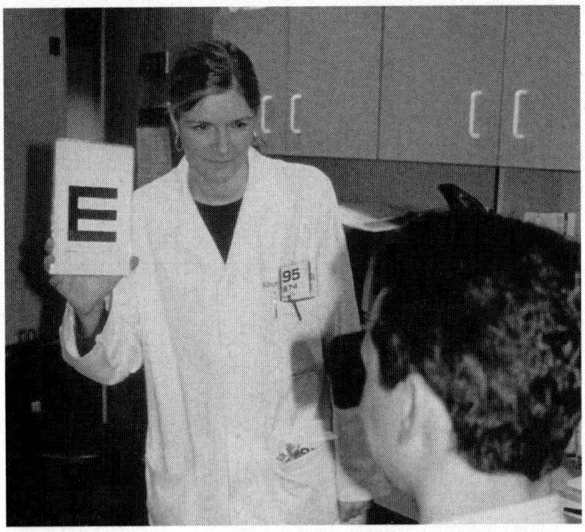

FIGURE 2–2. Determination of visual acuity using 200-size letters in an eye with worse than 20/200 but better than hand motions vision. The distance at which the patient can see the 20/200 E is determined. If this distance is three feet, then the visual acuity is recorded as "3/200."

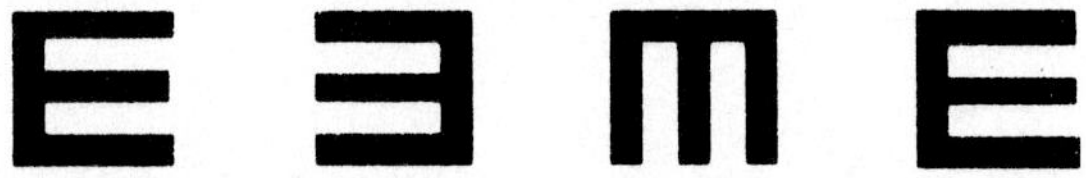

FIGURE 2–4. "Tumbling E's" for assessment of visual acuity in illiterate children. The child can be asked to indicate in which direction the E points (up, down, left, or right). The sizes of the E's correlate with the Snellen scale.

Rittler plates, both of which contain numbers or geometric shapes that the patient is asked to identify among different-colored dots (Fig. 2–8; see Color Plates 1 and 2). The result is recorded as a fraction of the color plates correctly identified ("8/10" or "8 out of 10," for instance), and defective color vision is termed *dyschromatopsia*. Their wide availability, ease of administration, and relatively low cost make the pseudoisochromatic plates a popular tool for detecting dyschromatopsias of all types, although they were originally designed to screen for congenital dyschromatopsias. Ishi-

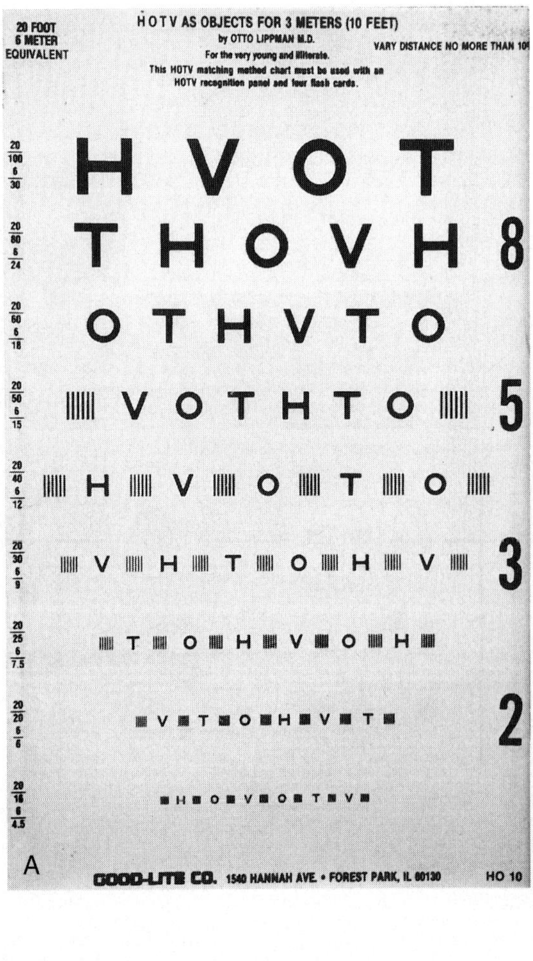

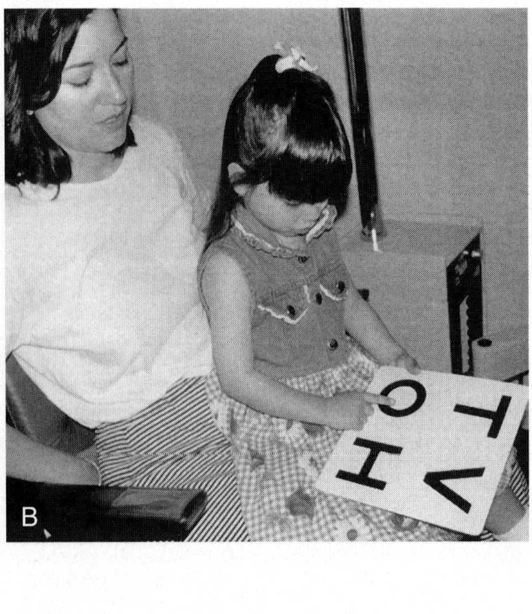

FIGURE 2–3. Determination of visual acuity using HOTV letters in a young child. **A.** The child is presented Snellen-like HOTV letters, and on this chart an examiner can point to the letter to be identified by the child. **B.** While the other eye patched, the child is asked to match the indicated letter on the chart with a hand-held card displaying the HOTV letters.

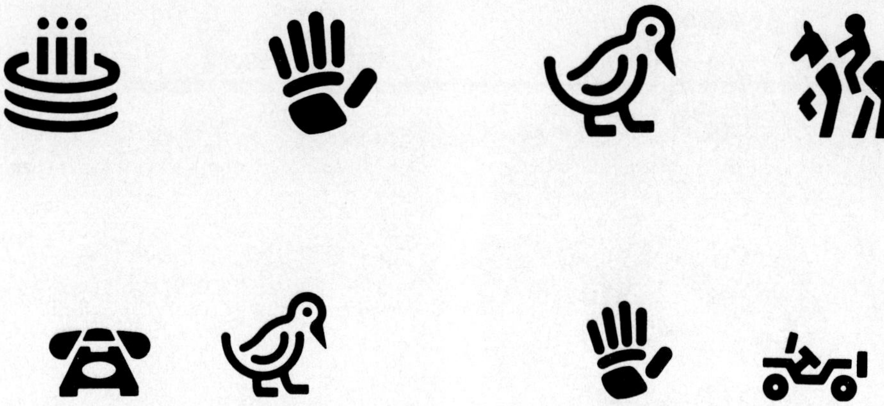

FIGURE 2–5. Allen figures for verbal but illiterate children. The child is asked to identify pictures drawn with high-contrast lines. The sizes of the pictures correlate with the Snellen scale.

hara color plates may be used, but Hardy–Rand–Rittler plates, which contain blue and purple figures, may be more helpful in detecting acquired dyschromatopsias due to optic neuropathy.[14]

Comparing the appearance of a red bottle top, for example, with each eye can test for qualitative intereye differences in color perception. A patient with monocular "red desaturation" may state that with the affected eye

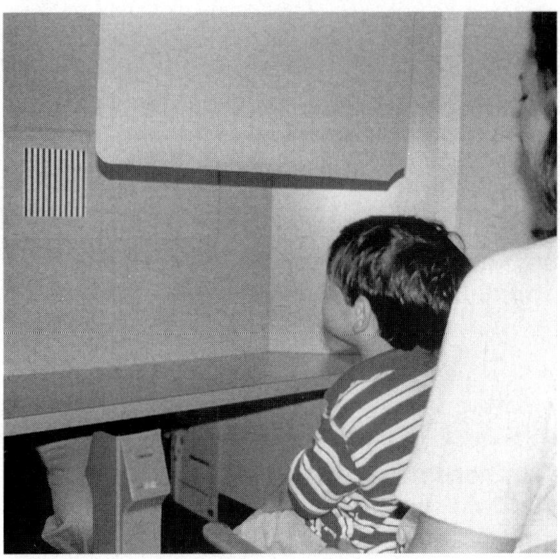

FIGURE 2–6. Teller acuity testing. Also known as a *preferential looking test,* the test is best used in infants and young children unable to identify the Allen figures. The child is held on the parent's lap, and the parent's eyes are shielded from the stimuli to prevent any influence upon the child. Gratings of various thicknesses are presented either to the child's right or left, and the examiner, who is behind the targets and looks through a peephole, records whether the child looked at the targets. The test assumes that a child would rather look at a pattern stimulus than a homogenous field.[6] The acuity is determined when the child has no visual preference and appears no longer to discern the stripes. Stripe thickness is measured in arcmins, and the results can be converted to Snellen equivalents.

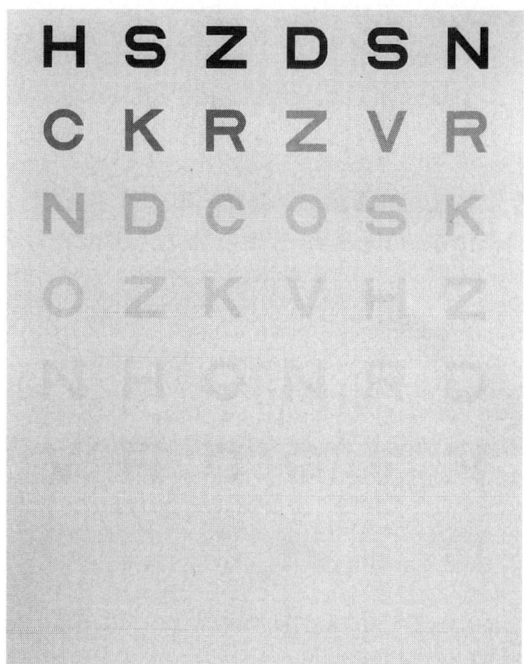

FIGURE 2–7. Contrast sensitivity. In this version, the Pelli–Robson test, each eye is evaluated separately, and the patient is asked to identify the letters across each row, starting at the top of the chart. The level of contrast sensitivity, recorded in log units, is determined when the patient reaches a group of three letters he or she can not identify.

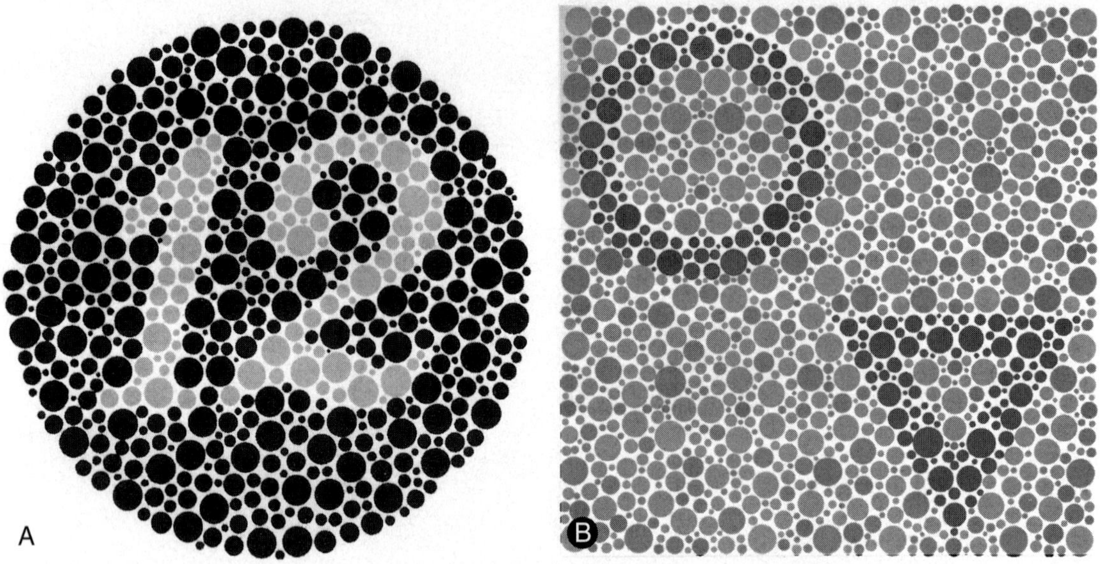

FIGURE 2–8. Pseudoisochromatic color plates. Each eye is tested separately. **A.** In standard pseudoisochromatic color plate testing, the patient is asked to identify the number seen within the colored dots. (*See Color Plate* 1.) **B.** Hardy–Rand–Rittler color plate. In this test, the patient is asked to identify the shape or symbol seen within the dots. (*See Color Plate* 2.)

the red bottle top appeared "washed out," "pink," or "orange."

Congenital dyschromatopsias are characterized by confusion between reds and greens (protan and deutan types) and blues and yellows (tritan type). They result from relative deficiencies in the red, green, and blue cone pigments. Congenital dyschromatopsias occur in approximately 8% to 9% of males[15] and slightly less than 1% of the females,[16] and they are typically symmetric, binocular, and stable.[17] The Farnsworth D-15 (dichotomous) panel test (Fig. 2–9; see Color Plate 3) or the larger Farnsworth–Munsell 100-hue test can be used to separate the various types. In both of these tests, patients are asked to arrange colored caps in linear sequence relative to reference caps. The D-15 is shorter and less cumbersome than the 100-hue test and can be performed quickly in the office with the proper lighting conditions.

Acquired dyschromatopsia may result from macular, retinal, optic nerve, or chiasmal lesions. Monocular acuity loss, deficits in color vision, and a relative afferent pupillary defect (see below) are highly characteristic of an ipsilateral optic neuropathy. Acquired optic nerve diseases typically produce a red/green color deficiency, but there are several notable exceptions, such as glaucoma.[17] Dyschromatopsias occurring in the setting of retinal disease, such as cone dystrophies, Stargardt disease, and toxic retinopathies, are usually associated with pigment migration or visible disturbances of the retinal pigment epithelium on funduscopic examination. Color vision loss combined with only mildly reduced acuity would be more suggestive of an optic neuropathy, while color deficits due to macular disease tend to associate with more severe acuity loss. Retrochiasmal disturbances can produce abnormal color vision in the defective visual field. An inferior occipital lobe lesion involving the lingual and fusiform gyri can cause defective color vision in the contralateral hemifield (see Chapter 9).[18]

Confrontation Visual Field Assessment

Testing the patient's visual fields can be accomplished at the bedside by finger confrontation methods in all four quadrants of each eye by asking the patient to fix on the examiner's nose then to "count the fingers" (Fig. 2–10A). Because of the over-representation of central vision in the nervous system, assessment of each quadrant within the central 10 degrees is more important than that of the periphery. One eye at a time is tested while the patient focuses on the examiner's nose. Sometimes, a visual field defect is best elicited

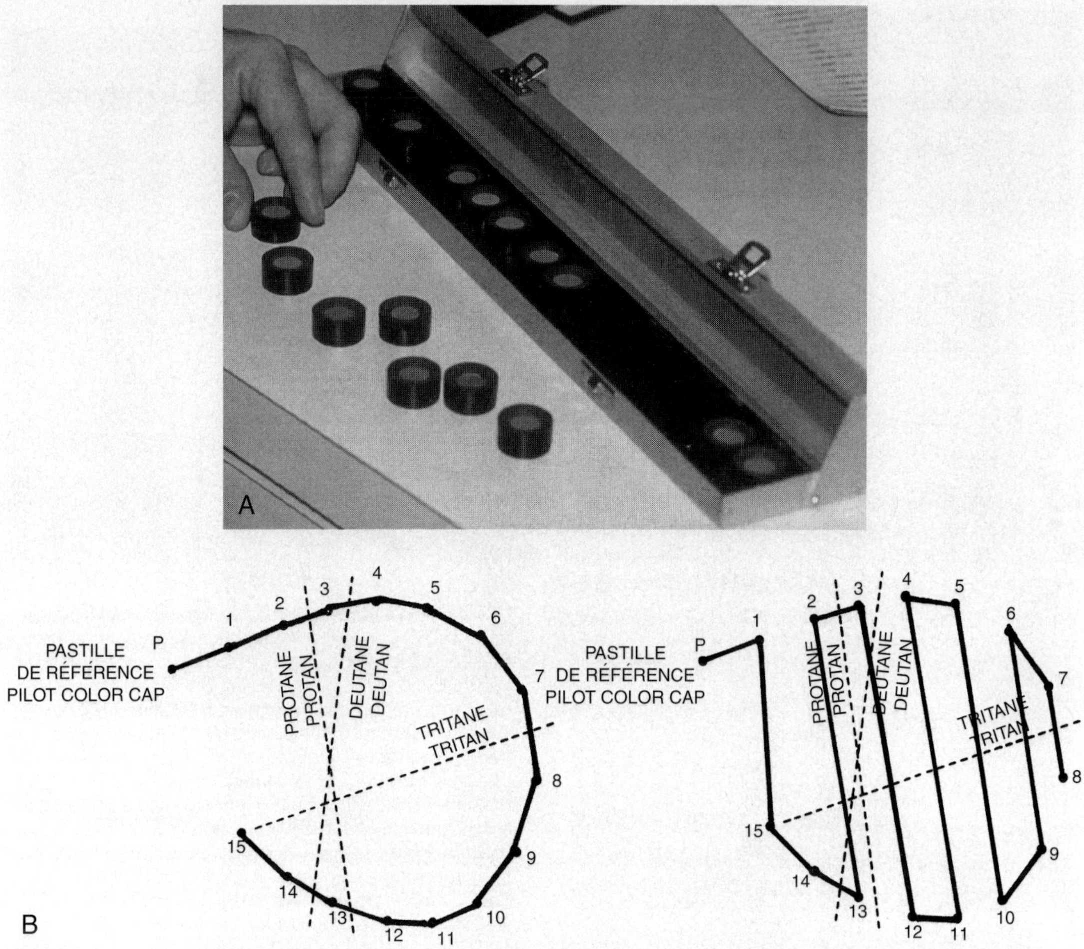

FIGURE 2–9. **A.** Farnsworth D-15 color test. The patient is asked to arrange colored discs in order of color similarity, starting with a reference disc (*See Color Plate* 3.) Again, each eye is tested separately. **B.** Each disc is numbered, and the results are recorded by connecting the numbers in the order in which the patient arranged the discs. Protanopes, deutanopes, and tritanopes tend to arrange them in incorrect but characteristic, easily identifiable patterns along one of three axes. A normal response is given on the left, while a protanope's response is depicted on the right.

by asking the patient if all parts of the examiner's face can be seen clearly: "Are the examiner's eyes equally clear?" If the patient does not see the nose clearly, a central scotoma should be suspected. Alternatively, the examiner can hold a finger over his nose and another finger a few degrees off center. If the patient sees the eccentric finger more clearly than the central one, again a central scotoma should be suspected. Testing of two separate quadrants of one eye enhances the yield of finding a field defect. Moving stimuli are almost always appreciated better than static ones, so the latter are preferable when screening for subtle field defects. Detection of finger wiggling is not as sensitive as finger counting, especially when the patient is asked to count fingers that are presented rapidly.

Color or subjective hand comparison is a useful adjunct to elicit defects respecting the vertical or horizontal meridians (Fig. 2–10B). Caution should be applied in patients with visual inattention or neglect, as they may exhibit a field defect during double simultaneous stimulation. However, these patients will exhibit no field defect when stimulated with single targets.

In a patient who is aphasic, uncooperative, intubated, sedated, or very young, responses such as finger mimicry, pointing to targets presented, visual tracking, or reflex blink to visual threat allow for a gross appraisal of visual field

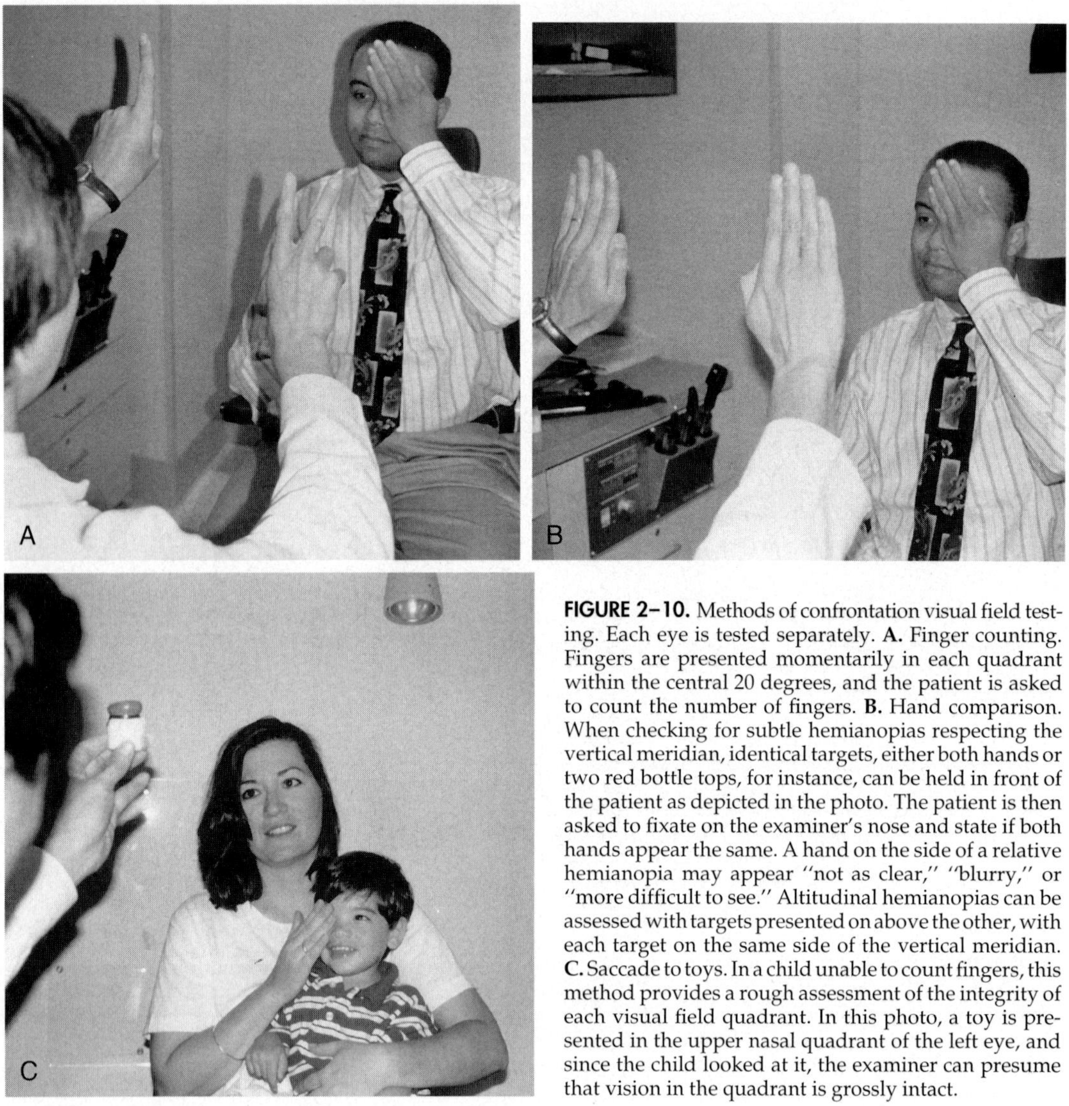

FIGURE 2–10. Methods of confrontation visual field testing. Each eye is tested separately. **A.** Finger counting. Fingers are presented momentarily in each quadrant within the central 20 degrees, and the patient is asked to count the number of fingers. **B.** Hand comparison. When checking for subtle hemianopias respecting the vertical meridian, identical targets, either both hands or two red bottle tops, for instance, can be held in front of the patient as depicted in the photo. The patient is then asked to fixate on the examiner's nose and state if both hands appear the same. A hand on the side of a relative hemianopia may appear "not as clear," "blurry," or "more difficult to see." Altitudinal hemianopias can be assessed with targets presented on above the other, with each target on the same side of the vertical meridian. **C.** Saccade to toys. In a child unable to count fingers, this method provides a rough assessment of the integrity of each visual field quadrant. In this photo, a toy is presented in the upper nasal quadrant of the left eye, and since the child looked at it, the examiner can presume that vision in the quadrant is grossly intact.

integrity. If the patient saccades to a visual stimulus in a given quadrant, the visual field in that area can be considered relatively intact (Fig. 2–10C). However, an absent reflex blink to visual threat, which depends on the intactness of the afferent visual pathway, including the occipital lobe, can be misleading. The reflex may be absent in very young normal infants and patients with Balint syndrome or neglect from right frontal and parietal lesions (see Chapter 9).[19] Care also should be taken so that the visual threat, usually a menacing hand gesture, does not move air onto the eye and elicit a corneal blink reflex (see below).

The results of confrontation visual field testing can be recorded in the chart within two circles. By convention, the visual field of the patient's right eye is drawn within the circle on the right, and the left eye's visual field in the circle on the left. Furthermore, the field is diagrammed from the patient's perspective. In Figure 2–11, examples of documentation of normal and abnormal confrontation fields are given. Because confrontation techniques produce only a gross estimation of the visual fields, more precise documentation requires a tangent screen, Goldmann perimeter, or automated threshold perimetry. These tests and their interpretation are discussed in great detail in Chapter 3.

The visual field can be altered by lesions anywhere in the afferent visual pathway; the

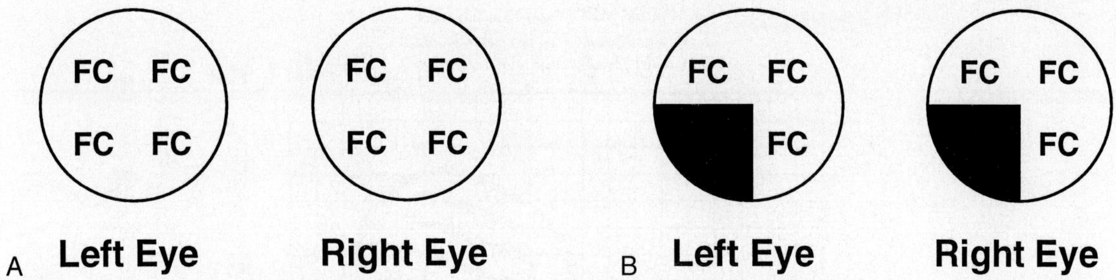

FIGURE 2–11. Schematic documentation of confrontation visual assessment. FC = finger counting. The fields are represented from the patient's point of view, and the right eye vision is recorded on the right, and the left eye vision on the left. **A.** Normal confrontational visual fields. The patient is able to count fingers in all four quadrants. **B.** Left lower quadrantanopsia. The defective field is documented by black, and the patient is able to count fingers in all other quadrants.

specific patterns of field loss and their relationship to neuroanatomic structures are also discussed in more detail in Chapter 3.

Amsler Grid Testing

To test central or macular vision, an Amsler grid (Fig. 2–12) (similar to a piece of graph paper with a central fixation point) can be viewed by the patient at near. The patient fixates on the central dot and is asked whether all the lines are straight and whether any parts are missing or blurry.

They may perceive abnormal areas on the grid that might correspond with visual field deficits. Amsler grid testing is particularly helpful in detecting central and paracentral field defects. Maculopathies typically produce a distortion in the grid pattern (*metamorphopsia*). The results of Amsler grid testing can be documented with a convention similar to that of confrontation visual field testing.

Photostress Test

Also not part of the routine neuro-ophthalmic examination, the photostress test has been advocated as a method of distinguishing retinal (macular) from optic nerve causes of visual loss.[20] After best corrected visual acuity is assessed, a bright light is shined into one eye for 10 seconds while the other eye is covered; a penlight, halogen transilluminator, or indirect ophthalmoscope held 2 to 3 cm from the eye can be used. The test should be performed with undilated pupils. Once the light is removed, acuity is retested continuously until the patient can read three letters on the Snellen line just larger than the baseline acuity (ie, 20/25 vs 20/20). The time to recovery is recorded, then the procedure is repeated with the other eye. Photostress recovery time is 27 seconds for normal eyes.[21] Optic neuropathies tend not to produce prolonged photostress recovery times, while macular disorders, such as macular edema, central serous retinopathy, and macular degeneration, may be associated with recovery times of several minutes.[21–23] The photostress recovery time is believed to be related to the amount of photopigment bleached by the light stimulus and the ability of rod and cone photoreceptors to convert photopigment back to the unbleached state.[24]

Higher Cortical Visual Function

Examination of visual attention, object recognition, and reading ability are important in patients with visual complaints unexplained by acuity or field loss. These functions and their neuroanatomic localization are discussed in greater detail in Chapter 9.

It is often difficult to separate a dense left hemianopia from dense neglect in a patient with a large right parietal lesion. In instances where the deficits are more subtle, the examiner can screen for visual inattention by presenting visual stimuli, such as fingers, separately in each hemifield, then together on both sides of midline (double simultaneous visual stimulation—similar to hand comparison (see Fig. 2–10B).[25] Individuals with subtle visual inattention but intact fields will see both stimuli when they are presented separately but may not see one of them when they are shown

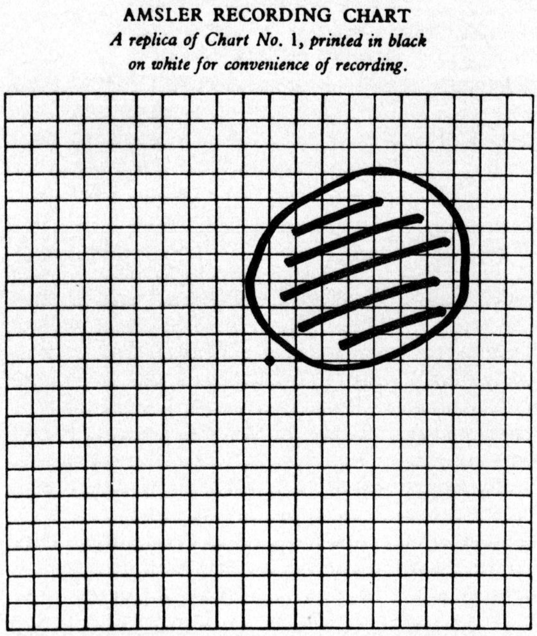

FIGURE 2–12. Amsler grid in a patient with central serous chorioretinopathy involving the macula inferiorly in the left eye. With the right eye covered, the patient was asked to look at the central dot and was asked if any of the lines were missing or wavy. She indicated the shaded area was blurry and distorted.

simultaneously. Other bedside tests include letter cancellation, in which the patient is asked to find a specific letter or shape within a random array.[26] Patients with left visual neglect may find the specified letter only when it appears on the right side of the page (Fig. 2–13A). The line cancellation test, in which the individual is asked to cross lines drawn in various locations at different angles throughout the page,[27] is similar. When patients with left neglect are asked to bisect a horizontal line, they may tend to "bisect" the lines to the right of the true center (Fig. 2–13B). Finally, when patients with left neglect are asked to copy a figure (a cube, flower, or Rey–Osterrieth complex figure, for example), they may incompletely or inaccurately copy the left side of the drawing.[28]

In patients suspected of visual agnosias, informal tests of visual recognition can be performed at the bedside using common objects such as a pen, cup, or book and asking the patient to name them.[29] An inability to recognize faces (*prosopagnosia*) can be tested with magazine or newspaper photos containing famous faces. Standardized facial and object recognition tasks are available during more formal neuropsychological testing. An inability to interpret complex scenes (*simultanagnosia*) can be tested with magazine pictures containing several elements or with a letter made up of smaller elements (Fig. 2–14). Simultanagnosia may be evident when the patient is tested with Ishihara color plates and is able to recognize the colors and trace the digits but is unable to recognize the number represented among the dots.[30]

Central achromatopsia, or difficulty perceiving colors because of a cortical lesion, may be detected by having the patient sort isoluminent threads or discs. The Farnsworth–Munsell 100-hue test may also be used for this purpose.

Errors in figure or clock drawing or copying are often nonspecific. However, these tasks sometimes can provide useful information, especially in patients with hemifield loss or hemineglect. When asked to copy a drawing, an individual with a hemianopia may duplicate only half of the figure (Fig. 2–15), while one with left hemineglect may show evidence of visuospatial difficulty. In a more difficult task, when the patient is asked to draw a clock face, visuospatial abnormalities associated with right parietal lesions may be more pronounced (Fig. 2–16). In a cautionary note, a normally drawn clock face does not exclude left unilat-

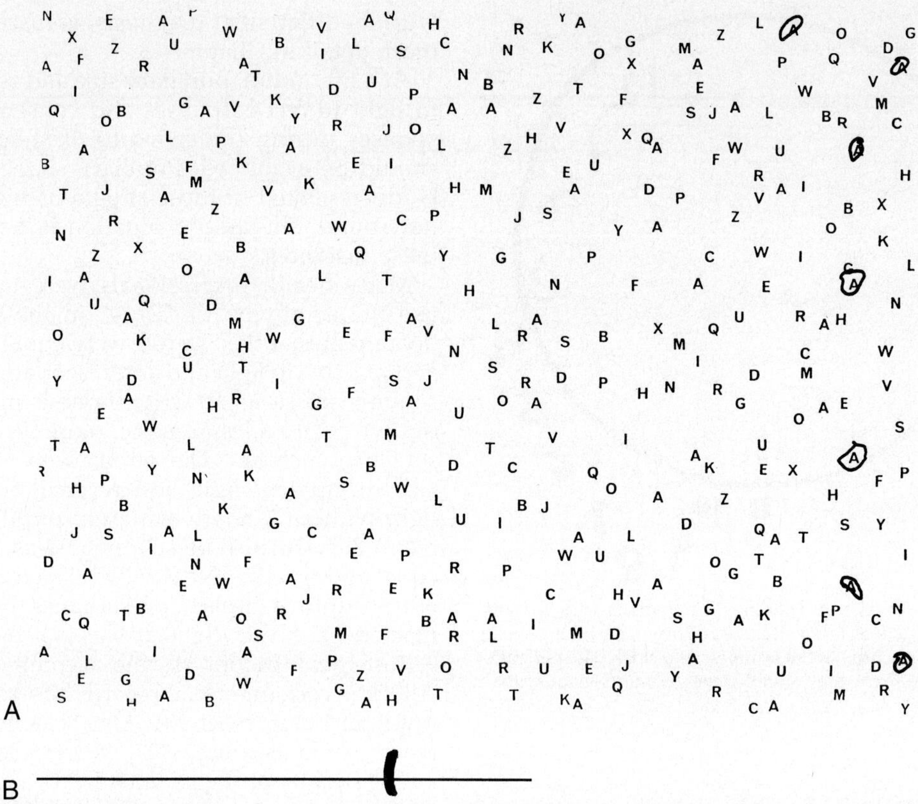

FIGURE 2–13. **A.** Letter cancellation. Patients are asked to identify the A's within the random array. This patient with severe left neglect found only those A's along the very right hand side of the page. (From Liu GT, Bolton AK, Price BH, Weintraub S: Dissociated perceptual-sensory and exploratory-motor neglect. J Neurol Neurosurg Psychiatr 1992;55:701-726, with permission.) **B.** Line bisection. Patients are asked to bisect a horizontal line. This patient with left neglect incorrectly thought the middle of the line was off to the right.

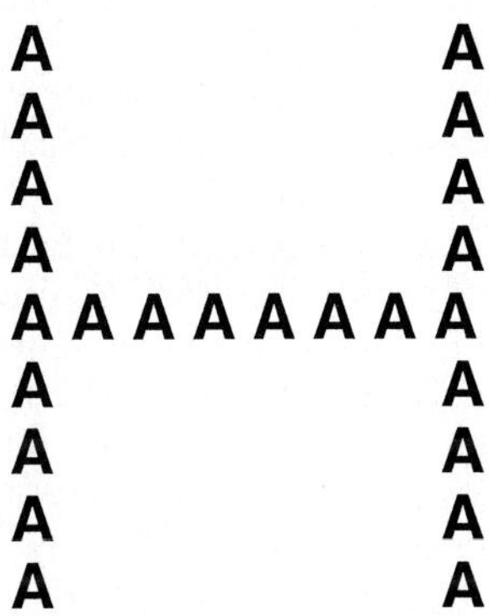

FIGURE 2–14. Simultanagnosia. The letter H is drawn by arranging multiple A's. A patient with simultanagnosia might be able to identify the A's but will not realize that the smaller elements together make an H.

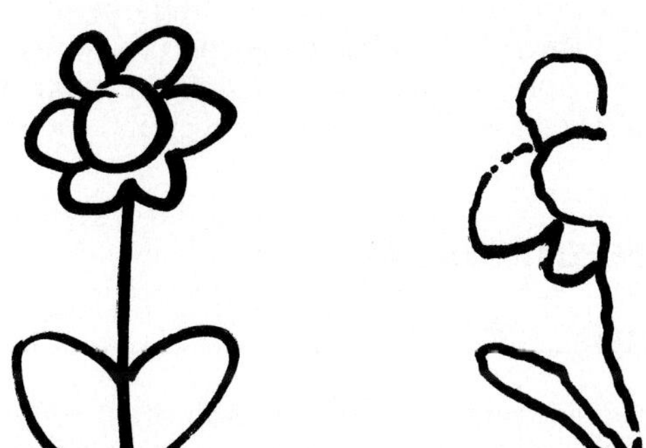

FIGURE 2–15. Copying a drawing. A flower was drawn by the examiner (*left*), and a patient with a right homonymous hemianopia was asked to copy it. The patient's drawing (*right*) included only elements from the left side of the figure.

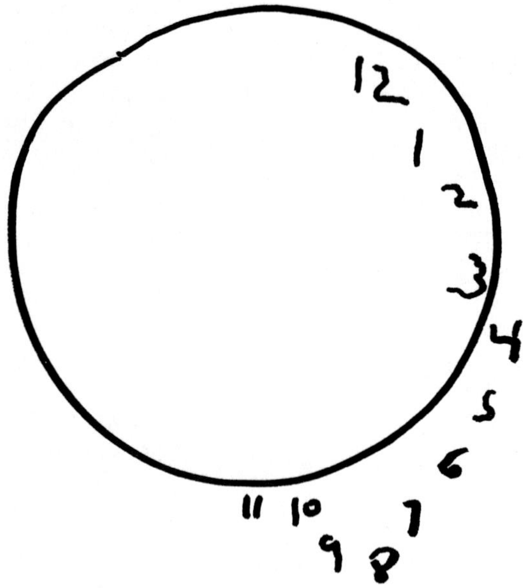

FIGURE 2–16. Clock drawing in a patient with a right parietal lesion. A large circle was drawn, and the patient was asked to draw in the numbers of a clock. The patient's response reflects the left-sided neglect and visuospatial difficulties.

eral spatial neglect.[31] The task can be performed with or without a predrawn circle, but if a circle is provided, the examiner should make sure it is large enough (2 or 3 inches in diameter) to make the test a useful one for evaluating visuospatial function. Interested readers are referred to the informative, detailed analysis of clock drawing by Freedman et al.[32]

The ability to read should be tested along with all the other main components of language function (see Mental Status Examination, below). An individual who can not read but is able to write (*alexia without agraphia*) likely has a lesion in the left occipital lobe.

EFFERENT SYSTEM

Pupils

Although pupillary dysfunction often reflects a lesion in the efferent parasympathetic pupillary pathway, abnormal pupillary reactivity also may be a sign of disorders affecting the afferent visual pathway. Some pupillary abnormalities are mentioned below in the context of the pupillary examination, but each, along with its differential diagnosis, is discussed in more detail in Chapter 13.

At a minimum, pupillary size and reactivity to light (direct responses and consensual responses during the swinging flashlight test) should be evaluated. Pupillary shape should be documented in those situations when it is not round; slit-lamp evaluation is helpful in these instances.

Many health professionals were taught to use the acronym "PERRLA" in the chart to document that the "pupils were equal, round, and reactive to light and accommodation." Acronyms are easier to write if one is in a rush, but we prefer a less generic, more descriptive sentence such as "The pupils were equal in size in ambient light and reacted briskly to light without a relative afferent pupillary defect." This can also be abbreviated as "Pupils: equal and reactive. No RAPD." The roundness of the pupils is implied, and because the pupils reacted briskly to light, it was not necessary to test their reaction during accommodation. Alternatively, one could record the size of each pupil and their reactivity. One scale for pupil reactivity is as follows: 3+ = brisk reaction, 2+ = slightly sluggish, and 1+ = very sluggish. Descriptions such as "brisk," "sluggish," or "unreactive" can also be used.

Pupillary Size. Pupillary size can be measured using the pupil gauge available on most near acuity cards (see Fig. 2–1B).[63] Usually the two pupils are equal in size, and each is located slightly nasal and inferior to the center of the cornea. Transient fluctuations in pupillary diameter are normal and are termed *hippus*. In infancy the pupils are usually small (2 to 3 mm), but they widen as the child grows older and achieve their largest sizes in adolescence. In adulthood they then become progressively more miotic.[33]

The term *anisocoria* refers to asymmetric pupillary sizes; in cases of anisocoria the amount of pupillary inequality in ambient light and dark should be compared. In the most common type of anisocoria, physiologic or essential, pupillary function is normal and the relative inequality is the same in light and dark. Long-standing pupillary inequality can be confirmed by viewing old photographs with the magnification of a slit lamp or 20-diopter lens.

Pathologic anisocoria suggests dysfunction in the efferent part of the pupillary pathway. Afferent pupillary dysfunction, due to optic nerve disease, for instance, does not produce anisocoria. In general, anisocoria greater in light implies the larger pupil has a parasympathetic abnormality, while anisocoria more prominent in the dark suggests the smaller pupil has oculosympathetic dysfunction (Horner syndrome). In the latter situation, the pupil will redilate slowly (dilation lag) when compared with the other pupil when the lights are turned down. To assess dilation lag, the examiner shines a dim light from below the patient's nose to provide minimal illumination before turning the room lights off. The size and speed of dilation are assessed for the first 5 seconds after the patient is placed in the dark. During this time, dilation lag should be maximal. Often the sympathetically denervated pupils will begin to catch up in size over the next 10 seconds of observation.

Light Reactivity—Direct and Consensual. Pupillary light reactivity (constriction) should be tested with a bright light such as a halogen transilluminator or indirect ophthalmoscope while the patient views a distant target (to prevent convergence-induced miosis) (Fig. 2–17) in a dimly lit room. We agree with Thompson et al[34] that "it is not necessary for the room to be as dark as a coal cellar or for the light to be of xenon-arc intensity." Fixation may be difficult in smaller children or uncooperative adults who may not hold still. With the light shined in one eye, the ipsilateral pupillary light reflex is the *direct response,* while that of the contralateral is the *consensual response.* Because light from one eye will reach both Edinger–Westphal nuclei symmetrically, normally both pupils react briskly when light is shined into just one eye (ie, the direct and consensual responses are equal) (Fig. 2–18A).

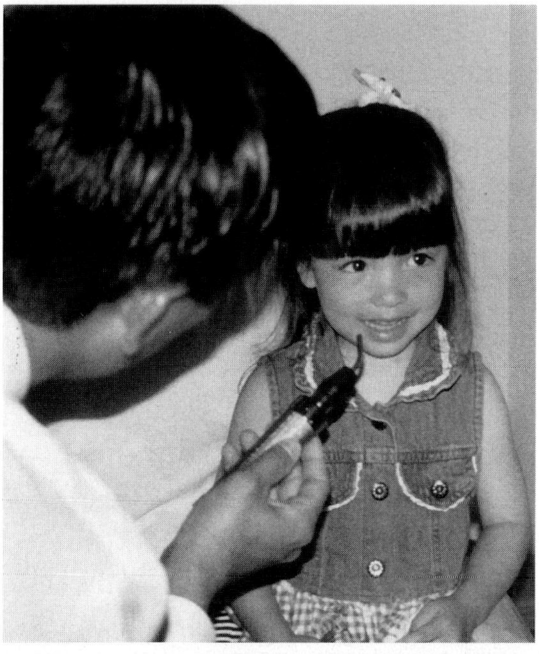

FIGURE 2–17. During examination of the pupils, the patient should fixate on a distance target to discourage accommodation and miosis.

The direct and consensual pupillary light responses may be diminished when light is directed in an eye with optic nerve or severe retinal dysfunction. Note that in these instances both pupils still have the same resting size, which is a reflection of the total amount of light reaching the midbrain pretectum from both eyes. In unilateral blindness (no light perception) due to optic nerve or retinal injury, both direct and consensual pupillary light reactions are absent (amaurotic or deafferented) when the light is shined in the blind eye. If the direct response is defective, but the consensual response is normal, it is likely that the ipsilateral pupil is paralyzed (efferent dysfunction).

Swinging Flashlight Test and Relative Afferent Pupillary Defects. The *swinging flashlight test* (*of Levitan*),[35] during which the light is alternately directed at each eye to compare each pupil's constriction to light, is an excellent method for evaluating relative optic nerve function. Testing of pupillary reactivity to light and the swinging flashlight test should be performed with a cadence. Rhythmic examination of the pupils, as well as pointing the light along the visual axis of each eye, promotes symmetric light exposure to both eyes. The light should be directed at each eye for about 1 second each ("one–one") to assess pupillary reactivity to light. Care should be taken to align the light along the visual axes, especially when the eyes are misaligned. Then the light should be alternated between each eye (without too much hesitation between eyes) for about 2 seconds each ("one–two–one–two"). Normally both pupils will exhibit symmetric constriction (Fig. 2–18A). Caution should be exercised in patients with anisocoria, in whom pupillary constriction may appear falsely asymmetric. In addition, testing with a light that is too bright or too dim may either mask or miss an asymmetric response.[36, 37] Occasionally, asymmetric pupillary responses are best detected by rapid (less than 1 second) swings of the flashlight. In this situation, one checks for any asymmetry in the initial pupillary constriction.

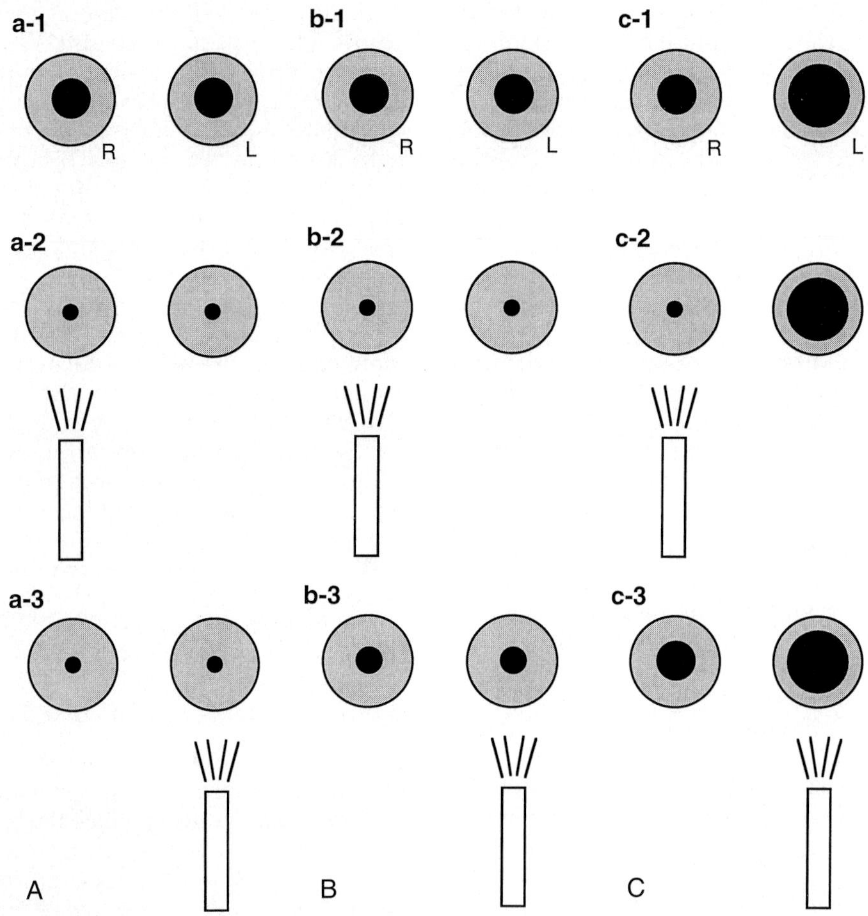

FIGURE 2–18. **A.** Normal swinging flashlight test, in which light directed in either eye elicits the same amount of pupillary constriction. **B.** Swinging flashlight test revealing a left relative afferent pupillary defect (LRAPD) in the hypothetical setting of visual loss in the left eye due to an optic neuropathy. (*b-1*) Pupillary sizes are equal at rest in ambient lighting. (*b-2*) Light stimulation of the good right eye results in brisk bilateral pupillary constriction. (*b-3*) Light stimulation of the defective left eye produces comparatively weaker pupillary constriction, and both pupils dilate. **C.** Left third nerve palsy and optic neuropathy. (*c-1*) The left pupil is fixed and dilated. (*c-2*) When the light is shined into the good right eye, the right pupil constricts normally. (*c-3*) However, when the light is shined into the left eye, the right pupil dilates because of the left optic neuropathy.

An asymmetric swinging flashlight test is highly suggestive of a unilateral optic neuropathy or severe retinal or macular abnormality. In these instances, when light is directed in the unaffected eye, both pupils will react normally. When the light is returned to the abnormal eye, both pupils will dilate because of the comparatively weaker pupillary constriction (*relative afferent pupillary defect* (RAPD) or *Marcus Gunn pupil*) (Fig. 2–18B). This finding reflects the difference in the amount of afferent input reaching the pretectal region of the midbrain.[64] Even if each pupil constricts to light, but a secondary redilation (*pupillary escape*[38]) occurs in one eye, the interpretation is the same[34]—this is what Marcus Gunn originally described.[39, 65] Hippus can be confused with an RAPD. However, an RAPD is suggested when there is an asymmetry of the pupillary response. Although RAPDs are most suggestive of unilateral optic nerve or retinal disease, they may also be seen in asymmetric chiasmal disorders, optic tract lesions,[40] amblyopia,[41] and rarely, pretectal disturbances.[42] The examiner should not ascribe an RAPD to a media opacity.

The swinging flashlight test requires only one working pupil (Fig. 2–18C). When one pupil is immobile, because of a third nerve palsy, for instance, one can still screen for an ipsilateral optic neuropathy by observing the consensual response in the fellow eye (with a second dim, obliquely directed light) during the swinging flashlight test. For example, a patient might present with a fixed and dilated pupil and poor vision in the left eye. When the light is brought back to the left eye, and the right pupil dilates, this suggests an optic neuropathy in the left eye. One should still call this a "left RAPD," but other terms include an "APD tested in a reverse fashion," "reverse Marcus Gunn pupil," or "reverse APD."

Methods of grading the RAPD vary. In the "number-plus system," a "1+ RAPD OS" refers to initial constriction, but early redilation of the left pupil; "2+" indicates no initial movement of the pupil, then dilation; "3+" means immediate redilation; while a "4+ RAPD" indicates an amaurotic pupil. The "number-plus system" is inherently subjective, and responses may vary from exam to exam depending on ambient lighting and intensity of the testing light.[43] Another method, which is similar but more descriptive, assigns asymmetric reponses on swinging flashlight tests into three groups: escape, amaurotic, and an "RAPD" as anything in between. Testing with computerized pupillography[44, 45] is more objective and reproducible, but these instruments are not widely used and are impractical as bedside tools. Thompson et al[34] advocate measuring the RAPD with neutral density filters, which are graded in log units. The filters are placed over the good eye during the swinging flashlight test until the pupillary responses are balanced and the RAPD is eliminated. However, again the end point is somewhat subjective. In general, useful clinical information comes simply from the knowledge of the presence or absence of an RAPD.

Accommodation. When a pupil has a sluggish reaction to light, accommodation should be tested, to see if the pupil will constrict to a near stimulus. Pupillary constriction may be elicited by having the patient actively view a near target, such as a toy for younger children or thumb, pen, or written material for older ones (Fig. 2–19). *Light-near dissociation* is the term applied to pupils that react poorly to light stimulation but constrict briskly during accommodation. If a pupil reacts to light, its reaction to near does not need to be tested, as pupils with intact light reactivity will also have normal constriction during accommodation.

Special Pupillary Considerations in Young Children

The pupils may be poorly reactive in a premature infant.[46] Pupillary constriction to light is usually absent before 29 weeks gestation but is invariably present by 31 weeks gestation.[47, 48] Infants born at 26 weeks gestation may have large pupils (5 mm), but by 30 weeks gestational age they should be approximately 3.5 mm.[49, 50]

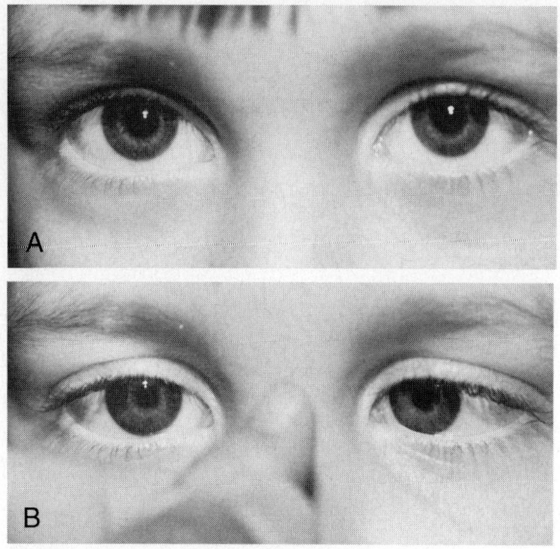

FIGURE 2–19. Pupillary constriction and convergence during the near response.

Eyelids

The neuro-ophthalmic evaluation of the eyelids requires assessment of their external appearance, position, and function. Eyelid disorders are discussed in Chapter 14.

Eyelid Appearance and Position. First, the eyelids and their position should be observed at rest with the eyes directed straight ahead. In an adult, normally the upper eyelid covers the top of the cornea (Fig. 2–20), while the lower eyelid lies at or just below the limbus (junction of cornea and sclera). In a neonate, the upper eyelid may be above the cornea, and the lower lid just above the limbus. Any obvious abnormalities in the shape or size of the lid should be noted. The *palpebral fissure,* the opening between the upper and lower eyelids, usually measures between 9 to 12 mm in height (in the middle) when the lids are open but relaxed. An upper eyelid above the limbus ("scleral show") implies the palpebral fissure is widened, and disorders causing lid retraction or poor eyelid closure should be considered. Fissure narrowing sug-

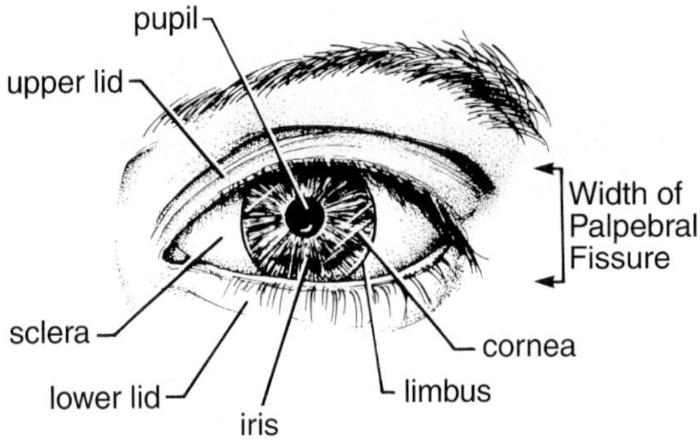

FIGURE 2–20. The normal left eye. (From Liu GT: Disorders of the eyes and eyelids. In Samuels MA, Feske S (eds): The Office Practice of Neurology, p 70. New York, Churchill Livingstone, 1996, with permission.)

gests either excessive orbicularis contraction or ptosis (eyelid drooping). When evaluating a ptotic eyelid, since lower lid position may vary greatly, it is often helpful to measure the distance between the pupillary light reflex and the upper lid margin. This number is referred to as the *margin reflex distance*, which typically measures 4 to 5 mm.[51] Whenever possible, eyelid appearance should be compared with that in old photographs.

The examiner should also note the position of the eyelid crease. It is usually approximately 10 mm from the lash margin and is formed by the skin insertion of the levator muscle. In levator dehiscence, for example, the distance from crease to lash margin increases.

Eyelid Function. The levator palpebrae superioris muscle lifts the eyelid, and its function can be assessed by manually fixing the brow and asking the patient to look downward.[52] A ruler is then placed at the lid margin and the number of millimeters of lid elevation is measured as the patient looks upward (Fig. 2–21).[53] Normal levator function is greater than 12 mm.[51] Ptosis produced by levator dehiscence and Horner syndrome is usually associated with normal levator function. In contrast, levator function is reduced in ptosis associated with myasthenia gravis, congenital ptosis, third nerve palsies, and myopathic conditions such as chronic progressive ophthalmoparesis and myotonic dystrophy. Findings characteristic of but not specific for myasthenic ptosis include fatiguability (drooping of the eyelids after an extended period of upgaze), curtaining (elevation of a ptotic eyelid causing drooping of the other eyelid), and Cogan's lid twitch (overshoot of the eyelid when moved from a relaxed to primary position).

Next the lids should be examined during eye movements. During horizontal conjugate gaze, the palpebral fissure widens in the abducting eye in approximately half of normal individuals, and in about 15% the lid elevates in the adducting eye as well. During upgaze, levator tone increases to lift the upper eyelid, while in downgaze, the eyelids should relax and follow the eyes smoothly. If the patient looks at a target moved downward and the eyelids lag behind (*lid lag*), thyroid eye disease, a dorsal midbrain lesion, or aberrant regeneration of the third nerve should be suspected.

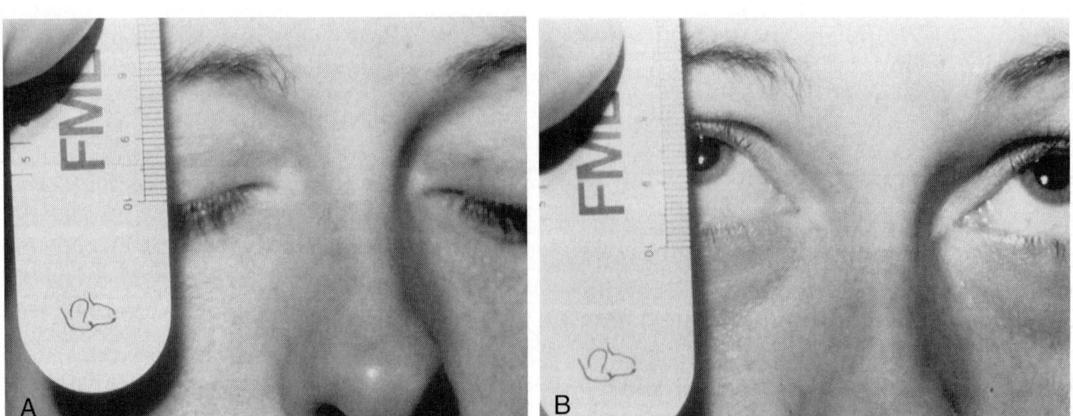

FIGURE 2–21. Measurement of eyelid function. **A.** To measure levator function a ruler is placed over the center of the eyelid as the patient gazes downward. **B.** The distance the lid travelled to reach upgaze is recorded. (From Galetta SL, et al: Neurol Clin 1996;14:201–222, with permission.)

Facial Nerve

The facial nerve (VII) supplies the muscles of facial expression. In addition, it has a parasympathetic component supplying the lacrimal gland and submandibular and sublingual salivary glands, and sensory components responsible for taste and sensation of the external ear, tongue, and palate. When facial nerve dysfunction is suspected, the major goal of the examination is to establish whether the process is supra- or infranuclear. Further details regarding anatomy and disorders of the facial nerve are discussed in Chapter 14.

Motor Evaluation. Assessment of facial nerve motor function begins by observing the patient at rest and noting any asymmetries of the face or blink pattern. Most supranuclear and infranuclear facial nerve palsies are associated with a flattened nasolabial fold and slightly widened palpebral fissure on the paretic side. Facial movement to emotional stimuli and voluntary command should also be assessed. A dissociation in response of spontaneous and voluntary movements is suggestive of supranuclear defects. Disease of the corticobulbar tracts tends to spare emotional facial responses, while those of the basal ganglia preserve voluntary movements. Preservation of forehead wrinkling, seen best in attempted upward gaze, is also characteristic of supranuclear lesions.[54]

Having the patient forcefully close the eyelids while the examiner attempts to open them can test the strength of the orbicularis oculi muscles. The examiner should note asymmetries in eyelash burying or *lagophthalmos,* that is, partial or total inability to close the lids. Having the patient smile should also be done to assess the integrity of lower part of the facial nerve. Excess contraction of the orbicularis oculi occurs in hemifacial spasm and blepharospasm. Small contractions around the eye giving the appearance of skin rippling could be myokymia, faciculations, or the result of aberrant reinnervation.

Taste. Taste is best tested using a cotton swab dipped in a sour, sweet, or bitter solution. Unilateral ageusia may be usefui in identifying a facial lesion as peripheral, but it should be noted that bedside tests are crude and often unreliable.[54]

Tear Function. Evaluation of tear function by observation alone, without actual testing, may lead to erroneous impressions (for example, that a patient with a facial palsy is tearing excessively). Testing for tearing is of limited diagnostic or prognostic value unless tear production is drastically reduced or absent on the involved side. Further, the results of actual tear testing may be similarly misleading. Increased tear flow (*epiphora*) noted by the history can be due to exposure irritation, paralytic ectropion, or failure of the lacrimal pump apparatus of the lower lid, and is not likely to be related to an irritative lesion of the greater superficial petrosal nerve. Similarly, decreased tearing may be due to corneal hypoesthesia rather than suggestive of a destructive process involving, for example, the greater superficial petrosal nerve.[54]

Tear testing usually involves Schirmer paper strips placed in the inferior conjunctival cul-de-sacs of each eye following topical anesthesia. To avoid erroneous results from pooled tears, the conjunctival tear lake should be dried prior to insertion of the paper strips. A Schirmer strip is inserted into the conjunctival sac of the uninvolved eye, and moments later a strip is placed in the involved eye. By following this sequence the reflex blepharospasm and tearing provoked by stimulating the normal eye does not influence the results in the contralateral eye.[54]

Approximately 10% of patients with Bell's palsy will have decreased or absent corneal sensation, usually from exposure hypoesthesia or as a form of adaptation. In such cases, prior to placing Schirmer strips, a topical anesthetic can be instilled into both eyes to eliminate the problem of selectively stimulating the eye with normal corneal sensation. The length of the moistened paper is compared on the two sides after a period of 5 minutes. In the event that one of the filter strips becomes completely moistened prior to the passage 5 minutes, both strips are removed and compared for results. Less than 5 mm of wetting is highly suggestive of tear deficiency, but this finding should be viewed in the context of the patient's clinical history and the results of the slit-lamp examination.[54]

Blink Reflexes. Simulation of either cornea with a cotton wisp or tissue corner will cause a bilateral blink (*corneal blink reflex*). The absence of blinking in either eye usually suggests a lesion within the ophthalmic division of the trigeminal nerve (V1), the afferent limb of the reflex. Asymmetric blinking implies facial nerve weakness on one side.[54]

The *reflex blink to visual threat,* described above in the section on visual field testing, tests the intactness of the afferent visual pathway as well as cortical attentional mechanisms.[19] A cardinal feature of cortical blindness, for instance, is an absent blink to visual threat. On the other hand, the *reflex blink to light or dazzle* requires only intact connections from eye to brain stem.

Physiologic Facial Synkineses. *Bell's phenomenon* is discussed in more detail below in the eye movement section. In some normal individuals, the ears will retract and flatten with conjugate lateral gaze; this is known as the *oculogyric auricular reflex* and is usually greater in the ear opposite the direction of lateral gaze. The presumed neural mechanism involves proprioceptive input from the extraocular muscles to the facial nuclear complex. In the nasolacrimal reflex, the secretion of tears may be induced by chemically stimulating the nasal mucosa with a dilute solution of ammonia or formaldehyde. The neural pathway for this reflex results from connections of the trigeminal nerve (V1) to the greater superficial petrosal nerve.

Ocular Motility and Alignment

The ocular motility examination consists of observation in primary gaze, evaluation of ductions and vergences, then detection of misalignment (strabismus). Monocular double vision that resolves with a pinhole is likely due to refractive error and not to an ocular motility abnormality.

Inspection. The presence of any obvious ocular misalignment or abnormal, spontaneous eye movements should be assessed first in primary gaze while the patient fixates on a distant target. *Esotropia* refers to the inward deviation of one eye relative to the other; while *exotropia* describes the outward deviation of one eye relative to the other. Any vertical misalignment is described by the laterality of the higher eye (eg, a left *hypertropia* indicates the left eye is higher than the right). Adjunctive observations should include the presence or absence of head turn or tilt.[55] When suspected but not visible with ordinary inspection, fine oscillations of the eye, such as superior oblique myokymia, may be seen more readily with the slit lamp or by witnessing movement of the optic disc during ophthalmoscopy.

Ductions. Ductions refer to monocular eye movements; rotations laterally are termed *abduction;* medially, *adduction;* upward, *elevation* (or *supraduction*); and downward, *depression* (or *infraduction*). Ductions can be tested by having the patient voluntarily direct gaze in the cardinal fields (up and right, up, up and left, right, left, down and right, down, and down and left). Ocular rotation can be recorded as a subjective percentage of normal (ie, 70% of normal). This should be documented in the chart from the examiner's perspective (Fig. 2–22A). In another scheme using numbers +4 to 0 to −4, 0 indicates a normal duction, +4 means severe overaction, while −4 signifies no movement (Fig. 2–22B).[56] The examiner should also observe the speed of the duction, which will typically be reduced with an ocular motor palsy but intact with a restrictive process.

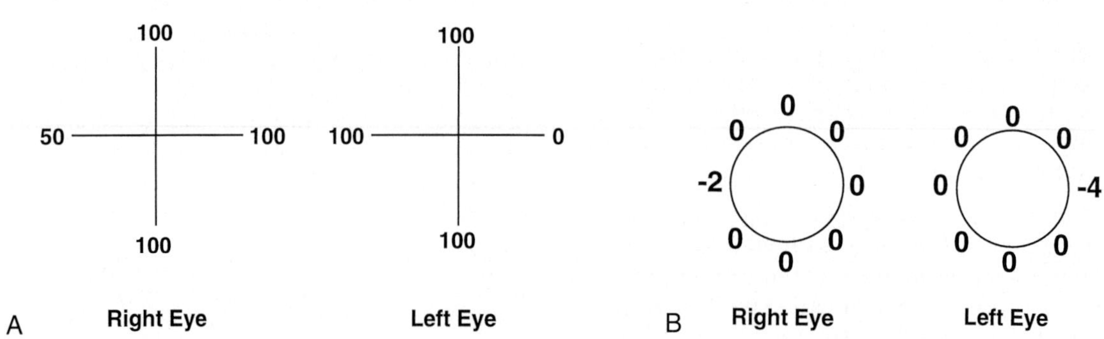

FIGURE 2–22. Recording ductions. **A.** In one method, the approximate percentages of the normal excursions in up, down, left, and right gazes are recorded. By convention, the diagrams are drawn from the examiner's view of the patient's eyes. In the example given, there is a partial abduction deficit of the right eye and no abduction of the left eye. **B.** In another method, ductions are graded from −4 to +4. Negative numbers indicate degrees of paralysis, while positive numbers indicate overaction. This example also diagrams a partial abduction deficit of the right eye and no abduction of the left eye.

Inability to move an eye despite pushing on the globe with a cotton-tip swab or pulling with forceps (following instillation of a topical anesthetic) suggests mechanical restriction (positive forced duction test) (Fig. 2–23B). In the forced generation test, the patient is asked to move the eye against the cotton-tip swab (Fig. 2–23C). Inability to do so usually indicates ocular motor nerve or muscle weakness. Patients with positive forced ductions but normal forced generations usually have a restrictive problem.

Bell's Phenomenon. *Bell's phenomenon* is the normal upward rotation of the globe elicited during forceful eyelid closure. This palpebral–oculogyric reflex, likely mediated by poorly defined brain stem connections between the seventh and third nerve nuclei, is easily visible in patients with peripheral facial nerve paralysis who attempt to shut their eyes (Fig. 2–24). In normal patients it can be observed by having the patient try to close his or her eyes while the examiner holds the lids open. Most commonly, the eyes rotate up and out, but the they may go up and in or straight up, and asymmetric left and right eye movements may be seen. However, in a study of 508 consecutive patients in an ophthalmic practice,[57] 42 (8%) had a downward response in one or both eyes, and in five (1%) the responses were horizontal.

Clinically, Bell's phenomenon can be helpful in two instances. (1) In an eye with defective voluntary supraduction, a normal Bell's phenomenon indicates a supranuclear defect with intact nuclear and infranuclear oculomotor nerve function for upgaze. For example, the reflex is preserved in upgaze paresis in Parinaud syndrome but defective in a complete third nerve palsy. (2) In patients with hemispheric defects, a stroke for example, both eyes may rotate contralateral to the lesion in a phenomenon known as *spasticity of conjugate gaze* (see Chapter 8).

Vergences. *Vergences* are binocular eye movements. *Convergence* can be evaluated by having

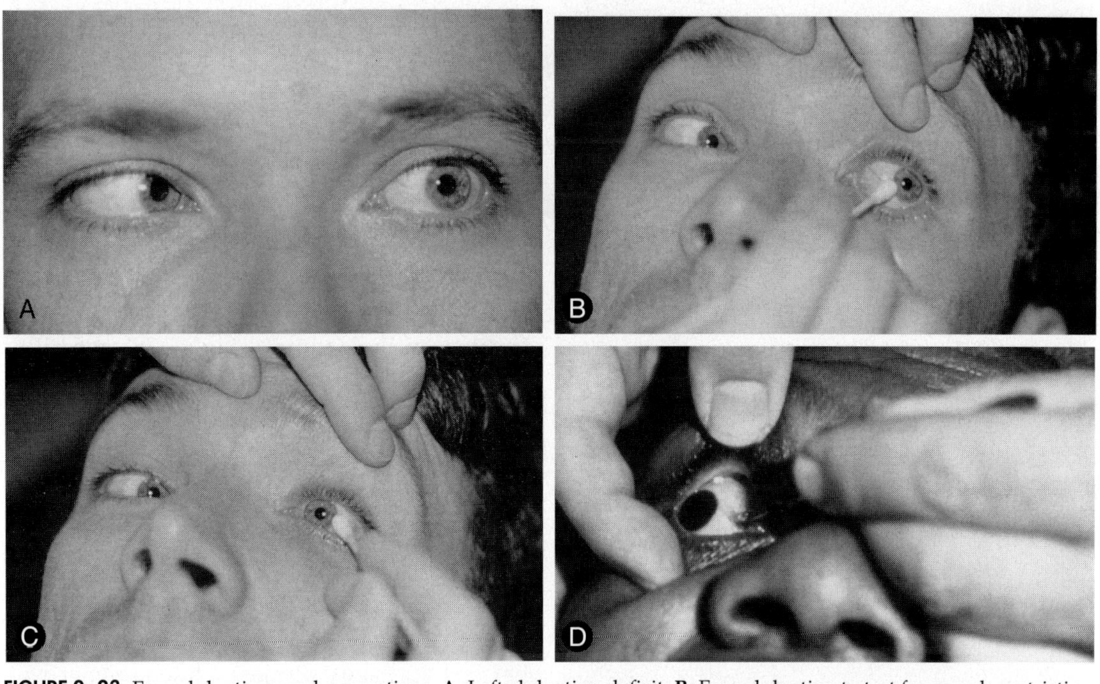

FIGURE 2–23. Forced ductions and generations. **A.** Left abduction deficit. **B.** Forced duction to test for muscle restriction. After instillation of topical anesthesia, an attempt is made at moving the eye laterally by pushing on it at the medial limbus with a sterile cotton swab. In this case the eye could be moved laterally, indicating the absence of restriction by the medial rectus muscle. This is *a negative forced duction test*. **C.** Forced generation to test for lateral rectus weakness. With the cotton swab on the lateral limbus, the patient is asked to abduct the eye. In this case the swab met no resistance, consistent with a lateral rectus palsy. This is a *positive forced generation test*. **D.** In an alternative method, forced ductions can be performed by pulling on the extraocular muscles with forceps. This patient had a right abduction deficit, and the medial rectus is manipulated.

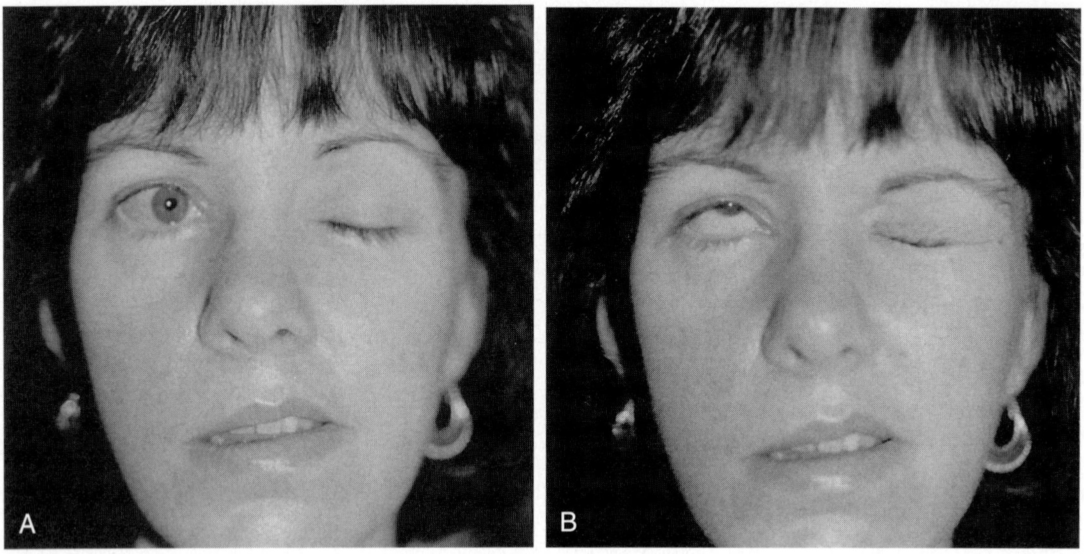

FIGURE 2–24. Bell's phenomenon. **A.** Traumatic right facial nerve palsy. **B.** Upon attempted eyelid closure, the right eye rotates upward.

the patient look at his or her thumb or other accommodative target as it is brought toward the nose; both eyes should adduct with pupillary constriction (see Fig. 2–19). *Pursuit movements* should then be tested by having the patient keep the head still and visually track a target moved slowly horizontally or vertically (Fig. 2–25). The speed and accuracy of *saccades,* which are high-velocity, conjugate eye movements, should be examined by having the patient look eccentrically then quickly refixate on a target in primary gaze (the examiner's nose, for instance) (Fig. 2–26).

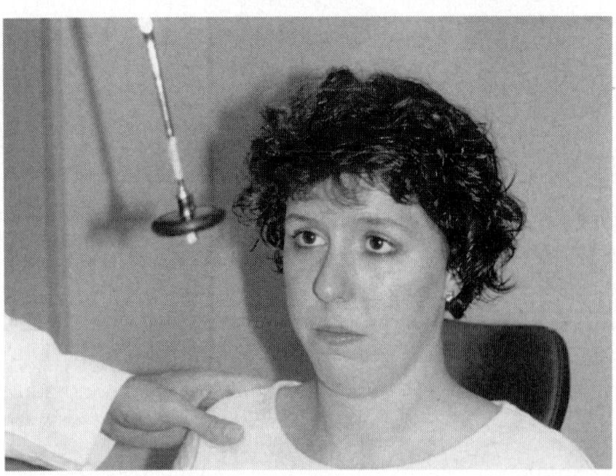

FIGURE 2–25. Testing pursuit. The patient is asked to fix and follow a slowly moving object, in this case, the end of a reflex hammer.

Oculocephalic responses can be evaluated by having the patient fix on a stationary target while the examiner gently rotates the head and extends and flexes the neck (Fig. 2–27). The stimulus is either from proprioceptive afferents in the neck or the vestibular system, or both. Abnormal eye movements that are overcome by oculocephalic stimulation are likely supranuclear (see Chapter 16). In addition, with an arm extended and the chair rotated, most patients should be able to maintain visual fixation on their thumb (Fig. 2–28); difficulty with this task, manifesting usually as nystagmus, suggests an inability to suppress the *vestibulo-ocular response* (VOR). This is usually a sign of central nervous system dysfunction. When rotated around the examiner, infants, normally with poor fixation, manifest a VOR with tonic eye deviation in the direction of rotation followed by quick corrective jerks.

Nystagmus is a rhythmic oscillation of the eyes; two major types are seen. *Jerk nystagmus* has fast and slow phases, while *pendular nystagmus* is more sinusoidal without a fast phase. Many normal individuals have physiologic jerk nystagmus in extremes of gaze. This type of nystagmus is a low-amplitude, high-frequency nystagmus that usually fatigues with prolonged eccentric gaze. Physiologic *op-*

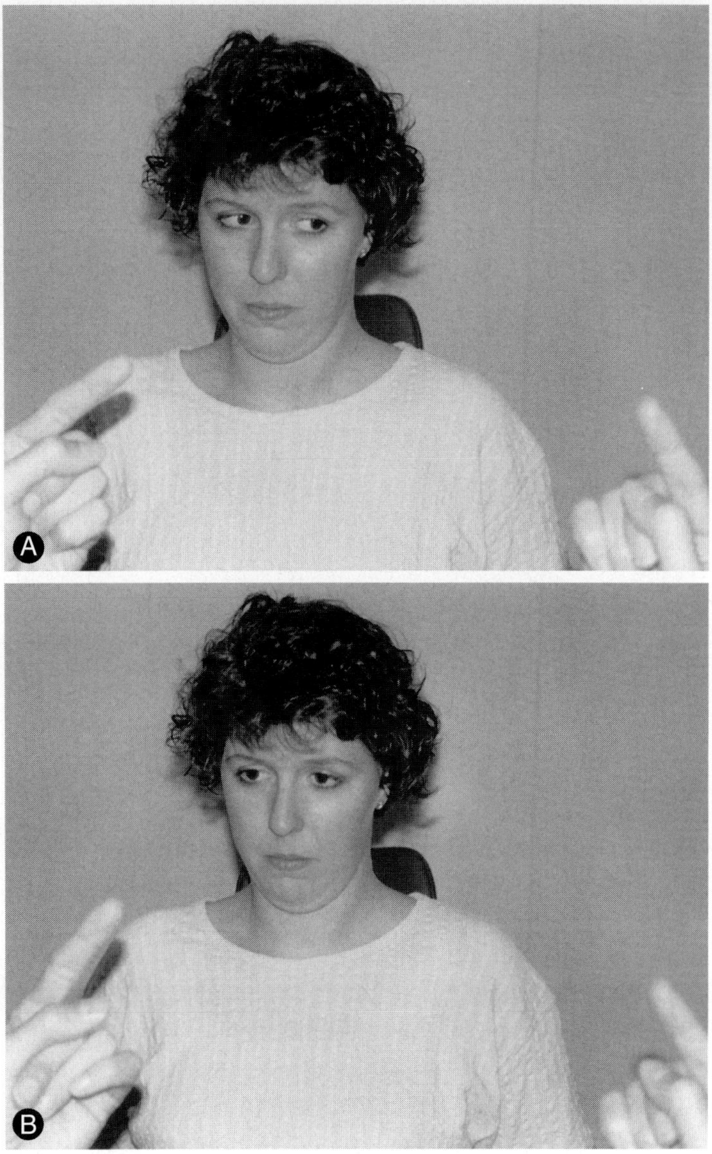

FIGURE 2–26. Testing saccades. **A.** The patient is asked to look at a target in the periphery. **B.** The speed and accuracy of the saccade is assessed as the patient is asked to look quickly at the target in front of his or her face.

tokinetic nystagmus (OKN) can be elicited by rotating a striped drum or moving a striped tape horizontally and vertically and asking the patient to "count the stripes as they go by" (Fig. 2–29). The slow phases of OKN are generated as the patient follows a target; the OKN fast phase is a corrective saccade to view the next target. Nystagmus and nystagmoid eye movements are discussed in Chapter 17.

Assessing Ocular Misalignment. Ophthalmoparesis often will be evident on evaluation of ductions alone, however, more subtle instances of misalignment may require cover or Maddox rod testing. Note both tests require sufficient vision in both eyes to view a distant target.

Two complementary cover tests, the cover–uncover and alternate cover, can be used to assess ocular misalignment. A *tropia* is a misalignment that is present at all times, while a *phoria* is a misalignment that occurs only when binocularity is interrupted. Cover–uncover testing is used to detect tropias, which are manifest by any refixation movement of the fellow eye after monocular occlusion while the patient fixates on a target in the distance (Fig. 2–30). An outward movement of the uncovered eye signifies an *esotropia,* an inward movement implies an *exotropia,* and a downward

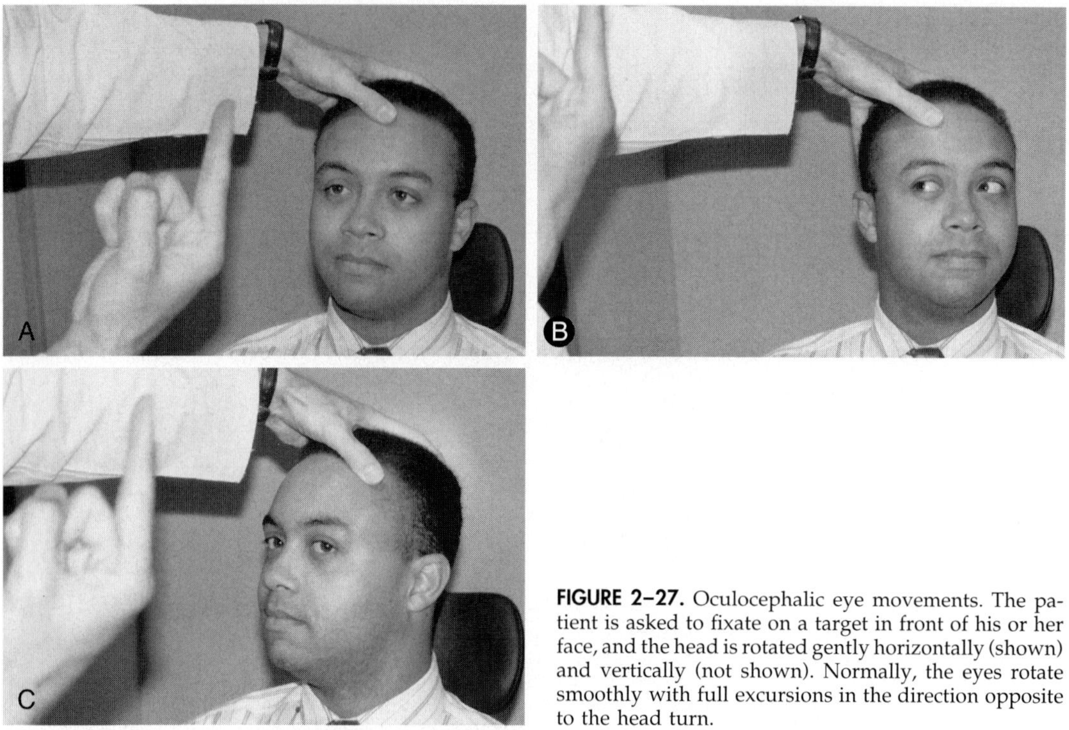

FIGURE 2–27. Oculocephalic eye movements. The patient is asked to fixate on a target in front of his or her face, and the head is rotated gently horizontally (shown) and vertically (not shown). Normally, the eyes rotate smoothly with full excursions in the direction opposite to the head turn.

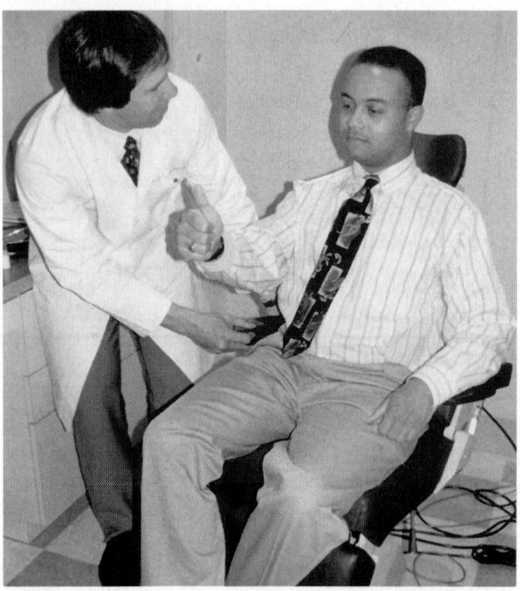

FIGURE 2–28. Suppressing the vestibulo-ocular response. The patient is asked to fixate on a target that will be stationary in relationship to the body, then the examination chair is rotated slowly. The eyes should remain still.

movement indicates a *hypertropia*. Regardless of which eye is vertically impaired, the side of the higher eye denotes the deviation. For instance, a right eye that is higher is called a right hypertropia. Then the occlusion is removed and the other eye tested. Alternate cover testing, achieved by alternately occluding each eye for about a second each, breaks binocular fusion. This test reveals the full deviation: any tropia plus any latent phoria. The refixation movement of the uncovered eye is interpreted in the same manner as in cover–uncover testing.

The ocular misalignment can be neutralized and quantified by placing a prism over one eye. Each eye is then alternately covered as the amount of prism, measured in diopters, is slowly increased (prism–alternate cover test) (Fig. 2–31). The apex of the prism points in the direction in which the eye is deviated. Thus, if an eye is exotropic, the prism is placed over the eye with the prism base in; if an eye is esotropic the prism is placed over the eye base out; if the eye is hypertropic, the prism is placed over the eye base down, while if the eye is hypotropic, the prism is placed over the eye with the base up. When the eyes no longer move on alternate cover testing, the deviation

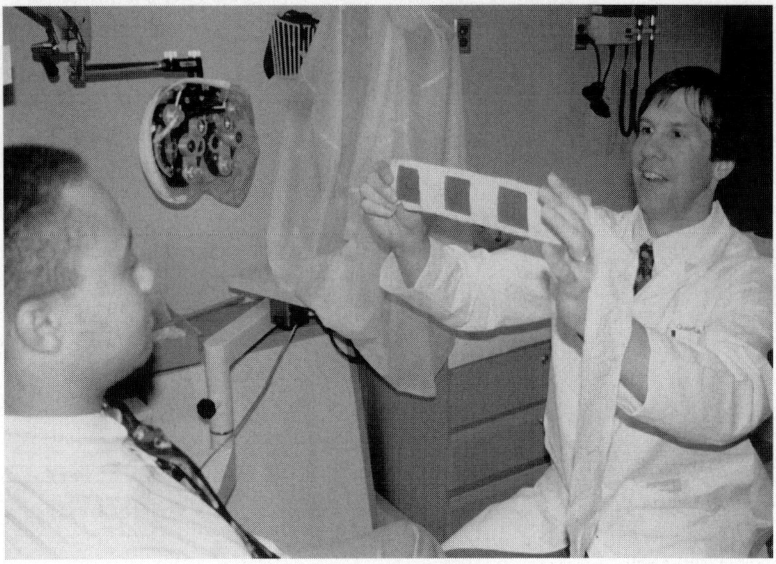

FIGURE 2–29. Eliciting optokinetic nystagmus. As the examiner moves a tape with red squares or other targets in the horizontal (shown) or vertical (not shown) direction, the patient is asked to "count the squares."

has been neutralized and the amount of prism required can be read off of the prism bar. Deviations should be measured in the cardinal positions and at near. Vertical deviations should also be evaluated with the head tilted toward the right and left shoulders. When one eye has extraocular muscle paralysis, the primary deviation refers to measurements taken when the prisms are placed over a nonfixing paretic eye, while the secondary deviation is the measurement taken with prisms placed over the fixing, nonparetic eye.[58]

The Maddox rod (Fig. 2–32A), containing parallel half-cylinders, can help detect small deviations but, by itself, does not identify the paretic eye. Maddox rod testing will reveal the full deviation: tropia plus latent phoria. If misalignment is detected, the direction of gaze that produces the greatest separation between images should be determined by moving the

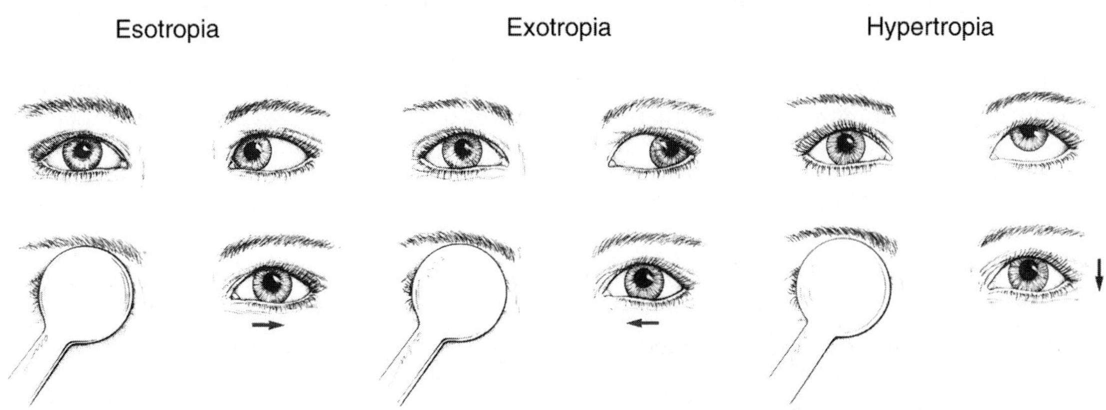

FIGURE 2–30. Cover testing for ocular misalignment. In each case the patient is fixing with the nonparetic right eye. Upon occlusion of the right eye, the misaligned left eye is forced to fixate. *Esotropic* eyes move laterally to fixate, while *exotropic* eyes move medially, and *hypertropic* eyes move downward to fixate. Thus the ocular deviations can be determined by direction of the fixation movements. (From Liu GT: Disorders of the eyes and eyelids. In Samuels MA, Feske S (eds): The Office Practice of Neurology, p 51. New York, Churchill Livingstone, 1996, with permission.)

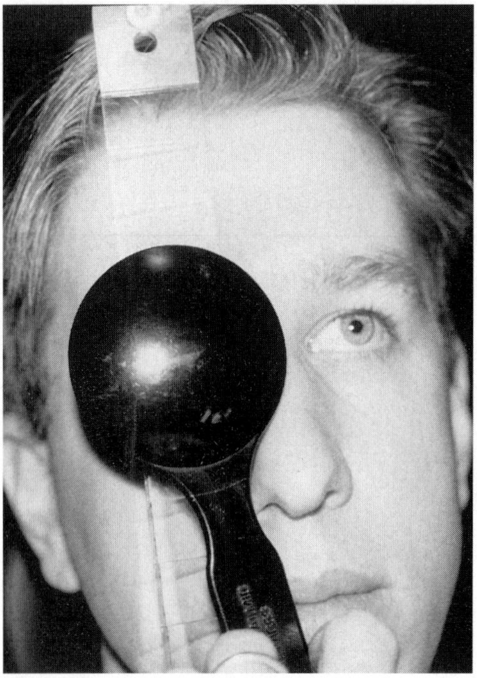

FIGURE 2–31. Prism–alternate cover testing for measurement of ocular misalignment. The prism bar contains a series of prisms of progressive strength (in diopters). Vertical prisms are used to measure hyperdeviations, while horizontal prisms are used in eso- and exodeviations. The patient fixates on a distant target, the eyes are alternately covered, and the prisms increased incrementally. The prism measurement is determined when the refixation movement, described in Figure 2–30, is neutralized.

fixation light in the cardinal positions of gaze. Similar to prism/cover techniques, the ocular misalignment in each position can be measured by placing a prism over either eye until the patient sees the line passing through the light (Fig. 2–32B). The red glass test is an analogous to the Maddox rod test except that the patient sees a red dot rather than a red line in the red glass test (Fig. 2–33).

In patients with monocular or binocular visual loss or in less cooperative patients such as children, the corneal light reflex can be used to assess ocular misalignment in the Hirschberg and Krimsky tests. In both, a bright light is directed toward the patient's face, and the patient is asked to try to look at the light; the relationship of the light's reflection and the center of the pupil is then observed. The Hirschberg test estimates the angle of misalignment (in degrees) based on the relationship of the light reflex and the iris (Fig. 2–34). In the Krimsky test, a variation of the Hirschberg test, and prism is placed over the deviated eye and increased or decreased until the light reflex is in the center of both pupils (Fig. 2–35). Both tests give only approximate measurements and are less accurate than alternate prism and cover tests.[59]

Measurements that are essentially the same in all cardinal positions of gaze define comitant strabismus, while in incomitant strabismus, the measurements differ. Incomitant measurements are more commonly associated with a paralyzed extraocular muscle or muscles (paralytic strabismus). On the other hand, comitant measurements are more frequently seen in long-standing deviations unassociated with extraocularmuscle palsies (nonparalytic strabismus).

EXTERNAL EXAMINATION

Any abnormalities of the periorbital region, such as ecchymoses or herniated fat, should be noted. When an orbital process is suspected, the eyes should be palpated and any resistance to retrodisplacement recorded. The amount of anterior protrusion of the globe can be assessed using an exophthalmometer (Hertel, for instance (Fig. 2–36)), which is indispensible when following proptosis in a patient with thyroid orbitopathy, for example.

Facial sensation within the three divisions of the trigeminal nerve (V) can be tested with a finger, tissue, or cold object. The examiner should pay particular attention to left/right asymmetries in sensation and differences between the three divisions. Corneal sensation, primarily a function of the first division of the trigeminal nerve (V1), can be evaluated with a wisp of cotton. The corneal blink reflex is described above in the facial nerve section. The masseter and pterygoid muscles are innervated by the motor division of V, which is contained in V3. Jaw strength can be tested by having the patient clench the teeth while the examiner palpates the masseter contraction. Opening and protruding the jaw tests the pterygoids; weakness of these muscles may cause lateral jaw deviation. Trigeminal nerve anatomy and disorders of facial sensation are discussed in Chapter 19.

SLIT-LAMP EXAMINATION

Slit-lamp examination (biomicroscopy) utilizes what essentially are a horizontally mounted microscope and a special light source to visualize directly the cornea, anterior chamber,

(Text continued on page 33)

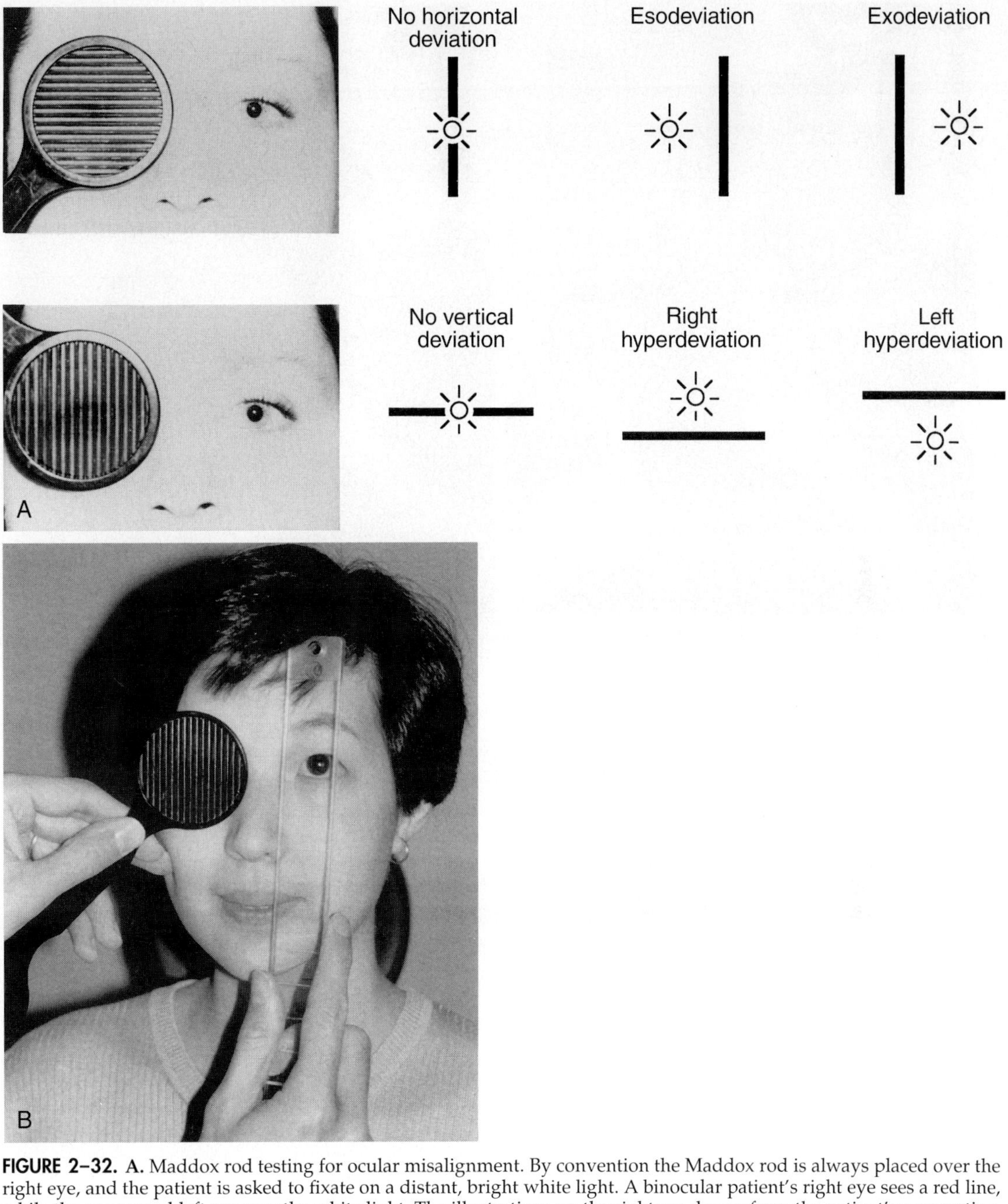

FIGURE 2–32. A. Maddox rod testing for ocular misalignment. By convention the Maddox rod is always placed over the right eye, and the patient is asked to fixate on a distant, bright white light. A binocular patient's right eye sees a red line, while the uncovered left eye sees the white light. The illustrations on the right are drawn from the patient's perspective. *Top row:* to evaluate horizontal ocular deviations, the bars on the Maddox rod are aligned horizontally, so the patient sees a vertical red line with the right eye. If there is no horizontal deviation, the patient perceives the red line passing through the white light. If the eyes are esodeviated, the red line, whose image would abnormally fall on nasal retina, appears to the right of the white light ("uncrossed diplopia"). Exodeviated eyes would result in the red line appearing to the left of the light ("crossed diplopia") because the red image would abnormally fall on temporal retina. *Bottom row:* to evaluate vertical deviations, the bars on the Maddox rod should be oriented vertically, so the patient will see a horizontal red line with the right eye. The red line passes through the white light when there is no vertical deviation, while a red line perceived below the light implies a right hyperdeviation, and a white light perceived below the red line indicates a left hyperdeviation (ie, the lower image corresponds to the hyperdeviated eye). Note that this test will characterize the ocular misalignment, but by itself it does not indicate which eye has the abnormal motility. (From Liu GT: Disorders of the eyes and eyelids. In Samuels MA, Feske S (eds): The Office Practice of Neurology, p 52. New York, Churchill Livingstone, 1996, with permission.) **B.** Prisms with Maddox rod. The correct prism measurement (in diopters) is arrived at when the patient indicates the red line passes through the light.

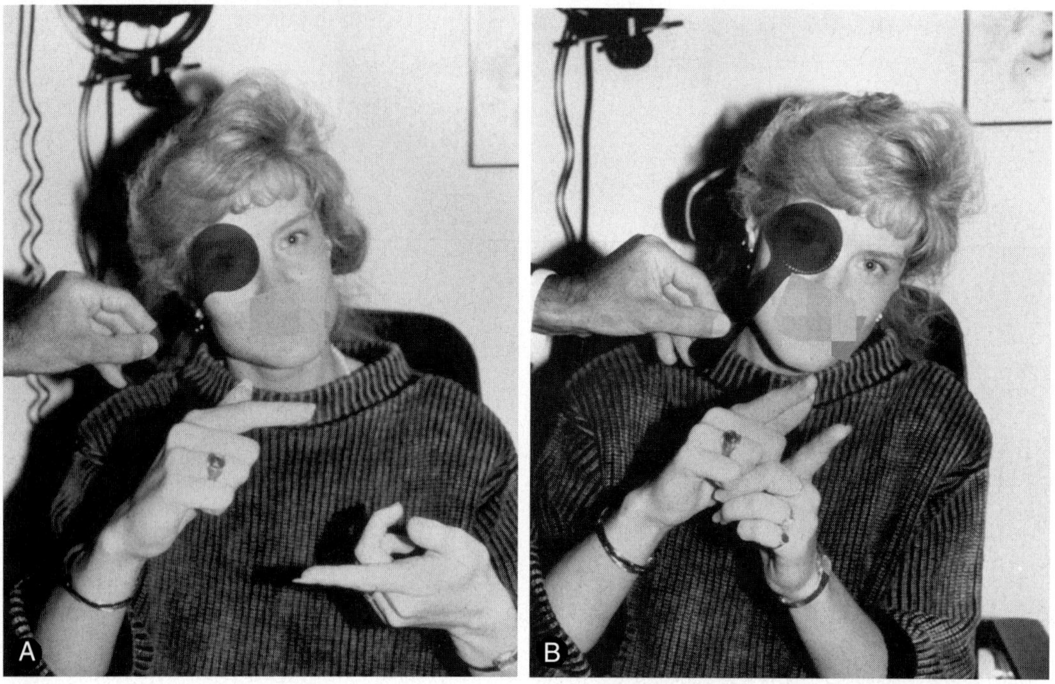

FIGURE 2–33. Red glass test in a patient with ocular misalignment. The patient fixes on a bright light source, and the right eye perceives a red light. The patient can express the perceived misalignment with his or her fingers. (Photos courtesy of Lawrence Gray, O.D.)

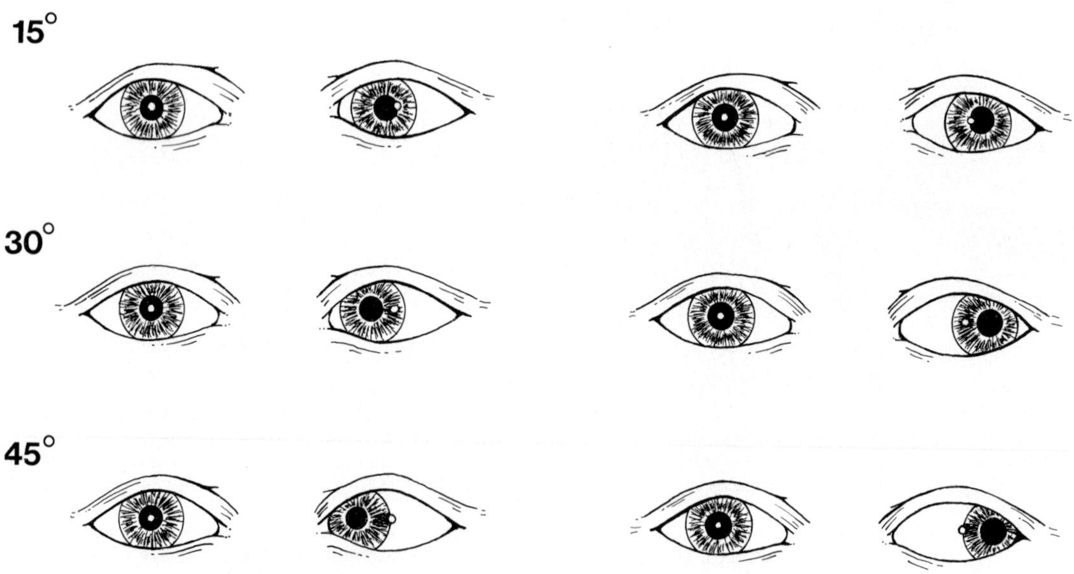

FIGURE 2–34. Hirschberg test. As the patient fixates on a bright light source, ocular misalignment in degrees can be estimated by observing the relationship of the corneal light reflection and the pupil and iris in the nonfixating, deviated eye. In these drawings the left eye is deviated. Light reflection at the pupillary margin = 15 degrees; in the middle of the iris = 30 degrees; and at the limbus = 45 degrees. These are approximations and obviously vary according to pupillary size.

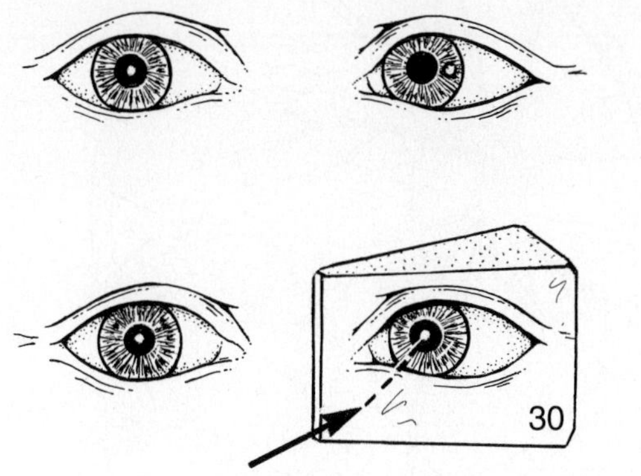

FIGURE 2–35. Krimsky test. As the patient fixates on a bright light source, ocular misalignment in prism diopters can be estimated when a prism moves the light reflection to the center of the cornea in the nonfixating, deviated eye.

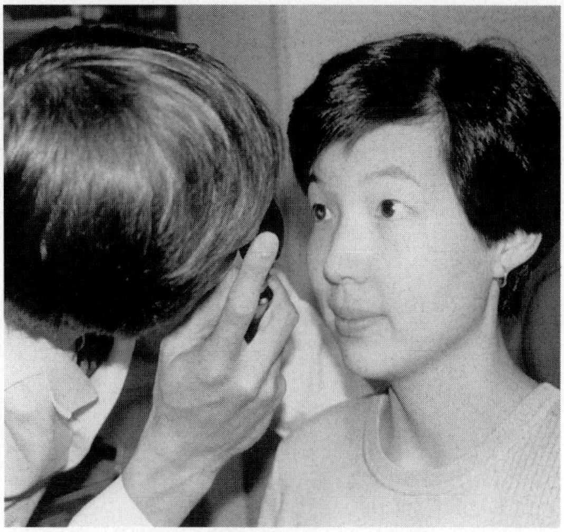

FIGURE 2–37. Direct ophthalmoscopy.

iris, and vitreous. Intraocular pressures should be measured by applanation. At the bedside, a halogen transilluminator and a magnifying lens (20-diopter lens, for instance), may substitute for a portable slit lamp.

FUNDUSCOPIC EXAMINATION

The posterior pole of the eye can be viewed with a direct ophthalmoscope (Fig. 2–37) through an undilated pupil, which allows the optic disc, retinal vasculature, macula, and peripapillary retina to be carefully examined (Fig. 2–38). Important details of the optic disc that should be noted include its color and contour and the cup-to-disc ratio as well as the clarity of the margins. The retinal vasculature should be evaluated in detail, with particular attention to the caliber of arteries and veins, branching patterns, and, when suspected, possible emboli. The macula, best observed by asking the patient to look at the direct ophthalmoscope's light, is examined for evidence of degeneration, lipid depo-

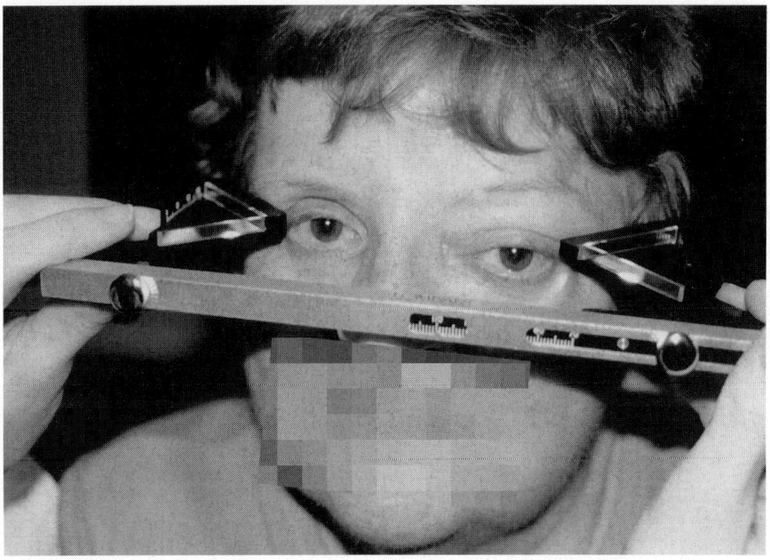

FIGURE 2–36. Hertel exophthalmometry. In this patient with the left eye protruding forward, the amount of relative proptosis can be measured.

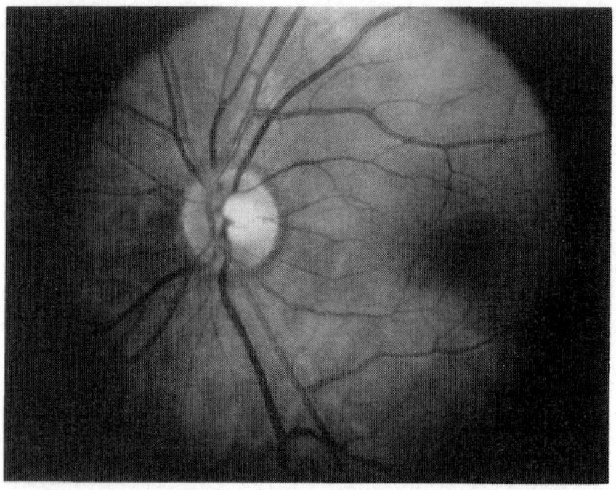

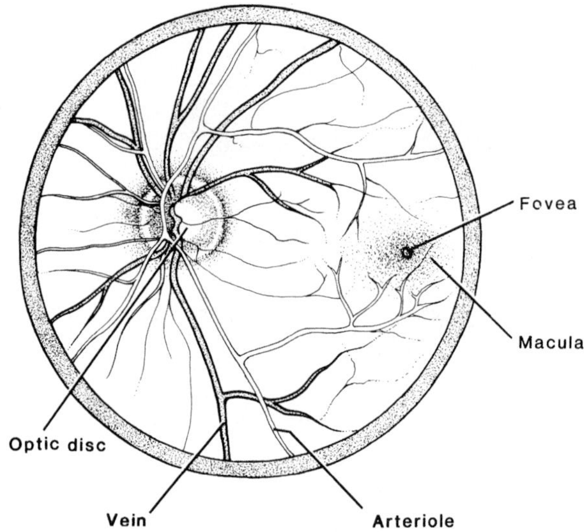

FIGURE 2–38. Photograph (*left*) of a normal left fundus. The corresponding illustration (*right*) labels important structures. (From Liu GT: Disorders of the eyes and eyelids. In Samuels MA, Feske S (eds): The Office Practice of Neurology, p 41. New York, Churchill Livingstone, 1996, with permission.)

sition, detachment, edema, or change in pigment color.

After pharmacologic dilation of the pupil with 1% tropicamide (an anticholinergic) and 2.5% phenylephrine (a sympathomimetic) topically, the disc and fundus can be evaluated using a 78- or 90-diopter lens with the slit lamp (Fig. 2–39), and the retinal periphery can be examined with a 20-diopter lens via indirect ophthalmoscopy (Fig. 2–40). Each technique permits a stereoscopic view of the fundus, which is especially important when evaluating disc swelling, disc contour, cup-to-disc ratio, and macular edema. In addition, both slit-lamp biomicroscopy and indirect ophthalmoscopy utilize very bright light sources, allowing greater visualization of structures in the back of the eye when there is a media opacity such as a cataract, corneal exposure, or vitritis, which may preclude direct ophthalmoscopy.

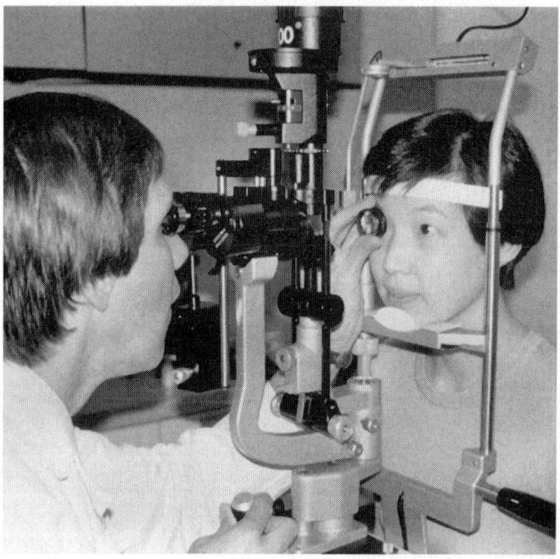

FIGURE 2–39. Slit-lamp biomicroscopic examination of the fundus with a 78-diopter lens.

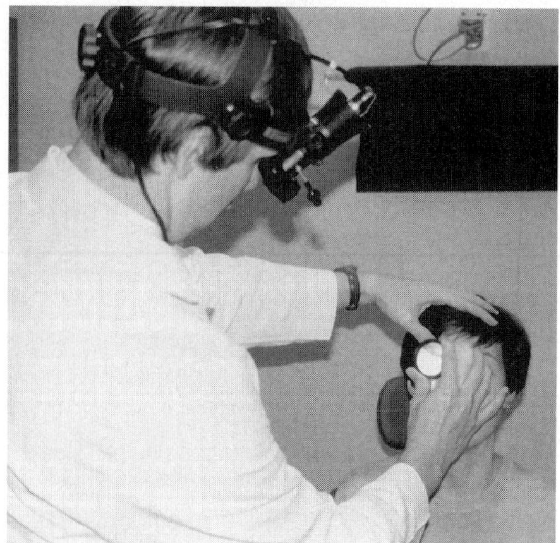

FIGURE 2–40. Indirect examination of the fundus with a 20-diopter lens.

The mydriatic effect of tropicamide peaks at 20 to 40 minutes and lasts 2 to 6 hours, while that of phenylephrine is maximum at 20 minutes and lasts 2 to 3 hours. Longer-acting mydriatics, such as cyclopentolate or atropine, are unnecessary unless a cycloplegic refraction is desired.

DIRECTED NEUROLOGIC EXAMINATION

Mental Status Evaluation

The level of the patient's consciousness, attention, and orientation should be documented. Verbal memory can be evaluated by requesting the patient to remember three unrelated words such as *car, Philadelphia,* and *honesty,* then after 5 minutes asking them to recite the list of items. The important components of language function (fluency, comprehension, reading, writing, repetition, and naming) should also be assessed.[29]

Abnormalities in these "cortically based" neurologic functions often provide clues regarding neuro-ophthalmic diagnosis. For instance, hemianopias that result from lesions of the optic radiations are often associated with mental status abnormalities. Temporal lobe lesions may be accompanied by personality changes, complex partial seizures, memory deficits, fluent aphasia (if the dominant side is involved), or Klüver–Bucy syndrome (hypersexuality, placidity, hyperorality, visual and auditory agnosia, and apathy) with involvement of the anterior temporal lobes bilaterally. A conduction aphasia, Gerstmann syndrome (finger agnosia, agraphia, acalculia, and right–left disorientation), and tactile agnosia, all suggest a dominant parietal lobe process. Left-sided neglect, topographic memory loss, and constructional and dressing apraxias, in association with a left hemianopia, suggest a nondominant, parietal lesion. More parieto-occipital or occipitally based visual disturbances such as Balint syndrome or cortical blindness may accompany dementia in Creutzfeld–Jacob disease, progressive multifocal leukoencephalopathy, or Alzheimer's disease.

Cranial Nerve Evaluation

The neuro-ophthalmic examination already assessed cranial nerves II to VII in detail, so in this part of the evaluation, the function of cranial nerves I and VIII to XII should be documented. Olfactory nerve (I) function can be tested in each nostril with coffee or perfume. The ability to discern whispers is an adequate screen of acoustic nerve (VIII) function. In the Weber test, a vibrating tuning fork (preferably 128 Hz) is placed in the middle of the forehead, and normally the patient will localize the vibration to the center of the head. In sensory-neural hearing loss the patient localizes the sound to the good ear, while in conductive hearing loss the patient localizes the sound in the affected ear. In the Rinne test, the vibrating tuning fork is placed on the mastoid process (testing bone conduction) then next to the auditory meatus (testing air conduction), and the patient is asked which is heard louder. In sensory-neural hearing loss, air and bone conduction are both reduced, or bone conduction is more affected. In conductive hearing loss, air conduction is reduced.

If the voice is not hoarse, the uvula is midline, and the palate elevates symmetrically, the general somatic efferent portions of the glossopharyngeal (IX) and vagus (X) nerves should be considered intact. The sternocleidomastoid and trapezius muscles, innervated by the accessory (XI) nerve, are responsible for head turning and shoulder shrugging, respectively. Tongue protrusion, a function of the hypoglossal (XII) nerve, should be symmetric. Hypoglossal nerve dysfunction causes ipsilateral tongue deviation when the tongue is extended.

Motor Function

The strength of the major muscle groups in the arms and legs should be tested. "0/5" indicates no muscle contraction, "3/5" means antigravity strength, while "5/5" indicates normal strength. If present, hypotonia, rigidity, or spasticity also should be noted.

Cerebellar Function

Important tests of cerebellar function include the finger–nose–finger and heel-to-knee-to-shin tasks. Difficulty with these is termed *dysmetria.* Dysdiadokinesia, also an indicator of cerebellar dysfunction, may be seen during testing of fine motor movements of the fingers, for instance, or rapid alternating movements such as tapping the hand against the thigh. Tandem walking also tests cerebellar function, and difficulty with this or a wide-based unsteady gait is termed *ataxia*.

Sensation

Sensory loss can accompany neuro-ophthalmic disease, especially visual loss due to cortical processes or nutritional optic neuropathies and ocular motility disorders associated with brain stem lesions. Modalities that should be tested include light touch, vibration, proprioception, pin prick (pain), and temperature. A homonymous field defect in combination with ipsilateral sensory loss, astereognosis (the inability to identify an object by palpation), decreased two-point discrimination, or graphesthesia (the inability to identify a number written on the hand) strongly suggests a parietal lesion. A process within the nondominant (usually right) parietal lobe can also produce a contralateral neglect syndrome or hemianopia, accompanied by contralateral sensory inattention. Pain or hemianesthesia and an ipsilateral homonymous field deficit implies co-involvement of the thalamus and optic radiations. In a lateral medullary (Wallenberg) stroke, Horner syndrome, lateropulsion, skew deviation, and nystagmus are often accompanied by ipsilateral facial and contralateral body numbness.

Gait

The patient should be asked to walk in relaxed fashion, and the examiner should observe the patient's posture, balance, mobility, and arm swing. Gait abnormalities can suggest the presence of an extrapyramidal disorder, hemiparesis, or cerebellar dysfunction.

Reflexes

Especially in patients with ocular motor palsies, hypoactive deep tendon reflexes may suggest more widespread neuropathies such as diabetic polyneuropathy, Guillain–Barré syndrome, or mononeuritis multiplex. A tonic pupil may be associated with absent reflexes, particularly at the ankles, in Adie syndrome. Hyperactive reflexes and extensor plantar responses (Babinski sign) suggest upper motor neuron dysfunction when a cortical, brain stem, or spinal cord lesion is suspected.

DIRECTED GENERAL EXAMINATION

A thorough but directed general examination of all patients can often provide important clues to neuro-ophthalmic diagnoses. It would be impossible to list all the abnormalities one might find; however, some examples are reviewed. The patient's general appearance might suggest an underlying chromosomal, endocrinologic, or metabolic disorder. For instance, the disfiguring frontal bossing and enlargement of the mandible and hands are characteristic of acromegaly associated with a growth hormone-secreting pituitary adenoma. Patients with pseudotumor cerebri tend to be young females with obesity or a history of recent weight gain. Skin lesions, such as erythema migrans (Lyme disease) or malar rash (systemic lupus erythematosus), and abnormal discolorations, such as café au lait spots and axillary freckling (neurofibromatosis), or hypopigmented ash-leaf spots (tuberous sclerosis), also may be helpful in guiding the evaluation of patients with visual disturbances.

Evaluation of the heart rate and blood pressure and auscultation of the carotid arteries and heart are important in any patient with a possible vascular process. Amaurosis fugax due to carotid disease may be associated with carotid bruits, which have approximately a 60% sensitivity and specificity for high-grade stenosis.[60] A cardiac murmur might suggest an embolic source. Cranial or ocular bruits might indicate an intracranial arteriovenous malformation or carotid–cavernous fistula. In some instances of visual loss due to anterior ischemic optic neuropathy, underlying giant cell arteritis is suggested by tender, cordlike temporal arteries and scalp sensitivity.

NEURO-OPHTHALMIC EXAMINATION IN COMATOSE PATIENTS

Plum and Posner[61] emphasize the evaluation of breathing pattern, pupillary function, eye movements, and motor responses in the neurologic assessment of comatose patients, especially with regard to brain stem localization and diagnosis. Thus, neuro-ophthalmic techniques are paramount in this clinical setting (Table 2–2). The ocular motility examination is especially important, because the pathways governing ocular motility traverse the entire brain stem, so pathology in this region often produces recognizable eye movement abnor-

TABLE 2–2. Neuro-ophthalmic Examination in a Comatose Patient

Pupils
Size
Shape
Reactivity

Eye movements
Position
Spontaneous eye movements
Elicited eye movements
  Oculocephalic
  Cold calorics (if oculocephalic responses absent)

Corneal reflexes

Funduscopy

malities. Conversely, if the eye movements are normal, likely the entire brain stem is intact as well.

The examiner of a comatose patient should decide, in a rostral–caudal fashion, which neuroanatomic structures have been affected by the disease process. In general, if the brain stem is intact in a comatose patient, bilateral hemispheric or thalamic disease should be suspected. If the brain stem is injured, the dysfunction should be localized to the midbrain, pons, or medulla.

In the neuro-ophthalmic assessment, pupillary size, shape, and reactivity should be evaluated first. If suspected, the absence of pupillary reaction to light should be confirmed with a magnifying lens. Unreactive pupils are suggestive of midbrain dysfunction or third nerve palsy, perhaps due to uncal herniation. Anisocoria may be due to unilateral Horner syndrome or a third nerve palsy. Bilaterally small pupils may be the result of a pontine hemorrhage or opiate toxicity. More detailed descriptions of these and other pupillary abnormalities in coma are given in Chapter 13.

Next, eye position and spontaneous eye movements should be observed. Overt misalignment such as an esotropia may suggest a sixth nerve palsy, while vertical or oblique mislignment may imply a third nerve palsy or skew deviation (see Chapter 15). Conjugate eye deviation may signify an ipsilateral hemispheric lesion, contralateral pontine process, or contralateral irritative seizure focus (see Chapter 16). Spontaneous roving eye movements in the vertical and horizontal direction indicate normal midbrain and pontine function. Rhythmic, repetitive vertical movements such as ocular bobbing or dipping may imply a pontine lesion (see Chapter 17).

Doll's eye or oculocephalic eye movements can be elicited by turning the head horizontally then vertically (Fig. 2–41). The eyes should deviate in the direction opposite to the head turn. A sixth nerve palsy, an internuclear ophthalmoplegia (see Chapter 15) or conjugate gaze paresis (see Chapter 16) may be evident this way. Oculocephalic eye movements are overly brisk in bilateral hemispheric disease, which can disinhibit the brain stem reflexes.[62] In the early stages of many drug intoxications and metabolic encephalopathy, the eye movements may be abnormal, but pupillary function is preserved. Oculocephalic maneuvers should not be performed in trauma patients with possible cervical spine injury.

If there are no oculocephalic eye movements, a stronger stimulus can be provided by applying ice cold water against the tympanic membranes, which provokes the vestibulo-ocular reflex (cold caloric test) (Fig. 2–41). The patient's head should be angled at 30 degrees to align the horizontal semicircular canals perpendicularly to the floor. After visual inspection to exclude rupture of the tympanic membrane, 30 to 60 cc of ice water can be irrigated into the external auditory canal using a large syringe and the tubing from a butterfly catheter or an angiocath without the needle (Fig. 2–42). A kidney basin should be placed under the ear to contain the overflow of ice water. The cold water creates convection currents in the endolymph of the horizontal semicircular canals, and inhibits the ipsilateral vestibular system. In the normal caloric response, the eyes move slowly and conjugately toward the tested ear, followed by a fast corrective phase in the opposite direction to reset the eyes, then the cycle repeats. The slow phase is produced by vestibulo-ocular connections from the unopposed contralateral ear, while the fast phase is mediated by the frontal eye fields. Warm water stimulation produces a contralateral slow phase and ipsilateral fast phase. The direction of the caloric response is named after the fast phase, and normal responses can be summarized in the pneumonic "COWS," which stands for "cold–opposite, warm–same." Caloric stimulation in the setting of a normal brain stem but bilateral hemispheric dysfunction would produce only an ipsilateral tonic slow phase. Complete brain stem injury would result in no slow or fast eye movements. The other ear can be tested after an interval of a few minutes. Bilateral caloric stimulation with cold water produces a downward slow

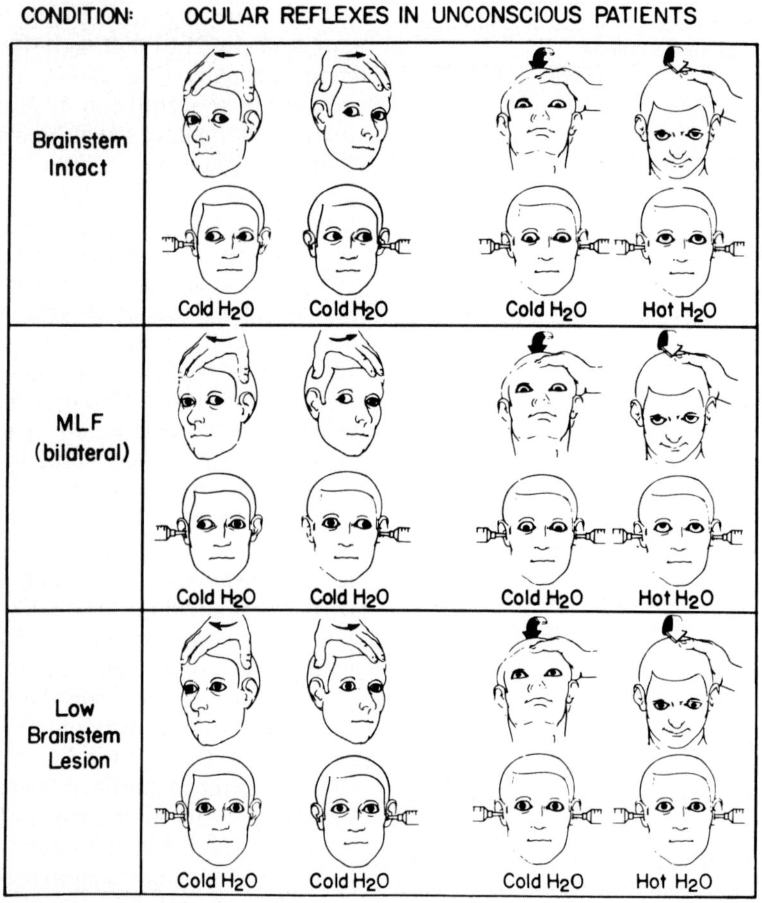

FIGURE 2–41. Ocular reflexes in unconscious patients. The upper section illustrates the oculocephalic (*above*) and oculovestibular (*below*) reflexes in an unconscious patient whose brain stem ocular pathways are intact. Horizontal eye movements are illustrated on the left and vertical eye movements on the right: lateral conjugate eye movements (*upper left*) to head turning are full and opposite in direction to the movement of the face. A stronger stimulus to lateral deviation is achieved by douching cold water against the tympanic membrane(s). There is a tonic conjugate deviation of both eyes toward the stimulus; the eyes usually remain tonically deviated for 1 or more minutes before slowly returning to the midline. Because the patient is unconscious, there is no nystagmus. Extension of the neck in a patient with an intact brain stem produces conjugate deviation of the eyes in the downward direction, and flexion of the neck produces deviation of the eyes upward. Bilateral cold water against the tympanic membrane likewise produces conjugate downward deviation of the eyes, whereas hot water (no warmer than 44°C) causes conjugate upward deviation of the eyes.

In the middle portion of the drawing, the effects of bilateral medial longitudinal fasciculus lesions on the oculocephalic and oculovestibular reflexes are shown. The left portion of the drawing illustrates that oculocephalic and oculovestibular stimulation deviates the appropriate eye laterally and brings the eye, which would normally deviate medially, only to the midline, since the medial longitudinal fasciculus, with its connection between the abducens and oculomotor nuclei, is interrupted (see Chapter 15). Vertical eye movements often remain intact.

The lower portion of the drawing illustrates the effects of a low brain stem lesion. On the left, neither oculocephalic nor oculovestibular movements cause lateral deviation of the eyes because the pathways are interrupted between the vestibular nucleus and the abducens area. Likewise, in the right portion of the drawing, neither oculocephalic nor oculovestibular stimulation causes vertical deviation of the eyes. (From Plum F, Posner JB: The diagnosis of stupor and coma, 3rd edition, p 55. Philadelphia, FA Davis, 1980, with permission.)

phase, while stimulation with warm water bilaterally results in an upward slow phase.

Other important neuro-ophthalmic observations in comatose patients include testing of the corneal reflexes and the funduscopic examination. The corneal reflexes can be evaluated with a sterile cotton swab as described above. Absent corneal reflexes suggest pontine dysfunction. The funduscopic examination is often normal, but papilledema would indicate elevated intracranial pressure, for instance, while a vitreous hemorrhage (Terson syndrome) may signify an aneurysmal subarachnoid hemorrhage. Because frequent monitor-

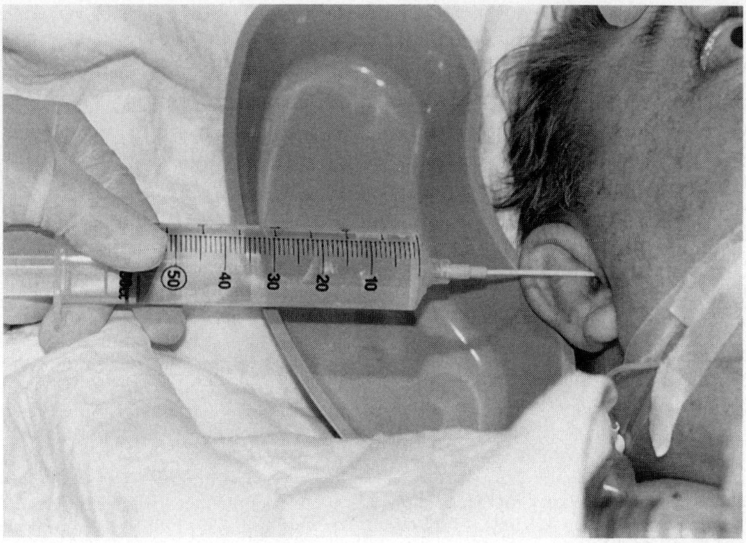

FIGURE 2–42. One method for performing cold caloric testing in a comatose patient. A 60-cc syringe filled with ice water (from a cup of water and ice) is connected to an angiocath with the needle removed. After excluding tympanic membrane rupture, water is injected into the inner ear canal. A kidney basin is used for water runoff. (From Liu GT, Coma. Neurosurg Clin N Am 1999;10:579–586, with permission.)

ing of the pupils is important in comatose patients, pharmacologic dilation of the pupils prior to funduscopic examination is not routinely recommended.

REFERENCES

1. Frisén L: Visual acuity. In: Clinical Tests of Vision, pp 24–39. New York, Raven Press, 1990.
2. Liu GT, Van Ostrand E, Newman NJ: CN II: Optic nerve and afferent visual pathway. In: Goetz GC, Pappert EJ (eds): Textbook of Clinical Neurology, pp 102–121. Philadelphia, WB Saunders, 1998.
3. Allen HF: Testing of visual acuity in preschool children. Pediatrics 1957;19:1093–1100.
4. Paine RS, Oppé TE: Neurological examination of children. Clin Dev Med 1966;20–21:99.
5. Hoyt CS, Nickel BL, Billson FA: Ophthalmological examination of the infant. Developmental aspects. Surv Ophthalmol 1982;26:177–189.
6. Lamkin JC: Can this baby see?: estimation of visual acuity in the preverbal child. Int Ophthalmol Clin 1992;32:1–23.
7. Quinn GE, Berlin JA, James M: The Teller acuity card procedure. Three testers in a clinical setting. Ophthalmology 1993;100:488–494.
8. Getz LM, Dobson V, Luna B, et al: Interobserver reliability of the Teller acuity card procedure in pediatric patients. Invest Ophthalmol Vis Sci 1996;37:180–187.
9. Eustis HS: Postnatal development. In: Wright KW (ed): Pediatric Ophthalmology and Strabismus, pp 45–59. St. Louis, CV Mosby, 1995.
10. Frisén L: The neurology of visual acuity. Brain 1980;103:639–670.
11. Comerford JP: Vision evaluation using contrast sensitivity functions. Am J Optom Physiol Opt 1983; 60:394–398.
12. Bodis-Wollner I: Detection of visual defects using the contrast sensitivity function. Int Ophthalmol Clin 1980;20:135–153.
13. Moseley MJ, Hill AR: Contrast sensitivity testing in clinical practice. Br J Ophthalmol 1994;78:795–797.
14. Aroichane M, Pieramici DJ, Miller NR, et al: A comparative study of Hardy–Rand–Rittler and Ishihara colour plates for the diagnosis of nonglaucomatous optic neuropathy. Can J Ophthalmol 1996;31:350–355.
15. Gouras P: Color vision. In: Kandel ER, Schwartz JH, Jessell TM (eds): Principles of Neural Science, pp 467–480. East Norwalk, CT, Appleton & Lange, 1991.
16. Hsia Y, Graham H: Color blindness. In: Graham CH (ed): Vision and Visual Perception. New York, John Wiley, 1965.
17. Hart WM: Acquired dyschromatopsias. Surv Ophthalmol 1987;32:10–31.
18. Zeki S: A century of cerebral achromatopsia. Brain 1990;113:1721–1777.
19. Liu GT, Ronthal M: Reflex blink to visual threat. J Clin Neuro-ophthalmol 1992;12:47–56.
20. Sadun AA: Distinguishing between clinical impairments due to optic nerve or macular disease. Metab Pediatr Syst Ophthalmol 1990;13:79–84.
21. Glaser JS, Savino PJ, Sumers KD, et al: The photostress recovery test in the clinical assessment of visual function. Am J Ophthalmol 1977;83:255–260.
22. Sloan PG: Clinical application of the photostress test. Am J Optom Arch Am Acad Optom 1968;45:617–623.
23. Wu G, Weiter JJ, Santos S, et al: The macular photostress test in diabetic retinopathy and age-related macular degeneration. Arch Ophthalmol 1990;108:1556–1558.
24. Zabriskie NA, Kardon RH: The pupil photostress test. Ophthalmology 1994;101:1122–1130.
25. Weintraub S, Mesulam M-M: Mental state assessment of young and elderly adults in behavioral neurology. In: Mesulam M-M (ed): Principles of Behavioral Neurology, pp 76–123. Philadelphia, FA Davis, 1985.

26. Weintraub S, Mesulam MM: Visual hemispatial inattention: stimulus parameters and exploratory strategies. J Neurol Neurosurg Psychiatr 1988;51:1481–1488.
27. Albert ML: A simple test of visual neglect. Neurology 1973;23:658–664.
28. Weintraub S, Mesulam M-M: Neglect: hemispheric specialization, behavioral components and anatomical correlates. In: Boller F, Grafman J (eds): Handbook of Neuropsychology, pp 76–123. Amsterdam, Elsevier Science, 1989.
29. Strub RL, Black FW: The mental status exam. In: Feinberg TE, Farah MJ (eds): Behavioral Neurology and Neuropsychology, pp 25–42. New York, McGraw–Hill, 1997.
30. Brazis PW, Graff-Radford NR, Newman NJ, et al: Ishihara color plates as a test for simultanagnosia. Am J Ophthalmol 1998;126:850–851.
31. Ishiai S, Sugishita M, Ichikawa T, et al: Clock-drawing test and unilateral spatial neglect. Neurology 1993;43:106–110.
32. Freedman M, Leach L, Kaplan E, et al: Clock drawing. A Neuropsychological Analysis, pp 3–8, 98–127. New York, Oxford University Press, 1994.
33. Miller NR: Walsh and Hoyt's Clinical Neuro-ophthalmology, 4th ed, pp 385–556. Baltimore, William & Wilkins, 1985.
34. Thompson HS, Corbett JJ, Cox TA: How to measure the relative afferent pupillary defect. Surv Ophthalmol 1981;26:39–42.
35. Levitan P: Pupillary escape in disease of the retina or optic nerve. Arch Ophthalmol 1959;62:768–779.
36. Borchert M, Sadun AA: Bright light stimuli as a mask of relative afferent pupillary defects. Am J Ophthalmol 1988;106:98–99.
37. Johnson LN: The effect of light intensity on measurement of the relative afferent pupillary defect. Am J Ophthalmol 1990;109:481–482.
38. Cox TA: Pupillary escape. Neurology 1992;42:1271–1273.
39. Burde RM, Landau WM: Clinical neuromythology XII. Shooting backward with Marcus Gunn: a circular exercise in paralogic. Neurology 1993;43:2444–2447.
40. Bell RA, Thompson HS: Relative afferent pupillary defect in optic tract hemianopsias. Am J Ophthalmol 1978;85:538–540.
41. Portnoy JZ, Thompson HS, Lennarson L, et al: Pupillary defects in amblyopia. Am J Ophthalmol 1983;96:609–614.
42. King JT, Galetta SL, Flamm ES: Relative afferent pupillary defect with normal vision in a glial brainstem tumor. Neurology 1991;41:945–946.
43. Browning DJ, Tiedeman JS: The test light affects quantitation of the afferent pupillary defect. Ophthalmology 1987;94:53–55.
44. Cox TA: Pupillography of a relative afferent pupillary defect. Am J Ophthalmol 1986;101:320–324.
45. Kawasaki A, Moore P, Kardon RH: Variability of the relative afferent pupillary defect. Am J Ophthalmol 1995;120:622–633.
46. Isenberg SJ, Molarte A, Vazquez M: The fixed and dilated pupils of premature neonates. Am J Ophthalmol 1990;110:168–171.
47. Robinson RJ: Assessment of gestational age by neurological examination. Arch Dis Child 1966;41:437–447.
48. Isenberg SJ, Dang Y, Jotterand V: The pupils of term and preterm infants. Am J Ophthalmol 1989;108:75–79.
49. Isenberg SJ: Clinical application of the pupil examination in neonates. J Pediatr 1991;118:650–652.
50. Liu GT: Abnormalities of the pupil: when should you worry? Contemp Pediatr 1995;12:83–98.
51. Nunery WR, Cepela M: Levator function in the evaluation and management of blepharoptosis. Ophthalmol Clin N Am 1991;4:1–16.
52. Sedwick LA: Ptosis. In: Margo C, Hamed L, Mames R (eds): Diagnostic Problems in Clinical Ophthalmology, pp 38–42. Philadelphia, WB Saunders, 1994.
53. Galetta SL, Liu GT, Volpe NJ: Diagnostic testing in neurology. Neuro-ophthalmology. Neurol Clin 1996;14:201–222.
54. May M, Galetta SL: The facial nerve and related disorders of the face. In: Glaser JS (ed): Neuro-Ophthalmology, pp. 239–278. Philadelphia, JB Lippincott, 1990.
55. Liu GT: Disorders of the eyes and eyelids: Disorders of the eye movements. In: Samuels MA, Feske S (eds): The Office Practice of Neurology, pp 50–60. New York, Churchill Livingstone, 1996.
56. Kaye SB, O'Donnell N, Holden R: Recording sensory and motor aspects of strabismus. J Pediatr Ophthalmol Strabis 1997;34:188–190.
57. Francis I, Loughhead J: Bell's phenomena: a study of 508 patients. Aust J Ophthalmol 1984;12:15–21.
58. Wright KW: Introduction to strabismus and the ocular-motor examination. In: Wright KW (ed): Pediatric Ophthalmology and Strabismus, pp 139–158. St. Louis, CV Mosby, 1995.
59. Choi R, Kushner BJ: The accuracy of experienced strabismologists using the Hirschberg and Krimsky tests. Ophthalmology 1998;105:1301–1306.
60. Sauve JS, Thorpe KE, Sackett DL, et al: Can bruits distinguish high-grade from moderate symptomatic carotid stenosis? The North American Symptomatic Carotid Endarterectomy Trial. Ann Intern Med 1994;120:633–637.
61. Plum F, Posner JB: The pathologic physiology of signs and symptoms of coma. In: The Diagnosis of Stupor and Coma, 3rd ed, pp 1–86. Philadelphia, FA Davis, 1980.
62. Ropper AH, Martin JB: Coma and other disorders of consciousness. In: Wilson JD (ed): Harrison's Principles of Internal Medicine, 12th ed, pp 193–200. New York, McGraw–Hill, 1991.
63. Litvan I, Saposnik G, Mauriño J, et al: Pupillary diameter assessment: need for a graded scale. Neurology 2000;54:530–531.
64. Lagrèze W-DA, Kardon RH: Correlation of relative afferent pupillary defect and estimated retinal ganglion cell loss. Graefe's Arch Clin Exp Ophthalmol 1998;236:401–404.
65. Enyedi LB, Dev S, Cox TA: A comparison of the Marcus Gunn and alternating light tests for afferent pupillary defects. Ophthalmology 1998;105:871–873.

PART II

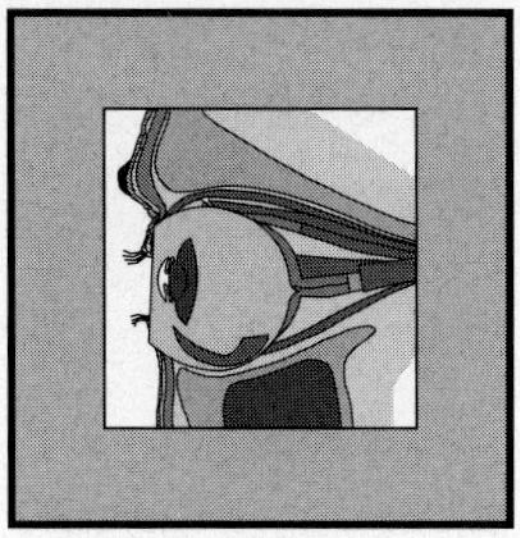

VISUAL LOSS AND OTHER DISORDERS OF THE AFFERENT VISUAL PATHWAY

CHAPTER 3

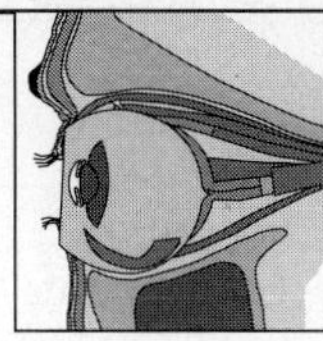

Visual Loss: Overview, Visual Field Testing, and Topical Diagnosis

The afferent visual pathways encompass structures which perceive, relay, and process visual information: the eyes, optic nerves (cranial nerve II), chiasm, tracts, lateral geniculate nuclei, optic radiations, and striate cortex (Fig. 3–1). In general, the visual abnormalities caused by lesions anterior to and including the chiasm cause acuity (clarity) loss, color deficits, and visual field defects (abnormal central or peripheral vision). From a neuro-ophthalmic standpoint, unilateral retrochiasmal (posterior to the chiasm) disturbances present primarily with homonymous (both eyes involved with the same laterality) visual field defects without acuity loss. Higher-order processing, instrumental in interpreting visual images, occurs in extrastriate association cortex. Abnormalities in these areas cause, for instance, deficits in object recognition, color perception, motion detection, and visual attention (neglect of visual stimuli in left or right hemifields).

This chapter will provide an overview of these structures, detail methods of visual field testing, then describe a framework for the localization and diagnosis of disorders affecting the afferent visual pathways. Determining *where* the lesion is first, then figuring out *what* it is second is the advocated approach. Further details regarding anatomy, blood supply, organization, neuro-ophthalmic symptoms, and differential diagnosis are detailed in Chapters 4 through 12.

NEUROANATOMY OF THE AFFERENT VISUAL PATHWAY—OVERVIEW

The Eye and Retina

The eyes are the primary sensory organs of the visual system. Before reaching the retina, light travels through the ocular media, consisting of the cornea, anterior chamber, lens, and vitreous. The size of the pupil, like the aperture of a camera, regulates the amount of light reaching the retina. The cornea and lens focus light rays to produce a clear image on the retina in the absence of refractive error, and the ciliary muscle can change the lens shape to adjust for objects at different distances (*accommodation*).

Retinal photoreceptors hyperpolarize in response to light. Cone photoreceptors are more sensitive to color and are concentrated in the middle of the retina, or macula, the center of which is the fovea. Rod photoreceptors, more important for night vision, predominate in the retinal periphery. Visual information is processed via horizontal, bipolar, and amacrine cells before reaching the ganglion cells, the axons of which make up the innermost portion of the retina and converge to form the optic disc and optic nerve. The optic disc represents the intraocular portion of the optic nerve anterior to the lamina cribrosa (see Fig. 2–38). The retina is normally transparent, and the orange-red color visible on funduscopy is due to the retinal pigment epithelium and choroidal circulation.

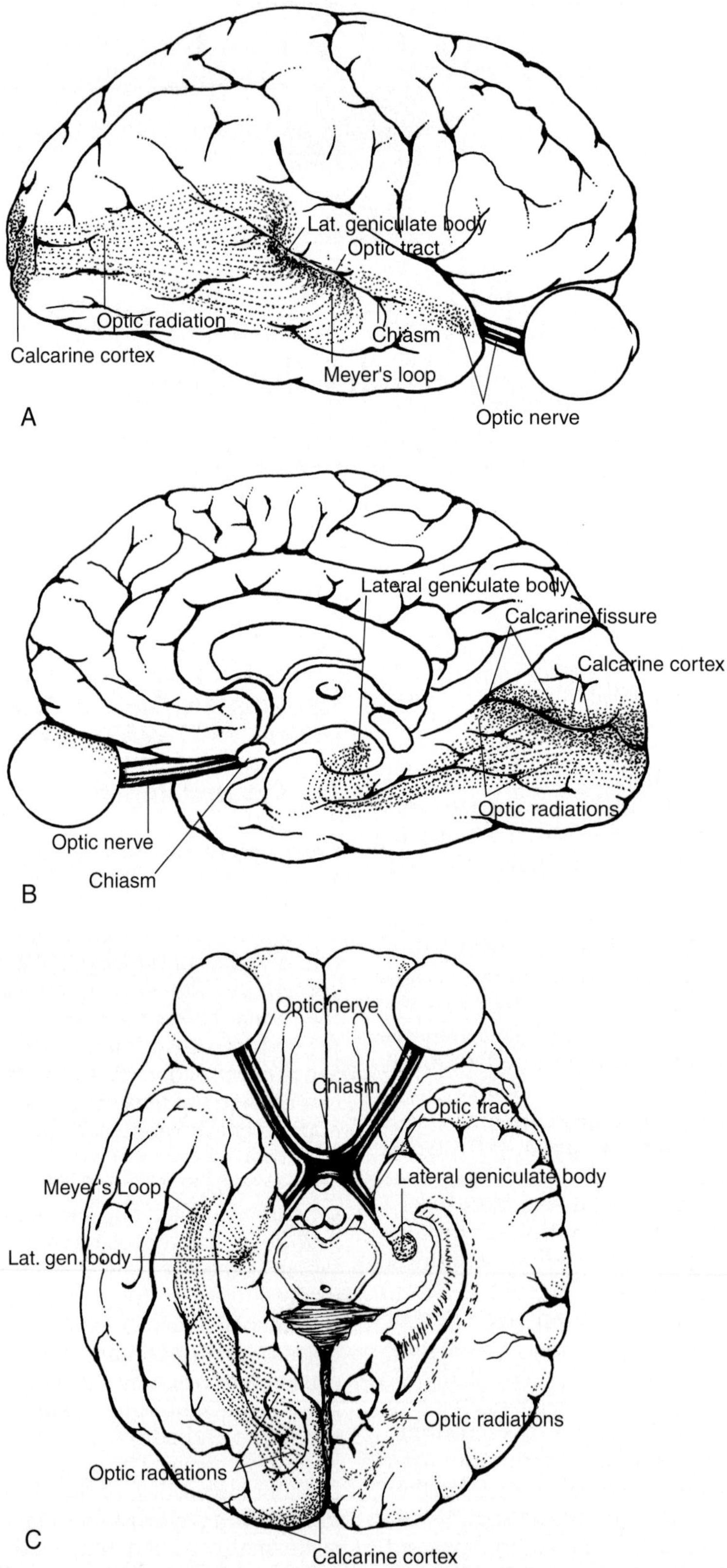

FIGURE 3–1. Afferent visual pathways. Major structures as viewed from (**A**) the lateral side, (**B**) the medial side, and (**C**) the underside of the brain. (Redrawn from Cushing H: Trans Am Neurol Assoc 1921:374–423.)

The retina nasal to the macula receives visual information from the temporal field, and the temporal retina from the nasal field (Fig. 3–2). The superior and inferior halves of the retina have a similar crossed relationship with respect to lower and upper fields of vision.

The ophthalmic artery, a branch of the internal carotid, provides most of the blood supply to the eye although there are external carotid anastomoses. The first major branch of the ophthalmic artery, the central retinal artery, pierces the dura of the optic nerve behind the globe, then travels within the nerve to emerge at the optic disc to supply the inner two thirds of the retina. The ophthalmic artery also gives rise to the posterior ciliary arteries, which supply the optic nerve head, choroid, and outer third of the retina.

Optic Nerve, Chiasm, and Tract

The optic nerve has four major portions: intraocular, intraorbital, intracanalicular, and intracranial. Posterior to the lamina cribrosa, optic nerve axons are myelinated by oligodendrocytes similar to those in white matter tracts in the brain and spinal cord.

Axons from the two optic nerves join at the optic chiasm, which lies in the suprasellar region, superior to the diaphragma sella and inferior to the third ventricle and hypothalamus. At the chiasm, fibers from nasal retina cross, and the most ventral axons from the inferior nasal retina bend into the most proximal aspect of the contralateral optic nerve (*Wilbrand's knee*), while the fibers from temporal retina remain ipsilateral in the lateral portion of the chiasm (Fig. 3–2). The ratio of crossed to uncrossed fibers is 53% : 47%. Ipsilateral temporal fibers and contralateral nasal fibers join to form the optic tracts.

Geniculocalcarine Pathway

At the lateral geniculate nucleus, a part of the thalamus located above the ambient cistern,

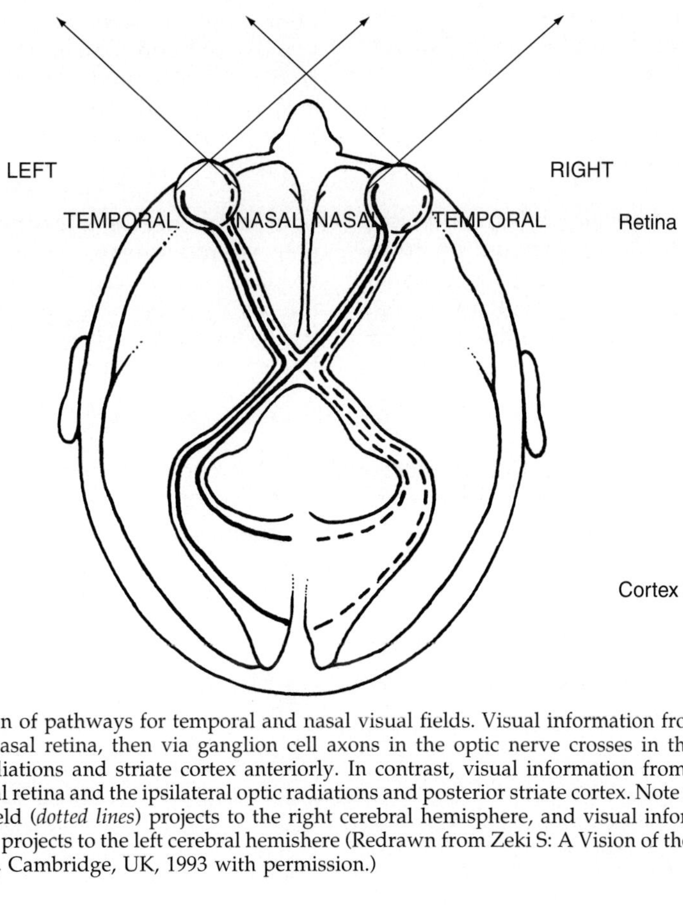

FIGURE 3–2. Separation of pathways for temporal and nasal visual fields. Visual information from the temporal visual field projects to the nasal retina, then via ganglion cell axons in the optic nerve crosses in the chiasm to reach the contralateral optic radiations and striate cortex anteriorly. In contrast, visual information from the nasal visual field projects to the temporal retina and the ipsilateral optic radiations and posterior striate cortex. Note that visual information from the left visual field (*dotted lines*) projects to the right cerebral hemisphere, and visual information from the right visual field (*solid lines*) projects to the left cerebral hemishere (Redrawn from Zeki S: A Vision of the Brain, p 23. Blackwell Scientific Publications, Cambridge, UK, 1993 with permission.)

the ganglion cell axons in the optic tract synapse with neurons destined to become the optic radiations. This latter structure is divided functionally and anatomically. Fibers coursing through the temporal lobe, termed *Meyer's loop,* subserve visual information from lower retina and connect to the inferior bank of the calcarine cortex. The parietal portion of the optic radiations relays information from upper retina to the superior bank of the calcarine cortex. Most of the optic radiations derive their blood supply from the middle cerebral artery. The mesial temporal section is supplied in part by branches of the posterior cerebral artery.

Striate Cortex

Brodmann area 17 (or V1, primary or striate cortex) is the end organ of the afferent visual system and is located within the calcarine cortex in the occipital lobe. Most of striate cortex, especially the portion situated posteriorly, is devoted to macular vision. Superior and inferior banks of calcarine cortex subserve contralateral inferior and superior quadrants, respectively. The majority of the occipital lobe is supplied by the posterior cerebral artery with a contribution from the middle cerebral artery in the occipital pole region.

Visual Association Areas

Higher processing of visual information occurs, for example, in the lingual and fusiform gyri bordering the inferior calcarine bank in structures believed to be equivalent to area V4 in monkeys, which is responsible for color vision. In an oversimplification, temporal lobe structures govern visual recognition and memory, while parietal lobe areas are responsible for motion and spatial analysis.

VISUAL FIELD TESTING

In patients with visual loss, the pattern of the visual field deficit can be highly localizing. Confrontation field testing, the techniques of which are detailed in Chapter 2, often provide extremely useful information. In general, the technique is specific, as field loss detected by confrontation is usually real.[1] However, confrontation is insensitive, as more subtle defects may be missed.[2]

More sensitive, reproducible, and precise visual field testing may be achieved by *automated or computerized threshold perimetry* or *kinetic testing with a Goldmann perimeter or tangent screen.*[3] Threshold computerized perimetry of the central 30 degrees of vision, although lengthy and tedious, in many instances is a more objective and more reproducible test for patients with optic neuropathies and chiasmal disturbances and those requiring serial testing. The kinetic techniques, because they are shorter and allow interaction with the examiner, may be more appropriate for screening and for patients with significant neurologic impairment. Computerized perimetry, owing to its wide availability and ease of administration, is currently the most popular test method.

Table 3–1 summarizes the advantages, disadvantages, and most appropriate neuro-ophthalmic uses of each modality. The examiner should always keep in mind that all modalities for visual field evaluation are inherently subjective and depend on the patient's level of alertness, cooperation, ability to fixate centrally, and response rapidity. In

TABLE 3–1. Advantages, Disadvantages, and Most Appropriate Neuro-ophthalmic Uses of Computerized Threshold, Goldmann Kinetic, and Tangent Screen Kinetic Perimetry

	Advantages	Disadvantages	Best Neuro-ophthalmic Uses
Computerized Threshold	Reproducible More objective More standardized Less reliance on a technician Intertechnician variability less important	Lengthy Tedious	Optic neuropathy Papilledema Chiasmal disorders Repeated follow-up
Goldmann Kinetic	Short Driven by technician or doctor	More subjective Depends on the skills of the perimetrist	Retrochiasmal disorders Neurologically impaired patients Severe visual loss
Tangent Screen Kinetic	Short Can be performed in the exam room	Central 30° only	Central field defects Functional visual loss

addition, astute patients feigning visual loss can voluntarily alter their visual fields during perimetric testing.

In most cases, the visual field is tested for each eye separately. Except in patients using miotic eye drops for glaucoma, for instance, field testing should take place before pharmacologic dilation of the pupils, which tends to worsen performance even if accommodative dysfunction has been corrected with lenses.[4, 5]

Visual fields are recorded so that the field of the right eye is on the right and the field of the left eye is on the left (see Fig. 2–10). The blind spot, caused by the absence of photoreceptors overlying the optic nerve, is located approximately 15 degrees temporal to and slightly below fixation and is drawn as an area without vision. As previously stated, *homonymous defects* are those present in both eyes with the same laterality. A *hemianopia* refers to loss of half of the visual field, respecting the vertical (usually) or horizontal meridian. *Congruity* refers to the symmetry of the field defect in both eyes.

The Hill of Vision Concept

Although the visual field is plotted on a piece of paper in two dimensions, it can be conceptualized three dimensionally as an "island or hill of vision in a sea of darkness" (Fig. 3–3).[6, 7] The z-axis value indicates visual sensitivity, while the location within the field of vision is plotted in the x,y plane. Foveal vision has the highest sensitivity but extends nasally and temporally only a few degrees. Thus, with increasing sensitivity (up on the z axis), the field of vision decreases in size, and the hill peaks at fixation ($x = 0$, $y = 0$). In contrast, at low sensitivities (lower on the z axis), the field of vision is much larger. The blind spot is depicted as an opening in the island temporal to the central peak,[8] and the opening extends all the way to the bottom of the island. Sensitivity falls more rapidly nasally than temporally. Outside of the x and y coordinates delimiting the bottom of the island, nothing is seen.

The major difference between threshold (static) and kinetic perimetry can be described using the hill of vision concept. Threshold perimetry determines the visual sensitivity (z-axis value) at any particular x,y point. On the other hand, kinetic perimetry plots the visual field (in the x,y plane) for a stimulus at a given sensitivity (z-axis) level. The plot of a kinetic field can be considered to be a two-dimensional representation of the hill of vision (Fig. 3–4).

When visual field defects occur, the corresponding part of the island is lost (Fig. 3–5). Visual field constriction can be conceptualized as the island of vision sinking into the sea of blindness. In these cases, the central peak occurs at a lower sensitivity level, and the field of vision at any particular sensitivity level is smaller.

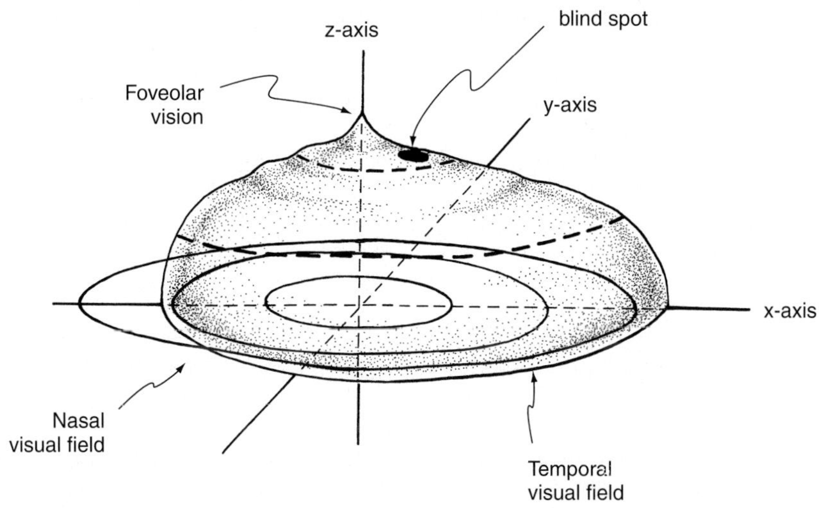

FIGURE 3–3. "Island of vision in a sea of blindness." This three-dimensional representation of the visual field plots visual sensitivity along the z-axis versus location within the x,y plane.

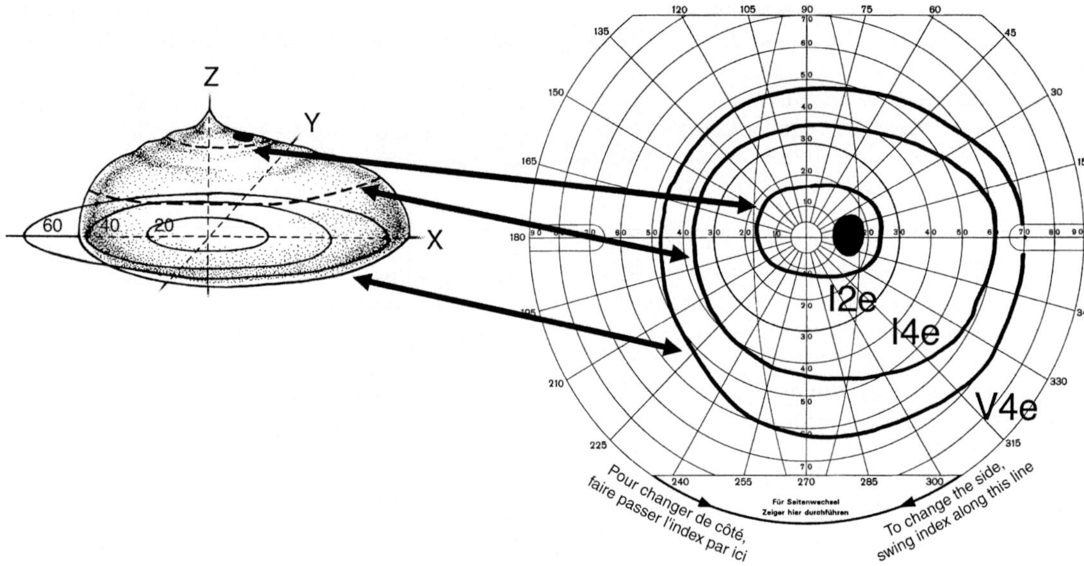

FIGURE 3–4. The island of vision (*left*) contains the information produced by kinetic perimetry (*right*). Kinetic perimetry plots the visual field (in the x,y plane) for a stimulus at a given sensitivity (z-axis) level. Thus each isopter (I4e plot, for instance) on the kinetic perimetry can be translated from the island of vision.

Computerized Threshold Perimetry

There are many types of computerized threshold perimetry in wide use, including Humphrey (Carl Zeiss), Octopus, and Dicon.[9] The major advantages of computerized perimetry over other forms are that they permit more standardized testing procedures,[10, 11] require less technician skill, and are affected less by inter-technician variability.[12] Some studies have also demonstrated that automated computerized perimetry may be more sensitive to subtle field loss than Goldmann perimetry.[12] The discussion in this section will highlight the testing features of the Humphrey perimeter (Fig. 3–6), which is the most popular.

In the Humphrey threshold 30-2 test, the computer presents white light stimuli against a white background within the central 30 degrees of vision of each eye. Lens correction for near is provided, and the patient looks at a central target and hits a buzzer when he or she sees the light. The stimulus size is kept the same, but the stimulus intensity is varied, and the computer records the intensity of the dimmest stimulus the patient saw at various points in the visual field. This *threshold intensity* is recorded in decibels, and the higher the number, the dimmer the stimulus and the higher the sensitivity. The computer also determines the location of the blind spot.

The test can be laborious and sometimes soporific, even for the most cooperative individuals. It is not unusual for each eye to be tested with over 450 points over approximately 15 minutes. FASTPAC software programs may save up to 40% of test time for a Humphrey field,[13] but the results may not be as accurate as with the regular full-threshold algorithm.[14] Patient reliability during a Humphrey field is reflected in the number and proportion of fixation losses, and false-positive and false-negative responses (Fig. 3–7). When the patient responds to a stimulus presented in the originally plotted blind spot, a *fixation loss* is thought to have occurred. A *false-positive* response happens when the patient hits the buzzer but no light stimulus was presented. When a patient does not hit the buzzer if a stimulus of identical location and greater intensity to one that was previously detected is presented, this is considered a *false-negative* response. Either a fixation loss rate of 20%, a false-positive rate of 33%, or a false-negative rate of 33% indicates an unreliable visual field.[15] Severe visual field loss may be associated with abnormally high false-negative rates.

The printout displays the visual field data in several ways (Fig. 3–7),[15, 16] including some with statistical analysis. The threshold intensities are presented in raw data form. The *grey*

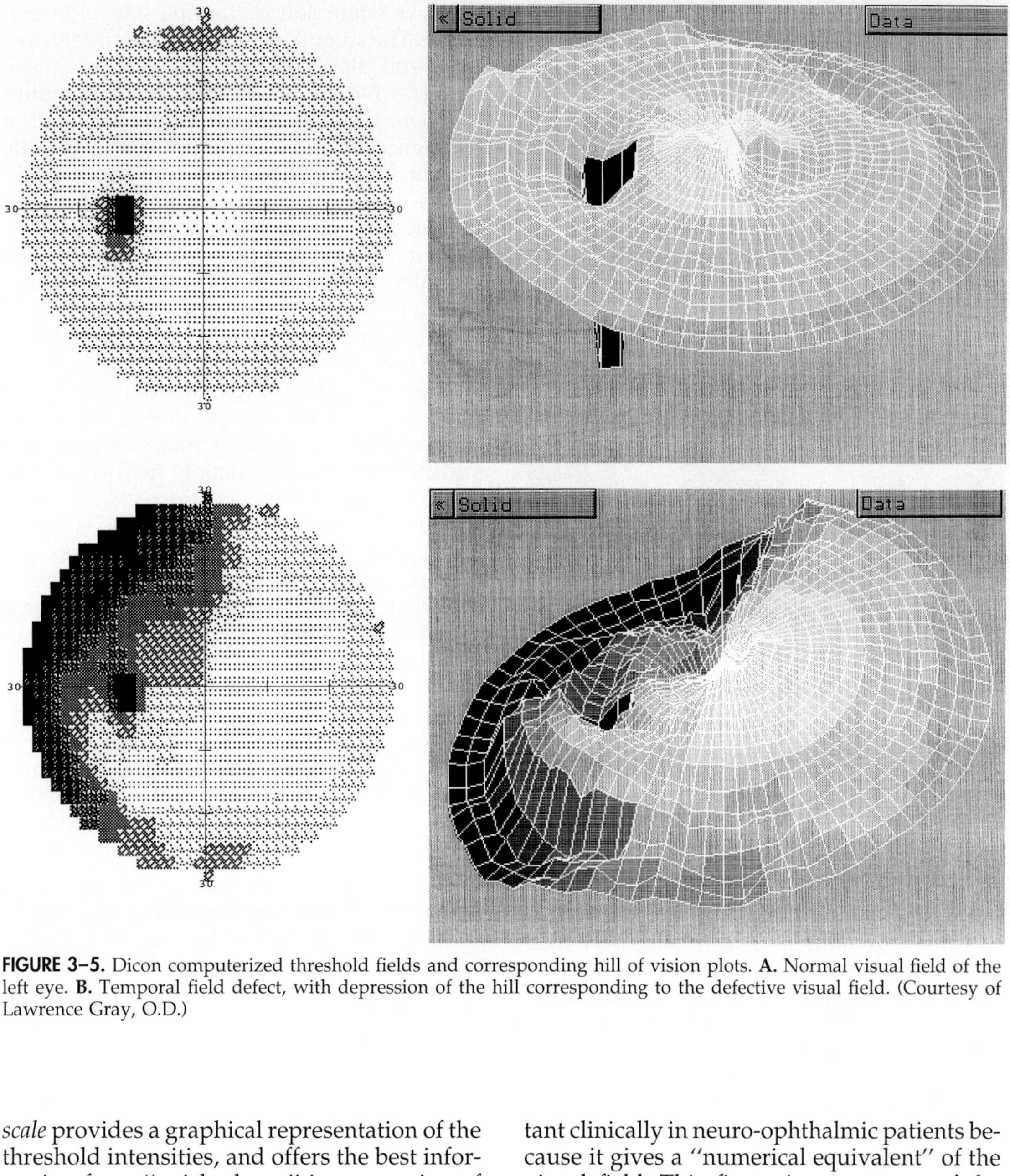

FIGURE 3–5. Dicon computerized threshold fields and corresponding hill of vision plots. **A.** Normal visual field of the left eye. **B.** Temporal field defect, with depression of the hill corresponding to the defective visual field. (Courtesy of Lawrence Gray, O.D.)

scale provides a graphical representation of the threshold intensities, and offers the best information for a "quick-glance" interpretation of the threshold visual field. The *total deviation map* plots the difference between each measured threshold value and those of age-matched normal values for each point in the visual field. The *pattern deviation map* accents local visual field defects after correcting for the overall height of the hill of vision. Diffuse field loss, as might occur with a cataract, are factored out this way. Probability displays are provided for the total deviation and pattern deviation maps. Of the global visual field indices, the *mean deviation* (MD) is the most important clinically in neuro-ophthalmic patients because it gives a "numerical equivalent" of the visual field. This figure is an average of the numbers in the total deviation plot, with each value weighted according to the normal range at that point. As a patient's visual field worsens, due to an enlarging scotoma for instance, the mean deviation becomes more negative. Serial visual fields can be compared by following the mean deviation.

Several factors may influence the patient's performance on this test. The learning curve is steep, and individuals undergoing threshold perimetry have a natural tendency to provide more reliable visual fields on subsequent test-

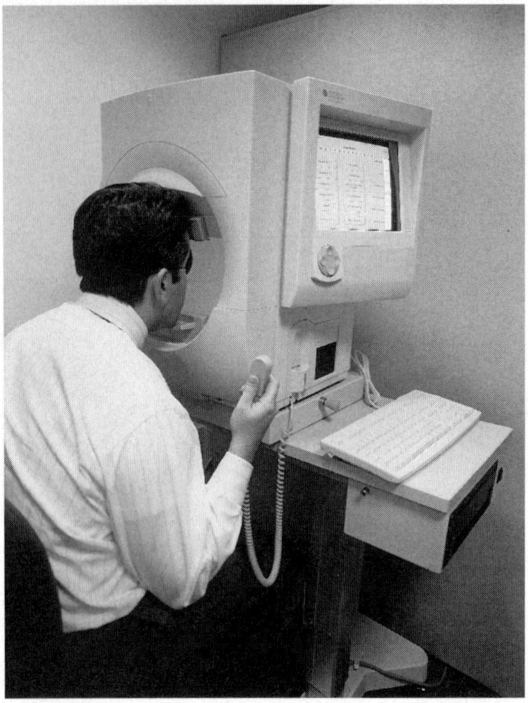

FIGURE 3–6. Humphrey computerized perimeter.

ing.[17] Mild ptosis may be associated with depression of the superior visual field,[18] and cataracts and pupillary miosis may cause diffusely decreased sensitivity.[19] The influence of age on the visual fields of normal individuals also has been studied, and a decrease in sensitivity with increasing age was found.[20, 21] There may also be some variability in performance over time in different disease states.[22]

During screening full field examinations such as 120-point ones, the computer presents static light stimuli of fixed size and intensity, and the patient presses the buzzer if he or she sees them. They are not typically threshold tests, and the plot depicts merely whether the light stimulus was seen or not. A "quantify defects" modification can be used to threshold test missed points. The full-field screens are helpful in detecting large field defects such as hemianopias or altitudinal field loss. However, because the points can be spread far apart, often the information provided is so vague that the test becomes unuseful.[23]

Goldmann Kinetic Perimetry

As the patient fixates on the central target in an illuminated bowl (Fig. 3–8), the perimetrist displays white dots of varying size and luminance. The stimuli are presented both centripetally and statically, and the patient hits a buzzer when he or she detects the stimulus. The perimetrist monitors the patient's fixation through a telescope, constantly reminds the patient to look straight ahead, and compliments good responses. This perimetrist–patient relationship makes the test ideal if the patient is young, has poor vision, or is neurologically impaired. Furthermore, Goldmann perimetry rarely requires more than 5 to 7 minutes per eye, and short breaks can be taken at the examiner's discretion. The test also can be tailored to the clinical situation: screening for chiasmal or hemianopic defects by paying particular attention to asymmetries along the vertical meridian,[24, 25] arcuate field defects in glaucoma, and infranasal defects in papilledema.[26] Since the whole visual field is tested, Goldmann perimetry will detect the rare peripheral visual field defects, due to anterior calcarine, temporal lobe, or early chiasmal compressive lesions, for instance, which may have been missed by computerized perimetry of the central 30 degrees.[27]

However, perimetrist bias can be a disadvantage, especially when Goldmann perimetry is used in serial follow-up. Another drawback to the technique is that the perimetrist needs a working knowledge of afferent visual pathway anatomy and related patterns of field loss.

The size of the stimulus (Fig. 3–9) is indicated by Roman numerals ranging from O to V, corresponding to dots measuring .062 mm^2 to 64 mm^2, respectively. Stimulus luminance is designated by an Arabic numeral from 1 to 4, in order of increasing brightness, together with a small letter from a to e, by convention usually held at e. The smallest, dimmest stimulus used in practice is labeled I1e, and the largest, brightest stimulus is designated by V4e. Usually the dots are white, but colored stimuli can be used in some situations, such as in the evaluation of hereditary optic neuropathies. Lens correction for near is given when targets are presented within the central 30 degrees.

The results are displayed from the patient's point of view (ie, what he or she sees). The area in which the stimulus was seen is called an *isopter,* which is labeled according to the stimulus size and luminance (Fig. 3–9). The normal temporal V4e field can extend at least 90 degrees, while the normal nasal V4e field

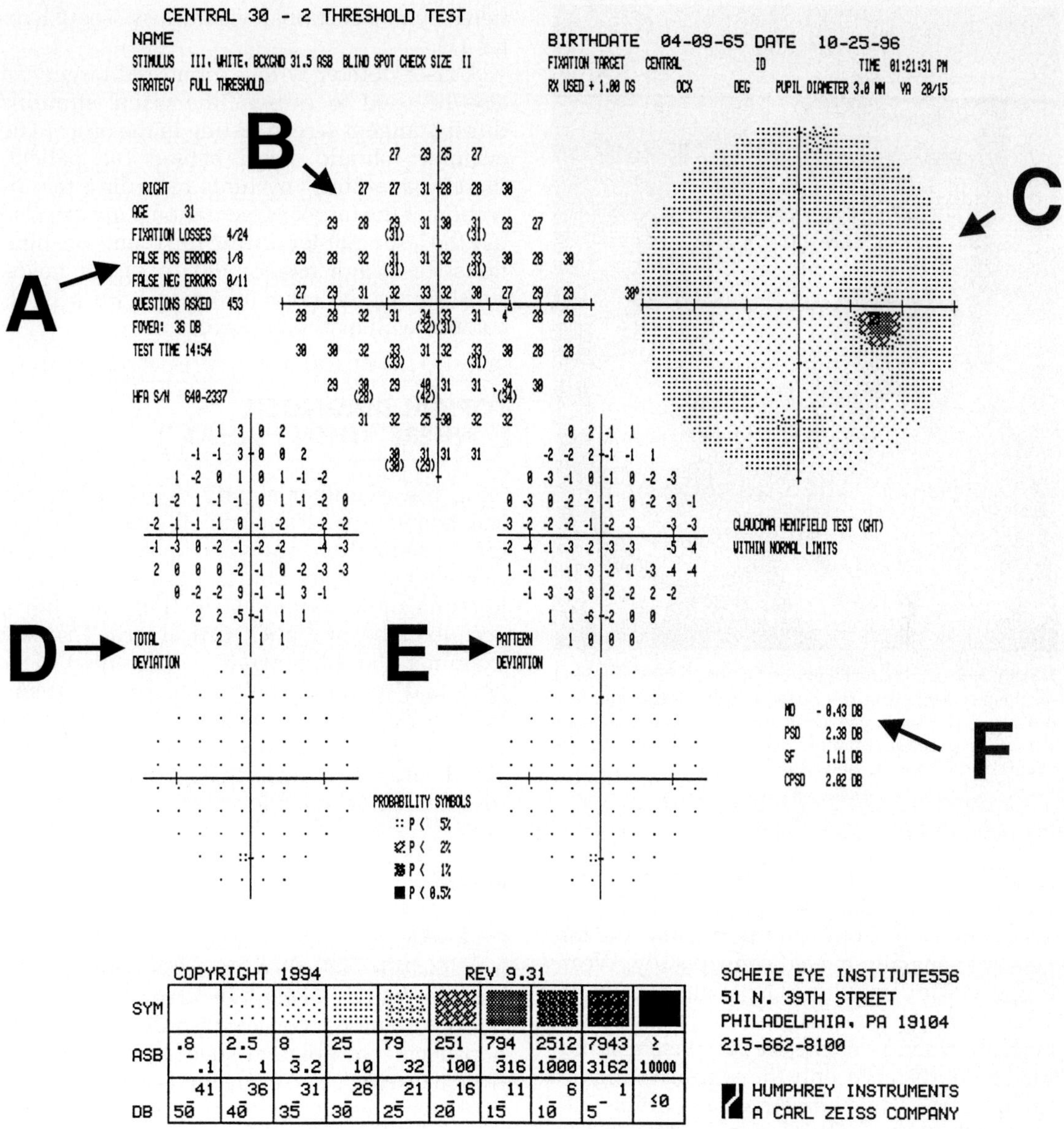

FIGURE 3–7. Normal Humphrey computerized 30-2 threshold visual field of the right eye. Note (**A**) the tabulation of the fixation losses and false-positive and -negative errors; (**B**) the raw data, recording the luminance, given in decibels (dB's), of the dimmest stimulus the subject saw at that position in the visual field; (**C**) the grey scale, containing a conversion of the raw data using the key at the bottom of the readout; (**D**) the total deviation; (**E**) the pattern deviation; and (**F**) the statistical analysis, including the mean deviation (MD).

can extend to at least 60 degrees. In normal individuals, it is sometimes sufficient to plot only the I4e isopter. The field using a test target that is either smaller or dimmer is always smaller than the field produced with a larger or brighter stimulus. *Scotomas,* circumscribed areas of visual field loss, are indicated by zones that are shaded in. The blind spot, the result of the absence of photoreceptors overlying the optic disc, is technically a scotoma and is temporal to fixation in all normal individuals.

Tangent Screen Visual Field Testing

This test can be performed quickly in any examination room equipped with a tangent screen hung on a wall.[23] The perimetrist moves

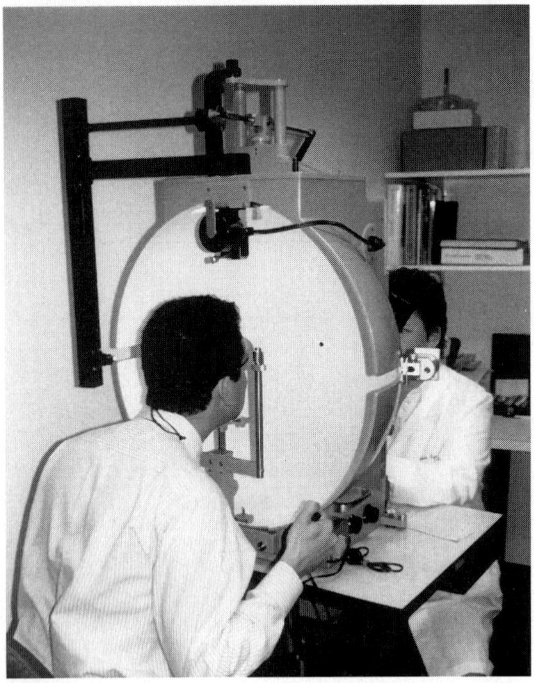

FIGURE 3–8. Goldmann kinetic perimetry. Note the subject has his head in a chin-rest in the middle of the spherical bowl and presses a buzzer in his right hand when he sees the presented stimulus. The tester administers the examination from the other side of the bowl.

round white or colored discs or spheres over a black or grey flat felt background (Fig. 3–10A), and as in Goldmann perimetry, the targets are generally moved centripetally. Wearing spectacle correction, the patient usually sits 1 meter away from the screen and indicates verbally when he or she sees the visual stimulus. At this distance, only the central 30 degrees can be tested. The perimetrist can outline with chalk where the patient saw the target, and the results can be recorded similar to the way confrontation fields are drawn (see Chapter 2). The isopters are designated as a fraction, such as 3w/1000, which indicates that a 3-mm white target was used at a distance of 1000 mm (1 meter).

Small central defects that may be missed by Goldmann perimetry or computerized field testing may be more evident with the tangent screen method. Subtle hemianopic deficits can be detected by holding two equivalent targets on both sides of fixation (Fig. 3–10B), and asking the patient if one appears different than the other. Perhaps the most common use of the tangent screen test is in the demonstration of nonphysiologic tubular visual fields in patients with functional visual loss (see Chapter 11).

A laser pointer with a round red target can also be used to present the visual stimulus during tangent screen testing in the office. The examiner should stand behind the patient, thereby avoiding any hints regarding the direction of the target presentation. One can also use the laser pointer during inpatient consultations for rough assessment of visual fields, substituting the tangent screen with a light-colored wall as the background.

TOPICAL DIAGNOSIS ("WHERE" THEN "WHAT")

First, the examiner should decide *where* the lesion is neuroanatomically. Based on the history, examination, and visual field testing, the examiner should be able to localize the process to retina, optic nerve, chiasm, tract, radiations, occipital lobe, or higher cortical area. Then the examiner should generate a differential diagnosis and attempt to determine *what* the lesion is. Historical features often guide the differential diagnosis, and then neuroimaging combined with other ancillary tests frequently narrow the list of possible causes.

History

Common complaints encountered with visual loss include so-called negative phenomena such as "blurry vision" or "grey vision." Patients with higher cortical disorders often have nonspecific complaints such as "I'm having trouble seeing" or "Focusing is difficult." Patients with lesions of the afferent visual pathway may also complain of positive phenomena, such as flashing or colored lights (*phosphenes* or *photopsias*), jagged lines, or formed visual hallucinations (a false perception that a stimulus is present). The complexity of positive phenomena does not specify localization.

The temporal profile of the visual loss will suggest possible diagnoses, and its monocularity or binocularity will help in localization. As a general rule, acute or subacute visual deficits result from ischemic or inflammatory injury to the optic nerve. Vitreous hemorrhage and retinal detachment are other important considerations. Chronic or progressive visual loss, in turn, may result from a compressive, infiltrative, or degenerative process. Cataracts, refrac-

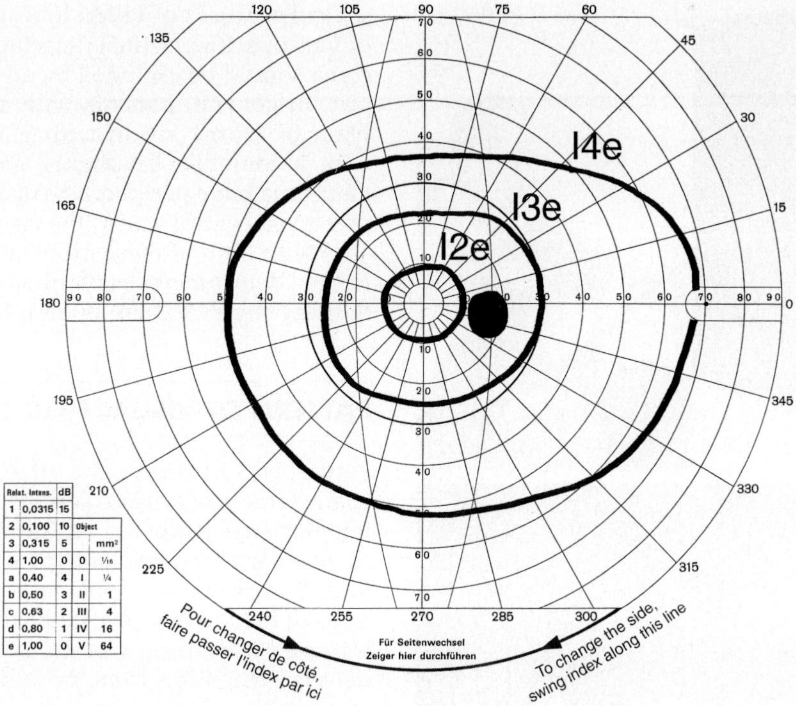

FIGURE 3–9. Normal Goldmann kinetic field of the right eye. The labels I4e, I3e, and I2e indicate the stimuli size and luminance (detailed in key on bottom left-hand side of the figure). The stimuli are presented in the periphery then directed radially to the center. The dark lines indicate the point at which the subject noticed the stimulus. Note the temporal location of the blind spot and that the temporal field is larger than the right.

tive error, open-angle glaucoma, and retinal disorders such as age-related macular degeneration or diabetic retinopathy also need to be considered when visual symptoms are insidious.

If a patient complains of monocular visual loss, a process in one eye or optic nerve should be considered. Painless transient visual loss characterized by a "grey shade" that encroaches on vision superiorly then resolves after seconds or minutes is typical of amaurosis fugax related to carotid disease. Painful monocular visual loss occurring over days is characteristic of an inflammatory or demyelinating optic neuropathy. With binocular visual loss, a lesion of both eyes or optic nerves, or of the chiasm, tract, radiations, or occipital lobe should be investigated. Further details regarding these specific complaints and their localizing value are provided in the respective chapters.

Associated neurologic deficits, such as motor or sensory abnormalities, will also assist in localization and often indicate a hemispheric abnormality. Medical conditions should always be investigated in the review of systems. Hypertension, diabetes, and smoking, for instance, predispose the patient to vascular disease, and a history of coronary artery disease should alert the examiner to the possibility of carotid artery insufficiency as well. Visual loss accompanied by endocrine symptoms, such as those consistent with hypopituitarism (amenorrhea, decreased libido, impotence, for example) or pituitary hypersecretion (galactorrhea, acromegaly, for example), suggests a chiasmal disorder.

Examination

Particular attention should be paid to assessment of acuity, color vision, confrontational visual fields, pupillary reactivity, and funduscopic appearance. Neuro-ophthalmic examination techniques are discussed in Chapter 2.

Monocular acuity loss, deficits in color vision, a central scotoma, a relative afferent pupillary defect, and optic disc swelling or pallor suggest an optic neuropathy. In an acute retrobulbar optic neuropathy, the optic disc may have a normal appearance. Monocular visual loss with a central scotoma, metamorphopsia, preserved color vision, and no afferent pupil-

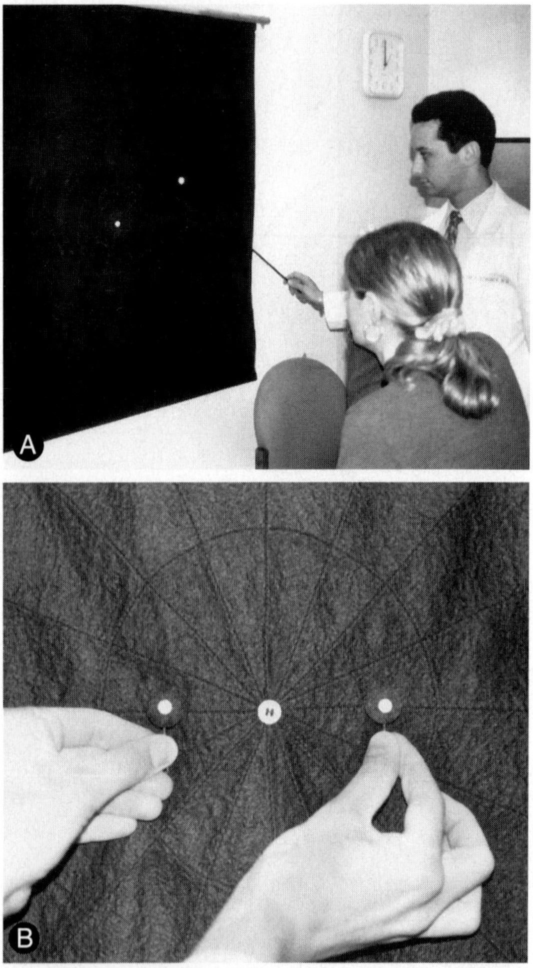

FIGURE 3–10. Tangent screen visual field test. Each eye is tested separately. **A.** The examiner moves a white or colored object in front of a black felt screen, and the patient points or verbalizes when he or she sees the target. The results can be recorded in white chalk on the felt, then transferred into the patient's record. **B.** Two equivalent targets can be presented while the patient fixates centrally to test for subtle central visual field defects respecting the vertical meridian.

lary defect makes a maculopathy more likely. Bilateral loss of acuity suggests bilateral optic nerve, chiasm, or bilateral retrochiasmal lesions. Homonymous hemianopic field loss with normal acuity, pupillary reactivity, and funduscopic appearance are normally associated with a retrogeniculate process. A hemianopia accompanied by an ipsilateral hemiparesis or sensory loss is likely to be the result of a parietal process, while an isolated hemianopia is more likely the result of an occipital lobe lesion.

Ocular causes of visual loss such as corneal or lens opacities, retinal detachments, or glaucoma should be excluded by an ophthalmologist. In general, patients with cataracts complain of blurry vision with glare, especially with automobile headlights, and those with glaucoma have peripheral visual field loss but preserved central acuity; the visual loss associated with both of these problems is insidious. Retinal detachments may present acutely with flashes of light, floaters, or peripheral field loss.

PATTERN OF VISUAL FIELD LOSS

Figure 3–11 illustrates the visual field deficits characteristic of various lesions within the afferent visual pathway. As alluded to earlier, monocular visual field defects most commonly localize to retina or optic nerve, and the patterns of field loss are typically altitudinal, central, cecocentral, or arcuate. Monocular field defects emanating from the blind spot, as in an arcuate scotoma, for instance, are almost always related to an optic nerve lesion or a retinal vascular occlusion.[28] A bitemporal hemianopia is very specific to the chiasm. Homonymous hemianopic deficits suggest a retrochiasmal lesion. Incongruous hemianopias tend to be more anterior, while congruous hemianopias, with or without macular sparing, are more characteristic of occipital disturbances. One possible explanation for this pattern is the closer grouping of retrochiasmal fibers from each eye as they proceed posteriorly. Complete homonymous hemianopias have no localizing value, because congruity can not be assessed. The particular patterns of visual field loss are discussed in greater detail in Chapters 4 through 8.

Ancillary Visual Testing

Electrophysiologic testing such as a visual evoked potential (VEP) or electroretinogram (ERG) can confirm the localization to optic nerve or retina, but these tests should never replace the clinical examination. VEPs measure the cortical activity in response to flash or patterned stimuli and are abnormal in the presence of a lesion in the afferent visual pathway. ERGs, which measure rod and cone photoreceptor function, are particularly helpful in sorting out the retinal dystrophies and degenerations.

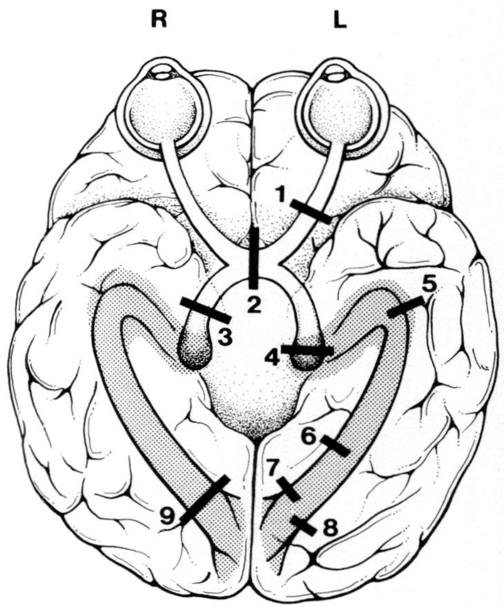

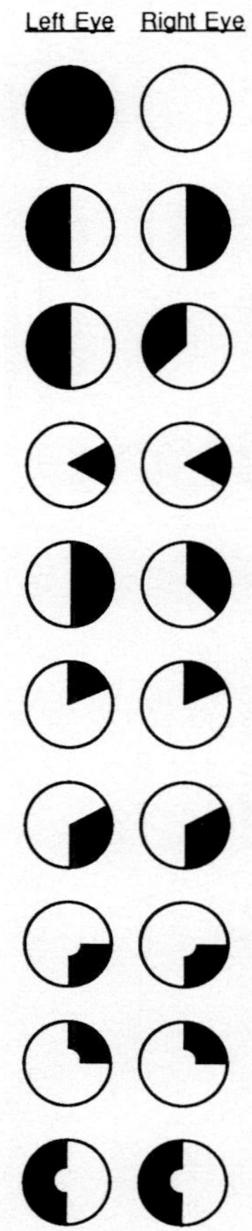

	Location	Field Defect: Comment
1	Left Optic Nerve	No light perception left eye
2	Chiasm	Bitemporal hemianopsia
3	Right Optic Tract	Incongruous left homonymous hemianopia
4	Left Lateral Geniculate Nucleus	Right homonymous sectoranopia (lateral choroidal artery) - or - Incongruous right homonymous hemianopia
5	Left Temporal Lobe	Right homonymous upper quadrant defect ("pie in the sky")
6	Left Parietal Lobe	Right homonymous defect, denser inferiorly
7	Left Occipital Lobe (upper bank)	Right homonymous lower quadrananopsia (macular sparing)
8	Left Occipital Lobe (lower bank)	Right homonymous upper quadrananopsia (macular sparing)
9	Right Occipital Lobe	Left homonymous hemianopia (macular sparing)

FIGURE 3–11. Visual pathways: correlation of lesion site and field defect, view of underside of the brain. *Homonymous* refers to a defect present in both eyes with the same laterality, while a *hemianopia* refers to visual loss respecting the vertical meridian. Congruous fields are symmetric in both eyes. Note that lesions of upper or lower occipital banks produce quadrantic defects, while lesions within temporal and parietal lobes cause field defects that tend not to respect the horizontal meridian.

TABLE 3–2. Topical Diagnosis: Various Causes of Visual Loss According to Lesion Site Within the Afferent Visual Pathway

Lesion Site	Common Causes	Findings
Ocular	Refractive error, media opacities	Vision may improve with pinhole; normal pupillary reactivity
Retina	Macular degeneration, central retinal artery occlusion, central retinal vein occlusion	Visible retinal abnormality on ophthalmoscopy
Optic nerve	Inflammatory lesions (idiopathic optic neuritis, sarcoid); ischemia (atherosclerotic, vasculitic); infiltrative/infectious (neoplastic, syphilis)	Afferent pupillary defect present if unilateral; central, centrocecal, or arcuate field defect; disc swelling may be visualized if optic nerve head involved
Chiasm	Sellar mass (pituitary adenoma, craniopharyngioma, meningioma, or aneurysm)	Bitemporal hemianopia; optic atrophy if chronic
Optic tract	Sellar mass	APD variable; incongruous hemianopia; "bow-tie" disc atrophy if long standing
Lateral geniculate	Stroke	Incongruous hemianopia, optic atrophy late; horizontal sectoranopia or quadruple quadrantanopia suggestive of infarction
Optic radiations (parietal)	Stroke, neoplasm	Inferior contralateral quadrantanopia; normal pupillary reactivity; defective optokinetic response with targets drawn toward the lesion
Optic radiations (temporal)	Stroke, neoplasm	Superior contralateral quadrantanopia; normal pupillary reactivity
Occipital	Stroke, neoplasm	Congruous contralateral hemianopia with or without macular sparing; normal pupillary reactivity; normal optokinetic response

Differential Diagnosis

Table 3–2 highlights examination findings, visual field abnormalities, and common causes to consider for various localizations within the afferent visual pathway. Optic neuropathies in young adults are typically inflammatory, while in older adults they are more commonly associated with vascular disease. The most common cause of a chiasmal syndrome is a compressive sellar mass. Strokes and neoplasms are the most common causes of retrochiasmal visual loss. The reader is referred to Chapters 4 through 8 for further details regarding the differential diagnoses and discussion of the various responsible causes.

REFERENCES

1. Shahinafar S, Johnson LN, Madsen RW: Confrontation visual field loss as a function of decibel sensitivity loss on automated static perimetry. Implications on the accuracy of confrontation visual field testing. Ophthalmology 1995;102:872–877.
2. Trobe JD, Acosta PC, Krischer JP, et al: Confrontation visual field techniques in the detection of anterior visual pathway lesions. Ann Neurol 1981;10:28–34.
3. Hupp SL: Visual fields in neuro-ophthalmology. J Ophthalmic Nurs Technol 1993;12:259–265.
4. Lindenmuth KA, Skuta GL, Rabbani R, et al: Effects of pupillary dilation on automated perimetry in normal patients. Ophthalmology 1990;97:367–370.
5. Kudrna GR, Stanley MA, Remington LA: Pupillary dilation and its effects on automated perimetry results. J Am Optom Assoc 1995;66:675–680.
6. Traquair HM: An Introduction to Clinical Perimetry, 5th edition, pp 1–16. London, Henry Kimpton, 1946.
7. Anderson DR: Introduction. In: Testing the Field of Vision, pp 1–17. St. Louis, CV Mosby, 1982.
8. Frisén L: The foundations of visual field testing. In: Clinical Tests of Vision, pp. 55–77. New York, Raven Press, 1990.
9. Wong AY, Dodge RM, Remington LA: Comparing threshold visual fields between the Dicon TKS 4000 automated perimeter and the Humphrey Field Analyzer. J Am Optom Assoc 1995;66:706–711.
10. American Academy of Ophthalmology: Automated perimetry. Ophthalmology 1996;103:1144–1151.
11. Johnson CA: Standardizing the measurement of visual fields. Ophthalmology 1996;103:186–189.
12. Katz J, Tielsch JM, Quigley HA, et al: Automated perimetry detects visual field loss before manual Goldmann perimetry. Ophthalmology 1995;102:21–26.
13. Mills RP, Barnebey HS, Migliazzo CV, et al: Does saving time using FASTPAC or suprathreshold testing reduce quality of visual fields? Ophthalmology 1994;101:1596–1603.
14. Mikelberg FS: The interpretation of automated visual fields. Can J Ophthalmol 1995;30:281–283.
15. Anderson DR: Automated perimetry. Trade secrets. Bascom Palmer Eye Institute, Miami, FL. Jan. 3, 1993;1–12.
16. Piltz-Seymour JR: Visual field conference. Scheie Eye Institute, Philadelphia, PA, Oct. 6, 1992;1–7.

17. Heijl A, Bengtsson B: The effect of perimetric experience in patients with glaucoma. Arch Ophthalmol 1996;114:19–22.
18. Meyer DR, Stern JH, Jarvis JM, et al: Evaluating the visual field effects of blepharoptosis using automated static perimetry. Ophthalmology 1993;100:651–658.
19. Harrington DO, Drake MV: Normal visual field. In: The Visual Fields. Text and Atlas of Clinical Perimetry, 6th edition, pp. 93–103. St. Louis, CV Mosby, 1990.
20. Haas A, Flammer J, Schneider U: Influence of age on the visual fields of normal subjects. Am J Ophthalmol 1986;101:199–203.
21. Jaffe GJ, Alvarado JA, Juster RP: Age-related changes of the normal visual field. Arch Ophthalmol 1986;104:1021–1025.
22. Wall M, Johnson CA, Kutzko KE, et al: Long- and short-term variability of automated perimetry result in patients with optic neuritis and healthy subjects. Arch Ophthalmol 1998;116:53–61.
23. Harrington DO, Drake MV: Manual perimeters: instruments and use. In: The Visual Fields. Text and Atlas of Clinical Perimetry, 6th edition, pp 13–34. St. Louis, CV Mosby, 1990.
24. Trobe JD, Acosta PC: An algorithm for visual fields. Surv Ophthalmol 1980;24:665–670.
25. Trobe JD, Acosta PC, Krischer JP: A screening method for chiasmal visual-field defects. Arch Ophthalmol 1981;99:264–271.
26. Wall M, George D: Visual loss in pseudotumor cerebri. Incidence and defects related to visual field strategy. Arch Neurol 1987;44:170–175.
27. Wirtschafter JD, Hard-Boberg A-L, Coffman SM: Evaluating the usefulness in neuro-ophthalmology of visual field examinations peripheral to 30 degrees. Trans Am Ophthalmol Soc 1984;82:329–357.
28. Larkin M: Visual fields interpretation. J Am Optom Assoc 1980;51:837–842.

CHAPTER 4

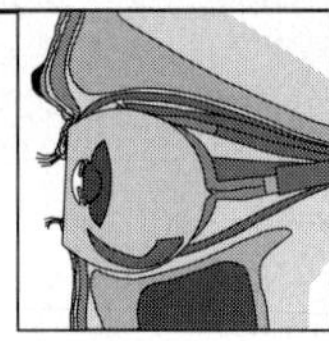

Vision Loss: Retinal Disorders of Neuro-Ophthalmic Interest

While a comprehensive review of all retinal disease is beyond the scope of this text, there are several entities that are particularly important in the neuro-ophthalmic differential diagnosis of visual loss. Patients with retinopathies may have symptoms and examination findings that overlap with patients with neuro-ophthalmic conditions. Both types of patients may manifest with visual acuity loss, visual field defects, and a paucity of findings on ophthalmoscopic examination. Certain retinal disorders may also provide invaluable clues to the existence of an underlying neurologic illness or systemic disease. In this chapter, we will examine the relevant retinal anatomy, the distinction between maculopathy and optic neuropathies, maculopathies that may mimic optic neuropathy, retinal vascular emboli and insufficiency, the photoreceptor disorders important in neuro-ophthalmic differential diagnosis (big blind spot syndrome, cancer-associated retinopathies), toxic retinopathies, heriditary retinopathies of neuro-ophthalmic interest, and the retinal manifestations of neurologic and systemic diseases and phakomatoses.

RETINAL ANATOMY

Cellular Elements of the Retina

The retina is a transparent structure that arises from the inner and outer layers of the embryologic optic cup. The outer layer consists of the retinal pigment epithelium (RPE) and the inner layer is a multicellular layer that makes up the neurosensory retina. The RPE consists of hexagonal cells extending from the optic nerve to the ora serata. The major functions of the RPE are to maintain the photoreceptors through vitamin A metabolism and phagocytosis of photoreceptor outer segements. Other functions include maintenance of the outer blood–retinal barrier, heat and light absorption, and production of extracellular matrix. Their basal sides form the inner layer of Bruch's membrane separating the retina from the choroid. Adjacent RPE cells have firm intracellular adhesions. Separation of the RPE from the neurosensory retina is called a *retinal detachment.*

The neurosensory retina consists of neural, glial, and vascular elements. The outermost layer (furtherest from the cornea and closet to the RPE) is the photoreceptor layer, consisting of rods and cones. The outer segments of the photoreceptors make contact with the RPE cells. The cell bodies of the photoreceptors make up the outer nuclear layer and are in contact with horizontal and bipolar cells through their process in the outer plexiform layer. The bipolar cells are oriented more vertically and bridge the connection to the inner plexiform layer where they synapse with ganglion cells and amacrine cells. The cell bodies of the bipolar cells, horizontal cells, and amacrine cells make up the inner nuclear layer located between the inner and outer plexiform layer. The ganglion cell axons run parallel to the surface of the retina and form the nerve fiber layer. The major glial cell of the retina is the Mueller cell, whose nucleus is in the inner nuclear layer and whose processes extend from the surface of the retina (inner limiting membrane) to the end of the outer nuclear layer (external limiting membrane). Together with some astrocytes and microglia these cells provide the nutritional and structural support to the retina.

Blood Supply

The first major branch of the internal carotid artery, the ophthalmic artery, provides the blood supply of the retina. It gives rise to the central retinal artery, which supplies the inner two thirds of the retina, and the posterior ciliary arteries, which supply the outer portions of the retina (Fig. 4–1). The temporal blood vessels arc above and below the macula in company with the arcuate nerve fiber bundles (ganglion cell axons). The vessels are found in the inner retinal layers and usually do not extend deeper than the inner plexiform layer. The outer retinal layers (photoreptors and RPE) receive their oxygen and nutrients through diffusion from the vascular supply in the choroid. There is a capillary-free zone of approximately 400 μm in the fovea called the *foveal avascular zone*. The absence of vascular elements is necessary for keen visual acuity. At artery and vein crossing points, the arteries lie over the veins and a basement membrane is shared. This crossing may be the basis for retinal vein occlusion. The density of retinal capillaries is greatest in the regions near the retinal veins. The central retinal vein lies temporal to the central retinal artery in the optic nerve head and eventually drains into the superior orbital vein and cavernous sinus. The retinal blood vessels, like the cerebral blood vessels, are responsible for maintenance of the blood retinal barrier. This is accomplished through tight junctions between endothelial cells. The retinal blood vessels do not have smooth muscles or an internal elastic lamina.

A cilioretinal artery arises from the choroidal circulation and is present in about 20% of individuals (see Fig. 4–9, below, for an example of a cilioretinal artery).[1] The blood supply of the choroid is from the ophthalmic artery via the branches of the anterior and posterior

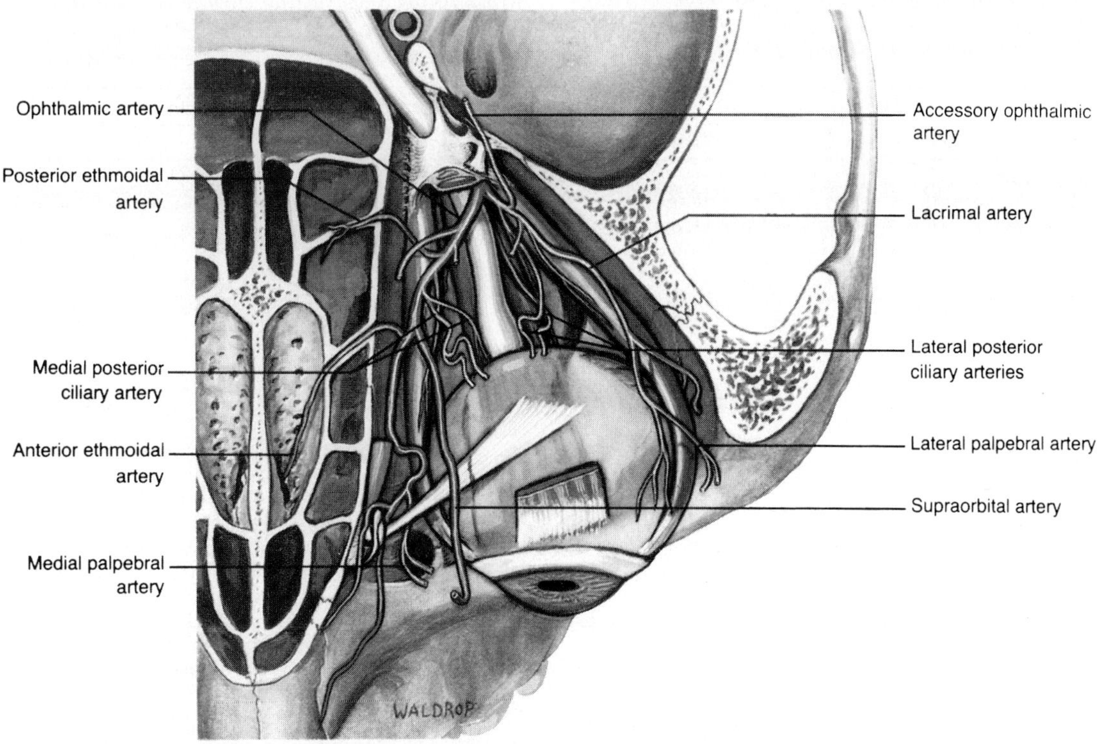

FIGURE 4–1. The orbital arteries as seen from above. The blood supply of the retina is from the ophthalmic artery and reaches the retina through the central retinal artery (not labeled; enters the optic nerve about 1 cm from the nerve globe junction) and the medial and lateral posterior ciliary arteries, which supply the choriocapillaris. (From Dutton JJ: Atlas of Clinical and Surgical Orbital Anatomy. Philadelphia, WB Saunders, 1994, with permission.)

ciliary arteries. Branches of these arteries form discrete capillary lobules of circulation. The choroid drains through the vortex veins and then into the superior and inferior orbital veins into the cavernous sinus. The separate drainage pathway for the retina (central vein) and choroid (vortex veins) is important to recognize. Many pathologic processes that cause central vein obstruction (eg, central retinal vein occlusion, optic nerve sheath meningioma) can cause collateral or "shunt" vessels to develop between the retinal veins at the optic nerve head and the choroidal circulation.

Other details of the internal carotid and ophthalmic artery blood supply are discussed in Chapters 5 and 10.

DISTINCTION BETWEEN MACULOPATHIES AND OPTIC NEUROPATHIES

Optic neuropathies and maculopathies may manifest with similar symptoms, such as central vision loss. When optic neuropathies or maculopathies take their classic forms they are not difficult to distinguish. However, some patients with reduced acuity will have normal-appearing optic nerves and maculae. In this setting, the combination of historical information, examination findings, and laboratory studies will aid in separating these entities (Table 4–1).

Symptoms

The presence of metamorphopsia or photopsia may be very helpful in localizing vision loss to the retina. Patients with metamorphopsia describe warping, bending, or crowding of the images, while those with photopsia complain of seeing sparkles of light. Both of these symptoms are very unusual in optic neuropathies. The complaint of light blindness or abnormal glare sensitivity also suggests the presence of retinal dysfunction and may be a prominent symptom in patients with cone dysfunction. In contrast, patients who detect a darkening of their vision or loss of color perception usually have optic nerve disease. Other symptoms that accompany the vision loss may provide distinguishing features. For instance, pain in association with vision loss is exceedingly uncommon in patients with retinal problems, but may ac-

TABLE 4–1. Clinical Distinction Between Optic Neuropathy and Maculopathy

Symptom, Sign, or Test	Optic Neuropathy	Maculopathy
Symptom		
Metamorphopsia	Rare	Common
Darkening of vision	Common	Rare
Recognition of peripheral field loss by patient	Common	Rare
Transient visual obscurations	Sometimes	Rare
Photopsia	Rare	Common
Glare or light sensitivity	Rare	Sometimes
Pain	Common in optic neuritis, rare in other optic neuropathies	Rare
Sign		
Reduced acuity	Common	Common
Dyschromatopsia	Severe	Mild
Amsler grid abnormality	Missing portions or gray spots	Distorted or bent lines
Afferent pupillary defect	Common	Rare (retinal disorder needs to be severe and asymmetric)
Visual field defects	Central, arcuate, nasal, altitudinal	Central scotoma and midperipheral defects in photoreceptor disease
Ophthalmoscopy	Swollen, pale, or normal optic nerve	Occasionally pale optic nerve; macular abnormality (pigment, atrophy, edema)
Photostress recovery	Normal	Abnormal
Test		
Electroretinography (ERG)	Normal	Normal or abnormal (especially focal ERG)
Ocular coherence tomography	Normal	Abnormal
Visual evoked response	Large latency delay	Small latency delay

company optic disease, particularly inflammatory conditions such as optic neuritis.

Signs

Reduction of visual acuity is commonly encountered in both macular and optic nerve disease. However, abnormalities of color vision help to distinguish macular disease from optic nerve dysfunction. For instance, when visual acuity is only mildly reduced but color vision is markedly impaired, optic nerve dysfunction is more likely. Similarly, when visual acuity is poor yet color vision is preserved, macular disease is much more likely. Two exceptions to this important clinical observation include patients with cone degenerations, who typically have very poor color vision, and patients with ischemic optic neuropathy, who may maintain excellent color vision in their intact visual field. Photostress testing can be helpful in identifying patients with maculopathies. In macular disease there can be a prolongation of the recovery time of the photoreceptor visual pigments after prolonged bright light exposure. The test, which is described in more detail in Chapter 2, is performed by shining a bright light in the eye and finding a prolonged recovery time for visual acuity in the affected eye compared to the unaffected eye. Patients with optic neuropathy will not have a prolonged recovery time after photostress.

The presence of an afferent pupillary defect also strongly suggests the presence of optic nerve disease. It usually takes rather extensive and asymmetric retinal lesions for such patients to develop a relative afferent pupil defect. In addition, visual field testing may be useful in distinguishing optic neuropathies and maculopathies. Both entities may be associated with central or centrocecal scotomas, although the presence of the latter field deficit favors optic nerve disease. Midperipheral ring-type scotomas are typical of retinal degenerations. Optic nerve-type field defects are reviewed in Chapter 5, and they usually assume characteristic patterns that respect the organization of the nerve fiber bundles. However, on automated visual field testing, both optic nerve and retinal disease may produce generalized depression of the visual field. This nonspecific type of field defect is usually unhelpful in distinguishing the two conditions.

Ophthalmoscopy is critical when distinguishing optic neuropathies from maculopathies. In general, abnormalities will be identified in almost all patients with significant macular or optic nerve disease, and it is only at the earliest stage of these visual problems that an abnormality may not be observed. Macular lesions that produce pigmentary changes, atrophy, or hemorrhage are usually observable on ophthalmoscopy. Optic nerve atrophy with or without nerve fiber layer dropout may be recognized on ophthalmoscopy, particularly when using the green filter light. Significant overlap may exist in the early phases of an optic neuropathy when pallor has not yet developed or in the later phases of retinal disease when mild optic disc pallor may be associated with the damaged retina.

Ancillary Testing

Ultimately, the examiner may need to rely on other diagnostic tests to identify and localize the cause of vision loss. Fluorescein angiography may be helpful in identifying occult macular problems. For instance, patients with diabetic macular ischemia might show capillary nonperfusion on fluorescein angiography with minimal findings on ophthalmoscopy. Fluorescein angiography may also be helpful in highlighting the pigmentary abnormalities that can occur with inherited retinal degenerations such as Stargardt's disease or the bull's eye pigmentary pattern common in toxic retinopathies.

Electroretinography is another useful diagnostic tool, particularly for patients with retinal degeneration, paraneoplastic retinopathy, or acute zonal occult outer retinopathy (see below). The ERG is usually recorded using a corneal contact lens and the signal recorded is evoked from the retina using a flash of light. The ERG is characterized by a negative waveform (a-wave) that represents the response of the photoreceptors and a positive waveform (b-wave) that is generated by a combination of cells including the Mueller and bipolar cells. The entire response takes less than 250 milliseconds. The ERG can be recorded under scotopic and photopic conditions to isolate the rod and cone responses. The cone-mediated response (photopic) is obtained by keeping the patient light adapted and using a bright flash to evoke the response. In this setting the rods are bleached out and do not contribute to the wave form. The rod-mediated response (scotopic) is recorded after a prolonged period of dark adaption and evoked with a dim light that is below the threshold of the cones. The a-wave is greatly reduced in scotopic conditions. Cone responses can also be isolated using a flickering light (30 cycles/second) since the rods cannot respond at that rate. When available, focal or multifocal ERG may provide additional information in subtle cases by examining a localized retinal flicker response. Multifocal ERGs are very helpful in creating a "topographic" representation of retinal sensitivity across the macula.

Electro-oculography is another test of retinal function and is based on the existence of an electrical potential across the retina. This potential seems to be dependent on the metabolic activity of the pigment epithelium, not the neurosensory retina. The oscillations in this potential can be increased by changing levels of illumination. A reduction in the ratio of light-adapted to dark-adapted potentials represents an abnormal electro-oculogram (EOG). The EOG generally parallels the ERG but certain exceptions exist, such as vitelliform macular dystrophy, in which the ERG is normal and the EOG is abnormal. Scanning laser ophthalmoscopes and ocular coherence tomography can be used to create a cross-sectional view of the retina and look for abnormal retinal thinning or degeneration.

Despite extensive evaluation, it may be impossible to localize the cause of the patient's vision loss. In this setting it is important to consider the possibility of nonorganic or functional vision loss. When doubt exists about the cause of the visual loss, one should consider screening the patient for the treatable causes of optic nerve dysfunction, including mass lesions, infectious, and nutritional processes.

MACULOPATHIES THAT MAY MIMIC OPTIC NEUROPATHY

The vast majority of patients with macular disease have findings on examination to make diagnosis sufficiently easy if careful ophthalmoscopy is performed. For instance, a patient with age-related macular degeneration and vision loss will almost always have abnormalities that can be seen in the macula (drusen, swelling, bleeding, or atrophy) to explain the symptoms. However, there are several macular conditions that are not well visualized and therefore optic neuropathy is suspected. These conditions are listed in Table 4–2 and summarized below. They are usually missed because the findings on clinical examination are subtle and overlooked or the clinical suspicion is not high enough and the correct diagnosis is never considered.

TABLE 4–2. Common Maculopathies That May Mimic Optic Neuropathies

Central serous maculopathy
Cystoid macular edema
Diabetic macular ischemia
Acute macular neuroretinopathy
Cone dystrophy
Toxic maculopathies
Idiopathic blind spot enlargement syndrome
Choroidal ischemia

Central Serous Chorioretinopathy

Central serous chorioretinopathy is a disorder that often affects young men, classically those with "type A" personalities. Other factors associated with central serous retinopathy include psychopharmocologic medication use, corticosteroid use, and systemic hypertension.[2] The patient may complain of sudden central visual loss and distortion. Metamorphopsia is a common feature. The condition results from abnormal leakage of fluid from the choroid into the subretinal spaces. On examination, there is reduced visual acuity and a central scotoma on visual field testing. Metamorphopsia is typically present on Amsler's grid testing. An afferent pupil defect is usually not seen. The diagnosis is established best by slit-lamp biomicroscopy examination of the fundus, during which exudative detachment of the macula will be evident (Fig. 4–2). The retinal elevation may be subtle and easily missed through an undilated pupil. Retrobulbar optic neuritis is the main differential diagnosis, although pain on eye movements is usually present in that setting. If necessary, fluorescein angiography will demonstrate the abnormal fluid leakage in the macula.

Cystoid Macular Edema

Patients with cystoid macular edema (CME) may be difficult to identify ophthalmoscopically and therefore are sometimes confused with those with optic nerve disease. CME most commonly occurs after cataract surgery but may occur in association with ocular inflammatory disease. Metamorphopsia is a common complaint. Small, shallow central visual field defects are frequently encountered and some

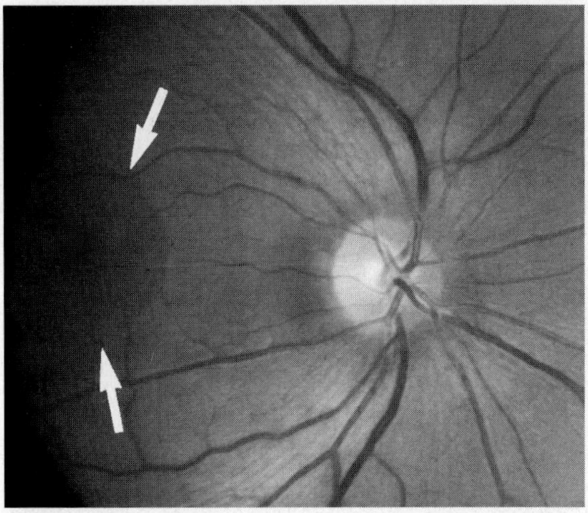

FIGURE 4–2. Fundus photograph of the right eye of a patient with central serous retinopathy. The white arrows delineate the edge of the small collection of fluid under the neurosensory retina. This view emphasizes how easily this condition can be missed when the fundus is examined with only a direct ophthalmoscope in the area of the optic nerve.

patients will struggle with the color plates, although they do not have true dyschromatopsia. CME may be "ophthalmoscopically occult." In these cases, the thickening or elevation of the macula may be very subtle, and the typical cysts may either be absent or difficult to see.

Fluorescein angiography is very helpful in identifying patients with CME not recognized by ophthalmoscopy. Patients with resolved CME may be difficult to diagnose because only mild pigmentary changes may be evident. Fluorescein angiography may be unhelpful in such cases. It is important to recognize CME because of the potential for effective treatment with anti-inflammatory agents.

Diabetic Ischemic Maculopathy

Ophthalmoscopically apparent macular edema is responsible for central vision loss in most patients with diabetic retinopathy. However, perfusion abnormalities causing macular ischemia may also cause vision loss. This usually occurs in patients with preproliferative or proliferative retinopathy. Closure of retinal capillaries is actually an early manifestation of the microvascular disease of diabetic retinopathy. Fortunately, this is usually not associated with significant vision loss. However, if the closure involves the arterioles, and the foveal avascular zone increases to 1000 μm, then acuity loss is common.[3] Although this type of vessel closure is easily seen on fluorescein angiography, other ophthalmoscopic clues include large dark retinal hemorrhages, multiple cotton-wool spots, and narrowed vessels.

However, the degree to which vision loss can be ascribed to this disorder may not correspond to the degree of ophthalmoscopic findings, and there are frequently confounding features. Patients with advanced diabetic retinopathy and vision loss may exhibit mild optic atrophy and pigmentary changes. The visual field loss that may occur following pan-retinal photocoagulation also complicates the clinical picture. The full-field and multifocal ERG may be useful in identifying retinal dysfunction in patients with diabetic retinopathy.[4,5] When unusual types of visual field defects are encountered, such as altitudinal defects or those respecting the vertical midline, then it is mandatory that alternative causes be considered, especially compressive optic nerve lesions.

Acute Macular Neuroretinopathy

This entity is also discussed below along with the big blind spot syndromes. It may be very difficult clinically to distinguish optic neuritis from this entity because of the tendency for it to cause central vision loss in young women. Classically, these patients have tiny, discrete central field defects, which are only apparent on Amsler's grid testing. An orange-brown petalloid retinal lesion may be observed on ophthalmoscopy (Fig. 4–3; see Color Plates 4 and 5). Again, this is another retinal diagnosis that is difficult to make without careful dilated funduscopy. The pathologic process occurs in the outer retinal layers but the cause is uncertain.

Two other maculopathies commonly encountered in neuro-ophthalmic differential diagnosis, cone dystrophies and toxic maculopathies, are also discussed in further detail below.

RETINAL VASCULAR EMBOLI AND INSUFFICIENCY

Retinal vascular insufficiency should be considered in the differential diagnosis of transient or permanent monocular visual loss. Emboli to the retinal vasculature, typically from the carotid artery bifurcation, are often the

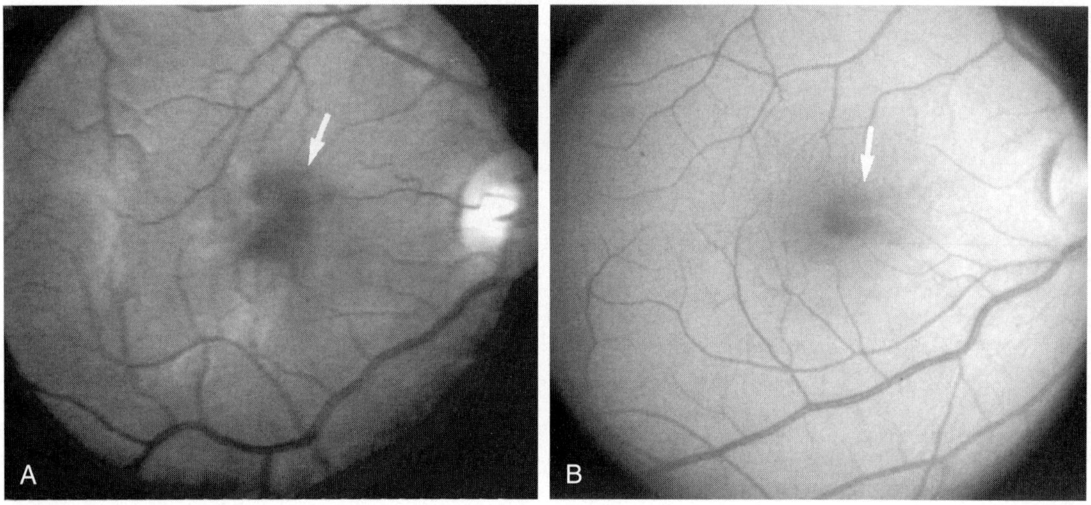

FIGURE 4–3. Fundus photographs of acute macular neuroretinopathy demonstrating subtle brownish discoloration of the retina. **A.** A "comma"-shaped area in the nasal parafoveal area (*white arrow*) is seen. **B.** A more striking petalloid, orange-brown lesion (*white arrow*) is seen in the nasal parafoveal retina. (See Color Plates 4 and 5.)

cause. On the other hand, asymptomatic retinal emboli are also frequently detected during ophthalmoscopy. In patients with either transient or permanent vision loss suspected to be a result of retinal vascular insufficiency or visible emboli on examination, a workup for either a carotid or a cardiac source of emboli must be pursued. This workup is detailed in Chapter 10, and usually includes a noninvasive carotid workup with ultrasound or magnetic resonance imaging-angiography and echocardiography. In younger patients or patients with unexplained recurrent symptoms or findings the workup can be expanded to include transesophageal echocardiography, a hematologic workup for hypercoaguable state, and occasionally conventional angiography.

Emboli

Types. There are three main types of retinal emboli: cholesterol, calcific, and platelet–fibrin.[6–9] The ophthalmoscopic differentiation of these types of emboli may be difficult. Sharma et al[8] found poor intra- and interobserver reliability in differentiating retinal emboli. The authors of this study cautioned against making decisions about workup based solely on the clinical impression of the embolus type. Other more rare types of emboli include those composed of amniotic fluid, bacteria, parasites, metastatic tumors, fat, air, and talc. These types of emboli are recognized within their specific settings (ie, talc with intravenous drug abuse, bacterial with endocarditis).

Cholesterol emboli (Hollenhorst plaques[10]) are the most common emboli and are copper-colored refractile bodies (Fig. 4–4; see Color Plate 6). Most cholesterol emboli lodge at bifurcations in the temporal retinal circulation. Platelet–fibrin emboli are grey and form cast-like elongated opacifications in retinal vessels

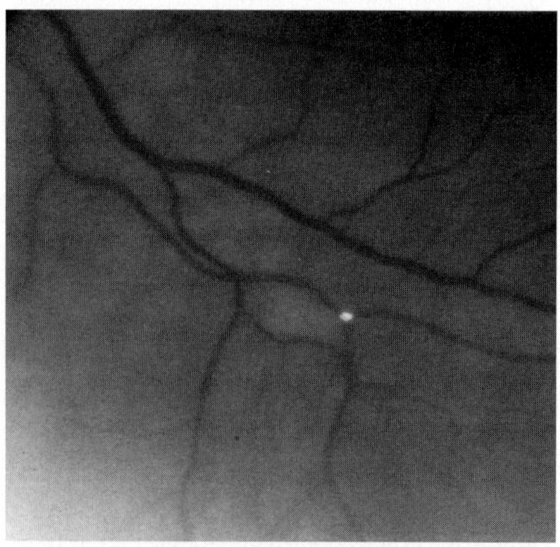

FIGURE 4–4. Hollenhorst plaque at the branch point of a temporal retinal artery. These emboli typically have a shiny yellow refractile appearance and are often seen without any evidence of retinal infarction. (From Volpe NJ, Liu GT, Galetta SL: Transient vision loss. Curr Conc Ophthalmol 1998;6:55-59, with permission.) (See Color Plate 6.)

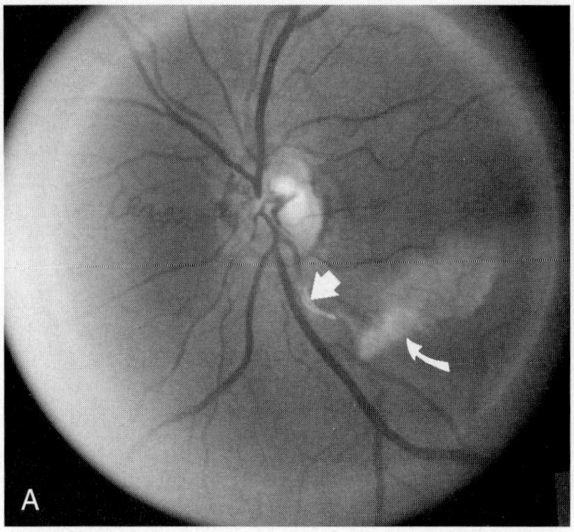

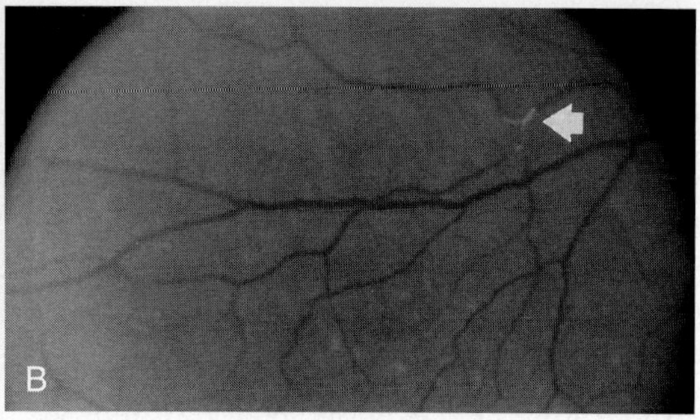

FIGURE 4–5. Platelet–fibrin emboli in retinal arteries. Note the yellow-grey, elongated, castlike nature of the emboli (*short white arrows*) within the retinal arteries. **A.** A twig branch retinal artery occlusion (*curved thin arrow*) is seen distal to the involved artery. **B.** A platelet–fibrin embolus without associated retinal infarction.

(Fig. 4–5). These emboli may follow acute carotid thrombosis or more rarely myocardial infarction. Calcific emboli are large, globoid, and white (Fig. 4–6). They tend to occur in the setting of cardiac valvular disease but may also originate from a carotid source.

Prevalence and Associations. The prevalence of retinal emboli in various populations has been reported to be approximately 1%.[11, 12] The 5-year incidence is 0.9%.[11] The prevalence increases with age, and they are more common in men. Emboli are associated with hypertension, smoking, vascular disease, and previous surgery.[12, 13] In one study emboli were not found in association with diabetes or obesity.[12] Cholesterol-type emboli are the most common type, followed by platelet–fibrin and calcific emboli.

Carotid Disease. In one series of patients with retinal emboli, 74 out of 207 underwent formal carotid angiography, and 18% of the asymptomatic patients were found to have significant stenosis (>75%).[14] The percentage was only slightly higher in symptomatic patients (21% with high-grade stenosis).[14] The stenosis was worse on the side of the embolus in 70% of patients. In patients with retinal arterial occlusion, the presence of a retinal embolus does not necessarily predict a higher degree of stenosis.[15] Furthermore, finding an embolus did not correlate with the presence of a structural cardiac lesion requiring intervention.[16] Asymptomatic patients with retinal emboli and carotid stenosis may in some cases benefit from carotid endarterectomy.[17] However, the decision for surgery should be made on an individual basis, as surgery for asymptomatic carotid stenosis is controversial (see Chapter 10).

Associated Morbidity and Mortality. Cholesterol and platelet–fibrin emboli are associated with an increased stroke risk,[11] similar to that of amaurosis fugax. Therefore patients with cholesterol emboli deserve a noninvasive evaluation (see Chapter 10). Pfaffenbach and Hollenhorst,[18] and Savino et al[19] were the first to report on the increase risk of stroke and death in patients with visible retinal emboli. In a more recent series, the annual stroke rate for patients with retinal emboli was 8.5% compared to 0.8% for controls.[20] Increased annual

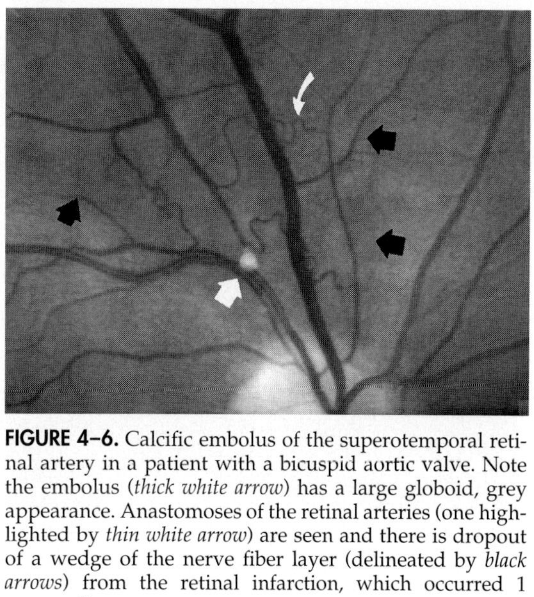

FIGURE 4–6. Calcific embolus of the superotemporal retinal artery in a patient with a bicuspid aortic valve. Note the embolus (*thick white arrow*) has a large globoid, grey appearance. Anastomoses of the retinal arteries (one highlighted by *thin white arrow*) are seen and there is dropout of a wedge of the nerve fiber layer (delineated by *black arrows*) from the retinal infarction, which occurred 1 year earlier.

rates of myocardial infarction also occurred in the embolus patients (7.7% versus 4.9%).[20] Patients with retinal emboli have a reduced life expectancy, likely reflecting their predisposition for stroke and cardiac events.[7]

Events Associated With Retinal Vascular Insufficiency

Amaurosis Fugax. Amaurosis fugax, or "fleeting" or transient monocular blindness, is usually sudden and is often described as a shade or curtain that obscures vision in one eye (see Chapter 10). Visual loss may be altitudinal, peripheral, central, or even vertical. As opposed to migrainous episodes of transient vision loss, there usually are no photopsias or positive visual phenomena. Most episodes last 10 minutes or less and are painless. Emboli from the carotid to the retinal vasculature are a common mechanism of amaurosis fugax. A nasal defect may suggest an embolic mechanism because of the tendency of these particles to lodge in the temporal retinal circulation. Some emboli lodge behind the lamina cribrosa and are not visible. Others that enter the retinal circulation break up and pass distally. Other causes include vasospasm, migraine, and antiphospholipid antibody syndrome.

Retinal Artery Occlusion. Permanent vascular disruption may cause a central artery occlusion (CRAO) or branch retinal artery occlusion (BRAO). Interestingly, CRAO is associated with visible emboli in 10% to 20% of patients, but BRAO has a higher rate, approaching 60% to 70%. Other mechanisms of retinal vascular occlusion are possible besides emboli, including local thrombosis, vasculitis, vasospasm and hypoperfusion. Although the frequency of operable carotid stenosis ipsilateral to a CRAO or BRAO varies from series to series, approximately 30% to 40% of patients will have >60% ipsilateral carotid stenosis.[21]

Central Retinal Artery Occlusion. An acute CRAO is a true emergency because the potential to restore vision may exist for the first 12 to 24 hours. Ophthalmoscopy reveals a cherry-red spot that results from the deep reddish color of the choroid showing through the surrounding, whitened retina (Fig. 4–7). Aggressive therapies should be offered to improve the delivery of oxygen to the retina. Although some patients spontaneously improve, the prognosis for visual improvement after CRAO is poor even with heroic measures such as paracentesis, inhalation of carbogen (95% oxygen, 5% carbon dioxide) for vasodilation and increased blood flow, lowering intraocular pressure with various drugs, and ocular massage. The efficacy of the these measures has never been proven, and one retrospective study suggested that the prognosis for visual recovery is not improved with these therapies.[22] Approximately 20% of patients develop iris neovascularization.[23] Recently, intra-

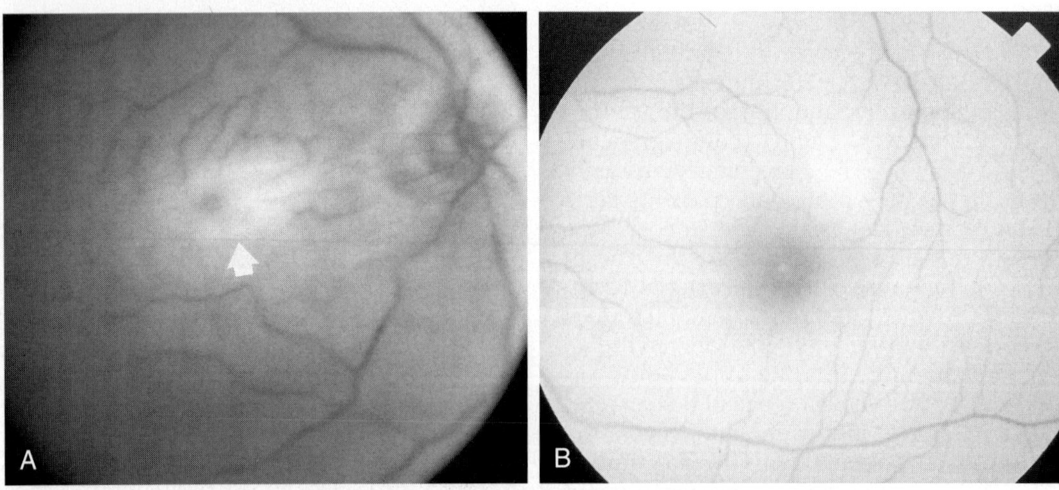

FIGURE 4–7. Cherry-red spots from a central retinal artery occlusion that can have a varied appearance depending on the time elapsed from the occlusion and the patient's pigmentation. **A.** An early cherry-red spot with a focal area of whitening (*arrow*) around a small dark area. **B.** Fully developed cherry-red spot with diffuse and marked retinal whitening and narrowed blood vessels.

arterial urokinase has been successfully used in patients with CRAO. Schmidt et al[24] treated 14 patients who had CRAO with urokinase. Four patients had marked improvement, and five had slight improvement. A control group of 41 patients had essentially no improvement.[24] In a followup study, the authors extended their experience with urokinase thrombolysis to 23 patients with CRAO.[25]

Branch Retinal Artery Occlusion. Patients with BRAO similarly represent a heterogenous group. Most patients present with and maintain better than 20/40 visual acuity. Ophthalmoscopy reveals retinal whitening involving a section of retina with a partial cherry-red spot (Fig. 4–8; see Color Plate 7). Nearly all BRAOs involve the temporal retinal arteries.[26] In the majority of cases, they occur in the setting of carotid artery disease, and the workup for carotid and cardiac sources of emboli should be pursued as in patients with CRAO. BRAO has also been described in a variety of other conditions, including infectious retinopathies (toxoplasmosis, cat scratch disease), internal carotid artery dissection,[27] antiphospholipid antibody syndrome, protein S deficiency,[28] Susac syndrome,[29] temporal arteritis,[30] and the presence of anticardiolipin antibody[31] and lupus anticoagulants.[32] One study suggested that the presence of a visible embolus and BRAO were factors correlated with a significantly worse survival compared to age-matched controls.[33] As in the management of CRAO, aggressive maneuvers to move the embolus by lowering intraocular pressure and using vasodilators have no proven benefit.[26]

Cilioretinal Artery Occlusions. Similar embolic events can lead to the obstruction of the cilioretinal artery. If present, a cilioretinal artery can protect macular vision when CRAO occurs. Isolated cilioretinal artery occlusions can occur as well with loss of central vision and preservation of peripheral vision.[34–36] Cilioretinal artery occlusions have also been described in systemic lupus erythematosis,[37] temporal arteritis,[38] antiphospholipid syndromes,[39] and sickle cell disease,[40] and in association with central retinal vein occlusions in young patients (Fig. 4–9).[41, 42]

Ocular Ischemic Syndrome. Hypoperfusion and subsequent ischemia of the globe associated with severe carotid disease may produce a variety of signs involving the posterior and anterior segments of the eye.[43–45] Patients may present with amaurosis fugax or gradual or sudden loss of vision.[43] In the posterior part of the eye, a venous stasis retinopathy characterized by midperipheral dot and blot hemorrhages may be evident.[43–45] Optic nerve disc swelling is typically not seen until the very late stages of posterior segment ischemia. Fluorescein angiography may reveal delayed retinal and choroidal perfusion.[45] The vascular occlusion is typically either in the ipsilateral internal carotid or in the ophthalmic arteries.

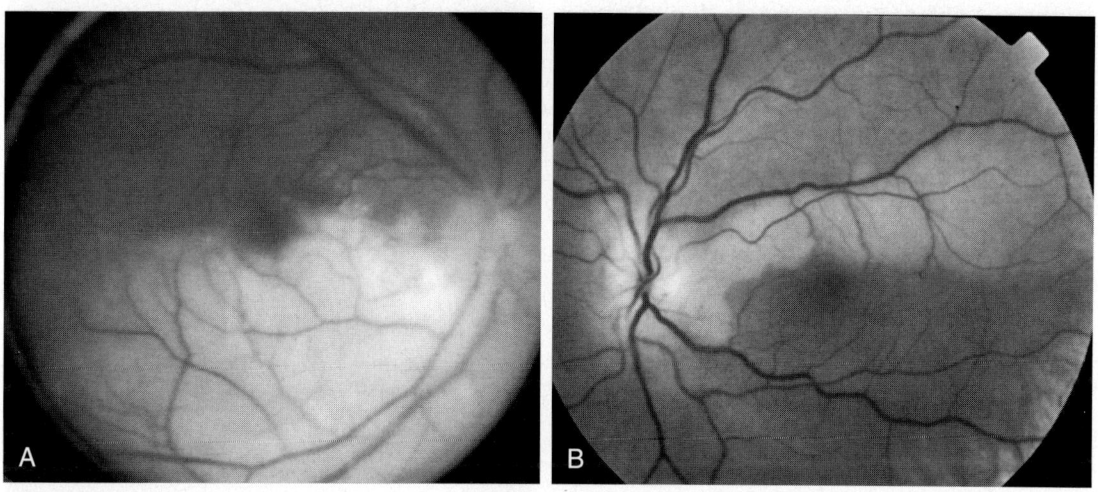

FIGURE 4–8. Branch retinal artery occlusions. **A.** Inferior branch retinal artery occlusion in a 14-year-old boy. There is a partial cherry-red spot. Extensive retinal whitening and swelling is seen. The optic nerve also appears slightly swollen. (See Color Plate 7.) **B.** Superior branch retinal artery occlusion with retinal whitening along the affected artery. This patient had temporal arteritis, and there is simultaneous swelling of the disc from ischemic optic neuropathy.

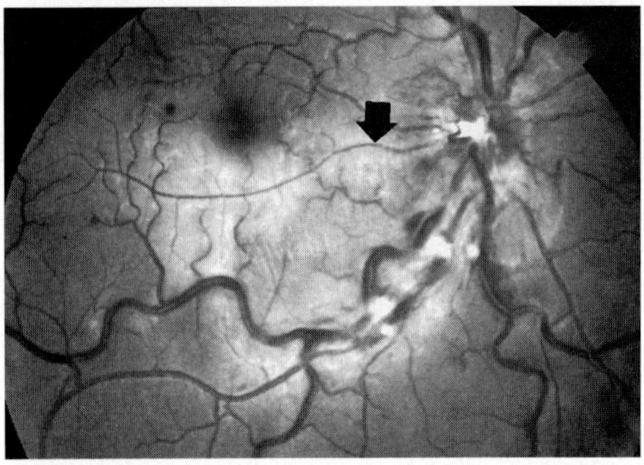

FIGURE 4–9. Nonischemic central retinal vein occlusion in a young man complicated by cilioretinal artery (*black arrow*) occlusion. Retinal whitening is seen extending around the affected cilioretinal artery. Visual acuity was normal but there was a dense superior paracentral scotoma.

Other manifestations of this condition are discussed in more detail with figures in Chapter 10.

Retinal Venous Occlusion

Occlusive disease of the retinal venous system (branch and central retinal vein occlusion) does not result from carotid disease and is not usually associated with optic neuropathy or other neurologic disease. However, retinal vein occlusion is a common cause of acute vision loss, photopsia, optic nerve swelling, cotton-wool spots, and retinal hemorrhages and therefore is important in the neuro-ophthalmic differential diagnosis. Retinal vein occlusion may also be associated with important systemic disorders. Retinal venous occlusive disorders are among the most common retinal disorders encountered in practice, occurring with an incidence of 5 per 1000.[46]

Central Retinal Vein Occlusion. Acute central retinal vein occlusion (CRVO) has a characteristic and dramatic appearance characterized by optic disc swelling, tortuosity and dilation of retinal veins, retinal edema, and intraretinal hemorrhages extending away from the disc into all four quadrants (Fig. 4–10). In milder and incomplete forms there may be only mild hemorrhages, mild venous dilation, and slight hyperemia of the disc. CRVOs are divided into two categories, ischemic and nonischemic, based on the degree of vision loss and the amount of capillary nonperfusion on fluorescein angiography. Nonischemic vein occlusions have prolonged circulation time and capillary permeability breakdown on fluorescein angiography. About half of these patients resolve the occlusion without significant vision loss, but 20% go on to complete occlusion.[47] Patients with ischemic CRVO are more likely to have poor vision at presentation and may develop rubeosis and require treatment with panretinal photocoagulation. An afferent pupillary defect is often present. Fluorescein angiography will reveal severe capillary nonperfusion and electroretinography will show a reduced b-/a-wave ratio.

The mechanism of CRVO is believed to be thrombosis of the central retinal vein although the actual cause of the thrombosis, and its relationship to atherosclerotic disease of the central retinal artery, is unknown.[48] Both ocular and systemic conditions have been associated with CRVO. Many patients with CRVO present with or develop open-angle glaucoma. Most studies find a high incidence of systemic hypertension and cardiovascular disease.[49] Elevated lipoprotein levels have been found in patients with retinal vein occlusion.[50] In younger patients collagen vascular disease may be a risk factor.[51] The association of vein occlusions with thrombotic states is discussed later in this chapter.

Branch Retinal Vein Occlusion. In branch retinal vein occlusion (BRVO) the findings of venous insufficiency develop in a portion of the retina. Such occlusions tend to occur at the

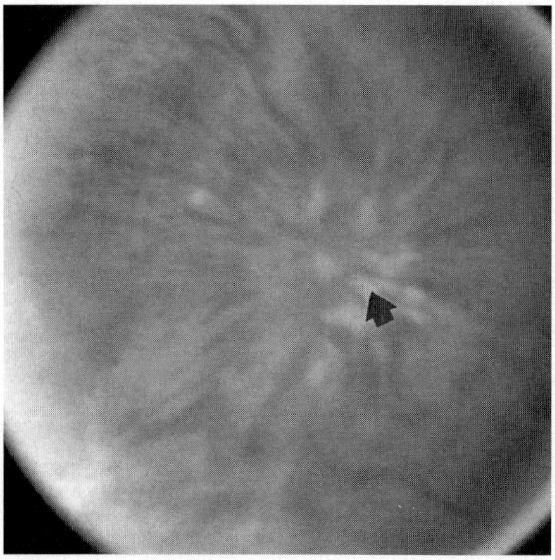

FIGURE 4–10. Massive optic disc edema (*black arrow*) and four-quadrant extensive intraretinal hemorrhages from central retinal vein occlusion.

point where the retinal artery and vein cross. The retinal findings typically occur in an arcuate pattern of hemorrhages, cotton-wool spots and retinal edema. Branch retinal vein occlusions usually occur in the superotemporal quadrant. The events leading to occlusion remain obscure but presumably include thrombosis of the vein perhaps caused by turbulent flow in the overlying artery, which shares the same adventitia as the vein. Fresh and recanalized thrombus has been identified in patients with BRVO.[52] Hypertension, male gender, hyperopia, diabetes and glaucoma may all be risk factors for BRVO.[53] BRVOs are commonly complicated by macular edema, which may result in central vision loss and may be treated by macular photocoagulation.[54] Neovascularization occurs in 20% to 30% of patients and may be prevented or treated with scatter photocoagulation.[55, 56]

PHOTORECEPTOR DISORDERS IMPORTANT IN NEURO-OPHTHALMOLOGY

Paraneoplastic retinopathy (PR) and the big blind spot syndromes are two subacute retinal disorders with a normal or minimally abnormal funduscopic appearance. Although these conditions are unrelated, they both are outer retinopathies (photoreceptor dysfunction) that are important in neuro-ophthalmic differential diagnosis because their presentation may mimic that of optic neuropathies. Retinal symptoms (photopsias) and retinal signs (midperipheral field defects or enlargement of the blind spot) occur in PR and the big blind spot syndromes and are important clues to their diagnosis.

Paraneoplastic Retinopathy

Primary malignancies and secondary tumors (metastatic and direct extension from adjacent structures) may produce vision loss by displacement, invasion, or compression of ocular tissues. However, ocular and neurologic dysfunction may evolve in patients with cancer without direct tumor involvement. These disorders are collectively termed *paraneoplastic syndromes*. They not only present a diagnostic challenge but may provide insight into the biologic behavior of tumors and their effect on the host immune system.[57, 58]

Sawyer, Selhorst, Zimmerman, and Hoyt[59] were the first to recognize the unusual features of a retinopathy occurring as a remote effect of cancer. *Paraneoplastic retinopathy* refers to a syndrome of subacute deterioration of vision and retinal function resulting from a nonmetastatic, remote effect of a malignancy. The clinical features of the paraneoplastic retinopathies are summarized in Table 4–3. This broader term encompasses several distinct entities, including cancer-associated retinopathy (CAR), which is the most common, cancer-associated cone dysfunction (CACD), melanoma-associated retinopathy (MAR), diffuse uveal melanocytic proliferation (DUMP), and paraneoplastic ganglion cell neuronopathy (PGCN). The exact prevalence of paraneoplastic retinal disorders is unknown.

Despite some fairly characteristic complaints and examination findings, the diagnosis of PR is rarely made at presentation. In addition, it is common for the syndrome to develop prior to recognition and diagnosis of the systemic malignancy.

Symptoms, Signs, and Electroretinography. Patients usually report decreased vision or a halo of missing peripheral vision. Common complaints also include the acute onset of photopsias (flashing lights) or positive visual phenomena. Differences in symptoms among the various entities correlate with the degree to which the rods versus cones are affected.

Visual acuity may be normal or markedly reduced. Other features on examination include abnormal color vision and prolonged photostress recovery time. An afferent pupil defect may be evident in cases with asymmetric retinal involvement. Goldmann visual fields may be more useful than automated perimetry since the scotomas usually begin in the midperiphery (Fig. 4–11). As the retinal degeneration evolves, the paracentral defects eventually connect to form a classic ring scotoma. Since the visual field defects result from retinal dysfunction, the "arcuate-type" defects typically do not respect the horizontal meridian. The outer retina does not have an anatomic demarcation along the horizontal meridian like the nerve fiber layer.

In general, there is usually a paucity of ocular findings compared to the symptoms and level of visual dysfunction. However, ocular examination may show a mild vitritis.[60] Attenuation of retinal vessels may be present.[60–65] Other findings described in these patients include optic disc pallor, granularity of the reti-

TABLE 4–3. Clinical Features of Paraneoplastic Syndromes

Disorder	Pathogenesis	Clinical manifestations and course
Cancer-associated retinopathy (CAR)	Antibodies to 23-kD antigen believed to be recoverin; other antibodies found, sometimes unknown	Subacute onset of photopsia and progressive visual field loss beginning as midperipheral scotoma Mild vitritis, narrowed retinal vessels Relentlessly progressive Diffuse loss of ERG Steroids may be helpful
Melanoma-associated retinopathy (MAR)	Antibodies to retinal bipolar cells in patients with metastatic melanoma	Onset of night blindness and dark adaption difficulties May have fixed nonprogressive defect ERG shows rod dysfunction (scotopic b-wave) and normal cone function ERG similar to congenital stationery night blindness
Paraneoplastic ganglion cell neuronopathy (PGCN)	Antibodies to retinal ganglion cells Immune deposits in the retina	Bilateral progressive loss of vision May have optic disc swelling Abnormal immunoglobulin levels in CSF Optic nerve demyelination may occur
Cancer-associated cone dysfunction (CACD)	Antibodies to CAR antigen and 50-kD protein Loss of cones in macula Infiltration by macrophages	Subacute onset of glare or photosensitivity ERG shows cone dysfunction with preservation of rod function Loss of color vision; central scotomas
Diffuse uveal melanocytic proliferation (DUMP)	Develops in women with reproductive tract cancers and men with cancers in retroperitoneal area	Bilateral subacute vision loss Primary tumor may not be known Subretinal proliferation of pigmentary cells and yellow orange lesions at level of retinal pigmented epithelium (RPE)

ERG = electroretinogram.

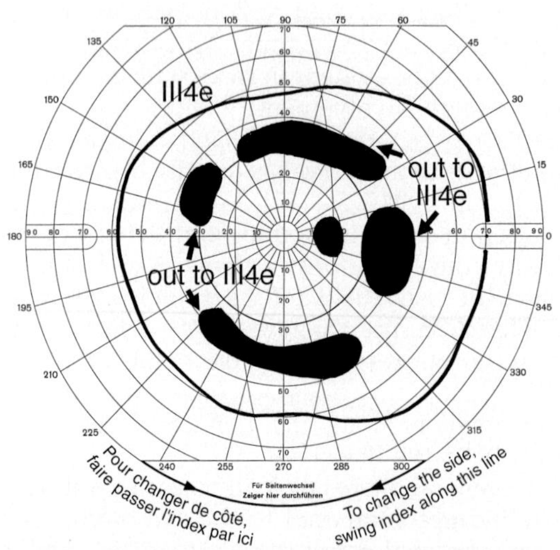

FIGURE 4–11. Goldmann visual field of the left eye of a patient with cancer-associated retinopathy. Photoreceptor dysfunction is manifested by midperipheral scotomas that do not respect the vertical or horizontal meridians. The scotomas are beyond 15 degrees of eccentricity.

nal pigment, and peripheral retinal pigmentation.

The diagnosis of PR is strongly suggested when an ERG shows evidence of diffuse retinal dysfunction in a patient with relatively precipitous visual loss. Most abnormal ERGs are found in patients with chronic retinal degenerations like retinitis pigmentosa. The ERG varies in PR depending on the particular syndrome.

Each subtype has several distinguishing signs and symptoms, ERG features, and systemic associations (Table 4–3):

Cancer-Associated Retinopathy. CAR patients, in whom rods are primarily affected, typically manifest with vision loss and night blindness (nyctalopia).[60, 61, 66] An abnormal scotopic ERG is usually found.

Several reports have described the histopathologic findings in CAR.[59, 61, 63, 73, 80–82] As expected, loss of photoreceptor inner and outer segments were present in each case. The degree of macular involvement was variable, and in general there was more rod than cone involvement.[61] Outer nuclear cell loss and the presence of inflammatory infiltrates were other notable features. Except in one case with phlebitis,[80] the retinal vasculature was typically reported as normal. The inner nuclear layer (ganglion cells) was always spared. In areas of photoreceptor loss, scattered melanophages and disruption of the retinal pigment epithelium have been observed.

Keltner and associates[73, 83] were the first to propose an autoimmune pathogenesis in CAR.[57, 58] They demonstrated antiretinal antibodies in a patient with cervical carcinoma in 1983.[73] These antibodies reacted with photoreceptors from normal human retina. Subsequently they performed enzyme-linked immunosorbent assay and Western blot testing in four patients with CAR and found a serum antibody that bound a 23-kD retinal antigen, which they termed the *CAR antigen*.[83] CAR antibodies are usually found only in patients with cancer who have experienced visual loss.

Most patients with CAR have antibodies to the 23-kD antigen, but some have other antibodies.[61, 62, 82] The specific circulating antibody responsible for CACD is unknown, but in one patient with CACD, 23-kD and 50-kD antibodies were identified.[84] The involved retinal antigen in patients with MAR appears to be distinct.[71] It is likely that several different antigens may elicit an immune response capable of causing retinal damage.

CAR is now believed to result from an antibody-mediated loss of photoreceptors. Presumably, antibodies are formed as part of an autoimmune reaction to tumor antigens. These antigens cross react with retinal antigens because of shared epitopes (antigenic mimicry). Tumor necrosis can expose antigens to immunologic surveillance and result in antibody production. The immune system may become "turned on" by the tumor, with a resultant nonspecific production of antibodies, some of which may cross react with retinal antigens. It is possible that the tumor cells themselves contain a retinal antigen (eg, recoverin, see below), which becomes exposed to immune surveillance.[82] Less likely, the tumor may produce the retinal antigen itself. The components of the activated immune response must then cross the blood–retinal barrier (presumably altered by focal or general cellular inflammation) and react with a photoreceptor antigen. The antibodies could also be synthesized in the central nervous system. Finally, the tissue-bound antibody–antigen complex must result in cell death or apoptosis. The antibody–antigen complex itself may be sufficient to poison the cells energy system or these immune complexes may bind complement and activate the complement cascade.

If patients with CAR are presumed to have antibody-mediated disease, then the involved antigen that is bound by antibody must play an important role in the biochemical function of the retina. Polans et al[85] found that antibodies in patients with CAR reacted with recoverin, a calcium channel photoreceptor protein (in the calmodulin family). In addition, serum antibodies from CAR patients have been used to isolate the gene that encodes the CAR antigen from a cDNA library of human retina. The resultant nucleotide sequence was shown to have been 90% homologous to the published sequence of bovine recoverin.[86] Recoverin is the CAR antigen in most patients. The exact mechanism by which the antibody–recoverin molecule complex causes cell death is unknown. An effect on energy production seems likely since the classic immune-mediated form of destruction that includes lymphocytic cellular infiltration is not observed in most cases.

Immunohistochemistry has been used to demonstrate that the serum antiretinal antibodies affect the outer retina.[61] The pattern observed respected the anatomic boundary between the outer plexiform and inner nuclear layers. A similar immunohistochemical staining pattern occurs with antibodies directed against recoverin. Outer retinal involvement on both histopathology and immunohistochemistry supports the theory that these antibodies have a role in the pathogenesis of the disease.

Cancer-Associated Cone Dysfunction. In contrast, CACD patients may complain of decreased acuity, dyschromatopsia, glare, photosensitivity, or reduced vision in bright light more suggestive of cone dysfunction. CACD is characterized by an abnormal cone ERG. Patients typically have color vision loss and central scotomas. Signs and symptoms are caused by loss of cones in the macula.[63]

Melanoma-Associated Retinopathy. Most patients with MAR have an established diagnosis of cutaneous melanoma and present uniformly with photopsias, night blindness, and floaters.[62, 65, 67, 68] A recent report described a patient with MAR and a primary melanoma in the maxillary sinus.[68] In some instances of MAR, at presentation metastatic melanoma is found.[62, 67, 69–71] Patients usually have better than

20/40 acuity at presentation, with dyschromatopsia and visual field defects (central scotomas, arcuate defects, and generalized constriction). Unlike patients with CAR, patients with MAR typically do not experience the relentless progression to blindness.

Patients with MAR have a highly specific ERG with the absence of b-waves under dark-adapted conditions and normal cone amplitudes, suggesting bipolar cell dysfunction.[62, 67, 68, 70, 71] The serum from patients with MAR can be shown by immunocytochemical techniques to react with retinal bipolar cells.[72] In most cases the a- and b-wave amplitudes are markedly reduced. Progressive visual loss has been correlated with progressive reduction of ERG amplitudes. Abnormal electro-oculograms have also been reported.[65, 73]

Bilateral Diffuse Uveal Melanocytic Proliferation. Bilateral DUMP manifests with subacute loss of vision that often develops prior to diagnosis of the primary neoplasm.[74–77] The most common primary tumors associated with this syndrome are carcinoma of the reproductive tract in women and cancers of the retroperitoneal area and the lungs in men. Funduscopic examination reveals bilateral proliferation of subretinal pigment and yellow-orange lesions at the level of the retinal pigment epithelium. The former retinal change may appear similar to choridal nevi. There may be serous detachments of the retina. Early-phase fluorescein angiography shows a pattern of hyperfluorescence, corresponding to the abnormalities observed at the level of the retinal pigment epithelium. Uveitis and a rapidly progressive cataract may occur.

Proliferation of nonmalignant cells has been shown on histopathology, and metastases have not been reported.[74, 76] The serous retinal detachments may respond to systemic corticosteroids or radiation. Treatment of the primary tumor may not alter the course of the progressive visual loss.

Paraneoplastic Ganglion Cell Neuronopathy. PGCN is essentially a form of paraneoplastic optic neuropathy. These conditions are discussed in Chapter 5. Suffice it to say that there have been scattered reports of patients with cancer presenting with demyelinating optic neuropathies without any evidence of cancer spread to the optic nerve or meninges. One report noted the presence of immune deposits in the retina and diffuse ganglion cell loss on histopathologic evaluation.[78]

Laboratory Findings. Fluorescein angiography occasionally shows periphlebitis.[79, 80] Standard laboratory testing (ie, blood chemistries and serum immunoglobulin levels) have no role in the diagnosis of PR. However, identification of serum antiretinal antibodies is an important diagnostic aid.

Systemic Evaluation. In individuals with suspected PR, a careful review of the patient's medical history and laboratory investigations should be undertaken to identify the underlying systemic malignancy. Approximately one half of the cases of PR are diagnosed prior to the discovery of the malignancy.[59, 61, 66, 73, 83] Like many of the other paraneoplastic syndromes, two thirds of patients with PR will have small cell carcinoma of the lung. Other associated tumors include melanoma in MAR,[62, 67, 69] breast carcinoma,[87] uterine carcinoma,[63, 81, 88] and cervical carcinoma.[73] In one reported patient there were three primary tumors (prostate, bladder, larynx).[65] PR has not been reported to occur with other paraneoplastic neurologic diseases.

Differential Diagnosis. PR must be distinguished from four broad categories of anterior visual pathway disease, including conditions that appear clinically similar but are not associated with systemic malignancy, conditions secondary to direct spread of tumor, toxic effects of chemotherapy, and other paraneoplastic conditions.[57, 58] Compressive or inflammatory lesions of the anterior visual pathway must be considered in all instances of subacute visual loss. Optic neuritis is a common misdiagnosis in patients ultimately shown to have PR.[61, 65] However, optic neuritis and ischemic optic neuropathy can usually be excluded on clinical grounds. Nearly all reported cases underwent neuroimaging of the anterior visual pathway to rule out a compressive lesion prior to diagnosis. Less common causes of subacute visual loss such as toxic, hereditary, and nutritional optic neuropathies should be considered and excluded based on historical and laboratory information. Ultimately, an abnormal ERG will distinguish PR from optic neuropathy.

The rapid rate of visual deterioration distinguishes PR from other retinal degenerations such as retinitis pigmentosa. The two conditions otherwise may mimic each other since both conditions result from photoreceptor dysfunction. In contrast to PR patients, most individuals with retinitis pigmentosa have abnormal fundi with pigmentary deposition.

Vision loss may develop by a variety of mechanisms in the cancer patient. Carcinomatous meningitis may produce an optic neuropathy. In this situation, the neuroimaging of the optic nerve and meninges and/or spinal fluid chemistry and cytology will typically be abnormal. Visual loss may also occur as a result of the toxic effects of chemotherapy. Chemotherapeutic agents including 1,3-bis (2-chlorethyl)-1-nitrosourea (BCNU), vincristine and cis-platinum have been reported to cause optic neuropathy. Radiation therapy may cause retrobulbar optic neuropathy months to years after treatment. The optic nerves or chiasm may show enhancement and enlargement on MRI. Paraneoplastic optic neuropathy (PON) has also been observed in patients with small cell carcinoma of the lung (see also Chapter 5).[89–92]

Antibody Testing. Testing for the 23-kD antibody or CAR antibody is now commercially available. However, the diagnosis of PR should still be based on clinical grounds.

Treatment. The therapy most often suggested has been immunosuppression to reduce systemic levels of antiretinal antibody. Treatment of the primary malignancy usually does not seem to alter the course of visual loss, although one reported patient had mild improvement.[79]

Therapy is with systemic corticosteroids.[93] Other systemic immunosuppressive drugs have not been tried systematically. Visual acuity and fields in PR patients have been reported to improve with steroids.[79, 80, 87, 93, 94] In one patient, visual acuity decreased each time the steroids were tapered and improved when they were reinstated.[73] Keltner et al[93] reported a patient with elevated serum antibodies that could be reduced with steroids. The elevated antibody titers were associated with further visual deterioration. Some patients fail to improve with corticosteroids.[59, 88] Plasmapheresis has been tried unsuccessfully in one case.[95]

Course. Patients with PR should be followed closely with serial acuities, visual fields, ERGs, and antiretinal antibody titers. The clinical course of PR is variable although rapid progression of CAR is the rule. Some MAR patients may remain stable. Development then worsening of a ring scotoma is characteristic of CAR. Patients are usually significantly visually impaired and progression to profound bilateral loss of vision occurs within weeks to months. Many patients die before they become totally blind. Retinal arterioles typically become more attenuated over time, and the electroretinographic responses progressively decline. The serum level of serum antiretinal antibodies may correlate with success of treatment and severity of the disease.

Big Blind Spot Syndromes

The term *big blind spot syndrome* has been used to describe several different entities, all of which present with an enlarged blind spot. These disorders include acute idiopathic blind spot enlargement (AIBSE) and multiple evanescent white dot syndrome (MEWDS). Enlargement of the blind spot is due either to optic nerve head swelling with displacement of the peripapillary retina or to dysfunction of the peripapillary retina when the optic nerve is ophthalmoscopically normal. Patients reported with AIBSE and MEWDS have a fairly uniform presentation, with the acute onset of a visual field defect around the physiologic blind spot with photopsias. These diseases are more common in women. Visual acuity is usually normal,[96, 97] and the visual field defects typically have steep borders. These disorders likely affect the outer retina and therefore may lie within the spectrum of a single disease.

Acute Idiopathic Blind Spot Enlargement. In 1988 Fletcher et al[98] described seven patients, age 25 to 39, with the acute onset of photopsias and enlargement of the blind spot without optic disc swelling. Two patients had abnormal multifocal ERGs, and the authors concluded that the syndrome resulted from peripapillary retinal dysfunction. Their patients had no abnormalities on fluorescein angiography, although two patients had peripapillary retinal pigment abnormalities. Two patients had recurrences, and three had recovery of their visual fields.

The moniker of AIBSE syndrome is now used to describe patients with the acute onset of positive visual phenomena and an enlarged blind spot without marked disc swelling. The field defects generally have steep borders and can mimic the temporal visual field defects of chiasmal disease Fig 4–12. Peripapillary pigmentary changes are common (Fig. 4–13).[99] Retinal pigment epithelial or choroidal abnormalities and disc staining on fluorescein angiography may be seen.[100, 101] Full-field ERGs are normal but focal ERGs directed at the peripapillary retina are abnormal.[98, 101] Photopsias tend to resolve over time although in most patients the visual field defect persists.[99]

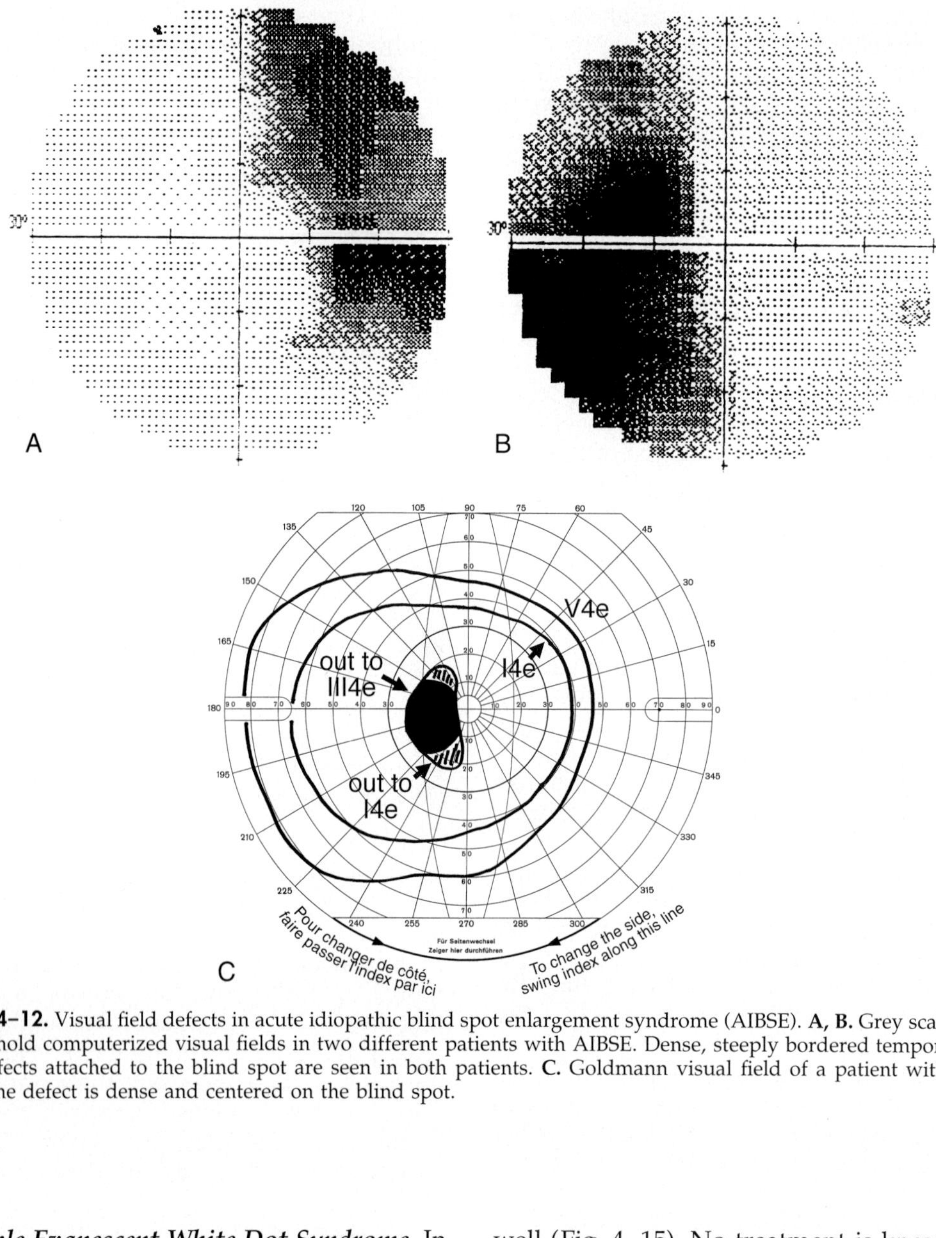

FIGURE 4–12. Visual field defects in acute idiopathic blind spot enlargement syndrome (AIBSE). **A, B.** Grey scale output of threshold computerized visual fields in two different patients with AIBSE. Dense, steeply bordered temporal visual field defects attached to the blind spot are seen in both patients. **C.** Goldmann visual field of a patient with AIBSE. Again the defect is dense and centered on the blind spot.

Multiple Evanescent White Dot Syndrome. In 1984, Jampol et al[102] and Takeda et al[103] described the multiple evanescent white dot syndrome (MEWDS). Jampol et al reported 11 patients (10 women) with acute unilateral vision loss, scotomas, and multiple evanescent white lesions at the level of the retinal pigment epithelium (Fig. 4–14; see Color Plate 8). Many of these and subsequently reported cases of MEWDS have had blind spot enlargement.[102, 104–106] Full-field electroretinographic abnormalities in patients with MEWDS have also been recognized.[102, 104–109] Fluroescein angiography can confirm the retinal pigment epithelial defects and sometimes reveal disc staining as well (Fig. 4–15). No treatment is known, and patients often have persistence of the visual field defect and recurrences.

The optic nerve sometimes may be involved in MEWDS. Dowdell[110] emphasized both the importance of MEWDS in the neuro-ophthalmic differential diagnosis and the possibility of direct inflammation of the optic nerve. While the extensive visual field loss on a retinal basis could cause an afferent pupil defect and dyschromatopsia, the possibility of simultaneous retinal ganglion cell and photoreceptor dysfunction needs to be considered. The optic nerve may also be involved by the presumed inflammatory process either pri-

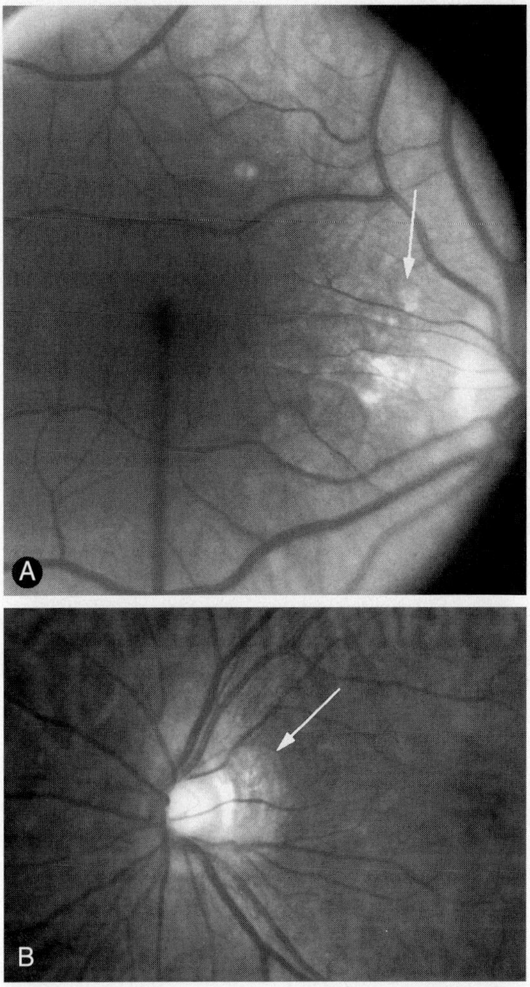

FIGURE 4–13. Peripapillary pigmentary changes in two patients with acute idiopathic blind spot enlargement syndrome (AIBSE). **A.** Areas of pigment atrophy (*arrow*) temporal to the optic nerve head. **B.** A grey halo of discoloration (*arrow*) around the disc in a patient acutely presenting with AIBSE.

marily or secondarily, from contiguous retinal or vascular inflammation. The white dots in MEWDS tend to extend centripetally away from the disc.

Differential Diagnosis. The high prevalence of initial misdiagnoses, the overlap with other common neuro-ophthalmic entities, and the variability of clinical findings make the big blind spot syndromes an important consideration in neuro-ophthalmic differential diagnosis. Photopsia may be incorrectly ascribed to migraine. The abrupt onset of a visual field defect in a young patient might suggest optic neuritis. The presence of the enlarged blind spot and disc hyperemia might suggest papilledema or a temporal defect from a chiasmal lesion.

Pathogenesis. Inflammatory changes, predisposition in women, sporadic occurrence, and relatively acute onset of symptoms suggest an autoimmune or infectious cause. Chung et al[111] have reported elevated levels of serum immunoglobulins in patients with MEWDS, although Jacobson et al[109] were unable to demonstrate histochemical evidence of retinal antibodies. Another variant of this group of conditions, termed *acute annular outer retinopathy,* has been described in which patients develop a visible greyish annular ring in the retina.[112, 113] Gass and Stern speculated that the greyish ring represented an immune ring at the leading edge of the inflammation.[112] Luckie et al's[113] patient seemed to respond to acyclovir, and they concluded that this implicated a herpes virus as the cause.

To date there have been no histopathologic studies of eyes of patients with AIBSE. No abnormal laboratory value has been consistently identified in patients with any of these syndromes. Members of the same family have been affected although there is no information to suggest a specific heritable pattern.

Overlapping Clinical Profiles. Since AIBSE shares many features with MEWDS, these conditions may lie within the spectrum of a single disease. In fact, Gass and Callanan[96, 97, 114] suggested the term *acute zonal occult outer retinopathy* (AZOOR) as an umbrella term for AIBSE, MEWDS, acute macular neuroretinopathy (AMN), and multifocal choroiditis. The clinical features of each of these conditions is summarized in Table 4–4. All four conditions are frequently characterized by acute, focal loss of outer retinal function associated with photopsias, occurrence predominantly in young woman, minimal or no initial fundus changes, and ERG abnormalities. As with patients with paraneoplastic retinopathy, the presence of photopsias suggests photoreceptor dysfunction.

As Gass suggested, the use of the umbrella term AZOOR would be supported by the frequent occurrence of enlarged blind spots in MEWDS.[102–106, 114–116] Enlargement of the blind spot has also been recognized in multifocal choroiditis but in these cases blind spot enlargement corresponds to funduscopic abnormalities of the peripapillary retina.[100, 101, 117] Since many patients with these retinal diseases are not evaluated with formal perimetry it is

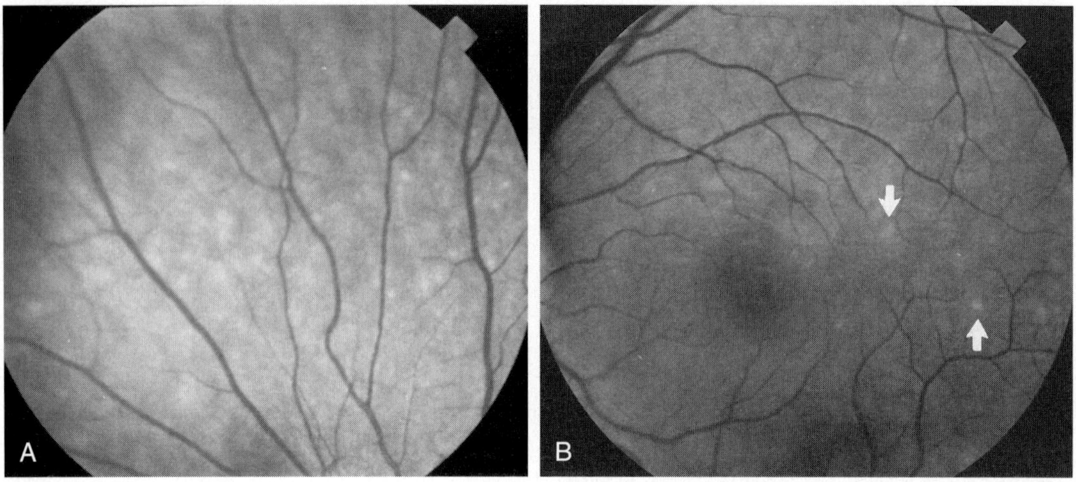

FIGURE 4–14. The multiple evanescent white dot syndrome (MEWDS) in two patients. **A.** Numerous white lesions are seen at the level of the RPE in the nasal periphery of one patient. (See Color Plate 8.) **B.** In another patient the white dots (*arrows*) are less easily seen.

possible that the prevalence of enlarged blind spots in these patients is even higher. It is certainly possible that the evanescent white dots of MEWDS are present but unrecognized or ophthalmoscopically obscure in some or all patients with AIBSE. The most compelling evidence that the conditions are the same are the reports of two different clinical presentations in the same patient. Patients with AIBSE and MEWDS have been reported to develop lesions typical of AMN.[96, 101] Patients with MEWDS and AIBSE have also been reported to develop multifocal active or atrophic fundus lesions more typical of multifocal choroiditis.[118–120]

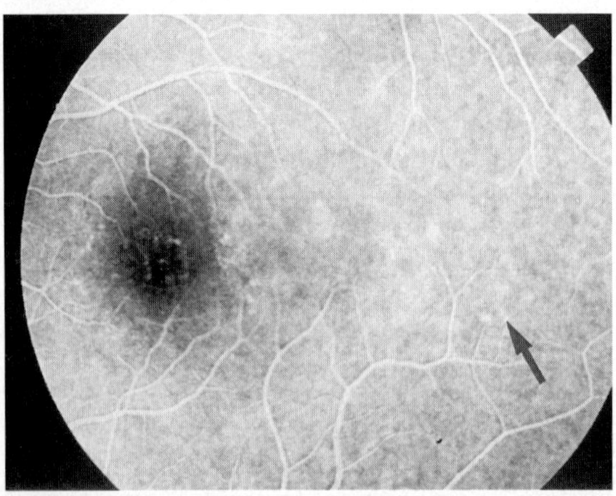

FIGURE 4–15. Late-phase fluorescein angiogram in a patient with multiple evanescent white dot syndrome (MEWDS). There are subtle late-staining lesions (*arrow*) at the level of the RPE.

However, several observations support splitting AIBSE from MEWDS, AMN, and multifocal choroiditis. The first and most striking is the highly variable appearance of the fundus at the time of presentation. The relative paucity of findings in the reported cases of AIBSE compared to the striking outer retinal reddish-orange lesion of AMN, the evanescent white dots at the level of the RPE in MEWDS, and the more persistent deep white pigmentary abnormalities of multifocal choroiditis suggest that all of these are indeed distinct abnormalities. It is not surprising that any condition associated with abnormalities of the outer retina would have a similar presentation (acute onset, photopsia, field defects, and abnormal ERG). In MEWDS and AMN visual field defects usually resolve, whereas in AIBSE the defects tend to persist. Unique features of the peripapillary retina (involved in AIBSE) such as the increased cone density, blood supply, and proximity to the optic nerve suggest it may be uniquely vulnerable to conditions that do not involve the remainder of the retina. Therefore, until a single cause is found for all of these conditions, it is reasonable to assume they are all distinct entities.

TOXIC RETINOPATHY

Because numerous systemic diseases and their treatment are encountered in neuro-ophthalmic practice, it is worthwhile to be aware of the toxic affects that medications can

TABLE 4–4. Clinical Features of the Outer Retinopathies*

Disorder	Distinctive Clinical Features	Ophtalmoscopic Findings
Acute idiopathic blind spot enlargement syndrome	Acute onset of photopsia Field defect centered on blind spot Photopsias resolve but field defect may persist	Mild disc hyperemia and staining on fluorescein angiography Peripapillary pigmentary changes
Multiple evanescent white dot syndrome	Acute onset of field defect Photopsia Generally resolves completely	Evanescent white dots
Acute macular neuroretinopathy	Sudden onset of small central or paracentral scotoma Some positive visual phenomena	Orange-brown petalloid lesion around the fovea
Acute zonal occult outer retinopathy	Bilateral Photopsia Permanent pigment changes in retina Abnormal electroretinogram	Pigmentary changes in retinal periphery

* For the purposes of highlighting the different features of each condition, the disorders are considered separately and distinctly.

have on the retina. These are summarized in Table 4–5. The best known retinal toxin is digoxin. Patients typically develop xanthopsia (yellow vision), scintillating scotomas, and paracentral scotomas.[121–123] Patients may have abnormalities in the cone (photopic) b-wave implicit times.[124] Color vision defects may be the earliest manifestation, and screening for digoxin toxicity with color vision testing has been suggested.[125] Patients may develop visual symptoms even when the digoxin level in the blood stream is in the therapeutic range.[126] Digoxin toxicity is discussed in more detail in Chapter 12.

TABLE 4–5. Ophthalmic Manifestations of Drugs Causing Retinal Toxicity

Drug	Ophthalmic Manifestations
Digoxin	Xanthopsia (yellow vision) Positive visual phenomena Decreased color vision
Tamoxifen	Crystalline deposits in the macula
Canthaxanthine	Crystalline deposits in the macula
Thioridazine	Pigmentary deposits on corneal and anterior lens capsule Pigmentary retinopathy
Isotretinoin	Decreased night vision
Chloroquine and hydroxychloroquine	Corneal whirl Bull's eye maculopathy
Nicotinic acid	Cystoid macular edema
Quinine	Retinal photoreceptor and ganglion cell toxicity
Vigabatrin	ERG abnormalities Visual field constriction

Quinine, used primarily in the treatment of malaria, is toxic to the retinal photoreceptors and ganglion cells. Several different drugs can cause a crystalline retinopathy. These include tamoxifen,[127–130] canthaxanthine,[131, 132] and methoxyflurane.[133] The deposits in the case of tamoxifen appear to be products of axonal degeneration.[127] The complication is sufficiently rare and has minimal affect on vision, so widespread screening is not recommended.[128] In the case of methoxyflurane, oxalosis results from metabolism of the drug. Various diuretics, nicotinic acid, and epinephrine can cause cystoid macular edema. Isotretinoin has been reported to affect retinal function and result in abnormal night vision.[134–137]

Chloroquine and hydroxychloroquine, used to treat malaria and collagen vascular disorders, cause a dose-related pigmentary retinopathy.[138–145] Other ocular findings include corneal whirl-type deposits and poliosis. The macular changes begin as a pigment mottling but then become a horizontally elongated bull's eye (Fig. 4–16). Patients slowly develop reduced central acuity and central visual field defects. Color vision testing and ERG give mixed results. It appears that the toxicity is dose related, and hydroxychloroquine dosages less than 6.5 mg/kg/day appear to be safe.[142] The drug is excreted very slowly, therefore toxicity can progress even after the drug is discontinued. Although it has been a subject of some debate, many experts feel that screening for retinopathy in patients taking hydroxychloroquine is unnecessary unless the daily dose exceeds 6.5 mg/kg/day or the patient has been on it for more than 10 years.[138, 139, 141] Hydroxychloroquine seems to be the safer of the two drugs.[145]

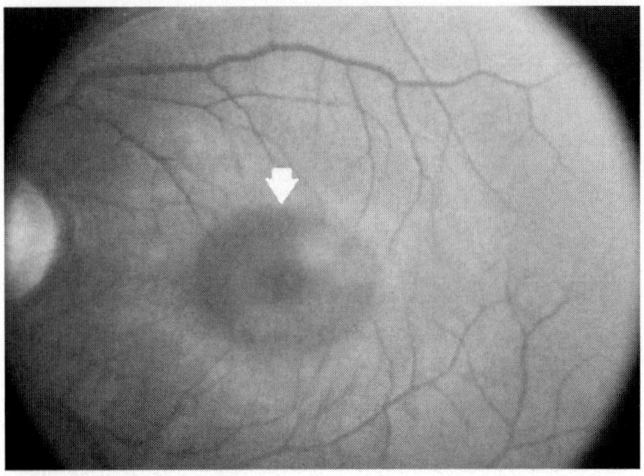

FIGURE 4–16. Fundus photography of a horizontally elongated "bull's eye" pigmentary abnormality (*arrow*) of the retina in a patient with chloroquine retinal toxicity.

Vigabitrin, an anticonvulsant, can cause ERG abnormalities and concentric visual field constriction in as many as half of patients taking the drug.[146, 147] This selective irreversible inhibitor of gamma-aminobutyric acid (GABA)-transaminase increases GABA available in central nervous system (CNS) synapses.

HEREDITARY RETINAL DYSTROPHIES IN NEURO-OPHTHALMIC DIFFERENTIAL DIAGNOSIS

The clinical spectrum of hereditary retinal degenerations includes a variety of presentations that overlap with common neuro-ophthalmic conditions. In particular, patients with hereditary retinal degenerations may present with insidious central vision loss, dyschromatopsia, and visual field defects. The vast majority of patients with typical retinitis pigmentosa present with a rod-dominated picture characterized by nyctalopia (night blindness), peripheral vision loss, and a characteristic bone-spicule pigmentation of the peripheral retina. Rarely patients present without any abnormal pigment accumulation. A subset of patients with heritable retinal degenerations have cone-dominated presentations that are characterized by light- or glare-induced blindness (hammarlopia), central vision loss, and dyschromatopsia. Prominent macular changes may be evident on ophthalmoscopy.

Cone or Cone–Rod Dystrophies

Cone dystrophies or cone–rod dystrophies usually present in middle age and have a variable inheritance pattern. The visual acuity and color vision may be moderately reduced at a time when the macular changes are subtle or absent on ophthalmoscopy. These disorders should be considered in all patients with bilateral subnormal acuity and color vision. It is not surprising that such cases are confused with optic neuropathies. In many cases the family history is not helpful. Perhaps this represents the existence of spontaneous mutations or the variable clinical expressivity of the disorder.

Classification. We use the term *cone dystrophy* to describe patients with progressive and heritable central vision loss who do not have a funduscopic appearance suggesting an alternative dystrophy (see Table 4–6). Cone dystrophies are a heterogeneous group of inherited disorders that result in dysfunction of the cone photoreceptors and their postreceptoral pathways. These disorders have been classified on the basis of the relative involvement of cones and rods and the relative involvement of central versus peripheral photoreceptors.[148] Based on their natural history, the cone dystrophies may also be divided into two groups: "stationary" and "progressive."[149] Based on careful study of several pedigrees, the genes responsi-

TABLE 4–6. Common Hereditary Macular Disorders With a Recognizable Fundus Appearance

Disease	Fundus Appearance
Best's disease (vitelliform dystrophy)	Egg yolk appearance; may develop scarring and neovascularization
Adult foveomacular dystrophy	Symmetric, oval, yellow subretinal lesion
Familial drusen	Numerous drusen may coalesce; choroidal neovascularization
Central areolar choroidal dystrophy	Early: pigment granularity Late: circular zone of RPE and choriocapillary atrophy
Myopic degeneration	Peripapillary atrophy, staphyloma, lacquer cracks
Stargardt's disease, (atrophic macular dystrophy with flecks) (fundus flavimaculatus)	Angulated flecks and atrophy in retina, "beaten bronze" appearance, dark "silent choroid" on fluorescein angiography
Juvenile retinoschisis	Foveal retinoschisis
Butterfly-shaped pattern dystrophy	Reticular butterfly-shaped pattern of pigmentation in macula

ble for some of these conditions have been elucidated.[150–153] Identification of the genotypes will ultimately lead to a proper classification system and better understanding of the phenotypic variability.

Clinical Features. Patients present with abnormal light sensitivity (photophobia or hammarlopia), photopsia, and reduced vision. Identifying the symptom of abnormal light sensitivity is critical to making the diagnosis. This light sensitivity may be erroneously interpreted as optical glare and lead to unnecessary cataract surgery. Symptoms typically develop over many years. Examination reveals reduced central acuity (20/30 to 20/400), dyschromatopsia, central scotomas on visual field testing, and pigmentary alterations in the macula (Fig. 4–17). Changes in color vision may be the first sign of the disease.[154] These patients have an abnormal ERG with cones affected more than rods, or only cones affected. Nonrecordable or abnormal (reduced b-wave amplitude or oscillatory potential), photopic (recorded in light, cone-mediated) responses on the ERG are likely to be detected. However, more specific information might be obtained from a focal or multifocal ERG that evaluates central retinal function.[155] An ERG may be used to follow these patients to determine the rate of disease progression.[156] Ocular coherence tomography may reveal thinning of the outer retina–choroid complex (ORCC)[157] (Fig. 4–18; see Color Plate 9). Optic disc pallor may also develop.[158]

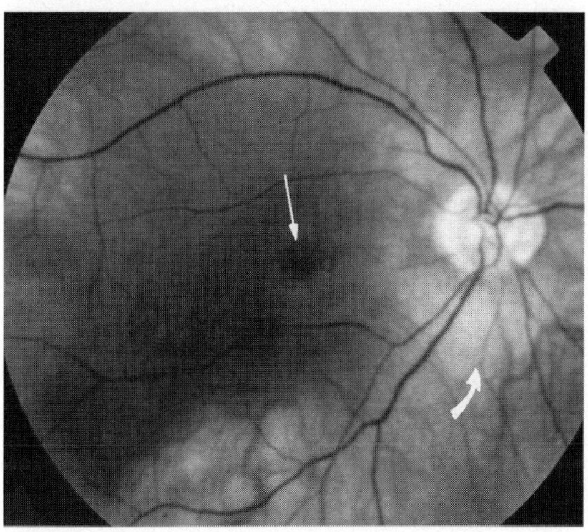

FIGURE 4–17. Fundus photograph of the right eye of a patient with cone dystrophy. In addition to fine granularity of the pigmentation in the macula (*thin arrow*) there is peripapillary pigment atrophy (*thicker curved arrow*). Macular pigmentary changes are often subtle and can be overlooked.

Hereditary Maculopathies With Obvious Ophthalmoscopic Abnormalities

Several heritable conditions affect the macula and result in a diagnostic fundus appearance. Some of the more common maculopathies are summarized in Table 4–6. Each has a characteristic fundus appearance and therefore would not be confused with an optic neuropathy. For instance, a patient with Stargardt's disease (Fig 4–19) would be recognized based on the abnormal fundus appearance and fluorescein angiography. However, early these conditions may be hard to recognize since symptoms of decreased central vision may precede the development of the typical fundus lesion.

Mitochondrial Diseases

Kearns–Sayre Syndrome. Retinal dystrophy or degeneration may be associated with chronic progressive external ophthalmoplegia (CPEO). Onset of retinopathy before age 20 combined with heart block, ataxia, and/or cerebrospinal fluid protein above 100 mg/dL is termed *Kearns-Sayre syndrome,* (KSS)[159] This condition is caused by mitochondrial DNA deletions.[160–164] Approximately one third of patients will have some type of pigmentary retinopathy.[165] Many patients have salt-and-pepper-type retinopathy with some macular dysfunction and ERG abnormalities. Other patients develop more widespread and progressive retinal dysfunction.[165, 166] CPEO and KSS are detailed in Chapter 14.

MELAS. Another important mitochondrial disorder is MELAS (mitochondrial encephalopathy with lactic acidosis and strokelike episodes). This condition frequently presents with strokelike episodes that may cause retrochiasmal visual loss. The condition usually results from a mutation at position 3243 of the mitochondrial DNA.[167] Like those with KSS, patients with MELAS can have a pigmentary abnormality in the retina. Visual symptoms related to the retina are usually absent or mild. Also, the pigmentary changes identified are subtle and occur primarily in the macula.[168, 169]

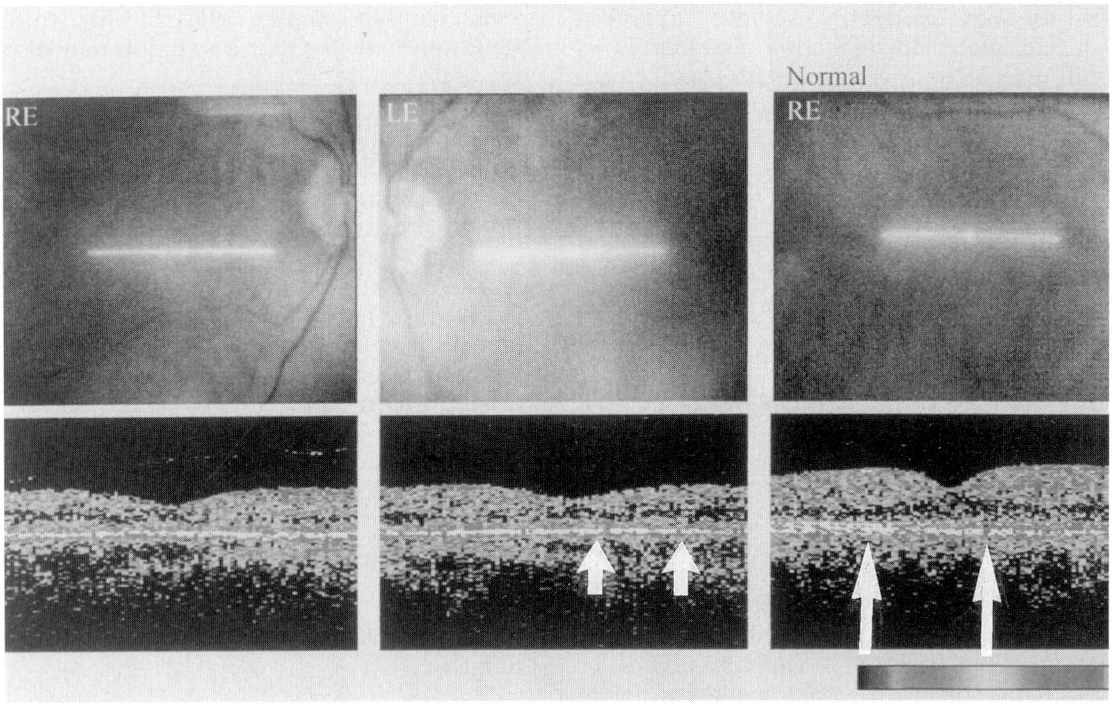

FIGURE 4–18. Ocular coherence tomography in a patient with cone dystrophy. In the upper row of the photograph, the scanning laser ophthalmoscope view is seen. The left and middle columns are from the right (RE) and left eyes (LE) of an affected patient. The column to the far right is from a normal subject. Overall thinning of the retina is seen in the patient compared to a normal control. In particular the outer retina choroid complex (red in Color Plate 9) is thinner in the cone dystrophy patient (*small arrows*) compared to normal (*large arrows*). (Photo courtesy of Arthur V. Cideciyan, Ph.D., and Samuel G. Jacobson, M.D.) (See Color Plate 9.)

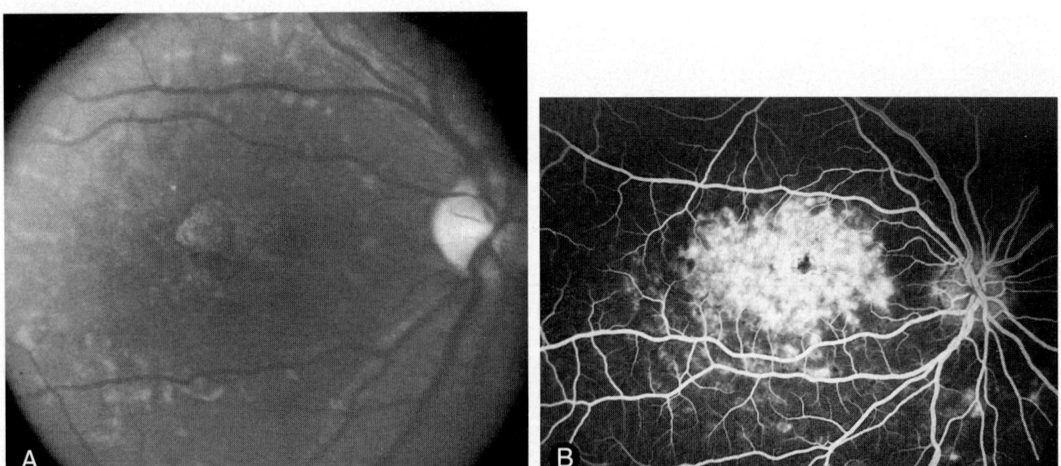

FIGURE 4–19. Fundus photograph and fluorescein angiogram in a patient with Stargardt's disease. **A.** Photograph demonstrating pigmentary atrophy in the macula and elongated subretinal yellow deposits. **B.** Late-phase fluorescein angiogram demonstrating a "silent" choroid that appears unusually dark and highlights the retinal vasculature. Late staining of the subretinal deposits is also seen.

Histopathologically, degeneration of photoreceptor outer segments in the macula has been identified.[170] MELAS is discussed further in Chapter 8.

NARP. This rare mitochondrial disorder is characterized by *n*europathy, *a*taxia, and *r*etinitis *p*igmentosa. Other clinical features include proximal muscle weakness, developmental delay, ataxia, seizures, and dementia.[171] The disease is maternally inherited, and a responsible mutation at position 8993 of the ATPase 6 gene has been identified.[172] This is the same gene identified in some patients with Leigh's disease (see Chapter 16).

OTHER DISEASES WITH RETINAL AND NEUROLOGIC MANIFESTATIONS

Vasculitis

Microangiopathy of the Brain, Retina, and Inner Ear (Susac Syndrome). This disorder predominantly affects young women.[173–177] It is also known as Susac syndrome to honor the man who recognized its characteristic features.[178] Recent reviews have identified about 60 patients in the literature.[179–181] Ninety percent of patients presented with retinal arterial occlusions and in 60% they are bilateral.[179–181] Mean age of onset is 30 years.[181] Although it resembles primary angiitis of the nervous system, it is the sensorineural hearing loss and retinal ischemic changes that mark it as a distinct entity. Hearing loss occurs in two thirds of patients.[179–181] Like primary CNS angiitis, the disorder is confined to the central nervous system. Global encephalopathy is common, occurring in 44% of patients.[181]

Involved areas of the brain demonstrate microinfarction of the grey and white matter. Inflammatory vessel changes have not been found in this disorder. Rather, involved segments have demonstrated vessel thickening or sclerosis.[176] Although the pathogenesis of this disorder is unknown, evidence points to autoimmune-related endothelial damage. In this regard, Notis et al[182] have demonstrated retinal vessel hyperfluorescence on fluorescein angiography 5 days prior to retinal infarction. Treatment with variable success has been achieved with corticosteroids and other immunosuppressive agents.[176] Anticoagulation has not been effective. One patient apparently responded to the combination of antiplatelet and calcium channel blocker therapy.[177] Vision loss in Susac syndrome has been successfully treated with hyperbaric oxygen.[29] Intravenous gamma globulin has also been anecdotally successful in treating this disorder. The prognosis is generally good as the disease tends to be self limited.[181]

Acute Posterior Multifocal Placoid Pigment Epitheliopathy. Acute posterior multifocal placoid pigment epitheliopathy (APMPPE) is a disorder first recognized by Gass in 1968.[183] This acute, but self-limiting disorder produces characteristic multifocal grey, white flat lesions at the level of the retinal pigment epithelium.[183] Pigment epithelial abnormalities seem to result from dysfunction of the choroidal vasculature.[184, 185] Neurologic manifestations have included headache, transient ischemic attacks, dysacusis, tinnitus, cerebral vasculitis, and stroke.[186–190] Stroke and aseptic meningitis are the two major pathologic substrates for the neurologic dysfunction seen in APMPPE. There have been nine previously reported cases of stroke with APMPPE.[191] Five patients had angiographic changes suggesting vasculitis. However, only two cases have had histologic proof of vasculitis. One patient had a positive muscle biopsy[187] and the other a brain biopsy that revealed granulomatosis inflammation of medium-sized arteries.[189] The infarcts have a tendency to involve the posterior circulation and the basal ganglia region. The strokes usually occur at the time of the visual loss, but may precede or follow the ocular manifestations.[191] Although cerebral vasculitis may remit spontaneously, aggressive immunosuppressive therapy has been suggested. Corticosteroids in combination with cyclophosphamide for 6 to 12 months is one proposed regimen.[191] The visual prognosis is generally good although initial involvement of the fovea and older age portend a worse visual outcome.[192]

Eale's Disease and Cogan Syndrome. Eale's disease and Cogan syndrome are primary vasculitic disorders of the eye but are infrequently associated with cerebral vasculitis. Both are distinguished from isolated CNS angiitis by their associated eye findings. Eale's disease is the disorder of young, healthy men who develop retinal vasculitis, vitreous hemorrhage, and peripheral nonperfusion of the retina with subsequent neovascularization.[193] Treatment is with laser photocoagulation. Besides the ocular manifestations, the central nervous system may be rarely affected. Patients have been reported with stroke, myelopathy and vascultis.[189, 194–199] Pathologically, both demyelinating and vasculitic changes have been noted within the CNS of patients with Eale's disease.[189] The prognosis for maintainence of good visual recovery is usually good but some patients have severe vision loss secondary to the neovascular complications.

Cogan syndrome is characterized by the presence of interstitial keratitis and vestibuloauditory dysfunction. Again the CNS may occasionally be affected. Reported manifestations include seizures, ataxia, cranial nerve palsies, stroke, and meningoencephalitis.[200]

CADASIL. Cerebral autosomal dominant arteriopathy with subcortical infarcts and leukoencephalopathy (CADASIL) is an arteriopathy affecting the small arteries and arterioles of the brain. CADASIL presents in young or middle adulthood with transient ischemic attacks, or stroke. Patients develop recurrent subcortical ischemic strokes, with characteristic MRI findings, leading to a stepwise decline and dementia with frontal lobe features. The histopathologic hallmark of CADISIL is a characteristic granular alteration of the arterial media that corresponds to the accumulation of electron-dense material surrounding the smooth muscle cells.[201] The presence of this granular material was originally described in brain vessels but identical electron microscopic findings have demonstrated similar findings in the media of peripheral tissue arteries. This allows for a pathologic diagnosis of the disease by a simple skin, muscle, or nerve biopsy. Ophthalmoscopically, thickening of the retinal arterioles can be observed, presumably as a result of similar deposition of granular material. The defective gene in CADASIL is Notch3 (chromosome 19), which encodes a large transmembrane receptor.[202]

Spinocerebellar Ataxias

The spinocerebellar ataxias (SCAs) are a group of conditions characterized by loss of neurons in the cerebellar cortex, basis pontis, and inferior olivary nucleus. Clinically, patients develop progressive ataxia with pyramidal and brain stem signs, and many patients develop supranuclear ophthalmoparesis (see Chapter 16 for further discussion). Patients with SCAs may have either optic atrophy or a pigmentary retinal degeneration.

In particular, patients with SCA-7 (autosomal dominant cerebellar ataxia (ADCA) type II) manifest with progressive ataxia and vision loss secondary to retinal degeneration. The genetic defect has been mapped to chromosome 3p.[203–205] The gene appears to be an abnormal CAG repeat that has been identified in pedigrees from around the world.[206–208] The onset of symptoms is usually in the second or third decade. Two thirds of patients will manifest with ataxia while one third present with ataxia with visual loss.[209] Vision loss may precede the development of ataxia but is often not recognized by the patient because of its insidious onset. Vision loss is bilateral and symmetric and mostly central.[210] Patients maintain relatively normal peripheral fields but develop reduced acuity, dyschromatopsia, and central scotomas with macular atrophy. Pigmentary changes at the macula may have a bull's eye appearance (Fig. 4–20; see Color Plate 10).[211] These pigmentary changes can extend into the periphery and over time optic atrophy may develop. The cone-derived, photopic, full-field ERG, or focal ERG or PERG (pattern electro retinogram) is reduced.[209] The rod responses are not affected until late in the disease. Severe atrophy of the retina has been demonstrated at autopsy.[212] About half of the patients develop supranuclear ophthalmoplegia (see Chapter 16).

Metabolic Diseases

Ophthalmologists must be aware of the various metabolic storage diseases and their manifestations, as ophthalmologic findings may

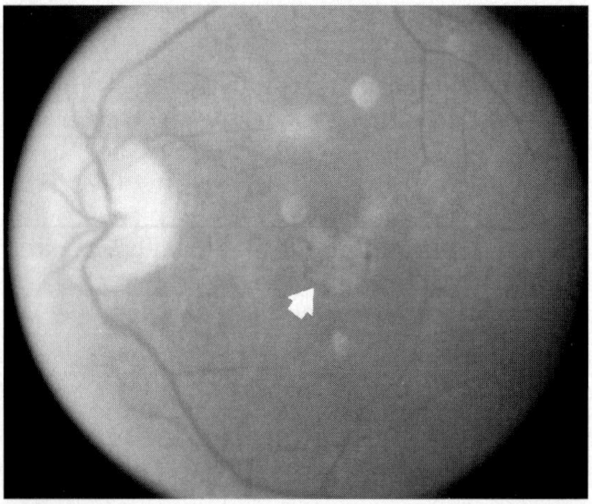

FIGURE 4–20. Macular pigmentary atrophy in bull's eye pattern (*arrow*) in a patient with spinocerebellar ataxia type 7 with pigmentary retinopathy. Circular white spots are photographic artifact. (See Color Plate 10.)

allow for early, accurate diagnosis. Ophthalmic manifestations are variable and can affect all parts of the eye. These are summarized in Table 4–7. These findings are present only in some of the patients and therefore the absence of a cherry-red spot or abnormal pigmentation in the neurologically impaired child or adult does not exclude these diagnoses.

Thrombotic Disorders (Hypercoaguable States)

Recently, a variety of thrombotic disorders have been recognized. These conditions include a variety of disorders that result from abnormalities of the clotting pathway and are characterized by abnormal clotting and ischemic events. They are generally more common in woman and may be associated with a number of systemic conditions, particular autoimmune disorders. Their ophthalmic presentations are fairly uniform and are characterized by amaurosis fugax from retinal ischemia, retinopathy associated with cotton-wool spots and intraretinal hemorrhages, and occasionally permanent deficits from choroidal ischemia, retinal artery occlusions, and ischemic optic neuropathy.

TABLE 4–7. Retinal Posterior Segment Manifestations of Metabolic Disorders

Storage Disorders With Cherry-Red Spot[320]
Tay–Sachs disease
Niemann pick disease
Metachromatic Leukodystrophy
Sialidosis
Infantile GM_2 gangliosidosis (Sandhoff's disease)
Farber disease
Retinal Pigmentary Degeneration
Mucopolysaccharidoses
Gaucher's
Refsum's disease (phytanic acid lipidosis)
Neuronal ceroid lipofuscinosis
Mucolipidosis
Cystinuria
Abetalipoproteinemia
Kearns–Sayre syndrome
Hallervorden–Spatz syndrome
Spinocerebellar ataxia type 7 (and occasionally type 1)
Usher syndrome
Cockayne disease
Optic Atrophy
Krabbe disease
Metachromatic leukodystrophy
Adrenoleukodystrophy
Alexander disease
Spinocerebellar ataxia type 1 and Friedreich's ataxia
Spongy degeneration
Pelizaeus–Merzbacher disease
Alper's disease

Antiphospholipid Antibody Syndrome. One of the best known of the thrombotic syndromes is the antiphospholipid antibody syndrome. The antiphospholipid antibodies directed against phospholipids include the lupus anticoagulants and anticardiolipin antibodies. Patients with antiphospholipid antibodies are more commonly women under age 50. There may be a history of lupus and repeated fetal loss. Many have a history of a strokelike event, transient ischemic attack, or arterial or venous thrombosis that is otherwise unexplained. Patients may be thrombocytopenic and the partial thromboplastin time may be prolonged. A variety of ocular symptoms and findings have been reported in patients with antiphospholipid syndrome.[32, 39, 213–215] Transient changes in vision are common.[32, 213] Occlusions of both retinal veins and arteries (Fig 4–21; see Color Plate 11) has been reported.[39, 213, 215] In a prospective series of 39 consecutive patients with antiphospholipid syndrome, Gelfand and associates[216] found 13 patients had symptoms and 12 complained of visual disturbances that were most often transient. Only two patients were found to have mild retinopathy. They concluded that the majority of transient visual symptoms described could be attributed to a central neurologic problem. Neurologic findings in these patients can be grouped into three clinical patterns: encephalopathy, multiple cerebral infarctions, and migraine-like headaches.[217, 218]

Other Thrombotic Disorders. There are other disorders of the clotting pathway that may lead to visual symptoms and signs. These in-

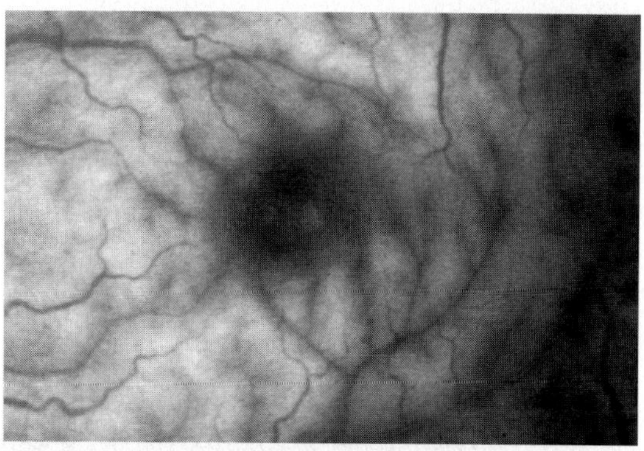

FIGURE 4–21. High-magnification fundus photograph demonstrating retinal whitening and ischemia in a patient with systemic lupus erythematosus and antiphospholipid antibodies. (See Color Plate 11.)

clude deficiencies of protein C, protein S, and antithrombin III[219] and hyperhomocysteinemia. Finally, activated protein C resistance can be seen with the factor V Leiden mutation, which has been reported in association with both retinal vein and retinal artery occlusions.[220–224] Until there is a more definitive understanding of the roles these factors play in retinal vascular occlusion, we recommend screening for these disorders in all patients under age 50 with amaurosis fugax or retinal arterial or venous occlusion.

Vogt–Koyanagi–Harada Syndrome

Vogt–Koyanagi–Harada (VKH) syndrome is the best-known uveomeningeal syndrome. It is a systemic disorder involving many organ systems, including the eye, skin, meninges, and ear. It is most common in Japan[225, 226] and parts of Latin American but is uncommon in the United States (except in American Indians) and in individuals of northern European ancestry.[227] There are many theories concerning the etiology of VKH syndrome that have focused on infectious and immune-mediated diseases. It seems most likely to result from a derangement of T-cell function.[228–230]

Patients usually present in the second to fourth decade although it has been described in children as young as 4 years old.[231–233] The disease usually develops in stages initially characterized by a flulike syndrome associated with headache, aseptic meningitis, dysacusis, and tinnitus. These symptoms may be present for several weeks. This is followed by the ocular symptoms of anterior and posterior uveitis, inferior exudative retinal detachments,[227] and disc hyperemia. The uveitis is usually bilateral and granulomatous in nature. Synechiae and cataract formation are common.[234] The anterior chamber may become shallow secondary to swelling of the ciliary processes.[235] About 40% of patients develop glaucoma, which may be open or closed angle.[236] The retinal pigmented epithelium (RPE) eventually becomes severely depigmented as the serous retinal detachments resolve. Subretinal yellow-white lesions may be seen in the peripheral retina. Neovascularization of the disc and retina with vitreous hemorrhage may also develop.[237] Hearing loss is common and patients complain of a peculiar sensitivity to touch of the hair and skin. In the later stages, patients develop depigmentation of the skin (vitiligo) and hair (poliosis) of any part of the body.

In the early stages, fluorescein angiography will reveal multiple pinpoint sources of leakage. Indocyanine green angiography may reveal patchy infiltrates, suggesting an inflammatory disorder of the choroid with subsequent circulatory compromise.[238] Echography reveals diffuse, low to medium reflective thickening of the choroid and serous retinal detachment.[239] MRI may demonstrate a similar thickening and enhancement of the choroid and retina.[240] During the early stages lumbar puncture will reveal a pleocytosis with lymphocytes and monocytes. Later in the course the spinal fluid may return to normal, and therefore a lumbar puncture should be performed early in the course if the diagnosis is suspected.

VKH syndrome is treated with corticosteroids.[241, 242] Incomplete responses and steroid dependency are commonly encountered.[243] Most patients require treatment for at least a year. Successful therapy with intravenous immune globulin has also been reported.[244] About 60% of patients maintain 20/30 or better vision.[227]

RETINAL MANIFESTATIONS OF SYSTEMIC INFLAMMATORY AND INFECTIOUS DISEASES

A variety of systemic infectious and inflammatory conditions may be associated with retinal manifestations. Retinal findings may take many different forms, including retinal phlebitis, retinal and choroidal granulomas, cotton-wool spots, and optic nerve head swelling. Patients may be asymptomatic with abnormalities detected on initial screening examinations. In other patients, ophthalmic symptoms and retinal abnormalities are the initial manifestations of the systemic disease.

Sarcoidosis

Sarcoidosis, a multisystem granulomatous disorder of unknown etiology, is the third most common cause of uveitis after idiopathic cases and cases associated with HLA B-27.[245] Most studies find about 30% of sarcoidosis patients have ophthalmic involvement.[246] However, in one series as many as 79% of sarcoidosis patients had ocular manifestations, and the most common was anterior uveitis.[247] Ophthalmic manifestations of sarcoidosis are listed in Table 4–8. Vitritis and retinal perivasculitis (seen in about two thirds of patients) and spotty retino-

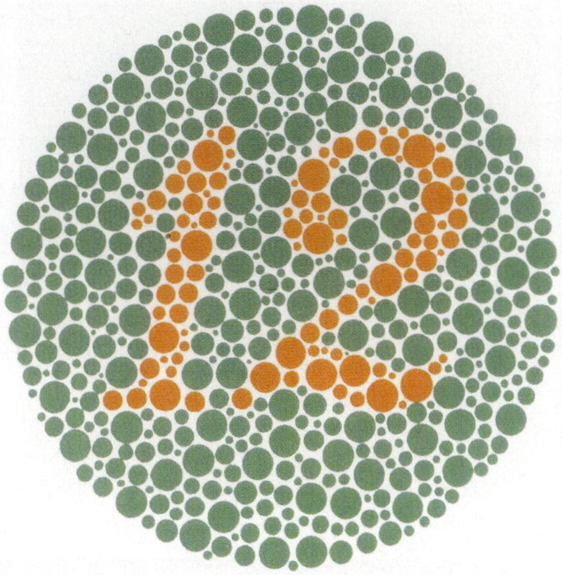

Color Plate 1

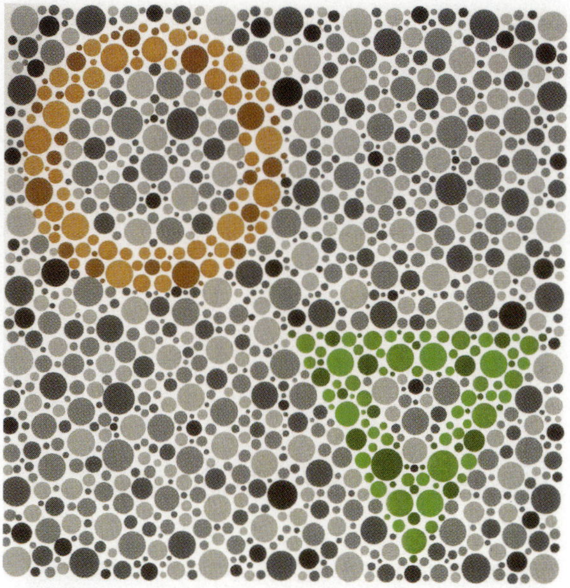

Color Plate 2

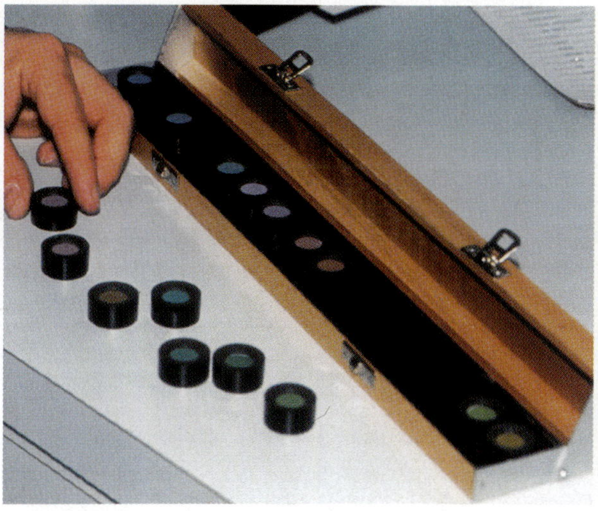

Color Plate 3

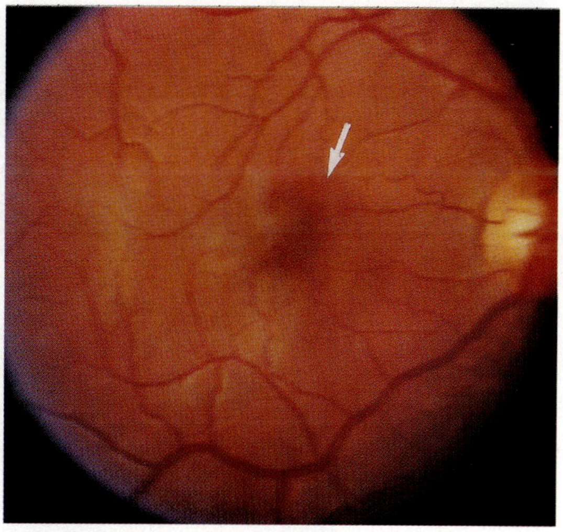

Color Plate 4

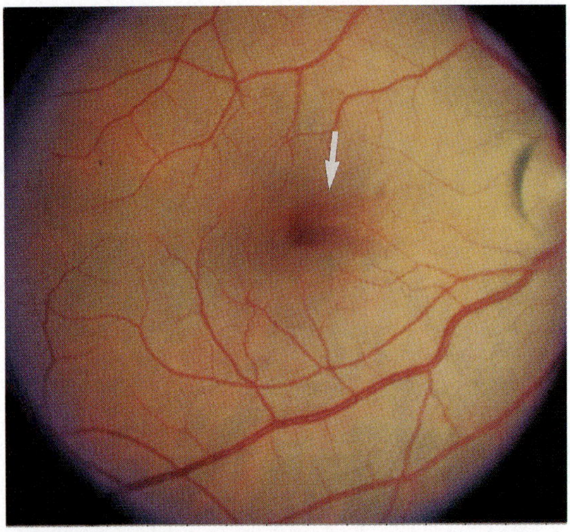

Color Plate 5

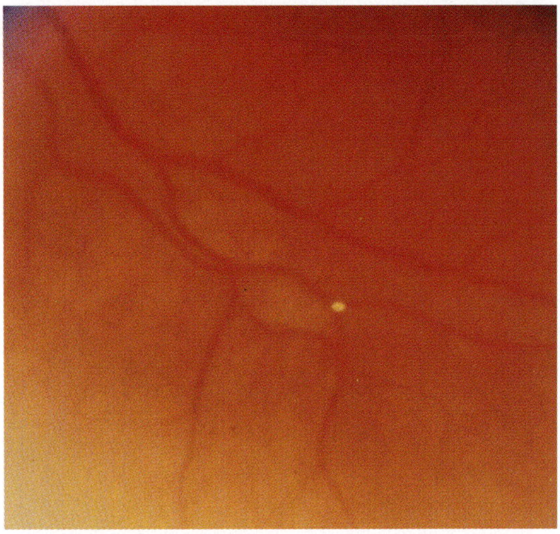

Color Plate 6

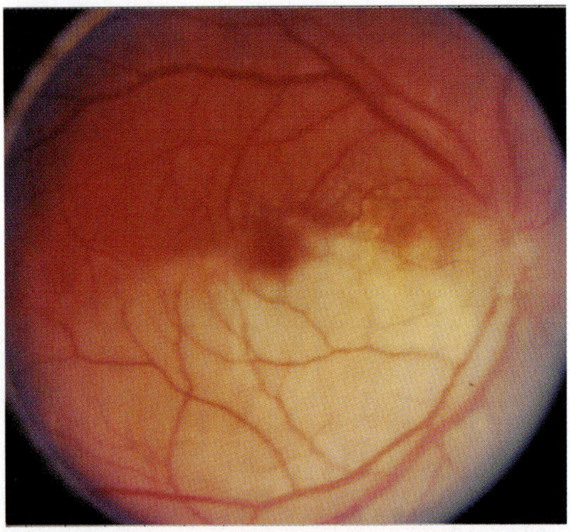

Color Plate 7

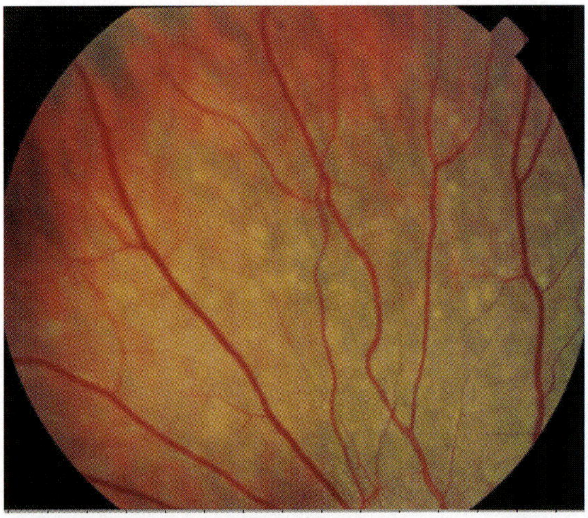

Color Plate 8

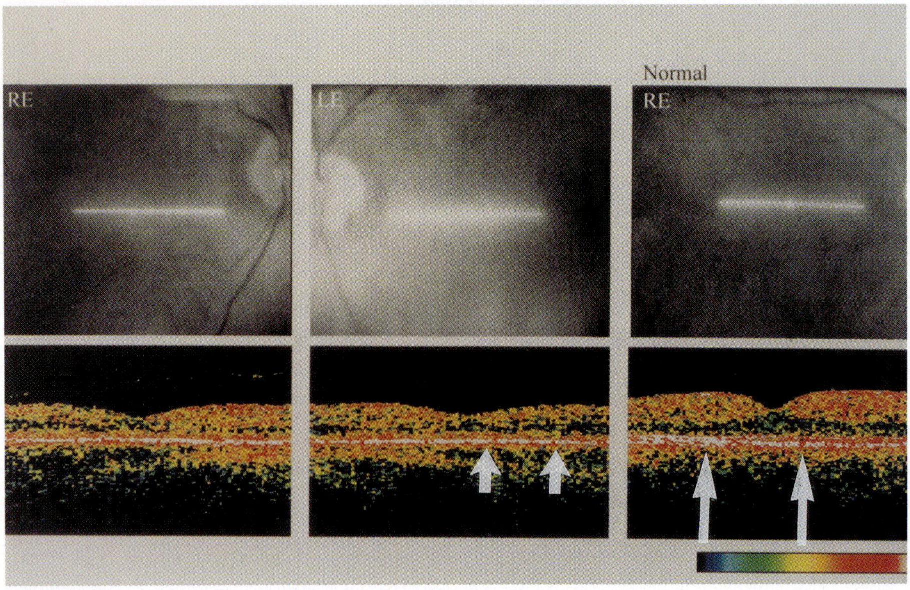

Color Plate 9

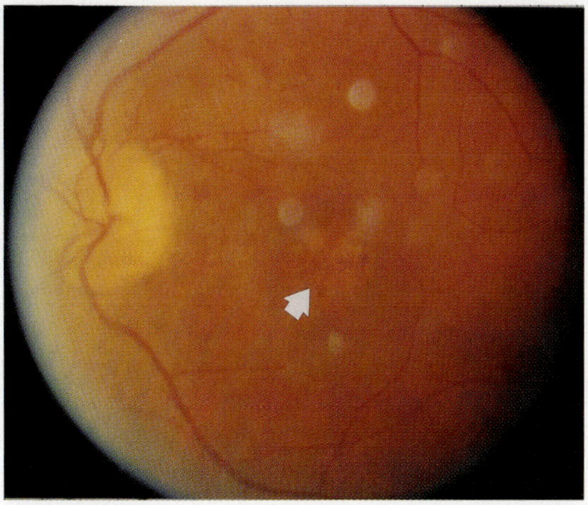

Color Plate 10

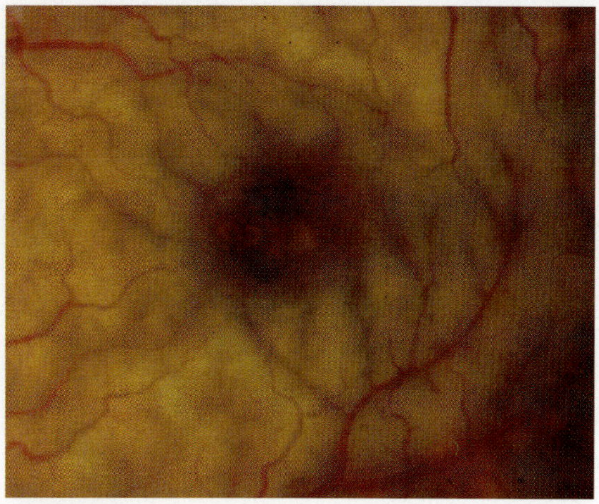

Color Plate 11

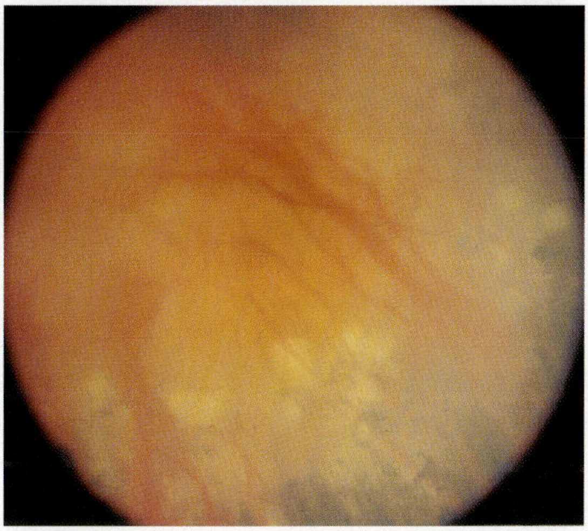

Color Plate 12

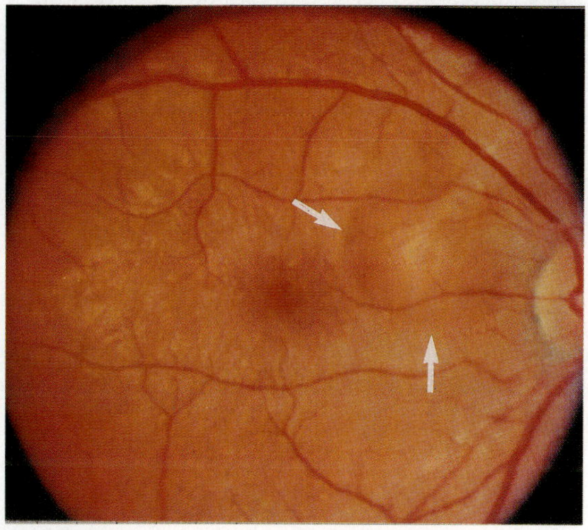

Color Plate 13

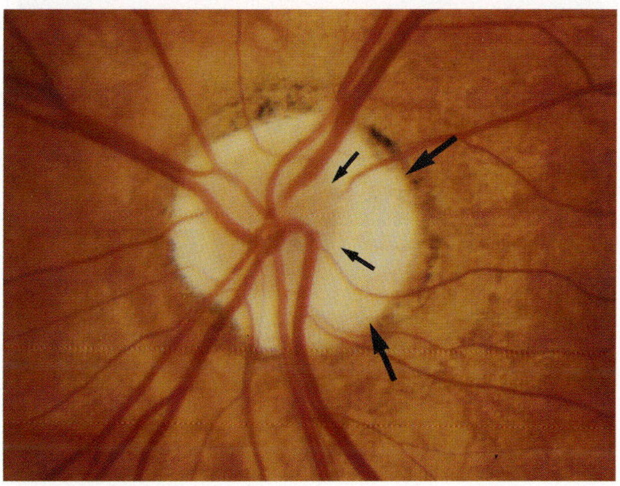

Color Plate 14

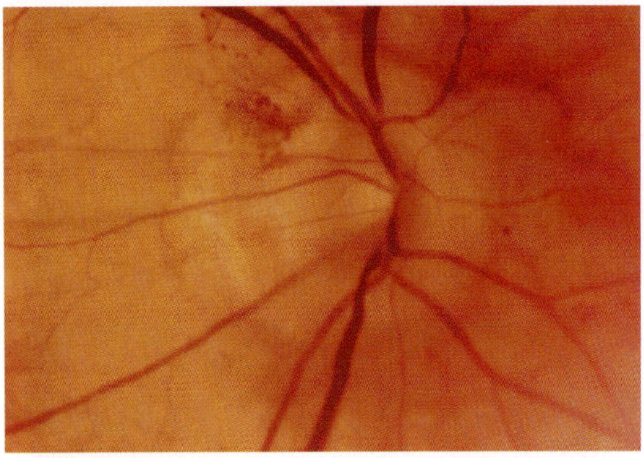
Color Plate 15

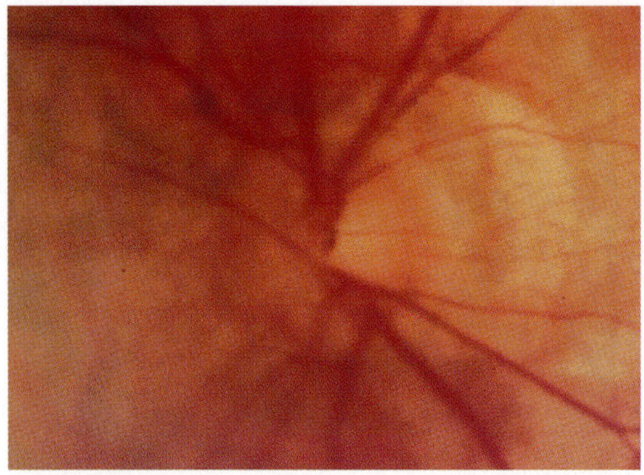
Color Plate 16

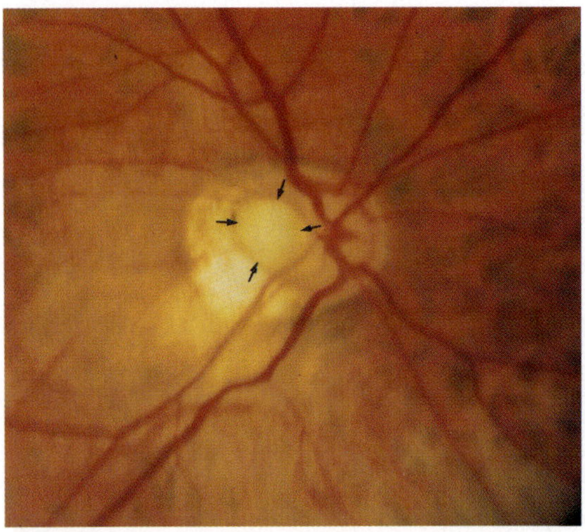
Color Plate 17

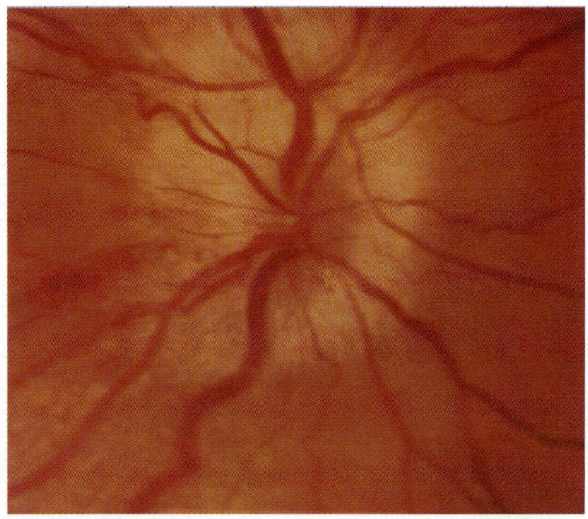
Color Plate 18

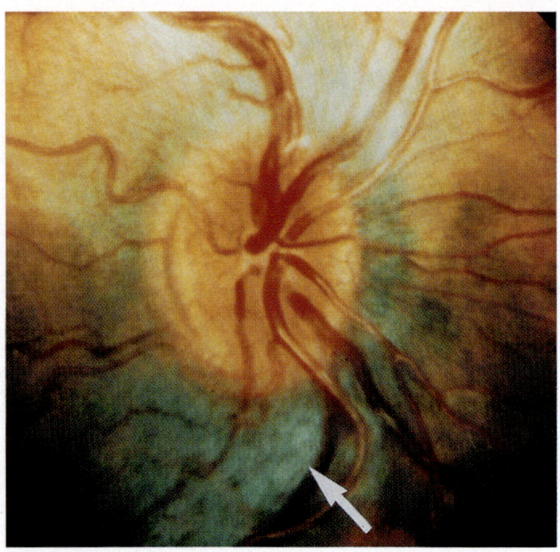
Color Plate 19

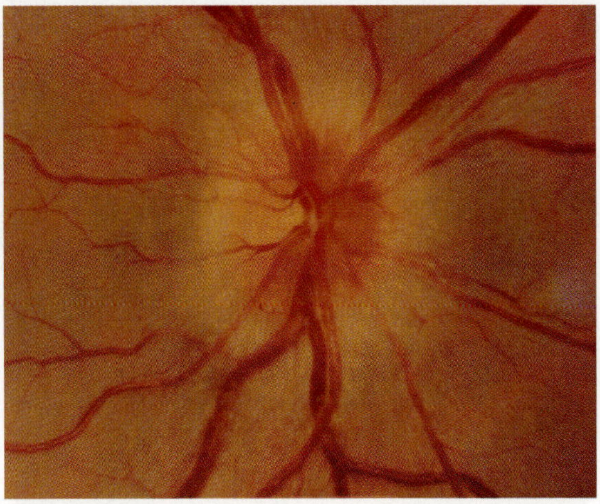

Color Plate 20

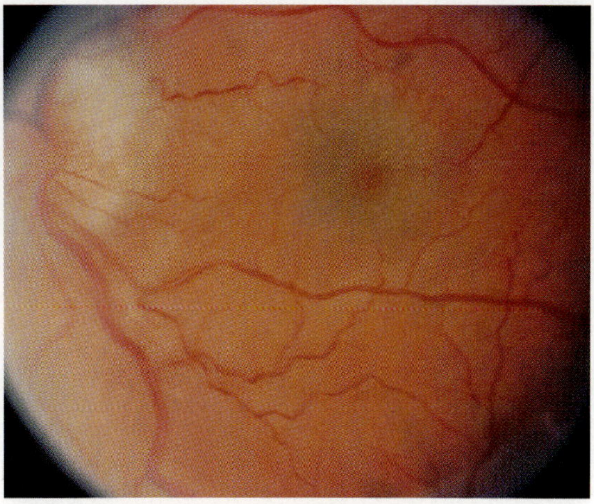

Color Plate 21

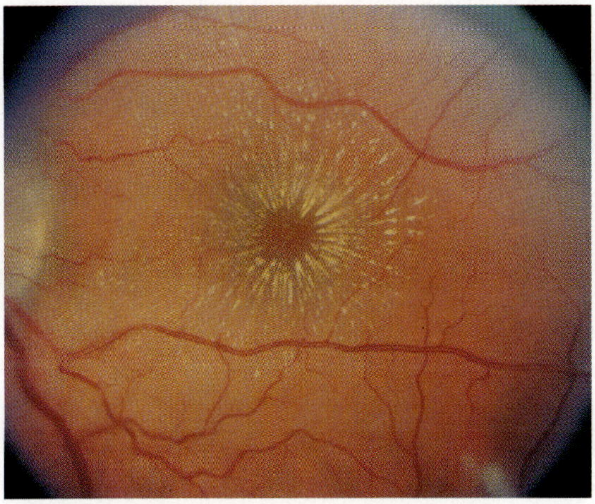

Color Plate 22

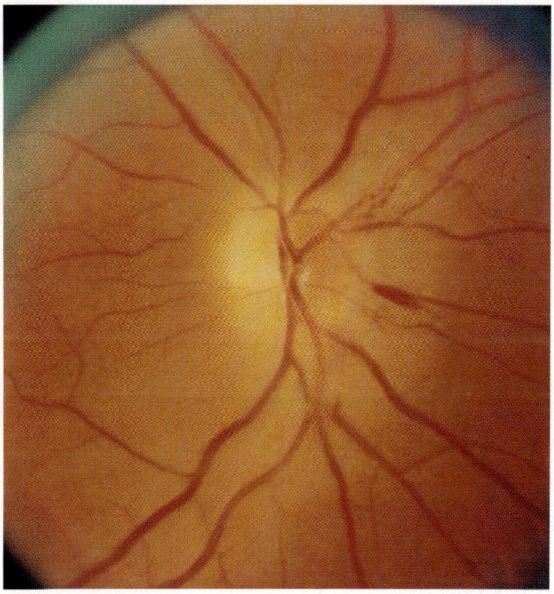

Color Plate 23

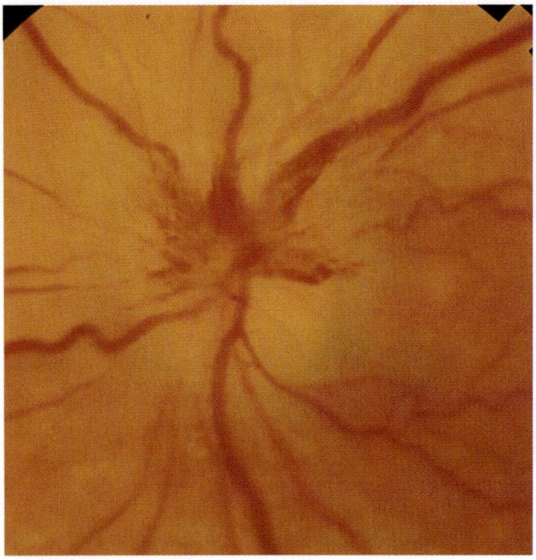
Color Plate 24

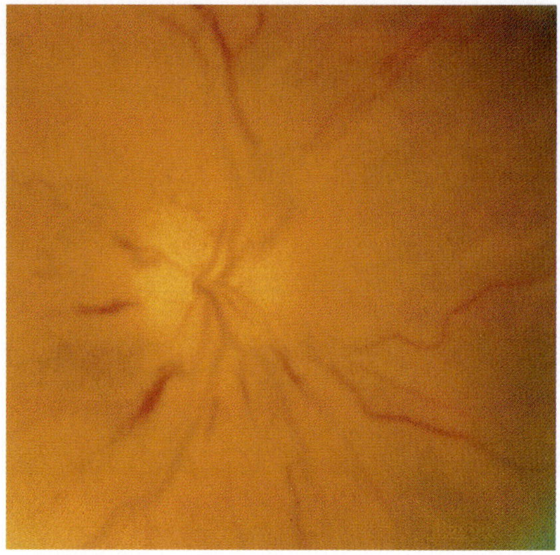
Color Plate 25

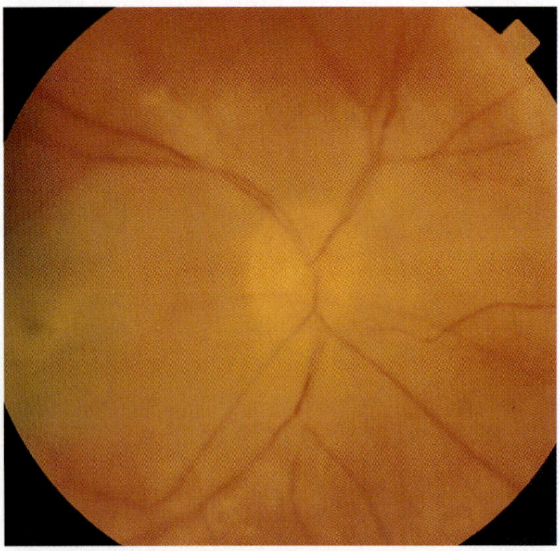
Color Plate 26

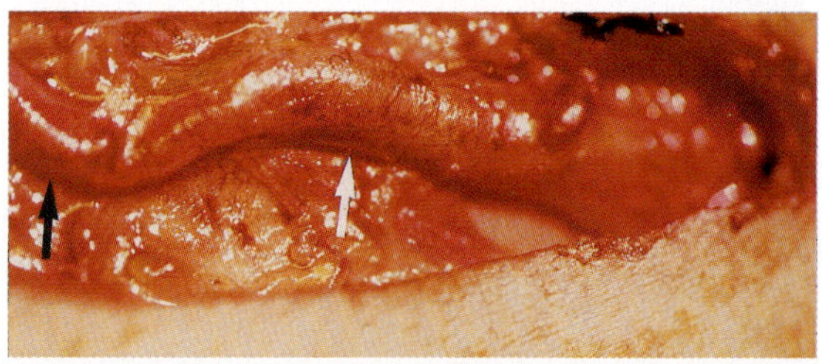
Color Plate 27

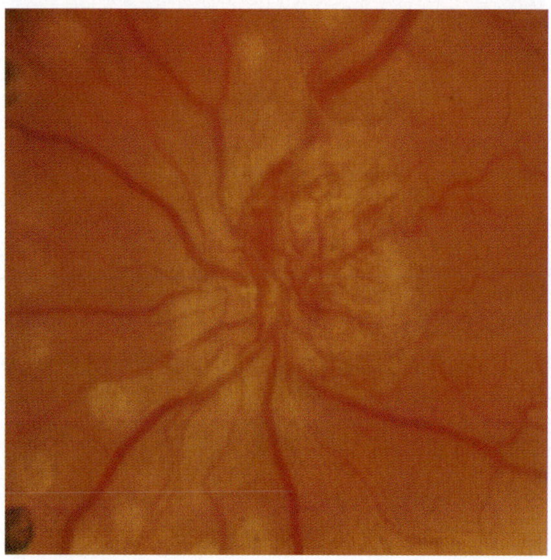
Color Plate 28

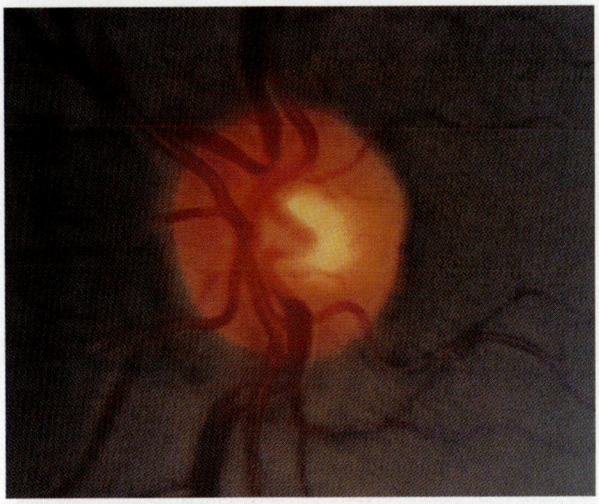

Color Plate 29

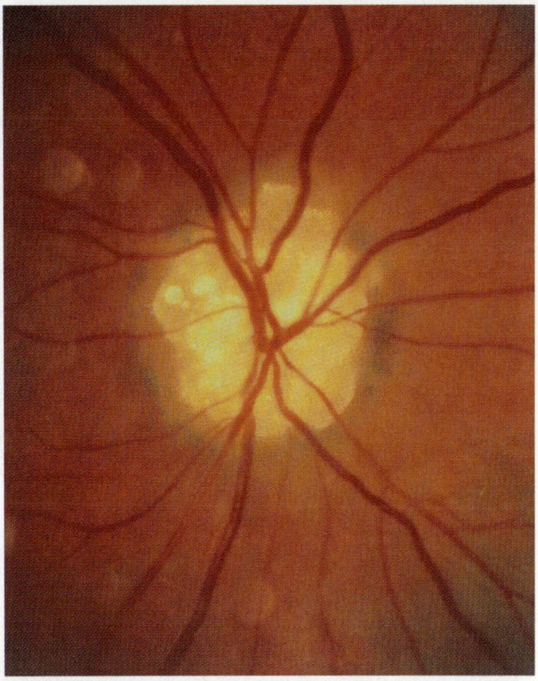

Color Plate 30

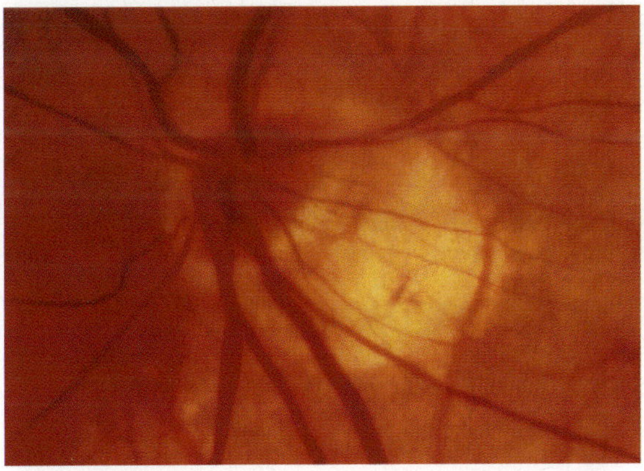

Color Plate 31

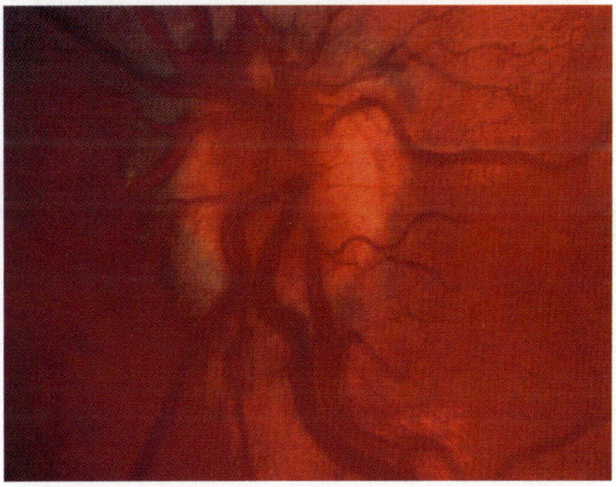

Color Plate 32

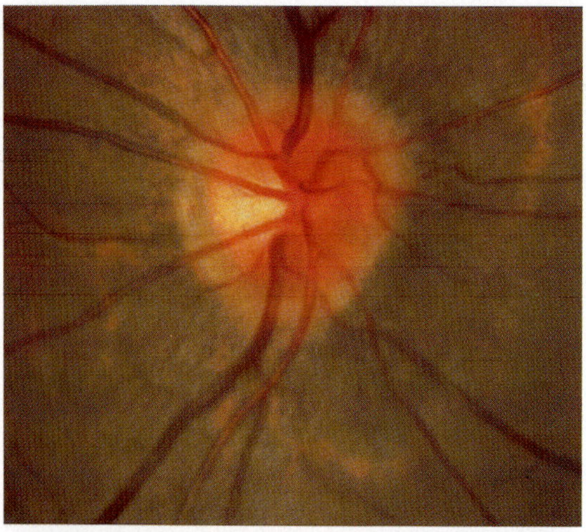

Color Plate 33

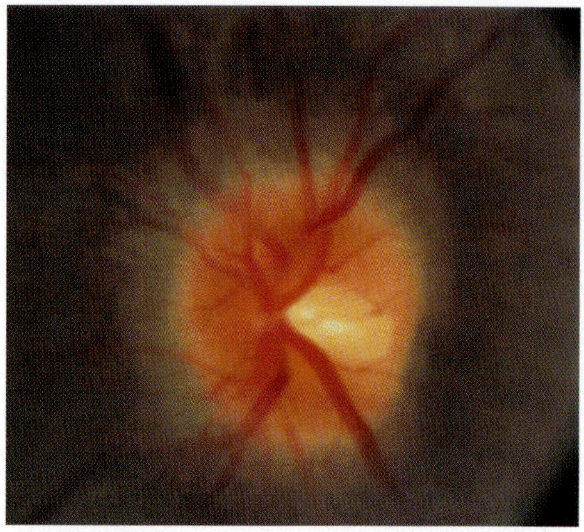

Color Plate 34

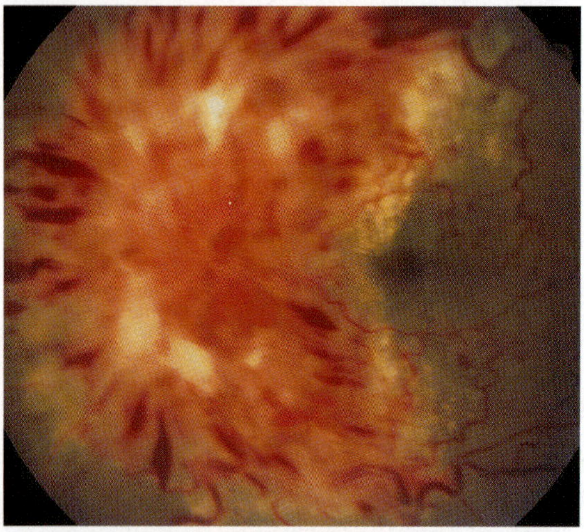

Color Plate 35

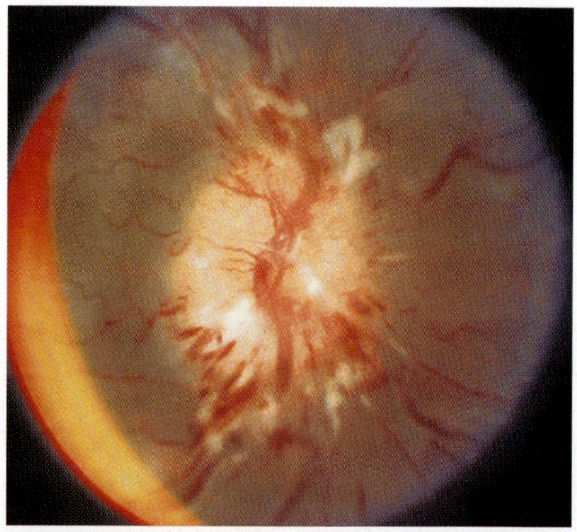

Color Plate 36

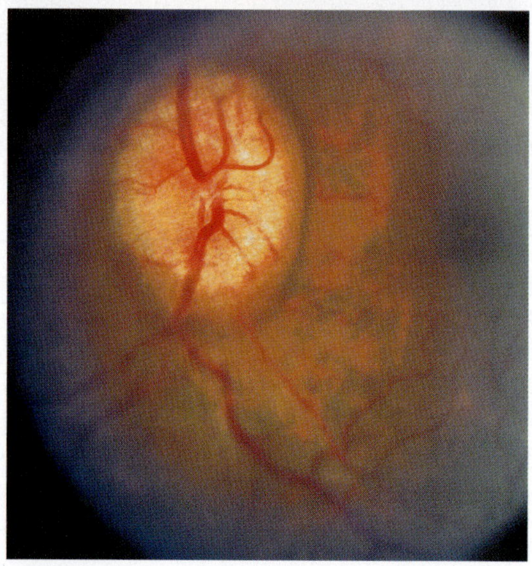

Color Plate 37

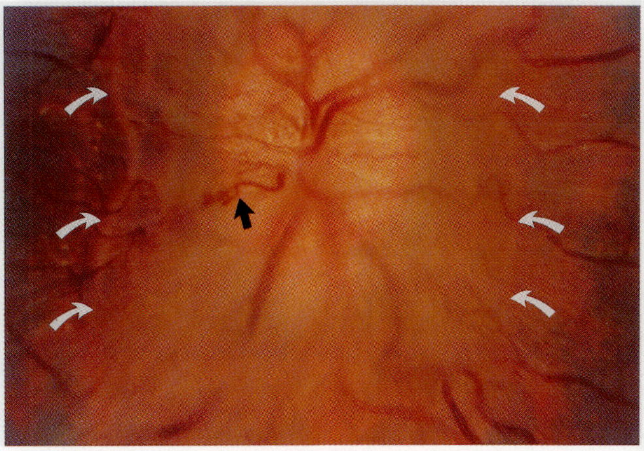

Color Plate 38

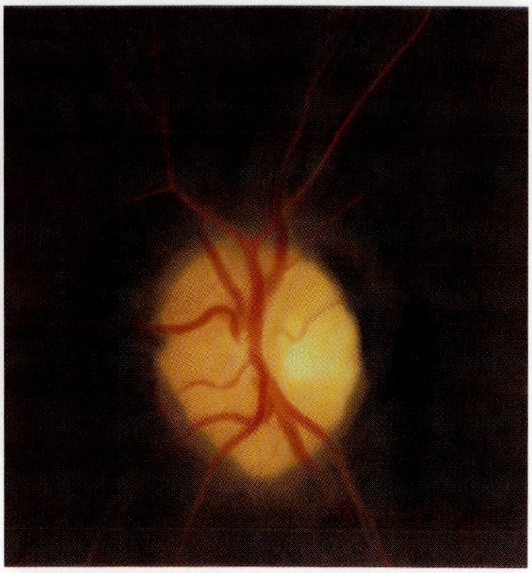

Color Plate 39

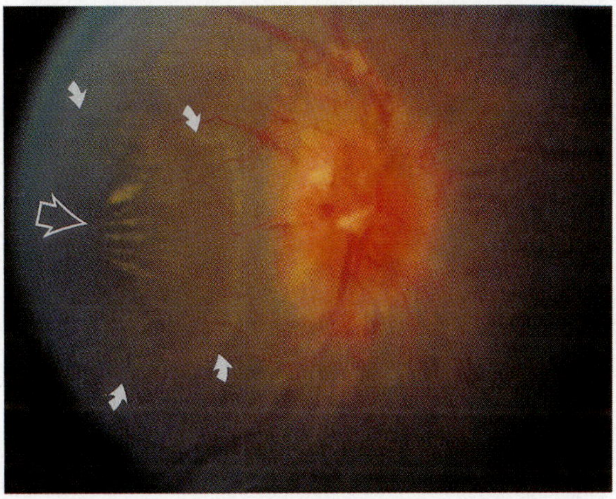

Color Plate 40

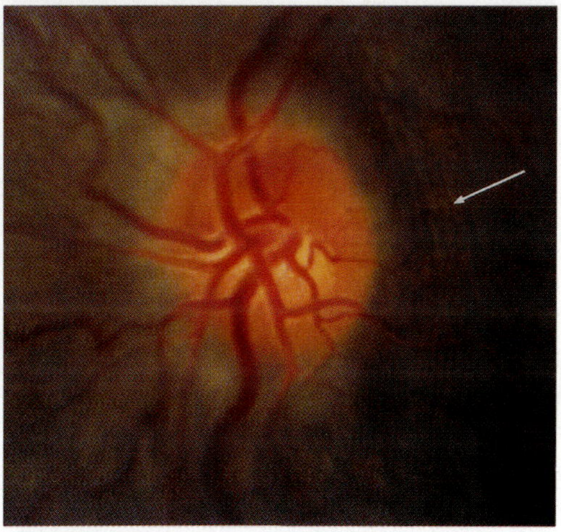

Color Plate 41

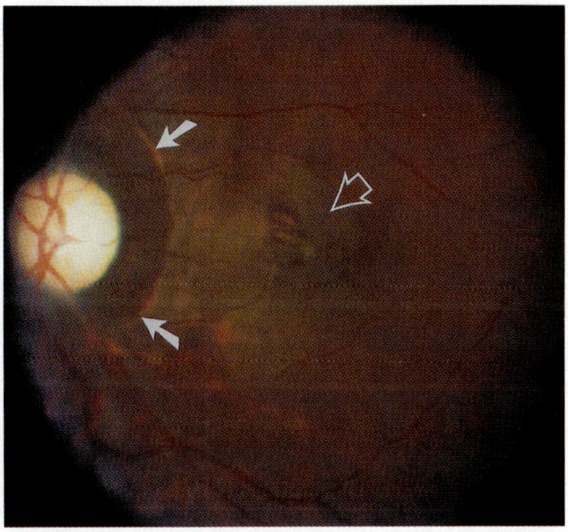

Color Plate 42

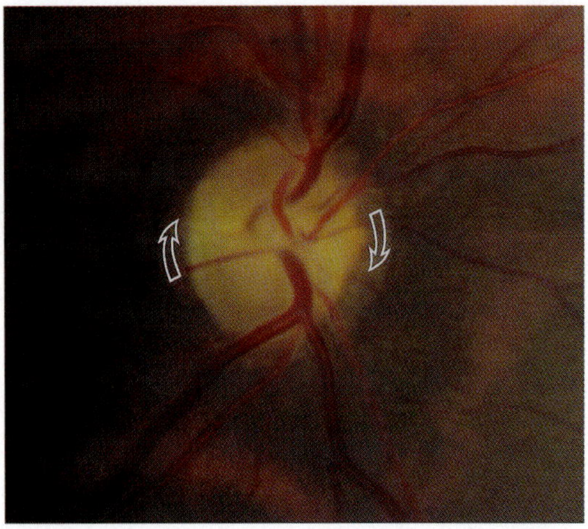

Color Plate 43

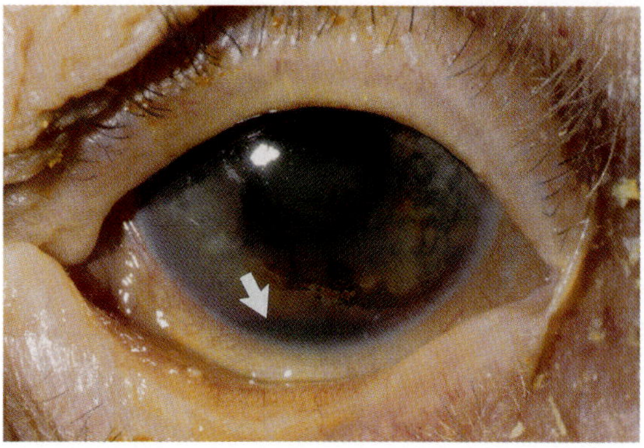

Color Plate 44

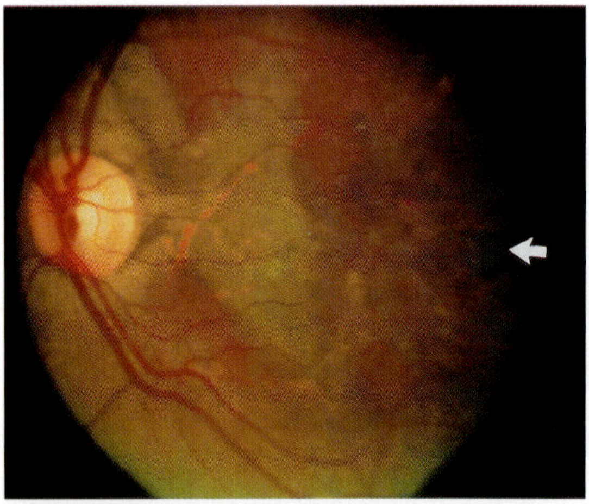

Color Plate 45

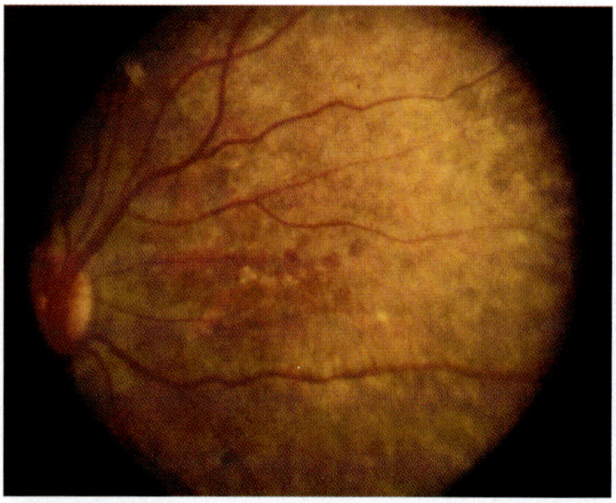

Color Plate 46

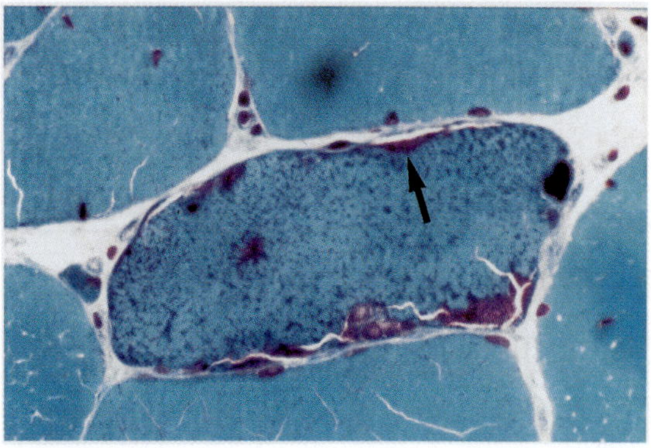

Color Plate 47

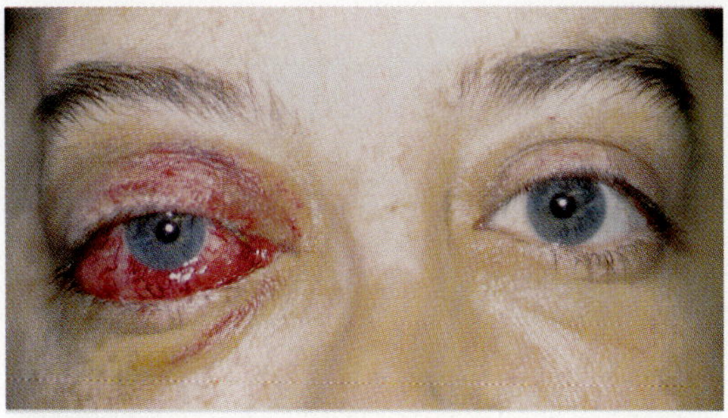

Color Plate 48

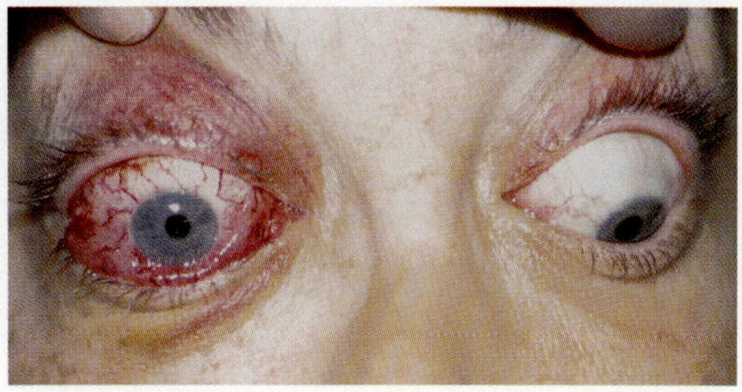

Color Plate 49

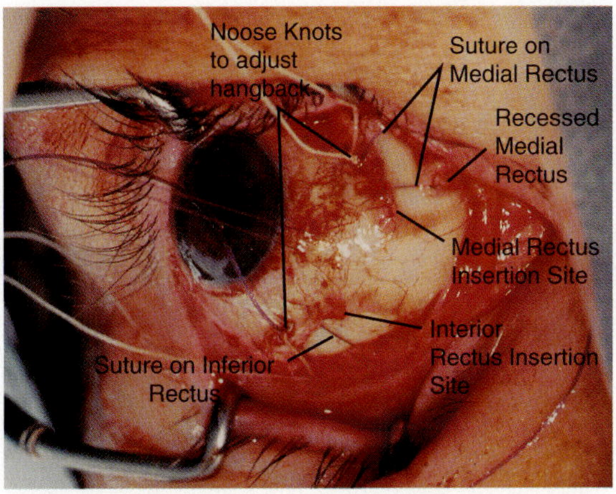

Color Plate 50

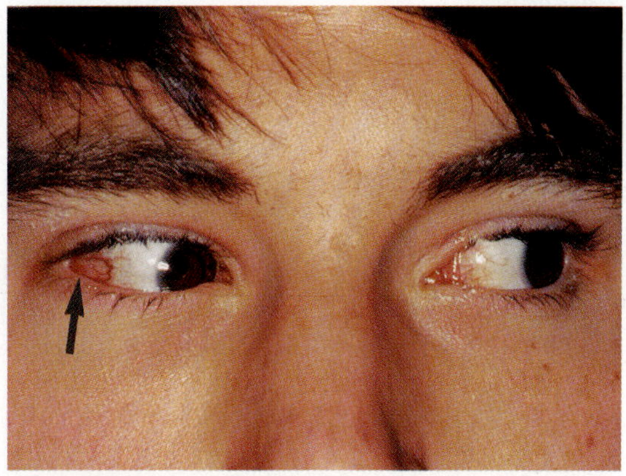

Color Plate 51

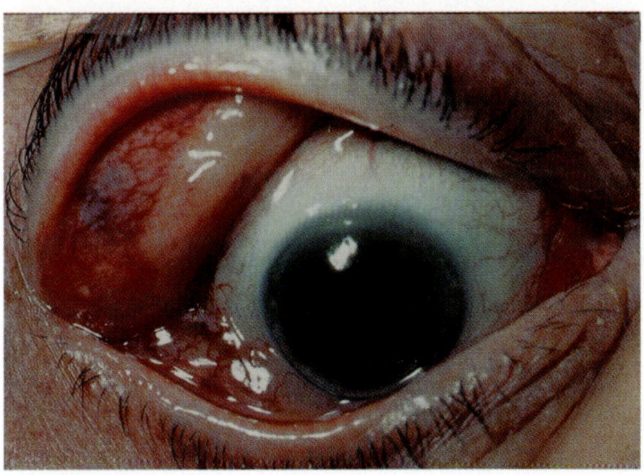

Color Plate 52

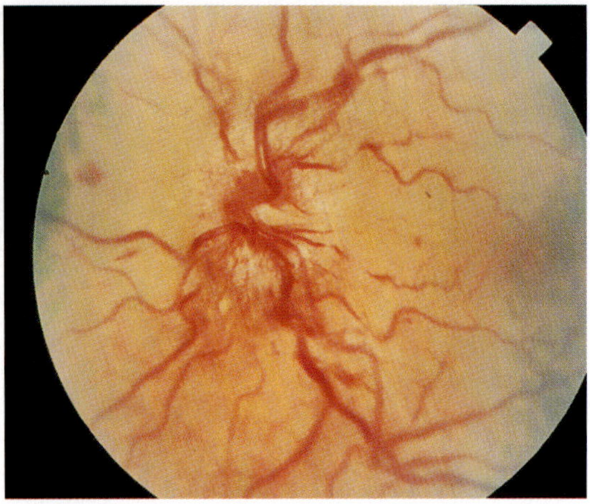

Color Plate 53

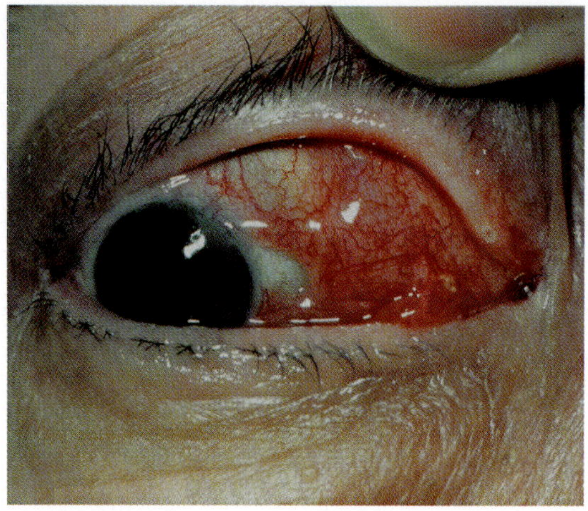

Color Plate 54

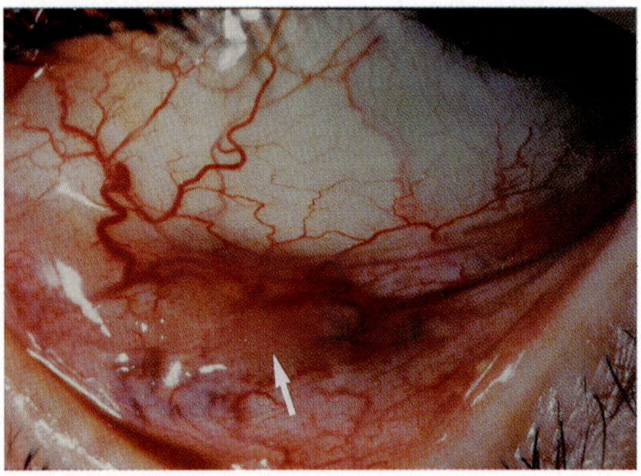

Color Plate 55

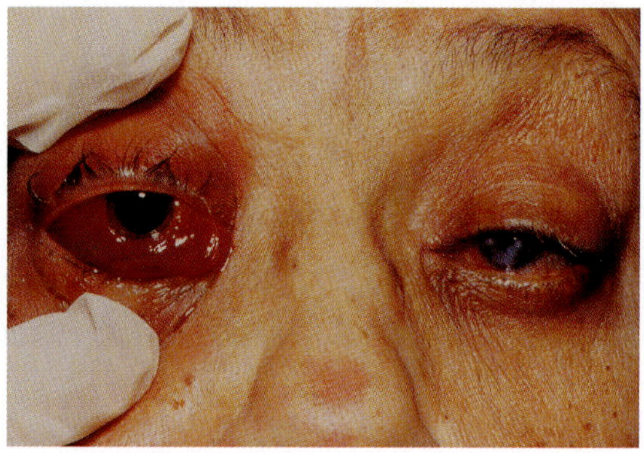

Color Plate 56

TABLE 4–8. Ophthalmic Manifestations of Sarcoidosis

Anterior Segment
Anterior uveitis
Iris nodules
Conjunctival granulomas
Interstitial keratitis
Band keratopathy
Posterior Segment/Retinal
Vitritis
Periphlebitis
Chorioretinitis
Choroidal nodules
Retinal neovascularization
Retinal vein occlusion
Optic Nerve/Chiasm
Optic perineuritis (see Chapter 5)
Optic disc edema (see Chapter 5)
Optic neuropathy (see Chapter 5)
Chiasmal/hypothalamic involvement (see Chapter 7)
Orbit/External
Lacrimal gland enlargement
Keratoconjunctivitis sicca
Orbital granuloma
Enlarged extraocular muscles

choroidal exudates (seen in about half of patients) are the most common posterior segment manifestations of sarcoidosis.[247–250] Vitreous inflammation may appear as a simple cellular infiltrate. Other patients will demonstrate the classic "snowballs" or "string of pearls" appearance (Fig. 4–22). Midperipheral phlebitis is seen and characterized by perivascular sheathing (Fig. 4–23). Periphlebitis may be more posterior and associated with disc edema.[248] Fluorescein angiography will highlight vessel wall staining (Fig. 4–24). More severe cases of periphlebitis are associated with the classic appearance of candle wax drippings. Retinal vein occlusion rarely complicates the periphlebitis.[251] Chorioretinal lesions may manifest as discrete infiltrates or nodules (Fig. 4–25),[322, 323] "punched-out" chorioretinal scars (Fig. 4–26; see Color Plate 12), or rarely as a large choroidal nodule (Fig. 4–25) simulating a metastatic tumor.[252] Indocyanine green angiography may show choroidal abnormalities before any lesions can be detected ophthalmoscopically.[253] Arterial macroaneurysms have also been described.[254] Neovascularization of the retina or optic nerve head is a rare complication of sarcoidosis. Optic nerve head involvement is discussed in Chapter 5.

Patients with suspected ocular sarcoidosis should be screened with chest roentgenography (or chest CT), angiotensin I-converting enzyme (ACE) levels, and occasionally gallium scanning. The diagnosis is often established by transbronchial biopsy.[255, 256] If there is an abnormal conjunctival appearance then conjunctival biopsy may be used to confirm the diagnosis.[257] Further details regarding diagnosing sarcoidosis are discussed in Chapter 5.

Treatment of the ocular complications of sarcoidosis is accomplished with topical steroids, injectable depot steroids, and systemic immunosuppression with steroids or steroid-sparing

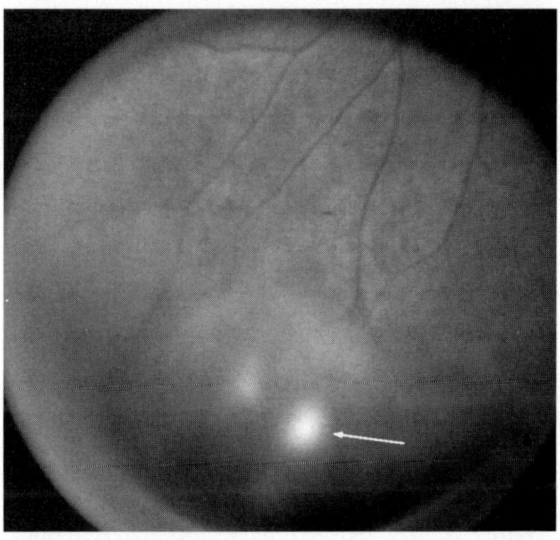

FIGURE 4–22. Fundus photograph of a patient with sarcoidosis. Vitritis and peripheral "snowball" collections of cells (*arrow*) are seen.

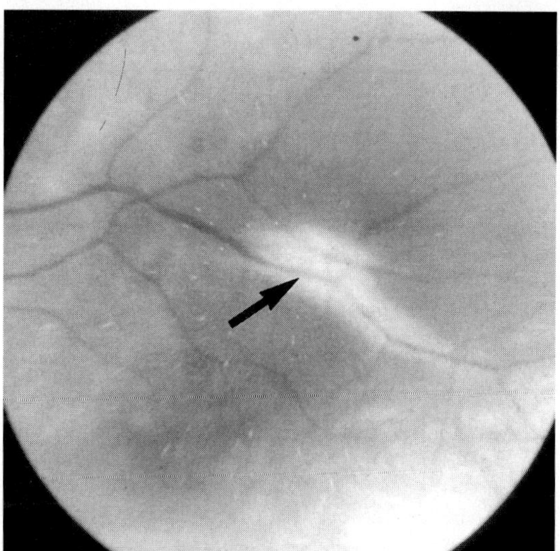

FIGURE 4–23. Perivascular cuffing (*black arrow*) and phlebitis in a patient with sarcoidosis.

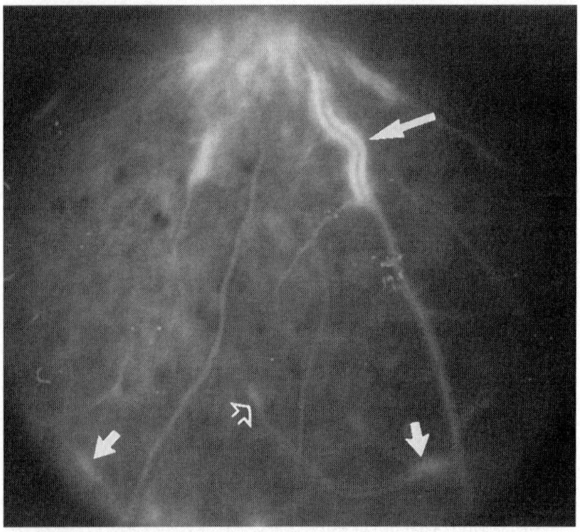

FIGURE 4–24. Vessel wall staining (*large arrow*) on fluorescein angiography in a patient with retinal phlebitis secondary to sarcoidosis. More subtle areas of vessel staining are seen on the inferior portion of the photograph (*small arrows*.)

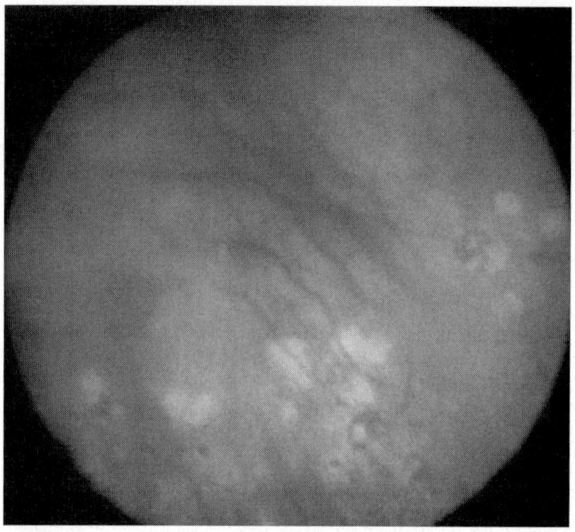

FIGURE 4–26. Punched-out, atrophic lesions in the retinal periphery of a patient with sarcoidosis. (See Color Plate 12.)

agents. Posterior segment manifestations usually require oral steroids. However, if there are no symptoms and only peripheral chorioretinitis is present, it is reasonable to observe the patient without treatment. Karma and associates[258] classified the course of ocular sarcoidosis into three categories: monophasic, relapsing, or chronic. The prognosis was poor for patients with the chronic form of the disease, with no patients retaining 20/30 vision or better. In contrast, 88% of patients in the monophasic group retained 20/30 vision or better.[258]

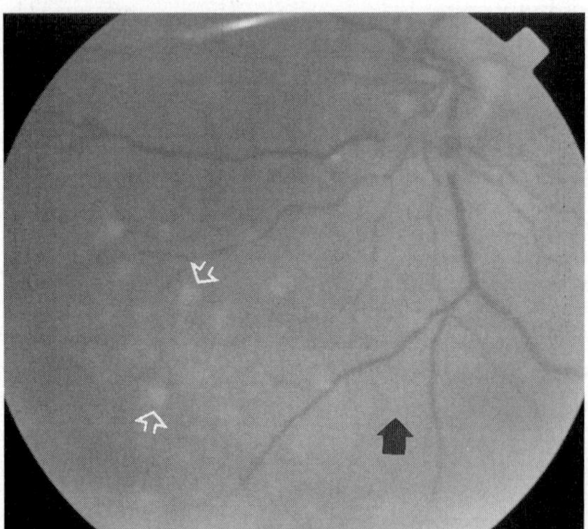

FIGURE 4–25. Small choroidal infiltrates (*white arrows*) in sarcoidosis. A larger and more confluent choroidal infiltrate (*black arrow*) simulating a metastatic choroidal tumor is also seen.

Systemic Lupus Erythematosus

In addition to the development of lupus anticoagulants (see above), patients with systemic lupus erythematosus (SLE) may develop a primary retinal vasculitis. Retinal findings were present in about 30% of patients in one series.[259] Retinal phlebitis may be most likely to occur when CNS lupus is present.[260] This manifests as perivascular cuffing by white blood cells or discrete focal leakage on fluorescein angiography.[259] Patients may develop retinal hemorrhage, exudates, and cotton-wool spots resulting from occlusion of small retinal blood vessels. Vasculitis affects arteries and veins and eventually leads to vaso-occlusive phenomena, including retinal infarction[261] (see Fig. 4–21) and subsequent neovascularization. A choroidopathy similar to that seen in eclampsia and characterized by serous retinal detachments has been described in patients with SLE.[262, 263]

Cat Scratch Disease

Cat scratch disease is a self-limited systemic illness caused by a gram-negative bacillus, *Bartonella henselae*. The organism is inoculated by the bite or scratch of an infected animal, but animal fleas may also transmit the disease. Patients subsequently develop lymphadenopathy, fever, and malaise. The most recognized ophthalmic manifestation of cat scratch disease is optic nerve head swelling and macular star formation (see Chapter 5). However, other patients with *Bartonella* infection manifest with vision loss as a result of uveitis and retinal infiltrates.[264] Discrete white retinal or choroidal lesions are the most common posterior-segment manifestation of cat scratch disease and may be observed in over 80% of patients.[264] Disc swelling and macular star formation were found in 63% of patients in the same series. Other findings may included arterial and venous occlusions. Because malignant hypertension (see below) may produce a similar funduscopic picture, blood pressure measurement should be carefully checked in all patients thought to have neuroretinitis from cat scratch disease.

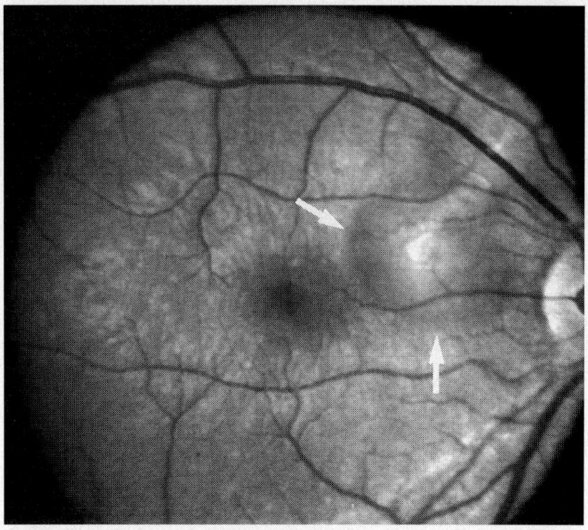

FIGURE 4–28. Serous detachment of the retina (*white arrows*) in a patient with vision loss and eclampsia. (See Color Plate 13.)

Malignant Hypertension and Eclampsia

Severe (malignant) hypertension leads to a breakdown of the blood–retinal barrier, with resultant optic disc edema, flame-shaped hemorrhages, cotton-wool spots, and lipid exudation into the retina (Fig. 4–27). Hayreh[265–268] studied hypertensive retinopathy in monkeys. The earliest ophthalmic manifestations were cotton-wool spots as a result of terminal retinal arteriole.[268] Lipid exudates may accumulate in Henle's layer, creating a picture similar to neuroretinitis.[269, 270] Disc edema may result from local optic nerve head ischemia and disrupted axonal transport or from elevated intracranial pressure that may accompany hypertensive encephalopathy. Malignant hypertension may also be associated with choroidopathy as a result of choriocapillaris occlusion. These patients have focal areas of opaque retinal pigment epithelium known as Elsching spots.[266] These areas may also demonstrate leakage on fluorescein angiography. Occasionally, patients with malignant hypertension develop exudative retinal detachments. Similar areas of focal fluid leakage and sensory retinal detachment may be seen as a manifestation of eclampsia even without other hypertension-related retinal changes (Fig. 4–28; see Color Plate 13).[271]

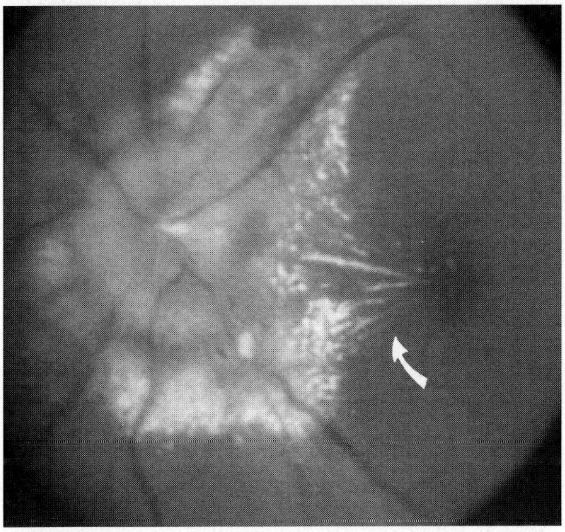

FIGURE 4–27. Optic disc swelling in malignant hypertension. Mild engorgement of the retinal veins is seen, as well as a cotton-wool spot along the inferotemporal vessel. In the rightmost portion of the photograph a few lipid exudates in a partial macular star pattern can be seen (*arrow*).

Blood Dyscrasias

A funduscopic picture very similar to malignant hypertension may be observed in anemia. Anemia only produces retinal ischemia when it is sudden or severe. In the setting of acute severe anemia the oxygen-carrying capacity of the blood is severely compromised and autoregulatory mechanisms have not yet compensated for the change. Patients may develop cotton-wool spots and intraretinal hemorrhages concentrated in the peripapillary region

(Fig. 4–29). The pattern is different in the hemoglobinopathies. Homozygous sickle cell anemia is the most common hemoglobinopathy to cause retinal manifestations. In this condition the abnormal shape of the red blood cells causes vascular occlusion in the retinal periphery. More posterior areas develop neovascularization, heralded by arteriovenous anastomoses that become shunt vessels with a characteristic fan-shaped appearance. The leukemias may also present with retinal findings by causing retinal ischemia. The retinal ischemia may develop as a consequence of the associated anemia, the increased viscosity of the blood, or the occlusion of vessels by large clumps of white cells. Patients with leukemia may also have intraretinal hemorrhages (some with white centers) preretinal hemorrhages and cotton-wool spots[272–274] (Fig. 4–30).

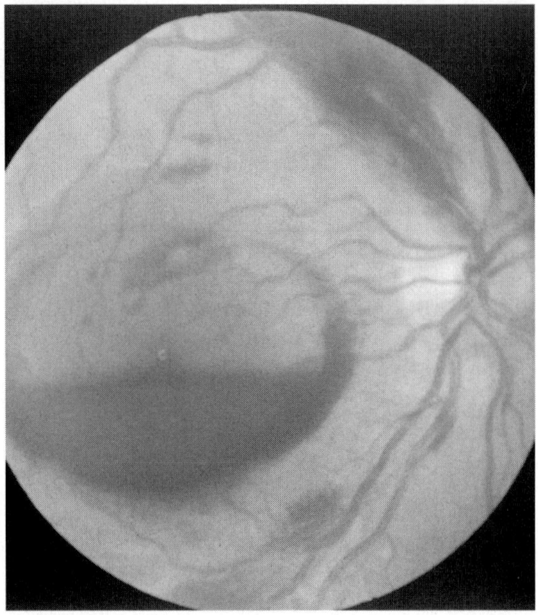

FIGURE 4–30. Intraretinal and preretinal (subhyloid, "boat"-shaped) hemorrhage in a patient with acute myelogenous leukemia.

PHAKOMATOSES

The phakomatoses are a group of hereditary conditions characterized by the presence of hamartomas of the skin, blood vessels, and nervous system (Table 4–9), and several have prominent retinal manifestations. The more common phakomatoses are neurofibromatosis type I and II, tuberous sclerosis (Bourneville's disease), encephalotrigeminal angiomatosis (Sturge–Weber syndrome), angiomatosis of the retina and cerebellum (von Hippel–Lindau disease), racemose angioma of the midbrain and retina (Wyburn–Mason syndrome), and ataxia telangiectasia (Louis–Bar syndrome). Except for the telangiectasia of the conjunctiva in Louis–Bar syndrome, all of these growths represent hamartomas (abnormal growth of mature cells). Telangiectasias of the conjunctiva are hamartias. Hamartias result from developmental abnormalities of the cells in the normal area of growth.

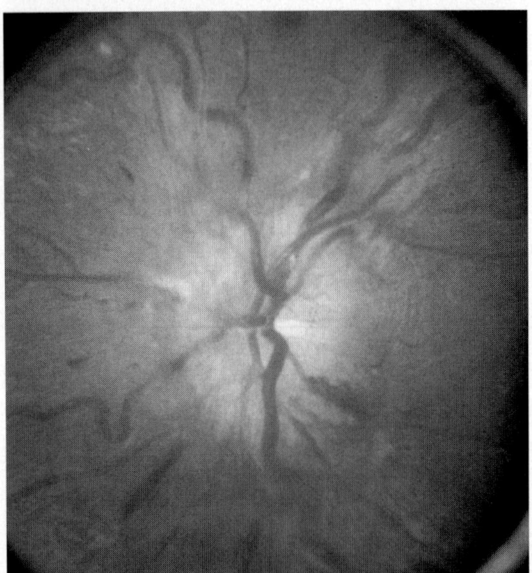

FIGURE 4–29. Fundus photograph of a patient with the acute onset of profound anemia. Disc swelling, retinal vein engorgement, and intraretinal hemorrhages are seen.

The phakomatoses with salient retinal manifestations will be discussed here. Neurofibromatosis type I is discussed in detail in Chapter 7, while ataxia telangiectasia is reviewed in Chapter 16.

Neurofibromatosis Type II

Neurofibromatosis type II (NF-2) was formerly called central NF. In 1987 it was shown to be a distinct disorder inherited in an autosomal domininant fashion. Unlike NF-1, which has been localized to chromosome 17, the gene for NF-2 is on chromosome 22 and encodes a 595-amino acid cytoskeletal protein.[275, 276] The incidence of NF-2 is 1 in 50,000, but the rate of mutation is unknown. The diagnosis of NF-2 requires bilateral acoustic neuromas or a unilateral acoustic neuroma and a first-degree rel-

TABLE 4–9. Clinical Features of the Major Phakomatoses

Disease	Inheritance	CNS Findings	Major Eye Findings	Skin Findings	Systemic Findings	Further Discussion
Neurofibromatosis type 1	Sporadic and dominant	Optic pathway gliomas T_2-weighted grey and white matter hyperintensies on MRI Secondary neoplasms Attention deficit and learning disorders	Iris Lisch nodules Optic nerve glioma Enlarged corneal nerves Eyelid neurofibromas Glaucoma Sphenoid wing dysplasia Retinal nevi and hypopigmentation	Café au lait spots Axillary/inguinal freckling Neurofibromas	Pheochromocytoma Neurofibromas Scoliosis Bony dysplasias	Chapter 7
Neurofibromatosis type 2	Dominant	Acoustic neuromas Gliomas Ependymomas Meningiomas Schwannomas	Posterior subcapsular cataracts Epiretinal membranes Retinal hamartomas Lisch nodules	Café au lait spots	None	Chapter 4
Tuberous sclerosis	Dominant	Seizures Cortical tubers Developmental delay Subependymal giant cell astrocytomas	Retinal astrocytomas	Facial angioma (adenoma sebacium) Periungual fibromas Shagreen patch Hypopigmented nodules	Renal angiomyolipoma Cardiac rhabdomyoma	Chapter 4
Von Hippel–Lindau disease	Dominant	Cerebellar hemangioblastoma	Retinal angiomas	None	Pheochromocytoma, renal cysts, renal carcinoma, hemangioblastoma of pancreas, liver, lung	Chapter 4
Ataxia–telangiectasia	Recessive	Cerebellar atrophy, ataxia, developmental delay	Telangiectasia of conjunctiva, ocular motor apraxia	None	Sinopulmonary infections, leukemia	Chapter 16
Sturge–Weber	Sporadic	Seizures Meningeal angiomas, intracranial calcifications Homonymous hemianopia Transient visual loss	Choroidal hemangioma, glaucoma	Facial angioma	None	Chapter 4 Chapter 8
Wyburn–Mason syndrome	Sporadic	Intracranial (midbrain) arteriovenous malformations	Retinal arteriovenous malformations	Cutaneous hemangiomata	Bone and soft tissue hypertrophy	Chapter 4

ative with bilateral acoustic neuromas. NF-2 is associated with other intracranial and intraspinal tumors, especially meningiomas. Prominent ocular findings are posterior subcapsular cataracts,[277] retinal hamartomata,[278–281] Lisch nodules,[282] epiretinal membranes,[278–281] and bilateral optic nerve sheath meningiomas (Fig. 4–31).[283] Early ophthalmologic evaluation may be helpful in establishing the diagnosis.[284]

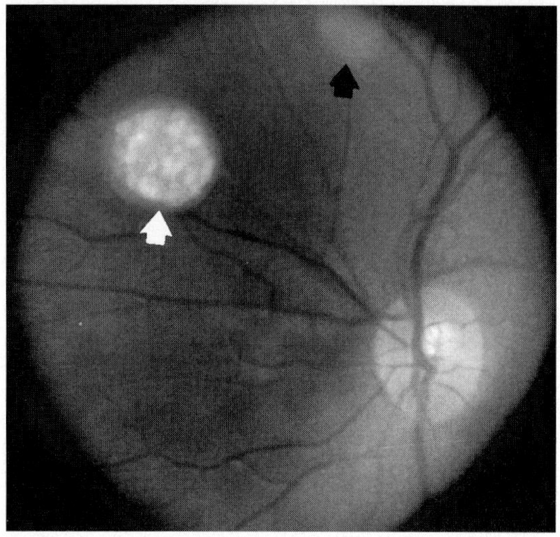

FIGURE 4–32. Fundus photograph of a patient with tuberous sclerosis and two types of retinal hamartomas. The first (*white arrow*) has a round, strikingly white-grey appearance with an irregular surface that resembles drusen. The other appears as a nerve fiber layer hamartoma that is only slightly elevated (*black arrow*).

Tuberous Sclerosis

The classic triad of tuberous sclerosis (TS) includes facial angioma (adenoma sebaceum), mental retardation, and seizures, but frequently there are also ocular, renal, and cardiac manifestations. The condition is dominantly inherited with a high rate of new mutations. We have seen several children with TS and parents who were unknowingly affected as well. Responsible defects in two genes, TSC1 (on chromosome 9, coding for hamartin) and TSC2 (on chromosome 16, coding for tuberin), have been identified, and either may cause TS.[285–290]

The most characteristic eye finding is a retinal astrocytic hamartoma, found in 50% to 90% of patients. Astrocytic hamartomas may occur anywhere in the fundus, but there are two major types, each with a different geographic predilection:

1. The most common reside in the posterior pole and are typically elevated, yellowish-white, and mulberry-like in appearance. These are often near the optic nerve (Fig. 4–32) and therefore may resemble giant optic disc drusen. Unlike drusen, however, they tend to obscure the underlying retinal vessels. These retinal lesions are similar in appearance to those observed in NF-2 and sarcoidosis of the optic nerve head.
2. Astrocytic hamartomas of the second type (Fig. 4–32) are smaller, flatter, whiter, and more translucent, and may mimic cotton-wool spots as they lie along the nerve fiber layer. Although these are also found in the posterior pole, they are more likely than the first type to be found further in the periphery.

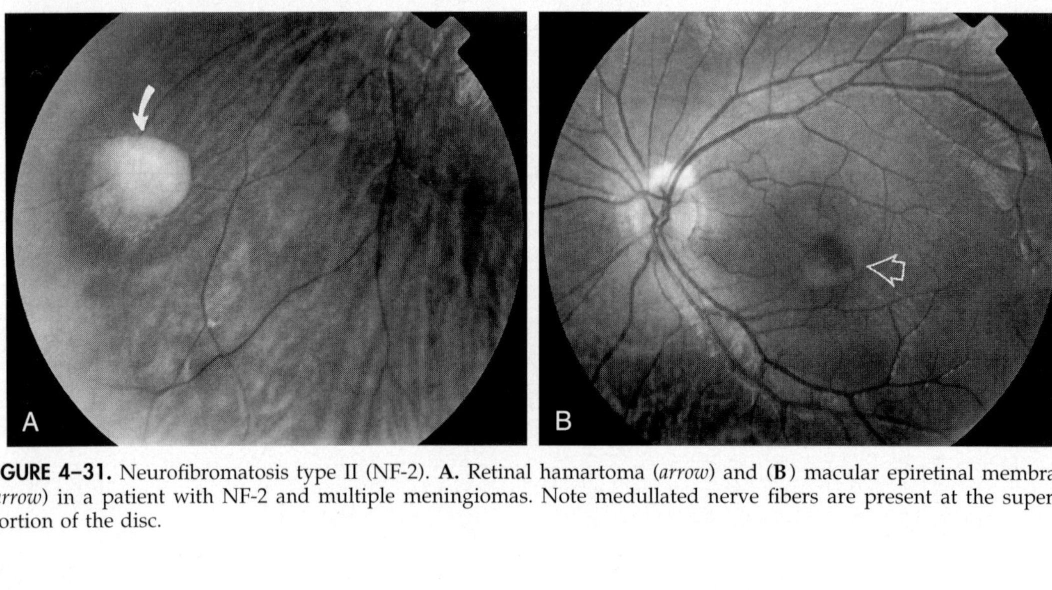

FIGURE 4–31. Neurofibromatosis type II (NF-2). **A.** Retinal hamartoma (*arrow*) and (**B**) macular epiretinal membrane (*arrow*) in a patient with NF-2 and multiple meningiomas. Note medullated nerve fibers are present at the superior portion of the disc.

There is also an intermediary type,[291] and we have also seen a rarely described exophytic retinal hamartoma.[292] The hamartomas arise from the retinal ganglion cell layer and are composed of astrocytes. Eventually they may involve all layers of retina. They contain large blood vessels and are not malignant. Retinal lesions in TS usually require no treatment as they rarely produce vision loss. However, we have seen large lesions involve the macula causing visual loss and leukocoria. The classic teaching is that most children have their full complement of mature retinal hamartomas by age 1, but lesions arising, enlarging, or calcifying later in life have been well documented.[293] In addition to the retinal hamartomas, other retinal findings include depigmented, punched-out lesions of the retina, colobomas, and optic atrophy. Papilledema, sometimes with associated visual loss,[294] can occur when there is hydrocephalus caused by obstruction of the foramen of Monro (see below). External findings are primarily eyelid angiofibromas.

Central nervous system manifestations include seizures, which eventually occur in 70% to 90% of patients and are the most common presenting symptom in TS.[295] The onset of seizures occurs in infancy usually manifesting as infantile spasms. Tonic clonic seizures may occur after the first year of life. Mental retardation, sometimes severe, is common, occurring in 50% to 60% of patients.

Neuroimaging techniques are helpful in identifying the typical cortical tubers, which produce high signal on T_2-weighted MRI (Fig. 4–33). They may also be seen as calcific opacities on CT. Subependymal nodules may lie along the ventricular surface. These nodules may continue to proliferate, at which point they are classified as subependymal giant cell astrocytomas. These are often found in patients between 5 and 18 years of age and rarely become malignant. They occur commonly near the foramen of Monro and can grow sufficiently large to obstruct CSF and cause hydrocephalus.[294]

The skin manifestations of TS occur in almost all patients.[296] Hypomelanotic macules (ash leaf patches, hypopigmented macules) are found in up to 90% of patients and can be single or multiple. They are usually 1 to 2 cm in diameter, but they may vary in size. Use of an ultraviolet light (Wood's lamp) in a dark room may help locate these macules, especially in lightly pigmented individuals. Facial angiomas (Fig. 4–34) are present in about 50% of patients and are usually first noted when the patient is between 3 and 5 years of age. Often confused for acne, they are small, but often confluent, pink or light brown, raised nodules typically located in the malar area and nasolabial folds. They may have a prominent vascular component and can cause recurrent bleeding. Other dermatologic manifestations include shagreen patches (leathery areas), ungual fibromas (Fig. 4–34), and forehead plaques. Other systemic findings include cardiac rhabdomyomas, kidney angiomyolipomas, renal cell carcinomas, and dental enamel pits.

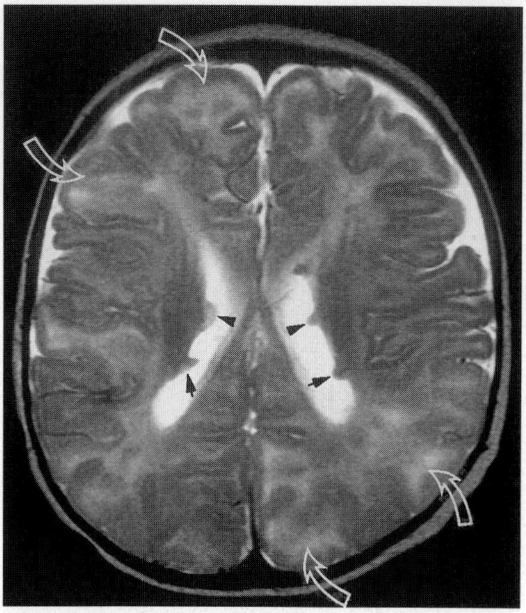

FIGURE 4–33. MRI scan in an infant with tuberous sclerosis. Note the normal immaturity of the myelin. However, cortical tubers, characterized by abnormal architecture of the cortex and underling white matter, may be seen (*white arrows*). Subependymal nodules (*dark arrows*) can be seen along the lining of the lateral ventricles.

Thus, all patients with TS should undergo neuro-ophthalmologic, and dermatologic examinations, head MRI, echocardiography, and ultrasound of the kidneys.

von Hippel-Lindau Disease

Von Hippel–Lindau (VHL) disease, or retinal angiomatosis, is an autosomal dominant condition with incomplete penetrance and variable expressivity. The defect is caused by mutations in VHL1, a tumor suppressor gene located on chromosome 3p.[297–299] The eponym of von Hippel disease is used when only the

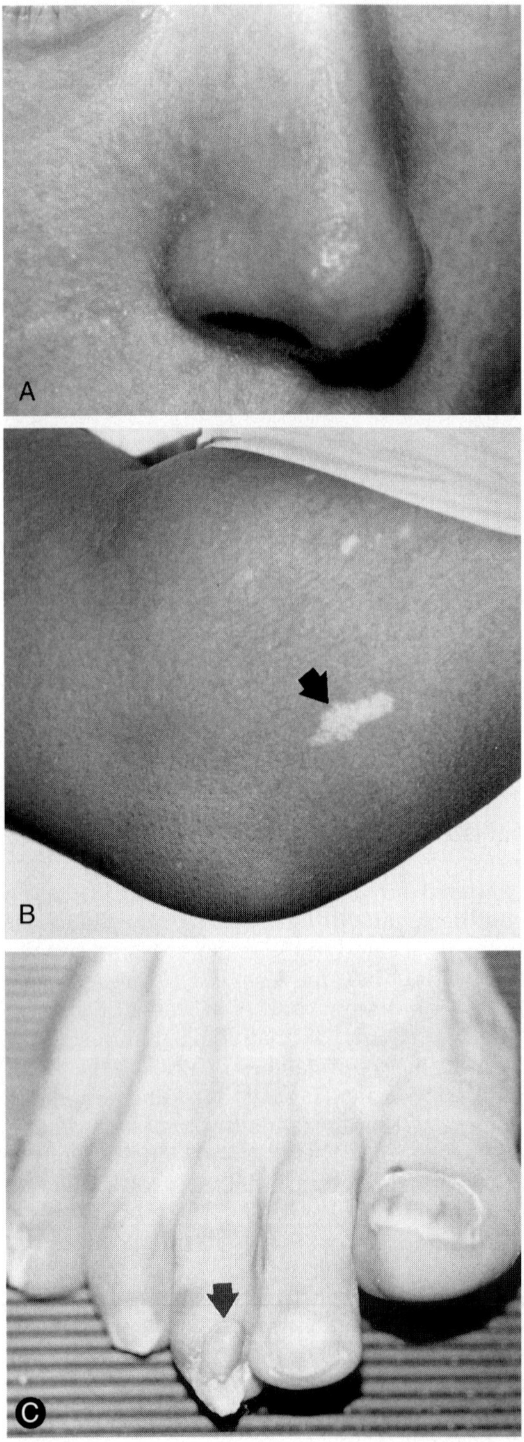

FIGURE 4–34. Common dermatologic manifestations of tuberous sclerosis. **A.** Facial angiomas (adenoma sebacium) **B.** Hypopigmented macule (*arrow*) in a darkly pigmented individual. **C.** Ungual fibromas (*arrow*).

retina is involved. VHL disease is the term used for those cases with both CNS and retinal involvement. Once again, the condition represents a dysgenesis of neuroectoderm and mesoderm, but the basic defect is not known. Features of the condition include angiomatosis of the retina, capillary hemangioblastomas of the CNS and cysts or tumors of the viscera. The disease may be lethal and careful monitoring is necessary to detect the associated renal cell carcinoma and pheochromocytoma. Cysts and angiomatous tumors involving the visceral organs are usually asymptomatic.

Angiomatosis retinae is found in 70% of patients and is usually the first observed manifestation of the condition.[300] These tumors are usually in a midperipheral location but occasionally are in the posterior pole or rarely in the intraorbital portion of the optic nerve. The lesions are bilateral in up to one half of the patients and multiple lesions are seen in one eye in one third of patients.[300, 301] The earliest lesion is a small capillary cluster the size and configuration of a diabetic microaneurysm. The fully developed classic lesions consists of an elevated, globular, pink retinal tumor that is often fed by a dilated tortuous retinal artery. Abnormal vessels on the disc may point to the anteriorly located tumor. Tumor enlargement is associated with lipid exudation and retinal detachment. Vision loss occurs in more than half of the patients with angiomatoses.[300, 301] Therapy for these lesions includes photocoagulation, cryotherapy, and diathermy, which are usually successful in obliterating small VHL angiomas. Argon laser can be used with small lesions and applied directly to the surface of the small angioma, with good long-term preservation of vision.[302] Cryotherapy and brachytherapy are useful in patients with larger tumors that are more anteriorly located and in eyes with media opacity.[303] Occasionally treatment of larger tumors can be followed by massive exudation and retinal detachment.

A cerebellar hemangioblastoma is the most common CNS finding and occurs in about half of patients. A typical hemangioblastoma consists of a small, highly vascular nodule within a much larger fluid-filled cyst. There can be striking hypertrophy of the feeding and draining vessels. Microscopically a hemangioblastoma is composed of fine capillaries within a matrix of lipid-laiden foam cells. Mitotic figures are not present. The retinal angioma has a similar histologic appearance but lacks the cystic component. The tumor has usually become symptomatic at the time of diagnosis and presents in the second to fourth decades of life with signs of hydrocephalus or cerebellar dysfunction. Although it is a resectable lesion, it is still a common cause of mortality. Medullary and spinal hemangioblastomas are relatively less common, but a medullary lesion may be lethal if it compresses vital brain stem structures. The spinal lesions most often appear in the upper cervical cord. Hemangioblastomas may also develop in the suprasellar cistern and cause a chiasmal syndrome.[304]

Renal cell carcinoma is recognized clinically in one third of patients and presents as hematuria, obstructive nephropathy, or an abdominal mass. Pheochromocytomas are usually asymptomatic and occur in less than 10% of patients.[305] These lesions tend to cluster in certain predisposed families. Polycythemia has been reported in up to 25% of VHL patients and particularly in those with cerebellar hemangioblastoma.

Encephalotrigeminal Angiomatosis (Sturge–Weber Syndrome)

Sturge–Weber syndrome (SWS) is characterized by the triad of skin, CNS, and ocular findings. Although the nevus flammeus (cutaneous hemifacial hemangioma) of the face is the most obvious sign, the major symptomatic manifestations are due to CNS involvement. The facial port wine stain (see Fig. 8–33) may occur with or without one of the other major manifestations: leptomeningeal angiomatosis, cerebral gyriform calcifications, and glaucoma. These are usually unilateral and ipsilateral. The syndrome shows no well-established genetic, sexual, or racial predilection.

Because the lesions are vascular, SWS was originally thought to be a mesodermal phakomatosis. However, the neural crest also seems to be important as it gives rise to the facial dermal connective tissue, the choroid of the eye, and the pia mater. Furthermore, the endothelial lining of vessels is still believed to be of mesodermal origin. Therefore, for full explanation of SWS it is necessary to postulate a defective interaction during embryogenesis between neural crest-derived elements and the vascular endothelium.

The ocular manifestations of SWS are choroidal hemangioma and glaucoma. Sixty percent of SWS patients develop glaucoma.[306] Of these patients, 60% have the disease prior to age two and can develop buphthalmos. Congenital glaucoma is most often associated with involvement of the upper lid by the facial hemangioma present at birth.[307] The actual cause of the glaucoma is not certain and several mechanisms may play a role. These include (1) outflow obstruction by an angle malformation and associated increased vascularity of the iris, (2) occlusion of the angle from anterior synechiae as a secondary phenomenon in patients with choroidal hemangioma and retinal detachment, (3) elevation of episcleral pressure, reducing outflow, (4) hypersecretion of aqueous, and (5) elevation of the intraocular pressure that results from increased permeability of the thin-walled vessels of the choroidal hemangioma. In general, patients with SWS have prominent iris processes that adhere to the trabecular meshwork on gonioscopy. This indicates a primary defect in the development of the angle. Trabeculotomy in infants and trabeculectomy in older patients are effective surgical therapies for patients with SWS and glaucoma.[308–310] Latanoprost may all be very effective in these patients.[311]

Choroidal hemangioma occurs in 55% of patients with SWS.[312] These hamangiomas are relatively flat, isolated lesions up to several millimeters in diameter and located in the posterior portion of the fundus. Occasionally, they may be diffuse and involve larger areas of choroid and in this case, appear similar to red velvet or catsup. Choroidal hemangioma is usually situated temporal to the optic disc, has its greatest height in the macular region, and is surrounded by dilated choroidal and retinal vessels. The lesions may be visible on MRI with gadolinium enhancement.[313] Typically choroidal hemangiomas cause no visual disturbance until early adulthood. During this slow-growth phase, they may be associated with cystoid degeneration of the overlying sensory retina, and they may eventually produce an exudative retinal detachment. Rarely calcifications occur in the angiomatous choroid. The hemangiomas have been successfully treated with irradiation,[314–317] but usually they are observed. Other ocular findings in SWS include heterochromia iridis, conjunctival angioma and dilation of episcleral vessels, tortuosity of retinal vessels, bilateral lens subluxation, anisocoria, and coloboma of the iris and optic nerve head.

The dermatologic manifestations include the nevus flammeus, which usually corresponds to the distribution of the ophthalmic, maxillary, and, more rarely, mandibular divisions of the trigeminal nerve. The lesion may extend to the region of the upper cervical nerves. Histopathologically, the skin vessels appear normal until late childhood, at which time they become widely dilated ectatic blood-filled capillaries. The deep dermal and subcutaneous vessels are affected in the more nodular lesions. The nevi do not regress and usually do not respond to local sclerosing agents or steroids.

The pathognomonic feature of the SWS is the CNS angioma of the pia and arachnoid mater (see discussion in Chapter 8). As a result of this angioma, the vascular circulation of the underlying cerebral cortex is often altered, leading to superficial calcification. The majority of patients will have intracranial calcifications on CT. On plain roentgenograms the calcifications appear as double curvilinear densities (tramlines). These cortical abnormalities result in focal or generalized seizures, contralateral hemiplegia, and mental retardation. The lesions can be identified in the first or second decade of life and may increase in size up until the second decade of life, at which point they remain stable.

Ataxia Telangiectasis, (Louis-Bar Syndrome)

Louis–Bar syndrome (LBS) is characterized by progressive cerebellar ataxia, cutaneous and conjunctival telangiectasias, and recurrent sinopulmonary infections. Unlike the other phakomatoses, it appears to be inherited in a recessive fashion, and the defect has been localized to chromosome 11. The conjunctival telangiectasias are similar to those seen in SWS but are bilateral and not associated with lesions of the choroid or the skin.

This phakomatosis is discussed in detail in Chapter 16.

Wyburn–Mason Syndrome

Patients with Wyburn–Mason syndrome (WMS) develop retinal and systemic arteriovenous malformations (AVMs). AVMs are direct communications between arteries and veins and involve the CNS, the ocular adnexa, and the nasopharynx. In WMS, AVMs have a predilection for the midbrain. Cerebral AVMs are discussed in detail in Chapter 8, and dural AVMs in Chapter 15.

Retinal AVMs are congenital, unilateral malformations that have a predilection for involvement of the vessels of the posterior pole and supratemporal quadrant. These lesions appear as arterial and venous dilations with marked tortuosity of a sector of the retinal circulation. Although most retinal AVMs are stable, several complications have been reported, including hemorrhage, vein occlusion, and neovascular glaucoma.[318, 319]

REFERENCES

1. Nipken LH, Schmidt D: Incidence, localization, length and course of the cilioretinal artery. Is there an effect on the course of temporal rental arteries? Klin Monatsbl Augenheilkd 1996;208:229–234.
2. Tittl MK, Spaide RF, Wong D, et al: Systemic findings associated with central serous chorioretinopathy. Am J Ophthalmol 1999;128:63–68.
3. Bresnick GH, Condit R, Syrjala S, et al: Abnormalities of the foveal avascular zone in diabetic retinopathy. Arch Ophthalmol 1984;102:1286–1293.
4. Fortune B, Schneck ME, Adams AJ: Multifocal electroretinogram delays reveal local retinal dysfunction in early diabetic retinopathy. Invest Ophthalmol Vis Sci 1999;40:2638–2651.
5. Tzekov R, Arden GB: The electroretinogram in diabetic retinopathy. Surv Ophthalmol 1999;44:53–60.
6. Arruga J, Sanders MD: Ophthalmologic findings in 70 patients with evidence of retinal embolism. Ophthalmology 1982;89:1336–1347.
7. Howard RS, Russell RW: Prognosis of patients with retinal embolism. J Neurol Neurosurg Psychiatry 1987;50:1142–1147.
8. Sharma S, Pater JL, Lam M, et al: Can different types of retinal emboli be reliably differentiated from one another? An inter- and intraobserver agreement study. Can J Ophthalmol 1998;33:144–148.
9. Younge BR: The significance of retinal emboli. J Clin Neuroophthalmol 1989;9:190–194.
10. Hollenhorst RW: Significance of bright plaques in the retinal arterioles. JAMA 1961;178:23–29.
11. Klein R, Klein BE, Jensen SC, et al: Retinal emboli and stroke. The Beaver Dam Eye Study. Arch Ophthalmol 1999;117:1063–1068.
12. Mitchell P, Wang JJ, Li W, et al: Prevalence of asymptomatic retinal emboli in an Australian urban community. Stroke 1997;28:63–66.
13. Bruno A, Russell PW, Jones WL, et al: Concomitants of asymptomatic retinal cholesterol emboli. Stroke 1992;23:900–902.
14. O'Donnell BA, Mitchell P: The clinical features and associations of retinal emboli. Aust NZ J Ophthalmol 1992;20:11–17.
15. Sharma S, Brown GC, Pater JL, et al: Does a visible retinal embolus increase the likelihood of hemodynamically significant carotid artery stenosis in patients with acute retinal arterial occlusion? Arch Ophthalmol 1998;116:1602–1606.
16. Sharma S, Brown GC, Cruess AF: Accuracy of visible retinal emboli for the detection of cardioembolic lesions requiring anticoagulation or cardiac surgery. Retinal Emboli of Cardiac Origin Study Group. Br J Ophthalmol 1998;82:655–658.

17. Executive Committee for the Asymptomatic Carotid Atherosclerosis Study: Endarterectomy for asymptomatic carotid artery stenosis. JAMA 1995;273:1421–1428.
18. Pfaffenbach DD, Hollenhorst RW: Morbidity and survivorship of patients with emboli crystals in the ocular fundus. Am J Ophthalmol 1973;75:66–72.
19. Savino PJ, Glaser JS, Cassidy J: Retinal stroke: is the patient at risk? Arch Ophthalmol 1977;95:1185–1189.
20. Bruno A, Jones WL, Austin JK, et al: Vascular outcome in men with asymptomatic retinal cholesterol emboli. A cohort study. Ann Intern Med 1995;122: 249–253.
21. Merchut MP, Gupta SR, Naheedy MH: The relation of retinal artery occlusion and carotid artery stenosis. Stroke 1988;19:1239–1242.
22. Atebara NH, Brown GC, Cater J: Efficacy of anterior chamber paracentesis and Carbogen in treating acute nonarteritic central retinal artery occlusion. Ophthalmology 1995;102:2029–2034.
23. Duker JS, Sivalingam A, Brown GC, et al: A prospective study of acute central retinal artery obstruction. The incidence of secondary ocular neovascularization. Arch Ophthalmol 1991;109:339–342.
24. Schmidt D, Schumacher M, Wakhloo AK: Microcatheter urokinase infusion in central retinal artery occlusion. Am J Ophthalmol 1992;113:429–434.
25. Schumacher M, Schmidt D, Wakhloo AK: Intra-arterial fibrinolytic therapy in central retinal artery occlusion. Neuroradiology 1993;35:600–605.
26. Ros MA, Magargal LE, Uram M: Branch retinal-artery obstruction: a review of 201 eyes. Ann Ophthalmol 1989;21:103–107.
27. McDonough RL, Forteza AM, Flynn HW, Jr: Internal carotid artery dissection causing a branch retinal artery occlusion in a young adult. Am J Ophthalmol 1998;125:706–708.
28. Greven CM, Weaver RG, Owen J, et al: Protein S deficiency and bilateral branch retinal artery occlusion. Ophthalmology 1991;98:33–34.
29. Li HK, Dejean BJ, Tang RA: Reversal of visual loss with hyperbaric oxygen treatment in a patient with Susac syndrome. Ophthalmology 1996;103:2091–2098.
30. Fineman MS, Savino PJ, Federman JL, et al: Branch retinal artery occlusion as the initial sign of giant cell arteritis. Am J Ophthalmol 1996;122:428–430.
31. Crofts JW, Nussbaum JJ, Levine SR, et al: Retinitis pigmentosa and branch retinal artery occlusion with anticardiolipin antibody. Case report. Arch Ophthalmol 1989;107:324.
32. Levine SR, Crofts JW, Lesser GR, et al: Visual symptoms associated with the presence of a lupus anticoagulant. Ophthalmology 1988;95:686–692.
33. De Potter P, Zografos L: Survival prognosis of patients with retinal artery occlusion and associated carotid artery disease. Graefes Arch Clin Exp Ophthalmol 1993;231:212–216.
34. Brown GC, Moffat K, Cruess A, et al: Cilioretinal artery obstruction. Retina 1983;3:182 187.
35. Gangwar DN, Grewal SP, Jain IS, et al: Cilioretinal artery occlusion: a case report. Ann Ophthalmol 1984;16:1022–1024.
36. Horton JC: Embolic cilioretinal artery occlusion with atherosclerosis of the ipsilateral carotid artery. Retina 1995;15:441–444.
37. el Asrar AM, Naddaf HO, al Momen AK, et al: Systemic lupus erythematosus flare-up manifesting as a cilioretinal artery occlusion. Lupus 1995;4:158–160.
38. Hayreh SS, Podhajsky PA, Zimmerman B: Ocular manifestations of giant cell arteritis. Am J Ophthalmol 1998;125:509–520.
39. Dori D, Gelfand YA, Brenner B, et al: Cilioretinal artery occlusion: an ocular complication of primary antiphospholipid syndrome. Retina 1997;17:555–557.
40. Kachmaryk MM, Trimble SN, Gieser RG: Cilioretinal artery occlusion in sickle cell trait and rheumatoid arthritis. Retina 1995;15:501–504.
41. Noble KG: Central retinal vein occlusion and cilioretinal artery infarction. Am J Ophthalmol 1994;118: 811–813.
42. Schatz H, Fong AC, McDonald HR, et al: Cilioretinal artery occlusion in young adults with central retinal vein occlusion. Ophthalmology 1991;98:594–601.
43. Mizener JB, Podhajsky P, Hayreh SS: Ocular ischemic syndrome. Ophthalmology 1997;104:859–864.
44. Costa VP, Kuzniec S, Molnar LJ, et al: Clinical findings and hemodynamic changes associated with severe occlusive carotid artery disease. Ophthalmology 1997;104:1994–2002.
45. Brown GC, Magargal LE: The ocular ischemic syndrome. Clinical, fluorescein angiographic and carotid angiographic features. Int Ophthalmol 1988;11: 239–251.
46. David R, Zangwill L, Badarna M, et al: Epidemiology of retinal vein occlusion and its association with glaucoma and increased intraocular pressure. Ophthalmologica 1988;197:69–74.
47. Zegarra H, Gutman FA, Zakov N, et al: Partial occlusion of the central retinal vein. Am J Ophthalmol 1983;96:330–337.
48. Green WR, Chan CC, Hutchins GM, et al: Central retinal vein occlusion: a prospective histopathologic study of 29 eyes in 28 cases. Trans Am Ophthalmol Soc 1981;79:371–422.
49. Rath EZ, Frank RN, Shin DH, et al: Risk factors for retinal vein occlusions. A case-control study. Ophthalmology 1992;99:509–514.
50. Dodson PM, Galton DJ, Hamilton AM, et al: Retinal vein occlusion and the prevalence of lipoprotein abnormalities. Br J Ophthalmol 1982;66:161–164.
51. Quinlan PM, Elman MJ, Bhatt AK, et al: The natural course of central retinal vein occlusion [see comments]. Am J Ophthalmol 1990;110:118–123.
52. Frangieh GT, Green WR, Barraquer Somers E, et al: Histopathologic study of nine branch retinal vein occlusions. Arch Ophthalmol 1982;100:1132–1140.
53. Johnston RL, Brucker AJ, Steinmann W, et al: Risk factors of branch retinal vein occlusion. Arch Ophthalmol 1985;103:1831–1832.
54. Finkelstein D: Argon laser photocoagulation for macular edema in branch vein occlusion. Ophthalmology 1986;93:975–977.
55. Hayreh SS, Rojas P, Podhajsky P, et al: Ocular neovascularization with retinal vascular occlusion—III. Incidence of ocular neovascularization with retinal vein occlusion. Ophthalmology 1983;90:488–506.
56. Argon laser scatter photocoagulation for prevention of neovascularization and vitreous hemorrhage in branch vein occlusion. A randomized clinical trial. Branch Vein Occlusion Study Group. Arch Ophthalmol 1986;104:34–41.
57. Rizzo JF, Volpe NJ: Cancer-associated retinopathy. In: Pepose JS, Holland G, Wilheimus K (eds): Ocular Infection and Immunity, pp 585–599. St. Louis, Mosby–Year Book, 1996.
58. Volpe NJ, Rizzo JF: Retinal disease in neuro-ophthalmology: Paraneoplastic retinopathy and the big

blindspot syndrome. Semin Ophthalmol 1995;10: 234–241.

59. Sawyer RA, Selhorst JB, Zimmerman LE, et al: Blindness casued by photoreceptor degeneration as a remote effect of cancer. Am J Ophthalmol 1976;81: 606–613.
60. Jacobson DM, Thirkill CE, Tipping SJ: A clinical triad to diagnose paraneoplastic retinopathy. Ann Neurol 1990;28:162–167.
61. Rizzo JF, Gittinger JW: Selective immunohistochemical staining in the paraneoplastic retinopathy syndrome. Ophthalmology 1992;99:1286–1295.
62. Rush JA: Paraneoplastic retinopathy in malignant melanoma. Am J Ophthalmol 1993;115:390–391.
63. Cogan DG, Kuwabara T, Currie J, et al: Paraneoplastic retinopathy simulating cone dystrophy with achromatopsia. Klin Monatsbl Augenheilk 1990;197: 156–158.
64. Hammerstein W, Jurgens H, Gobel U: Retinal degeneration and embryonal rhabdomyosarcoma of the thorax. Fortschr Ophthalmol 1991;88:463–465.
65. Matsui Y, Mehta MC, Katsumi O, et al: Electrophysiological findings in paraneoplastic retinopathy. Graefes Arch Clin Exp Ophthalmol 1992;230:324–328.
66. Chung SM, Selhorst JB: Cancer-associated retinopathy. Ophthalmol Clin North Am 1992;5:587–596.
67. Berson EL, Lessell S: Paraneoplastic night blindness with malignant melanoma. Am J Ophthalmol 1988; 106:307–311.
68. Singh AD, Milam AH, Shields CL, et al: Melanoma associated retinopathy. Am J Ophthalmol 1995;119: 369–370.
69. Andreasson S, Ponjavic V, Ehinger B: Full-field electroretinogram in a patient with cutaneous melanoma-associated retinopathy. Acta Ophthalmol 1993;71: 487–490.
70. Alexander KR, Fishman GA, Peachy NS, et al: "On" response defect in paraneoplastic night blindness with cutaneous malignant melanoma. Invest Ophthalmol Vis Sci 1992;33:477–483.
71. Milam AH, Saari JC, Jacobson SG, et al: Autoantibodies against retinal bipolar cells in cutaneous melanoma-associated retinopathy. Invest Ophthalmol Vis Sci 1993;34:91–100.
72. Potter MJ, Thirkill CE, Dam OM, et al: Clinical and immunocytochemical findings in a case of melanoma-associated retinopathy. Ophthalmology 1999;106:2121–2125.
73. Keltner JL, Roth AM, Chang RS: Photoreceptor degeneration: possible autoimmune disorder. Arch Ophthalmol 1983;101:564–569.
74. Borruat FX, Othenin-Girard P, Uffer S, et al: Natural history of diffuse uveal melanocytic proliferation. Ophthalmology 1992;99:1698–1704.
75. Margo CE, Pavan PR, Gendelman D, et al: Bilateral melanocytic uveal tumors associated with systemic nonocular malignancy: malignant melanomas or benign paraneoplastic syndrome. Retina 1987;7: 137–141.
76. Leys AM, Dierick HG, Sciot RM: Early lesions of bilateral diffuse melanocytic proliferation. Arch Ophthalmol 1991;109:1590–1594.
77. Ryll DL, Campbell RJ, Robertson DM, et al: Pseudometastatic lesions of the choroid. Ophthalmology 1980;87:1181–1186.
78. Grunwald GB, Kornguth SE, Towfighi J, et al: Autoimmune basis for visual paraneoplastic syndrome in patients with small cell lung carcinoma. Retinal immune deposits and ablation of retinal ganglion cells. Cancer 1987;60:780–786.
79. Oohira A, Tamaki Y, Nagahara K, et al: A case of paraneoplastic retinopathy. Jpn J Ophthalmol 1993; 37:28–31.
80. Ohnishi Y, Ohara S, Sakamoto T, et al: Cancer-associated retinopathy with retinal phlebitis. Br J Ophthalmol 1993;77:795–798.
81. Campo E, Brunier MN, Merino MJ: Small cell carcinoma of the endometrium with associated ocular paraneoplastic syndrome. Cancer 1992;69:2283–2288.
82. Adamus G, Guy J, Schmied JL, et al: Role of anti-recoverin autoantibodies in cancer-associated retinopathy. Invest Ophthalmol Vis Sci 1993;34:2626–2633.
83. Thirkill CE, Roth AM, Keltner JL: Cancer-associated retinopathy. Arch Ophthalmol 1987;105:372–375.
84. Jacobson DM, Thirkill CE: Paraneoplastic cone dysfunction: an unusual visual remote effect of cancer [letter]. Arch Ophthalmol 1995;113:1580–1582.
85. Polans AS, Burton MD, Haley TL, et al: Recoverin, but not visinin, is an autoantigen in the human retina identified with a cancer-associated retinopathy. Invest Ophthalmol Vis Sci 1993;34:81–90.
86. Thirkill CE, Tait RC, Tyler NK, et al: The cancer-associated retinopathy antigen is a recoverin-like protein. Investi Ophthalmol Vis Sci 1992;33:2768–2772.
87. Klingele TG, Burde RM, Rappazzo JA, et al: Paraneoplastic retinopathy. J Clin Neuroophthalmol 1984;4:239–245.
88. Crofts JW, Bachynski BN, Odel JG: Visual paraneoplastic syndrome associated with undifferentiated endometrial carcinoma. Can J Ophthalmol 1988; 23:128–132.
89. Boghen D, Sebag M, Michaud J: Paraneoplastic optic neuritis and encephalomyelitis. Report of a case. Arch Neurol 1988;45:353–356.
90. Pillay N, Gilbert JJ, Ebers GC, et al: Internuclear ophthalmoplegia and "optic neuritis": paraneoplastic effects of bronchial carcinoma. Neurology 1984; 34:788–791.
91. Waterston JA, Gilligan BS: Paraneoplastic optic neuritis and external ophthalmoplegia. Aust NZ J Med 1986;16:703–704.
92. Malik S, Furlan AJ, Sweeney PJ, et al: Optic neuropathy: a rare paraneoplastic syndrome. J Clin Neuro-ophthalmol 1992;12:137–141.
93. Keltner JL, Thirkill CE, Tyler NK, et al: Management and monitoring of cancer-associated retinopathy. Arch Ophthalmol 1992;110:48–53.
94. Jacobson DM: Acute zonal occult outer retinopathy and central nervous system inflammation. J Neuro-ophthalmol 1996;16:172–177.
95. Thirkill CE, Fitzgerald P, Sergott RC, et al: Cancer-associated retinopathy (CAR syndrome) with antibodies reacting with retinal, optic-nerve, and cancer cells. N Engl J Med 1989;321:1589–1594.
96. Gass JDM, Hamed LM: Acute macular neuroretinopathy and multiple evanescent white dot syndrome occurring in the same patients. Arch Ophthalmol 1989;107:189–193.
97. Callanan D, Gass JD: Multifocal choroiditis and choroidal neovascularization associated with the multiple evanescent white dot and acute idiopathic blind spot enlargement syndrome. Ophthalmology 1992; 99:1678–1685.
98. Fletcher WA, Imes RK, Goodman D, et al: Acute idiopathic blindspot enlargement. A big blindspot

syndrome without optic disc edema. Arch Ophthalmol 1988;106:44–49.
99. Volpe NJ, Rizzo JF, Lessell S: Acute idiopathic blind-spot enlargement syndrome: A review of 27 new cases. Arch Ophthalmol (in press).
100. Khorram KD, Jampol LM, Rosenberg MA: Blind spot enlargement as a manifestation of multifocal choroiditis. Arch Ophthalmol 1991;109:1403–1407.
101. Singh K, deFrank MP, Shults WT, et al: Acute idiopathic blind spot enlargement. A spectrum of disease. Ophthalmology 1991;98:497–502.
102. Jampol LM, Sieving PA, Pugh D, et al: Multiple evanescent white dot syndrome. I. Clinical findings. Arch Ophthalmol 1984;102:671–674.
103. Takeda M, Kimura S, Tamiya M: Acute disseminated retinal pigment epitheliopathy. Folia Ophthalmol Japan 1984;35:2613–2620.
104. Hamed LM, Glaser JS, Gass JDM, et al: Protracted enlargement of the blind spot in the multiple evanescent white dot syndrome. Arch Ophthalmol 1989;107:194–198.
105. Aaberg TM, Campo RV, Joffe L: Recurrences and bilaterality in the multiple evanescent white-dot syndrome. Am J Ophthalmol 1985;100:29–37.
106. Nakao K, Isashiki M: Multiple evanescent white dot syndrome. Jpn J Ophthalmol 1986;30:376–384.
107. Leys A, Leys M, Jonckheere P, et al: Multiple evanescent white dot syndrome (MEWDS). Bull Soc Belge Ophtalmol 1990;236:97–108.
108. Borruat FX, Othenin GP, Safran AB: Multiple evanescent white dot syndrome. Klin Monatsbl Augenheilkd 1991;198:453–456.
109. Jacobson SG, Morales DS, Sun XK, et al: Pattern of retinal dysfunction in acute zonal occult outer retinopathy. Ophthalmology 1995;102:1187–1198.
110. Dodwell DG, Jampol LM, Rosenberg M, et al: Optic nerve involvement associated with the multiple evanescent white-dot syndrome. Ophthalmology 1990;97:862–868.
111. Chung YM, Yeh TS, Liu JH: Increased serum IgM and IgG in the multiple evanescent white dot syndrome. Am J Ophthalmol 1987;104:187–188.
112. Gass JDM, Stern C: Acute annular outer retinopathy as a variant of acute zonal occult outer retinopathy. Am J Ophthalmol 1995;119:330–334.
113. Luckie A, Ai E, Piero ED: Progressive zonal outer retinitis. Am J Ophthalmol 1994;118:583–588.
114. Gass JD: Acute zonal occult outer retinopathy. Donders Lecture: The Netherlands Ophthalmological Society, Maastricht, Holland, June 19, 1992. J Clin Neuro Ophthalmol 1993;13:79–97.
115. Kimmel AS, Folk JC, Thompson HS, et al: The multiple evanescent white dot syndrome with acute blind spot enlargement. Am J Ophthalmol 1989;107:425–426.
116. Tejada PP, Pina HE, Mendez RM: Multiple evanescent white dot syndrome. Ann Ophthalmol 1993;25:216–218.
117. Reddy CV, Brown J, Jr., Folk JC, et al: Enlarged blind-spots in chorioretinal disorders. Ophthalmology 1996;103:606–617.
118. Dreyer RF, Gass JDM: Multifocal choroiditis and panuveitis: a syndrome that mimics ocular histoplasmosis. Arch Ophthalmol 1984;102:1776–1784.
119. Morgan CM, Schatz H: Recurrent multifocal choroiditis. Ophthalmology 1986;93:1138–1147.
120. Watzke RC, Packer AJ, Folk JC, et al: Punctate inner choroidopathy. Am J Ophthalmol 1984;98:572–584.
121. Piltz JR, Wertenbaker C, Lance SE, et al: Digoxin toxicity. Recognizing the varied visual presentations. J Clin Neuro-ophthalmol 1993;13:275–280.
122. Johnson LN: Digoxin toxicity presenting with visual disturbance and trigeminal neuralgia. Neurology 1990;40:1469–1470.
123. Closson RG: Visual hallucinations as the earliest symptom of digoxin intoxication. Arch Neurol 1983;40:386.
124. Weleber RG, Shults WT: Digoxin retinal toxicity. Clinical and electrophysiological evaluation of a cone dysfunction syndrome. Arch Ophthalmol 1981;99:1568–1572.
125. Chuman MA, LeSage J: Color vision deficiencies in two cases of digoxin toxicity. Am J Ophthalmol 1985;100:682–685.
126. Wolin MJ: Digoxin visual toxicity with therapeutic blood levels of digoxin. Am J Ophthalmol 1998;125:406–407.
127. Kaiser Kupfer MI, Kupfer C, Rodrigues MM: Tamoxifen retinopathy. A clinicopathologic report. Ophthalmology 1981;88:89–93.
128. Heier JS, Dragoo RA, Enzenauer RW, et al: Screening for ocular toxicity in asymptomatic patients treated with tamoxifen. Am J Ophthalmol 1994;117:772–775.
129. Ah Song R, Sasco AJ: Tamoxifen and ocular toxicity. Cancer Detect Prev 1997;21:522–531.
130. Lee AG: Tamoxifen retinopathy. J Neuro-ophthalmol 1998;18:276.
131. Espaillat A, Aiello LP, Arrigg PG, et al: Canthaxanthine retinopathy. Arch Ophthalmol 1999;117:412–413.
132. Sharkey JA: Idiopathic canthaxanthine retinopathy. Eur J Ophthalmol 1993;3:226–228.
133. Novak MA, Roth AS, Levine MR: Calcium oxalate retinopathy associated with methoxyflurane abuse. Retina 1988;8:230–236.
134. Maclean H, Wright M, Choi D, et al: Abnormal night vision with isotretinoin therapy for acne [letter]. Clin Exp Dermatol 1995;20:86.
135. Lerman S: Ocular side effects of accutane therapy. Lens Eye Toxic Res 1992;9:429–438.
136. Weleber RG, Denman ST, Hanifin JM, et al: Abnormal retinal function associated with isotretinoin therapy for acne. Arch Ophthalmol 1986;104:831–837.
137. Denman S, Weleber R, Hanifin JM, et al: Abrmal night vision and altered dark adaptometry in patients treated with isotretinoin for acne [letter]. J Am Acad Dermatol 1986;14:692–693.
138. Block JA: Hydroxychloroquine and retinal safety. Lancet 1998;351:771.
139. Levy GD, Munz SJ, Paschal J, et al: Incidence of hydroxychloroquine retinopathy in 1,207 patients in a large multicenter outpatient practice. Arthritis Rheum 1997;40:1482–1486.
140. Mavrikakis M, Papazoglou S, Sfikakis PP, et al: Retinal toxicity in long term hydroxychloroquine treatment. Ann Rheum Dis 1996;55:187–189.
141. Mazzuca SA, Yung R, Brandt KD, et al: Current practices for monitoring ocular toxicity related to hydroxychloroquine (Plaquenil) therapy. J Rheumatol 1994;21:59–63.
142. Spalton DJ, Verdon Roe GM, Hughes GR: Hydroxychloroquine, dosage parameters and retinopathy. Lupus 1993;2:355–358.
143. Weiner A, Sandberg MA, Gaudio AR, et al: Hydroxychloroquine retinopathy. Am J Ophthalmol 1991;112:528–534.

144. Easterbrook M: Chloroquine retinopathy. Arch Ophthalmol 1991;109:1362.
145. Finbloom DS, Silver K, Newsome DA, et al: Comparison of hydroxychloroquine and chloroquine use and the development of retinal toxicity. J Rheumatol 1985;12:692–694.
146. Miller NR, Johnson MA, Paul SR, et al: Visual dysfunction in patients receiving vigabatrin. Clinical and electrophysiologic findings. Neurology 1999;53: 2082–2087.
147. Kälviäinen R, Nousiainen I, Mäntyjärvi M, et al: Vigabatrin, a gabaergic antiepileptic drug, causes concentric visual field defects. Neurology 1999;53:922–926.
148. Szlyk JP, Fishman GA, Alexander KR, et al: Clinical subtypes of cone–rod dystrophy. Arch Ophthalmol 1993;111:781–788.
149. Simunovic MP, Moore AT: The cone dystrophies. Eye 1998;12:553–565.
150. Meire FM, Bergen AA, De Rouck A, et al: X linked progressive cone dystrophy. Localisation of the gene locus to Xp21-p11.1 by linkage analysis. Br J Ophthalmol 1994;78:103–108.
151. Balciuniene J, Johansson K, Sandgren O, et al: A gene for autosomal dominant progressive cone dystrophy (CORD5) maps to chromosome 17p12-p13. Genomics 1995;30:281–286.
152. Nakazawa M, Kikawa E, Chida Y, et al: Autosomal dominant cone-rod dystrophy associated with mutations in codon 244 (Asn244His) and codon 184 (Tyrl 184Ser) of the peripherin/RDS gene. Arch Ophthalmol 1996;114:72–78.
153. Kelsell RE, Gregory Evans K, Payne AM, et al: Mutations in the retinal guanylate cyclase (RETGC-1) gene in dominant cone-rod dystrophy. Hum Mol Genet 1998;7:1179–1184.
154. Mantyjarvi MI: Color vision defect as first symptom of progressive cone-rod dystrophy. J Clin Neuro-ophthalmol 1990;10:266–270.
155. Kretschmann U, Seeliger M, Ruether K, et al: Spatial cone activity distribution in diseases of the posterior pole determined by multifocal electroretinography. Vision Res 1998;38:3817–3828.
156. Birch DG, Anderson JL, Fish GE: Yearly rates of rod and cone functional loss in retinitis pigmentosa and cone-rod dystrophy. Ophthalmology 1999;106: 258–268.
157. Huang Y, Cideciyan AV, Papastergiou GI, et al: Relation of optical coherence tomography to microanatomy in normal and rd chickens. Invest Ophthalmol Vis Sci 1998;39:2405–2416.
158. Krauss HR, Heckenlively JR: Visual field changes in cone-rod degenerations. Arch Ophthalmol 1982; 100:1784–1790.
159. Kearns TP, Sayre GP: Retinitis pigmentosa, external ophthalmoplegia and complete heart block. Arch Ophthalmol 1958;60:280–289.
160. Schon EA, Rizzuto R, Moraes CT, et al: A direct repeat is a hotspot for large-scale deletion of human mitochondrial DNA. Science 1989;244:346–349.
161. Mita S, Schmidt B, Schon EA, et al: Detection of "deleted" mitochondrial genomes in cytochrome-c oxidase-deficient muscle fibers of a patient with Kearns–Sayre syndrome. Proc Natl Acad Sci USA 1989;86:9509–9513.
162. Vazquez Acevedo M, Coria R, Gonzalez Astiazaran A, et al: Characterization of a 5025 base pair mitochondrial DNA deletion in Kearns–Sayre syndrome. Biochim Biophys Acta 1995;1271:363–368.
163. Brockington M, Alsanjari N, Sweeney MG, et al: Kearns–Sayre syndrome associated with mitochondrial DNA deletion or duplication: a molecular genetic and pathological study. J Neurol Sci 1995; 131:78–87.
164. Zeviani M, Moraes CT, DiMauro S, et al: Deletions of mitochondrial DNA in Kearns–Sayre syndrome. 1988 [classical article]. Neurology 1998;51:1525 and 1528 pages following.
165. Mullie MA, Harding AE, Petty RK, et al: The retinal manifestations of mitochondrial myopathy. A study of 22 cases. Arch Ophthalmol 1985;103:1825–1830.
166. Francois J: Metabolic tapetoretinal degenerations. Surv Ophthalmol 1982;26:293–333.
167. Fang W, Huang CC, Lee CC, et al: Ophthalmologic manifestations in MELAS syndrome. Arch Neurol 1993;50:977–980.
168. Isashiki Y, Nakagawa M, Ohba N, et al: Retinal manifestations in mitochondrial diseases associated with mitochondrial DNA mutation. Acta Ophthalmol Scand 1998;76:6–13.
169. Sue CM, Mitchell P, Crimmins DS, et al: Pigmentary retinopathy associated with the mitochondrial DNA 3243 point mutation. Neurology 1997;49:1013–1017.
170. Rummelt V, Folberg R, Ionasescu V, et al: Ocular pathology of MELAS syndrome with mitochondrial DNA nucleotide 3243 point mutation. Ophthalmology 1993;100:1757–1766.
171. Johns DR: Mitochondrial DNA and disease. N Engl J Med 1995;333:638–644.
172. Holt IJ, Harding AE, Petty RKH, et al: A new mitochondrial disease associated with mitochoindrial DNA heteroplasmy. Am J Hum Genet 1990;46: 428–433.
173. Coppeto JR, Currie JN, Monteiro ML, et al: A syndrome of arterial-occlusive retinopathy and encephalopathy. Am J Ophthalmol 1984;98:189–202.
174. Monteiro ML, Swanson RA, Coppeto JR, et al: A microangiopathic syndrome of encephalopathy, hearing loss, and retinal arteriolar occlusions. Neurology 1985;35:1113–1121.
175. Bogousslavsky J, Gaio JM, Caplan LR, et al: Encephalopathy, deafness and blindness in young women: a distinct retinocochleocerebral arteriolopathy? J Neurol Neurosurg Psychiatry 1989;52:43–46.
176. Susac JO: Susac's syndrome: the triad of microangiopathy of the brain and retina with hearing loss in young women. Neurology 1994;44:591–593.
177. Wildemann B, Schulin C, Storch Hagenlocher B, et al: Susac's syndrome: improvement with combined antiplatelet and calcium antagonist therapy [letter]. Stroke 1996;27:149–151.
178. Susac JO, Hardman JM, Selhorst JB: Microangiopathy of the brain and retina. Neurology 1979;29:313–316.
179. Petty GW, Engel AG, Younge BR, et al: Retinocochleocerebral vasculopathy. Medicine (Baltimore) 1998;77:12–40.
180. Papo T, Biousse V, Lehoang P, et al: Susac syndrome. Medicine Baltimore 1998;77:3–11.
181. O'Halloran HS, Pearson PA, Lee WB, et al: Microangiopathy of the brain, retina, and cochlea (Susac syndrome). A report of five cases and a review of the literature. Ophthalmology 1998;105:1038–1044.
182. Notis CM, Kitei RA, Cafferty MS, et al: Microangiopathy of brain, retina, and inner ear. J Neuroophthalmol 1995;15:1–8.
183. Gass JD: Acute posterior multifocal placoid pigment epitheliopathy. Arch Ophthalmol 1968;80:177–185.

184. Park D, Schatz H, McDonald HR, et al: Acute multifocal posterior placoid pigment epitheliopathy: a theory of pathogenesis. Retina 1995;15:351–352.
185. Howe LJ, Woon H, Graham EM, et al: Choroidal hypoperfusion in acute posterior multifocal placoid pigment epitheliopathy. An indocyanine green angiography study. Ophthalmology 1995;102:790–798.
186. Weinstein JM, Bresnick GH, Bell CL, et al: Acute posterior multifocal placoid pigment epitheliopathy associated with cerebral vasculitis. J Clin Neuroophthalmol 1988;8:195–201.
187. Bewermeyer H, Nelles G, Huber M, et al: Pontine infarction in acute posterior multifocal placoid pigment epitheliopathy. J Neurol 1993;241:22–26.
188. Althaus C, Unsold R, Figge C, et al: Cerebral complications in acute posterior multifocal placoid pigment epitheliopathy. Ger J Ophthalmol 1993;2:150–154.
189. Wilson CA, Choromokos EA, Sheppard R: Acute posterior multifocal placoid pigment epitheliopathy and cerebral vasculitis. Arch Ophthalmol 1988;106:796–800.
190. Kersten DH, Lessell S, Carlow TJ: Acute posterior multifocal placoid pigment epitheliopathy and late-onset meningo-encephalitis. Ophthalmology 1987;94:393–396.
191. Comu S, Verstraeten T, Rinkoff JS, et al: Neurological manifestations of acute posterior multifocal placoid pigment epitheliopathy. Stroke 1996;27:996–1001.
192. Roberts TV, Mitchell P: Acute posterior multifocal placoid pigment epitheliopathy: a long-term study. Aust NZ J Ophthalmol 1997;25:277–281.
193. Moyenin P, Grange JD: Eales' syndrome. Clinical aspects, therapeutic indications and course of 29 cases. J Fr Ophtalmol 1987;10:123–128.
194. Kutsal YG, Altioklar K, Atasu S, et al: Eales' disease with hemiplegia. Clin Neurol Neurosurg 1987;89:283–286.
195. Gordon MF, Coyle PK, Golub B: Eales' disease presenting as stroke in the young adult. Ann Neurol 1988;24:264–266.
196. Katz B, Wheeler D, Weinreb RN, et al: Eales' disease with central nervous system infarction. Ann Ophthalmol 1991;23:460–463.
197. Atabay C, Erdem E, Kansu T, et al: Eales disease with internuclear ophthalmoplegia. Ann Ophthalmol 1992;24:267–269.
198. Phanthumchinda K: Eales' disease with myelopathy. J Med Assoc Thai 1992;75:255–258.
199. Weber F, Conrad B: Chronic encephalitis and Eales disease. J Neurol 1993;240:299–301.
200. Bicknell JM, Holland JV: Neurologic manifestations of Cogan's syndrome. Neurology 1978;28:278–281.
201. Rubio A, Rifkin D, Powers JM, et al: Phenotypic variability of CADASIL and novel morphologic findings. Acta Neuropathol Berl 1997;94:247–254.
202. Joutel A, Vahedi K, Corpechot C, et al: Strong clustering and stereotyped nature of Notch3 mutations in CADASIL patients. Lancet 1997;350:1511–1515.
203. Jobsis GJ, Weber JW, Barth PG, et al: Autosomal dominant cerebellar ataxia with retinal degeneration (ADCA II): clinical and neuropathological findings in two pedigrees and genetic linkage to 3p12–p21.1. J Neurol Neurosurg Psychiatry 1997;62:367–371.
204. Holmberg M, Johansson J, Forsgren L, et al: Localization of autosomal dominant cerebellar ataxia associated with retinal degeneration and anticipation to chromosome 3p12–p21.1. Hum Mol Genet 1995;4:1441–1445.
205. Gouw LG, Kaplan CD, Haines JH, et al: Retinal degeneration characterizes a spinocerebellar ataxia mapping to chromosome 3p. Nat Genet 1995;10:89–93.
206. Johansson J, Forsgren L, Sandgren O, et al: Expanded CAG repeats in Swedish spinocerebellar ataxia type 7 (SCA7) patients: effect of CAG repeat length on the clinical manifestation. Hum Mol Genet 1998;7:171–176.
207. David G, Durr A, Stevanin G, et al: Molecular and clinical correlations in autosomal dominant cerebellar ataxia with progressive macular dystrophy (SCA7). Hum Mol Genet 1998;7:165–170.
208. David G, Abbas N, Stevanin G, et al: Cloning of the SCA7 gene reveals a highly unstable CAG repeat expansion. Nat Genet 1997;17:65–70.
209. Enevoldson TP, Sanders MD, Harding AE: Autosomal dominant cerebellar ataxia with pigmentary macular dystrophy. A clinical and genetic study of eight families. Brain 1994;117:445–460.
210. Hamilton SR, Chatrian GE, Mills RP, et al: Cone dysfunction in a subgroup of patients with autosomal dominant cerebellar ataxia. Arch Ophthalmol 1990;108:551–556.
211. Duinkerke Eerola KU, Cruysberg JR, Deutman AF: Atrophic maculopathy associated with hereditary ataxia. Am J Ophthalmol 1980;90:597–603.
212. Martin JJ, Van Regemorter N, Krols L, et al: On an autosomal dominant form of retinal–cerebellar degeneration: an autopsy study of five patients in one family. Acta Neuropathol Berl 1994;88:277–286.
213. Castanon C, Amigo MC, Banales JL, et al: Ocular vaso-occlusive disease in primary antiphospholipid syndrome. Ophthalmology 1995;102:256–262.
214. Asherson RA, Merry P, Acheson JF, et al: Antiphospholipid antibodies: a risk factor for occlusive ocular vascular disease in systemic lupus erythematosus and the 'primary' antiphospholipid syndrome. Ann Rheum Dis 1989;48:358–361.
215. Kleiner RC, Najarian LV, Schatten S, et al: Vaso-occlusive retinopathy associated with antiphospholipid antibodies (lupus anticoagulant retinopathy). Ophthalmology 1989;96:896–904.
216. Gelfand YA, Dori D, Miller B, et al: Visual disturbances and pathologic ocular findings in primary antiphospholipid syndrome. Ophthalmology 1999;106:1537–1540.
217. Levine SR, Welch KM: The spectrum of neurologic disease associated with antiphospholipid antibodies. Lupus anticoagulants and anticardiolipin antibodies. Arch Neurol 1987;44:876–883.
218. Briley DP, Coull BM, Goodnight SH, Jr: Neurological disease associated with antiphospholipid antibodies. Ann Neurol 1989;25:221–227.
219. Iijima H, Gohdo T, Imai M, et al: Thrombin-antithrombin III complex in acute retinal vein occlusion. Am J Ophthalmol 1998;126:677–682.
220. Price DT, Ridker PM: Factor V Leiden mutation and the risks for thromboembolic disease: a clinical perspective [see comments]. Ann Intern Med 1997;127:895–903.
221. Gottlieb JL, Blice JP, Mestichelli B, et al: Activated protein C resistance, factor V Leiden, and central retinal vein occlusion in young adults. Arch Ophthalmol 1998;116:577–579.
222. Tayyanipour R, Pulido JS, Postel EA, et al: Arterial vascular occlusion associated with factor V Leiden gene mutation. Retina 1998;18:376–377.

223. Spagnolo BV, Nasrallah FP: Bilateral retinal vein occlusion associated with factor V Leiden mutation. Retina 1998;18:377–378.
224. Talmon T, Scharf J, Mayer E, et al: Retinal arterial occlusion in a child with factor V Leiden and thermolabile methylene tetrahydrofolate reductase mutations [see comments]. Am J Ophthalmol 1997;124:689–691.
225. Kotake S, Furudate N, Sasamoto Y, et al: Characteristics of endogenous uveitis in Hokkaido, Japan. Graefes Arch Clin Exp Ophthalmol 1996;234:599–603.
226. Murakami S, Inaba Y, Mochizuki M, et al: A nationwide survey on the occurrence of Vogt–Koyanagi–Harada disease in Japan. Jpn J Ophthalmol 1994; 38:208–213.
227. Moorthy RS, Inomata H, Rao NA: Vogt–Koyanagi–Harada syndrome. Surv Ophthalmol 1995;39:265–292.
228. Maezawa N, Yano A, Taniguchi M, et al: The role of cytotoxic T lymphocytes in the pathogenesis of Vogt–Koyanagi–Harada disease. Ophthalmologica 1982;185:179–186.
229. Maezawa N, Yano A: Two distinct cytotoxic T lymphocyte subpopulations in patients with Vogt–Koyanagi–Harada disease that recognize human melanoma cells. Microbiol Immunol 1984;28: 219–231.
230. Norose K, Yano A, Wang XC, et al: Dominance of activated T cells and interleukin-6 in aqueous humor in Vogt–Koyanagi–Harada disease. Invest Opthalmol Vis Sci 1994;35:33–39.
231. Rathinam SR, Vijayalakshmi P, Namperumalsamy P, et al: Vogt–Koyanagi–Harada syndrome in children. Ocul Immunol Inflamm 1998;6:155–161.
232. Cunningham ET, Jr, Demetrius R, Frieden IJ, et al: Vogt–Koyanagi–Harada syndrome in a 4-year old child. Am J Opthalmol 1995;120:675–677.
233. Gruich MJ, Evans OB, Storey JM, et al: Vogt–Koyanagi–Harada syndrome in a 4-year-old child. Pediatr Neurol 1995;13:50–51.
234. Moorthy RS, Rajeev B, Smith RE, et al: Incidence and management of cataracts in Vogt–Koyanagi–Harada syndrome. Am J Ophthalmol 1994;118:197–204.
235. Kawano Y, Tawara A, Nishioka Y, et al: Ultrasound biomicroscopic analysis of transient shallow anterior chamber in Vogt–Koyanagi–Harada syndrome. Am J Ophthalmol 1996;121:720–723.
236. Forster DJ, Rao NA, Hill RA, et al: Incidence and management of glaucoma in Vogt–Koyanagi–Harada syndrome. Opthalmology 1993;100:613–618.
237. Moorthy RS, Chong LP, Smith RE, et al: Subretinal neovascular membranes in Vogt–Koyanagi–Harada syndrome. Am J Ophthalmol 1993;116:164–170.
238. Oshima Y, Harino S, Hara Y, et al: Indocyanine green angiographic findings in Vogt–Koyanagi–Harada disease. Am J Ophthalmol 1996;122:58–66.
239. Forster DJ, Cano MR, Green RL, et al: Echographic features of the Vogt–Koyanagi–Harada syndrome. Arch Ophthalmol 1990;108:1421–1426.
240. Ibanez HE, Grand MG, Meredith TA, et al: Magnetic resonance imaging findings in Vogt–Koyanagi–Harada syndrome. Retina 1994;14:164–168.
241. Hayasaka S, Okabe H, Takahashi J: Systemic corticosteroid treatment in Vogt–Koyanagi–Harada disease. Graefes Arch Clin Exp Ophthalmol 1982;218:9–13.
242. Sasamoto Y, Ohno S, Matsuda H: Studies on corticosteroid therapy in Vogt–Koyanagi–Harada disease. Ophthalmologica 1990;201:162–167.
243. Limon S, Girard P, Bloch Michel E, et al: Current aspects of the Vogt–Koyanagi–Harada syndrome. Apropos of 9 cases. J Fr Ophtalmol 1985;8:29–35.
244. Helveston WR, Gilmore R: Treatment of Vogt–Koyanagi–Harada syndrome with intravenous immunoglobulin. Neurology 1996;46:584–585.
245. Rodriguez A, Calonge M, Pedroza Seres M, et al: Referral patterns of uveitis in a tertiary eye care center. Arch Ophthalmol 1996;114:593–599.
246. Jabs DA, Johns CJ: Ocular involvement in chronic sarcoidosis. Am J Ophthalmol 1986;102:297–301.
247. Ohara K, Okubo A, Sasaki H, et al: Intraocular manifestations of systemic sarcoidosis. Jpn J Ophthalmol 1992;36:452–457.
248. Thorne JE, Galetta SL: Disc edema and retinal periphlebitis as the initial manifestation of sarcoidosis. Arch Neurol 1998;55:862–863.
249. Spalton DJ, Sanders MD: Fundus changes in histologically confirmed sarcoidosis. Br J Ophthalmol 1981; 65:348–358.
250. Brinkman CJ, Rothova A: Fundus pathology in neurosarcoidosis. Int Ophthalmol 1993;17:23–26.
251. Kimmel AS, McCarthy MJ, Blodi CF, et al: Branch retinal vein occlusion in sarcoidosis. Am J Ophthalmol 1989;107:561–562.
252. Tingey DP, Gonder JR: Ocular sarcoidosis presenting as a solitary choroidal mass. Can J Ophthalmol 1992; 27:25–29.
253. Wolfensberger TJ, Herbort CP: Indocyanine green angiographic features in ocular sarcoidosis. Ophthalmology 1999;106:285–289.
254. Rothova A, Lardenoye C: Arterial macroaneurysms in peripheral multifocal chorioretinitis associated with sarcoidosis. Ophthalmology 1998;105:1393–1397.
255. Kosmorsky GS, Meisler DM, Rice TW, et al: Chest computed tomography and mediastinoscopy in the diagnosis of sarcoidosis-associated uveitis. Am J Ophthalmol 1998;126:132–134.
256. Ohara K, Okubo A, Kamata K, et al: Transbronchial lung biopsy in the diagnosis of suspected ocular sarcoidosis. Arch Ophthalmol 1993;111:642–644.
257. Nichols CW, Eagle RC, Jr, Yanoff M, et al: Conjunctival biopsy as an aid in the evaluation of the patient with suspected sarcoidosis. Ophthalmology 1980;87: 287–291.
258. Karma A, Huhti E, Poukkula A: Course and outcome of ocular sarcoidosis. Am J Ophthalmol 1988;106: 467–472.
259. Lanham JG, Barrie T, Kohner EM, et al: SLE retinopathy: evaluation by fluorescein angiography. Ann Rheum Dis 1982;41:473–478.
260. Jabs DA, Fine SL, Hochberg MC, et al: Severe retinal vaso-occlusive disease in systemic lupus erythematous. Arch Ophthalmol 1986;104:558–563.
261. Hall S, Buettner H, Luthra HS: Occlusive retinal vascular disease in systemic lupus erythematosus. J Rheumatol 1984;11:846–850.
262. Abu el Asrar AM, Naddaf HO, Mitwali A: Choroidopathy in a case of systemic lupus erythematosus. Lupus 1995;4:496–497.
263. Benitez del Castillo JM, Castillo A, Fernandez Cruz A, et al: Persistent choroidopathy in systemic lupus erythematosus. Doc Ophthalmol 1994;88:175–178.
264. Solley WA, Martin DF, Newman NJ, et al: Cat scratch disease. Posterior segment manifestations. Ophthalmology 1999;106:1546–1553.
265. Hayreh SS, Servais GE, Virdi PS: Fundus lesions in malignant hypertension. IV. Focal intraretinal peri-

arteriolar transudates. Ophthalmology 1986;93: 60–73.
266. Hayreh SS, Servais GE, Virdi PS: Fundus lesions in malignant hypertension. VI. Hypertensive choroidopathy. Ophthalmology 1986;93:1383–1400.
267. Hayreh SS, Servais GE, Virdi PS, et al: Fundus lesions in malignant hypertension. III. Arterial blood pressure, biochemical, and fundus changes. Ophthalmology 1986;93:45–59.
268. Hayreh SS, Servais GE, Virdi PS: Cotton-wool spots (inner retinal ischemic spots) in malignant arterial hypertension. Ophthalmologica 1989;198:197–215.
269. Leavitt JA, Pruthi S, Morgenstern BZ: Hypertensive retinopathy mimicking neuroretinitis in a twelve-year-old girl. Surv Ophthalmol 1997;41:477–480.
270. Noble KG: Hypertensive retinopathy simulating Leber idiopathic stellate neuroretinitis [letter]. Arch Ophthalmol 1997;115:1594–1595.
271. Oliver M, Uchenik D: Bilateral exudative retinal detachment in eclampsia without hypertensive retinopathy. Am J Ophthalmol 1980;90:792–796.
272. Karesh JW, Goldman EJ, Reck K, et al: A prospective ophthalmic evaluation of patients with acute myeloid leukemia: correlation of ocular and hematologic findings. J Clin Oncol 1989;7:1528–1532.
273. Perazella MA, Magaldi J: Images in clinical medicine. Retinopathy in leukemia. N Engl J Med 1994;331:922.
274. Wiznia RA, Rose A, Levy AL: Occlusive microvascular retinopathy with optic disc and retinal neovascularization in acute lymphocytic leukemia. Retina 1994;14:253–255.
275. Rouleau GA, Merel P, Lutchman M, et al: Alteration in a new gene encoding a putative membrane-organizing protein causes neuro-fibromatosis type 2. Nature 1993;363:515–521.
276. Trofatter JA, MacCollin MM, Rutter JL, et al: A novel moesin-, ezrin-, radixin-like gene is a candidate for the neurofibromatosis 2 tumor suppressor. Cell 1993;72:791–800.
277. Kaiser Kupfer MI, Freidlin V, Datiles MB, et al: The association of posterior capsular lens opacities with bilateral acoustic neuromas in patients with neurofibromatosis type 2. Arch Ophthalmol 1989;107: 541–544.
278. Mautner VF, Hazim W, Pohlmann K, et al: Ophthalmologic spectrum of neurofibromatosis type 2 in childhood. Klin Monatsbl Augenheilkd 1996;208: 58–62.
279. Meyers SM, Gutman FA, Kaye LD, et al: Retinal changes associated with neurofibromatosis 2. Trans Am Ophthalmol Soc 1995;93:245–252; discussion 252–247.
280. Landau K, Yasargil GM: Ocular fundus in neurofibromatosis type 2. Br J Ophthalmol 1993;77:646–649.
281. Sivalingam A, Augsburger J, Perilongo G, et al: Combined hamartoma of the retina and retinal pigment epithelium in a patient with neurofibromatosis type 2. J Pediatr Ophthalmol Strabismus 1991;28:320–322.
282. Garretto NS, Ameriso S, Molina HA, et al: Type 2 neurofibromatosis with Lisch nodules. Neurofibromatosis 1989;2:315–321.
283. Cunliffe IA, Moffat DA, Hardy DG, et al: Bilateral optic nerve sheath meningiomas in a patient with neurofibromatosis type 2. Br J Ophthalmol 1992; 76:310–312.
284. Evans DG, Huson SM, Donnai D, et al: A genetic study of type 2 neurofibromatosis in the United Kingdom. II. Guidelines for genetic counselling. J Med Genet 1992;29:847–852.
285. Kandt RS, Haines JL, Smith M, et al: Linkage of an important gene locus for tuberous sclerosis to a chromosome 16 marker for polycystic kidney disease. Nat Genet 1992;2:37–41.
286. Haines JL, Short MP, Kwiatkowski DJ, et al: Localization of one gene for tuberous sclerosis within 9q32–9q34, and further evidence for heterogeneity. Am J Hum Genet 1991;49:764–772.
287. Fryer AE, Chalmers A, Connor JM, et al: Evidence that the gene for tuberous sclerosis is on chromosome 9. Lancet 1987;1:659–661.
288. Fahsold R, Rott HD, Lorenz P: A third gene locus for tuberous sclerosis is closely linked to the phenylalanine hydroxylase gene locus. Hum Genet 1991; 88:85–90.
289. Crino PB, Henske EP: New developments in the neurobiology of the tuberous sclerosis complex. Neurology 1999;53:1384–1390.
290. Smith M, Smalley S, Cantor R, et al: Mapping of a gene determining tuberous sclerosis to human chromosome 11q14–11q23. Genomics 1990;6:105–114.
291. Williams R, Taylor D: Tuberous sclerosis. Surv Ophthalmol 1985;30:143–154.
292. Wolter JR, Mertus JM: Exophytic retinal astrocytoma in tuberous sclerosis. J Pediatr Ophthalmol 1969; 6:186–190.
293. Zimmer Galler IE, Robertson DM: Long-term observation of retinal lesions in tuberous sclerosis. Am J Ophthalmol 1995;119:318–324.
294. Dotan SA, Trobe JD, Gebarski SS: Visual loss in tuberous sclerosis. Neurology 1991;41:1915–1917.
295. Webb DW, Fryer AE, Osborne JP: Morbidity associated with tuberous sclerosis: a population study. Dev Med Child Neurol 1996;38:146–155.
296. Webb DW, Clarke A, Fryer A, et al: The cutaneous features of tuberous sclerosis: a population study. Br J Dermatol 1996;135:1–5.
297. Maher ER, Bentley E, Yates JR, et al: Mapping of the von Hippel–Lindau disease locus to a small region of chromosome 3p by genetic linkage analysis. Genomics 1991;10:957–960.
298. Latif F, Tory K, Gnarra J, et al: Identification of the von Hippel–Lindau disease tumor suppressor gene. Science 1993;260:1317–1320.
299. Maher ER, Bentley E, Yates JR, et al: Mapping of von Hippel–Lindau disease to chromosome 3p confirmed by genetic linkage analysis. J Neurol Sci 1990; 100:27–30.
300. Webster AR, Maher ER, Moore AT: Clinical characteristics of ocular angiomatosis in von Hippel–Lindau disease and correlation with germline mutation. Arch Ophthalmol 1999;117:371–378.
301. Moore AT, Maher ER, Rosen P, et al: Ophthalmological screening for von Hippel–Lindau disease. Eye 1991;5:723–728.
302. Rosa RH, Jr., Goldberg MF, Green WR: Clinicopathologic correlation of argon laser photocoagulation of retinal angiomas in a patient with von Hippel–Lindau disease followed for more than 20 years. Retina 1996;16:145–156.
303. Kreusel KM, Bornfeld N, Lommatzsch A, et al: Ruthenium-106 brachytherapy for peripheral retinal capillary hemangioma. Ophthalmology 1998;105: 1386–1392.
304. Balcer LJ, Galetta SL, Curtis M, et al: von Hippel–Lindau disease manifesting as a chiasmal syndrome. Surv Ophthalmol 1995;39:302–306.
305. Atuk NO, Stolle C, Owen JA, Jr, et al: Pheochromocytoma in von Hippel–Lindau disease: clinical presen-

tation and mutation analysis in a large, multigenerational kindred. J Clin Endocrinol Metab 1998;83: 117–120.

306. Sujansky E, Conradi S: Outcome of Sturge-Weber syndrome in 52 adults. Am J Med Genet 1995;57: 35–45.
307. Phelps CD: The pathogenesis of glaucoma in Sturge–Weber syndrome. Ophthalmology 1978;85:276–286.
308. Awad AH, Mullaney PB, Al Mesfer S, et al: Glaucoma in Sturge-Weber syndrome. J AAPOS 1999;3:40–45.
309. Agarwal HC, Sandramouli S, Sihota R, et al: Sturge–Weber syndrome: management of glaucoma with combined trabeculotomy–trabeculectomy. Ophthalmic Surg 1993;24:399–402.
310. Iwach AG, Hoskins HD, Jr., Hetherington J, Jr, et al: Analysis of surgical and medical management of glaucoma in Sturge–Weber syndrome. Ophthalmology 1990;97:904–909.
311. Yang CB, Freedman SF, Myers JS, et al: Use of latanoprost in the treatment of glaucoma associated with Sturge–Weber syndrome. Am J Ophthalmol 1998; 126:600–602.
312. Sullivan TJ, Clarke MP, Morin JD: The ocular manifestations of the Sturge-Weber syndrome. J Pediatr Ophthalmol Strabismus 1992;29:349–356.
313. Griffiths PD, Boodram MB, Blaser S, et al: Abnormal ocular enhancement in Sturge–Weber syndrome: Correlation of ocular MR and CT findings with clinical and intracranial imaging findings. AJNR: Am J Neuroradiol 1996;17:749–754.
314. Zografos L, Bercher L, Chamot L, et al: Cobalt-60 treatment of choroidal hemangiomas. Am J Ophthalmol 1996;121:190–199.
315. Schilling H, Sauerwein W, Lommatzsch A, et al: Long-term results after low dose ocular irradiation for choroidal haemangiomas. Br J Ophthalmol 1997;81:267–273.
316. Gottlieb JL, Murray TG, Gass JD: Low-dose external beam irradiation for bilateral diffuse choroidal hemangioma [letter]. Arch Ophthalmol 1998;116:815–817.
317. Zografos L, Egger E, Bercher L, et al: Proton beam irradiation of choroidal hemangiomas. Am J Ophthalmol 1998;126:261–268.
318. Shah GK, Shields JA, Lanning RC: Branch retinal vein obstruction secondary to retinal arteriovenous communication. Am J Ophthalmol 1998;126:446–448.
319. Effron L, Zakov ZN, Tomsak RL: Neovascular glaucoma as a complication of the Wyburn-Mason syndrome. J Clin Neuroophthalmol 1985;5:95–98.
320. Kivlin JD, Sanborn GE, Myers GG: The cherry-red spot in Tay–Sachs and other storage diseases. Ann Neurol 1985;17:356–360.
321. Kerrison JB, Newman NJ: The phacomatoses. Neurosurg Clin North Am 1999;10:775–787.
322. Cook BE, Robertson DM: Confluent choroidal infiltrates with sarcoidosis. Retina 2000;20:1–7.
323. Thorne JE, Brucker AJ: Choroidal white lesions as an early manifestation of sarcoidosis. Retina 2000; 20:8–15.

CHAPTER 5

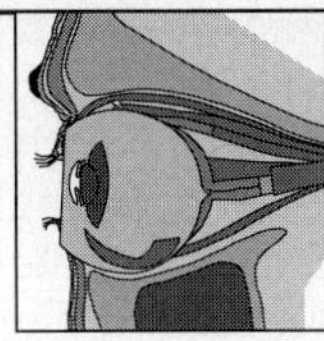

Visual Loss: Optic Neuropathies

The diagnosis of optic neuropathy is usually considered under two circumstances: (1) when visual loss is associated with an anomalous, swollen, or pale optic disc, and (2) when the fundus exam is normal but deficits in acuity, color, and visual field are accompanied by an afferent pupillary defect. In each of these situations, the examiner must rely on historical information, examination findings, and diagnostic testing first to confirm the presence of optic nerve dysfunction, then to determine its cause.

A solid understanding of optic nerve anatomy and physiology is important when approaching patients with optic nerve dysfunction, and this chapter will review these topics. Typical clinical features of optic neuropathies will then be detailed. The subsequent discussion will suggest an approach to the patient with an optic neuropathy and then outline a strategy used to sort between the various optic neuropathies. The features (presentation, examination, and management) of the different causes of optic nerve dysfunction will then be addressed.

OPTIC NERVE ANATOMY AND PHYSIOLOGY

The optic nerve is composed of 1.2 million retinal ganglion cell axons.[1–3] The axons form the nerve fiber layer and eventually synapse in the lateral geniculate body, the pretectum, the superior colliculus, the accessory optic nuclei, and the suprachiasmatic nuclei in the hypothalamus. The supporting cells and blood supply of the optic nerve change throughout its course, which is generally divided into four sections: intraocular, intraorbital, intracanalicular, and intracranial. In fact, the optic nerve is more like a brain tract and less like the other cranial nerves. The optic nerve, like all other parts of the central nervous system (CNS), is invested by the meninges, including the dura, (which blends into the sclera) arachnoidal, and pial membranes. It is myelinated by oligodendrocytes beyond the lamina cribosa and is supported by astrocytes like the white matter in the brain and spinal cord. This is unlike peripheral nerves, which are myelinated by Schwann cells. In addition, the optic nerve has virtually no capacity for regeneration.

Ganglion Cells and the Intraocular Optic Nerve

The cell bodies of retinal ganglion cells and dendrites synapse with amacrine and bipolar cells in the inner plexiform layer of the retina. There are different types of retinal ganglion cells and each type may have a specific visual function. There is currently no agreed-on classification. The concept of parallel processing was introduced to recognize that different types of visual information are processed in parallel streams throughout the pre- and postgeniculate visual pathways.[4–7] Two broad pathways are generally thought to exist. The first is largely responsible for high spatial resolution, color vision, and fine stereopsis and is referred to as the *parvocellular (P) pathway* based on the layers in the lateral geniculate body (LGB) to which they project. The second (*magnocellular, M,* or *luminance*) pathways are responsible for low spatial resolution, motion, and coarse stereopsis. For the purposes of understanding retinal neurophysiology, ganglion cell types generally can be divided into these two different broad categories, M (large) and P (small) cells.[8] M cells project to the magnocellular layer and P cells project to the parvocellular layer of the LGN. As would be expected, the macula (fine spatial resolution) contains mostly P cells; in the peripheral retina the difference in numbers of each type of cell is much less. These two distinct populations of cells persist throughout the retrogeniculate pathways into the striate cortex, where magnocellular axons synapse from the LGN in layer 4c-alpha and parvocellular axons synapse in layer 4c-beta. The relationship between magnocellular and parvocellular pathways and higher cortical areas is discussed in Chapter 9.

Each of the retinal ganglion cells projects to a specific portion of the LGN to preserve the strict point-to-point correspondence (retinotopy). Temporal retinal nerve fibers are arranged on either side of the horizontal raphe and arch around the fovea (arcuate bundles) to divert the retinal elements, except the photoreceptors, away from the fovea (Fig. 5–1). These fibers enter the superior and inferior poles of the disc. Immediately adjacent to the disc, the nerve fiber layer reaches its maximal thickness of 200 μm. The horizontal raphe divides the superior and inferior retinal fibers and is the anatomic basis for several types of visual field defects (eg, nasal steps, altitudinal defects). Nasal macula ganglion cells travel directly to the disc in the papillomacular bundle. Ganglion cells from the central 5 degrees of visual field comprise approximately one third of the total number of axons at the disc. Fibers from the retina nasal to the disc enter the nasal portion of the optic nerve. As they enter the optic nerve head, ganglion cell axons reorganize so that the axons from peripheral ganglion cells are most superficial in the nerve fiber layer and form the more peripheral portions of the optic nerve and macular ganglion cell axons form the center of the nerve.[9]

As they turn to exit the eye at the scleral canal, the optic nerve fibers are supported by the lamina cribosa. Astrocytes make up a large portion of these supporting cells, and they are intertwined, creating a basketlike structure through which the optic nerve axons pass. The astrocytes extend from the lamina cribosa, and their processes are in intimate contact with the axons. Presumably they support the axons physiologically in this area before the axons pass the lamina where oligodendrocytes assume the major supportive role.

The main structural support of the optic nerve as it exits the globe is the lamina cribrosa. The lamina cribrosa contains plates of collagen

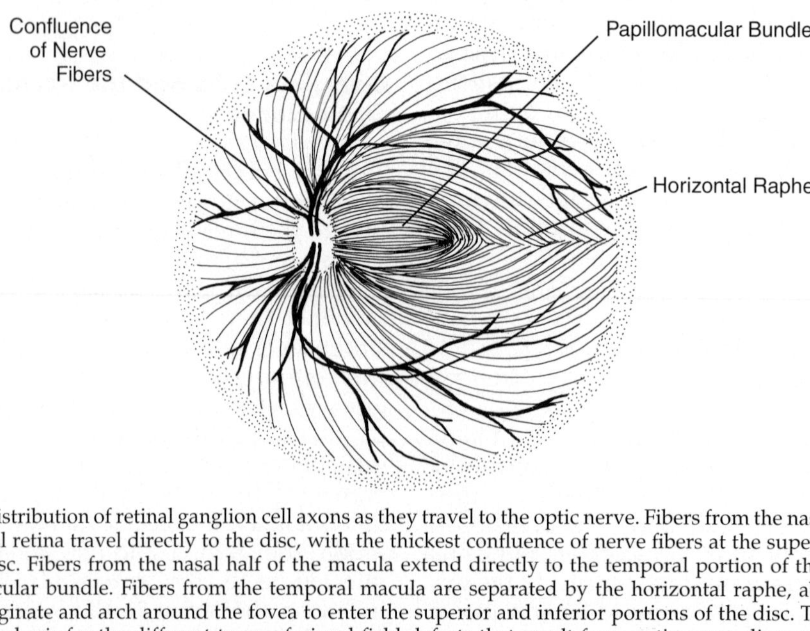

FIGURE 5–1. Distribution of retinal ganglion cell axons as they travel to the optic nerve. Fibers from the nasal, superonasal, and inferonasal retina travel directly to the disc, with the thickest confluence of nerve fibers at the superior and inferior poles of the disc. Fibers from the nasal half of the macula extend directly to the temporal portion of the optic nerve in the papillomacular bundle. Fibers from the temporal macula are separated by the horizontal raphe, above and below which they originate and arch around the fovea to enter the superior and inferior portions of the disc. These nerve fiber bundles are the basis for the different types of visual field defects that result from optic nerve disease.

(types I, III, V, and VI) with interspersed elastin fibers.[10–13] This combination provides both structure and elastic resiliency along the laminar beams, and astrocytes provide metabolic support. Differences exist in the size and thickness of the lamina beams. The largest holes (most axons, least structural support) are in the superior and inferior portions of the disc (arcuate bundles), and this may be one explanation why these fibers might be the most vulnerable to changes in intraocular pressure.[14]

All of the blood supply to the optic nerve is ultimately derived from the ophthalmic artery. The nerve fiber layer of the retina receives its blood supply from branches of the central retinal artery, and when present, cilioretinal arteries also contribute to the peripapillary nerve fiber layer. A capillary bed from the central retinal artery provides the blood flow to the superficial optic nerve head. Branches of the short posterior ciliary arteries are the major blood supply to the optic nerve head below its surface. The area of the nerve served by each posterior ciliary artery is variable and segmental. Since anastomoses between the posterior ciliary arteries are scant, the optic nerve head can be a watershed area. The nature of the blood supply by the posterior ciliary arteries to the optic nerve head is the likely explanation for the segmental disc swelling and/or atrophy that often accompanies ischemic processes. Branches of the posterior ciliary arteries reach the capillary plexus in the area of the lamina choroidalis and lamina cribrosa through branches of the intrascleral circle of Zinn–Haller and from branches of choroidal vessels that supply the choriocapillaris (Fig. 5–2).[15, 16] Capillaries in the region of the lamina cribrosa are within the laminar beams and surround the nerve fiber bundles.

Intraorbital Optic Nerve

Several environmental changes occur as the axons pass through the lamina cribrosa, which is essentially at the level of the sclera. Optic nerve myelination begins (oligodendrocytes) and the pressure gradient on the axons increases as they subjected first to intraocular pressure, then to the intracranial pressure, which is transmitted through the subarach-

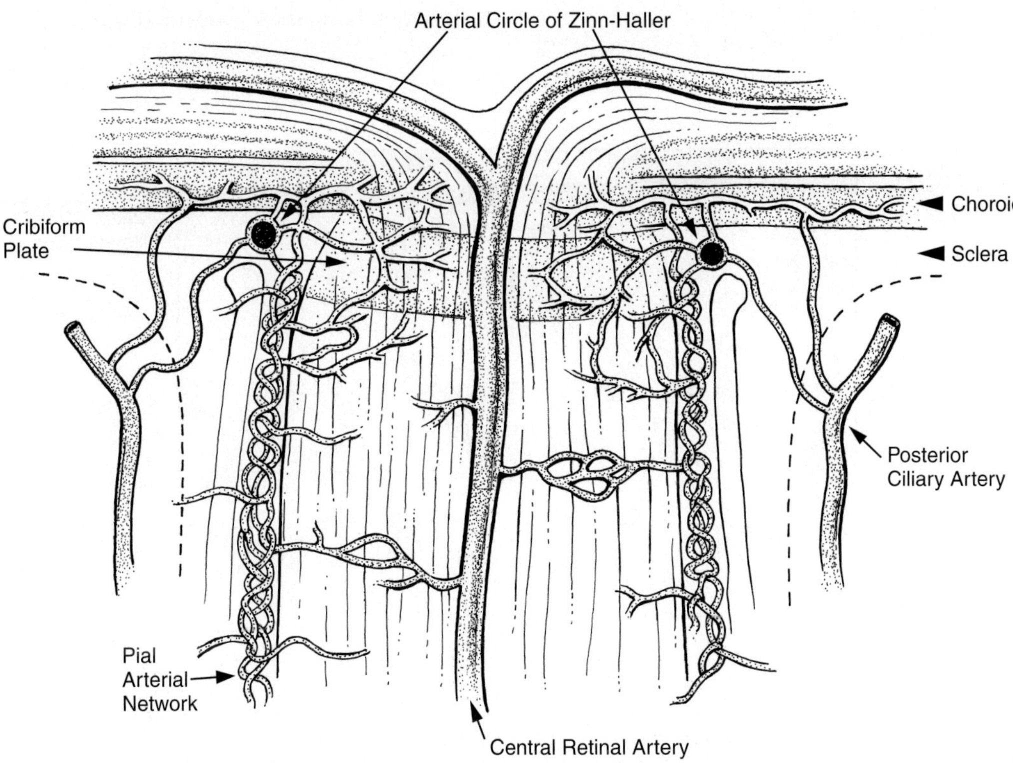

FIGURE 5–2. The circulation of the optic nerve head. The blood is derived primarily from the arteriolar anastamotic circle of Zinn-Haller, which is supplied by the posterior ciliary arteries, the pial arteriole plexus, and the peripapillary choroid. (Redrawn from Hayreh SS: Br J Ophthalmol 1963:47, with permission.)

noid space all the way up to the nerve-globe junction. The intraorbital optic nerve is between 20 and 30 mm in length and is always longer than the distance from the globe to the orbital apex. Therefore there is always slack (the nerve usually takes on an S shape) to allow for unrestricted eye movements. Each axon is surrounded by myelin and glial cells, which provide metabolic support at the nodes of Ranvier. The entire nerve is surrounded by closely adherent pia mater. Arachnoid trabeculae connect the pia to the surrounding dura, which at the apex of the orbit is contiguous with the annulus of Zinn. The optic nerve is divided into septae by collagenous connective tissue, which also contains the centripetally penetrating capillaries from the pia. These are supplied largely by recurrent branches of the short posterior ciliary arteries and capillary branches of the ophthalmic artery. Capillaries are also supplied anteriorly by branches from the central retinal artery, which pierces the optic nerve 10 to 15 mm from the nerve–globe junction. There may also be collateral circulation to the intraorbital optic nerve through anastomotic branches from the external carotid artery. These branches can be supplied from the middle meningeal, superficial temporal, and transverse facial arteries.

Nerve fiber orientation within the optic nerve is highly specific. In the first third of the optic nerve, macular fibers lie temporally and then move to occupy the central portion of the optic nerve. Nasal retinal fibers remain in the nasal portion of the intraorbital optic nerve. The superior temporal fibers are located above the temporally located macular fibers and the inferior fibers are located below the macula fibers.

Intracanalicular Optic Nerve

After leaving the orbit, the optic nerve enters the optic canal, which sits within the two bases of the lesser wing of the sphenoid bone (Fig. 5–3). The medial wall of the canal forms the lateral wall of the sphenoid sinus and in some patients is absent with meninges in direct contact with sinus mucosa.[17] The thickest bones of the canal are located at the orbital apex. The orbital plate of the frontal bone separates the canal from the overlying frontal lobe. Contained within the canal are also the ophthalmic artery, the meninges, and the sympathetic plexus. The dura and therefore the optic nerve are fixed to the periosteum throughout the canal, which is usually around 10 mm in length.

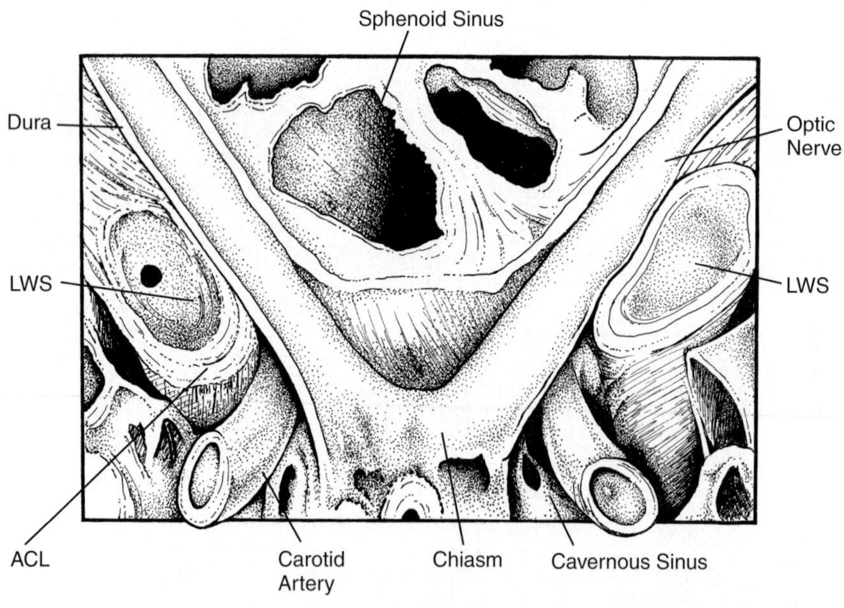

FIGURE 5–3. Axial view of the proximal optic nerves within the optic canal. The optic canal sits between the two bases of the lesser wing of the sphenoid bone (*LWS*) and contains the optic nerve, meninges, sympathetic plexus, and ophthalmic artery. Anteriorly, the dura coalesces to form the annulus of Zinn. The space is tight and the dura is fixed to the bone. The spehoid sinus forms the medial wall of the canal. The chiasm sits behind the sphenoid sinus and the intracranial opening of the canal is formed by the anterior clinoid process (*ACL*). Lateral to the chiasm is the cavernous sinus, which contains the carotid artery.

This tight space makes the optic nerve particularly vulnerable to trauma and small space-occupying lesions in this area. The two optic canals run medially toward each other and rise at a 45-degree angle. In the optic canal, the blood vessels of the pial plexus are usually supplied by the internal carotid artery.

Intracranial Optic Nerve

The length of the intracranial optic nerve is variable (4 to 15 mm) depending on the position of the chiasm in relationship to the sella turcica (above the sella, prefixed, or postfixed; see Chapter 7). The course of the intracranial optic nerve is upward at a 45-degree angle to reach the chiasm. Immediately above the nerves lie the anterior cerebral and anterior communicating arteries, and above these lie the olfactory nerves and frontal lobes. Just lateral to each nerve lies the internal carotid artery, and the ophthalmic artery arises from the internal carotid just below the optic nerve. Just under each optic nerve and above the pituitary gland lies the planum sphenoidale. Blood supply to the pial plexus of vessels supplying the optic nerve can arise from branches of the internal carotid artery, the anterior cerebral arteries, or from the anterior communicating artery.

Optic Nerve Physiology

Maintenance of the ganglion cell axons' structure, clearance of expired organelles, and energy supply to the synapse is accomplished through axoplasmic transport. Axoplasmic flow disruption has been demonstrated in experimental papilledema[18] and secondary to acute elevation of intraocular pressure.[19–22] In addition, many pathologic processes (ischemia, compression, inflammation, and toxins) can result in impaired axoplasmic transport. Therefore some believe that impaired axoplasmic transport may be the final common pathway for optic nerve damage in most disease processes.[23]

The diameter of a ganglion cell axon is approximately 100 times larger than the cell body, and the maintenance of axonal health is dependent on effective axonal transport. *Orthograde axonal transport* refers to movement away from the cell body (toward the lateral geniculate body) and *retrograde transport* occurs toward the cell body. Orthograde transport occurs at both slow and fast speeds and is dependent on the cytoskeleton of the axon (microtubules, neurofilaments, and microfilaments). Transported materials include proteins and transmitters, and these are transported in smooth surface vesicles at a rate of about 400 mm/day (5 hours to the LGB). The elements of the cytoskeleton (microtubules, neurofilaments) are transported at a slower rate of 1 to 4 mm/day.[24] Retrograde transport (toward the cell body) of pinocytic vesicles and lysosomes occurs at a rate of about 200 mm/day. Movement of vesicles along the cytoskeleton is dependent on actin, kinesin, and dynein. How these motor proteins accomplish transport along the microtubule is not clear, but it may occur in a fashion similar to the sliding-filament system seen in muscles. The transport process is dependent on availability of oxygen and energy (ATP), which is delivered by mitochondria moving constantly in orthograde and retrograde fashions. Disruption of axonal transport by energy deprivation, anoxia, or compression will therefore result in optic nerve dysfunction.

Information from ganglion cells to the LGB is provided by varying the rate of action potentials. Light stimulates the retinal photoreceptors, and in turn signals are modified by the horizontal, bipolar, and amacrine cells before reaching the ganglion cells. There are many more photoreceptors than ganglion cells (approximately 130 : 1) and the input to an individual ganglion cell is thought to be organized in a center/surround fashion. This is the initial coding system for visual information. Some ganglion cells have on-center receptive fields, and increase their action potential firing rate when the visual stimulus is a circle of light in the middle, surrounded by darkness. Off-center ganglion cells prefer stimuli with darkness in the middle, surrounded by light. The various rates (eg, sustained firing versus transient firing) at which ganglion cells produce action potentials in response to stimulation is the basis for the distinction between cells believed to be responsible for fine spatial resolution versus those responsible for motion detection and initiation of visual reflexes.[25]

HISTORY

The cause of many optic neuropathies can be correctly identified after reviewing the patient's history. The temporal profile of the visual loss is most important. Details in this regard include rapidity of visual loss (sudden versus insidious, episodic versus gradual), presence of premonitory visual symptoms, and the period of time to visual nadir. Next, attention should be given to associated symptoms, both ocular and nonocular. Some related ocular symptoms that should be considered include pain (in particular pain worsened by eye movements), bulging, fullness or proptosis of the globe, redness, photophobia, and positive visual phenomenon. Nonocular neurologic symptoms would include headache, anosmia, facial paresthesias or numbness, facial weakness, bladder incontinence, transient weakness or numbness, hearing loss, and audible intracranial noises. Clues to any underlying systemic illness should be sought, as well as evidence of recent infection or ongoing rheumatologic symptoms. Risk factors for vasculopathic disease should be identified in addition to systemic medications that may have secondary effects on the optic nerve. A careful family history should attempt to identify relatives with decreased vision or with degenerative neurologic illness, glaucoma, or migraine.

EXAMINATION

Most patients with optic neuropathy can be identified by the characteristic combination of acuity loss, color deficiency, visual field defect, an afferent pupillary defect, and an abnormal-appearing optic nerve on funduscopy (anomalous, swollen, or pale). Along with the historical review, the qualities of each parameter are sometimes helpful in identifying the particular cause of optic nerve dysfunction. Specific examination techniques are detailed in Chapter 2.

Systemic Evaluation

The examination of the patient with suspected optic neuropathy begins with the general evaluation of the patient's physical health, mental status, and vital signs. Markedly elevated blood pressure in a patient with swollen discs suggests the presence of malignant hypertension. An irregular pulse from atrial fibrillation suggests that an acutely acquired visual field defect might be the result of an embolic arterial occlusion. A rapid pulse might suggest hyperthyroidism, and obesity and recent weight gain would point to idiopathic intracranial hypertension. Profound cachexia might suggest cancer spread, temporal arteritis, or nutritional amblyopia. Odd behavior might suggest early on the possibility of nonorganic or functional visual loss.

Visual Acuity

Although visual acuity is commonly reduced in optic neuropathies, the finding is highly variable. In fact, visual acuity is the least sensitive of all the tested functions and is not always helpful in identifying the presence of optic neuropathy or its cause. For instance, profound optic nerve dysfunction with an afferent pupillary defect, dyschromatopsia, and visual field loss may be present with 20/15 visual acuity. Furthermore, virtually any of the causes of optic nerve dysfunction can be associated with any level of visual acuity loss.

Color Vision

Dyschromatopsia and in particular the mismatch of good acuity and poor color vision are very important and sensitive indicators of optic nerve dysfunction. The basis for this mismatch is not completely understood. It may reflect the fact that the optic nerve is largely composed of ganglion cell axons arising in the macular region, and these axons have a one-to-one relationship with the high density of cones in this region. However, there are many patients with profound optic nerve dysfunction who may do relatively well with color plate testing and notice only a mild difference in color saturation between the two eyes.

Contrast Sensitivity

Abnormal contrast sensitivity is another sign of optic nerve dysfunction. Some patients with optic neuropathy have good acuity but may have reduced contrast sensitivity thresholds. It is also helpful in patients with congenital dyschromatopsia who are suspected to have an optic nerve problem in whom color plate testing can not be used. Less commonly, it can be used to document recovery in optic neuritis, which is almost always associated with a profound reduction in contrast sensitivity.

Pupils

The identification of a relative afferent pupil defect (RAPD) is very helpful in localizing vision loss to the optic nerve and is the hallmark of asymmetric disease of the anterior visual pathway. The swinging flashlight test is described in more detail in Chapter 2.

Pulfrich Phenomenon

Pulfrich described a phenomenon that is occasionally reported as a symptom in patients with optic neuropathy. It can be tested for in the office. The Pulfrich phenomenon is a stereo illusion in which a to-and-fro motion in the plane facing the subject is seen as an elliptical movement by an individual with an unilateral optic neuropathy.[26] An object (ball on a string or pen) is swung in front of both eyes.[27] For example, from the eye with a unilateral optic neuropathy, the information is delayed in reaching the cortex, relative to the normal fellow eye. This delay in time between the two eyes is interpreted by the cortex as a separation in space, creating the stereo illusion. Movement is always perceived as toward the diseased eye (ie, right eye, counterclockwise and left eye, clockwise). Affected patients may report difficulty with driving, walking, or performing tasks in the household utilizing stereopsis.[28] Treatment may consist of placing a filter in front of the normal eye.[28] The Pulfrich phenomenon is only infrequently seen in patients with decreased vision due to media opacities or retinal disease.

Visual Fields

The hallmark of an optic neuropathy is an abnormal visual field. Concepts of visual field testing and the various types and their advantages and disadvantages are discussed in Chapter 3. Patients with optic neuropathy have visual field defects that generally fall into three different categories. These are (1) generalized constriction, (2) central defects, and (3) nerve fiber bundle defects.

Generalized Constriction. This type of field defect (Fig. 5–4) is the least specific and the hardest to localize. In these patients, kinetic perimetry shows reduced size of the peripheral isopters, and on automated perimetry peripheral rim defects are seen. The examiner must be careful in interpreting fields with generalized constriction as there are many non-neuro-ophthalmic causes of this type of defect, including media opacities, small pupils, poor patient cooperation, retinal degenerations, and nonorganic visual loss. However, diffuse suppression of the visual field on automated perimetry is in fact the most common defect in patients with optic neuritis.[29]

Central Defects. These include central scotomas, paracentral defects, and centrocecal scotomas (Fig. 5–4). These three types of visual fields are related and imply involvement of the central portion of the optic nerve. They are the most common types of defects in patients with nutritional and toxic optic neuropathies, but are also seen in any of the optic neuropathies. Any patient who has reduced central visual acuity must have a central scotoma by definition, although such defects are not always measurable on perimetry. Central field defects are also the rule in patients with macular disease.

Nerve Fiber Bundle Defects. The third category includes arcuate defects, altitudinal defects, and nasal steps (Fig. 5–4). These defects, as they are so named, imply a localization to a particular group of nerve fibers. In general, they respect the horizontal meridian because of the anatomic boundary of the horizontal raphe. These field defects occasionally may also respect the vertical meridian, but this finding should be considered atypical, and patients with such fields should be investigated for the possibility of intracranial disease (see Fig. 7–11). The nerve fiber bundle types of visual field defects can be seen in all of the different optic neuropathies but certain patterns are common. For instance, altitudinal defects are the most common defects in ischemic optic neuropathy. In general, visual field defects will help to confirm the presence of an optic neuropathy but will not be diagnostic of a specific cause.

Funduscopy

Disc Swelling The normal optic nerve (Fig. 5–5; also see Color Plate 29) has a pinkish-orange color with sharp margins.[30] The nerve fiber layer is best seen at the 6 and 12 o'clock positions, where it is thickest. A central cup is identifiable and the vessels can be seen clearly as they cross the margin of the disc. Optic neuropathies are frequently associated with disc swelling or edema. Ophthalmoscopic features include hyperemia, elevation of the optic nerve head, and edema of the nerve fiber layer blurring the disc margins. The cup may be

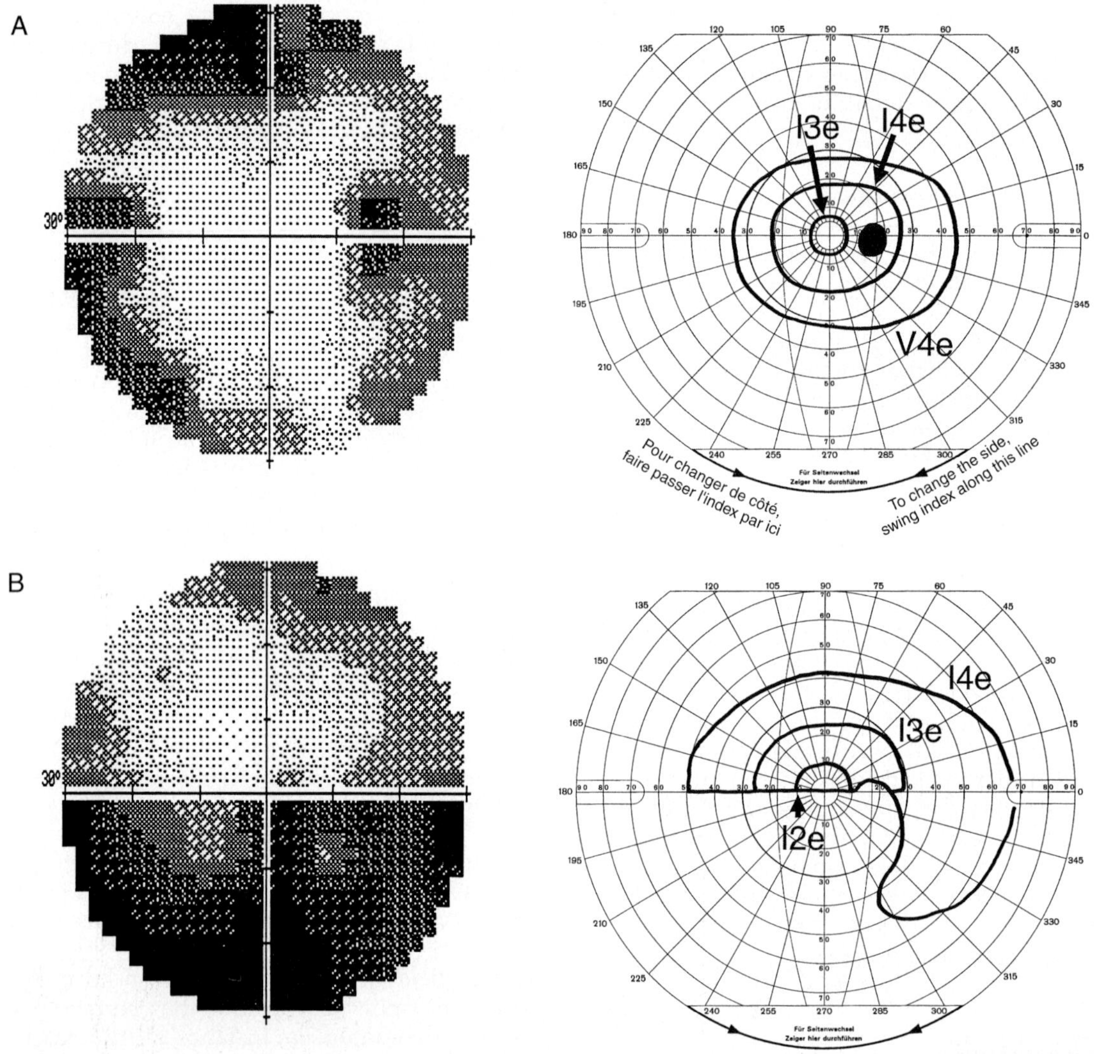

FIGURE 5–4. Paired examples of static threshold perimetry grey-scale (*left*) and kinetic perimetry visual fields (*right*) seen in optic neuropathies. Note that the threshold and kinetic perimetries have different scales. The first pair of fields (**A**) demonstrates generalized constriction, which is the least specific and hardest to localize type of visual field defect. It can also be seen with media opacities and retinal disease, or simply from slow reactions during testing. Altitudinal (**B**), nasal step (**C**), and arcuate (**D**) defects are characteristic of optic neuropathies and represent nerve fiber bundle defects. Central scotomas (**E**) and centrocecal defects (**F,** central defects attached to the blind spot) are also commonly seen with optic neuropathies.

obliterated, and there may be associated retinal or choroidal folds. There may be venous dilation, associated splinter hemorrhages, dilated capillaries, exudates, or cotton-wool spots. Swollen optic nerves resulting from anterior visual pathway compressive lesions may have features that suggest chronicity (absence of hemorrhages, pseudodrusen from axoplasmic stasis) or collateral vessels from retinal to ciliary circulation ("shunt vessels").

Disc Atrophy or Pallor. Although this technically implies a histopathologic diagnosis, the term *optic atrophy* is often substituted for the ophthalmoscopic observation of optic nerve head pallor or loss of pinkness which commonly accompanies permanent damage to the optic nerve. A combination of the loss of the superficial capillary bed along with the loss of tissue volume and astrocytic proliferation is responsible for this change in optic nerve head

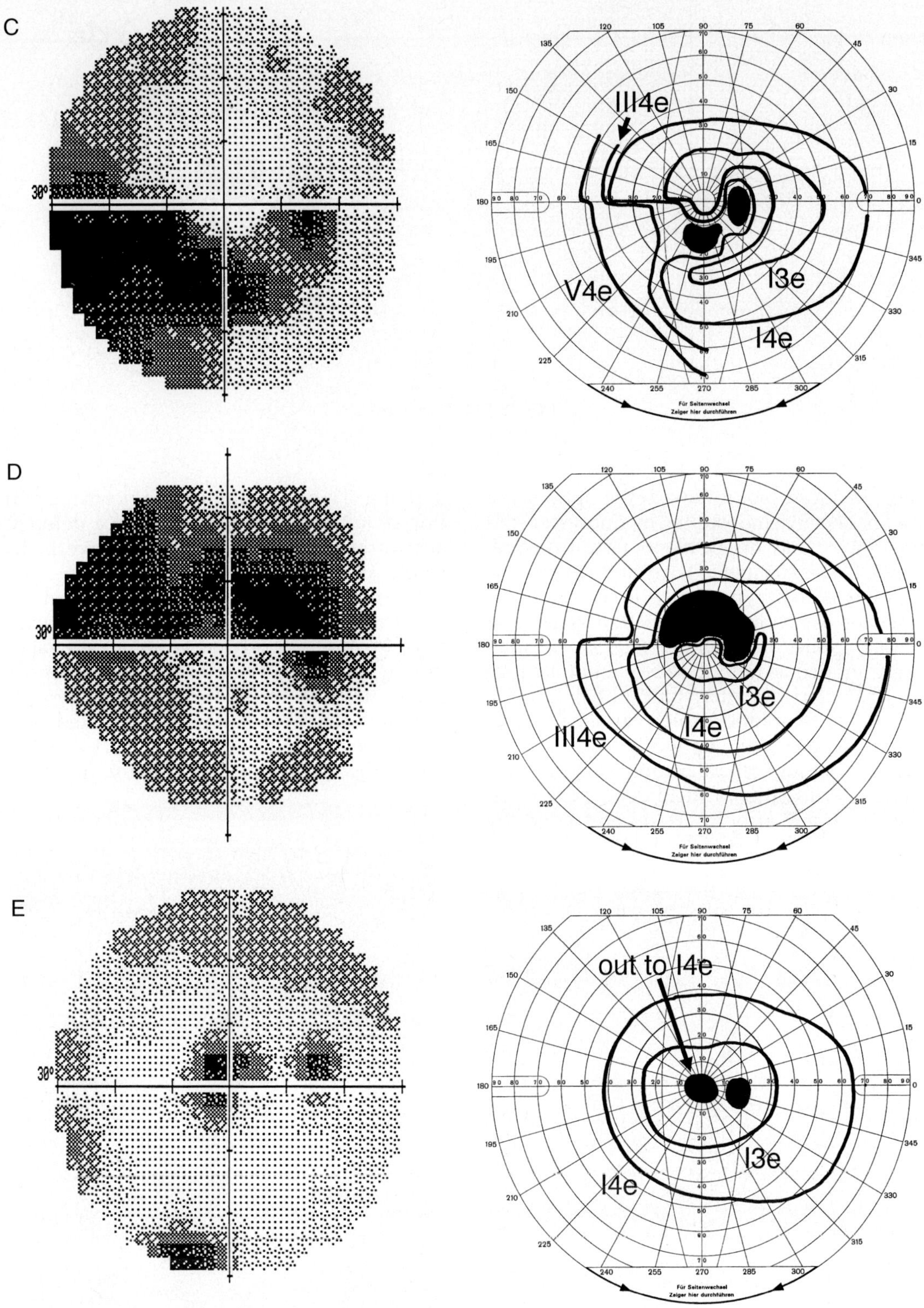

FIGURE 5–4. *Continued*

F

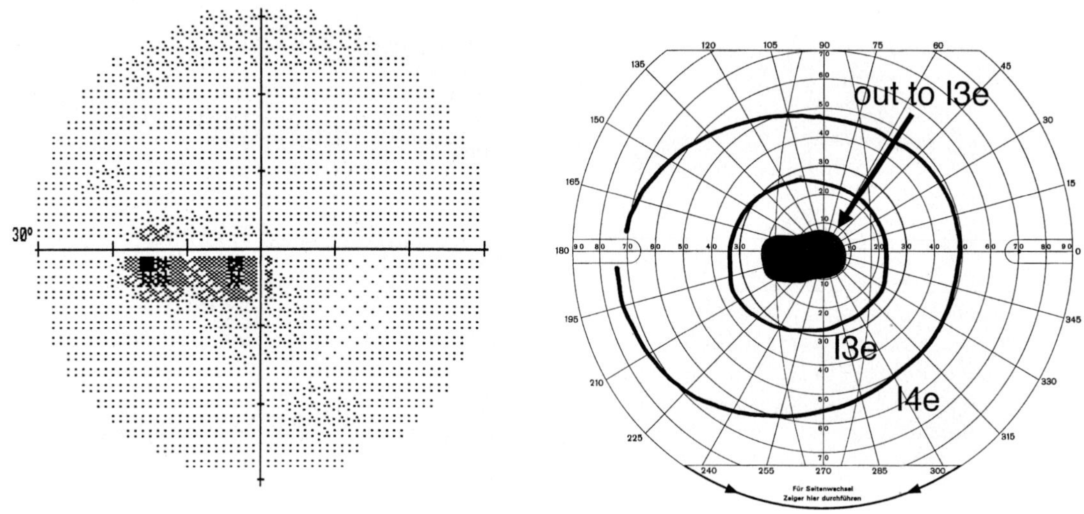

FIGURE 5–4. *Continued*

color. Reduced blood flow to the optic nerve head has been demonstrated by fluorescein angiography[31] and direct blood flow measurements.[32] When using the term *optic atrophy*, the examiner is identifying ganglion cell death, not reduction or involution of function as the term *atrophy* applies in other conditions. Atrophy can be graded as mild to severe and may take on a characteristic pattern (altitudinal, sectoral, bow tie, or temporal), which can be a clue to disease pathogenesis or localization. For instance, superior sectoral atrophy might be associated with inferior field loss. Not infrequently, optic atrophy is accompanied by cupping. This may simply be a normal evolution of appearance or may reflect a defective structural integrity of the optic nerve in the setting of atrophy.[22, 33]

Primary optic atrophy occurs without significant swelling or reactive gliosis. Secondary atrophy implies previous swelling and subsequent gliotic reaction that accompanies the nerve atrophy. In the former (primary optic atrophy) the disc pallor is associated with sharp disc margins and easily visible details on the disc surface and vasculature (Fig. 5–6).

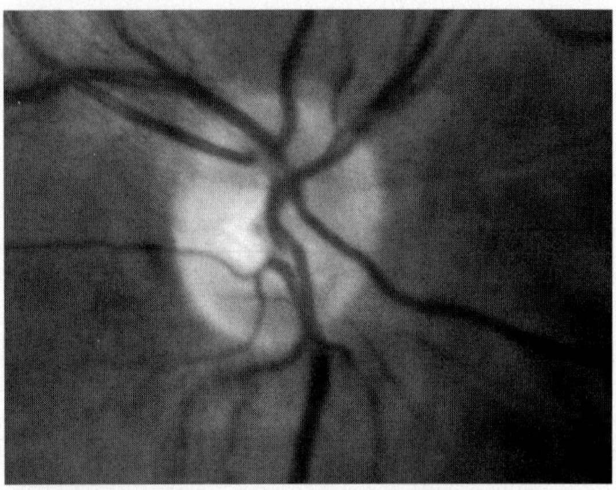

FIGURE 5–5. The normal-appearing optic nerve. Margins are sharp and color is diffusely pink. Nerve fiber striations are seen best at the 10 to 12 o'clock and 6 to 8 o'clock positions just beyond the disc edge. Despite this, the vessels are clearly seen traversing the nerve fiber layer and are not obscured by these fibers. (Also see Color Plate 29.)

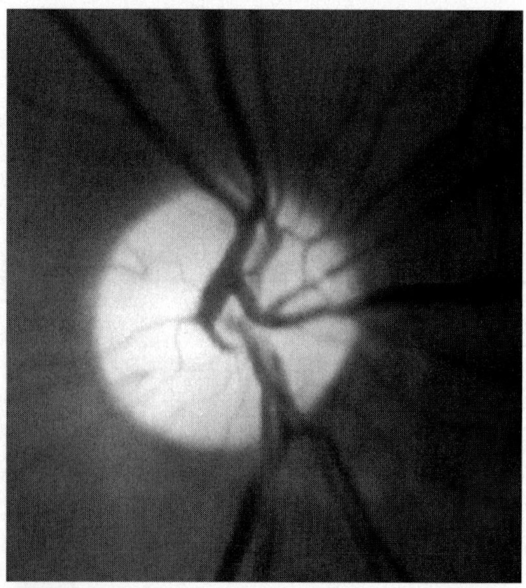

FIGURE 5–6. Primary optic atrophy. The disc is diffusely pale and has sharp, distinct margins.

Most patients (even those with some swelling initially) with acute optic neuropathies later develop primary optic atrophy. In the latter case (secondary optic atrophy) there is a haze to the disc surface or overlying nerve fiber layer that obscures the disc margin and the ophthalmoscopic view of the disc's surface details (Fig. 5–7). The typical setting for secondary optic atrophy is either atrophic papilledema (see Chapter 6) or severe inflammatory disc edema. In some cases, pallor of the disc might not yet be evident but the examiner can identify defects in the nerve fiber layer. In this setting there is a sharp cutoff from the normal appearing nerve fibers to an area with an absence of fibers (Fig. 5–8). These defects can be more easily seen with red-free light (Fig. 5–9) and when there is a pattern of defects alternating with more normal nerve fibers is often describes as "rakelike."

Related Retinal Lesions. When the disc is swollen, other funduscopic findings may aid in the diagnosis. For instance, dilated and tortuous retinal veins accompanied by retinal hemorrhages suggests a retinal vein occlusion, while macular lipid deposition suggests neuroretinitis. When the disc is normal, the examiner should be absolutely certain a macular lesion is not mimicking an optic neuropathy.

Slit Lamp Examination

Other causes of visual acuity loss, such as corneal, lens, or vitreous opacities, should be excluded. The presence of iritis or uveitis would suggest an inflammatory disorder.

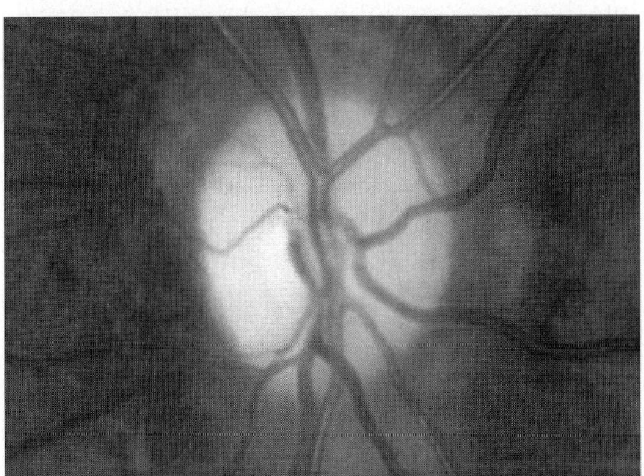

FIGURE 5–7. Secondary optic atrophy. As with primary atrophy, the disc is pale but there is a haziness to the area of the disc margin from previous swelling and reactive gliosis.

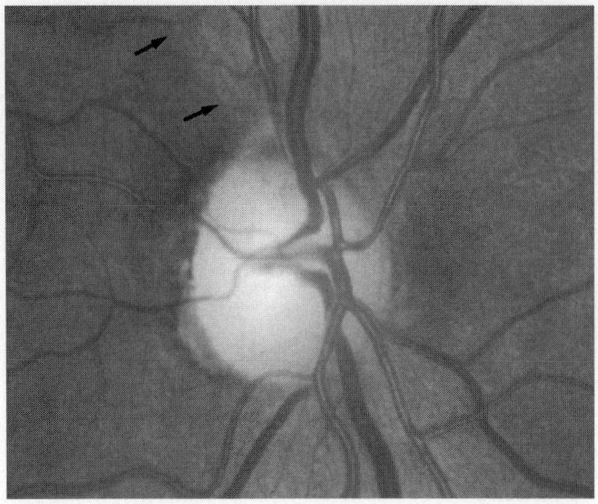

FIGURE 5–8. Right optic nerve with minimal temporal pallor and a sharp cutoff (*arrows*) in the nerve fiber layer demarcating corresponding atrophy of ganglion cell axons.

APPROACH TO PATIENTS WITH OPTIC NEUROPATHY

When the history and examination are typical of optic neuropathy (visual acuity and color vision loss, decreased contrast sensitivity, afferent pupillary defect, and typical visual field defect), four different diagnostic groups should be considered, based on the funduscopic appearance of the disc: *anomalous, swollen, normal,* and *pale.* Clinically, there is considerable overlap among these four groups of

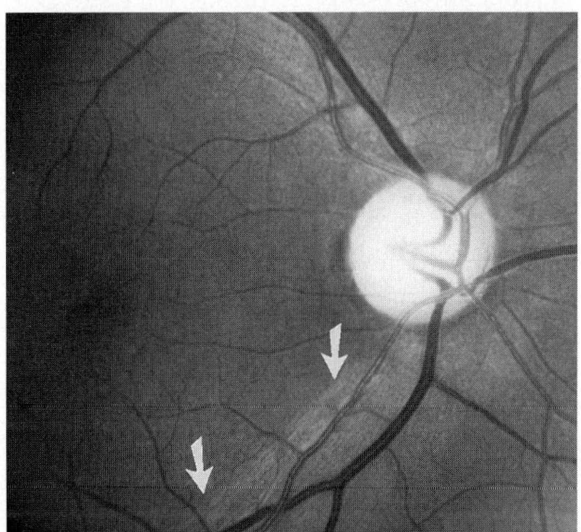

FIGURE 5–9. Red-free photograph of optic disc pallor with nerve fiber layer defect. The area of normal striations of the nerve fiber layer are clearly demarcated (*arrows*).

patients, although we believe distinguishing between them serves as a useful framework when considering the differential diagnoses of an optic neuropathy. For instance, patients with anterior ischemic optic neuropathy always have abnormal-appearing (swollen) optic nerves, and occult compressive lesions are important to consider in the setting of visual loss and a normal fundus. The appearance of congenital disc anomalies are usually distinct. However, when the disc is swollen, normal, or atrophic, usually the examiner will have to rely heavily on the clinical presentation, historical details, and the rest of the examination to make the correct diagnosis.

Anomalous Discs

These are due to congenital anomalies, and they are listed in Table 5–1.

Swollen Optic Nerves

Table 5–2 lists optic neuropathies that may present with disc swelling. The most common diagnoses to consider here are anterior ischemic optic neuropathy and optic neuritis. Patients with anterior ischemic optic neuropathy will generally be older and have vasculopathic risk factors such as diabetes and hypertension. Those with optic neuritis are typically younger and often have periocular pain exacerbated by eye movements.

Papilledema or disc edema from elevated intracranial pressure is discussed elsewhere (Chapter 6), but it is important to note the relative mismatch between the amount of disc swelling and visual function in papilledema. A markedly swollen optic nerve with relatively preserved visual acuity is the hallmark of papilledema in its early stages. Acuity loss and central field defects would be more characterisitic of optic neuropathy.

In more rare circumstances other features of the examination will help identify the cause of the swollen disc with vision loss. The presence of vitritis would suggest the possibility of infectious disc swelling, as in syphilitic uveitis with optic neuropathy. The presence of a macular star makes neuroretinitis the most likely diagnosis. Other infiltrative conditions such as leukemia might be associated with retinal hemorrhages or a distinct mass in the optic nerve head.

TABLE 5–1. Congenital Disc Anomalies

Optic nerve hypoplasia
Tilted discs
Optic pits
Optic disc colobomas
Morning glory disc anomaly
Staphyloma
Pseudopapilledema
Optic disc drusen

TABLE 5–2. Common Optic Neuropathies That Can Present With Disc Swelling

Idiopathic optic neuritis
Anterior ischemic optic neuropathy
Diabetic papillopathy
Optic nerve tumors
Optic nerve glioma
Optic nerve sheath meningioma
Inflammatory optic neuropathies
Sarcoidosis
Optic perineuritis
Infectious optic neuropathies
Syphilitic optic neuropathy
Lyme-associated optic neuropathy
Radiation-induced optic neuropathy
Toxic optic neuropathy (eg, amiodarone associated)
Infiltrative optic neuropathy
Lymphoma/leukemia
Metastatic tumor
Uveitis-associated optic neuropathy
Acute and chronic papilledema

Normal-Appearing Optic Nerves

In retrobulbar optic neuropathies, the normal fundus appearance acutely implies that the disease process is occurring in the optic nerve behind the lamina cribrosa in its intraorbital, intracanalicular, or intracranial portion. Entities that can commonly present with a normal-appearing fundus are listed in Table 5–3. The examiner should be aware of overlap in certain conditions, such as optic neuritis, in which one third of patients will have a swollen optic nerve head; Leber's hereditary optic neuropathy, in which the nerve can have a pseudoswollen appearance; and radiation-induced optic

TABLE 5–3. Acute Optic Neuropathies That Commonly Present With Normal-Appearing Optic Nerves (Retrobulbar Optic Neuropathies)

Optic neuritis
Traumatic optic neuropathy
Compressive optic neuropathy (early)
Posterior ischemic optic neuropathy
Radiation-induced optic neuropathy

neuropathy, in which stigmata of radiation retinopathy may be present and/or the optic nerve may be acutely swollen. Whenever the optic nerve appears normal in a suspected optic neuropathy the macula region should be carefully examined. Chapter 4 contains a discussion of the differentiation between optic neuropathy and maculopathy.

Optic Disc Pallor

Optic atrophy may be evident on the initial examination or can evolve on subsequent evaluations. All of the conditions listed in Tables 5–2 and 5–3, when associated with permanent visual dysfunction, will be accompanied ultimately by the development of optic atrophy. In this setting, the examiner will identify a history of a previous episode consistent with the clinical picture (eg, a previous inflammatory, ischemic, or traumatic injury to the optic nerve). In some instances, patients become suddenly aware of their visual loss at a time after the process began and in this setting (pseudosudden onset), their initial examination will reveal optic atrophy. Entities that commonly present in this fashion are listed in Table 5–4. Most importantly, chronic progressive visual loss accompanied by disc pallor strongly suggests a compressive lesion.

In summary, in most cases of suspected optic neuropathy, careful consideration of historical details, the general examination, and the ophthalmoscopic appearance of the optic nerve head will lead to the correct diagnosis long before any ancillary tests are ordered. The specific optic neuropathies will now be discussed in greater detail.

CONGENITAL DISC ANOMALIES

In this category are included a variety of disorders (Table 5–1) whose hallmark is an abnormal-appearing optic nerve, each with a pathognomonic or distinct "diagnostic appearance." These anomalies take many different forms, and generally for the congenital condition represent an embryologic mishap with resulting malformation. Occasionally, systemic associations will be identified to point the examiner to the correct optic nerve anomaly.

TABLE 5–4. Optic Neuropathies Commonly Presenting With Optic Disc Pallor at Initial Evaluation

Compressive optic neuropathy
Toxic/nutritional optic neuropathy
Infectious (syphilitic) optic neuropathy
Hereditary (dominant) optic atrophy

The level of visual loss associated with congenital disc anomalies ranges from minimal visual dysfunction to total blindness. In children, the most common ophthalmic presentation of a unilateral disc anomaly is strabismus (usually sensory eso- or exotropia), while those with bilateral disc anomalies more frequently present with poor vision or nystagmus.[34] In some adults, a routine eye examination may demonstrate acuity or visual field and funduscopic examination will disclose the previously unrecognized disc anomaly. Many such patients are unaware of long-standing defects or arbitrarily ascribe visual problems to "a lazy eye," for example. Some patients with congenital anomalies will become acutely aware of their visual deficit, confusing the examiner since the visual field defect that, by its nature, must have predated the onset of the symptomatic awareness of reduced vision. Usually the visual deficit is static. However, it is important to recognize that some congenital or developmental abnormalities may be associated with newly acquired vision loss. For example, macular detachment may complicate a congenital optic pit or optic disc drusen may be associated with anterior ischemic optic neuropathy.

Hypoplasia

Optic nerve hypoplasia is a variable condition that can be associated with either minimal or marked visual dysfunction, can be unilateral or bilateral, and may or may not be associated with a more widespread neurologic developmental disorder. This is the most common congenital optic nerve abnormality. Embryologically, the reduced number of functioning axons may result from the exaggeration of a normal developmental process. That is, early on at 16 to 17 weeks there are approximately 3 million optic nerve axons, which ultimately are reduced to approximately 1 million at the time of birth. Hypoplasia may therefore be an overdone but normal process of involution.[35]

Affected patients can have any level of visual function, ranging from minimal acuity or field loss to no light perception (NLP), and they may have unilateral or bilateral optic nerve hypoplasia. Ophthalmoscopically, the optic nerve appears small with a reduced diameter (Fig. 5–10; see Color Plate 14). This finding may be subtle and hard to recognize, and sometimes the loss of nerve fiber layer is viewed best using red-free light during ophthalmoscopy.[36] The appearance of hypoplastic nerves can be quite variable, and the key to making the diagnosis is identifying the true edge of the optic nerve (Fig. 5–11). In young infants, the diagnosis of a mild degree of hypoplasia can be extremely difficult and can often be made only subjectively. In general, more severely hypoplastic nerves are associated with poorer vision,[37] because a smaller disc has fewer ganglion cell axons passing through it. Classically, but seen only in a minority of cases, there is a ring of visible sclera and pigmentation surrounding the optic nerve. This creates a peripapillary halo, or the so-called double-ring sign (Fig. 5–10).[38] One study[39] suggested optic nerve hypoplasia associated with tortuosity of the retinal veins might be a marker of endocrinopathy (see below). Magnetic resonance imaging (MRI) frequently demonstrates thin optic nerves and chiasm.

Optic nerve hypoplasia may occur in isolation or in combination with other midline developmental abnormalities that share the same embryologic forebrain derivation. In *de Morsier syndrome,* or septo-optic dysplasia, optic nerve hypoplasia is associated with absence of the septum pellucidum (see Fig. 7–39). A dysgenetic, thin, or absent corpus callosum

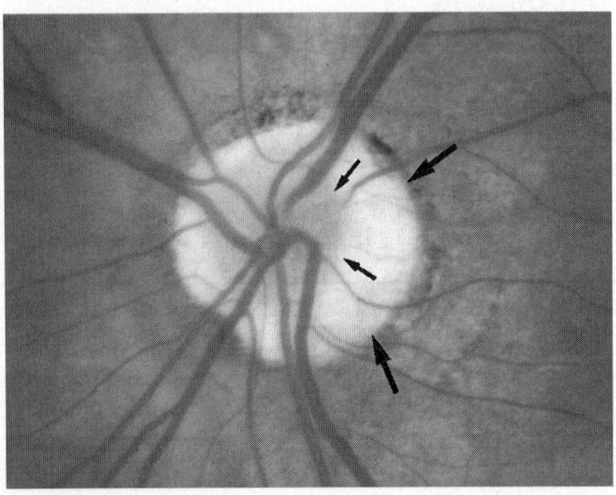

FIGURE 5–10. Optic nerve hypoplasia. The edge of the nerve is marked by the small arrows. The nerve is about one third of the normal size when judged by the vessels, which are of normal caliber. The classic double-ring sign is present and is the result of the white ring of visible bare sclera (*large arrows*) bordered by the pigment epithelium that surrounds the optic nerve. (See Color Plate 14.)

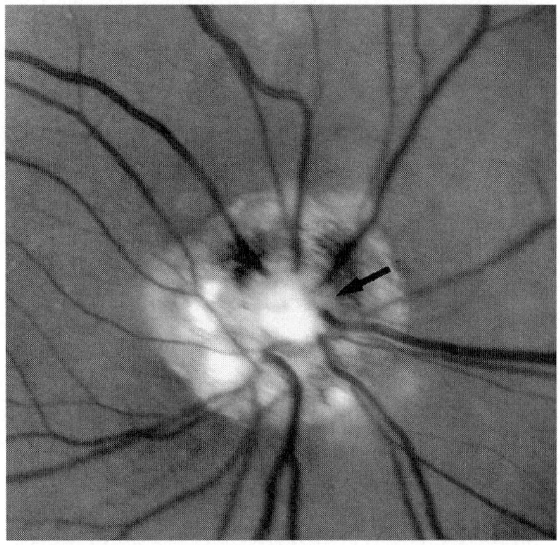

FIGURE 5–11. Optic nerve hypoplasia (*arrow on nerve edge*) accompanied by peripapillary pigmentary abnormalities and anomalous "spoke-like" takeoff of the retinal vessels.

may also be seen in this disorder. In addition, in 1970 Hoyt and colleagues[40] reported the association of septo-optic dysplasia and pituitary dwarfism. Since then, the symptom complex of optic nerve hypoplasia and hypopituitarism has been well recognized and well studied.[41] Growth hormone (GH) deficiency is the most common endocrinologic abnormality, but decreased secretion of thyroid stimulating hormone (TSH), corticotropin (ACTH), luteinizing hormone (LH), follicular stimulating hormone (FSH), and antidiuretic hormone (ADH) may be seen individually or in combination.[42, 43] Although hypopituitarism occurs only in a minority of patients with optic nerve hypoplasia, the consequences can be devastating. In one series of patients with bilateral optic nerve hypoplasia,[44] 11.5% had panhypopituitarism. In addition, at least five cases of sudden death have been reported,[45] each attributed to the affects of corticotropin deficiency, thermoregulatory disturbances, and diabetes insipidus. Hypopituitarism often correlates neuroradiologically with the presence of posterior ectopic pituitary tissue, usually seen as an abnormal area of hyperintensity at or near the tuber cinereum on T_1-weighted MR images (Fig. 5–12),[46] or absence of the normal posterior pituitary bright spot.[47] In one purported mechanism,[34] posterior pituitary ectopia is attributed to a perinatal insult to the hypophyseal portal system, resulting in necrosis of the infundibulum. However, other au-

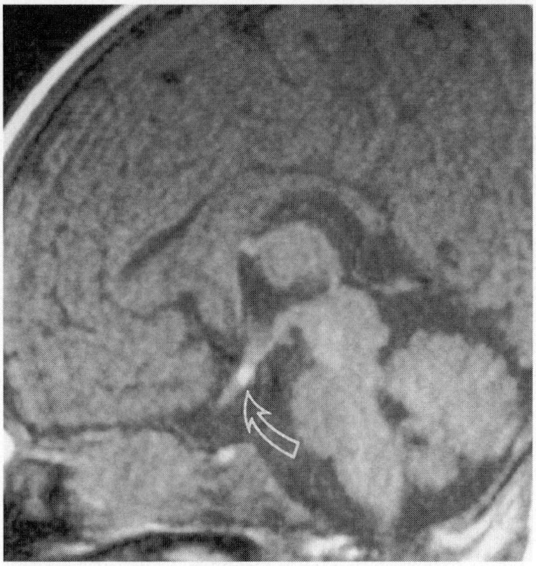

FIGURE 5–12. Ectopic pituitary tissue in a patient with septo-optic dysplasia. Note the increased signal intensity (*arrow*), indicating ectopic posterior pituitary tissue, at the tuber cinereum.

thors have suggested an earlier dysembryogenesis of the developing optic nerves and pituitary stalk.[48]

Septo-optic dysplasia is also associated with schizencephaly, a cortical migrational abnormality producing cerebral clefts extending from and including the ventricular lining to cortical surface (Fig. 5–13). Schizencephaly may manifest clinically with developmental delay, contralateral hemiparesis, and seizures. Kuban et al.[49] have suggested that the combination of septo-optic dysplasia and schizencephaly may result from a perinatal insult at or around the sixth week of embryogenesis, at which time cerebral morphogenesis, development of the eye, and delineation of the lamina terminalis, which forms the septum pellucidum, take place. Other associated cortical migrational abnormalities seen in association with optic nerve hypoplasia include cortical heterotopias and pachygyria.[46] An in-utero vascular insult, involving the distribution of the proximal trunk of the anterior cerebral artery, has also been proposed as a mechanism.[50]

A wide variety of congenital ocular syndromes have been recognized to occur with optic nerve hypoplasia. These include colobomas, Duane's syndrome, albinism, aniridia, Goldenhar syndrome, Aicardi syndrome, hemifacial atrophy, Klippel–Trenaunay–Weber syndrome, microphthalmos, and blepharophimosis.[51] Optic nerve hypoplasia may also occur in association with congenital suprasellar tumors such as craniopharyngiomas, chiasmal/hypothalamic gliomas,[52] and teratomas.[53] The mechanism in these cases is thought to be tumor compression of the visual pathways early in life, precluding normal optic nerve development. Optic nerve hypoplasia has also been recognized as a consequence of maternal use of alcohol (fetal alcohol syndrome), cocaine, phenytoin, and lysergic acid diethylamide (LSD).

A peculiar variant is superior segmental optic nerve hypoplasia, which can occur for unclear reasons in children of diabetic mothers.[54] One study[55] found 8.8% of offspring at risk had this condition, but it may also occur without a history of maternal diabetes.[56] Inferior visual field defects are detected in patients who are usually asymptomatic or perhaps have a long history of tripping or bumping into objects at their feet. The field defect corresponds to the segmental superior hypoplasia of the optic nerve (Fig. 5–14). Typically the superior rim of the disc is thin and the central retinal artery appears to arise out of the superior portion of the disc (Fig. 5–15). There may also be abnormal peripapillary pigment superiorly.[57]

In addition, rarely, the optic nerves fail to form at all in a condition known as *optic nerve aplasia*.[58] The disorder may be uni- or bilateral, and in monocular cases is often associated in the same eye with microphthalmos in an otherwise healthy individual.[59]

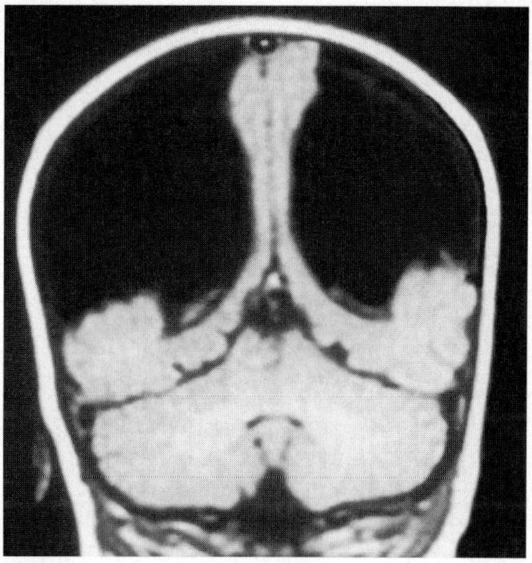

FIGURE 5–13. Coronal T_1-weighted MR images with large dark schizencephalic clefts extending to the cortical surface in a patient with septo-optic dysplasia.

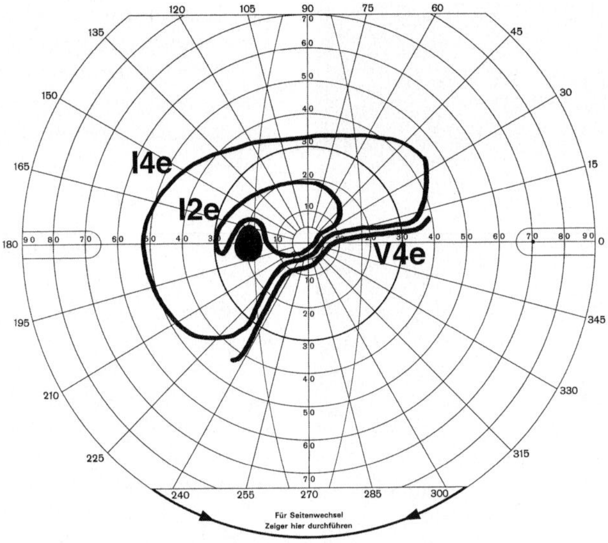

FIGURE 5–14. Kinetic Goldmann visual field from the left eye of a patient with superior segmental hypoplasia of the optic nerve head demonstrating characteristic inferior visual field loss. The patient's mother was diabetic.

Finally, the term *hypoplasia* has also been applied to the entity of homonymous hemiopic hypoplasia. This condition results from transsynaptic atrophy of the optic nerve in patients with congenital hemispheric lesions (often also associated with hemiplegia). The disc classically takes on a pattern of bow-tie atrophy in the eye contralateral to the hemispheric lesion and of subtle hypoplasia on the side of the hemispheric lesion.[60] Transsynaptic degeneration of ganglion cell axons is probably also responsible for optic nerve hypoplasia or pallor associated with periventricular leukomalacia[61] or more severe encephalomalacia due to in-utero or perinatal injury (see Chapter 8).[46]

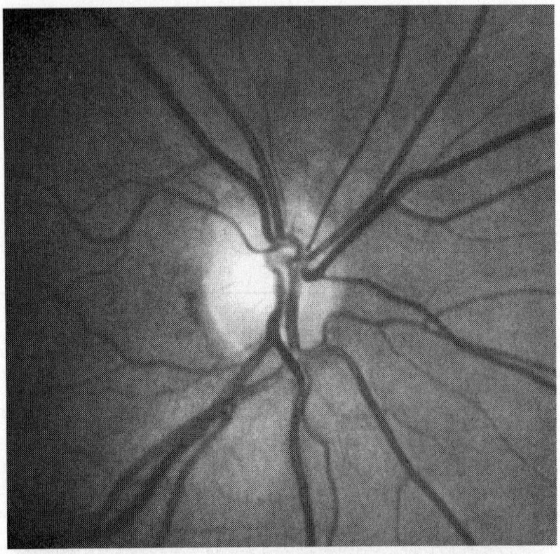

FIGURE 5–15. Optic nerve in a patient with superior segmental hypoplasia of the optic disc demonstrating only a small thin area of nerve tissue superiorly. The retinal vessels seem to arise out of the superior portion of the disc.

Evaluation. In young children, because the new diagnosis of optic nerve hypoplasia has several potential ophthalmologic, neurologic, developmental, and endocrinologic implications, in many cases a thorough clinical and radiologic assessment is mandated. Pediatric ophthalmologic evaluations are necessary for assessment and management of possible visual impairment, amblyopia, refractive error, nystagmus, and strabismus. Some authors[62] have suggested neuroradiologic and endocrinologic evaluations only in children with bilateral optic nerve hypoplasia and poor vision. However, Brodsky and Glasier's[46] careful clinicoradiologic study demonstrated that some children with unilateral optic nerve hypoplasia, who seem normal otherwise, may have absence of the septum pellucidum or posterior pituitary ectopia evident on MRI. Furthermore, these authors believed that radiographically evident pituitary ectopia could predict hypopituitarism, and callosal and hemispheric abnormalites could predict neurodevelopmental problems.

Therefore, in one approach,[46] all young children with optic nerve hypoplasia, whether uni- or bilateral, should undergo MRI with attention to the pituitary region and cortex. Those with evidence of pituitary ectopia should be referred to a pediatric endocrinologist for complete hormone screening. Radiographic demonstration of cortical migrational abnormalities or intrauterine hemispheric injury should prompt an evaluation by a pediatric neurologist. Otherwise normal adults with newly detected optic nerve hypoplasia without historical evidence of endocrinologic, neurologic, or developmental abnormalities usually need no further workup because any radiographic anomalies will be incidental.

Tilted Disc Anomaly

Tilted discs arise when the optic nerve enters the sclera at an oblique angle, and the typical crescent creates a disparity in the opening of the retina compared to the sclera. A tilted disc is common in high myopes and can associated with temporal visual field defects that do not respect the vertical meridian. On the same spectrum is nasal hypoplasia of the disc, which is not associated with any systemic condition or any specific risk factors. The discs typically appear tilted and the vessels seem to arise out of the nasal edge of the disc (Fig. 5–16; see Color Plates 15 and 16). The corresponding temporal visual field defects are important to distinguish from acquired bitemporal hemianopias. They usually demonstrate dense temporal field defects that attach to the blind spots but do not approach the vertical midline as in the field defects associated with chiasmal disease (Fig. 5–17).[63]

Optic Pits and Colobomas

Faulty closure of the embryonic fetal fissure of the optic stalk and cup may cause incomplete formation, termed a *coloboma,* of the iris, optic nerve, retina, and choroid. The anatomic defects are usually located inferiorly. Colobomatous involvement of the optic disc is highly variable, but can affect the entire nerve head. Alternatively, only the peripapillary retinal pigment epithelium and choroid are involved. Ophthalmoscopically, the typical finding is an excavated disc with sparing of the superior rim and preservation of the normal retinal vasculature (Fig. 5–18).[38] Optic disc colobomas are frequently associated with fundus colobomas.[64] Acuity and visual field loss, often superiorly, may be evident. Patients with colobomas should be investigated radiographically for the possibility of other forebrain abnormalities, especially basal encephaloceles (see below).[65, 66]

Optic pits (Fig. 5–19; see Color Plate 17) are small excavations of the neural retinal rim of the optic disc usually involving the inferotemporal portion of the optic nerve. The area of "missing" disc is often associated with a corresponding superior arcuate field defect.[67] These temporal disc abnormalities can lead to serous detachment of the macula and decreased central acuity.[68] In this setting it is believed that fluid flows from the vitreous cavity through the pit to elevate the sensory retina.

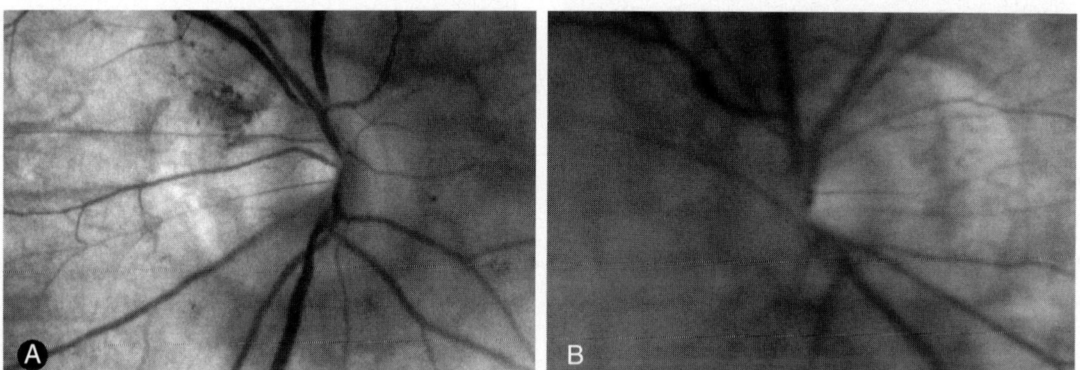

FIGURE 5–16. Right (**A**) and left (**B**) discs of a patient with nasal hypoplasia of the disc. The discs appear tilted, with the vessel origin appearing to be from the nasal portion of the disc. A peripapillary nerve fiber hemorrhage is present on the right temporal disc margin and the nasal margin of the left disc is difficult even to identify. (See Color Plates 15 and 16.)

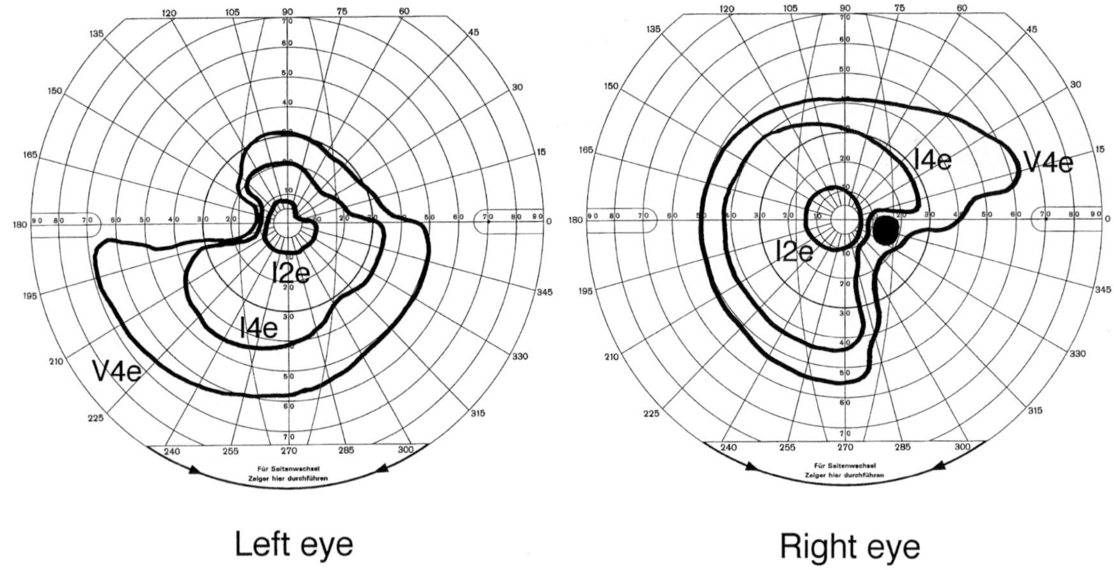

FIGURE 5–17. Goldmann visual fields of a patient with nasal hypoplasia of the discs whose fundi are pictured in Figure 5–16. There is a "pseudo-bitemporal hemianopia," as the field defects arise from or attach to the blindspot and do not respect the vertical meridian. Note the superior nasal field constriction in the left eye field.

Acquired "pit"-like defects have been described involving the temporal disc rim in patients with open angle glaucoma.[69]

It has been suggested that optic pits and colobomas share the same embryologic mechanism, with the former representing a milder variant of the latter.[38]

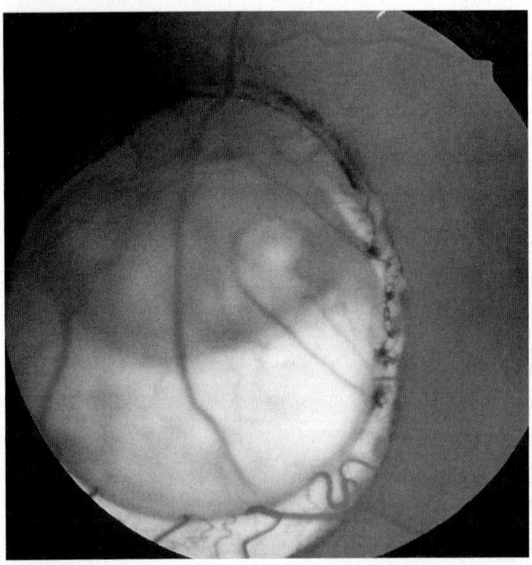

FIGURE 5–18. Extensive coloboma involving the peripapillary posterior pole. The optic nerve is seen at the superior edge of the coloboma within the excavated area.

Morning Glory Disc Anomaly

The morning glory disc is a congenital anomaly named after the flower that it resembles (Fig. 5–20). A congenital funnel-shaped excavation of the posterior fundus typically incorporates the optic disc. Other characteristic features include disc enlargment, orange color, and surrounding choroidal pigmentary disturbances.[38] The retinal vessels curve from the disc edge and travel radially, producing a

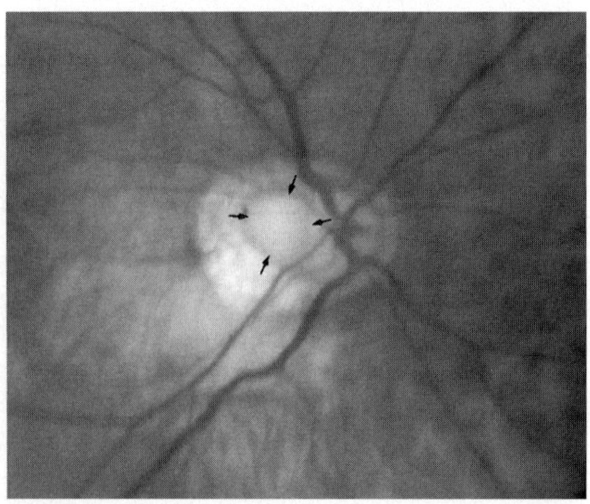

FIGURE 5–19. Optic pit appears as a grey excavation (*outlined by arrows*) in the temporal portion of the optic nerve head (see Color Plate 17).

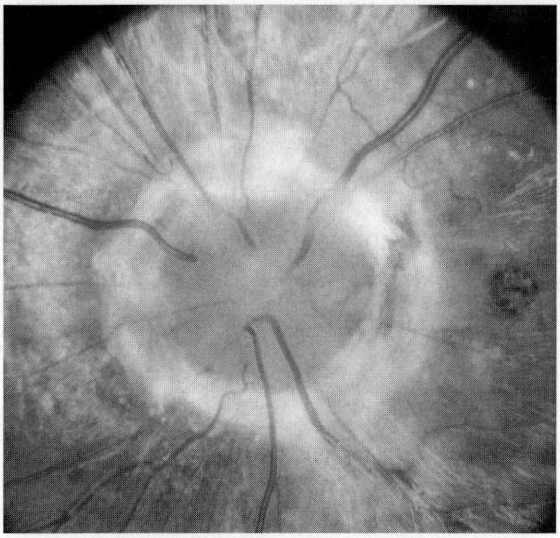

FIGURE 5–20. "Morning-glory" disc anomaly with associated retinal detachment. Note the spokelike configuration of the blood vessels and the absence of a normal central retinal artery. (See Color Plate 17.)

spokelike vessel configuration.[70] The normal central retinal vasculature is conspicuously absent ophthalmoscopically. Arteriovenous connections may branch between the major retinal vessels, sometimes creating a rosette or arcade appearance on fluorescein angiography.[71] The disc excavation is often filled with white glial tissue and vascular remnants. The vision is usually poor in the affected eye, but retinal detachments associated with the anomaly may lead to acquired visual loss (Fig. 5–20).[38]

The anomaly is likely related to defective closure of the embryonic fissure, similar to a coloboma, but others purport a mesenchymal abnormality.[38, 72] The glial and vascular abnormalities are thought to result from primary neuroectodermal dysgenesis.[38, 72]

In addition, there have been three reports[73–75] of patients with morning glory disc anomaly and moyamoya disease, which is a rare idiopathic cerebrovascular disorder characterized by progressive bilateral stenosis or occlusion of the distal internal carotid arteries and formation of a collateral vascular network in the basal ganglia region. *Moyamoya* is Japanese term for "puff of smoke," which describes the angiographic appearance of the abnormal vessels. The association of morning glory disc and moyamoya disease suggests the disc anomaly may in some cases result from intracranial vascular dysgenesis.

Morning glory disc anomaly is also associated with transsphenoidal basal encephalocele,[76] a condition that encompasses a complex series of malformations characterized by herniation of the chiasm, hypothalamus, pituitary, and anterior cerebral arteries through a bony defect in the anterior skull base. Other abnormalities include hypertelorism, depressed nasal bridge, midline upper lid notch, cleft palate, panhypopituitarism, and callosal agenesis. Herniated tissue may present as a pulsatile posterior nasal mass, and surgical removal, because of potential disasterous vascular, endocrine, and visual consequences, is for the most part contraindicated.[38] Morning glory discs are also seen in neurofibromatosis type 2.[630]

Evaluation. Patients with morning glory disc should undergo MRI to exclude a basal encephalocele, and magnetic resonance angiography should also be considered to exclude moyamoya vessels, which may place the individual at risk for cerebrovascular ischemia. Neuroimaging often demonstrates the widened, excavated nature of the optic nerve head and distal optic nerve.[77]

Staphyloma

In addition to disc colobomas and morning glory disc anomaly, staphylomas should also be considered in the differential diagnosis of excavated disc anomalies. The entire disc lies within a deep peripapillary excavation, but features that distinguish it from the other two related anomalies include a relatively normal disc, preservation of the normal retinal vasculature, and absence of a central glial tuft.[38] There are no commonly associated CNS abnormalities.

Optic Neuropathy Asssociated With Optic Disc Drusen

Pseudopapilledema, optic nerve head drusen, and their distinction from true papilledema are discussed in detail in Chapter 6. However, because visual loss associated with disc drusen is truly an optic neuropathy, it will be reviewed here.

Many patients with disc drusen are completely asymptomatic, although about 70% will have visual field defects.[78, 79] Although most patients will be identified during a funduscopic examination (Fig. 5–21), some are detected after an abnormal visual field test is obtained in the setting of vague, progressive (insidious) vision loss. Contact between disc

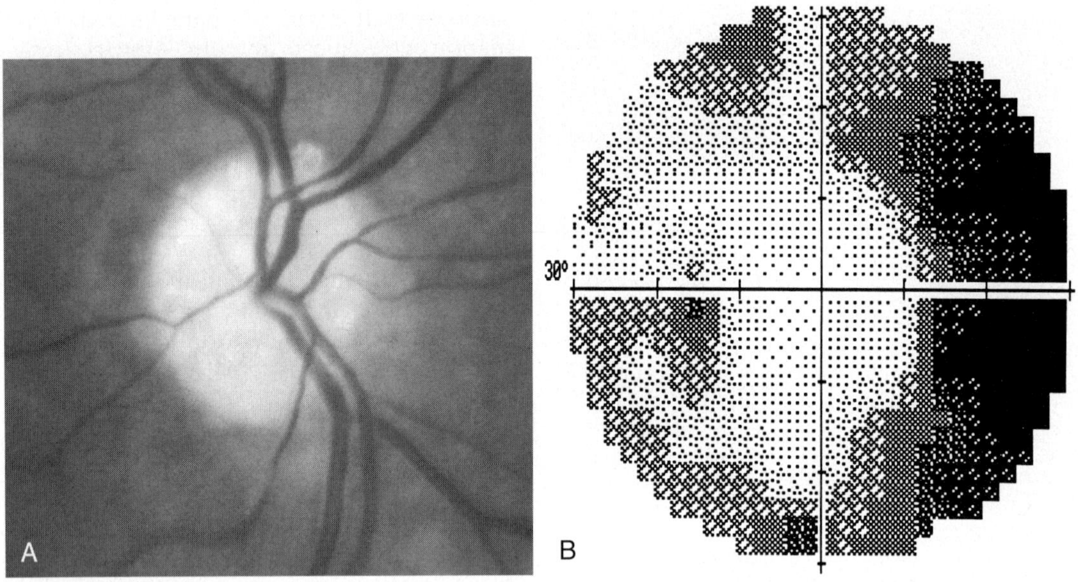

FIGURE 5–21. Field loss due to optic disc drusen. **A.** Drusen are evident and optic disc pallor has developed. **B.** Static perimetry demonstrating visual field constriction.

drusen and nearby nerve fibers presumably results in nerve fiber layer thinning[80] and axonal dysfunction. Optic nerve-type visual field defects are produced that may be progressive, but are almost never associated with central vision loss. Thus, all patients with central visual acuity loss and optic nerve head drusen should be investigated. Typical nerve fiber bundle-type defects are seen, including arcuate defects and nasal steps and optic disc pallor may develop (Fig. 5–21).

On rare occasions patients present with sudden and more catastrophic vision loss. This is most often on the basis of a superimposed ischemic optic neuropathy, which may or may not be associated with true disc edema and splinter hemorrhages (Fig 5–22; see color Plate 18).[81–86] Other ocular ischemic conditions have been observed in association with optic nerve head drusen, including central retinal artery, branch retinal artery, and central vein occlusions.

Treatment. There is no known treatment for visual loss associated with optic disc drusen. Repeat computerized visual fields over years will generally show only slight changes, and therefore can be done to comfort and reassure the patient on an annual basis. However, serial visual fields in asymptomatic patients with optic disc drusen are unnecessary. Generally, a lower threshold for glaucoma treatment should be applied in patients who coincidentally have elevated intraocular pressure and optic disc drusen. Some neuro-ophthalmologists have advocated the use of intraocular pressure-lowering agents even in the presence of a normal intraocular pressure. Optic nerve sheath fenestration appears to convey no benefit in the treatment of this disorder, but experience has been limited.

HEREDITARY OPTIC NEUROPATHIES

These represent a heterogenous group of diseases that are characterized by an inheritance pattern that may be spontaneous, recessive, dominant, or mitochondrial, and in which vision loss occurs as the result of optic nerve dysfunction. Hereditary optic neuropathies may manifest as monosymptomatic lesions or may accompany other CNS disease. They can present as subtle fixed deficits in early life (Kjer's dominant optic atrophy) or as catastrophic sequential vision loss in early adulthood (Leber's hereditary optic neuropathy (LHON)). They will be recognized in the setting of the appropriate family history, the highly suggestive clinical presentations, and, in some cases, by specific genetic testing. A variation on this theme includes patients who develop optic atrophy in association with heritable neuronal lipid storage diseases. The examiner is best served by working within a

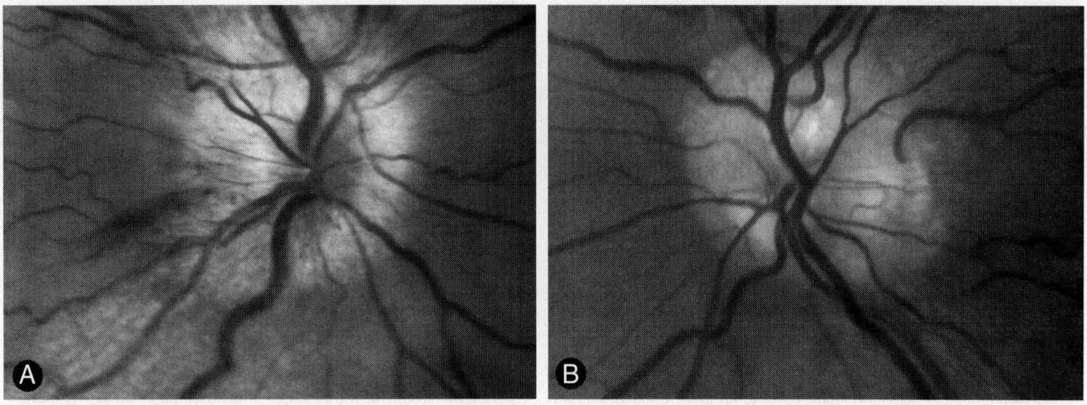

FIGURE 5–22. Optic disc drusen with associated anterior ischemic optic neuropathy. **A.** The right optic nerve is hyperemic with nerve fiber layer edema and associated splinter hemorrhages. (See Color Plate 18.) **B.** Buried disc drusen can be seen in the patient's uninvolved left eye.

framework that defines these entities on a clinical basis. Their modes of presentation and examination findings are unique. As molecular genetics continues to evolve, we will have a better understanding of the pathogenesis of these conditions, more accurate classifications, and ultimately effective gene-directed therapy.

Leber's Hereditary Optic Neuropathy

Leber's hereditary optic neuropathy typically causes a subacute, sequential optic neuropathy with visual loss in young, healthy individuals. Since the disorder was described in 1871 by Leber,[87] the clinical profile of LHON has been well established, although it is highly variable in members of the same pedigree. Men are affected more often than women and the disease usually presents in the second or third decade. Characteristic funduscopic changes are recognized in many cases, including circumpapillary telangiectatic microangiopathy, pseudoedema of the nerve fiber layer, and absence of fluorescein angiographic staining of the disc.[88] Spontaneous visual recovery may occur in some cases.[89] With knowledge of these characteristics alone, clinicians have been able to diagnose LHON with considerable accuracy.

However, it became clear from numerous pedigrees that the disease was maternally inherited. This prompted Wallace and associates to search for a cytoplasmic determinant of inheritance, and attention was focused on the mitochondrial DNA (mtDNA). A mtDNA mutation in which a nucleotide substitution occurred at position 11778 was identified in 9 of 11 families.[90, 91]

Demographics. Eighty to ninety percent of affected individuals are males.[92–95] Newman and associates found that 82% of genetically proven cases of LHON from 49 different pedigrees occurred in men.[92] The reason for this male predominance is unclear. In Newman's series, the age at onset was from age 8 to 60, with a mean of 27.6 years and with the vast majority between 26 and 37. Woman develop the disease at an older age than men in the same pedigree, however, the age at which initial symptoms occur varies.

Neuro-ophthalmic Symptoms. Leber's hereditary optic neuropathy causes an acute or subacute failure of vision in one or both eyes. The average interval between first and second eye involvement is several months, with a range from simultaneous presentation (which occurred in 55% of cases) to 9 months.[92] Many simultaneous cases may represent sequential involvement of the eyes in which the attack in the first eye went unrecognized. The vision loss is usually painless although headache occasionally occurs. Uhthoff's symptom (worsening of vision associated with elevation of body temperature, see optic neuritis, below) has been reported in LHON.[88, 92]

Neuro-ophthalmic Signs. Patients present with signs of an acute optic neuropathy, with loss of central vision and dyschromatopsia. Visual acuity measurements reflect the dense central field defect, are typically between 5/200 and 20/200, and only rarely are reduced to the hand movements or light perception level. Total blindness from LHON is exceedingly unusual. Visual field testing shows a central or centrocecal scotoma in virtually all cases. Although pupillary light reflexes had been thought to be normal, more definitive studies have demonstrated that afferent pupillary defects are typically present when visual loss is unilateral or asymmetric.[96, 97] This issue is still controversial, however, as some investigators have suggested that pupillary afferent fibers are relatively spared compared to those mediating vision.[631]

The classic disc appearance in patients with acute LHON was emphasized by Smith, Hoyt and Susac in 1973.[88] Leber commented on tortuosity of vessels and "white-striated opacity" in the peripapillary region. Findings also include circumpapillary telangiectatic microangiopathy, pseudoedema, or swelling with hyperemia of the nerve fiber layer around the disc (Fig 5–23; see Color Plate 19), and the absence of true edema or staining of the disc on fluorescein angiography. If these features are identified, the physician can confidently diagnose LHON, confirm this with genetic testing, and spare the patient additional invasive testing looking for other acute causes of optic neuropathy. These findings can also be used to identify patients within a family at risk for developing the disease as they are present in a subset of patients who are in the preclinical phase of the disease.[93, 95, 98] About two thirds of the male and one third of the female asymptomatic descendants of affected females have the characteristic fundus changes.

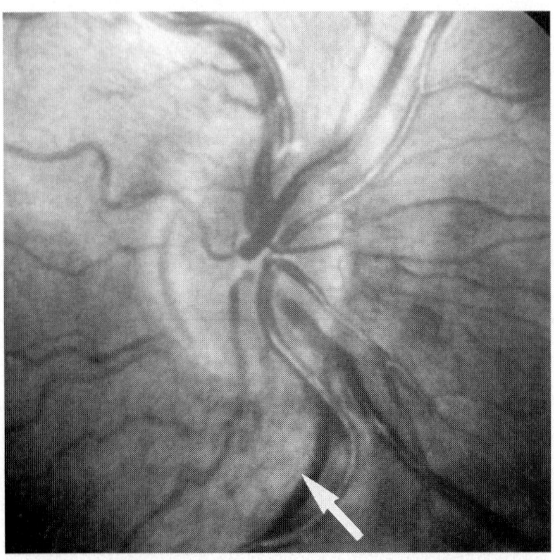

FIGURE 5–23. The typical appearance of the optic nerve in acute Leber's hereditary optic neuropathy. The disc appears hyperemic with dilated surface capillaries and haziness to the nerve fiber layer best seen inferiorly (*arrow*). (See Color Plate 19.)

However, there are many cases in which the acute nerve fiber layer and vascular changes are absent, and the disc may have a normal appearance. LHON patients subsequently develop optic atrophy regardless of the fundus appearance acutely. After the onset of optic atrophy, it is difficult to identify patients with LHON because pseudopapilledema and telangiecstasis have resolved (Fig. 5–24). Trobe and associates[33] showed fundus photographs of nine different categories of optic atrophy to ophthalmologists and found that in the 16 cases of LHON the diagnostic accuracy ranged from 0% to 38%. Therefore, because the acute changes are often absent and the late changes are not diagnostic, the diagnosis of LHON should never be dismissed solely on the basis of the appearance of the nerve. Fortunately, improvement of vision is not rare and occurs with different frequencies depending on the specific mutation (see below). The reported frequency of visual recovery is between 4% and 32%.[92, 93]

Cerebrospinal fluid (CSF) analysis and electroretinography are not helpful. Visual evoked responses showed prolonged latency and reduced amplitude and have been reported to also be abnormal in some asymptomatic relatives of LHON patients.[95]

Other Associated Signs and Symptoms. The ophthalmoscopically visible local changes have led many to conclude that there are unique features that place the intraocular optic nerve and perhaps only the papillomacular bundle ganglion cells at greatest risk for damage in LHON. However, the association of LHON with other conditions and the results of ancillary testing suggest alternatively that more may be occurring than is seen ophthalmoscopically. Magnetic resonance imaging, particularly with short-time inversion recovery (STIR) sequences, demonstrated optic nerve high-signal abnormalities in each of eight patients examined with this technique.[99] The MR images of the brains in these patients were all normal. However, nonspecific white matter lesions have been observed on MRI scans of other affected individuals. Gadolinium enhancement of the optic nerve can occur but is unusual.[648]

Although rare, comitant neurologic disease has been asociated with LHON. A disease resembling multiple sclerosis has also been re-

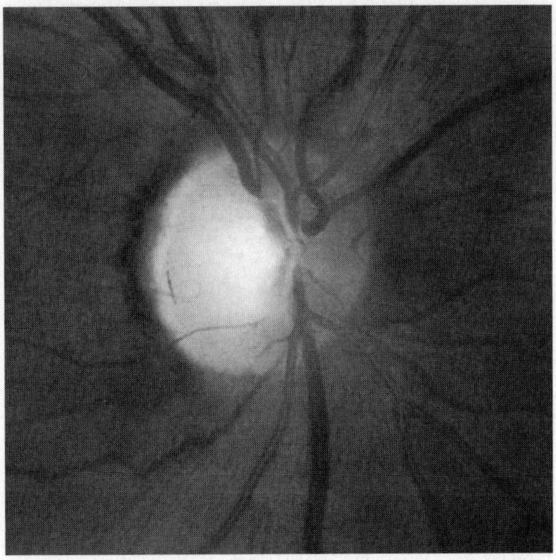

FIGURE 5–24. The right atrophic optic nerve of a patient with Leber's hereditary optic neuropathy who had presented 6 months earlier. There is typically temporal pallor with loss of nerve fibers in the papillomacular bundle.

ported to occur with LHON.[98, 100, 101] In Newman's series,[92] 3 of 72 LHON patients also had a peripheral neuropathy.

Cardiac conduction defects and arrhythmias and skeletal deformities have been associated with LHON. Abnormal electrocardiograms (ECGs), specifically, conduction abnormalities, have been convincingly demonstrated in various pedigrees.[102, 103] Wolff–Parkinson–White and Lown–Ganong–Levine were the most common abnormalities found. Other ECG abnormalities included, Q waves, atrial fibrillation, bundle branch blocks and ventricular hypertrophy. In Newman's series,[92] 17 patients had ECGs, 14 were normal, 1 had supraventricular tachycardia, 1 premature ventricular contractions, and 1 a short QT interval.[92] It is important to recognize that cardiac disease is often asymptomatic and can be found in patients with no evidence of optic neuropathy. LHON patients have been found to have skeletal deformities, including congenital hip dislocation, arachnodactyly, pes cavus, talipes equinovarus, kyphoscoliosis, arched palate, and spondyloepiphyseal dysplasia.

Mitochondrial Genetics. Because mothers transmit LHON vertically to all their offspring, and males do not pass on the disease, mitochondrial inheritance became the most plausible explanation. Mitochondria are intracytoplasmic organelles and because the oocyte contributes all the cytoplasm of the developing zygote, all mitochondria are inherited from the mother. Only daughters will pass on the mitochondria to their descendants. Mitochondria are unique among cellular organelles because they contain their own DNA. The mitochondrial matrix, in addition to containing enzymes and an apparatus for transcription and translation, has 2 to 10 copies of a double-stranded circular DNA of about 16.5 kilobases and contains 37 genes that are essential to the respiratory chain. Mitochondria contain ribosomes and therefore are able to synthesize the proteins encoded by their DNA.

Examination of the mitochondrial genome in patients with LHON led to the discovery of a point mutation by Wallace and associates in 1988.[91] The guanine to adenine substitution results in a subtle change of the basic amino acid arginine to histidine. The result is an abnormal subunit 4 (ND4) of the NADH dehydrogenase:coenzyme Q1 reductase subunit (complex I), which is the first enzyme in the pathway of oxidative phosphorylation. The 11778 mutation has been identified in numerous other pedigrees and singleton cases. These seemingly unrelated pedigrees and the sporadic, nonfamilial occurrence of LHON suggest that the mutation can arise spontaneously. However, the 11778 mutation alone is not a sufficient explanation for all cases of LHON. Since that time, causative mutations at position 3460 and 14484 have been identified.[104–106] These mutations affect the ND1 and ND6 subunit genes of complex I, respectively.[107–109]

Alone, these mutations do not explain the variable occurrence of the disease within the same pedigree, its wide spectrum of phenotypic expression, and the susceptibility of male offspring. Variable phenotypic expression of the mtDNA mutation is, as of now, unexplained. The three theories that have been advanced to explain this are: (1) heteroplasmy (coexistence of mutant and normal mtDNA), (2) a second genetic factor possibly on the X chromosome, and finally, (3) environmental factors. It is most likely that all of these factors contribute to the phenotypic expression of the disease. Consideration should therefore be given to tissue-specific factors and environmental contributions to optic atrophy. The nerve cells of the eye and CNS are most dependent on mitochondrial ATP. Ganglion cell axons may have a point at which energy is insufficient to run cellular pumps and allow for adequate protein synthesis. External factors capable of damaging oxidative phosphorylation, such as cyanide poisoning (cigarette smoking), alcohol, and environmental toxins, may also contribute to the onset of visual loss. None of these predictably accompany the acute visual deterioration in affected individuals, but it seems feasible that they can alter "genetically programmed" cell death.

Treatment. There is no known effective treatment or prophylaxis for the visual loss that occurs with LHON. Steroids, cyanide antagonists, and hydroxycobalamin have been tried without effect. Some physicians recommend that family members in LHON pedigrees and patients affected in one eye with LHON avoid tobacco and heavy alcohol use. Some success has been reported in other diseases that affect mitochondrial energy production with the use of cofactors such as succinate and coenzyme Q.[110–112] However, their value in treating or preventing of LHON remains to be proved.

Genetic Testing. The discovery of the mtDNA mutation that is responsible for LHON has raised as many questions as it has answered. The test is highly specific, with no false positives. Definitive molecular genetic diagnosis can help to avoid the emotional pain and expense of extensive diagnostic evaluations and treatment in patients with LHON. This can be particularly helpful in sporadic cases. The precise genetic testing will help us to define better the clinical profile of LHON patients. It is well recognized that the rate of spontaneous recovery is highest in patients with the 14484 mutation and lowest in those with the 11778 mutation.

Awareness of the specific defect in energy production may help in the development of specific therapies aimed at bypassing or lessening the impact of the defect. Genetic counseling can be offered if the mutation is identified. Finally, the discovery of the mutation in LHON will serve as a model for investigation of other diseases suspected of being transmitted by mtDNA.

Dominant Optic Atrophy

In his description of 19 affected families, Kjer reported the details of a dominantly inherited optic neuropathy that now bears his name.[113] Patients typically present before the end of the first decade of life with the insidious onset of bilateral (although often asymmetric) vision loss. Acuities range from 20/20 to 20/200, and patients typically have central and centrocecal visual field defects with intact peripheral isopters.[114] Forty percent of patients retain acuity, of 20/60 or better.[113] Presentation with nystagmus is uncommon. Visual loss usually does not progress once the patient reaches the second decade of life.[115] Color vision loss typically occurs along the blue–yellow or tritanopic axis (see Chapter 2).[116, 117] The associated optic disc pallor often takes on a striking wedgelike appearance with temporal excavation of the neuroretinal rim (Fig. 5–25), although the whole disc sometimes is pale.

Since the disease is dominantly inherited, examination of first-degree relatives often aids in the diagnosis of patients suspected of having dominant optic atrophy. Because of the highly variable degree of visual dysfunction, seemingly asymptomatic adult and child relatives can often be identified if visual acuity or color loss or optic atrophy is present. Recently pedigree analysis has identified the gene implicated in Kjer's. First, linkage analyses mapped the defect to the chromosome 3q region.[118] More recently this has been confirmed at the 3q27-3q28 chromosome.[119, 120] This has allowed for more accurate identification of symptomatic and asymptomatic carriers.[114, 121, 122] A much less common locus on 18q12.2-12.3 has also been identified.[123, 632]

Treatment. There is no known effective treatment at this time. Histopathologic studies have demonstrated diffuse loss of retinal ganglion cells, suggesting primary ganglion cell death as the mechanism of disease.[124] Spontaneous improvement has not been reported. Patients should be screened for sensory neural hearing

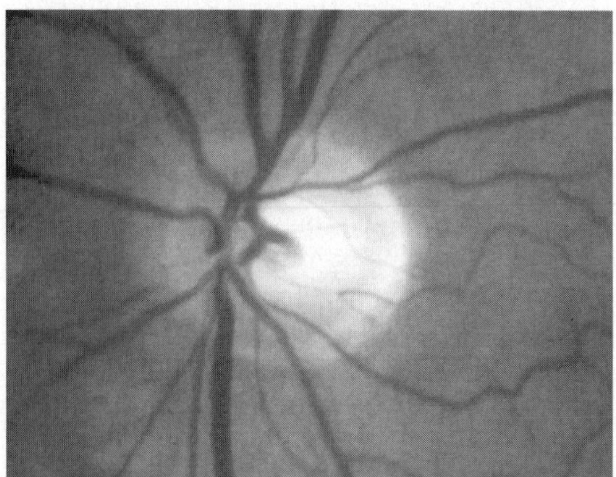

FIGURE 5–25. Optic nerve appearance in dominantly inherited optic neuropathy (Kjer's) with a wedge of pallor and excavation involving the temporal portion of the optic nerve.

loss as this occurs with increased frequency in this subgroup of patients.[117] When dominant optic atrophy is considered in children without affected family members, compressive lesions and other causes of optic neuropathy with pallor should be excluded.

Recessive Optic Atrophy

Both simple (isolated) and complex (associated defects) forms of recessively inherited optic neuropathy exist. As is typical of most genetic conditions, the recessive form of hereditary optic atrophy is generally much more severe than the dominant form. Patients present in early childhood (age 2 to 4) with more profound visual acuity loss and searching nystagmus.[125] There is often a history of parental consanguinity. Visual acuity is usually stable, and whether this occurs congenitally is unknown. There is usually diffuse disc pallor and attenuation of retinal vessels. Distinction from photoreceptor dysfunction in Leber's congenital amaurosis can be accomplished with electroretinography, which should be normal in recessive optic atrophy. Complicated, recessive optic atrophy, when associated with spinocerebellar degeneration, cerebellar ataxia, pyramidal tract dysfunction, and mental retardation, is termed *Behr syndrome*.[126] Some regard this as part of the continuum of optic atrophy associated with hereditary ataxias.[127]

Wolfram (DIDMOAD) Syndrome

Wolfram syndrome or DIDMOAD (*d*iabetes *i*nsipidus, *d*iabetes *m*ellitus, *o*ptic *a*trophy, and *d*eafness) syndrome encompasses the above findings and presents in childhood or adolescence.[128, 129] There is a great degree of variability in presentation but the hallmark is optic atrophy with progressive vision and hearing loss in a juvenile-onset diabetic. Other reported abnormalities include ptosis, ataxia, seizures, mental retardation, nystagmus, abnormal electroretinogram, abnormal CSF protein, and short stature. Neuropathologic studies have demonstrated atrophy of the optic, chiasm, brain stem, and cerebellum.[130, 131] The inheritance pattern is autosomal recessive or sporadic, but the possibility that Wolfram syndrome is a mitochondrial disorder has also been suggested.

Optic Atrophy Associated With Neurologic and Metabolic Disease

Optic atrophy and progressive visual dysfunction frequently accompanies a variety of other inherited, degenerative neurologic conditions (Table 5–5). In each of these conditions progressive visual loss occurs, with dyschromatopsia, central or centrocecal field defects, and optic atrophy. Visual loss progresses along with the systemic neurologic syndrome but vision loss usually remains moderate. Optic atrophy occurs in conjunction with spinocerebellar degenerations (see Chapter 16), ataxias, and sensory motor peripheral neuropathies. Friedreich's ataxia[132, 133] and Charcot–Marie–Tooth disease[134] are classic neurologic syndromes associated with optic atrophy. Progressive optic atrophy is also recognized in patients with congenital deafness.[135, 136] More recently, primary retinal degenerations have been recognized to occur in conjunction with these inherited ataxias (see Chapter 4).

Lysosomal storage diseases (inherited deficiency of an enzyme required for normal metabolism of lysosomal macromolecules) are associated with a variety of ocular manifestations. In particular, optic atrophy results from ganglion cell damage from these accumulated materials. The conditions most commonly associated with optic atrophy are the mucopolysaccharidoses (Hurler and Scheie syndromes) and the lipidoses (gangliosidosis, Tay–Sachs, Niemann–Pick (see Chap-

TABLE 5–5. Metabolic and Degenerative Neurologic Diseases Associated With Optic Atrophy

Ataxias[623]
Spinocerebellar degenerations (SCAs—see Chapter 15)[624]
Friedreich's ataxia
Charcot–Marie–Tooth disease
Olivopontocerebellar atrophy
Mucopolysaccharidoses
Hurler
Scheie
Hunter A, B
Sanfilippo A, B
Morquio
Maroteaux-Lamy A
Lipidoses
Tay–Sachs
Adrenoleukodystrophy
Metachromatic leukodystrophy
Generalized gangliosidosis
Juvenile gangliosidosis
Niemann–Pick A
Krabbe's disease
Pelizaeus–Merzbacher disease

ter 16), adrenoleukodystrophy (see Chapter 8), and metachromatic leukodystrophy). These are also discussed in Chapter 4.

INFLAMMATORY OPTIC NEUROPATHIES

The inflammatory optic neuropathies represent a heterogeneous group of conditions characterized by acute or subacute, often painful, vision loss that results from inflammation of the optic nerve. Inflammatory optic neuropathies are the most common causes of optic neuropathy in young adults. The term *optic neuritis* has come to have an even more specific implication: inflammatory optic neuropathy that accompanies demyelinating disease. Other inflammatory optic neuropathies include contiguous spread of inflammation from meninges, sinuses, and orbital soft tissues. These processes may be immune mediated, granulomatous, or infectious. Some patients may be labeled as having papillitis (a nonspecific term) when the inflammatory process leads to optic nerve-head swelling.

Optic Neuritis

The vast majority of patients with inflammatory optic neuropathy have optic neuritis, a nerve inflammation secondary to demyelination. In many patients optic neuritis is the heralding manifestation of multiple sclerosis.[137]

The Optic Neuritis Treatment Trial (ONTT)[138] has provided the best prospective data regarding the clinical presentation, outcome with respect to treatment, and development of multiple sclerosis in patients with optic neuritis. The benefit of treatment with oral or intravenous (IV) steroids had never been investigated by a randomized, prospective, masked trial. Along with the answer to this question came the most accurate and detailed recording of the clinical symptoms and measured visual function in patients with optic neuritis.

The study was multicentered and entered 448 patients that were treated either with oral placebo, IV steroids followed by an oral steroids taper, or oral steroids alone. Each patient had a detailed history review and a careful ophthalmic and neurologic examination. Visual acuity, color vision, contrast sensitivity, and Humphrey and Goldmann visual fields were recorded for each patient. Every patient had blood work for syphilis and lupus, and a fraction that consented underwent lumbar puncture. Patients were followed for all four of the measurable visual parameters and for the development of clinically definite multiple sclerosis.

Demographics. Patients with optic neuritis are typically young, with a peak incidence in the third and fourth decade (9 to 60), and more women than men are affected.[139, 140] In the ONTT, 77% of the patients were women, 85% were white, and the mean age was 32. The prevalence of optic neuritis varies to some extent based on geography and race. Several studies have looked at the incidence of optic neuritis, and in general the range is between 1 and 6 new cases per year per 100,000 population.[141, 142] In the US study (Rochester, Minn.) the rate was 6.4 new cases annually per 100,000 population.[141] It is clear that rates vary with race, geography, and latitude, with whites of northern European ancestry at latitudes away from the equator being most susceptible. Whites of Mediterranean ancestry are less commonly affected, and in African-Americans and Asians the condition is relatively uncommon. Some studies have demonstrated a seasonal pattern to its incidence.[633]

Neuro-ophthalmic Symptoms. Vision loss is rapid in onset, generally being recognized over a period of hours to a few days. Symptoms commonly reported by optic neuritis patients are summarized in Table 5–6. Vision loss can progress for up to 1 to 2 weeks. Reduced color vision invariably accompanies the vision loss in optic neuritis. Patients frequently report a darkening or reduced vividness of color. Red objects may be described as either pinker or browner in patients with dyschromatopsia.

Characteristic pain precedes the vision loss by a few days and is present in the majority of patients (92% in the ONTT).[140] Globe tenderness and worsening of pain on eye movements

TABLE 5–6. Common Symptoms in Optic Neuritis

Decreased vision
Visual field defects
Reduced color vision
Uhthoff's symptom
Decreased depth perception
Pain
Phosphenes
Movement induced
Sound induced

are typical.[143] The exact origin of the pain is unknown but presumably pain is the result of the pulling on the dura (in contact with the inflamed nerve) by the eye muscle origin from the annulus of Zinn. Because this pain characteristically disappears after 3 to 5 days, pain persisting for longer then 7 days should be considered atypical and prompt an investigation for other causes of pain and optic neuropathy such as a systemic inflammatory condition, scleritis, malignant glioma, orbital inflammatory syndrome, aneurysm, or a sinus mucocele.

Phosphenes or flashing lights described by patients with optic neuritis generally take a variety of forms, including lights, sparkles, and shifting squares. They may be exacerbated by eye movements or loud noises.[144, 145] These symptoms were present in 30% of patients in the ONTT.[140] These phosphenes can accompany the acute loss of vision and can also persist for months after resolution. They are not unique to inflammatory optic neuropathies but can occur in the setting of compressive lesions as well. The presence of phosphenes should also raise the possibility of concomitant retinal disease, as in neuroretinitis.

Uhthoff's symptom is transient visual obscuration associated with elevation in body temperature.[146–148] The symptom can be provoked by as little as hot food or cooking but most typically is brought on by physical exertion or a hot shower.[147] Vision loss generally takes the form of blurring, greying, or reduced color vision and begins minutes after exposure to heat. Minutes to 1 hour later, vision returns to baseline without residua. This symptom is not unique to optic neuritis patients and has been described in hereditary, toxic, compressive,[149] and sarcoid[150] optic neuropathies. Uhthoff's symptom tends to relapse and remit, and return of the symptom after a period of time does not necessarily herald the onset of recurrent inflammation. For unclear reasons, the presence of Uhthoff's symptom may be a poor prognostic indicator as it correlates with white matter lesions on MRI and with the subsequent development of multiple sclerosis and recurrent optic neuritis.[147]

Neuro-ophthalmic Signs (Table 5–7). Patients typically have reduced visual acuity ranging from nearly normal to NLP. In the ONTT,[138, 140] 10% of patients had 20/20 vision, 25% had between 20/25 and 20/40 acuity, 29% were 20/50 to 20/190 and 36% were between 20/200 and NLP.

TABLE 5–7. Common Examination Findings in Optic Neuritis

Visual acuity loss
Dyschromatopsia
Reduced contrast sensitivity
Reduced stereoacuity
Visual field loss
Global reduced sensitivity
Central or centrocecal defects
Altitudinal defects
Afferent pupillary defect
Normal or swollen optic nerve

Dyschromatopsia can usually easily identified by testing with pseudoisochromatic color plates and noting asymmetry between the eyes. More sensitive and extensive testing can be done with the Farnsworth–Munsell 100-hue test, but in clinical practice this is unnecessary. In one series, dyschromatopsia was detected in all patients using the 100-hue test compared to only half of the patients tested with the Ishihara plates.[151] However, in the ONTT the 100-hue test was only modestly more sensitive than the Ishihara plates in detecting dyschromatopsia (88% abnormal by plates and 94% abnormal by the 100-hue test).[140] Further analysis of these data identified certain trends concerning the type of color vision loss (blue/yellow versus red/green at presentation and then after recovery). Ultimately Katz[152] concluded that no specific type of color defect was predictably associated with optic neuritis and that the type of defect can change in the course of recovery. Subjective intereye differences can usually be brought out by asking patients to describe their perception of these plates or a red test object.

Contrast sensitivity was measurably abnormal in 98% of patients in the ONTT when compared to age-matched controls.[140] In fact, contrast sensitivity in optic neuritis was found to be the most sensitive indicator of visual dysfunction in acute and recovered optic neuritis.[153]

Patients with optic neuritis almost always have some visual field loss. On manual kinetic perimetry, the most common visual field defects in optic neuritis are central scotomas. The ONTT used computer static threshold perimetry as their standard and found 45% of the patients had diffuse field loss and 55% had local defects.[29] Of these localized visual field defects, the most common were altitudinal defects (29%) and "three-quadrant defects" (14%). Combined, central, and centrocecal defects occurred in 16% of patients. Overall these patterns of visual field loss represent the full spectrum of "optic nerve"-type field defects and do not aid the examiner in distinguishing optic neuritis from other causes of optic nerve dysfunction.[154]

The ONTT carefully studied fellow eye abnormalities in patients with acute unilateral optic neuritis.[155] Visual field defects were the most common (48% of patients) although abnormalities in acuity, color vision, and contrast sensitivity were also identified. Most of these deficits resolved over several months. Because all of the abnormal visual function parameters tended to improve with time, they were not thought to be false positives or spurious results. The question remains as to whether these represent subtle simultaneous bilateral attacks or unrecognized previous attacks. Also, whether these patients with bilateral findings are at increased risk of developing multiple sclerosis is uncertain.

On the fundus examination about one third of patients have mild optic nerve-head swelling[140, 156] (Fig. 5–26; see Color Plate 20). This finding is generally much less marked than the swelling in papilledema, and it is less sectoral and unassociated with the capillary dilation and splinter hemorrhages typical of anterior ischemic optic neuropathy.[140] Less than 5% of patients have retinal exudates, phlebitis, or vitreous cells.[140] Extensive vitritis and retinal vein sheathing is unusual in optic neuritis and in this setting alternative diagnoses such as sarcoidosis and syphilis should be considered. Patients with typical optic neuritis do not later develop a macular "star." Such stars are more consistent with neuroretinitis (see below), a condition that is believed not to be a precursor of multiple sclerosis.

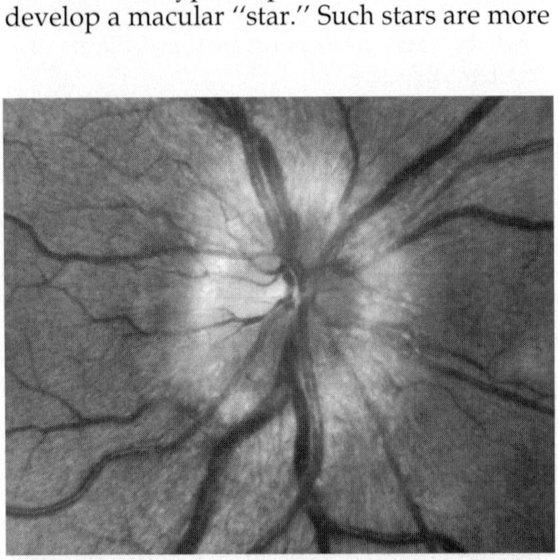

FIGURE 5–26. Optic nerve appearance in a patient with optic neuritis. Note the mild diffuse swelling and the absence of hemorrhages, cotton-wool spots, and exudates. (See Color Plate 20.)

Diagnostic Studies. The ONTT demonstrated that in typical patients (young patients with subacute vision loss and pain on eye movements), no laboratory test (blood studies, lumbar puncture, or MRI) aided in the diagnosis of idiopathic optic neuritis. These tests were done on patients entering the study, and they did not alter the course, treatment, or ultimate visual outcome of any of the patients.[140] However, the study did demonstrate a potential value for MRI in identifying patients at increased risk of developing multiple sclerosis.

Magnetic resonance imaging scan abnormalities consistent with plaques in the white matter of patients with optic neuritis are well recognized (Fig. 5–27).[157, 158] Abnormalities and enhancement are the result of breakdown of the blood–brain barrier. In the ONTT, 59% of patients with a previous normal neurologic history had clinically silent white matter lesions.[159] The most typical findings are small, T_2 hyperintense lesions in the periventricular white matter, subcortical white matter, and pons.[160] Enhancement of the lesions on T_1 images indicates active plaques. These findings may be nonspecific and have been seen in "normal" patients and patients with other systemic inflammatory conditions. They are present in approximately 90% of patients with clinically definite multiple sclerosis.[161, 162] To some extent, the presence and number of white matter lesions depends on the MR technique used. New modifications include the use of STIR (short-term inversion recovery) and FLAIR (fluid level attenuated inversion recovery) sequences, which increase the sensitivity of detecting these white matter lesions.[163–165] In the ONTT,[159] patients' MRI scans were graded from 0 to IV depending on the number of typical white matter signal abnormalities. Only, 41% of patients had normal studies. The significance of the baseline MRI scans is discussed below in the section on optic neuritis' relationship to multiple sclerosis.

Over 80% of patients with optic neuritis have demonstrable lesions in the affected optic nerve using STIR sequences with fat-suppressed views of the orbit and a orbital surface coil[158] (Fig. 5–28). It has been shown that poor visual prognosis may correlate with optic nerve lesion size and location in the optic canal.[158, 166] The lesions in the canal may be the most damaging because the tight bony canal

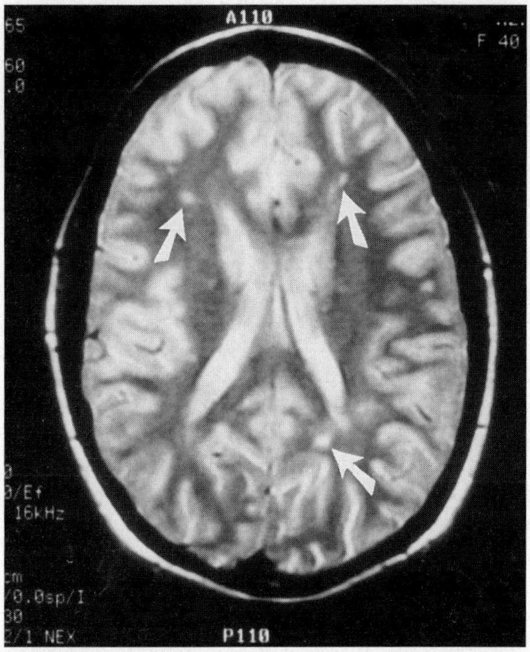

FIGURE 5–27. Axial T_2-weighted MRI scan of the brain in a patient with acute optic neuritis demonstrating numerous bright signal abnormalities (*arrows*), consistent with demyelination, in the periventricular white matter.

causes secondary compression as the nerve swells. This site is relatively uncommon, as the anterior and mid orbital portions of the optic nerve are most frequently involved. Enhancement of the lesion with gadolinium indicates an active process. When recovery occurs with the restoration of the blood–brain barrier, the nerve no longer enhances with gadolinium.

Visual evoked potentials (VEPs) are only an extension of the neuro-ophthalmic examination and should not be used to make a diagnosis of optic neuritis in the setting of unexplained vision loss. Although changes in the VEPs can provide objective information to help confirm the diagnosis of optic neuritis, the diagnosis will always be a clinical one. In general, the occipital pattern VEPs will show marked latency changes with amplitude changes that generally correlate with the level of acuity loss. Usually the hallmark of optic neuritis would be markedly prolonged latency (p100) with relative preservation of amplitude. Other optic neuropathies (presumably with more direct axonal injury) generally have lower amplitudes with less effect on latency. Despite these generalizations there is significant overlap and variability,[167, 168] and therefore, we never use or recommend VEPs in the routine diagnosis or management of acute optic neuropathies. Recovery of the latency and improved conduction speed reflect recovery of the blockade due to inflammatory changes and edema. Recovery is not believed to be on the basis of remyelination.[169]

Although popular in the past, lumbar punctures and CSF analysis were found to be unnecessary in the initial evaluation of patients with typical isolated optic neuritis because they neither changed the diagnosis nor added to information garnered from MRI in predicting the future development of multiple sclerosis.[170] Among the 83 patients in the ONTT who had spinal fluid analysis, the protein and glucose were usually normal, and only one third of patients had a pleocytosis usually between 6 to 27 WBC/mm^3. Myelin basic protein was detected in about one fifth of patients, and IgG synthesis in about two fifths. Oligoclonal banding occurred in approximately half of the patients and was associated with the future development of clinically definite multiple sclerosis. However, oligoclonal banding usually occurred in the presence of white matter lesions on MRI, which is less invasive and had a greater predictive value. Another study found the combination of an abnormal MRI scan and the presence of oligoclonal banding to be strongly associated with the development of multiple sclerosis.[171]

Course and Recovery. The ONTT clearly demonstrated that the visual prognosis in optic neuritis without treatment was the same when either oral or IV steroids were given.[172] The same study demonstrated that IV steroids increased the rate at which vision recovered, but at 1 year all treatment groups tested similarly.

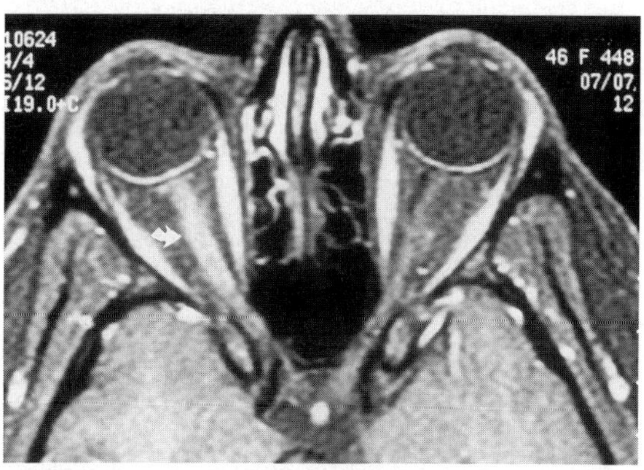

FIGURE 5–28. Axial T_1-weighted, fat-suppressed, gadolinium-enhanced orbital MRI scan in a patient with acute optic neuritis in the right eye. Diffuse enhancement of the right optic nerve (*arrow*) is present.

This finding was confirmed in another study[173] that compared IV methylprednisolone with placebo in patients with either short or long segments of optic nerve enhancement on MRI. In the ONTT, oral prednisone increased the rate of recurrent optic neuritis.[138] The mechanism for this is unclear, but this phenomenon continued to be observed at the 5-year follow-up.[174]

Recovery from optic neuritis is fairly prompt and usually nearly complete. In almost all of the patients in the ONTT (regardless of treatment type), recovery began within 1 month.[175] The ONTT and other reports[176] have shown that patients with initial poor acuity (20/400—NLP) have a poorer prognosis although most still improve to better than 20/40 vision.

However, there is great variability in the quality of the "20/20" vision that remains. Recovery to 20/20 vision does not truly capture the types of visual dysfunction and the symptomatology that many patients report following recovery from optic neuritis.[177, 178] In the ONTT, 63% of patients thought that their vision had not recovered to normal, although only a few reported any difficulty carrying on daily activities. Among 215 patients who reported their vision to be somewhat or much worse than it was before their optic neuritis, 43% had either normal results or only one abnormal result on all four measures of visual function tested (acuity, color, contrast, field).[178] Stereoacuity (despite normal Snellen acuity) was found to be abnormal in 85% of 27 patients in an earlier study.[177]

One study suggested that visual loss in optic neuritis in African-Americans was more severe at onset and after 1 year of follow-up compared with that in Caucasians.[179]

Multiple Sclerosis. Because of the close association between optic neuritis and multiple sclerosis, the features and treatment of MS will be summarized before their relationship is discussed below.

Multiple sclerosis is characterized by transient neurologic dysfunction, lasting days or weeks, owing to focal demyelination in the CNS. In addition to optic neuritis, other common clinical manifestations include double vision due to involvement of the medial longitudinal fasciculus (internuclear ophthalmoplegia (INO)) (see Chapter 15), ataxia and nystagmus due to cerebellar white matter tract involvement (see Chapter 17), extremity weakness, bladder difficulty, and sensory abnormalities. Rarely, patients may also have uveitis (pars planitis and panuveitis).[180] Multiple sclerosis primarily affects young adults, most often women, but children and older adults may also develop the disease.

In most individuals the initial course of multiple sclerosis is relapsing-remitting, with neurologic exacerbations separated by weeks, months, or years. Spontaneous recovery or near-recovery is the rule at this stage. Unfortunately, more severely affected patients may exhibit a progressive form of the disorder. This is manifested by a continuous decline in neurologic function that may have a profound effect on vision, ambulation, and cognition. Although the observations have been inconsistent and the reasons unclear, there may be an increased risk of attacks in the initial 6-month postpartum period in women with relapsing-remitting disease.[181–183]

Pathologically, new demyelinative plaques are characterized by perivascular inflammatory cell infiltration by CD4+ T cells.[184] Chronically, the plaques typically exhibit myelin destruction, disappearance of oligodendrocytes, intact axons, and astrocyte proliferation. Recent pathologic evidence[185] suggests axonal transection may be seen in some instances, perhaps explaining the irreversibility of some neurologic deficits. Radiographically, the white matter lesions are typically periventricular and often project perpendicularly from the ventricular surface. However, recent attention has been directed at MRI demonstration of brain atrophy and spectographic evidence of neuronal cell loss in MS.[635]

The cause is unclear, but multiple sclerosis is likely an autoimmune process that occurs in genetically susceptible individuals following an environmental exposure.[186] An immune cross reaction to viral antigens has been implicated.[187] A greater incidence of multiple sclerosis in Caucasians and first-degree relatives of affected individuals supports the notion that genetic factors may also play a role. The possibility of an environmental factor is also supported by the proponderance of cases in northern latitudes. The diagnosis is primarily a clinical one (Table 5–8), established formally when the Poser criteria[188] are satisfied.

Traditionally, most treatment options in MS have been symptomatic. Although most exacerbations are self-limited, those causing severe weakness or incoordination may require a short course of high-dose IV methylprednisolone. Other treatment options for attacks in relapsing-remitting disease include intra-

TABLE 5–8. Diagnostic Criteria for Multiple Sclerosis

Category	Attacks	Clinical Evidence of Attacks		Paraclinical Evidence (MRI, EP)
Clinically definite	2	2		
	2	1	and	1

(Courtesy of Dennis Kolson, MD, PhD.) MRI = white matter lesions on magnetic resonance imaging; EP = abnormal visual, somatosensory, or brain-stem auditory evoked potentials.

muscular (IM) adrenocorticotropic hormone (ACTH) and IV immune globulin. Cyclophosphamide, plasma exchange, methotrexate, azathioprine, and cyclosporine can be used in chronic-progressive forms of the disease, but their benefit is marginal.[186]

Recently, however, three medications—interferon beta-1b, interferon beta-1a, and copolymer 1—have been shown to alter the natural history of multiple-sclerosis and have been approved for use in patients with relapsing-remitting multiple sclerosis.[186, 634] In large controlled studies, each decreased the frequency of exacerbations, and interferon beta-1b and -1a slowed the rate of appearance of new white matter lesions on MRI.[189–194, 636, 637]

1. Interferon beta-1b (Betaseron, Berlex Laboratories, Richmond, Calif.) is an immune modulator that decreases production of interferon gamma, decreases activation of T lymphocytes, and affects antigen presentation.[195, 196] The medication is given subcutaneously every other day.
2. Interferon beta-1a (Avonex, Biogen, Cambridge, Mass.), also an immune modulator, is administered by a weekly IM injection. In contrast to interferon beta-1b and copolymer, interferon beta-1a was the only drug shown, with statistical significance, to delay the progression of sustained neurologic disability when compared with placebo.[193, 197] Furthermore, interferon beta-1a has been shown to have a large impact in delaying the subsequent development of MS in high risk (MR showing other white matter lesions) monosymptomatic patients. This study further emphasizes the importance of early treatment in multiple sclerosis patients or those monosymptomatic patients with high risk for this disorder.
3. Glatiramer acetate (Copaxone, Teva Marion Partners, Kansas City, Mo.), formerly known as copolymer 1, is a synthetic protein composed of amino acid copolymers intended to simulate those of myelin basic protein.[198] By inducing immune tolerance, copolymer 1 in animals prevents the development of experimental allergic encephalomyelitis, a disorder related to multiple sclerosis and believed to be caused by immunoreactivity to myelin basic protein. The medication is given subcutaneously every day. Glatiramer acetate also has a positive effect on neurologic disability, but this benefit is not sustained as demonstrated for interferon beta-1a.[199]

Recently, the chemotherapuetic agent mitoxantrone (Novantrone, Immunex, Seattle, Wash.) has been recommended for approval in patients with secondary progressive multiple sclerosis.

The Relationship Between Optic Neuritis and Multiple Sclerosis. Optic neuritis can occur in patients who have already developed multiple sclerosis, or it can be the first manifestation. Most patients with multiple sclerosis will have optic neuritis at some time during the course of their illness. The clinical features of optic neuritis are indistinguishable in patients with or without MS.

Several prospective studies have examined the risk of developing MS after the first attack of optic neuritis (Table 5–9). Some authors have suggested that most, if not all, patients with optic neuritis will eventually develop multiple sclerosis during their lifetime.[137, 169, 200–202]

In previously normal patients with optic neuritis, the most reliable predictor for the future development of multiple sclerosis is the presence of white matter lesions on MRI.[203] In Jacob's series,[204] 38% of patients with abnormal MRI scans developed multiple sclerosis, while only 16% with normal MRI scans developed multiple sclerosis. In the 5-year follow-up in the ONTT,[205] the ratio was 51% to 16% (Table 5–9). In the ONTT,[205] MS did not develop in any patient with a normal MRI scan who had (1) painless visual loss, (2) severe optic disc

TABLE 5–9. Prospective Studies Examining the Risk of Developing Multiple Sclerosis (MS) After a First Attack of Optic Neuritis

Study	Location	Follow-up (years)	Proportion Developing MS	Comments
Landy (1983)[625]	Australia	Range 1–29	71%	
Francis et al (1987)[200]	UK	Mean 11.6	57%	By life-table analysis, probability of MS by 15 years was 75%
Rizzo & Lessell (1988)[137]	New England (USA)	Mean 14.9	58%	By life-table analysis, probability of MS by 15 years was 74% for women and 34% for men
Sandberg-Wollheim et al (1990)[626]	Sweden	Mean 12.9	38%	By life-table analysis, probability of MS by 15 years was 45%
Morrissey et al (1993)[160]	UK	Mean 5.3	Normal MRI: 6%; abnormal MRI: 82%	MRI white matter lesions were associated with development of MS
Jacobs et al (1997)[204]	New York (USA)	Range 4 months to 19 years	Normal MRI: 16%; abnormal MRI: 38%	MRI white matter lesions were associated with development of MS
Optic Neuritis Study Group (ONTT) (1997)[205]	USA and Canada	5	Normal MRI: 16%; abnormal MRI: 51%	MRI white matter lesions were associated with development of MS

edema, (3) disc or peripapillary hemorrhage, or (4) macular exudate. Patients with isolated spinal cord or brain stem syndromes and white matter lesions on brain MRI also have an increased risk for developing multiple sclerosis.[206] Although less predictive, the following other tests are also associated with the development of multiple sclerosis if positive at the time of the first attack of optic neuritis: CSF oligoclonal bands,[207, 208] increased CSF IgG synthesis,[204] HLA-DR2 antigen,[171, 209] and somatosensory evoked potentials.

The ONTT demonstrated that a course of IV steroids given at the time of an acute attack of optic neuritis, particularly in patients with abnormal MRI scans, reduced the rate of development of clinically definite multiple sclerosis in the first 2 years.[203] Although controversial, these findings led to the broad recommendation that patients with optic neuritis and abnormal MRI scans should be treated with steroids to reduce the risk of developing multiple sclerosis.[210] Subsequently, after 3 years that beneficial effect disappeared.[211]

Evaluation of Optic Neuritis in Typical Cases. In typical cases of optic neuritis (acute or subacute monocular visual loss with pain on eye movements in a young adult), MRI scanning of the brain is the only requisite test. The predictive value of MRI is important in patient counselling, and some patients with abnormal MRI scans may desire treatment to reduce the relative risk of early conversion to multiple sclerosis (see below). Serum serologies, lumbar punctures, and evoked potentials are unnecessary. Typical patients should be followed within the first week or two to document the visual nadir, then at four weeks to insure that vision starts to recover spontaneously. Those with disc swelling should be observed for development of a macular star (see neuroretinitis).

Evaluation of Optic Neuritis in Atypical Cases. Criteria for atypical optic neuritis include (1) marked disc swelling, (2) vitritis, (3) progression of visual loss after 1 week, (4) lack of partial recovery within 4 weeks of onset of visual loss, and (5) persistent pain. A suggested workup with diagnostic considerations in these cases is given in Table 5–10. Compressive lesions will have been excluded by MRI.

Treatment in Typical Cases. Many patients, especially those with normal MRI scans, will not require any treatment and vision usually improves spontaneously. However, IV corticosteroids followed by a short course of oral steroids may be considered in two instances:

1. In patients with white matter lesions on MRI, steroid treatment should be offered to reduce the risk of developing MS for the first 2 years.
2. We have a low threshold for IV corticosteroid treament in patients with severe unilateral or bilateral visual loss because of their slightly poorer visual prognosis and because steroids may hasten recovery.

Methylprednisolone 250 mg IV qid is given for 3 days, followed by prednisone 1 mg/kg

TABLE 5–10. Suggested Diagnostic Considerations, Laboratory Evaluation, and Distinguishing Features in *Atypical* Cases of Optic Neuritis

Entity	Laboratory Test	Comment
Optic nerve compression	MRI	Progressive loss of vision beyond 10 days
Carcinomatous meningitis	CSF cytology	Systemic tumor almost always present
Syphilis	MHATP	Papillitis with hemorrhage Optic perineuritis Uveitis
Lyme	Serum Lyme titer	Endemic area Erythema chronicum migrans Optic perineuritis
Sarcoid	ACE CXR	Optic nerve granuloma Uveitis Periphlebitis
Anterior ischemic optic neuropathy	ESR	Age > 50 Segmental disc swelling Disc hemorrhage
Lupus	ANA	Arthritis Antiphospholipid antibody syndrome
Nutritional	B_{12} level	Progressive optic atrophy Pernicious anemia Ileum dysfunction
Leber's hereditary optic neuropathy	Mitochondrial analysis	Males > females Pseudo-edematous disc Telangiectasias

ACE = angiotensin converting enzyme, ANA = antinuclear antibody, CSF = cerebrospinal fluid, CXR = chest x-ray, ESR = erythrocyte sedimentation rate, MHATP = Microhemagglutination–*Treponema pallidum,* MRI = magnetic resonance imaging.

qd for days 4 through 14, then 20 mg of prednisone on day 15, and 10 mg on days 16 and 18. At home, IV steroids can be administered safely, and if there are no relative contraindications such as diabetes, peptic ulcer disease, or coronary artery disease, the risk is small.[212] Hospitalization may be required in older individuals and in those with the aforementioned medical illnesses. Because of the increased risk of recurrent episodes, patients with optic neuritis should not be given oral prednisone alone.[638]

The use of oral methylprednisolone in acute optic neuritis has been studied but has not become standard practice.[213] In patients with unresolved visual loss due to visual loss, there have been anecdotal reports of using IV immunoglobulin.[214] However, routine use of such an expensive therapy will require more rigorous investigation. At this time, we can not recommend its use in patients with stable visual loss from optic neuritis.

Neuromyelitis Optica (Devic's Disease)

Neuromyelitis optica, or Devic's disease, is a variant of optic neuritis in which patients develop bilateral optic neuritis in association with transverse myelitis. It tends to occur in young adults, but is also well recognized in children. Both monophasic illnesses and recurrent attacks have been described.[639] Patients tend to present with visual loss and evidence of spinal cord dysfunction within 8 weeks of each other.

Spinal fluid abnormalities, including increased protein and pleocytosis, have been described. Periventricular white matter changes on the MRI scan are less consistent than in routine multiple sclerosis.[640] One report of eight patients with Devic's disease found no radiographically evident cerebral white matter lesions.[215] Autopsy studies have demonstrated typical demyelinating plaques (like multiple sclerosis) in some patients, while in others a necrotizing myelitis (unlike multiple sclerosis) with thickened blood vessel walls was found.[215, 216] Astrocytosis, reactive gliosis, and microcavitation may be seen pathologically in the optic nerves.[215]

Because of the necrotizing nature of the lesions, the prognosis for recovery may be worse from both a visual and neurologic standpoint, especially in elderly patients. In a review of the literature,[217] 22% of the reported cases developed respiratory failure, 16% died in the acute stages, 14% had a poor neurologic outcome, and 70% of patients improved neurologically. Older age was a poor prognostic factor along with CSF pleocytosis and more severe myelitis. In this same study, 42% of the patients had a recurrence of a demyelinating event suggestive of multiple sclerosis with the other 58% having a monophasic illness without recurrence.[217] Many patients in the latter group had prodromal symptoms suggestive of a viral illness and a course suggestive of a postinfectious encephalomyelitis.

Neuromyelitis optica is also well recognized in children and has been purported to have an excellent prognosis for recovery. In one study,[218] all patients had a preceding viral syndrome, 90% had bilateral visual loss, and all patients had disc swelling. In this same study,[183] vision in all patients recovered to 20/20 (some with optic atrophy), and no patients had recurrences of neurologic illness. However, our experience is less sanguine, and we have treated some children with multiple exacerbations and permanent visual loss.

Other systemic conditions may be associated with Devic's disease. These include systemic lupus erythematosus,[219] other connective tissue diseases, and pulmonary tuberculosis.[220, 221]

Treatment usually consists of high-dose IV or oral corticosteroids, sometimes in combination with other immunosuppressants or immune modulators.[222]

Pediatric Optic Neuritis

In many cases, inflammatory disease of the optic nerve in children is quite different from that in adults. While there are some children and adolescents who have unilateral attacks of demyelinating optic neuritis and go on to develop multiple sclerosis, there are many others with an illness that seems to be quite distinct from the adult variety of the disease. Like adults, most children experience acute loss of vision associated with an afferent pupil defect and visual field defects. Unlike adults, children have a much higher likelihood of having bilateral involvement (50% to 75%) and disc swelling (50% to 75%).[223–225, 641]

There have been no formal studies evaluating the optimal treatment of childhood optic neuritis. However, because of the patients' young ages, we favor more aggressive evaluation and treatment when visual loss is unilateral and severe or bilateral at any level. Workup includes MRI, serologies, and lumbar puncture to exclude other causes. Hospitalization and 3 to 5 days of IV methylprednisolone (4 mg/kg qid) therapy is initiated, followed by an oral prednisone taper (starting at 1 mg/kg, then reduced over 2 to 4 weeks). Prognosis for recovery in children is generally excellent, with vision in greater than 80% of children returning to 20/20 or better.[223–225, 642] Good et al, however, reported that in a series of 10 children, the vision of 7 remained at 20/200 or worse.[226]

Etiologic considerations in childhood optic neuritis suggest there may be two distinct subsets of patients. One group has their neurologic event (immune mediated) as a postinfectious acute disseminated encephalomyelitis, with or without radiographically demonstrable white matter lesions. This group of patients has a monophasic illness with recovery and without recurrence. The second group may have "idiopathic" (genetic predisposition with environmental trigger) demyelination, recover, but later develop recurrent neurologic illness suggestive of multiple sclerosis. The possibility that these two groups are linked and that viral illness or vaccinations are important triggers of multiple sclerosis has also been proposed.[227] For instance, cases of childhood optic neuritis and multiple sclerosis have been reported after viral illnesses and chicken pox.[227–230] Overall, between 10% and 50% of children with optic neuritis eventually develop multiple sclerosis.[225, 226, 231–233]

Sarcoidosis

Sarcoidosis is a multisystem disorder of unknown etiology, characterized pathologically by noncaseating epithelioid cell granulomas. It is much more common in African-Americans and slightly more common in women than men. The initial onset of the systemic illness may be an isolated visual or neurologic presentation, or there may be systemic symptoms including rash, fevers, night sweats, diarrhea, pulmonary symptoms, and lymphadenopathy. Most patients will have hilar adenopathy detectable on chest roentgenography, as extrapulmonary sarcoidosis without hilar adenopathy is rare. CNS involvement in sarcoidosis occurs in about 5% of cases.[234, 235] The most common neurologic involvement is seventh nerve palsy (see Chapter 14), followed by other cranial nerve involvement, aseptic meningitis, and peripheral neuropathy.

On the other hand, ocular involvement in chronic sarcoidosis occurs in about 25% of patients.[236] In the vast majority this takes the form of a relapsing and remitting anterior uveitis, often associated with ocular hypertension. In patients with posterior segment involvement, sarcoidosis most commonly presents with retinal vasculitis, vitreous infiltrates, and choroidal lesions, often with associated disc swelling (see Chapter 4).

Optic nerve involvement in the setting of sarcoidosis can take many different forms. Some patients present with a syndrome similar to idiopathic optic neuritis. Other patients have optic nerve head granuloma (Fig. 5–29) while others may have a swollen nerve (due to either optic nerve or optic nerve sheath infiltration).[237] Less common is a pure retrobulbar presentation with a normal-appearing optic nerve head. Sarcoidosis is also a well-recognized cause of perineuritis.

Patients can present with progressive vision loss, and in general have less pain than patients with idiopathic optic neuritis. Vision loss initially may be steroid responsive. Other patients have a relentless downhill course despite the use of steroids and develop profound visual impairment. Cases with spontaneous improvement and isolated disc swelling without optic nerve dysfunction have been reported.[238] Sarcoidosis with optic nerve involvement must be considered in all patients thought to have inflammatory or compressive disease of the anterior visual pathway (also see Chapter 7). Important clues are the presence of a steroid-responsive optic neuropathy and findings atypical for ordinary optic neuritis such as significant vitritis, retinal vasculitis, or enlargement of the optic nerve on MRI. Sarcoidosis can also present as an orbital inflammatory syndrome (see Chapter 18).

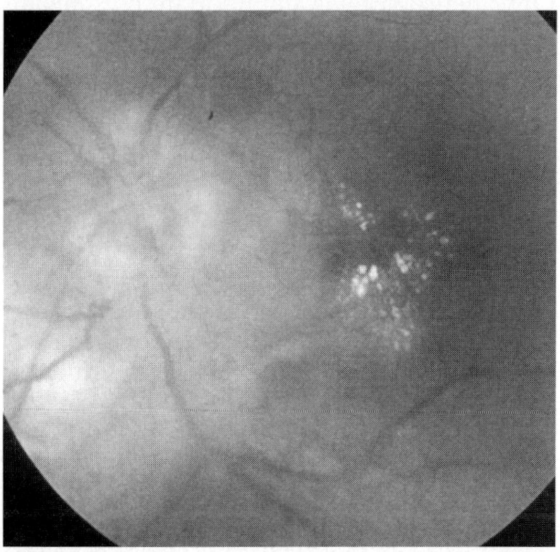

FIGURE 5–29. Optic nerve head appearance in a patient with sarcoidosis and a granuloma of the optic nerve head and peripapillary subretinal area. There are exudates in the macular region.

Diagnostic Studies/Evaluation. Presentation with a markedly thickened optic nerve sheath on the MRI scan mimicking optic nerve sheath meningioma is well recognized.[239–242] MRI is often helpful by demonstrating periventricular multifocal white matter lesions in CNS sarcoidosis.[243]

When sarcoidosis is suspected, a chest film, an angiotensin converting enzyme level (ACE) and, if necessary, a gallium scan should be obtained. Whenever possible, diagnosis should be confirmed by biopsy (often pulmonary via bronchoscopy or of hilar nodes via mediastinoscopy). On occasion, conjunctival or lacrimal gland biopsies, which are less invasive than the pulmonary or hilar biopsies, can be used and are diagnostic.[244, 245] In general we do not favor blind biopsies of any tissue but prefer to biopsy tissue that either appears abnormal or had been shown to be abnormal on roentgenography or gallium scanning. Finally, it is reasonable to consider sarcoidosis in all cases of unexplained optic neuropathy, and screening with chest roentgenography and ACE levels will occasionally point to the diagnosis.

Treatment. Treatment with systemic steroids is likely to be required for a protracted time (weeks to months).[246] Other patients require chronic immunosuppression with alternative cytotoxic drugs.[246] Treatment is generally with systemic steroids, and cyclosporine has been reported to be effective as well.[247]

Other neuro-ophthalmic presentations of sarcoidosis are described elsewhere in the textbook.

Optic Perineuritis and Orbital Inflammatory Syndromes

Patients with optic perineuritis present with an inflammatory optic neuropathy that presumably primarily involves the optic nerve sheath as the focus of the inflammatory reaction. In many cases the cause is unknown. Histopathologically, these patients have been shown to have nonspecific chronic inflammation, occasionally granulomatous and often associated with varying degrees of fibroplasia and collagen deposition.[248–251]

In our experience, patients with this condition fall into three broad categories. The first are patients with other evidence of an acute orbital inflammatory syndrome (orbital pseudotumor) such as proptosis, eyelid swelling, eye muscle involvement, and posterior scleritis. In these patients there is clinical evidence of optic neuropathy. Neuroimaging reveals orbital inflammatory changes as well as optic nerve sheath enhancement. This entity is discussed in more detail in Chapter 18. The second group of patients have optic perineuritis in the setting of a systemic condition, most commonly sarcoidosis, syphilis, Lyme disease, or tuberculosis. In the final group the condition is idiopathic, with no evidence of orbital disease or systemic infection.

The distinction of optic neuritis from optic perineuritis is largely based on clinical presentation and radiographic demonstration of optic nerve sheath thickening or enhancement. Vision loss may be mild initially in perineuritis and is commonly bilateral. The optic nerve head is often swollen, with secondary retinal venous stasis changes, dilation of vessels, and peripheral retinal hemorrhages. Clinically it must be distinguished from papilledema since both share the clinical features of bilateral disc swelling and relatively good visual function. In most patients with perineuritis, the CSF exhibits a normal opening pressure with a mild pleocytosis. Patients may also have an acute presentation that mimics optic neuritis, or they may present with an insidiously progressive optic neuropathy.

Diagnostic Studies/Evaluation. The presence of associated vitreous cells and infiltrates is suggestive of a systemic condition associated with the perineuritis, and extensive workup for sarcoidosis, syphilis, Lyme disease, and tuberculosis should be initiated. Optic nerve sheath thickening can be documented with orbital ultrasound and either computed tomography (CT) or MRI. Enhancement of the sheath is more prominent than the enhancement of the nerve itself with contrast studies. Radiographically, perineuritis can be difficult to distinguish from optic nerve sheath meningioma.[250] If there is more widespread evidence of meningeal involvement, syphilitic, cryptococcal, tuberculosis, and carcinomatous meningitis are more likely. If papilledema is considered, patients with headache should undergo lumbar puncture to rule out elevated intracranial pressure.

Treatment. Treatment for perineuritis is directed at the systemic infection and involves systemic steroids. In our experience, in the setting of infectious perineuritis, patients are often successfully treated with good recovery of vision. The idiopathic form, or that associated with orbital inflammation, can, however, take a chronic form that is resistant to steroid treatment and is associated with significant fibrosis of the optic nerve sheath.

Uveitis-Associated Disc Swelling

Patients with uveitis, particularly with posterior segment involvement, can have disc swelling. A nonspecific process resulting from simple breakdown of the blood–retinal barrier in posterior uveitis should be distinguished from an inflammatory process involving the optic nerve itself. The former is more common. These are patients, for instance with pars planitis, who develop disc swelling often accompanied by cystoid macular edema. In this setting, there is usually only enlargement of the blind spot without evidence of optic neuropathy. In the second group of patients, an inflammatory or infectious process, often granulomatous (commonly sarcoid or syphilis), involves the nerve itself, and significant visual dysfunction with optic neuropathy is often present. Optic disc swelling can also accompany hypotony, which may occur with chronic uveitis.

Optic Neuropathy Related to Systemic Lupus Erythematosus

Optic neuropathy is an important but uncommon neuro-ophthalmic complication of systemic lupus erythematosus.[252] Optic neuropathy was found in only 2 of 150 (1.3%) patients with lupus in the Johns Hopkins series.[253] Jabs et al[253] reported seven such cases and reviewed 24 other cases reported in the literature. Interestingly, 13 of the 24 (54%) cases of lupus-related optic neuropathy were associated with transverse myelitis. This pattern of optic neuropathy with transverse myelitis mimics Devic's neuromyelitis optica (see above).[219]

The optic neuropathy can appear similar to anterior ischemic optic neuropathy (AION, see below) with disc swelling and exudates (Fig. 5–30) or retrobulbar optic neuritis. The pathogenesis is unclear, but is related either to demyelination or to varying degrees of small-vessel vaso-occlusive disease. These patients require initial treatment with high-dose IV methylprenisolone, and many require chronic steroids.

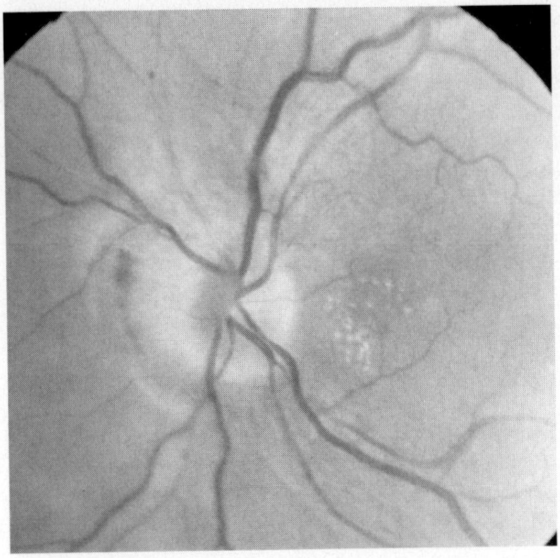

FIGURE 5–30. Optic nerve appearance in a patient with systemic lupus erythematosis and optic neuritis. Chronic disc swelling and retinal exudates are present.

Other neuro-ophthalmic complications of lupus are detailed in Chapter 8.

Autoimmune Optic Neuropathy

This distinct variety of optic nerve inflammation is similar to lupus optic neuropathy. However, in these patients no specific connective tissue diagnosis can be made using strict clinical or serologic criteria, despite extensive searching. The entity of autoimmune optic neuropathy is believed to be a chronic autoimmune condition characterized by recurrences of visual loss and steroid dependency.[254, 255] Its similarity to lupus optic neuropathy suggests an optic nerve antigen may be susceptible to an autoimmune attack. An alternative possibility is that optic nerve dysfunction arises in the setting of autoimmune disease as a result of small-vessel occlusion from immune complex deposition or a hypercoaguable state. Some cases have had abnormal skin biopsies, with perivascular infiltrate and immune complex deposition within the dermis.[256] Affected patients are generally adults aged 25 to 55, but the condition probably occurs at any age. Bee-sting optic neuropathy is thought to be a unique autoimmune-type optic neuropathy.[257, 258, 643]

Evaluation and Treatment. We recommend a search for an autoimmune condition in any patient that has "optic neuritis" that worsens for more than 1 week after initial steroid therapy, or in any patient who fails to begin to improve by the third week after onset of visual loss (see atypical optic neuritis, above). Continued efforts, such as a rheumatologic consultation, consideration of a skin biopsy to exclude vasculitis, and serologies, should be made in these patients to try to identify a systemic autoimmune condition. Early recognition can lead to successful treatment with high doses of steroids. Other immunosuppressive therapies are often required to supplement steroid therapy in this chronic and relapsing condition.[255, 259]

INFECTIOUS OPTIC NEUROPATHIES

Sinusitis and Mucoceles

For decades it was believed that the vast majority of cases of optic neuritis resulted from contiguous disease and inflammation in the paranasal sinuses. Subsequently, it has been shown that the radiographic presence of sinus inflammation and mucosal thickening is fairly ubiquitous, and that most cases of optic neuritis result from demyelination. Nevertheless, it is clear that paranasal sinus disease can cause (1) a condition not dissimilar in presentation to optic neuritis (acute optic neuropathy plus pain on eye movements), or (2) progressive optic neuropathy from chronic compression.

In the many cases the optic neuropathy results from compression or inflammation from a nearby mucocele.[260–262] In other cases contiguous inflammation in the posterior ethmoid and sphenoid sinus causes optic nerve dysfunction without mass effect.[263, 264] This may occur more commonly in patients with no medial wall of the optic canal (meninges in direct contact with sinus mucosa), an anatomic variant that occurs in about 4% of normal patients.[17]

Evaluation and Treatment. This diagnosis should be entertained in all cases of acute optic neuropathy that are atypical for optic neuritis in any way. In particular, it should be suspected in elderly patients and patients with a history of severe sinus disease, when there are associated fevers or ophthalmoplegia, or when progression of optic neuritis occurs beyond 2 weeks.

When significant sinusitis is identified on MRI in these patients, particularly in the posterior ethmoid and sphenoid sinuses, or when a mucocele is present, prompt otolaryngologic consultation should be sought. Then antibiotic and often surgical therapy can be arranged. In this setting, visual loss can often be totally reversed.

Neuroretinitis

The term *neuroretinitis* refers to optic neuropathy associated with the unique combination of disc edema and peripapillary or macular hard exudates, which form a star or sunburst pattern around the fovea (Fig. 5–31; see Color Plates 21 and 22). The condition was first described by Leber and is therefore frequently referred to as *Leber's stellate neuroretinitis.*[265] Several series have described this somewhat heterogenous group,[266, 267] and there are several important observations that have been made. Neuroretinitis is frequently a manifestation of a systemic infection, so a cause should be sought when the diagnosis is made. Although the initial presentation can be very similar to that of idiopathic (demyelinating) optic neuritis, a macular star associated with optic neuritis is not associated with an increased risk of developing multiple sclerosis.

The macular star results from fluid leakage from optic disc capillaries into Henle's layer (outer plexiform), which retains the lipid precipitates. All of the leakage is believed to be from the disc since the retinal vasculature does not leak on fluorescein angiography. In fact, the presence of these exudates can be a nonspecific finding in any patient with disc swelling.[268–270] For instance, at least a partial star can occasionally be seen in patients with a variety of different causes of optic disc swelling, such as ischemic optic neuropathy or papilledema (see Chapter 6).

Therefore, we group patients with the finding of optic disc edema with a macular lipid star into two groups:

1. *Idiopathic or infectious neuroretinitis.* Patients in this group present with decreased vision and a swollen optic nerve, and initially a diagnosis of optic neuritis may be made, but within 1 to 2 weeks the macular star is evident. Patients in this group are generally aged 10 to 50, and there is no sex predilection. Occasionally they have pain around the eye or bilateral involvement.[266, 267] Neuroretinitis has been reported in children and behaves similarly to the disease in adults.[271] In up to 50% of patients with neuroretinitis, a preceding viral illness is reported.

   The examination is notable for moderate acuity loss (usually 20/40 to 20/200) but can be as poor as light perception. Typical features of optic nerve dysfunction are present, with decreased color vision, nerve fiber defects on visual field testing, and afferent pupil defects. Vitreous cells are present in about 90%.[266, 267] The disc swelling can either be focal or diffuse, and sometimes the disc has a pale quality. Development of the lipid star is often preceded by serous detachment of the macula or evidence of inflammation in the peripheral retina. The prognosis for visual recovery is excellent although recurrent neuroretinitis with poor visual outcome has been reported.[272]

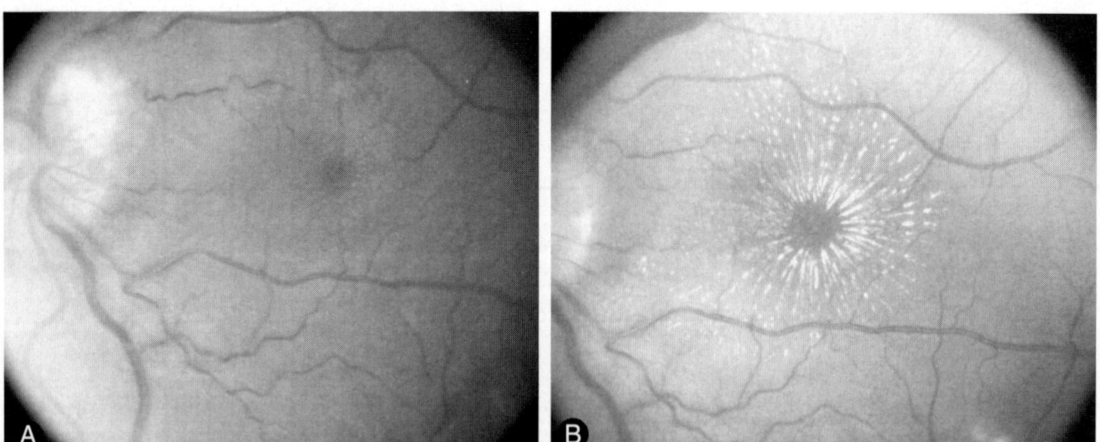

FIGURE 5–31. Fundus appearance in a patient with neuroretinitis. **A.** Acutely there is pale disc swelling. Fine yellow spots are seen on careful inspection of the macular region. **B.** Within 1 week the more classic macular star developed. (See Color Plates 21 and 22.)

Important infectious causes of neuroretinitis include cat scratch disease (*Bartonella henselae* bacillus),[273, 274] syphilis,[275, 276] Lyme disease,[277, 278] and toxoplasmosis.[279, 280] Patients with *Bartonella* infection frequently will describe cat scratches and a recent viral illness with fever and adenopathy.[281] Endocarditis has been reported as a complication of *Bartonella henselae* infection, and encephalopathy and meningitis in patients with concurrent human immunodeficiency virus (HIV) infection have been described.[273, 282]

2. *Macular star due to other causes of disc swelling.* These patients have a fairly typical presentation of an optic neuropathy associated with disc edema (ischemic optic neuropathy,[283] for example) and, curiously, usually a few weeks after presentation, develop a macular star. In these patients the original diagnosis may be rethought and consideration should be given to papilledema associated with increased intracranial pressure or malignant hypertension as the cause of the swelling and exudates. As in the first group of patients, development of a macular star is often preceded by serous macular detachment.

Evaluation and Treatment. At the time of diagnosis of neuroretinitis, appropriate historic review and laboratory tests (including *Bartonella* titers) should be ordered to rule out the infectious causes listed above. Appropriate antibiotic therapy is indicated when syphilis, Lyme disease, or toxoplasmosis is diagnosed. Many cases will be either titer negative and presumably idiopathic or the result of *Bartonella* infection (cat scratch disease).[284] Reed and associates reported seven patients, all with positive *Bartonella* titers.[285] *Bartonella* infection is considered to be self-limited and no treatment has been proven to be beneficial in cat scratch-associated neuroretinitis. Reed and associates reported that treatment with doxycycline and rifampin seemed to shorten the course when compared to historic controls.[285] We consider using doxycycline if visual loss is severe or disc swelling persists beyond 3 weeks. Most patients recover but many are left with residual visual symptoms secondary to optic nerve dysfunction.

Syphilis

Syphilitic involvement of the optic nerves represents a heterogenous group of conditions. Optic neuropathy is not uncommon in patients with secondary syphilis. Patients can develop retrobulbar optic neuritis, papillitis with retinal vasculitis (Fig. 5–32), and perineuritis and neuroretinitis in the setting of secondary lues. The severity of the visual symptoms is variable and depends on the site of the infection. Patients with syphilitic perineuritis tend to have milder visual loss (sometimes none at all) as compared to patients with direct optic nerve involvement. Bilateral disease is nearly almost always present, often with other evidence of secondary syphilis such as rash, uveitis, and mild signs of meningeal inflammation.[286] MRI in perineuritis shows diffuse thickening and enhancement of the optic nerve sheath.[287] In contrast, progressive vision loss with optic atrophy can also been seen as a manifestation of tertiary syphilis. This is a slowly progressive (generally not episodic) visual deterioration not associated with other active inflammation of the eye.

Diagnostic Studies/Evaluation. Syphilitic optic neuropathy can almost always be diagnosed with appropriate serum and CSF serologies except in the setting of HIV, which can alter test results in a seronegative disease.[288] In the non-HIV-infected individual, the serum microhemaglutten assay for *Treponema pallidum* (MHA-TP) or the fluorescent treponemal antibody absorption test (FTA-ABS) should almost always be positive in the patient with neuro-ophthalmic signs and symptoms suggestive of syphilis. The serum Venereal Disease Research Laboratory (VDRL) and rapid plasma reagent (RPR) tests are also useful screening tests but they may be negative in neurosyphilis. Although a positive CSF VDRL is confirmatory of a diagnosis of neurosyphilis, it is often negative and therefore can not be used solely to exclude this diagnosis. Often, one relies on the presence of a positive serum test and the presence of elevated CSF white blood cell count or protein concentration to determine disease activity. Since the presentation of syphilitic optic neuropathy is quite variable, the clinical suspicion for this condition must exist in all cases of atypical inflammatory optic neuropathy and unexplained progressive optic atrophy.

Treatment. Treatment of syphilitic optic neuropathy with positive CSF VDRL and presumed tertiary syphilis must be with IV aqueous penicillin.[275, 276] Secondary syphilis with perineuritis and normal CSF has been treated successfully with IM procaine penicillin.[276] The

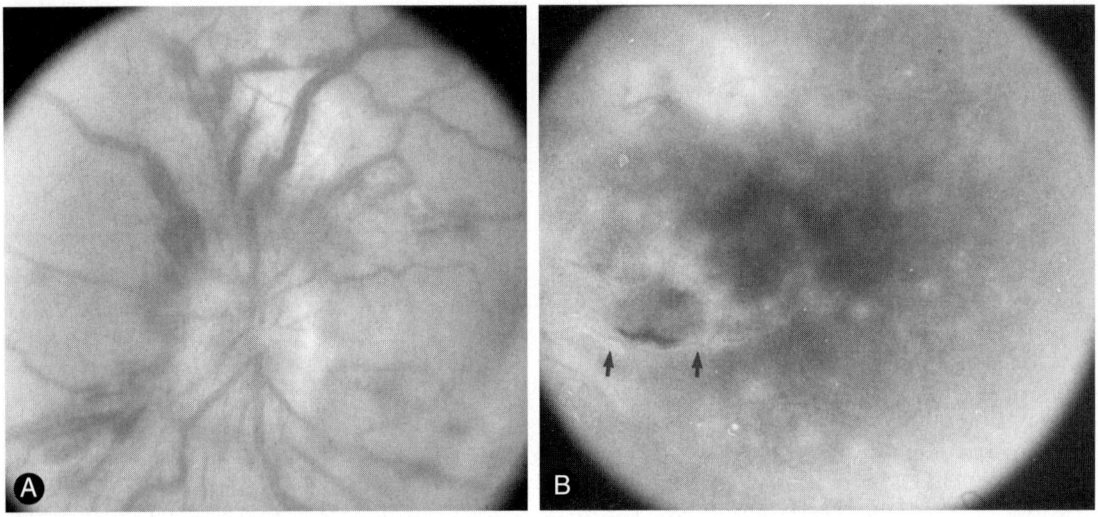

FIGURE 5–32. A. Fundus appearance in acute syphilitic papillitis and retinal vasculitis. Extensive intraretinal hemorrhage and venous dilation are compatible with papillophlebitis. **B.** Fluorescein angiogram of the same patient demonstrating staining of vessel walls (*arrows*) and leakage of dye into the retina.

disease in patients with HIV is similar. Syphilitic optic nerve involvement has been reported as an initial manifestation of HIV infection and tends to have an excellent prognosis with appropriate treatment.[289]

Lyme Disease

The neurologic manifestations of Lyme disease are protean,[290] and the neuro-ophthalmic manifestations have recently been extensively reviewed.[291] Lyme-associated optic neuritis and perineuritis are rare, and the diagnosis should be made primarily in patients who have a history of erythema migrans, a bout of arthritis, and positive titers in serum and CSF whenever possible. Many of the reported cases of Lyme-associated optic neuritis and ischemic optic neuropathy are circumspect. They were based simply on recent exposure and presence of serum titers, neither of which is adequate to implicate Lyme as the definite cause of optic nerve dysfunction.[291] We recommend that a positive serum lyme titer be confirmed by Western blot testing since there is a relatively high rate of false positives seen with conventional serum antibody titer level testing. Lyme is also an important cause of low-grade meningitis associated with elevated intracranial pressure and a pseudotumor cerebri-like presentation (see Chapter 6).[277, 291] When the optic nerve is involved, the picture is usually one of uveitis-associated neuroretinitis and unusual fluorescein angiographic characteristics, including neuroretinal edema and patchy and diffuse hyperfluorescence.[278] It some patients, neuroretinitis can be resistant to antibiotic treatment.[278]

HIV-Associated Optic Neuropathy

The setting of systemic immunosuppression is an important risk factor for primary infection of the optic nerve from a variety of pathogens.[292] In the acquired immunodeficiency syndrome (AIDS) infectious optic neuropathy may result from primary HIV infection of the nerve, cytomegalovirus infection, or acute retinal necrosis associated with herpes virus. In addition, optic neuropathy can develop in the setting of granulomatous inflammation of the meninges associated with cryptococcus, toxoplasmosis, tuberculosis, aspergillus, or syphilis. These can also cause elevated intracranial pressure with papilledema and associated progressive visual loss. Primary HIV optic neuropathy can be an acute retrobulbar optic neuritis with pain on eye movements or a slowly progressive condition.[293] Treatment with steroids or antivirals may be effective. The condition likely results from direct HIV infection of the optic nerve or alternatively nerve damage can result from the immune reaction directed against the infected optic nerve.

Cytomegalovirus (CMV) infection is the most common opportunistic infection to involve the posterior segment of the eye. The majority of patients develop retinitis with associated hemorrhagic necrosis. This herpes virus can primarily infect the optic nerve and cause a papillitis or the optic nerve can be involved secondarily by contiguous spread from adjacent retina.[294–296] Papillitis occurs in about 4% of patients with CMV retinitis. Patients require management with high and prolonged doses of IV foscarnet or ganciclovir, and the prognosis for visual recovery is very variable.[294]

Fungal disease can involve the optic nerves through granulomatous inflammation of the meninges. Cryptococcus is the most common fungal infection of the CNS and most common cause of optic neuropathy.[297, 298] Patients can present with either sudden vision loss or progressive vision loss from papilledema associated with elevated intracranial pressure. The mechanisms for vision loss include direct fungal invasion and adhesive arachnoiditis along with elevated intracranial pressure. Optic nerve sheath fenestration may be beneficial in some patients along with systemic treatment with amphotericin B (see Chapter 6).

Herpes Zoster

Optic neuropathy can occur in patients with recent herpes zoster ophthalmicus. It must be very rare given the paucity of reported cases compared to the prevalence of the condition. Vision loss can take the form a catastrophic ischemic event perhaps from an angiitis or behave more like an inflammatory optic neuropathy from zoster infection of the nerve.[299, 300] This condition is well recognized in both immunocompetent and immune incompetent patients.[301–303] In immunocompromised patients varicella zoster optic neuritis can precede retinitis and result in severe permanent vision loss.[303–305] Presentation occurs soon after the onset of the rash but may also be delayed by weeks. Vision loss is usually unilateral and severe. There may be papillitis with a macular star or the fundus may be normal. Treatment with acyclovir and steroids can be attempted with variable results. An optic neuritis-like illness has also been described after primary varicella infection (chicken pox).[306]

ISCHEMIC OPTIC NEUROPATHIES

Ischemic optic neuropathy (ION) is an acute, presumably vascular optic neuropathy unrelated to inflammation, demyelination, or compression. Sudden, often catastrophic "strokelike" vision loss in elderly patients with vasculopathic risk factors is typical of this condition. ION is classified as nonarteritic or arteritic.

The nonarteritic variety is almost always anterior with optic nerve head swelling, by definition. Thus the term *nonarteritic anterior ION* (AION) is applied to this group. The majority of these patients are elderly, have diabetes and/or hypertension, and are particularly at risk if they have a small, cupless, crowded optic nerve head (Fig. 5–33). Other systemic conditions that have been reported in association with AION include antiphospholipid antibody syndrome, previous radiation therapy, juvenile diabetes, shock, severe hypertension, and migraine.

Arteritic ION is usually due to temporal arteritis. Patients in this group can present either with disc swelling (arteritic AION) or without disc swelling. The latter presentation is termed *arteritic posterior ischemic optic neuropathy* (PION) and should remain a diagnosis of exclusion because of its rarity. When arteritic ION is a heralding manifestation of temporal arteritis, other generalized symptoms are usually present.

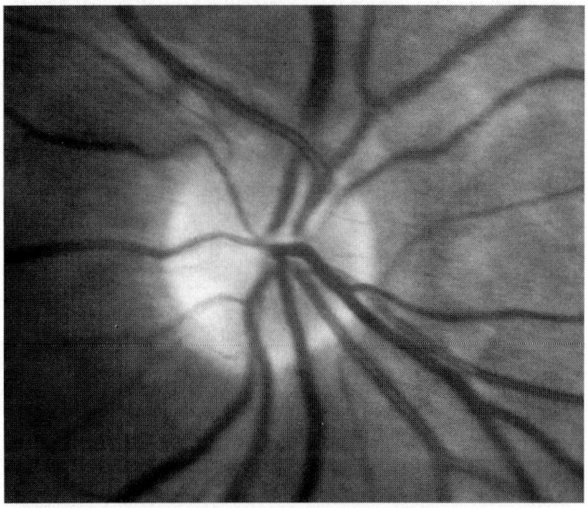

FIGURE 5–33. The typical appearance of the "disc at risk" for development of anterior ischemic optic neuropathy. The nerve is small and there is no cup.

The remainder of this section will discuss the diagnosis and management of nonarteritic and arteritic ION in detail and also highlight some of the other less common varieties.

Nonarteritic Ischemic Optic Neuropathy

Nonarteritic AION is the most common cause of unilateral optic nerve swelling and optic neuropathy in adults over age 50.[307] The term *ischemic optic neuropathy* was used in 1966 to describe 11 patients with the characteristic triad of vision loss, afferent pupil defect, and a swollen optic nerve.[308]

Demographics. The majority of patients are 60 to 70 years of age, but there is no absolute age range. In the Bascom Palmer series, Boghen and Glaser described 37 patients with nonarteritic AION, and the age range was 40 to 80.[309] Although there was a minimum age requirement of 50 for eligibility, the recently completed Ischemic Optic Neuropathy Decompression Trial (IONDT) found a mean age of 66 ± 8.7.[310] This study randomized patients with AION and visual acuity worse than 20/64 to either optic nerve sheath decompression or observation.

Population studies of patients 50 years or older suggest an annual incidence rate of 2.3/100,000 population/year and an increased rate in Caucasians compared to African-Americans or Hispanic individuals.[307] There is an increased risk in patients with diabetes mellitus, hypercholesterolemia, ischemic heart disease, and systemic hypertension.[311, 312, 354] In the IONDT 47% of the patients had hypertension and 24% had diabetes mellitus.[310] The prevalence of these systemic risk factors was lower in patients who were not randomized because their affected eye had vision better than 20/64. This suggests hypertension and diabetes may be risk factors for more significant vision loss.

Nocturnal hypotension, in some cases due to the treatment of arterial hypertension, may be a separate and distinct risk factor which may explain the high rate of vision loss that occurs upon awakening.[313, 314] Nocturnal hypotension has been demonstrated in patients with progressive vision loss.[315, 316] Another important risk factor is the disc at risk or crowded optic nerve head.[317–320] The fellow eye is often found to have a small or absent cup. Other studies have shown hyperopic refractive errors and smoking to be possible risk factors as well.[321, 322] Patients with nonarteritic ION do not have increased incidence of hypercoagulable states[354] or of carotid disease on the affected side compared to age-matched controls.[323]

Neuro-ophthalmic Symptoms. Most patients describe a sudden onset of monocular visual loss, often upon awakening (40% in the IONDT study[310]). It is maximal when noted, and often does not progress. There are usually no prodromal ocular symptoms and no associated systemic symptoms. The presence of prodromal amaurosis fugax or diplopia should increase the suspicion for temporal arteritis. Pain is rare but can occur in about 10% of patients.[324]

Neuro-ophthalmic Signs. Exam findings are typical of an optic neuropathy with reduced acuity (at any level), dyschromatopsia, an afferent pupil defect, visual field loss that is most often inferior altitudinal,[154, 309, 325] and (again by definition) disc edema that is often pale and sectoral with splinter hemorrhages and dilated capillaries on the disc surface (Fig. 5–34; see Color Plates 23 and 24). In the IONDT, 49% of patients had better than 20/64 visual acuity at the time of presentation and 34% were worse than 20/200.[310] Patients typically have dyschromatopsia. However, many patients will identify color plates correctly, and the dyschromatopsia is detected only by subjective comparison between the eyes. An afferent pupillary defect should be present unless the other eye had a similar previous problem. Visual field defects can take any "optic nerve" type in addition to the classic altitudinal field loss. Up to one quarter of patients will have central scotomas.[154] Vitritis is not usually present and its presence should increase the clinical suspicion for alternative inflammatory and infectious diagnoses.

The characteristic disc appearance (Fig. 5–34) has sectoral swelling and splinter hemorrhages, often with attenuation of the peripapillar arterioles.[326] If a previous attack in the other eye resulted in a pale disc, the term *pseudo-Foster Kennedy* syndrome applies with ischemic swelling in the newly affected eye and old atrophy in the other eye (Fig. 5–35, also see Chapter 6).[327] Sequential attacks of ischemic optic neuropathy are distinguished from the true Foster Kennedy syndrome by the nature of the field loss and the reduction of the visual acuity in the eye with the swollen optic nerve.

Diagnostic Studies/Evaluation. Usually no further diagnostic studies need be obtained

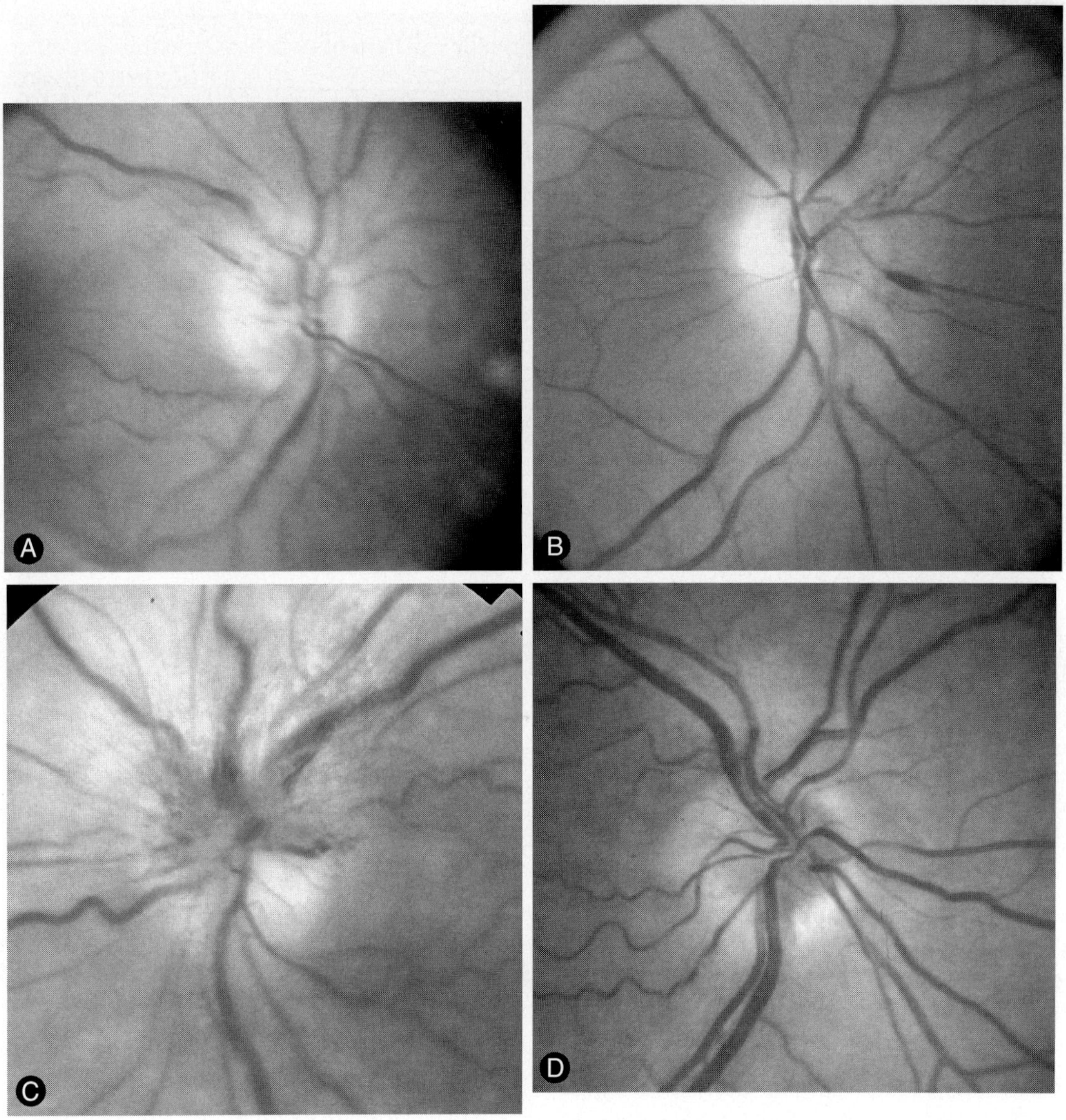

FIGURE 5–34. Typical appearances of the optic nerve in acute anterior ischemic optic neuropathy. In each case there is disc edema. Other commonly associated findings are (**A**) splinter hemorrhages and dilated capillaries on the disc surface, (**B**) sectoral disc pallor (See Color Plate 23), (**C**) sectoral swelling (see Color Plate 24). In **D**, the swelling is very mild.

although the erythrocyte sedimentation rate (ESR) and c-reactive protein levels should be checked to screen for temporal arteritis (see below). However, carefully timed fluorescein angiography may be able to distinguish ION disc swelling from other causes of disc swelling by demonstrating delayed optic nerve head filling.[328, 329] MRI does not have a role in the diagnosis of acute ION but on occasion is necessary to exclude compressive and infiltrative conditions mimicking simple ION. Gadolinium enhancement of the optic nerve may occur but is unusual.[649] Patients with nonarteritic ION have been shown to have an increased number of white matter ischemic changes compared to age- and disease-matched controls.[330] This likely reflects the presence of vasculopathic risk factors.

Clinical Course. The majority of patients have a fixed deficit, but a variable course with a significant incidence of progressive vision loss in the first month and high rate of spontaneous recovery can occur. A small percentage progress or recur.[331–333] One of the surprising outcomes of IONDT was the high rate of spontaneous improvement. Forty-three percent of the

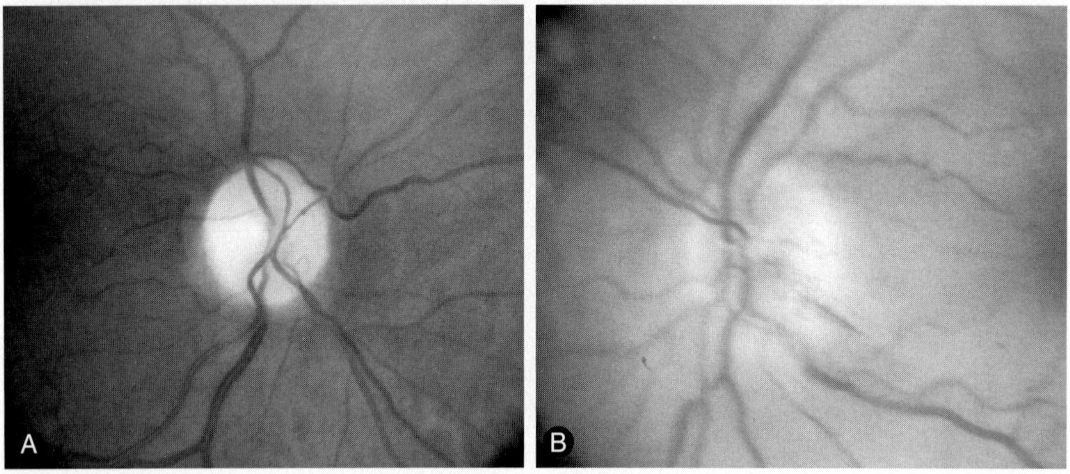

FIGURE 5–35. Right and left optic nerves of a patient with pre-existing optic neuropathy and disc pallor in the right eye (**A**) and acute vision loss in the left eye associated with disc swelling (**B**). The appearance of pallor in one eye and swelling in the other commonly results from sequential attacks of ischemic optic neuropathy and is termed the *pseudo-Foster Kennedy* syndrome.

patients who received no treatment recovered three or more lines of vision.[334] Other studies have also demonstrated spontaneous visual improvement.[331, 335] Optic atrophy develops as the disc edema resolves and there may be "luxury perfusion" or presumed upregulated capillaries on the surface of the ischemic disc.[336]

Some patients will be examined during a peculiar asymptomatic phase of the disease in which no visual dysfunction is measured but the disc is swollen. This premonitory phase of disc swelling often progresses to cause visual loss but may also resolve spontaneously.[337, 338]

There is a lifetime risk of 30% to 40% of patients having second-eye involvement.[339] The cumulative incidence rates are even higher in older patients and patients with diabetes and hypertension. Although one study suggested an increased risk of cerebrovascular and cardiovascular disease in ION patients,[340] this study has been criticized, and many believe that there is probably no increased risk for these conditions in patients with ION. Two recent studies examined the correlation between the visual dysfunction between the two eyes to determine if the result in one predicted the outcome of the other.[341, 342] In one study there was high correlation and in the other there was not.

Pathogenesis. Hayreh has provided much of the information concerning the presumed pathogenesis of ION.[343] AION may result from insufficiency in the posterior ciliary artery circulation and branches of peripapillary choroidal artery system. They may occlude with subsequent infarction of the ganglion cell axons where they coalesce to form the optic nerve head.[344] How systemic microvascular disease, a crowded optic nerve head, and possibly nocturnal hypotension ultimately lead to optic nerve head infarction is not certain.[345] Intuitively it is postulated that microvascular, atherosclerotic capillary disease compromises already narrowed lumens (from the crowded disc). Ultimately relative poor perfusion and catastrophic infarction occurs when perfusion pressure is reduced below a critical level. Experimental occlusion of the posterior ciliary arteries in monkeys results in a similar clinical appearance to ION with pale disc swelling.[346] There is limited evidence to suggest that an embolic event may cause nonarteritic ION.[347]

Several other factors support a vascular occlusive cause: sudden onset, association with diabetes, hypercholesterolemia, and hypertension, lack of evidence of inflammation, similarities in presentation to the arteritic variety, and a similar syndrome can be created in animals with an experimental vascular occlusion. However, there are several factors that cast some doubt on a simple vaso-occlusive pathogenesis in nonarteritic AION[345]:

1. There is no good autopsy evidence of occluded vessels.
2. The cilioretinal and choroidal circulations are usually spared.
3. Occurrence soon after cataract surgery is well recognized.[348, 349] Half of these patients

have involvement of the second eye if operated regardless of anesthesia type.

4. AION is only rarely associated with carotid disease.
5. Sequential attacks in two eyes are separated by months or years without intervening evidence of vascular occlusion affecting other organs.
6. Patients may have months of premonitory disc edema prior to visual loss.[337, 338]
7. One cause for ION is major blood loss (see below). In this setting there may be a delay of days to weeks before vision loss occurs.[350]
8. There are well-recognized cases of progression over weeks.[331–333]
9. ION is rarely encountered as a consequence of known embolic disorders such as atrial fibrillation.
10. Repeated attacks in the same eye are unusual. A protective effect from the first attack is certainly atypical for other kinds of vaso-occlusive disease such as stroke or myocardial infarction.

Other Systemic Associations With Nonarteritic AION. In addition to the general atherosclerotic risk factors of diabetes and hypertension, ION has been reported in the setting of other systemic afflictions. A hypercoagulable state secondary to antiphospholipid antibodies has been reported to occur in patients with AION, thus "young" patients with ION should be investigated for this possibility.[351–353] However, prothrombotic states in general are not associated with AION.[354] Patients with uremia have been described with vision loss and optic nerve swelling presumably on an ischemic basis.[355, 356] Visual loss is bilateral and improvement with hemodialysis has been reported. A possible component to the disc swelling from elevated intracranial pressure has been postulated.[355] Other patients with acute hypertensive crisis as in the setting of pre-eclampsia have been reported to develop ION.[357] Although perhaps an example of two common, unrelated conditions occurring in the same patient, typical migrainous episodes followed by AION have been reported.[358, 359]

Treatment. There is no known effective therapy. Steroids were used in the past but are now generally thought to be ineffective. Recently, optic nerve sheath fenestration or decompression was used and seemed to improve vision in some progressive cases.[360–362] Other series did not support the findings of these authors,[363, 364] and ultimately the IONDT was undertaken to answer the question definitively. The study concluded that the surgery was not beneficial and may be harmful since the group receiving surgery had a lower rate of visual recovery and a higher rate of loss of three or more lines of acuity.[334]

Hyperbaric oxygen[365] and aspirin[366] have also been shown to be ineffective in altering the early course of ischemic optic neuropathy. Heparin and warfarin are also unhelpful. Interestingly, levodopa and carbidopa have been shown to improve visual acuity in patients with even long-standing vision loss from ischemic optic neuropathy.[367] In this prospective, double-masked trial with 20 subjects, no effect on color vision or mean deviation of visual field was observed. Whether this ultimately becomes an important treatment for nonarteritic ION remains to be seen, however. A method of heparin-induced extracorporeal LDL/fibrinogen precipitation (HELP) designed to increase blood flow improved some visual function parameters in ION patients.[368] Finally, the protective effect of a previous attack of ION is powerful, as recurrence within a previously affected eye is rare. This has led Burde to suggest prophylactic, induced but controlled optic atrophy by panretinal photocoagulation.[320]

There is also no effective prophylaxis for second-eye involvement. For this purpose we often place patients with nonarteritic AION on aspirin 325 mg/day, if tolerated, but there is no prospective proof of its efficacy.[369, 370]

Clinical Distinction Between Optic Neuritis and Ischemic Optic Neuropathy. The clinical profile of these two groups of patients can overlap significantly, particularly in adults between the ages of 30 and 50, when they present with disc swelling but without pain on eye movements.[154] There are no laboratory tests to distinguish the two entities. However, in most instances the distinction is easily made based on consideration of the patient's age, associated symptoms, and exam findings. Patients under age 40 almost never get ION. The presence of pain is common in optic neuritis, while it is present in less than 10% of ION patients, and generally is not exacerbated by eye movements.[324] Also, a normal appearing nerve is common in optic neuritis and by definition not seen in AION. Warner et al[326] found that altitudinal swelling, pallor, arterial attenuation, and hemorrhage were more common in AION than in optic neuritis. Factors that are not helpful in distinguishing the two entities are sex, presenting visual acuity, and laboratory tests. Depending on the type of defect, the visual fields may be helpful in identifying typical ION from optic neuritis, as patients with ION typically have inferior altitudinal field loss.[371] However, there is enough overlap to make the distinction based on field criteria alone impossible. Maximal visual loss within 24 hours is not uncommon in optic neuritis and progression for up to 10 days can occur with ION.

Temporal Arteritis and Ischemic Optic Neuropathy

Visual symptoms due to temporal (giant cell, cranial, granulomatous, Horton's) arteritis are a neuro-ophthalmic emergency. Acute vision loss, the most feared complication of this disorder, occurs in between 7% and 60% of patients.[372] The most common mechanism is arteritic ION, referring to sudden optic nerve infarction due to vessels narrowed by vasculitis. A nonocular cause of visual loss in temporal arteritis, occipital lobe infarction, is reviewed in Chapter 8. Since many cases of blindness in giant cell arteritis are preventable with immediate administration of corticosteroids, suspected patients require emergent recognition and intervention.

Demographics. There is an increased incidence in women (3 : 1). Most affected individuals are Caucasian, but patients in other racial groups may be affected. The prevalence of giant cell arteritis increases with age, and it affects 1 in 1000 patients over age 80.[373–376] Most patients are over age 70, and cases below age 50 are exceedingly rare,[377] making patients with AION due to giant cell arteritis on average older than patients with nonarteritic AION.

Pathology. The vasculitis involves large and mid-sized arteries containing an elastic lamina. For the most part, these vessels tend to be extradural. The arteritis has a predilection for the superficial temporal, vertebral, ophthalmic, and posterior ciliary arteries.[378] This distribution explains the high frequency of blindness and the occasional cerebellar, brain stem, and occipital lobe strokes observed in this disorder. Optic nerve infarction typically occurs at a retrolaminar or prelaminar/retrolaminar watershed zone supplied by branches of the short ciliary arteries and branches of the ophthalmic artery.[379] Other vessels less commonly involved include the internal carotid, external carotid, and central retinal arteries. In addition, dissection due to involvement of the proximal aorta and myocardial infarction from vasculitis in the coronary arteries have both been reported.[380]

Histologically, early cases are characterized by lymphocytes limited to the internal or external elastic lamina or adventitia of the vessel wall, with destruction of those layers. More marked involvement is typified by involvement of all vascular layers. Necrosis and granulomas containing multinucleated histiocytic and foreign-body giant cells, histiocytes, and lymphocytes may be seen.[381] Inflammation of the arterial wall narrows the vessel lumen and allows thrombosis and vascular occlusion.[382]

Pathogenesis. The greater incidence in Caucasians and an association with HLA antigens DR3, DR4, DR5, DRB1, and Cw3 suggests giant cell arteritis may have a genetic component.[381, 383] Immunologic studies have demonstrated involvement of humoral and cellular immunity, particularly of T-cells.[383] Tissue and T-cell production of interferons and macrophage secretion of interleukins are also likely important.[384] The simultaneous occurrence of giant cell arteritis in a husband and wife supports a possible environmental exposure or infectious cause.[385]

Neuro-ophthalmic Symptoms. Patients may have premonitory episodes of transient monocular blindness prior to visual loss (sometimes when rising from a supine position) related to impaired ocular blood flow.[386] Another complaint may be bright-light amaurosis, caused by the increased metabolic demands of photoreceptors for which blood flow is unavailable.[387] Transient episodes of binocular diplopia[388] and formed visual hallucinations[389] may occur as well.

Visual loss is usually sudden and severe, and sometimes there is accompanying pain. Simultaneous bilateral vision loss occurs in 20% to 62% of patients with temporal arteritis.[388, 390–394] In untreated patients, one study found second-eye involvement occurs in approximately 75% of patients within days, and usually within a week.[391]

In contrast, simultaneous presentation with nonarteritic ION is rare and usually occurs only as a complication of surgery or with significant blood loss. Table 5–11 contrasts the clinical presentations of arteritic and nonarteritic ION.

Neuro-ophthalmic Signs. The neuro-ophthalmic complications of giant cell arteritis have been

TABLE 5–11. The Clinical Distinction Between Nonarteritic and Arteritic Ischemic Optic Neuropathy

Criteria	Nonarteritic	Arteritic
Age (years)	Any, usually 60–70	Rare under 50, most over 70
Race	No difference	More common in Caucasians, less common in African-Americans
Sex	No difference	More common in women
Preceding systemic symptoms	None	Common
Preceding ocular symptoms	None	Common, transient visual loss or diplopia
Pain	Rare	Common
Vision loss	Minimal to severe	Usually severe
Simultaneous involvement of eyes	Extremely rare	Occasional
Second-eye involvement	30%–40% in months or years	75% within days or weeks
Disc appearance	Sectoral edema	Normal or chalky white swelling
Sedimentation rate	< 40	Any; usually > 90
Fluorescein angiogram	Normal; can have delayed optic nerve head filling	Choroidal filling defects
Anatomic predisposition	Small, crowded optic nerve head	None
Other signs of ocular ischemia	Never	Occasional
Late optic atrophy	Simple pallor	Can have cupping
Response to steroids	None	Systemically—definite Vision—sometimes

the topic of several reviews.[383, 395–397] AION is the most common (80% to 90%) cause of vision loss in temporal arteritis (Table 5–12).[388, 391–393, 398] Visual loss is usually profound and in general is more severe than in nonarteritic ION.[309, 388, 394] Hand motion and NLP vision, which are uncommon in the nonarteritic version, occurred in 24% of eyes in one series (Fig. 5–36).[388]

The disc edema of arteritic AION is classically described as chalky white and may extend away from the disc (Fig. 5–37; see Color Plate 25). Alternatively, the infarction may be posterior or retrobulbar without disc swelling (posterior ischemic optic neuropathy (PION), see below). Cotton-wool spots may be an early sign (Fig. 5–38).[399] Vision loss may also occur on the basis of choroidal ischemia[400] or branch or central retinal artery occlusion (Fig. 5–39; see Color Plate 26). The simultaneous presence of AION and retinal arterial occlusion indicate ophthalmic artery involvement. Since few other disorders cause both of these together in the same eye, this combination makes the diagnosis arteritis until proven otherwise. Later in the course when optic atrophy supervenes, it is often associated with cupping.[401]

There may also be signs of ocular ischemia.[402, 403] Motility disturbances may also occur and result either from ischemia of the ex-

TABLE 5–12. Etiology of Visual Loss ($N = 63$ eyes) in One Study of 45 Patients With Biopsy-Proven Giant-Cell Arteritis

Anterior ischemic optic neuropathy (AION)*	55 (88%)
Posterior ischemic optic neuropathy (PION)	2 (3%)
Central retinal artery occlusion (CRAO)	3 (5%)
Branch retinal artery occlusion (BRAO)	3 (5%)
Choroidal infarction	4 (6%)
Optic atrophy (exact etiology unclear)	3 (5%)

* AION and CRAO, one eye; AION and BRAO, two eyes; AION and choroidal infarct, four eyes.

(From Liu GT et al, Ophthalmology 1994;101:1779–1785, with permission.)

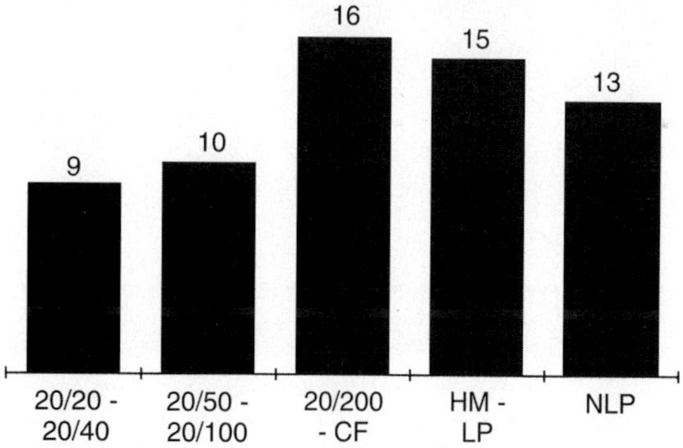

FIGURE 5–36. Initial visual acuities ($N = 63$ eyes) in one study of 45 patients with biopsy-proven giant cell arteritis and visual symptoms. (From Liu GT et al, Ophthalmology 1994;101:1779–1785, with permission.)

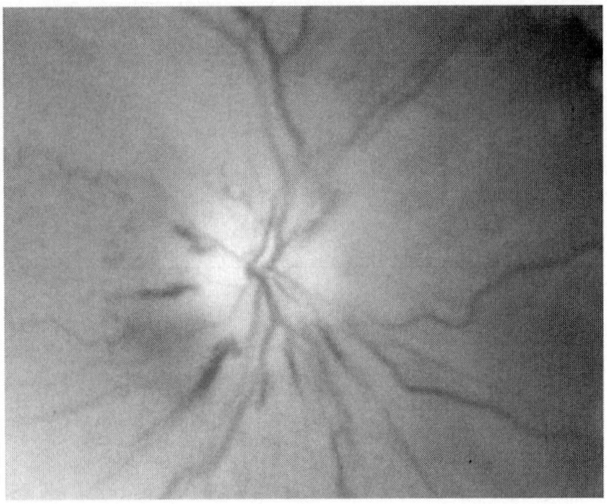

FIGURE 5–37. Acutely swollen optic nerve from arteritic ischemic optic neuropathy. Swelling has a chalky white appearance. (See Color Plate 25.)

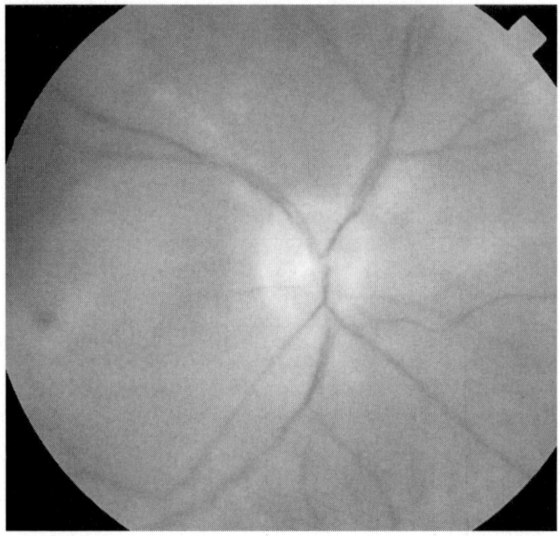

FIGURE 5–39. Central retinal artery occlusion from temporal arteritis. A macular cherry-red spot is present and there is no visible occlusive embolus. (See Color Plate 26.)

traocular muscles, ischemic ocular motor nerve palsies, or brain-stem stroke (see Chapter 15).[404]

Systemic Symptoms and Signs. Most patients with visual complications due to giant cell arteritis will have premonitory systemic symptoms (Table 5–13) for days or years prior to or accompanying their visual symptoms. Patients may have polymyalgia rheumatica (proximal muscle ache, stiffness, and arthralgias), headache, scalp tenderness, jaw claudication when chewing or talking, fever, malaise, or weight loss. Most of these symptoms are due to end-organ ischemia. Headaches and jaw claudication are the most common symptoms, and jaw claudication may predict a higher risk for vision loss.[388, 390, 405] In fact the new onset of headache in any elderly patient should raise this diagnostic possibility. Less common systemic complications include scalp necrosis[406, 407] and tongue or swallowing claudication. Between 16% and 26% of patients with visual complications due to giant cell arteritis will have an "occult" form[391, 408–410] with ophthalmic complaints but no systemic symptoms.

Physical examination will generally show an ill-appearing patient. Cachexia and pallor may

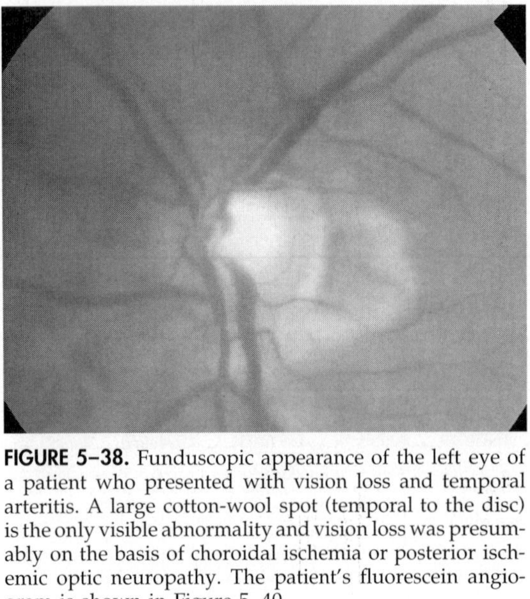

FIGURE 5–38. Funduscopic appearance of the left eye of a patient who presented with vision loss and temporal arteritis. A large cotton-wool spot (temporal to the disc) is the only visible abnormality and vision loss was presumably on the basis of choroidal ischemia or posterior ischemic optic neuropathy. The patient's fluorescein angiogram is shown in Figure 5–40.

TABLE 5–13. Systemic Symptoms Prior to Ophthalmic Presentation in One Study of 45 Patients With Biopsy-Proven Giant Cell Arteritis and Visual Symptoms

Symptom	%
Headache	58%
Jaw claudication	53%
Weight loss	31%
Malaise	22%
Polymyalgia rheumatica	22%
Anorexia	20%
Fever	11%
Neck pain	11%
Scalp tenderness	11%
Anemia	9%
Dementia	4%
Swallowing claudication	4%
Confusion, facial pain, periorbital edema, somnolence, tinnitus, vertigo	Each 2%

(From Liu GT et al, Ophthalmology 1994;101:1779–1785, with permission.)

be evident. The temporal artery may be tender, prominent, cordlike, and pulseless.

The neurologic complications of giant cell arteritis,[411] which include cerebrovascular symptoms[412] and other cranial nerve palsies,[413] are discussed further in Chapters 8 and 15.

Making the Diagnosis. In our experience, patients with AION or central retinal artery occlusion due to giant cell arteritis can be identified by any combination of (1) age over 50, (2) typical fundus appearance (disc swelling with or without retinal infarction), (3) typical systemic symptoms, (4) high erythrocyte sedimentation rate (ESR), (5) positive temporal artery biopsy, (6) high C-reactive protein, and (7) abnormal fluorescein angiography. When systemic symptoms are absent in so-called occult temporal arteritis,[409] the ESR is almost always elevated.[388] If the ESR is normal, systemic symptoms are almost always present. In other words, visual loss due to giant cell arteritis with a normal ESR and without systemic symptoms would be extremely unusual. Although more strict criteria for the diagnosis of giant cell arteritis have been published,[414] we have found the above guidelines to be extremely helpful in clinical practice.

The discussion below details the various laboratory tests.

Blood Tests. Normal ESRs can be estimated by the following formula: age × 0.5 for males, and (age + 10) × 0.5 for females. The ESR is usually elevated in giant cell arteritis and often is above 90 mm/hr. However, elevated ESRs are nonspecific, since a number of normal elderly patients have increased ESRs and half of those with ESRs over 50 have no explanation found.[415, 416] In addition, as many as 22% of patients with temporal arteritis and visual symptoms can have normal ESRs.[373, 388, 417]

In a recent study, an elevated C-reactive protein (>2.45 mg/dl), another acute phase reactant, was more sensitive (100%) than the ESR (>47 mm/hr) for the diagnosis of giant cell arteritis.[405] The combination of an elevated ESR and C-reactive protein yielded a specificity of 97% for the diagnosis of giant cell arteritis.

Chronic mild to moderate normochromic anemia also may be evident.[381]

Fluorescein Angiography. Fluorescein or indocyanine angiography may show delayed choroidal filling and focal, patchy perfusion defects (Fig. 5–40).[418–421] We have found this test to be extremely useful because of its relative sensitivity and specificity for giant cell arteritis when those angiographic features are demonstrated.

Temporal Artery Biopsy. If temporal arteritis is clinically suspected, a temporal artery biopsy should be performed (Fig. 5–41). The procedure rarely results in significant complications, and therefore a low threshold to perform biopsy should exist. A high ratio of negative to positive results is acceptable. Skip lesions are often present, so generally long segments (>3 cm) are recommended.[422–424] Grossly, at the

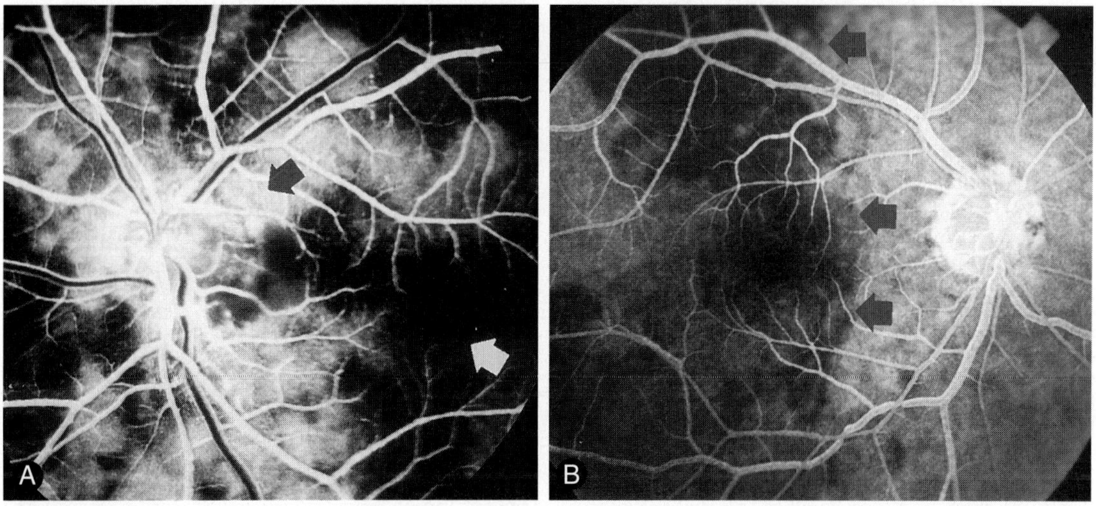

FIGURE 5–40. Fluorescein angiograms in two patients with temporal arteritis and vision loss. The angiogram in **A** corresponds to the eye in Figure 5–38. Normal choroidal perfusion (*large black arrow*) is accompanied by large patchy areas of nonperfusion (*large white arrow*). Similar findings are seen in another patient (**B**) with a large area of choroidal nonperfusion (*large black arrows*).

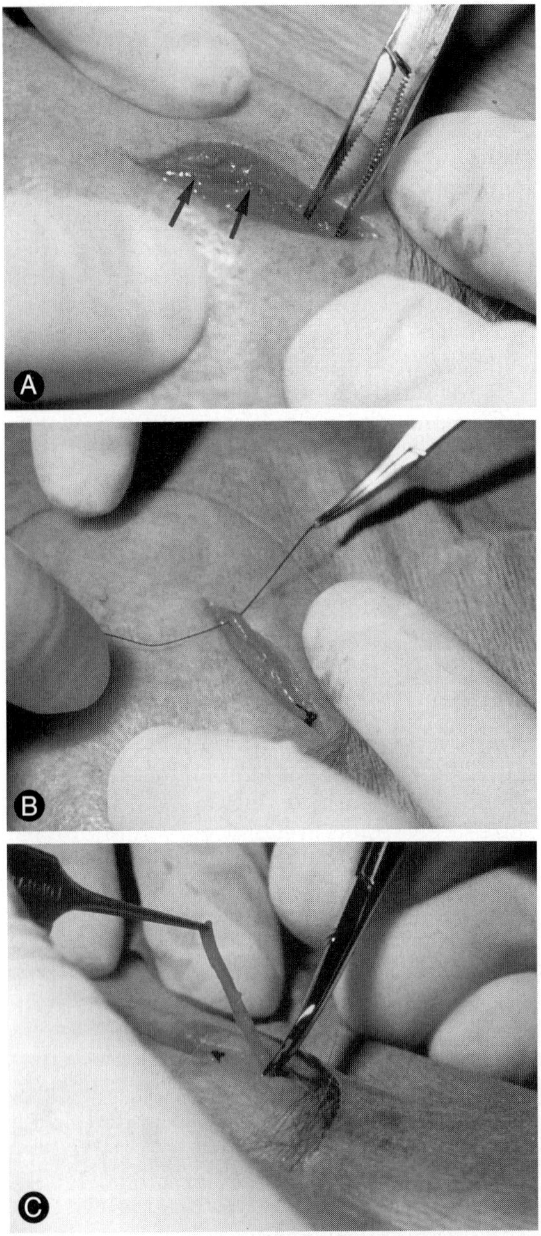

FIGURE 5–41. Sequence of steps used to perform temporal artery biopsy, which can be performed in the office under local anesthesia. Location of the artery either by palpation of the pulse or with doppler is critical. An incision is made directly over the artery through the skin and subcuticular layers. **A.** The dissection is carried through the subcutaneous fat with cautery exposing the artery in the superficial temporal fascia (arrows point to artery). Blunt dissection is used to separate the artery from the surrounding fascia. **B.** A silk suture ligature is tied around either end of the artery. **C.** The segment of artery between the two sutures is then removed through sharp dissection away from the rest of the fascia.

time of surgery, arterial abnormalities are often present and consist of irregular thickening, stiffness, and a mottled grey appearance (Fig. 5–42; see Color Plate 27). Multiple transverse sections should be made of each segment. Histopathologic evaluation (Fig. 5–43) reveals transmural inflammation, with destruction of the internal elastic lamina, obliteration of the lumen, and characteristic epithelioid cell and giant cells. False-positive temporal artery biopsies are rare, but have been seen in Wegener's granulomatosis[425] and sarcoidosis,[426] for example. A rarely necessary but alternative biopsy site is the occipital artery.[427]

The issue of whether to obtain a bilateral or unilateral temporal artery biopsy remains controversial. In many cases the initial biopsy can be seen to be grossly abnormal at the time of surgery (see Fig. 5–42) and only unilateral biopsy need be performed. We obtain bilateral biopsies when the initial biopsy is negative or equivocal and clinical suspicion for giant cell arteritis remains high. In a series of 186 patients who had bilateral biopsies, only 6 (3%) had a different pathology between the two sides.[428] In three cases, the findings were consistent with healed arteritis and in the other three cases early arteritis was suggested. Thus, the added value of a second contralateral temporal biopsy is relatively low.

There is no reason to withhold treatment while waiting to do a biopsy. Histopathologic evidence of arteritis can be seen at least 1 week after treatment with steroids.[429] It is also now well established that biopsies in some chronic cases can still reflect diagnostic pathology several weeks and maybe even years after steroid therapy has begun.[388, 430–432]

Only rarely, based on clinical grounds, is a diagnosis of biopsy-negative temporal arteritis made. We caution against making this diagnosis routinely and as well against making a di-

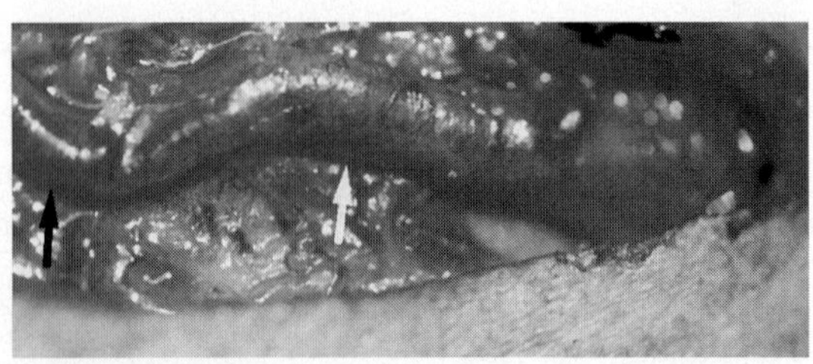

FIGURE 5–42. Gross abnormalities in the appearance of the superficial temporal artery at the time of biopsy in a patient with temporal arteritis. The thinner, more normal-appearing artery is seen to the left (*black arrow*) and the thickened, grey, more mottled artery is seen in the middle (*white arrow*). (See Color Plate 27.)

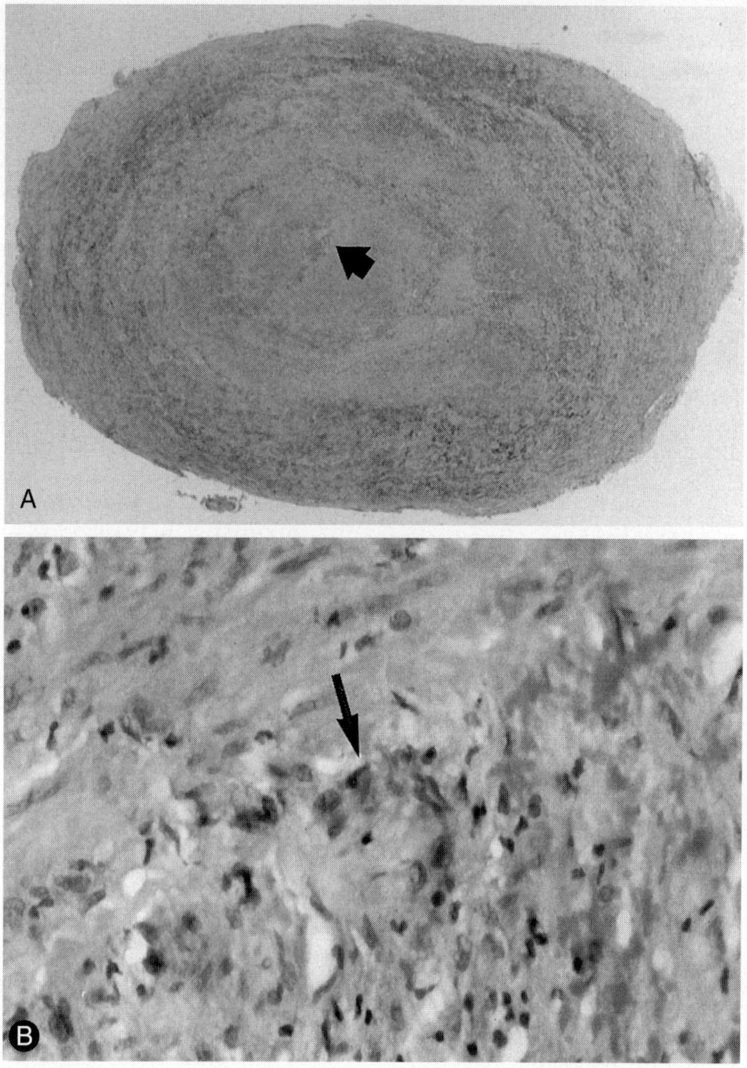

FIGURE 5–43. Histopathology of superficial temporal artery biopsy. **A.** Low-power view demonstrating transmural inflammation and obliteration of the arterial lumen (*arrow*). **B.** Higher-power view demonstrating giant cell (*arrow*). (Courtesy of Dr. Laura Balcer.)

agnosis without biopsy on a presumptive basis. Too often, months down the line, during steroid treatment, with devastating side effects for the patient,[433] the clinician is left in a quandary because no tissue diagnosis was made.

Noninvasive Vascular Studies. Abnormal ocular perfusion may be noted with ocular pneumoplethysmography. Color doppler may demonstrate abnormal flow within the ophthalmic, central retinal, and short posterior ciliary arteries,[434] and temporal artery wall abnormalities may also be seen with this modality.[435] Currently these tests are not part of our usual workup.

Management/Treatment. When patients present with vision loss, successful prevention of second-eye involvement is the goal of prompt and accurate diagnosis. There is also a risk for neurologic and cardiac complications in untreated patients. Evidence from anecdotal and retrospective studies suggest that (1) corticosteroids retard the progression of visual loss, (2) corticosteroids may diminish the risk of fellow-eye involvement, (3) on occasion (15% to 34%) steroids may restore some vision, sometimes dramatically, and (4) IV steroids may be more effective than oral steroids in protecting the fellow eye and enhancing visual prognosis, in part because of a higher IV corticosteroid dose and greater bioavailability.[388, 390,

[436–442] Alternatively, some authors have argued that IV steroids are no more effective than oral regimens.[443, 444] However, it is our impression that while systemic symptoms may respond to oral doses, patients with visual symptoms due to giant cell arteritis require larger doses of corticosteroids given intravenously.

Therefore, in the absence of prospective data, in cases in which diagnosis is strongly suspected and visual symptoms or signs are present, we recommend immediate IV steroid therapy (methylprednisolone 250 mg qid) for 3 to 5 days with ulcer prophylaxis. The high ESR and systemic symptoms usually improve immediately. Following the IV treatment, prednisone 1 mg/kg per day is given orally. The steroid dose should remain high for the first month; then, as long as the ESR stays normal and systemic symptoms are absent, the dose can be tapered slowly over 6 to 12 months. Many individuals require a small daily or every other day maintenance dose beyond this period. Side effects from chronic steroid usage are common in this age group,[445] therefore a physician knowledgeable and experienced in the use of steroids should supervise steroid dosing and management of side effects.

Cases of giant cell arteritis refractory to corticosteroids are extremely challenging.[403] Some patients demonstrate flow-related ophthalmologic and neurologic phenomena, requiring Tredelenburg positioning or heparinization.[387, 446] In addition, some patients' symptoms recur many months or even years after initial corticosteroid treatment.[388, 447] Repeat temporal artery biopsies can demonstrate persistent or recurrent arteritis in these cases.[448] In these instances, steroid-sparing, anti-inflammatory, and immunomodulating therapy such as methotrexate or dapsone[449, 450] can be considered.

Visual Prognosis. The prognosis for visual improvement in giant cell arteritis is relatively poor.[391, 451] Many studies[393, 451, 452] reported absolutely no recovery in NLP eyes, an observation the Bascom Palmer series[388] supported with the exception of one case. Progressive vision loss can also occur despite steroid therapy, oral or IV, in 9% to 14% of patients.[388, 390, 453, 454]

However, there are several anecdotal reports of patients with giant cell arteritis and AION[379, 436, 438, 440, 441] or central retinal artery occlusion[439] who enjoyed remarkable visual improvement. Literature reviews and institutional series demonstrate that as many as 15% to 34% of patients may experience some recovery of vision.[388, 390, 455] Relatively higher rates of improvement have been attributed to the use of IV versus oral corticosteroids, as a greater percentage of patients (9 of 23 (39%) versus 5 of 18 (28%)) improved after IV treatment in the Bascom Palmer series.[388] However, this difference was not statistically significant, and as alluded to earlier, the advantages of IV over oral treatment are controversial.[443, 444] Visual recovery without steroid treatment is rare.[455]

Relationship Between Polymyalgia Rheumatica and Temporal Arteritis. It is possible these two entities represent the same rheumatologic disorder, except the term *temporal arteritis* is used to describe cases with involvement of the arterities of the head. Patients with polymyalgia rheumatica may develop temporal arteritis and visual loss despite years of corticosteroid treatment.[388] The best treatment regimen (ie, low-dose versus high-dose corticosteroids or some alternative medication) for preventing ophthalmic complications in polymyalgia rheumatica and in cases of temporal arteritis without previous ocular symptoms has not been established.[456–460]

Posterior Ischemic Optic Neuropathy

Posterior ION (PION), presumably due to infarction of the retrolaminar optic nerve, should prompt a thorough systemic workup. In contrast to nonarteritic AION, nonarteritic PION is exceedingly unusual. The diagnosis of a retrobulbar ischemic optic neuropathy in an elderly patient demands immediate investigation for giant cell arteritis, inflammatory causes, and an infiltrative process associated with carcinomatous meningitis or CNS infection, for example. Blood loss and surgery, discussed below, should also be considered. Inflammatory conditions such as lupus, polyarteritis nodosa, and herpes zoster have been reported in association with PION.[461] Sickle cell disease has also been reported as a cause.[462] Neuroimaging is also required to exclude the sudden presentation of a compressive mass lesion such as pituitary apoplexy or an ophthalmic artery aneurysm.

Recently migraine has also been reported as a cause of PION.[463] One series identified diabetes, hypertension, and carotid stenosis as risk factors for PION,[464] but in our experience such cases are exceedingly rare.

Ischemic Optic Neuropathy Associated With Surgery or Blood Loss

In so-called shock-associated ischemic optic neuropathy, an additional risk factor of anemia, atherosclerosis, or severe blood loss must be present in order for low blood pressure to cause infarction of the optic nerve.[465, 466] The patients that Drance reported were middle aged to elderly, and most had a history of significant blood loss.[467] Visual loss, often profound, may be delayed for hours to days following the hypotensive event, suggesting an abnormal autoregulatory mechanism may be responsible.[350, 468] When disc swelling occurs, it tends to be pallid.

Either anterior or posterior ischemic optic neuropathy can occur during or following surgery.[469] Reported procedures have included lumbar spine surgery, neck surgery, open heart surgery, and surgical procedures complicated by blood loss.[468, 470–475] One case was reported in association with peritoneal dialysis.[644]

The visual prognosis in shock or postoperative ischemic optic neuropathy is poor. High-dose steroids may be tried but in general are unhelpful.

Diabetic Papillopathy

The spectrum of disc swelling in diabetic patients ranges from the typical older patient with diabetes as a risk factor for common AION to the young juvenile diabetic with benign disc swelling that resolves without residua. This is a continuum, as some young patients can develop mild optic neuropathy and some older diabetics can have transient optic nerve swelling without vision loss.

The type I or juvenile-onset, insulin-dependent diabetic patients are generally diagnosed with benign diabetic papillopathy or papillophlebitis.[476–478] The onset is usually between age 20 and 40, and patients have generally had diabetes for years. Mild visual loss to approximately 20/40 is not uncommon, and there is often corresponding enlargement of the blind spot with occasional arcuate or central field defects. Typically prominent telangiectactic vascular dilation (Fig. 5–44; see Color Plate 28) is evident on the disc surface, and contiguous swelling may extend into the macula.[477] Disc edema may be bilateral and may be prolonged with a highly variable course. Patients have an increased risk for subsequent disc neovascularization.[477, 479] Visual recovery begins weeks to months after onset and may precede the resolution of the disc swelling. Mild optic atrophy can develop. The pathogenesis of this condition is poorly understood but most likely represents blood flow disruption to the optic disc surface, sufficient enough to cause swelling and interfere with axoplasmic transport but insufficient to cause impaired nerve function. In the setting of bilateral disc swelling, it is important to distinguish this condition from papilledema.

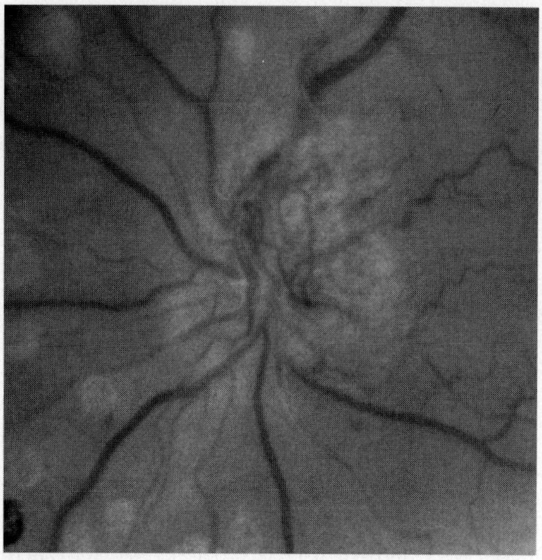

FIGURE 5–44. Appearance of the optic nerve in acute diabetic papillopathy. In addition to disc swelling there are dilated vessels on the disc surface. Round lesions in the retinal periphery are the result of previous panretinal photocoagulation. (See Color Plate 28.)

COMPRESSIVE OPTIC NEUROPATHIES

Compressive lesions can be identified by their typical presentation with slowly progressive visual loss and optic nerve atrophy. Although less common, compressive optic neuropathy should still be considered in patients with acute vision loss, and in addition most individuals with unexplained vision loss should undergo MRI to exclude this potentially treatable cause.

Causes. Compressive optic neuropathy can result in the setting of benign or malignant neoplasms, contiguous sinus (mucocele) lesions or osseous processes (fibrous dysplasia), enlarged extraocular muscles, or abnormal vascular structures such as aneurysms. This condition can develop intrinsically from the nerve substance or from adjacent structures. More rarely they are the result of infiltrative processes or from spread of mass lesions from different sites as with metastatic tumors. Table 5–14 summarizes the important causes of compressive optic neuropathy.

Symptoms. Ophthalmic and nonophthalmic symptoms generally evolve subacutely or insidiously (Table 5–15). Sudden vision loss can be superimposed on a chronic compressive problem, such as hemorrhage into a lymphangioma (chocolate cyst) or in a pituitary tumor (apoplexy), expansion of a cystic lesion as with craniopharyngioma, rapid enlargement of a parainfectious lesion such as a mucocele, and finally, rapid expansion of an aneurysm. Other associated symptoms are outlined in Table 5–15.

Neuro-ophthalmic Signs. Patients usually present with reduced acuity, color vision, and visual field defects typical of an optic neuropathy (central, centrocecal, or nerve fiber bundle). The optic nerve may appear normal, pale, or swollen. Optic disc swelling can result from compression and axoplasmic stasis, elevated intracranial pressure, or direct nerve infiltration. Compression will only result in optic nerve head swelling when the lesion is intraorbital and is not a consequence of intracanalicular or intracranial lesions, which more typically result directly in optic atrophy. Papilledema is an unusual cause for disc swelling in the setting of compressive optic neuropathy except with large subfrontal meningiomas and with massive lesions that compress the third ventricle and cause obstructive hydrocephalus. When a large frontal lobe lesion compresses one optic nerve with resultant ipsilateral optic atrophy and elevates intracranial pressure to cause contralateral papilledema, this is the Foster Kennedy syndrome (see Chapter 6).[480] Swelling may be accompanied by collateral ("shunt") vessels (Fig. 5–45) which bypass the central retinal vein and allow blood to flow from the retinal circulation directly into the ciliary circulation. They are common with optic nerve sheath meningioma but also occur with gliomas and chronic papilledema. Visual loss in the setting of extrinsic compression of the optic nerve results from a combination of Wallerian (ascending or beginning at the cell body) axonal degeneration, demyelination, and axonal dysfunction.

Diagnostic Studies/Neuroimaging. The diagnosis of compressive lesions of the anterior visual pathways requires neuroimaging. The best modality for the orbits and brain is

TABLE 5–14. Compressive Lesions of the Optic Nerve

Intraorbital
Primary orbital tumors (see Chapter 18)
Cavernous hemangioma
Schwannoma
Secondary orbital tumors (see Chapter 18)
Sinus tumor
Metastatic tumors
Enlarged extraocular muscles (see Chapter 18)
Intraorbital/Intracanalicular/Intracranial
Optic nerve neoplasms (primary)
Optic nerve glioma (juvenile benign)
Malignant optic nerve glioma
Optic nerve sheath meningioma
Optic nerve neoplasms (metastatic)
Carcinomatous meningitis
Optic nerve metastasis
Lymphoma
Leukemia
Myeloma
Intracanalicular/Intracranial
Nontumor sinus causes
Mucocele
Paraclinoid tumors
Meningioma
Vascular causes
Aneurysm
Ectatic carotid arteries
"Chiasmal" lesions (see Chapter 7)
Pituitary adenoma
Craniopharyngioma
Suprasellar meningioma
Other causes
Fibrous dysplasia

TABLE 5–15. Common Ophthalmic and Nonophthalmic Symptoms Associated With Compressive Optic Neuropathy

Ophthalmic
Reduced vision
Subacute progression
"Pseudosudden" onset from unrecognized disease
Decreased color vision
Gaze evoked amaurosis
Pain on eye movement
Orbital fullness
Proptosis
Ptosis
Nonophthalmic
Headache (mass effect or dural involvement)
Facial numbness or paresthesias (trigeminal nerve involvement)
Reduced sense of smell (olfactory nerve involvement)
Endocrine abnormalities (hypothalamic/pituitary axis involvement)

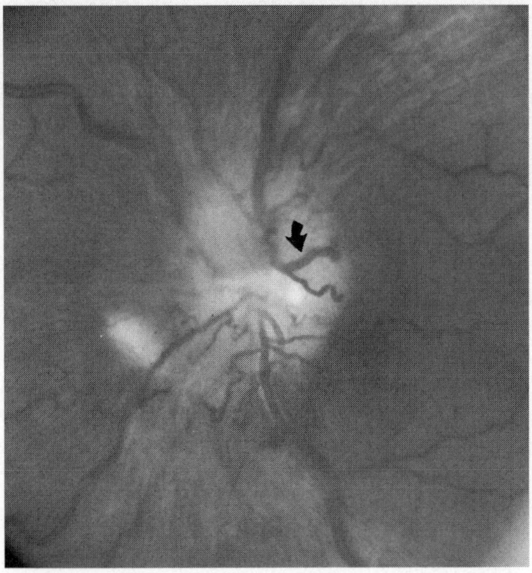

FIGURE 5–45. Chronic disc swelling from a subfrontal meningioma with disc collateral vessel (*arrow*) that connects the retinal venous system to the choroid, thereby bypassing the central retinal vein.

MRI with fat-saturated orbital views and gadolinium-DPTA enhancement (Fig. 5–46). This technique offers excellent views of the globe, optic nerve head, optic nerve, optic nerve sheath, extraocular muscles, and orbital apex. It is far superior to CT in the evaluation of the intracranial portion of the optic nerve, the chiasm, and the cavernous sinus. CT serves an ancillary role and is helpful in evaluating bony changes, tumor calcification, and paranasal sinus disease.

The remaining discussion highlights the various compressive causes. However, primarily orbital processes, such as Graves or thyroid eye disease, are covered in Chapter 18, metastatic lesions are summarized later in this chapter in the section discussing cancer, and sellar processes that can cause intracranial compression of the optic nerve are discussed in Chapter 7.

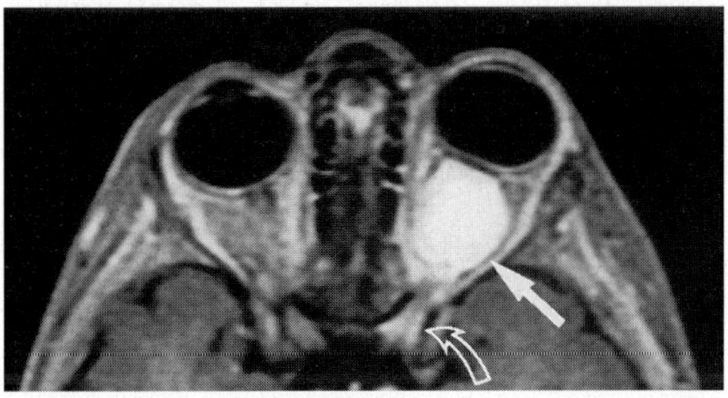

FIGURE 5–46. Axial T_1-weighted, fat-saturated, gadolinium-enhanced MRI scan of the orbits demonstrating normal anatomic detail of the right orbit (globe, optic nerve, extraocular muscles and orbital apex) and an optic nerve glioma in the left orbit. The intraorbital portion (*straight white arrow*) of the left optic nerve is bulbous and enhances, while the intracranial portion (*curved white open arrow*) is only slightly thickened, but also enhances.

Primary Optic Nerve Neoplasms: Optic Nerve Glioma (Juvenile, Benign)

Primary gliomas of the anterior visual pathways are of two different varieties. The first is the juvenile, benign, pilocytic astrocytoma. The second is the rare malignant glioblastoma of adulthood.

The benign optic gliomas of childhood generally present in the first decade of life with proptosis and slowly progressive painless vision loss (Fig. 5–47).[481] The disc may be swollen or pale and secondary strabismus often accompanies the vision loss. Visual field defects are generally central scotomas but temporal or bitemporal field defects may occur if the prechiasmatic portion of the nerve is involved.[482] Rare ophthalmic complications include congenital glaucoma with buphthalmos ("ox eye"), central retinal vein occlusion, iris rubeosis with neovascular glaucoma, and ocular ischemic syndrome.

Demographics. Most patients present in childhood, before age 10. About one quarter (range 10% to 70%, depending on series) of the patients with optic nerve and chiasmal glioma have neurofibromatosis (NF) type 1.[483] In contrast, about 15% of patients with NF-1 develop anterior visual pathway gliomas, and in two thirds of this subset, the neuro-ophthalmologic

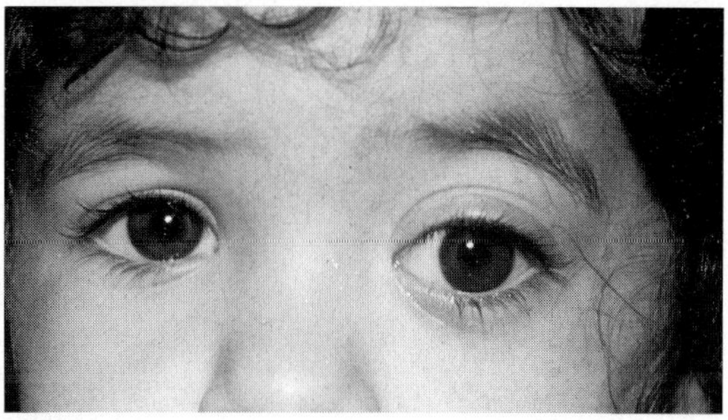

FIGURE 5–47. A young girl who presented with decreased vision and proptosis of the left eye from an optic nerve glioma. The corresponding MRI scan is demonstrated in Figure 5–46.

examination is normal without visual loss or optic atrophy.[484] The relationship between NF-1 and optic pathway gliomas is discussed in more detail in the section on chiasmal/hypothalmic gliomas in Chapter 7.

Diagnostic Studies/Neuroimaging. Neuroimaging typically reveals fusiform enlargement, kinking, and enhancement of the optic nerve (see Fig. 5–46).[485, 486] MRI is better than CT in this setting because of its superiority in evaluating the possibility of intracranial extension. At the time of detection about half of the tumors already exhibit chiasmal involvement.[487] The diagnosis is generally a clinical and radiographic one, and tumor biopsy of a suspected optic nerve glioma is almost never needed, especially in the setting of NF-1. In our experience, bilateral optic nerve enlargement without chiasmal involvement is virtually pathognomonic of NF-1.

Pathology. Histologically the tumors are generally juvenile pilocytic astrocytomas. They are usually confined to the subarachnoid space, occasionally invade the optic nerve, and only rarely extend outside the optic nerve sheath. The tumors appear benign without mitosis, cellular atypia, or necrosis. Occasionally proliferation of arachnoid around the tumor may simulate meningioma.

Clinical Course. The clinical course is highly variable. Most tumors grow only very slowly and may have self-limited growth. Many patients with tumors confined to the orbit will maintain good vision and in some rare instances even improve spontaneously.[481] Alvord and Lofton[487] projected, however, that all tumors eventually grow, with 70% showing progression within 3 years and 7% of patients dying of their disease. Some believe that the prognosis is worse in non-NF cases, and this has been our impression as well.

Optic nerve gliomas presenting without radiographic demonstration of chiasmal or hypothalamic involvement, which subsequently extend posteriorly, are uncommon. To our knowledge, there has been only one published, well-documented report.[488] However, this case was examined with CT only, and it is possible that microscopic infiltration of the chiasm in the initial study was missed. Using modern gadolinium-enhanced MRI, with thin, high-resolution sections through the chiasm and proximal optic nerve, we have yet to see any patient with an optic nerve glioma with unequivocal sparing of the chiasm at presentation who later developed chiasmal involvement.

Treatment. It cannot be overemphasized that in younger children, an optic nerve tumor is amblyogenic. Therefore, in children under age 8 with monocular vision loss from an optic pathway tumor, part-time occlusion therapy (patching) of the unaffected eye is recommended under the direction of a pediatric ophthalmologist.[489] This is an attempt to reverse any possible amblyopic component of visual loss complicating that due to optic neuropathy. In many patients we have been able to regain several lines of visual acuity within weeks of diagnosis. Thus, in terms of visual recovery, we consider patching the most effective therapy.

Usually serial neuro-ophthalmic examinations and MRI are performed to exclude clinical or radiographic progression. Either is an indication for more aggressive treatment, and options include chemotherapy, radiation, or surgical removal of the tumor. Chemotherapy would be first-line treatment in a child under 6, while radiation of the optic nerve tumor would be the primary option in an older child. Both of these modalities appear to have some efficacy in halting progression, at least temporarily. They are discussed in more detail in the glioma section in Chapter 7.

Surgical removal of the prechiasmatic portion of the optic nerve is a better option than chemotherapy or radiation when the eye is almost blind and the proptosis is severe and cosmetically unacceptable, or when the tumor appears on serial scanning to be encroaching upon a previously uninvolved chiasm.[490, 491] The procedure requires a combined approach by an orbital surgeon, to excise the intraorbital portion, and a neurosurgeon, to remove via craniotomy, the intracanalicular and intracranial portion. The extraocular muscles and the nerves supplying them are spared.

Primary Optic Nerve Neoplasms: Malignant Optic Nerve Glioma (Glioblastoma)

Malignant optic nerve glioblastoma represents a much rarer, distinct condition that affects middle-age to older adults. Patients present with unilateral or bilateral (chiasmal involvement) vision loss, headache, and pain on eye movements that is similar to that in optic neuritis. Patients often have disc swelling, and the fundus appearance may mimic that of venous stasis retinopathy.[492, 493] Patients can progress to bilateral blindness within weeks. With intraorbital involvement there is proptosis and conjunctival chemosis, and there can be progression to neovascular glaucoma. The tumor spreads intracranially and often involves the diencephalon. Death usually occurs within months. Radiation therapy may be associated with some preservation of vision and prolongation of life. Early in the course transient visual improvement may occur when steroids are used empirically before the correct diagnosis is made.

Involvement of the chiasm is discussed in Chapter 7.

Meningiomas of the Optic Nerve Sheath

Compressive optic neuropathy may result from meningiomas arising primarily from the intraorbital optic nerve sheath. These primary optic nerve sheath meningiomas (ONSMs) occur primarily in middle-aged women (2:1 men) and are usually unilateral. Bilateral and multifocal cases occur in NF type II.[494]

Pathology and Growth Characteristics. The tumors arise from meningothelial cells in the arachnoid villi. ONSMs surround the optic nerve and result in impaired axonal transport and interfere with the pial blood supply to the optic nerve. Growth of these tumors is usually indolent over many years, but the rate may increase with pregnancy.[495]

Neuro-ophthalmic Symptoms and Signs. Patients usually present with slowly progressive vision loss, and other visual complaints include double vision, transient visual obscurations, and gaze evoked amaurosis.[496–498] On occasion they are aware of headache or notice proptosis.

Patients have moderate to severe acuity loss, with 15% to 50% having better than 20/40 and 20% to 60% having less than 20/200 acuity.[496–498] Dyschromatopsia is usually present, and visual field defects commonly seen include central scotomas, enlarged blind spots, and generalized constriction. The optic disc essentially always appears abnormal, with about half the patients having optic atrophy and half having disc swelling.[496–498] Optociliary collateral vessels are present in 15% to 33% of patients and are commonly seen in both swollen and atrophic nerves.[645] Most patients have measurable proptosis.

Diagnostic Studies/Neuroimaging. Neuroimaging is usually diagnostic, showing diffuse, tubular optic nerve enlargement (Fig. 5–48). On CT, calcification or a "tram track sign," referring to two parallel lines along the length of the nerve, is often seen.[486, 497] MRI is now the procedure of choice to identify and determine the extent of ONSMs (Fig. 5–48).[499, 500] The tumor is isointense with brain on T_1- and T_2-weighted images and smoothly enhances with gadolinium.[501] Often the MRI scan will show the tumor to be separate from the optic nerve proper on coronal views, and exquisite demonstration of the details of the intracanalicular optic nerve helps to identify intracranial extension.

The pattern of fusiform enlargement overlaps with optic nerve glioma but kinking is not seen with meningioma. The diagnosis is

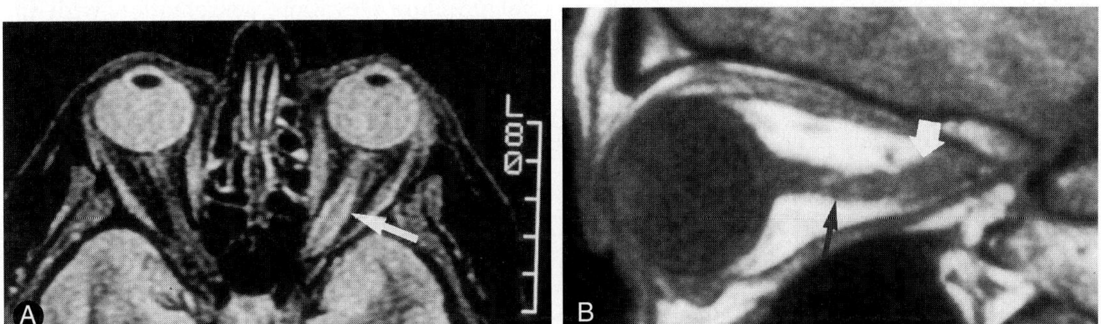

FIGURE 5–48. Neuroimaging in optic nerve sheath meningiomas. **A.** Axial, T_2-weighted MRI scan showing left optic nerve sheath meningioma with diffuse enlargement of the posterior portion of the intraorbital optic nerve (*arrow*). **B.** In another example, on a sagittal T_1-weighted image, the beginning of the diffuse, isointense, sheath enlargement is clearly seen (*black arrow*) and widens (*white arrow*) toward the orbital apex.

therefore established on clinical and radiographic grounds and like glioma, tumor biopsy is almost nerve needed. The radiographic appearance of ONSMs also can be simulated by orbital pseudotumor (particularly the sclerosing variety), optic perineuritis,[287] sarcoid infiltration, and lymphomatous and carcinomatous meningitis. All of these conditions present with much more rapidity than ONSMs and are often associated with pain.

Clinical Course. These tumors progress insidiously, sometimes causing complete blindness of the eye. Fortunately, intracranial extension of optic nerve sheath meningioma is quite rare.

Treatment. In the rare equivocal case, biopsy is required to establish the diagnosis. This is recommended only in an eye with poor vision after serial lumbar punctures to exclude inflammation and neoplasm were normal, and after steroids failed to improve vision.

The mainstay of management for optic nerve sheath meningioma is radiation therapy.[498, 502–504] This modality is generally reserved for adult patients with salvageable vision. If visual function is good, better than 20/40 with mild field loss, then observation alone can be used until progression is documented. Radiation therapy can be offered when vision loss progresses.

Surgical excision is not recommended as a method of improving vision but is used to treat blind, uncomfortable, or unsightly eyes and as well to reduce the risk of intracranial extension. In patients with intracranial extension, surgery and radiation have been tried. Surgical results are poor,[496] although radiation has been shown to be of some benefit.[505] The potential benefit of surgery, however, is much greater in ONSMs than in surgical decompression (not necessarily excision) of meningiomas arising secondarily from sphenoid wing and paraclinoid meningiomas.[506, 507]

Meningiomas of the Skull Base

Alternatively, meningiomas arising from the planum sphenoidale or olfactory groove may involve the optic nerve in its intraorbital or intracanalicular portions (Table 5–16). Suprasellar, tuberculum sellae, parasellar, and sphenoid wing meningiomas can also cause optic neuropathy, but because suprasellar and tuberculum sellae meningiomas more commonly cause chiasmal compression, and the other two are more likely lead to eye movement disorders, they are discussed in more detail in Chapters 7 and 15, respectively. The section on meningiomas in Chapter 7 also provides an overview of the pathology, associations, and neuroimaging characteristics of skull base meningiomas.

TABLE 5–16. Specific Neuro-ophthalmic Presentations in Meningiomas at the Base of Skull[627]

Tumor Location	Neuro-ophthalmic Findings
Planum sphenoidale and olfactory groove	Optic neuropathy, Foster Kennedy syndrome
Tuberculum sellae	Unilateral or bilateral vision loss, often with chiasmal involvement
Optic canal and anterior clinoid process	Unilateral or chiasmal vision loss, orbital extension
Medial sphenoid wing	Optic neuropathy and ophthalmoplegia
Lateral sphenoid wing	Proptosis and ophthalmoplegia without optic neuropathy
Diaphragma sellae	Chiasmal syndrome

Planum Sphenoidale and Olfactory Groove Meningiomas. Tumors that involve only the olfactory groove do not cause vision loss as they are not in contact with the optic nerve or chiasm. However, this is a site at which tumors can grow to a sufficiently large size without causing many other neurologic symptoms. Patients may present with papilledema from mass effect, and further historical review reveals anosmia and behavior suggestive of frontal lobe dysfunction. The tumors grow posteriorly over the planum sphenoidale to reach the superior aspect of the intracranial optic nerves and cause direct compression and symptoms of decreased vision. In this setting, with compression of one optic nerve as well as intracranial pressure elevation, presentation with the Foster Kennedy syndrome is possible.

Visual symptoms most often develop insidiously and are sometimes isolated. Patients are generally found to have moderate to severe vision loss and either a normal-appearing optic nerve or optic atrophy. Neuroimaging is usually sufficient to make the diagnosis of skull-base meningiomas (Fig. 5–49) and therefore biopsy is rarely needed. MRI features include isointense, smoothly enhancing masses (Figs. 5–49 and 5–50) with dural tails (Fig. 5–50).

Treatment and Visual Outcome. The clinical course is usually one of insidious progression. Older patients with only mild to moderate

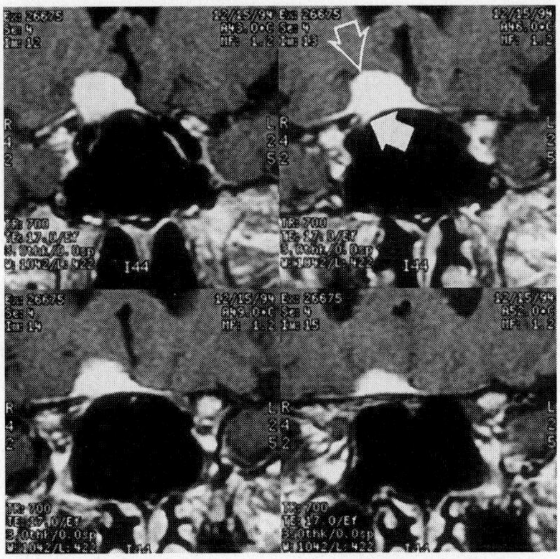

FIGURE 5–49. Serial coronal, T_1-weighted, gadolinium-enhanced MRI scans of a planum sphenoidale meningioma. Smooth enhancement of the mass (*open arrow*) is seen in all four images and contact with the optic nerve can be seen (*solid arrow*).

symptoms who are not necessarily good surgical candidates can be observed with serial visual field examinations and MRI scans. Currently chemotherapy is not generally used to treat meningiomas, although some preliminary work has suggested that progesterone receptor antagonists may be useful. The mainstay of management of these basal meningiomas is surgery and radiation, which are often used in combination. With microsurgical techniques patients have an excellent chance (44% to 62%) for improvement of vision, and this is the procedure of choice in patients well enough to undergo craniotomy.[506–509] Unfortunately, in these same series up to 25% of patients worsen after surgery, and mortality rates are as high as 10%. Radiation has been shown in one series to improve vision,[505] and should be used in patients who are poor surgical risks or in whom there is significant residual tumor. Less than 45 cGy should be used so as to avoid the late complication of radiation-induced damage to the chiasm or optic nerves.[510]

Aneurysms

The intracranial optic nerve is closely related to the anterior cerebral artery, the anterior communicating artery, the ophthalmic artery, and the supraclinoid portion of the internal carotid artery in the anterior aspect of the circle of Willis (see Fig. 7–2). Both saccular (berry) aneurysms and fusiform (atherosclerotic) aneurysms are well-known causes of compressive optic neuropathy. Berry aneurysms typically arise from pre-existing defects in the media and elastica of arteries at the site of arterial bifurcations. They are rare in children and develop with increasing frequency related to age. They range in size from a few millimeters up to 5 or 6 cm. The very small and very large aneurysms have a very low risk for rupture and bleeding.[511] It is the large or giant aneurysms that are generally associated with compression of the anterior visual pathways.

Giant aneurysms arising from the ophthalmic artery, the carotid ophthalmic junction, and the supraclinoid carotid artery can all present with unilateral compressive optic neuropathy or chiasmal syndrome (see Chapter 7). In particular, aneurysms in the supraclinoid region characteristically present with a nasal scotoma.[512] Patients with compressive optic neuropathy from aneurysms may often have fluctuating vision, perhaps related to aneurysm size changes that occur spontaneously or to vascular spasm. MRI (Fig. 5–51) and magnetic resonance angiography are the procedures of choice in patients suspected of having an aneurysm, but the gold standard for diagnosis is formal cerebral angiography. Radiographic features of aneurysms in this area are reviewed in Chapter 7.

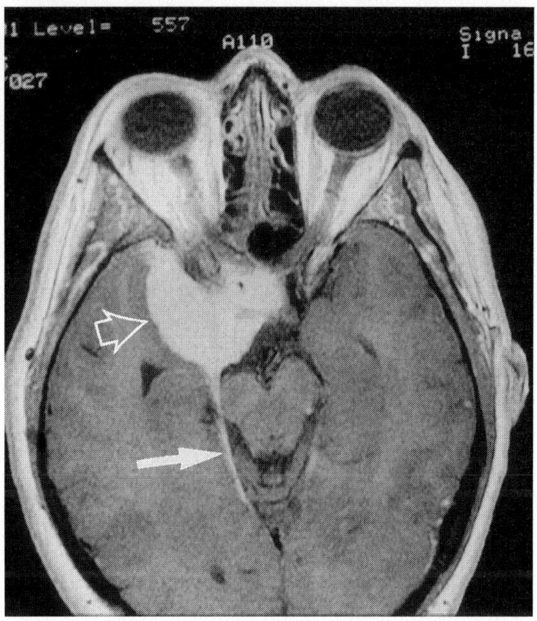

FIGURE 5–50. Contrast-enhanced, axial, T_1-weighted MRI scan of a smoothly enhancing sphenoid wing meningioma (*open arrow*) with a dural tail (*solid arrow*).

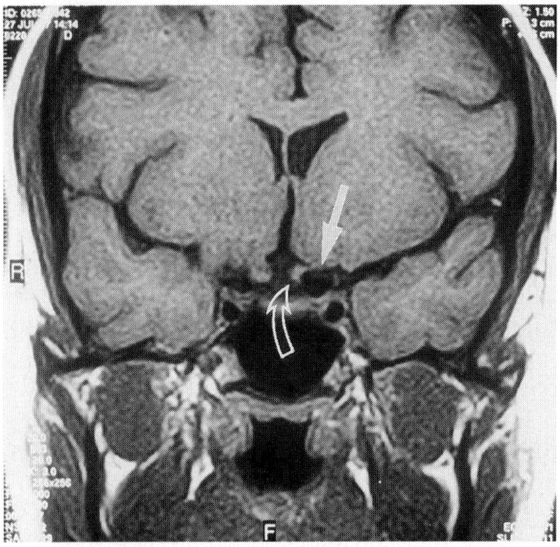

FIGURE 5–51. Coronal, T_1-weighted MRI scan demonstrating an aneurysm (*solid arrow*) in contact with the left optic nerve (*open arrow*).

Clinical Course/Treatment. The natural history of these lesions is generally unfavorable, as many untreated patients later develop subarachnoid hemorrhage, blindness, dementia, or homonymous hemianopia.[513] Treatment of aneurysms in this area is either surgical or endovascular,[513–515] and is reviewed in more detail in Chapter 7.

Fusiform aneurysms or ectatic dilation of the carotid artery may also compress the intracranial optic nerve or chiasm. This has been postulated as one of the causes of optic neuropathy in elderly patients and is thought to have a possible role in the pathogenesis of some cases of low-tension glaucoma.[516, 517] However, Jacobson has recently demonstrated that contact between the carotid artery and optic nerve or chiasm is seen in 70% of asymptomatic patients.[518] True compression by a dolichoectatic artery significant enough to produce vision loss is relatively rare.[646]

LOW-TENSION GLAUCOMA AND OPTIC NERVE CUPPING

The distinction between glaucomatous optic neuropathy and alternative causes of optic neuropathy is rarely difficult. Patients with glaucoma are usually easily identified by their high intraocular pressures. However, in glaucoma with low or normal pressures or in optic neuropathies with optic nerve cupping, the clinical distinction may be very complicated. Since making this separation is critical in order to avoid missed diagnoses and unnecessary treatment, these two common scenarios will be reviewed.

Low- or Normal-Tension Glaucoma

Low- or normal-tension glaucoma (LTG) is a condition in which glaucoma-like field defects, optic nerve head cupping, and normal intraocular pressures are present. The prevalence of LTG varied in large series of glaucoma patients from 7% to 70%.[519] In the Baltimore Eye Survey, 16.7% of glaucomatous eyes never had a recorded intraocular pressure >21 mm Hg, the usual upper limit of normal.[520] LTG probably includes several different subsets of patients. Some patients have unrecognized (undocumented) elevated intraocular pressure or have secondary causes of glaucoma that are currently inactive such as uveitis, intermittent narrow angle, or traumatic angle recession. Some patients have normal pressures with visual field progression but had higher pressures in the past. The term *burned-out glaucoma* has often been applied to these patients. Finally, perhaps the most interesting subset of patients have a progressive optic neuropathy characterized by cupping of the optic nerve head without ever having elevated intraocular pressures. Many believe that these patients have a truly unique disease, perhaps of an ischemic or vascular nature.

Studies have shown an increase in the incidence of migraine and ischemic white matter disease on the MRI scan in patients with LTG.[521, 522] While this information supports a vascular, non-intraocular-pressure-related theory for the cause of LTG, most LTG patients studied behave much more like patients with primary open angle glaucoma and elevated intraocular pressure than patients with "vascular optic neuropathies" such as ION. Slow and relentless progression over years (nonepisodic visual loss) is the rule with relatively symmetric disease between the eyes, along with preservation of central and color vision. LTG patients tend to have more focal atrophy and cupping of the disc, disc hemorrhages, and more dense visual field defects extending closer to fixation than those with high-tension glaucoma. There is still sufficient overlap with high-pressure glaucoma to make the two entities, in most situations, clinically indistinguishable except for the absence of elevated intraocular pressure.

Other Causes of Optic Neuropathy With Optic Nerve Cupping

Several common scenarios occur in which optic nerve cupping due to high- or normal-tension glaucoma is considered, but alternative causes of optic neuropathy are more likely. These situations are: (1) progressive vision loss in the setting of an established diagnosis of glaucoma and normal pressure; (2) visual field loss, optic nerve head cupping, and pallor of the neuroretinal rim without elevated intraocular pressure, and (3) glaucoma complicated by episodic or rapidly progressive vision loss.

Alternative causes of *acquired cupping of the optic nerve* include anterior visual pathway compression by meningiomas, craniopharyngiomas, pituitary adenomas, and aneurysms.[33,523] Cupping has also been described in previous anterior and posterior ischemic optic neuropathy, optic neuritis, shock- or hypotension-induced optic neuropathy, syphilitic optic neuropathy, traumatic optic neuropathy, dominantly inherited optic atrophy, Leber's hereditary optic neuropathy, and methanol-induced optic neuropathy.[524]

Based on careful review of historical information, the examiner should be able to identify most patients with these alternative diagnoses. However, on historical features alone, compressive lesions may be less obvious.

We suggest four criteria that in our experience are positive predictors of these other causes of optic neuropathy. These include: (1) the presence of headache or other neurologic symptoms, (2) atypical visual field defects (those respecting the vertical meridian, central or centrocecal scotomas), (3) atypical rate of progression of visual field loss, and finally, (4) pallor beyond the cupping of the optic nerve (ie, the nerve rim pallor, especially nasally) (Fig. 5–52). In Bianchi-Marzoli et al's series of 29 patients with cupping from compressive anterior visual pathway lesions, only one had cupping and field loss as an isolated manifestation of their optic neuropathy.[523] All others had reduced acuity, dyschromatopsia, and an afferent pupillary defect. Other clinical features more commonly seen in compressive lesions, for instance, and less frequently associated with LTG include presentation under age 50, symptoms of decreased vision, and fluctuating vision. In another series,[525] acuity worse than 20/40 was another feature more associated with cupping due to an intracranial mass lesion.

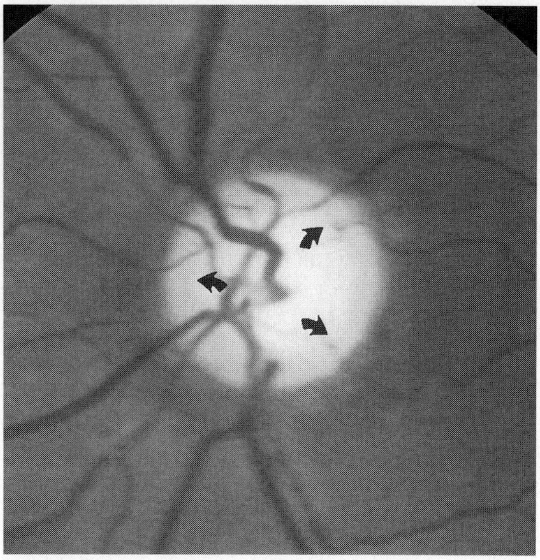

FIGURE 5–52. Pallor beyond cupping in a patient with nonglaucomatous optic neuropathy. Although the cup (*arrows*) is enlarged, significant pallor of the neuroretinal rim is seen.

Evaluation. Our workup of atypical patients would include MRI of the brain and orbits with gadolinium, syphilis serology and, in patients with central field defects, B_{12} and folate levels. In some situations additional testing for sarcoidosis and other autoimmune conditions is indicated based on patient history and demographics.

Episodic or rapidly progressive vision loss may occur in some patients with a well-established history of glaucoma. Some of these patients have a subtype of LTG in which abrupt loss of vision presents like ischemic optic neuropathy. However, optic nerve head swelling is absent and there is often a splinter hemorrhage at the disc margin (Fig. 5–53). This area of the disc often develops focal atrophy and cupping. Workup of these patients is generally unrevealing, but screening for vasculitis (ESR, antinuclear antibodies, rheumatoid factor) is indicated as is careful blood pressure monitoring for episodes of systemic hypotension. These patients may have a true vascular optic neuropathy. A second subtype of patients in this group has both glaucoma and a superimposed distinct cause of vision loss such as ischemic optic neuropathy or a compressive lesion. Any patient who reliably describes sudden or rapidly progressive vision loss in the setting of glaucoma should also be evaluated for other causes of optic neuropathy.

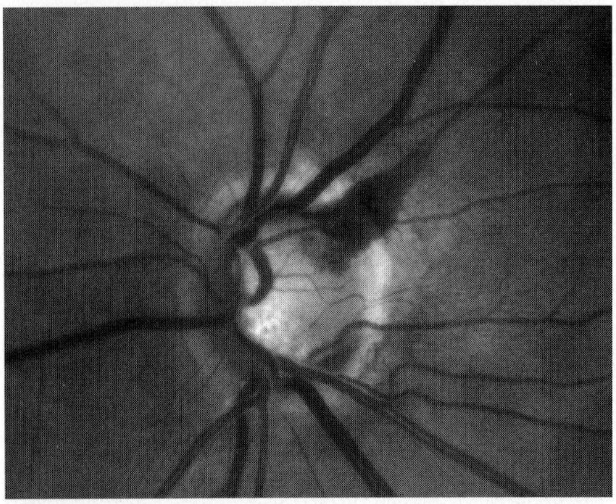

FIGURE 5–53. Cupping of the optic nerve associated with a splinter hemorrhage at the disc margin.

OPTIC NEUROPATHIES ASSOCIATED WITH CANCER

A history of cancer in a patient with neuro-ophthalmic symptoms raises important diagnostic considerations. Several important entities must be considered in patients with vision loss or eye movement problems. The secondary effects of cancer are typically the result of local invasion, metastases, or the consequences of asthenia. The direct effects of cancer on the eye, its adnexa, and the CNS are well known. Primary ocular malignancies and secondary tumors (metastatic and direct extension from adjacent structures) as well as parasellar tumors (primary and secondary) cause vision loss because of displacement or compression of the eye or optic nerve. In the past two decades, unusual instances of organ failure, not resulting from the direct affect of cancer on the organ, have been observed in patients with cancer and have been collectively termed *paraneoplastic syndromes*. These syndromes not only present diagnostic challenges but also provide insight into the biologic behavior of tumors and their effect on the host immune system. Finally, toxicity of antineoplastic drugs and previous irradiation can result in vision loss.

Carcinomatous Meningitis

Carcinomatous meningitis is a common cause of multiple cranial neuropathies secondary to multifocal seeding of the leptomeninges. It is typically a late manifestation of cancer, and the third and sixth nerves are the most commonly involved. Next most commonly involved are the facial, trigeminal, and acoustic nerves. Common primary tumors metastasizing to the meninges include those of the breast and lung. Optic neuropathy in these patients can mimic posterior ischemic neuropathy with acute or subacute vision loss with normal fundus. Alternatively, the nerve may be swollen as in ischemic optic neuropathy. The mechanism of optic nerve dysfunction may be infiltrative, ischemic, demyelinative, or compressive.[526–529] The diagnosis must be suspected and usually can be made based on the presence of abnormal CSF with increased protein and neoplastic cells. It may require three to six CSF examinations to make the diagnosis. Although MRI (Fig. 5–54) might reveal thickening of the optic nerve or abnormal meningeal enhancement, it may also been normal initially.

Optic Nerve Metastases

Isolated metastases to the optic nerve are uncommon but well recognized. Reported primary neoplasms include those of the breast, lung, stomach, and pancreas.[530, 531] Ophthalmoscopically there may be a visible mass invading the optic nerve head. Vascular compression may result in a central retinal vein or artery occlusion.[532] Alternatively, the fundus acutely may be normal if the metastasis is situated more posteriorly, and the clinical scenario may mimic retrobulbar optic neuritis. Radiographically, the optic nerve may exhibit fusiform enlargement, like an intraorbital optic nerve meningioma or glioma.[532–534] Corticosteroids, radiation, and chemotherapy may be indicated. The overall associated mortality is high.

The choroid and orbit are more common sites for metastasis to the eye, and the optic nerve may be involved from secondary extension from these structures. Compressive optic neuropathy may result from metastases to the bony optic canal.[535]

Lymphoma and Leukemia

Optic neuropathies associated with lymphoma or leukemia are rare but can result from a variety of different causes. Cases of direct infiltration of the optic nerve head in both diseases have been reported. As well, with lymphoma, optic neuropathy can be part of the presentation of lymphomatous meningitis.[536, 537] In this

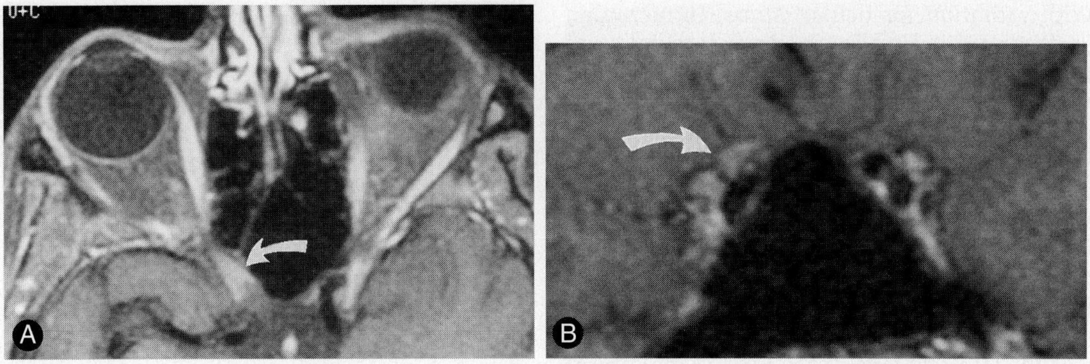

FIGURE 5–54. Axial (**A**) and coronal (**B**) T_1-weighted gadolinium-enhanced MRI scans of a patient with carcinomatous meningitis and right optic nerve involvement. Abnormal enhancement (*arrows*) of the intracranial right optic nerve can be seen.

setting lymphoma causes vision loss by direct invasion via the pial septae.[538] Lymphoma can also present as a mass lesion in the orbit,[539] and MRI can demonstrate abnormal optic nerve enhancement.[536] In some instances it is impossible to determine whether the optic neuropathy results from tumor infiltration or as a side effect of treatment with radiation or chemotherapy. Optic neuropathy has been reported as a manifestation of lymphoma thought to be in remission.[540]

A similar spectrum exists in patients with leukemic optic neuropathy. Direct infiltration of the optic nerve head can cause massive swelling, and there may be associated retinal infiltration with hemorrhages. Optic neuropathy usually accompanies other manifestations of CNS involvement. Histopathologic studies reveal direct infiltration of the optic nerve via pial septae.[541, 542] Vision loss results from vascular compromise or chronic axoplasmic stasis from swelling. Patients with chronic lymphocytic leukemia have been reported to have a more insidious course with progressive visual field loss associated with optic atrophy.[543] Careful consideration should be given to the possibility that vision loss is a consequence of chemotherapy as opposed to leukemic infiltration, particularly in patients treated with vincristine.[544] Radiation is the mainstay of treatment for patients with progressive vision loss and optic nerve involvement from leukemia and lymphoma.

Paraneoplastic Optic Neuropathy

Paraneoplastic processes are conditions in which distant organ failure develops in the setting of cancer but not as a result of direct invasion, metastatic spread, or treatment. The process is mediated by an antibody directed against a tumor antigen and cross reacts with a host (nontumor) antigen. Although paraneoplastic retinopathy (photoreceptor dysfunction, see Chapter 4) is the most common type of paraneoplastic process causing vision loss, rare cases of paraneoplastic optic neuropathy have been described.

Paraneoplastic optic neuropathy (PON) has been reported in patients with carcinoma of the lung.[545–551] Patients develop visual loss and commonly have optic nerve swelling. Vision loss can precede the presentation of the systemic malignancy and generally progresses over a period of weeks. Spontaneous visual recovery and improvement on steroids have been observed. Many patients have a concurrent paraneoplastic cerebellar syndrome characterized by dysarthria and ataxia.[549, 550] Neuropathologic examinations have demonstrated simultaneous involvement of the brain stem with findings typical of paraneoplastic encephalomyelitis. Based on histopathologic demonstration of perivascular lymphocytic infiltration, gliosis, and demyelination of the optic nerves, the condition is thought to be inflammatory and might be more accurately termed *paraneoplastic optic neuritis*.[546, 547] No consistent autoantibody has been demonstrated, but abnormal serum antibodies against cytoplasm of the central neurons and glia of the CNS,[548] anti CV-2 antibodies,[550] and autoantibodies to optic nerve and retina have been found.[549]

Radiation Optic Neuropathy

Delayed radiation damage to the anterior visual pathways has been reported in association with radiation for ocular, sinus, intracranial, and intraorbital malignancies.[552] It is believed to result from cumulative damage to glial and vascular endothelial cells[647] and typically occurs 18 to 36 months after a total dose of 50 Gy. Optic nerve dysfunction results from microvasculopathy and occlusive endarteritis with subsequent optic nerve ischemia. There may also be a component of direct neuronal demyelination and degeneration before vascular changes are seen.

When radiation is likely to include the anterior visual pathways in the field, a maximum total dose of 5000 to 6000 cGy in fractions under 200 cGy is considered to have with an acceptably low risk. Radiation optic neuropathy (RON) occurs most frequently with irradiation of pituitary adenoma but has been documented with treatment of parasellar meningioma, craniopharyngioma, sinus carcinoma, nasopharyngeal carcinoma, skull base tumors such as chordoma, and intraocular tumors. It has been described with gamma knife stereotactic radiosurgery in addition to conventional external beam irradiation.[553, 554]

The differential diagnosis of RON includes recurrent tumor, secondary empty sella syndrome (including optic nerve and chiasmal arachnoiditis), and rarely, radiation-induced parasellar tumors. In fact, tumor recurrence is the most common cause of late visual deterioration after CNS tumor excision and radiation.

Neuro-ophthalmic Signs. Radiation optic neuropathy typically presents with acute, painless visual loss in one or both eyes. There is no correlation to patient age, and vision loss is often severe. The majority of cases occurs within 3 years after completion of radiation therapy, with a peak incidence at 1 to 1.5 years. Vision loss from optic neuropathy can either include disc swelling (Fig. 5–55) or be retrobulbar. Disc swelling can be nonspecific but may also be accompanied by stigmata of radiation retinopathy, including cotton-wool spots and intraretinal vascular abnormalities and hemorrhages. Unfortunately, progression of visual loss over weeks to months is common. Spontaneous recovery is extremely rare. Chiasmal syndromes from radiation optic neuropathy are discussed in Chapter 7.

Evaluation. Computed tomographic images of CNS radionecrosis may show regions of decreased attenuation in white matter and slight enhancement with contrast. With MRI the optic nerves may appear slightly swollen but otherwise normal on unenhanced studies, and usually demonstrate focal contrast enhancement with T_1-weighted gadolinium-DTPA images (Fig. 5–56). The enhancement may resolve after the acute phase of visual loss.[555] MRI is the study of choice to distinguish radiation optic neuropathy from recurrent tumor.

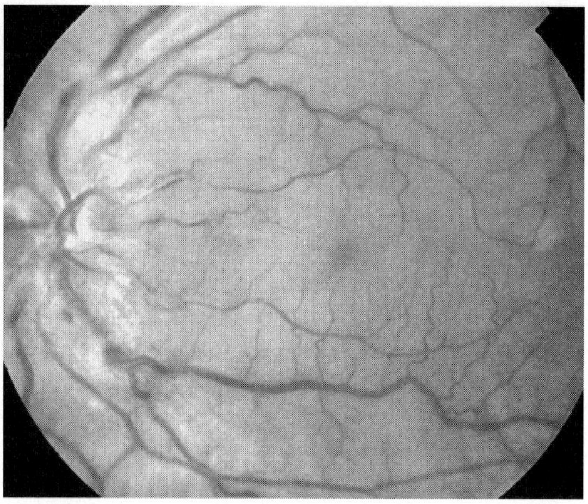

FIGURE 5–55. Funduscopic appearance in acute radiation-induced optic neuropathy associated with disc swelling.

Treatment. There is no proven effective treatment for RON, but occasionally systemic corticosteroids are successful. Their mechanism of action is not clear, but steroids may reduce overall tissue edema and retard demyelination. Hyperbaric oxygen has been used in the treatment of RON with mixed results.[556–558] More recently heparin followed by prolonged coumadinization has been used successfully in the treatment of cerebral radionecrosis, myelopathy, and plexopathy.[559] Although there are some anecdotal reports of its success in treating RON,[560] the role of anticoagulation in this disorder requires further investigation.

NUTRITIONAL AND TOXIC OPTIC NEUROPATHIES

Toxic and nutritional optic neuropathies are often described together because they both frequently present with slowly progressive, bilateral vision loss with dyschromatopsia, and central or centrocecal scotomas. Diagnostic criteria proposed by Lessell are summarized in Table 5–17.[561] These entities are uncommon but frequently are considered in the differential diagnosis of unexplained vision loss. Care must be taken to distinguish these conditions from hereditary optic neuropathies, retinopathies, and nonorganic visual loss.

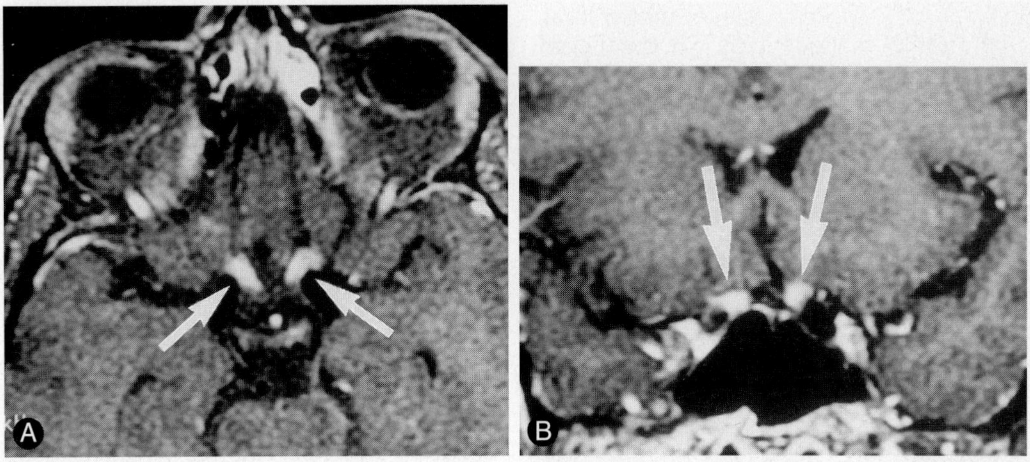

FIGURE 5–56. Axial (**A**) and coronal (**B**) T_1-weighted, gadolinium-enhanced MRI scans of the optic nerves in a patient with bilateral radiation-induced optic neuropathy. Both optic nerves (*arrows*) in their intracranial portions enhance with gadolinium.

Toxic optic neuropathies are usually recognized by the patient's exposure history. Patients commonly encounter these substances either through therapy with antibiotics or chemotherapeutic agents, recreational drug abuse, or industrial exposure. Therefore toxic optic neuropathy might limit the usefulness of a drug or be hazardous in the work place. Deficiency or nutritional optic neuropathies typically arise in individuals who are malnourished, have a malabsorption problem, or are involved in a widespread epidemic limiting adequate nutrition.[562]

B_{12} Deficiency

This vitamin is found in milk, eggs, meat, and cheese and must be ingested. Vitamin B_{12} deficiency, which takes years to develop, generally arises in three different clinically settings. The first and most common is pernicious anemia. This autoimmune condition results in gastric atrophy, reduced intrinsic factor production by gastric parietal cells, and B_{12} malabsorption. It affects middle-aged individuals and can cause a megaloblastic anemia. An associated neurologic condition, subacute combined degeneration of the spinal cord, can develop. In this setting patients develop both a peripheral neuropathy with numbness, tingling, and decreased deep tendon reflexes, and leg weakness with extensor plantar responses from myelopathy. The second setting is in patients with a previous history of partial or complete removal of the stomach or ileum, rendering them unable to absorb B_{12}. The third setting, simple lack of B_{12} in the diet as might occur with a strict vegan, is the rarest.

TABLE 5–17. Diagnostic Criteria for Toxic and Nutritional Optic Neuropathies[561]

Gradual painless progression
Bilateral
Dyschromatopsia
Centrocecal field defects
Vision better than hand movements
Optic disc appearance normal initially
Absence of metamorphopsia
Absence of hallucinations
Improvement with treatment or removal of offending toxin

A 1959 review identified 29 cases of B_{12} optic neuropathy in the world literature, suggesting the condition is very rare.[563] Although several cases have been added, the modern literature still contains few such cases.[564] Patients present as outlined above with slowly progressive vision loss with dyschromatopsia and centrocecal scotomas. The optic nerve may be normal or may demonstrate pallor and nerve fiber defects (Fig. 5–57). Vision loss may precede the recognition of the anemia or the other neurologic symptoms.[563] Visual evoked response abnormalities have been found in patients without visual symptoms.[565] The diagnosis is confirmed by low serum B_{12} levels or elevated methylmalonic acid or homocysteine,[566] both of which require B_{12} for their metabolism. Treatment is with parental hydroxycobalamin, and with prompt therapy, vision loss may be reversible.

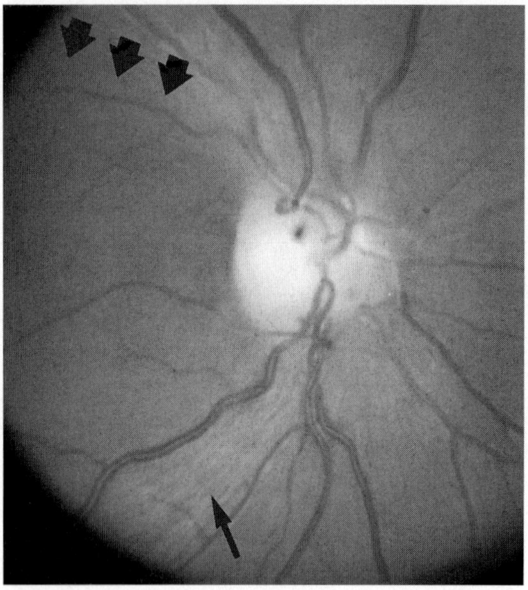

FIGURE 5–57. Funduscopic appearance in B_{12} deficiency. There is temporal pallor of the optic nerve head, nerve fiber dropout in the papillomacular bundle (*large arrows*), and rakelike defects in the nerve fiber layer (*single arrow*).

Optic neuropathy has been shown in primate studies to be the result of demyelination involving the papillomacular bundle.[567, 568] The pathogenesis remains unclear, but may result from build up of toxic levels of cyanide (especially in cigarette smokers) or improper fatty acid synthesis leading to myelin dysfunction. More recently Rizzo proposed that adenosine triphosphate deficiency may be a final common pathway for B_{12} optic neuropathy, Leber's hereditary optic neuropathy, and tobacco–alcohol amblyopia.[564]

Other Vitamin Deficiencies: Deficiencies in thiamine (B_1), pyridoxine (B_6), folic acid, niacin, and riboflavin (B_2) have all been suggested causes of optic neuropathy. Deficiency in thiamine typically results in beri beri or Wernicke's encephalopathy. Neuropathy developing in prisoners of war is one purported example of thiamine optic neuropathy, as the visual deficits in this group improve with thiamine supplementation.[569] Ketogenic and high-protein, low-carbohydrate diets may also put a patient at risk for developing thiamine deficiency. In the case of pyridoxine there has not been a causal relationship established between the deficiency state and optic neuropathy. However, certain drugs, like isoniazide, bind pyridoxine, and the toxicity of this drug has been attributed to altered pyridoxine availability. For riboflavin, niacin, and folic acid, cases of deficiency-associated optic neuropathy were reported in the first half of the century but were largely speculative. These are not important causes of nutritional amblyopia, and their causative role in the development of optic neuropathy remains suspect.

Tobacco–Alcohol Amblyopia

The most commonly recognized nutritional or toxic optic neuropathy may actually be a combination of both a nutritional deficiency state and a toxic effect from tobacco smoking. Small series of patients with this so-called tobacco–alcohol amblyopia or optic neuropathy have been reported.[570–573] Patients typically complain of an insidiously progressive loss of central vision and dyschromatopsia. Acute changes in the appearance of the fundus have been described and include peripapillary dilated vessels and hemorrhages.[574, 575]

The exact role of the nutritional component and the toxic affects of alcohol are debated. Patients often under-report their daily alcohol intake and are malnourished. Since neither ethyl alcohol nor tobacco have been found to be directly toxic to the anterior visual pathways, it is generally believed that poor nutrition is central to the development of decreased vision. Cyanide intoxication may play a role as well. Similar conditions can occur in patients that abuse either alcohol or tobacco. Histopathologic evaluation has shown prominent loss of both papillomacular bundle nerve fibers as well as diffuse nerve fiber loss.[576]

Specific vitamin deficiencies are infrequently identified, but testing for B_{12} and folate levels should be performed. All attempts should be made to convince the patient to reduce alcohol intake. Even if they are unsuccessful, recovery may result if a nutritious diet with B-vitamin supplementation (including hydroxycobalamin parenterally) is instituted.[570, 572]

Cuban and Tropical Optic Neuropathies

An epidemic of optic neuropathy with features similar to toxic and nutritional optic neuropathy occurred in Cuba. Numerous reports characterized these patients, who developed optic and peripheral neuropathies.[577–584] Between 1991 to 1993, epidemic optic and peripheral neuropathy affected more than 51,000 people in Cuba. A study by Cuban and US investigators characterized and identified risk factors for the optic neuropathy.[581] In 123 patients with severe optic neuropathy, prominent clinical features included subacute loss of vision with field defects, dyschromatopsia, optic nerve pallor, and decreased vibratory and temperature sense in the legs. Tobacco use, particularly cigar smoking, increased the risk of optic neuropathy. High dietary intakes of methionine, vitamin B_{12}, and riboflavin reduced the risk. They concluded that the epidemic of optic and peripheral neuropathies in Cuba between 1991 and 1993 appeared to be linked to tobacco use and the malnutrition caused by Cuba's economic situation. Some have suggested a role for mitochondrial mutations, in particular the mutations associated with Leber's hereditary optic neuropathy, but this remains controversial.[578–580, 584] Improvement in visual symptoms occurred with the initiation of vitamin supplementation in the population.[583]

Other groupings of possible toxic and or nutritional optic neuropathies include tropical amblyopia and Jamaican optic neuropathy. The pathogenesis of these conditions remains unproved, and they may represent the same condition or even a hereditary optic neuropathy. The largest series of patients with tropical amblyopia was reported by Osuntokun and Osuntokon.[585] Two hundred and eighty-eight patients were examined with ataxia and optic neuropathy. Other features included peripheral neuropathy and decreased hearing. An unusual feature was the presence of peripheral field constriction without central defects in most patients. The role of poor nutrition and the ingestion of cassava (cyanide source) was unclear. Jamaican optic neuropathy is similar although the condition tends to affect teenagers and is unaccompanied by other neurologic symptoms.[586] Similar pathogenic mechanisms have been considered, including a genetic defect, treponemal infection, nutritional defects, and toxic by-products in homemade "bush teas." A similar syndrome has been described in patients in Tanzania.[587]

Specific Toxic Optic Neuropathies

Methanol. Methanol is a well-recognized optic nerve toxin and can cause profound vision loss even in small doses. The presentation is quite different from that of other toxic optic neuropathies because patients may develop sudden vision loss with disc swelling, and they may be comatose with metabolic acidosis. Patients are typically inebriated, then within 18 to 48 hours develop headache, dyspnea, vomiting, abdominal pain, and bilateral visual blurring. Visual symptoms initially may be transient. Patients may have ingested methanol in a suicide attempt or as an inadvertent contaminant in home made alcohols. Benton and Calhoun[588] reported the largest series of patients ($N = 320$) who ingested methanol as a contaminant of bootleg whiskey.

The acute optic disc edema is indistinguishable from papilledema. Disc swelling has been demonstrated in experimental methanol poisoning in monkeys,[589] and results from axoplasmic stasis secondary to demyelination and axoplasmic obstruction.[590] The pathogenesis of these changes is presumed to be a histotoxic anoxia occurring in a vascular watershed.[590] Although the majority of the damage is believed to result from demyelination of the retrolaminar optic nerve,[590, 591] electrophysiologic studies suggest additional widespread photoreceptor and Mueller cell dysfunction.[592] Treatment is aimed at the acidosis and includes dialysis and IV ethyl alcohol, which interferes with methanol metabolism. Morbidity is high, and the prognosis for visual recovery is poor. Optic atrophy develops and can be accompanied by cupping.[524]

Ethambutol. Ethambutol causes a dose-related optic neuropathy and was recognized as an optic nerve toxin soon after its introduction as a treatment for tuberculosis. The toxicity is thought to result from its chelating properties. A typical presentation includes either central field defects with loss of acuity and dyschromatopsia or well-preserved central visual function with peripheral visual field loss.[593] Chiasmal-type central bitemporal field loss may also occur. Vision loss is not accompanied by other neurologic symptoms. Doses less than 15 mg/kg/day are thought to be safe but in patients taking between 15 and 25 mg/kg/day visual symptoms generally develop over a period of months.[593, 594] More severe and irreversible vision loss has been reported in patients treated with ethambutol for renal tuberculosis.[595] Dyschromatopsia (particularly for green) and loss of contrast sensitivity are reported to be early signs of visual loss.[596] Some recovery usually occurs with discontinuation of the drug but abnormalities in the visual fields and contrast sensitivity may persist.[597] Older patients may be less likely to recover.[598]

Amiodarone. An optic neuropathy with disc swelling very similar to anterior ischemic optic neuropathy has been reported in patients taking the antiarrhythmia drug amiodarone.[599–603] Debate still exists as to whether this is a true toxic optic neuropathy caused by amiodarone versus ordinary ischemic optic neuropathy. The patient population taking the drug is likely to be vasculopathic and at risk for ordinary ION, further clouding the issue. However, some clinical features may distinguish amiodarone associated optic neuropathy from ION. For instance, visual loss may be insidious over months, often with bilateral simultaneous involvement of the eyes, and is usually less severe then in ordinary ION.[599, 601, 604, 605] The disc swelling may last for months, and some recovery can be associated with discontinuation of the drug.[603] Abnormal lamellar inclusions in optic nerve axons have been identified on histopathologic study.[600]

Halogenated Hydroxyquinolines. Halogenated hydroxyquinolines have been implicated in the development of myelopathy and optic neuropathy (subacute myelooptic neuropathy, SMON). The drug was used to prevent diarrhea when traveling and for other gastrointestinal symptoms. The condition has largely been reported in Japan.[606] Patients develop optic atrophy with severe vision loss that may be partially reversible with discontinuation of the drug.

Other Toxic Optic Neuropathies. As more and more drugs are developed to treat neoplasms, an increasing number of optic nerve toxins have been identified. In some instances multiple-drug regimens for chemotherapy and bone marrow transplantation are associated with optic neuropathy, and the specific cause cannot be identified.[607] The list of other drugs reported to cause toxic optic neuropathy is long and is summarized in Table 5–18. The table does not describe every reported optic nerve toxin but supplements the discussion above with some of the more commonly encountered ones.

TABLE 5–18. Other Drugs (Not Discussed in Detail in the Text) That Can Cause Toxic Optic Neuropathy[561, 628, 629]

Drug	Clinical Features
Arsenicals	Irreversible
Busulfan	Also causes cataract
Carmustine (BCNU)	Also causes retinal degeneration
Chloramphenicol	Disc swelling, associated peripheral neuropathy
Cisplatin	May cause disc swelling, associated peripheral neuropathy, and ototoxicity
Cytosine arabanoside	Optic nerve toxicity when given intrathecally
Digitalis	Likely more prominent effect is on the retina
Disulfiram	Rapid vision loss and recovery when discontinued; acetaldehyde may cause optic neuropathy
Ethylene glycol	Acute vision loss, disc swelling; similar course as with methanol-induced optic neuropathy
Fludarabine	Encephalopathy
Hydrogen sulfide	Blindness and hearing loss
Interferon	Disc edema and decreased vision
Isoniazide	Sensory neuropathy reversible with pyridoxine; disc swelling, retinal hemorrhages
Lead	Disc edema, retinal pigment epithelium changes
Methotrexate	Disc edema, idiosyncratic
Organophosphates	Chronic exposure, reduced number of ganglion cells
Quinine	Ganglion cell damage
Toluene	Industrial exposure, reversible
Vincristine	Demyelination; also ophthalmoplegia and cortical blindness

TRAUMATIC OPTIC NEUROPATHY

Of the various forms of vision loss due to trauma, optic nerve injuries are some of the most difficult to diagnose and treat. Hippocrates may have been the first to recognize this condition when he identified the phenomenon of acute and delayed vision loss after injuries placed to and slightly above the brow. In truth he may have identified patients with traumatic glaucoma or cataracts, but he clearly highlighted the brow as the point of impact. It is now recognized that the brow and other facial eminencies are most frequently the site of impact in patients with posterior indirect traumatic optic neuropathy (TON) (see below).

Traumatic optic neuropathy can take many forms. *Direct* injuries are caused by projectiles or penetrating objects that enter the orbit. *Indirect* injuries are caused by forces that are transmitted to the optic nerve from the globe and orbit. Examples of this type include posterior indirect traumatic optic neuropathy, which is discussed in more detail below, and optic nerve avulsion. The latter may occur with only minor damage to the front of the eye if it is rotated forcefully, causing separation of the optic nerve as it exits the globe.[608] Funduscopically, avulsion is often accompanied by intraocular hemorrhages that may preclude viewing the nerve head.[609, 610] The visual prognosis following optic nerve avulsion is poor.[611] Also recognized are a traumatic form of ION and optic nerve dysfunction due to optic nerve sheath or orbital hemorrhages.

Posterior Indirect Traumatic Optic Neuropathy

Posterior indirect TON is traumatic loss of vision that occurs without external or initial ophthalmoscopic evidence of injury to the eye or the nerve. This condition occurs in patients of all ages, and, as with any traumatic condition, it is most common in young men. It is estimated that 2% to 5% of patients with head injuries have TON, and therefore, based on the incidence of head injuries, there are 4 to 5 cases of TON/100,000 population per year. Frontal blows are most common and one study showed a high rate in patients involved in falls from bicycles.[612] Patients need not have loss of consciousness, and the entity certainly occurs in situations of relatively minor head trauma.

Neuro-Ophthalmic Signs. As with any optic neuropathy, there is loss of acuity and color vision, an afferent pupil defect, and visual field defects of any type although central scotomas and altitudinal defects are most common. The fundus is normal.

Mechanism. The mechanism of injury in posterior indirect TON is uncertain but likely multifactorial. In part, the injury to the optic nerve probably occurs as the head hits a hard surface and suddenly decelerates, but the eyeball continues forward. This creates shearing forces that damage the optic nerve's canalicular portion, which is tightly fixed by dural attachments. In addition, holographic interferometric studies performed by Anderson[613] have shown that forces to the facial eminencies are focally manifested around the optic foramen. The combination of these two factors lead to compressing, stretching, and contusing of the optic nerve. These injuries may then cause the nerve to swell, and in the tight bony optic canal there is no room for expansion. Therefore, delayed visual loss may result from further compression from edema within the optic canal.

Diagnostic Studies/Neuroimaging. Optic canal fractures are identified in only approximately one third of patients (Fig. 5–58), and therefore identification of a fracture is *not* necessary for diagnosis.[612] Coronal CT images are best for identifying these fractures. The optic canal is located in the superior posterior lateral aspect of the sphenoid sinus.

Differential Diagnosis. Admittedly, funduscopic evaluation is difficult in patients with altered consciousness, as their pupils cannot be dilated while pupillary status is monitored. Important entities that need to be considered in the differential diagnosis include preexisting optic neuropathy, traumatic retinal injury, and factitious visual loss since many patients are seeking secondary gain in the setting of the injury. The absence of an afferent pupillary defect would support nonphysiologic visual loss.

Treatment. Review of several series reveals that 25% to 50% of patients improve spontaneously.[612–617] There are two available options for treatment. Corticosteroids can be used to treat optic nerve swelling and inflammation. Alternatively, since the nerve is swollen within the confines of a tight bony canal, removal of those bones to decompress the canal and prevent compression may also improve the condition.

Several retrospective studies have shown that steroids, particularly at "megadoses" in studies performed by Seiff and Spoor, can increase the percentage of patients who improve to 66%.[616] The use of megadose steroids is extrapolated from traumatic spinal cord injury studies. Bracken and Braughler in The National Acute Spinal Cord Injury Trial showed that megadose steroids were effective in reducing permanent deficits in patients with spinal cord injury.[618, 619] Glucocorticoid activity is less important in the purported mechanism than

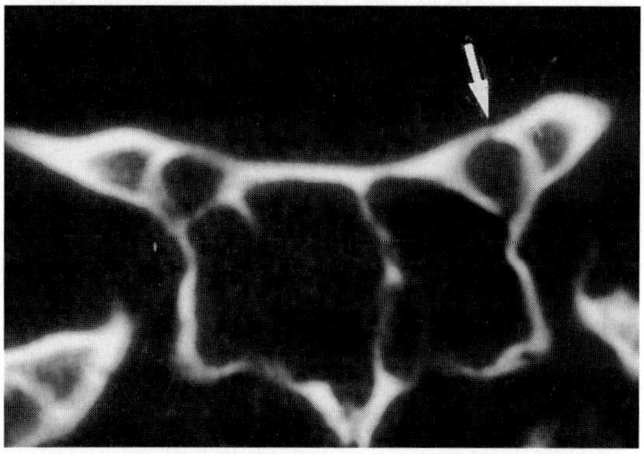

FIGURE 5–58. Coronal bone window CT scan demonstrating a fracture (*arrow*) of the left optic canal.

the ability of these agents in high doses to scavenge free radicals and prevent lipid peroxidation, perhaps a final pathway in white matter injury. They may also enhance blood flow. Methylprednisolone is the most effective, and the dose of 30 mg/kg is about 8 to 10 times higher than a normal IV pulse, as in the optic neuritis treatment trial, for example.

Experimental work is currently being conducted to examine the ability of NMDA receptor antagonists, lazaroids, or 21-aminosteroids with and without vitamin E analogs, calcium channel blockers, and GM1 gangliosides to prevent lipid peroxidation and free-radical damage in nerve tissue. These compounds may some day prove to be effective medical treatments of TON.

Both transcranial and extracranial surgical decompression of the optic canal have also shown promise. Uncontrolled and retrospective studies have demonstrated an approximately 70% improvement rate in patients who have extracranial surgery performed via a transethmoidal transsphenoidal route.[615, 620] Endoscopic approaches are also available. The complication rate is very low, with no major morbidity or death. However, since the carotid canal sits next to the optic canal, this procedure should not be performed by inexperienced surgeons.

In a comparative, nonrandomized study[621] comparing observation with treatment with corticosteroids or optic canal decompression, no clear benefit was found for either of these modalities. Vision improved by three Snellen lines in 57% of the untreated group, 32% of the surgery group, and 52% of the steroid group. A randomized, controlled, prospective study comparing these interventions to no treatment has not been performed because of the difficulty of performing such a study.

Each institution should try to identify a team including an ophthalmologist, neuroradiologist, and otolaryngologist to care for patients with TON. In the absence of prospective, randomized data, treatment should be made on an individualized basis, with the following guidelines[622]:

1. When the diagnosis is made, megadoses of IV methylprednisolone (30 mg/kg load followed by 5 mg/kg/hr) can be given, ideally within 8 hours of injury. This regimen can be given for 48 hours, and extended to 96 hours if improvement is observed. An oral prednisone taper for 2 weeks can follow.
2. Once the patient is on steroids, surgical optic canal decompression can be considered if: (i) there is severe loss of visual field or acuity, (ii) there is no improvement after 24 hours, or (iii) the patient deteriorates. Extracranial surgery is preferable. Unless patients are undergoing other craniofacial surgery or there is an obvious bony fragment or hematoma impinging on the nerve, surgery should not be performed on unconscious patients who can not understand the risks and benefits of the procedure.
3. Patients who are initially NLP should not be treated differently, because recovery from NLP has been reported.

REFERENCES

1. Kupfer C, Chumbley L, Downer JC: Quantitative histology of optic nerve optic tract and lateral geniculate nucleus of man. J Anat 1967;101:393–401.
2. Potts AM, Hodges D, Sherman CB, et al: Morphology of the primate optic nerve: I–III. Invest Ophthalmol Vis Sci 1972;11:980–1016.
3. Oppel O: Mikroskopische Untersuchungen uber die Anzahl und Kaliber der markhaltigen Nervenfasern im fasciculus Opticus des Menshen. Arch Ophthalmol 1963;166:19–27.
4. Maunsell JHR: Functional visual streams. Curr Opin Neurobiol 1992;2:506–510.
5. Merigan WH, Maunsell JHR: How parallel are the primate visual pathways? Ann Rev Neurosci 1993;16:369–402.
6. Shapley R: Visual sensitivity and parallel retinocortical channels. Ann Rev Psychol 1990;41:635–658.
7. Sadun AA: Parallel processing in the human visual system: A new perspective. Neuro-ophthalmology 1986;6:351–352.
8. Kaplan E, Shapley RM: The primate retina contains two types of ganglion cells with high and low contrast sensitivity. Proc Natl Acad Sci USA 1986;83:2755–2757.
9. Ogden TE: Nerve fiber layer of the macaque retina: retinotopic organization. Invest Ophthalmol Vis Sci 1983;24:85–98.
10. Hernandez MR, Luo XX, Igoe F, et al: Extracellular matrix of the human lamina cribrosa. Am J Ophthalmol 1987;104:567–576.
11. Hernandez MR, Igoe F, Neufeld AH: Extracellular matrix of the human optic nerve head. Am J Ophthalmol 1986;102:139–148.
12. Morrison JC, Jerdan JA, L'Hernault NL, et al: The extracellular matrix composition of the monkey optic nerve head. Invest Ophthalmol Vis Sci 1988;29:1141–1150.
13. Morrison JC, Jerdan JA, Dorman ME, et al: Structural proteins of the neonatal and adult lamina cribrosa. Arch Ophthalmol 1989;107:1220–1224.
14. Quigley HA: Regional differences in the structure of the lamina cribrosa and their relationship to glaucomatous visual field loss. Arch Ophthalmol 1981; 99:137–143.
15. Hayreh SS: The 1994 Von Sallman Lecture: the optic nerve head circulation in health and disease. Exp Eye Res 1995;61:259–272.

16. Onda E, Cioffi GA, Bacon DR, et al: Microvasculature of the human optic nerve. Am J Ophthalmol 1995;120:92–102.
17. Maniscalo JE, Habal MB: Microanatomy of the optic canal. J Neurosurg 1978;48:402–406.
18. Minckler DS, Tso MO: Experimental papilledema produced by cyclocryotherapy. Am J Ophthalmol 1976;82:577–589.
19. Minckler DS, Bunt AH, Johanson GW: Orthograde and retrograde axoplasmic transport during ocular hypertension in the monkey. Invest Ophthalmol Vis Sci 1977;16:426–441.
20. Quigley HA, Anderson DR: The dynamics and location of axonal transport blockade by acute intraocular pressure elevation in primate optic nerve. Invest Ophthalmol Vis Sci 1976;15:606–616.
21. Quigley HA, Guy J, Anderson DR: Blockade of rapid axonal transport: effect of intraocular pressure elevation in primate optic nerve. Arch Ophthalmol 1979;97:525–531.
22. Quigley HA, Flower RW, Addicks EM, et al: The mechanism of optic nerve damage in experimental acute intraocular pressure elevation. Invest Ophthalmol Vis Sci 1980;19:505–517.
23. Morrison JC: Anatomy and physiology of the optic nerve. In: Kline LB (ed): Optic Nerve Disorders, pp 1–20. San Francisco, American Academy of Ophthalmology and Palace Press, 1996.
24. Hoffman PN, Lasek RJ: The slow component of axonal transport: identification of major structural polypeptides of the axon and their generality among mammalian neurons. J Cell Biol 1975;66:351–366.
25. Ikeda H, Wright MJ: Receptive field organization of "sustained" and "transient" retinal ganglion cells which subserve different functional roles. J Physiol (London) 1972;222:769–800.
26. Diaper CJM: Pulfrich revisited. Surv Ophthalmol 1997;41:493–499.
27. Mojon DS, Rosler KM, Oetliker H: A bedside test to determine motion stereopsis using the Pulfrich phenomenon. Ophthalmology 1998;105:1337–1344.
28. Diaper CJM, Dutton GN, Heron G: The Pulfrich phenomenon: its symptoms and their management. J Neuro-ophthalmol 1999;12:12.
29. Keltner JL, Johnson CA, Spurr JO, et al: Baseline visual field profile of optic neuritis. The experience of the optic neuritis treatment trial. Optic Neuritis Study Group. Arch Ophthalmol 1993;111:231–234.
30. Jonas JB, Budde WM, Panda-Jonas S: Ophthalmoscopic evaluation of the optic nerve head. Surv Ophthalmol 1999;43:293–320.
31. Frisén L, Claesson M: Narrowing of the retinal arterioles in descending optic atrophy: a quantitative clinical study. Ophthalmology 1984;91:1342–1346.
32. Sebag J, Delori FC, Feke GT, et al: Anterior optic nerve blood flow decreases in clinical neurogenic optic atrophy. Ophthalmology 1986;93:858–865.
33. Trobe JD, Glaser JS, Cassady JC: Optic atrophy: differential diagnosis by fundus observation alone. Arch Ophthalmol 1986;98:1040–1041–1045.
34. Brodsky MC, Baker RS, Hamed LM: Congenital optic disc anomalies. In: Pediatric Neuro-Ophthalmology, pp 42–75. New York, Springer-Verlag, 1996.
35. Hoyt CS, Good WV: Do we really understand the difference between optic nerve hypoplasia and optic atrophy? Eye 1992;6:201–204.
36. Manor RS, Korczyn AD: Retinal red-free light photographs in two congenital conditions: a case of optic hypoplasia and a case of congenital hemianopia. Ophthalmologica 1976;173:119–127.
37. Borchert M, McCulloch D, Rother C, et al: Clinical assessment, optic disk measurements, and visual-evoked potential in optic nerve hypoplasia. Am J Ophthalmol 1995;120:605–612.
38. Brodsky MC: Congenital optic disk anomalies. Surv Ophthalmol 1994;39:89–112.
39. Hellström A, Wiklund L-M, Svensson E, et al: Optic nerve hypoplasia with isolated tortuosity of the retinal veins. Arch Ophthalmol 1999;117:880–884.
40. Hoyt WF, Kaplan SL, Grumbach MM, et al: Septo-optic dysplasia and pituitary dwarfism. Lancet 1970;1:893–894.
41. Morishima A, Aranoff GS: Syndrome of septo-optic pituitary dysplasia: the clinical spectrum. Brain Dev 1986;8:233–239.
42. Margalith D, Tze WJ, Jan JE: Congenital optic nerve hypoplasia with hypothalamic–pituitary dysplasia. Am J Dis Child 1985;139:361–366.
43. Costin G, Murphree AL: Hypothalamic–pituitary function in children with optic nerve hypoplasia. Am J Dis Child 1985;139:249–254.
44. Siatkowski RM, Sanchez JC, Andrade R, et al: The clinical, neuroradiographic, and endocrinologic profile of patients with bilateral optic nerve hypoplasia. Ophthalmology 1997;104:493–496.
45. Brodsky MC, Conte FA, Taylor D, et al: Sudden death in septo-optic dysplasia. Report of 5 cases. Arch Ophthalmol 1997;115:66–70.
46. Brodsky MC, Glasier CM: Optic nerve hypoplasia: clinical significance of associated central nervous system abnormalities on magnetic resonance imaging. Arch Ophthalmol 1993;111:66–74.
47. Sorkin JA, Davis PC, Meacham LR, et al: Optic nerve hypoplasia: absence of posterior pituitary bright signal on magnetic resonance imaging correlates with diabetes insipidus. Am J Ophthalmol 1996;122: 717–723.
48. Brodsky MC: Optic nerve hypoplasia with posterior pituitary ectopia: male predominance and nonassociation with breech delivery. Am J Ophthalmol 1999; 127:238–239.
49. Kuban KCK, Teele RL, Wallman J: Septo-optic-dysplasia-schizencephaly. Radiographic and clinical features. Pediatr Radiol 1989;19:145–150.
50. Lubinsky MS: Hypothesis: septo-optic dysplasia is a vascular disruption sequence. Am J Med Genet 1997;69:235–236.
51. Frisén L, Holmegaard L: Spectrum of optic nerve hypoplasia. Br J Ophthalmol 1978;62:7–15.
52. Taylor D: Congenital tumours of the anterior visual system with dysplasia of the optic disc. Br J Ophthalmol 1982;66:455–463.
53. Lee JT, Hall TR, Bateman JB: Optic nerve hypoplasia secondary to intracranial teratoma. Am J Ophthalmol 1997;124:705–706.
54. Kim RY, Hoyt WF, Lessell S, et al: Superior segmental optic hypoplasia: a sign of maternal diabetes. Arch Ophthalmol 1989;107:1312–1315.
55. Landau K, Bajka JD, Kirchschläger BM: Topless optic disks in children of mothers with type I diabetes mellitus. Am J Ophthalmol 1998;125:605–611.
56. Hashimoto M, Ohtsuka K, Nakagawa T, et al: Topless optic disk syndrome without maternal diabetes mellitus. Am J Ophthalmol 1999;128:111–112.
57. Nelson M, Lessell S, Sadun AA: Optic nerve hypoplasia and maternal diabetes mellitus. Arch Neurol 1986;43:20–25.

58. Scott IU, Warman R, Altman N: Bilateral aplasia of the optic nerves, chiasm, and tracts. Am J Ophthalmol 1997;124:409–410.
59. Margo CE, Hamed LM, Fang E, et al: Optic nerve aplasia. Arch Ophthalmol 1992;110:1610–1613.
60. Hoyt WF, Rios-Montenegro EN, Behrens MM, et al: Homonymous hemioptic hypoplasia. Br J Ophthalmol 1972;56:537–545.
61. Jacobson L, Hellström A, Flodmark O: Large cups in normal-sized optic discs. A variant of optic nerve hypoplasia in children with periventricular leukomalacia. Arch Ophthalmol 1997;115:1263–1269.
62. Lambert SR, Hoyt CS, Narahara MH: Optic nerve hypoplasia. Surv Ophthalmol 1987;32:1–9.
63. Buchanan TAS, Hoyt WF: Temporal visual field defects associated with nasal hypoplasia of the optic disc. Br J Ophthalmol 1981;65:636–640.
64. Gopal L, Badrinath SS, Kuma KS, et al: Optic disc in fundus coloboma. Ophthalmology 1996;103:2120–2127.
65. Apple DJ, Rabb MF, Walsh PM: Congenital anomalies of the optic disc. Surv Ophthalmol 1982;27:3–41.
66. Pagen RA: Ocular colobomas. Surv Ophthalmol 1981;25:223–236.
67. Brown GC, Shields JA, Goldberg RE: Congenital pits of the optic nerve head. II: clinical studies in humans. Ophthalmology 1980;87:51–65.
68. Kranenburg EW: Crater-like holes in the optic disc and central serous retinopathy. Arch Ophthalmol 1960;64:912–924.
69. Cashwell LF, Ford JG: Central visual field changes associated with acquired pits of the optic nerve. Ophthalmology 1995;102:1270–1278.
70. Kinder P: Morning glory syndrome: unusual congenital optic disk anomaly. Am J Ophthalmol 1970;69:376–384.
71. Brodsky MC, Wilson RS: Retinal arteriovenous communications in the morning glory disc anomaly. Arch Ophthalmol 1995;113:410–411.
72. Pollock S: The morning glory disc anomaly: contractile movement, classification, and embryogenesis. Doc Ophthalmol 1987;65:439–460.
73. Hanson RR, Price RL, Rothner AD, et al: Developmental anomalies of the optic disc and carotid circulation: a new association. J Clin Neuro-ophthalmol 1985;5:3–8.
74. Massaro M, Thorarensen O, Liu GT, et al: Morning glory disc anomaly and moyamoya vessels. Arch Ophthalmol 1998;116:253–254.
75. Bakri SJ, Siker D, Masaryk T, et al: Ocular malformations, moyamoya disease, and midline cranial defects: a distinct syndrome. Am J Ophthalmol 1999;127:356–357.
76. Goldhammer Y, Smith JL: Optic nerve anomalies in basal encephalocele. Arch Ophthalmol 1975;93:115–118.
77. Murphy BL: Optic nerve coloboma (morning glory syndrome): CT findings. Radiology 1994;91:59–61.
78. Lorentzen SE: Drusen of the optic disc. A clinical and genetic study. Acta Ophthalmol 1966;Suppl 90:1–180.
79. Savino PJ, Glaser JS, Rosenberg MA: A clinical analysis of pseudopapilledema. II: visual field defects. Arch Ophthalmol 1979;97:71–75.
80. Roh S, Noecker RJ, Schuman JS, et al: Effect of optic nerve head drusen on nerve fiber layer thickness. Ophthalmology 1998;105:878–885.
81. Gittinger JW, Lessell S, Bondar RL: Ischemic optic neuropathy associated with disc drusen. J Clin Neuro-ophthalmol 1984;4:79–84.
82. Michaelson C, Behrens M, Odel J: Bilateral anterior ischemic optic neuropathy associated with optic disc drusen and systemic hypotension. Br J Ophthalmol 1989;73:762–764.
83. Moody TA, Irvine AR, Cahn PH, et al: Sudden visual field constriction associated with optic disc drusen. J Clin Neuro-ophthalmol 1993;13:8–13.
84. Sarkies NJ, Sanders MD: Optic disc drusen and episodic visual loss. Br J Ophthalmol 1987;71:537–539.
85. Beck RW, Corbett JJ, Thompson HS, et al: Decreased visual acuity from optic disc drusen. Arch Ophthalmol 1985;103:1155–1159.
86. Newman WD, Dorrell ED: Anterior ischemic optic neuropathy associated with disc drusen. J Neuro-ophthalmol 1996;16:7–8.
87. Leber T: Ueber hereditare und congenital angelegte Sehnervenleiden. Graefes Arch Klin Exp Ophthalmol 1871;17:249–291.
88. Smith JL, Hoyt WF, Susac JO: Ocular fundus in acute Leber optic neuropathy. Arch Ophthalmol 1973;90:349–354.
89. Lessell S, Gise RL, Krohel GB: Bilateral optic neuropathy with remission in young men: variation on a theme by Leber? Arch Neurol 1983;40:2–6.
90. Singh G, Lott MT, Wallace DC: A mitochondrial DNA mutation as a cause of Leber's hereditary optic neuropathy. N Engl J Med 1989;320:1300–1305.
91. Wallace DC, Singh G, Lott MT, et al: Mitochondrial DNA mutation associated with Leber's hereditary optic neuropathy. Science 1988;242:1427–1430.
92. Newman NJ, Lott MT, Wallace DC: The clinical characteristics of pedigrees of Leber's hereditary optic neuropathy with the 11778 mutation. Am J Ophthalmol 1991;111:750–762.
93. Nikoskelainen E, Hoyt WF, Nummelin K: Ophthalmoscopic findings in Leber's hereditary optic neuropathy: I. Fundus findings in asymptomatic family members. Arch Ophthalmol 1982;100:1597–1602.
94. Nikoskelainen EK, Savontaus ML, Wanne OP: Leber's hereditary optic neuroretinopathy, a maternally inherited disease: a genealogical study in four pedigrees. Arch Ophthalmol 1987;105:665–671.
95. Carroll WM, Mastaglia FL: Leber's optic neuropathy: a clinical and visual evoked potential study of affected and asymptomatic members of a six generation family. Brain 1979;102:559–580.
96. Jacobson DM, Stone EM, Miller NR, et al: Relative afferent pupillary defects in patients with Leber hereditary optic neuropathy and unilateral visual loss. Am J Ophthalmol 1998;126:291–295.
97. Lüdtke H, Kriegbaum C, Leo-Kottler B, et al: Pupillary light reflexes in patients with Leber's hereditary optic neuropathy. Graefe's Arch Clin Exp Ophthalmol 1999;237:207–211.
98. Nikoskelainen E, Sogg RL, Rosenthal AR, et al: The early phase in Leber hereditary optic atrophy. Arch Ophthalmol 1977;95:969–978.
99. Kermode AG, Moseley IF, Kendall BE, et al: Magnetic resonance imaging in Leber's optic neuropathy. J Neurol Neurosurg Psychiat 1989;52:671–674.
100. Palan A, Stehouwer A, Went LN: Studies on Leber's optic neuropathy III. Doc Ophthalmol 1989;71:77–87.
101. Bhatti MT, Newman NJ: A multiple sclerosis-like illness in a man harboring the mtDNA 14484 mutation. J Neuro-ophthalmol 1999;19:28–33.
102. Rose FC, Bowden AN, Bowden P: The heart in Leber's optic atrophy. Br J Ophthalmol 1970;54:388–393.
103. Nikoskelainen E, Wanne O, Dahl M: Pre-excitation syndrome and Leber's hereditary optic neuropathy. Lancet 1985;1:696.

104. Howell N, Kubacka I, Xu M, et al: Leber hereditary optic neuropathy: involvement of the mitochondrial NDI gene and evidence for an intragenic suppressor mutation. Am J Hum Genet 1991;48:935–942.
105. Johns DR, Neufield MJ: An ND-6 mitochondrial DNA mutation associated with Leber's hereditary optic neropathy. Biochem Biophys Res Commun 1992; 187:1551–1557.
106. Johns DR, Smith KH, Savino PJ, et al: Leber's hereditary optic neuropathy: Clinical characteristics of the 15257 mutation. Ophthalmology 1993;100:981–986.
107. Pezzi PP, De Negri AM, Sadun F, et al: Childhood Leber's hereditary optic neuropathy (ND1/3460) with visual recovery. Pediatr Neurol 1998;19: 308–312.
108. Cock HR, Tabrizi SJ, Cooper JM, et al: The influence of nuclear background on the biochemical expression of 3460 Leber's hereditary optic neuropathy. Ann Neurol 1998;44:187–193.
109. Carelli V, Ghelli A, Bucchi L, et al: Biochemical features of mtDNA 14484 (ND6/M64V) point mutation associated with Leber's hereditary optic neuropathy. Ann Neurol 1999;45:320–328.
110. Bresolin N, Bet L, Binda A, et al: Clinical and biochemical correlations in mitochondrial myopathies treated with coenzyme Q10. Neurology 1988;38: 892–899.
111. Shoffner JM, Lott MT, Voljavec AS, et al: Spontaneous Kearns–Sayre/chronic external ophthalmoplegia plus syndrome associated with a mitochondrial DNA deletion: a slip-replication model and metabolic therapy. Proc Natl Acad Sci USA 1989;86:7952–7956.
112. Wallace DC: Mitochondrial DNA mutations and neuromuscular disease. Trends Genet 1989;5:9–13.
113. Kjer P: Infantile optic atrophy with dominant mode of inheritance: a clinical and genetic study of 19 Danish families. Acta Ophthalmol 1959;suppl 54:1–46.
114. Votruba M, Fitzke FW, Holder GE, et al: Clinical features in affected individuals from 21 pedigrees with dominant optic atrophy. Arch Ophthalmol 1998;116:793–800.
115. Elliot D, Traboulsi EI, Maumenee IH: Visual prognosis in autosomal dominant optic atrophy. Am J Ophthalmol 1993;115:360–367.
116. Kline LB, Glaser JS: Dominant optic atrophy: the clinical profile. Arch Ophthalmol 1979;97:1680–1686.
117. Hoyt CS: Autosomal dominant optic atrophy: a spectrum of disability. Ophthalmology 1980;87:245–251.
118. Eiberg H, Kjer B, Kjer P, et al: Dominant optic atrophy (OPA1) mapped to chromosome 3q region, I: linkage analysis. Hum Mol Genet 1994;3:977–980.
119. Johnston RL, Burdon MA, Spalton DJ, et al: Dominant optic atrophy, Kjer type. Linkage analysis and clinical features in a large British pedigree. Arch Ophthalmol 1997;117:100–103.
120. Brown J, Finger JH, Taylor CM, et al: Clinical and genetic analysis of a family affected with dominant optic atrophy (OPA1). Arch Ophthalmol 1997;115: 95–103.
121. Wiggs JL: Genomic mapping of Kjer dominant optic atrophy. Arch Ophthalmol 1997;115:115–116.
122. Johnston RL, Seller MJ, Behnam JT, et al: Dominant optic atrophy. Refining the clinical diagnostic criteria in light of genetic linkage studies. Ophthalmology 1999;106:123–128.
123. Votruba M, Moore AT, Bhattacharya SS: Clinical features, molecular genetics, and pathophysiology of dominant optic atrophy. J Med Genet 1998;35: 793–800.
124. Johnston PB, Glaser RN, Smith VC, et al: A clinicopathologic study of autosomal dominant optic atrophy. Am J Ophthalmol 1979;88:868–875.
125. Waardenburg PJ: Different types of hereditary optic atrophy. Acta Genet Statist Med 1957;7:287–290.
126. Behr C: Die Komplizierte, Hereditar-familare Optikusatrophie des Kindesalters: Ein bisher nicht beschriebener Symptomkomplex. Klin Monatsbl Augenheilkd 1909;47:138–160.
127. Horoupian DS, Zuker DK, Moshe S, et al: Behr Syndrome: A clinicopathologic report. Neurology 1979; 29:323.
128. Wolfram DJ: Diabetes mellitus and simple optic atrophy among siblings. Mayo Clin Proc 1938;13:715–717.
129. Lessell S, Rosman NP: Juvenile diabetes mellitus and atrophy. Arch Neurol 1977;34:759–765.
130. Genís D, Dávalos A, Molins A, et al: Wolfram syndrome: a neuropathological study. Acta Neuropathologica 1997;93:426–429.
131. Barrett TG, Bundey SE, Fielder AR, et al: Optic atrophy in Wolfram (DIDMOAD) syndrome. Eye 1997;11:882–888.
132. Carroll WM, Kriss A, Baraitser M, et al: The incidence and nature of visual pathway involvement in Friedreich's ataxia: a clinical and visual evoked potential study of 22 patients. Brain 1980;103:413–434.
133. Livingstone IR, Mastaglia FL, Edis R, et al: Visual involvement in Friedreich's ataxia and hereditary spastic ataxia: A clinical and visual evoked response study. Arch Neurol 1981;38:75–79.
134. Hoyt WF: Charcot–Marie–Tooth disease with primary optic atrophy. Arch Ophthalmol 1960;64: 925–928.
135. Konigsmark BW, Knox DL, Hussels IE, et al: Dominant congenital deafness and progressive optic nerve atrophy. Occurrence in four generations of a family. Arch Ophthalmol 1974;91:99–103.
136. Kollarits CR, Pinheiro ML, Swann ER, et al: The autosomal dominant syndrome of progressive optic atrophy and congenital deafness. Am J Ophthalmol 1979;87:789–792.
137. Rizzo JF, Lessell S: Risk of developing multiple sclerosis after uncomplicated optic neuritis. Neurology 1988;38:185–190.
138. Beck RW, Cleary PA, Anderson MM, et al: A randomized, controlled trial of corticosteroids in the treatment of acute optic neuritis. N Engl J Med 1992;326:581–588.
139. Wray SH: Optic Neuritis. In: Albert DM, Jakobiec FA (eds): Principles and Practice of Ophthalmology, pp 2539–2568. Philadelphia, WB Saunders, 1994.
140. Optic Neuritis Study Group: The clinical profile of optic neuritis. Experience of the Optic Neuritis Treatment Trial. Arch Ophthalmol 1991;109:1673–1678.
141. Percy AK, Nobrega FT, Kurland LT: Optic neuritis and multiple sclerosis. An epidemiologic study. Arch Ophthalmol 1972;87:135–139.
142. Wikstrom J: The epidemiology of optic neuritis in Finland. Acta Neurol Scand 1975;52:196–206.
143. Lepore FE: The origin of pain in optic neuritis. Arch Neurol 1991;48:748–749.
144. Lessell S, Cohen MM: Phosphenes induced by sound. Neurology 1979;29:1524–1526.
145. Davis FA, Bergen D, Schauf C, et al: Movement phosphenes in optic neuritis: a new clinical sign. Neurology 1976;26:1100–1104.
146. Parkin PJ, Hierons R, McDonald WI: Bilateral optic neuritis: a long term follow up. Brain 1984;107: 951–964.

147. Scholl GB, Song HS, Wray SH: Uhthoff's symptom in optic neuritis: Relationship to magnetic resonance imaging and development of multiple sclerosis. Ann Neurol 1991;30:180–184.
148. Uhthoff W: Untersuchungen uber die bei der multiplen Herdsklerose vorkommenden Augenstorungen. Arch Psychiatry 1889;21:303.
149. Lepore FE: Uhthoff's symptom in disorders of the anterior visual pathways. Neurology 1994;44:1036–1038.
150. Haupert CL, Newman NJ: Prolonged Uhthoff phenomenon in sarcoidosis. Am J Ophthalmol 1997; 124:564–566.
151. Griffin JF, Wray SH: Acquired color vision defects in retrobulbar neuritis. Am J Ophthalmol 1978;86: 193–201.
152. Katz B: The dyschromatopsia of optic neuritis: a descriptive analysis of data from the optic neuritis treatment trial. Trans Am Ophthalmol Soc 1995;93: 685–708.
153. Trobe JD, Beck RW, Moke PS, et al: Contrast sensitivity and other vision tests in the optic neuritis treatment trial. Am J Ophthalmol 1996;121:547–553.
154. Rizzo JF, Lessell S: Optic neuritis and ischemic optic neuropathy: Overlapping clinical profiles. Arch Ophthalmol 1991;100:1668–1672.
155. Beck RW, Kupersmith MJ, Cleary PA, et al: Fellow eye abnormalities in acute unilateral optic neuritis. Experience of the optic neuritis treatment trial. Ophthalmology 1993;100:691–697.
156. Nikoskelainen E: Symptoms, signs and early course in optic neuritis. Acta Ophthalmol 1975;53:254–272.
157. Merandi SF, Kudryk BT, Murtagh FR, et al: Contrast enhanced MR imaging of optic nerve lesions in patients with acute optic neuritis. AJNR 1991;12: 923–926.
158. Miller DH, Newton MR, van der Pool JC: Magnetic resonance imaging of the optic nerve in optic neuritis. Neurology 1988;38:175–179.
159. Beck RW, Arrington J, Murtagh FR: Brain MRI in acute optic neuritis. Experience of the Optic Neuritis Study Group. Arch Neurol 1993;8:841–846.
160. Morrissey SP, Miller DH, Kendall BE, et al: The significance of brain magnetic resonance imaging abnormalities at presentation with clinically isolated syndromes suggestive of multiple sclerosis. Brain 1993;116:135–146.
161. Lukes SA, Crookes LE, Aminoff MJ, et al: Nuclear magnetic resonance imaging in multiple sclerosis. Ann Neurol 1983;13:592.
162. Young IR, Hall AS, Pallis CA, et al: Nuclear magnetic resonance of the brain in multiple sclerosis. Lancet 1981;2:1063–1066.
163. Gass A, Moseley IF, Barker GJ, et al: Lesion discrimination in optic neuritis using high-resolution fat-suppressed fast spin-echo MRI. Neuroradiology 1996;38:317–321.
164. Onofrj M, Tartaro A, Thomas A, et al: Long echo time STIR sequence MRI of optic nerves in optic neuritis. Neuroradiology 1996;38:66–69.
165. Tourbah A, Deschamps R, Stievenart JL, et al: Magnetic resonance imaging using FLAIR pulse sequence in white matter diseases. J Neuroradiol 1996; 23:217–222.
166. Dunker S, Wiegand W: Prognostic value of magnetic resonance imaging in monosymptomatic optic neuritis. Ophthalmology 1996;103:1768–1773.
167. Bobak P, Bodis-Wollner I, Harnois C, et al: Pattern electroretinograms and visual evoked potentials in glaucoma and multiple sclerosis. Am J Ophthalmol 1983;96:72–83.
168. Halliday AM, Halliday E, Kriss A, et al: The pattern evoked potential in compression of the anterior visual pathways. Brain 1976;99:357–361.
169. McDonald WI: The significance of optic neuritis. Trans Ophthalmol Soc UK 1983;103:230–235.
170. Rolak LA, Beck RW, Paty DW, et al: Cerebrospinal fluid in acute optic neuritis: experience of the optic neuritis treatment trial. Neurology 1996;46:368–372.
171. Söderström M, Ya-Ping J, Hillert J, et al: Optic neuritis. Prognosis for multiple sclerosis from MRI, CSF, and HLA findings. Neurology 1998;50:708–714.
172. Beck RW, Cleary PA, the Optic Neuritis Study Group: Optic neuritis treatment trial. One year follow-up results. Arch Ophthalmol 1993;111:773–775.
173. Kapoor R, Miller DH, Jones SJ, et al: Effects of intravenous methylprednisolone on outcome in MRI-based prognostic subgroups in acute optic neuritis. Neurology 1998;50:230–237.
174. Optic Neuritis Study Group: Visual function five years after optic neuritis: experience of the Optic Neuritis Treatment Trial. Arch Ophthalmol 1997; 115:1545–1552.
175. Beck RW, Cleary PA, Backlund JC, et al: The course of visual recovery after optic neuritis. Experience of the optic neuritis treatment trial. Ophthalmology 1994;101:1771–1778.
176. Slamovits TL, Rosen CE, Cheng KP, et al: Visual recovery in patients with optic neuritis and visual loss to no light perception. Am J Ophthalmol 1991;111:209–214.
177. Fleishman JA, Beck RW, Linares OA, et al: Deficits in visual function after resolution of optic neuritis. Ophthalmology 1987;94:1029–1035.
178. Cleary PA, Beck RW, Bourque LB, et al: Visual symptoms after optic neuritis. Results from the Optic Neuritis Treatment Trial. J Neuro-ophthalmol 1997; 17:18–23.
179. Phillips PH, Newman NJ, Lynn MJ: Optic neuritis in African Americans. Arch Neurol 1998;55:186–192.
180. Biousse V, Trichet C, Bloch-Michel E, et al: Multiple sclerosis associated with uveitis in two large clinic-based series. Neurology 1999;52:179–181.
181. Sadovnick AD, Eisen K, Hashimoto SA, et al: Pregnancy and multiple sclerosis. A prospective study. Arch Neurol 1994;51:1120–1124.
182. Damek DM, Shuster EA: Pregnancy and multiple sclerosis. Mayo Clin Proc 1997;72:977–989.
183. Confavreux C, Hutchinson M, Hours MM, et al: Rate of pregnancy-related relapse in multiple sclerosis. N Engl J Med 1998;339:285–291.
184. Lucchinetti CF, Rodriguez M: The controversy surrounding the pathogenesis of the multiple sclerosis lesion. Mayo Clin Proc 1997;72:665–678.
185. Trapp BD, Peterson J, Ransohoff RM, et al: Axonal transection in the lesions of multiple sclerosis. N Engl J Med 1998;338:278–285.
186. Rudick RA, Cohen JA, Weinstock-Guttman B, et al: Management of multiple sclerosis. N Engl J Med 1997;337:1604–1611.
187. Arnason BGW: Pathophysiology of multiple sclerosis: finding the mechanisms of demyelination. Adv Neuroimmunol 1996;3:13–18.
188. Poser CM, Paty DW, Scheinberg L, et al: New diagnositic criteria for multiple sclerosis: guidelines for research protocols. Ann Neurol 1983;13:227–231.
189. The IFNB Multiple Sclerosis Study Group: Interferon beta-1b is effective in relapsing–remitting multiple

sclerosis. I. Clinical results of a multicenter, randomized, double-blind, placebo-controlled trial. Neurology 1993;43:655–661.

190. Paty DW, Li DKB, the UBC MS/MRI Study Group, et al: Interferon beta-1b is effective in relapsing–remitting multiple sclerosis. II. MRI analysis results of a multicenter, randomized, double-blind, placebo-controlled trial. Neurology 1993;43:662–667.
191. The IFNB Multiple Sclerosis Study Group and the University of British Columbia MS/MRI Analysis Group: Interferon beta-1b in the treatment of multiple sclerosis. Final outcome of the randomized controlled trial. Neurology 1995;45:1277–1285.
192. Johnson KP, Brooks BR, Cohen JA, et al: Copolymer 1 reduces relapse rate and improves disability in relapsing–remitting multiple sclerosis: results of a phase III multicenter, double-blind, placebo-controlled trial. Neurology 1995;45:1268–1276.
193. Jacobs LD, Cookfair DL, Rudick RA, et al: Intramuscular interferon beta-1a for disease progression in relapsing multiple sclerosis. Ann Neurol 1996; 39:285–294.
194. Simon JH, Jacobs LD, Campion M, et al: Magnetic resonance studies of intramuscular interferon beta-1a for relapsing multiple sclerosis. Ann Neurol 1998;43:79–87.
195. Arnason BGW: Interferon beta in multiple sclerosis (editorial). Neurology 1993;43:621–643.
196. Yong VW, Chabot S, Stuve O, et al: Interferon beta in the treatment of multiple sclerosis. Mechanisms of action. Neurology 1998;51:682–689.
197. Rudick RA, Goodkin DE, Jacobs LD, et al: Impact of interferon beta-1a on neurologic disability in relapsing multiple sclerosis. Neurology 1997;49:358–363.
198. Wolinsky JS: Copolymer 1: a most reasonable alternative therapy for early relapsing–remitting multiple sclerosis with mild disability (editorial). Neurology 1995;45:1245–1247.
199. Johnson KP, Brooks BR, Cohen JA, et al: Extended use of glatiramer acetate (Copaxone) is well tolerated and maintains its clinical effect on multiple sclerosis relapse rate and degree of disability. Neurology 1998;50:701–708.
200. Francis DA, Compston DAS, Batchelor JR, et al: A reassessment of the risk of multiple sclerosis developing in patients with optic neuritis after extended follow up. J Neurol Neurosurg Psychiatr 1987;50: 758–765.
201. Miller DH, Ormerod IEC, McDonald WI, et al: The early risk of multiple sclerosis after optic neuritis. J Neurol Neurosurg Psychiatr 1988;51:1569–1571.
202. Miller DH, Ormerod IEC, Rudge P, et al: The early risk of multiple sclerosis following acute syndromes of the brainstem and spinal cord. Ann Neurol 1989;26:635–639.
203. Beck RW, Cleary PA, Trobe JD, et al: The effect of corticosteroids for acute optic neuritis on the subsequent development of multiple sclerosis. N Engl J Med 1993;329:1764–1769.
204. Jacobs LD, Kaba SE, Miller CM, et al: Correlation of clinical, magnetic resonance imaging, and cerebrospinal fluid findings in optic neuritis. Ann Neurol 1997;41:392–398.
205. Optic Neuritis Study Group: The 5-year risk of MS after optic neuritis: experience of the Optic Neuritis Treatment Trial. Neurology 1997;49:1404–1413.
206. O'Riordan JI, Thompson AJ, Kingsley DPE, et al: The prognostic value of brain MRI in clinically isolated syndromes of the CNS. A 10-year follow-up. Brain 1998;121:495–503.
207. Cole SR, Beck RW, Moke PS, et al: The predictive value of CSF oligoclonal banding for MS 5 years after optic neuritis. Optic Neuritis Study Group. Neurology 1998;51:885–887.
208. Tumani H, Tourtellotte WW, Peter JB, et al: Acute optic neuritis: combined immunological markers and magnetic resonance imaging predict subsequent development of multiple sclerosis. The Optic Neuritis Study Group. J Neurol Sci 1998;155:44–49.
209. Frederiksen JL, Madsen HO, Ryder LP, et al: HLA typing in acute optic neuritis. Relation to multiple sclerosis and magnetic resonance imaging findings. Arch Neurol 1996;54:76–80.
210. Kupersmith MJ, Kaufman D, Paty DW: Megadose corticosteroids in multiple sclerosis. Neurology 1994;44:1–4.
211. Beck RW: The optic neuritis treatment trial. Three year follow up results. Arch Ophthalmol 1995;113: 136–137.
212. Chrousos GA, Kattah JC, Beck RW, et al: Side effects of glucocorticoid treatment. Experience in the optic neuritis treatment trial. JAMA 1993;269:2110–2112.
213. Sellebjerg F, Nielsen HS, Frederiksen JL, et al: A randomized, controlled trial of oral high-dose methylprednisolone in acute optic neuritis. Neurology 1999;52:1479–1484.
214. van Engelen BGM, Hommes OR, Pinkers A, et al: Improved vision after intravenous immunoglobulin in stable demyelinating optic neuritis (letter). Ann Neurol 1992;32:834–835.
215. Mandler RN, Davis LE, Jeffrey DR, et al: Devic's neuromyelitis optica: a clinicopathological study of 8 patients. Ann Neurol 1993;34:162–168.
216. Lefkowitz D, Angelo JN: Neuromyelitis optica with unusual vascular changes. Arch Neurol 1984; 41:1103–1105.
217. Whitham RH, Brey RL: Neuromyelitis optica: two new cases and review of the literature. J Clin Neuro-ophthalmol 1985;5(4):263–269.
218. Jeffery AR, Buncic JR: Pediatric Devic's neuromyelitis optica. J Pediatr Ophthalmol Strabismus 1996; 33:223–229.
219. April RS, Vansonnenberg E: A case of neuromyelitis optica (Devic's syndrome) in systemic lupus erythematosus. Neurology 1976;26:1066–1070.
220. O'Riordan JI, Gallagher HL, Thompson AJ, et al: Clinical, CSF, and MRI findings in Devic's neuromelitis optica. J Neurol Neurosurg Psychiatr 1996;60: 382–387.
221. Silber MH, Willcox PA, Bowen RM, et al: Neuromyelitis optica (Devic's syndrome) and pulmonary tuberculosus. Neurology 1990;40:934–938.
222. Mandler RN, Ahmed W, Dencoff JE: Devic's neuromyelitis optica: a prospective study of seven patients treated with prednisone and azathioprine. Neurology 1998;51:1219–1220.
223. Kriss A, Francis DA, Cuendet B: Recovery of optic neuritis in childhood. J Neurol Neurosurg Psychiatr 1988;51:1253–1258.
224. Kennedy C, Carroll FD: Optic neuritis in children. Arch Ophthalmol 1960;63:747–755.
225. Riikonen R, Donner M, Erkkila H: Optic neuritis in children and its relationship to multiple sclerosis: a clinical study of 21 children. Dev Med Child Neurol 1988;30(3):349–359.
226. Good WV, Muci-Mendoza R, Berg BO, et al: Optic neuritis in children with poor recovery of vision. Aust N Z J Ophthalmol 1992;20:319–323.

227. Riikonen R: The role of infection and vaccination in the genesis of optic neuritis and multiple sclerosis in children. Acta Neurol Scand 1989;80:425–431.
228. Farris BK, Pickard DJ: Bilateral postinfectious optic neuritis and intravenous steroid therapy in children. Ophthalmology 1990;97:339–345.
229. Stevenson VL, Acheson JF, Ball J, et al: Optic neuritis following measles/rubella vaccination in two 13-year-old children (letter). Br J Ophthalmol 1996; 80:1110–1111.
230. Purvin V, Hrisomalos N, Dunn D: Varicella optic neuritis. Neurology 1988;38:501–503.
231. Visudhiphan P, Chiemchanya S, Santadusit S: Optic neuritis in children: recurrence and subsequent development of multiple sclerosis. Pediatr Neurol 1995;13:293–295.
232. Kennedy C, Carter S: Relation of optic neuritis to multiple sclerosis in children. Pediatrics 1961;28: 1253–1258.
233. Lucchinetti CF, Kiers L, O'Duffy A, et al: Risk factors for developing multiple sclerosis after childhood optic neuritis. Neurology 1997;49:1413–1418.
234. Stern BJ, Krumholz A, Johns C, et al: Sarcoidosis and its neurological manifestations. Arch Neurol 1985; 42:909–917.
235. Delaney P: Neurologic manifestations in sarcoidosis. Review of the literature with a report of 23 cases. Ann Intern Med 1977;87:336–345.
236. Jabs DA, Johns CJ: Ocular involvement in chronic sarcoidosis. Am J Ophthalmol 1986;102:297–301.
237. Beardsley TL, Brown SVL, Sydnor CF, et al: Eleven cases of sarcoidosis of the optic nerve. Am J Ophthalmol 1984;97:62–77.
238. Galetta SL, Schatz NJ, Glaser JS: Acute sarcoid optic neuropathy with spontaneous recovery. J Clin Neuro-ophthalmol 1989;9:27–32.
239. Ing EB, Garrity JA, Cross SA, et al: Sarcoid masquerading as optic nerve sheath meningioma. Mayo Clin Proc 1997;72:38–43.
240. Graham EM, Ellis CJ, Sanders MD, et al: Optic neuropathy in sarcoidosis. J Neurol Neurosurg Psychiatr 1986;49:756–763.
241. Beck AD, Newman NJ, Grossniklaus HE, et al: Optic nerve enlargement and chronic visual loss. Surv Ophthalmol 1994;38:555–556.
242. Carmody RF, Mafee MF, Goodwin JA, et al: Orbital and optic pathway sarcoidosis: MR findings. AJNR Am J Neuroradiol 1994;15:775–783.
243. Miller DH, Kendall BE, Barter S, et al: Magnetic resonance imaging in central nervous system sarcoidosis. Neurology 1988;38:378–383.
244. Weinreb RN: Diagnosing sarcoidosis by transconjunctival biopsy of the lacrimal gland. Am J Ophthalmol 1984;97:573–576.
245. Nichols CW, Eagle RC, Yanoff M, et al: Conjunctival biopsy as an aid in the evaluation of the patient with suspected sarcoidosis. Ophthalmology 1980;87: 287–291.
246. Gelwan MJ, Kellen RI, Burde RM, et al: Sarcoidosis of the anterior visual pathway: successes and failures. J Neurol Neurosurg Psychiatr 1988;51:1473–1480.
247. Bielory L, Frohman LP: Low-dose cyclosporine therapy of granulomatous optic neuropathy and orbitopathy. Ophthalmology 1991;98:1732–1736.
248. Krohel GB, Charles H, Smith RS: Granulomatous optic neuropathy. Arch Ophthalmol 1981;99:1053–1055.
249. Kennerdell JS, Dresner SC: The non-specific orbital inflammatory syndromes. Surv Ophthalmol 1984; 29:93–103.
250. Dutton JJ, Anderson RL: Idiopathic inflammatory optic neuritis simulating optic nerve sheath meningioma. Am J Ophthalmol 1985;100:424–430.
251. Margo CE, Levy MH, Beck RW: Bilateral idiopathic inflammation of the optic nerve sheaths. Ophthalmology 1989;96:200–206.
252. Lessell S: The neuro-ophthalmology of systemic lupus erythematosus. Doc Ophthalmol 1979;47:13–42.
253. Jabs DA, Miller NR, Newman SA, et al: Optic neuropathy in systemic lupus erythematosus. Arch Ophthalmol 1986;104:564–568.
254. Dutton JJ, Burde RM, Klingele TG: Autoimmune retrobulbar optic neuritis. Am J Ophthalmol 1982; 94:11–17.
255. Kupersmith MJ, Burde RM, Warren FA, et al: Autoimmune optic neuropathy: evaluation and treatment. J Neurol Neurosurg Psychiatr 1988;51:1381–1386.
256. Riedel P, Wall M, Grey A, et al: Autoimmune optic neuropathy (letter). Arch Ophthalmol 1998;116:1121–1124.
257. Song HS, Wray SH: Bee sting optic neuritis. A case report with visual evoked potentials. J Clin Neuro-ophthalmol 1991;11:45–49.
258. Berrios RR, Serrano LA: Bilateral optic neuritis after a bee sting. Am J Ophthalmol 1994;117:677–678.
259. Unsold R: Neuropathies of the optic nerve in inflammatory systemic diseases and vasculitis. A frequently misdiagnosed early symptom. Ophthalmology 1994;91:251–262.
260. Slavin ML, Liebergall DA: Acute unilateral visual loss in the elderly due to retrobulbar optic neuropathy. Surv Ophthalmol 1996;41:261–267.
261. Johnson LN, Hepler RS, Yee RD, et al: Sphenoid sinus mucocele (anterior clinoid variant) mimicking diabetic ophthalmoplegia and retrobulbar neuritis. Am J Ophthalmol 1986;102:111–115.
262. Dunya IM, Frangieh GT, Heilman CB, et al: Anterior clinoid mucocele masquerading as a retrobulbar neuritis. Ophthal Plast Reconstr Surg 1996;12:171–173.
263. Galati LT, Baredes S, Mauriello J, et al: Visual loss reversed after treatment of acute bacterial sinusitis. Laryngoscope 1996;106:148–151.
264. Rothstein J, Maisel RH, Berlinger NT, et al: Relationship of optic neuritis to disease of the paranasal sinuses. Laryngoscope 1984;94:1501–1508.
265. Casson RJ, O'Day J, Crompton JL: Leber's idiopathic stellate neuroretinitis: differential diagnosis and approach to management. Aust NZ J Ophthalmol 1999;27:65–69.
266. Dreyer RF, Hopen G, Gass JD, et al: Leber's idiopathic stellate neuroretinitis. Arch Ophthalmol 1984;102: 1140–1145.
267. Maitland CG, Miller NR: Neuroretinitis. Arch Ophthalmol 1984;102:1146–1150.
268. Leavitt JA, Pruthi S, Morgenstern BZ: Hypertensive retinopathy mimicking neuroretinitis in a twelve year old girl. Surv Ophthalmol 1997;41:477–480.
269. Brazis PW, Lee AG: Optic disc edema with a macular star. Mayo Clin Proc 1996;71:1162–1166.
270. Verm A, Lee AG: Bilateral optic disc edema with macular exudates as the manifesting sign of a cerebral arteriovenous malformation. Am J Ophthalmol 1997;123:422–424.
271. Weiss AH, Beck RW: Neuroretinitis in childhood. J Pediatr Ophthalmol Strab 1989;26:198–203.
272. Purvin VA, Chioran G: Recurrent neuroretinitis. Arch Ophthalmol 1994;112:365–371.
273. Drancourt M, Birtles R, Chaumentin G, et al: New serotype of Bartonella henselae in endocarditis and cat scratch disease. Lancet 1996;347:441–443.

274. Wong MT, Dolan MJ, Lattuada CP, et al: Neuroretinitis, aseptic meningitis, and lymphadenitis associated with Bartonella (Rochalimaea) henselae infection in immunocompetent patients and patients infected with human immunodeficiency virus type 1. Clin Infect Dis 1995;21:352–360.
275. Folk JC, Weingeist TA, Corbett JJ, et al: Syphilitic neuroretinitis. Am J Ophthalmol 1983;95:480–486.
276. Arruga J, Valentines J, Mauri F, et al: Neuroretinitis in acquired syphilis. Ophthalmology 1985;92:262–270.
277. Lesser RS, Kornmehl EW, Pachner AR, et al: Neuro-ophthalmologic manifestations of Lyme disease. Ophthalmology 1990;97:699–706.
278. Karma A, Stenborg T, Summanen P, et al: Long-term follow-up of chronic Lyme neuroretinitis. Retina 1996;16:505–509.
279. Fish RH, Hoskins JC, Kline LB: Toxoplasmosis neuroretinitis. Ophthalmology 1993;100:1177–1182.
280. Burnett AJ, Shortt SG, Isaac-Renton J, et al: Multiple cases of acquired toxoplasmosis retinitis presenting in an outbreak. Ophthalmology 1998;105:1032–1037.
281. Guauri RR, Lee AG, Purvin V: Optic disk edema with a macular star. Surv Ophthalmol 1998;43:270–274.
282. Marra CM: Neurologic complications of Bartonella henselae infection. Curr Opin Neurol 1995;8:164–169.
283. Tomsak RL, Zakov ZN: Nonarteritic anterior ischemic optic neuropathy with macular edema: visual improvement and fluorescein angiographic characteristics. J Neuro-ophthalmol 1998;18:166–168.
284. Wear DJ, Marglieth AM, Hadfield TL, et al: Cat scratch disease. A bacterial infection. Science 1983;221:1403–1405.
285. Reed JB, Scales DK, Wong MT, et al: Bartonella henselae neuroretinitis in cat scratch disease. Diagnosis, management and sequelae. Ophthalmology 1998;105:459–466.
286. Weinstein JM, Lexow SS, Ho P, et al: Acute syphilitic optic neuritis. Arch Ophthalmol 1981;99:1392–1395.
287. Frohman L, Wolansky L: Magnetic resonance imaging of syphilitic optic neuritis/perineuritis. J Neuro-ophthalmol 1997;17:57–59.
288. Johns BR, Tierney M, Felsustein D: Alteration in the natural history of neurosyphilis by the concurrent infection with the human immunodeficiency virus. N Engl J Med 1987;316:1569–1572.
289. Mcleish WM, Pulido JS, Holland S, et al: The ocular manifestations of syphilis in the human immunodeficiency virus type-1 infected host. Ophthalmology 1990;97:196–203.
290. Finkel M: Lyme disease and its neurologic complications. Arch Neurol 1988;45:99–104.
291. Balcer LJ, Winterkorn JM, Galetta SL: Neuro-ophthalmic manifestations of Lyme disease. J Neuro-ophthalmol 1997;108:108–121.
292. Winward KE, Hamed LM, Glaser JS: The spectrum of optic nerve disease in human immunodeficiency virus infection. Am J Ophthalmol 1989;107:373–380.
293. Newman NJ, Lessell S: Bilateral optic neuropathies with remission in two HIV positive men. J Clin Neuro-ophthalmol 1992;12:1–5.
294. Patel SS, Rutzen AR, Marx JL, et al: Cytomegalovirus papillitis in patients with acquired immune deficiency syndrome. Visual prognosis of patients treated with ganciclovir and/or foscarnet. Ophthalmology 1996;103:1476–1482.
295. Baglivo E, Leuenberger PM, Kraus KH: Presumed bilateral cytomegalovirus-induced optic neuropathy in an immunocompetent person. A case report. J Neuro-ophthalmol 1996;16:14–17.
296. Mansor AM, Li HK: Cytomegalovirus optic neuritis: characteristics, therapy and survival. Ophthalmologica 1995;209:260–266.
297. Cohen DB, Glasgow BJ: Bilateral optic nerve cryptococcosis in sudden blindness in patients with acquired immune deficiency syndrome. Ophthalmology 1993;100:1689–1694.
298. Lipson BK, Freeman WR, Beniz J: Optic neuropathy associated with cryptococcal arachnoiditis in AIDS patients. Am J Ophthalmol 1989;107:523–527.
299. Jensen J: A case of herpes zoster ophthalmicus complicated with neuroretinitis. Acta Ophthalmol 1948;26:551–555.
300. Gunduz K, Ozdemir O: Bilateral retrobulbar optic neuritis following unilateral herpes zoster ophthalmicus. Ophthalmologica 1994;208:61–64.
301. Deane JS, Bibby K: Bilateral optic neuritis following herpes zoster. Arch Ophthalmol 1995;113:972–973.
302. Litoff D, Catalano RA: Herpes zoster optic neuritis in human immunodeficiency virus infection. Arch Ophthalmol 1990;108:782–783.
303. Shayegani A, Odel JG, Kazim M, et al: Varicella zoster virus retrobulbar optic neuritis in a patient with human immunodeficiency virus. Am J Ophthalmol 1996;122:586–588.
304. Lee MS, Cooney EL, Stoessel KM, et al: Varicella zoster virus retrobulbar optic neuritis preceding retinitis in patients with acquired immune deficiency syndrome. Ophthalmology 1998;105:467–471.
305. Meenken C, van den Horn GJ, de Smet MD, et al: Optic neuritis heralding varicella zoster virus retinitis in a patient with acquired immunodeficiency syndrome. Ann Neurol 1998;43:534–536.
306. Selbst RG, Selhorst JB, Harbison JW, et al: Parainfectious optic neuritis. Report and review following varicella. Arch Neurol 1983;40:347–350.
307. Johnson LN, Arnold AC: Incidence of nonarteritic and arteritic anterior ischemic optic neuropathy. Population-based study in the state of Missouri and Los Angeles County, California. J Neuro-ophthalmol 1994;14:38–44.
308. Miller GR, Smith JL: Ischemic optic neuropathy. Am J Ophthalmol 1966;62:103–115.
309. Boghen DR, Glaser JS: Ischaemic optic neuropathy. The clinical profile and natural history. Brain 1975;98:689–708.
310. Ischemic Optic Neuropathy Decompression Trial Study Group: Characteristics of patients with nonarteritic anterior ischemic optic neuropathy eligible for the Ischemic Optic Neuropathy Decompression Trial. Arch Ophthalmol 1996;114:1366–1374.
311. Hayreh SS, Joos KM, Podhajsky PA, et al: Systemic diseases associated with nonarteritic anterior ischemic optic neuropathy. Am J Ophthalmol 1994; 118:766–780.
312. Jacobson DM, Vierkant RA, Belongia EA: Nonarteritic anterior ischemic optic neuropathy. A case-control study of potential risk factors. Arch Ophthalmol 1997;115:1403–1407.
313. Hayreh SS, Podhajsky PA, Zimmerman B: Nonarteritic anterior ischemic optic neuropathy: time of onset of visual loss. Am J Ophthalmol 1997;124:641–647.
314. Hayreh SS, Podhajsky P, Zimmerman MB: Role of nocturnal arterial hypotension in optic nerve head ischemic disorders. Ophthalmologica 1999;213: 76–96.
315. Landau K, Winterkorn JM, Mailloux LU, et al: 24 hour blood pressure monitoring in patients with anterior

ischemic optic neuropathy. Arch Ophthalmol 1996;114:570–575.
316. Hayreh SS, Zimmerman MB, Podhajsky P, et al: Nocturnal arterial hypotension and its role in optic nerve head and ocular ischemic disorders. Am J Ophthalmol 1994;117:603–624.
317. Doro S, Lessell S: Cup : disc ratio and ischemic optic neuropathy. Arch Ophthalmol 1993;103:1143–1144.
318. Beck RW, Servais GE, Hayreh SS: Anterior ischemic optic neuropathy. IX. Cup-to-disc ratio and its role in pathogenesis. Ophthalmology 1987;94:1502–1508.
319. Beck RW, Savino PJ, Repka MX, et al: Optic disc structure in anterior ischemic optic neuropathy. Ophthalmology 1984;91:1334–1337.
320. Burde RM: Optic disc risk factors for non arteritic ischemic optic neuropathy. Am J Ophthalmol 1993;115:759–763.
321. Katz B, Spencer WH: Hyperopia as a risk factor for nonarteritic anterior ischemic optic neuropathy. Am J Ophthalmol 1993;15:754–758.
322. Chung SM, Gay CA, McCrary JA: Nonarteritic ischemic optic neuropathy. The impact of tobacco use. Ophthalmology 1994;101:779–782.
323. Fry CL, Carter JE, Kanter MC, et al: Anterior ischemic optic neuropathy is not associated with carotid artery atherosclerosis. Stroke 1993;24:539–542.
324. Swartz NG, Beck RW, Savino PJ, et al: Pain in anterior ischemic optic neuropathy. J Neuro-ophthalmol 1995;15:9–10.
325. Repka MX, Savino PJ, Schatz NJ, et al: Clinical profile and long-term implications of anterior ischemic optic neuropathy. Am J Ophthalmol 1983;96:478–483.
326. Warner JEA, Lessell S, Rizzo JF, et al: Does optic disc appearance distinguish ischemic optic neuropathy from optic neuritis. Arch Ophthalmol 1997;115:1408–1410.
327. Schatz NJ, Smith JL: Non-tumor causes of the Foster Kennedy syndrome. J Neurosurg 1967;27:37–44.
328. Arnold AC, Hepler RS: Fluorescein angiography in acute nonarteritic anterior ischemic optic neuropathy. Am J Ophthalmol 1994;117:222–230.
329. Arnold AC, Badr MA, Hepler RS: Fluorescein angiography in nonischemic optic disc edema. Arch Ophthalmol 1996;114:293–298.
330. Arnold AC, Hepler RS, Hamilton DR, et al: Magnetic resonance imaging of the brain in nonarteritic ischemic optic neuropathy. J Neuro-ophthalmol 1995; 15:158–160.
331. Arnold AC, Hepler RS: Natural history of nonarteritic ischemic optic neuropathy. J Neuro-ophthalmol 1994;14:66–69.
332. Borchert M, Lessell S: Progressive and recurrent nonarteritic anterior ischemic optic neuropathy. Am J Ophthalmol 1988;106:433–449.
333. Kline LB: Progression of visual field defects in ischemic optic neuropathy. Am J Ophthalmol 1988; 106:199–203.
334. The Ischemic Optic Neuropathy Decompression Trial Research Group: Optic nerve decompression surgery for nonarteritic ischemic optic neuropathy (NAION) is not effective and may be harmful. JAMA 1995;273:625–632.
335. Barrett DA, Glaser JS, Schatz NJ, et al: Spontaneous recovery of vision in progressive anterior ischaemic optic neuropathy. J Clin Neuro-ophthalmol 1992; 12:219–225.
336. Friedland S, Winterkorn JM, Burde RM: Luxury perfusion following anterior ischemic optic neuropathy. J Neuro-ophthalmol 1996;16:163–171.
337. Hayreh SS: Anterior ischemic optic neuropathy. V: Optic disc edema an early sign. Arch Ophthalmol 1981;99:1030–1040.
338. Gordon RN, Burde RM, Slamovits T: Asymptomatic optic disc edema. J Neuro-ophthalmol 1997;17:29–32.
339. Beri M, Klugman MR, Kohler JA, et al: Anterior ischemic optic neuropathy. VII. Incidence of bilaterality and various influencing factors. Ophthalmology 1987;94:1020–1028.
340. Guyer DR, Miller NR, Auer CL, et al: The risk of cerebrovascular disease in patients with anterior ischemic optic neuropathy. Arch Ophthalmol 1985; 103:1136–1142.
341. WuDunn D, Zimmerman K, Sadun AA, et al: Comparison of visual function in fellow eyes after bilateral nonarteritic anterior ischemic optic neuropathy. Ophthalmology 1997;104:104–111.
342. Boone MI, Massry GG, Frankel RA, et al: Visual outcome in bilateral nonarteritic ischemic optic neuropathy. Ophthalmology 1996;103:1223–1228.
343. Hayreh SS: Anterior ischemic optic neuropathy. I. Terminology and pathogenesis. Br J Ophthalmol 1974;58:955–963.
344. Hayreh SS: Anterior ischaemic optic neuropathy. Differentiation of arteritic from non-arteritic type and its management. Eye 1990;4:25–41.
345. Lessell S: Nonarteritic anterior ischemic optic neuropathy: enigma variations (editorial). Arch Ophthalmol 1999;117:386–388.
346. McLeod D, Marshall J, Kohner EM: Role of axoplasmic transport in the pathophysiology of ischaemic disc swelling. Br J Ophthalmol 1980;64:247–261.
347. Liebermann MF, Shahi A, Green WR: Embolic ischemic optic neuropathy. Am J Ophthalmol 1978; 86:206–210.
348. Cullen JF: Ischaemic optic neuropathy. Trans Ophthalmol Soc UK 1967;87:759–774.
349. Hayreh SS: Anterior ischemic optic neuropathy. IV: Occurrence after cataract extraction. Arch Ophthalmol 1980;98:1410–1416.
350. Hayreh SS: Anterior ischemic optic neuropathy. VIII. Clinical features and pathogenesis of posthemorrhagic amaurosis. Ophthalmology 1987;94: 1488–1502.
351. Galetta SL, Plock GL, Kushner MJ, et al: Ocular thrombosis associated with antiphospholipid antibodies. Ann Ophthalmol 1991;23:207–212.
352. Bertram B, Remky A, Arend O, et al: Protein C, protein S, and antithrombin III in acute ocular occlusive diseases. Ger J Ophthalmol 1995;4:332–335.
353. Rosler DH, Conway MD, Anaya JM, et al: Ischemic optic neuropathy and high-level anticardiolipin antibodies in primary Sjogren's syndrome. Lupus 1995;4:155–157.
354. Salomon O, Huna-Baron R, Kurtz S, et al: Analysis of prothrombotic and vascular risk factors in patients with nonarteritic anterior ischemic optic neuropathy. Ophthalmology 1999;106:739–742.
355. Hamed LM, Winward KE, Glaser JS, et al: Optic neuropathy in uremia. Am J Ophthalmol 1989;108:30–35.
356. Knox DL, Hanneken AM, Hollows FC: Uremic optic neuropathy. Arch Ophthalmol 1988;106:50–54.
357. Beck RW, Gamel JW, Willcourt RJ, et al: Acute ischemic optic neuropathy in severe preeclampsia. Am J Ophthalmol 1980;90:342–346.
358. Katz B: Bilateral sequential migrainous ischemic optic neuropathy. Am J Ophthalmol 1985;99:489.
359. O'Hara M, O'Connor PS: Migrainous optic neuropathy. J Clin Neuro-ophthalmol 1984;4:85–90.

360. Sergott RC, Cohen MS, Bosley TM, et al: Optic nerve decompression may improve the progressive form of non arteritic ischemic optic neuropathy. Arch Ophthalmol 1989;107:1743–1754.
361. Spoor TC, McHenry JG, Lau-Sickon L: Progressive and static nonarteritic ischemic optic neuropathy treated by optic nerve sheath decompression. Ophthalmology 1993;100:306–311.
362. Kelman SE, Elman MJ: Optic nerve sheath decompression for nonarteritic ischemic optic neuropathy improves multiple visual function measurements. Arch Ophthalmol 1991;109:667–671.
363. Glaser JS, Teimory M, Schatz NJ: Optic nerve sheath fenestration for progressive ischemic optic neuropathy. Results in second series consisting of 21 eyes. Arch Ophthalmol 1994;112:1047–1050.
364. Yee RD, Selky AK, Purvin VA: Outcomes of optic nerve sheath decompression for nonarteritic ischemic optic neuropathy. J Neuro-ophthalmol 1994;14: 70–76.
365. Arnold AC, Hepler RS, Lieber M, et al: Hyperbaric oxygen therapy for nonarteritic anterior ischemic optic neuropathy. Am J Ophthalmol 1996;122:535–541.
366. Botelho PJ, Johnson LN, Arnold AC: The effect of aspirin on the visual outcome of nonarteritic anterior ischemic optic neuropathy. Am J Ophthalmol 1996;121:450–451.
367. Johnson LN, Gould TJ, Krohel GB: Effect of levodopa and carbidopa on recovery of visual function in patients with nonarteritic anterior ischemic optic neuropathy of longer than six months' duration. Am J Ophthalmol 1996;121:77–83.
368. Haas A, Walzi M, Jesenik F, et al: Application of HELP in nonarteritic anterior ischemic optic neuropathy: a prospective, randomized, controlled study. Graefes Arch Clin Exp Ophthalmol 1997;235:14–19.
369. Beck RW, Hayreh SS, Podhajsky P, et al: Aspirin therapy in nonarteritic anterior ischemic optic neuropathy. Am J Ophthalmol 1997;123:212–217.
370. Kupersmith MJ, Frohman L, Sanderson M, et al: Aspirin reduces the incidence of second eye NAION: a retrospective study. J Neuro-ophthalmol 1997;17: 250–253.
371. Gerling J, Meyer JH, Kommerell G: Visual field defects in optic neuritis and anterior ischemic optic neuropathy: distinctive features. Graefes Arch Clin Exp Ophthalmol 1998;236:188–192.
372. Goodman BW: Temporal arteritis. Am J Med 1979;67:839–852.
373. Biller J, Asconape J, Weinblatt ME, et al: Temporal arteritis associated with a normal sedimentation rate. JAMA 1982;247:486–487.
374. Bengtsson B-A, Malmvall B-E: The epidemiology of giant cell arteritis including temporal arteritis and polymyalgia rheumatica. Incidences of different clinical presentations and eye complications. Arth Rheum 1981;24:899–904.
375. Hauser WA, Ferguson RH, Holley KE, et al: Temporal arteritis in Rochester, Minnesota, 1951 to 1967. Mayo Clin Proc 1971;46:597–602.
376. Huston KA, Hunder GG, Lie JT, et al: Temporal arteritis: a 25-year epidemiologic, clinical, and pathologic study. Ann Intern Med 1978;88:162–167.
377. Shah P, Murray PI, Harry J: An unusual case of giant cell arteritis. Am J Ophthalmol 1993;115:393–394.
378. Wilkinson IMS, Russell RWR: Arteries of the head and neck in giant cell arteritis. A pathological study to show the pattern of arterial involvement. Arch Neurol 1972;27:378–391.
379. Kattah JC, Mejico L, Chrousos GA, et al: Pathologic findings in a steroid-responsive optic nerve infarct in giant-cell arteritis. Neurology 1999;53:177–180.
380. Säve-Söderbergh J, Malmvall B-E, Andersson R, et al: Giant cell arteritis as a cause of death. JAMA 1986;255:493–496.
381. Hunder GG: Giant cell arteritis and polymyalgia rheumatica. In: Kelley WN, Harris ED, Ruddy S, Sledge CB (eds): Textbook of Rheumatology, 3rd edition, pp 1200–1208. Philadelphia, WB Saunders, 1989.
382. McDonnell PJ, Moore GW, Miller NR, et al: Temporal arteritis. A clinicopathologic study. Ophthalmology 1986;93:518–530.
383. Ghanchi FD, Dutton GN: Current concepts in giant cell (temporal) arteritis. Surv Ophthalmol 1997; 42:99–123.
384. Weyand CM, Bartley GB: Giant cell arteritis: new concepts in pathogenesis and implications for management. Am J Ophthalmol 1997;123:392–395.
385. Galetta SL, Raps EC, Wulc AE, et al: Conjugal temporal arteritis. Neurology 1990;40:1839–1842.
386. Finelli P: Alternating amaurosis fugax and temporal arteritis. Am J Ophthalmol 1997;123:850–851.
387. Galetta SL, Balcer LJ, Liu GT: Giant cell arteritis with unusual flow related neuro-ophthalmologic manifestations. Neurology 1997;49:1463–1465.
388. Liu GT, Glaser JS, Schatz NJ, et al: Visual morbidity in giant cell arteritis: clinical characteristics and prognosis for vision. Ophthalmology 1994;101:1779–1785.
389. Hart CT: Formed visual hallucinations: a symptom of cranial arteritis. Br Med J 1967;3:643–644.
390. Aiello PD, Trautmann JC, McPhee TJ, et al: Visual prognosis in giant cell arteritis. Ophthalmology 1993;100:550–555.
391. Jonasson F, Cullen JF, Elton RA: Temporal arteritis. A 14-year epidemiological, clinical and prognostic study. Scot Med J 1979;24:111–117.
392. Graham E: Survival in temporal arteritis. Trans Ophthalmol Soc UK 1980;100:108–110.
393. Wagener HP, Hollenhorst RW: The ocular lesions of temporal arteritis. Am J Ophthalmol 1958;45:617–630.
394. Eshaghian J: Controversies regarding giant cell (temporal, cranial) arteritis. Doc Ophthalmol 1979; 47:43–67.
395. Cullen JF, Coleiro JA: Ophthalmic complications of giant cell arteritis. Surv Ophthalmol 1976;20:247–260.
396. Keltner JL: Giant-cell arteritis. Signs and symptoms. Ophthalmology 1982;89:1101–1110.
397. Mehler MF, Rabinowich L: The clinical neuro-ophthalmologic spectrum of temporal arteritis. Am J Med 1988;85:839–843.
398. Hayreh SS, Podhajsky PA, Zimmerman B: Ocular manifestations of giant cell arteritis. Am J Ophthalmol 1998;125:509–520.
399. Melberg MS, Grand MG, Dieckert JP, et al: Cotton wool spots and the early diagnosis of giant cell arteritis. Ophthalmology 1995;102:1611–1614.
400. Slavin ML, Barondes MJ: Visual loss caused by choroidal ischemia preceding anterior ischemic optic neuropathy in giant cell arteritis. Am J Ophthalmol 1994;117:81–86.
401. Sebag J, Thomas JV, Epstein DL, et al: Optic disc cupping in arteritic anterior ischemic optic neuropathy resembles glaucomatous cupping. Ophthalmology 1986;93:357–361.
402. Hamed LM, Guy JR, Moster ML, et al: Giant cell arteritis in the ocular ischemic syndrome. Am J Ophthalmol 1992;113:702–705.

403. Hwang JM, Girkin CA, Perry JD, et al: Bilateral ocular ischemic syndrome secondary to giant cell arteritis progressing despite corticosteroid treatment. Am J Ophthalmol 1999;127:102–104.
404. Barricks ME, Traviesa DB, Glaser JS, et al: Ophthalmoplegia in cranial arteritis. Brain 1977;100:209–221.
405. Hayreh SS, Podhajsky PA, Raman R, et al: Giant cell arteritis: validity and reliability of various diagnostic criteria. Am J Ophthalmol 1997;123:285–296.
406. Dudenhoefer EJ, Cornblath WT, Schatz MP: Scalp necrosis with giant cell arteritis. Ophthalmology 1998;105:1875–1878.
407. Rudd JC, Fineman MS, Sergott RC: Ischemic scalp necrosis preceding loss of visual acuity in giant cell arteritis. Arch Ophthalmol 1998;116:1690–1691.
408. Simmons RJ, Cogan DG: Occult temporal arteritis. Arch Ophthalmol 1962;68:8–18.
409. Cullen JF: Occult temporal arteritis. A common cause of blindness in old age. Br J Ophthalmol 1967; 51:513–525.
410. Hayreh SS, Podhajsky PA, Zimmerman B: Occult giant cell arteritis: ocular manifestations. Am J Ophthalmol 1998;125:521–526.
411. Caselli RJ, Hunder GG, Whisnant JP: Neurologic disease in biopsy proven giant cell (temporal) arteritis. Neurology 1988;38:352–359.
412. Thielen KR, Wijdicks EFM, Nichols DA: Giant cell (temporal arteritis): involvement of the vertebral and internal carotid arteris. Mayo Clin Proc 1998; 73:444–446.
413. Gout O, Viala K, Lyon-Caen O: Giant cell arteritis and Vernet's syndrome. Neurology 1998;50:1862–1864.
414. Hunder GG, Bloch DA, Michel BA, et al: The American College of Rheumatology 1990 criteria for the classification of giant cell arteritis. Arthritis Rheum 1990;33:1122–1128.
415. Milne JS, Williamson J: The ESR in older people. Gerontol Clin 1972;14:36–42.
416. Miller A, Green M, Robinson D: Simple rule for calculating normal erythrocyte sedimentation rate. Br Med J Clin Res Ed 1983;286:266.
417. Jacobson DM, Slamovitz TL: Erythrocyte sedimentation rate and its relationship to hematocrit in giant cell arteritis. Arch Ophthalmol 1987;105:965–967.
418. Mack HG, O'Day J, Currie JN: Delayed choroidal perfusion in giant cell arteritis. J Clin Neuro-ophthalmol 1991;11:221–227.
419. Quillen DA, Cantore WA, Schwartz SR, et al: Choroidal non-perfusion in giant cell arteritis. Am J Ophthalmol 1993;116:171–175.
420. Siatkowski RM, Gass JDM, Glaser JS, et al: Fluorescein angiography in the diagnosis of giant cell arteritis. Am J Ophthalmol 1993;115:57–63.
421. Sadun F, Pece A, Brancato R: Fluorescein and indocyanine green angiography in arteritic anterior ischaemic optic neuropathy (letter). Br J Ophthalmol 1998;82:1344–1345.
422. Klein RG, Campbell RJ, Hunder GG, et al: Skip lesions in temporal arteritis. Mayo Clin Proc 1976;51: 504–510.
423. Chambers WA, Bernadino VB: Specimen length in temporal artery biopsies. J Clin Neuro-ophthalmol 1988;8:121–125.
424. Albert DM, Ruchman ML, Keltner JL: Skip areas in temporal arteritis. Arch Ophthalmol 1976;94:2072–2077.
425. Nishino H, DeRemee RA, Rubino FA, et al: Wegener's granulomatosis associated with vasculitis of the temporal artery: report of five cases. Mayo Clin Proc 1993;68:115–121.
426. Levy MH, Margo CE: Temporal artery biopsy and sarcoidosis. Am J Ophthalmol 1994;117:409–410.
427. Kattah JC, Cupps T, Manz HJ, et al: Occipital artery biopsy: a diagnostic alternative in giant cell arteritis. Neurology 1991;41:949–950.
428. Boyev LR, Miller NR, Green WR: Efficacy of unilateral versus bilateral temporal artery biopsies for the diagnosis of temporal arteritis. Am J Ophthalmol 1999;128:211–215.
429. Allison MC, Gallagher PJ: Temporal artery biopsy and corticosteroid treatment. Ann Rheum Dis 1984;43:416–417.
430. Achkar AA, Lie JT, Hunder GG, et al: How does previous corticosteroid therapy affect the biopsy findings in giant cell (temporal) arteritis? Ann Intern Med 1994;120:987–992.
431. To KW, Enzer YR, Tsiaras WG: Temporal artery biopsy after one month of corticosteroid therapy. Am J Ophthalmol 1994;117:265–267.
432. Guevara RA, Newman NJ, Grossniklaus HE: Positive temporal artery biopsy 6 months after prednisone treatment. Arch Ophthalmol 1998;116:1252–1253.
433. Wiggins RE: Invasive aspergillosis. A complication of treatment of temporal arteritis. J Neuro-ophthalmol 1995;15:36–38.
434. Ho AC, Sergott RC, Regillo CD, et al: Color doppler hemodynamics of giant cell arteritis. Arch Ophthalmol 1994;112:938–945.
435. Schmidt WA, Kraft HE, Vorpahl K, et al: Color duplex ultrasonography in the diagnosis of temporal arteritis. N Engl J Med 1997;337:1336–1342.
436. Model DG: Reversal of blindness in temporal arteritis with methylprednisolone (letter). Lancet 1978;1:340.
437. Lipton RB, Solomon S, Wertenbaker C: Gradual loss and recovery of vision in temporal arteritis. Arch Intern Med 1985;145:2252–2253.
438. Rosenfeld SI, Kosmorsky GS, Klingele TG, et al: Treatment of temporal arteritis with ocular involvement. Am J Med 1986;80:143–145.
439. Matzkin DC, Slamovits TL, Sachs R, et al: Visual recovery in two patients after intravenous methylprednisolone treatment of central retinal artery occlusion secondary to giant-cell arteritis. Ophthalmology 1992;99:68–71.
440. Diamond JP: Treatable blindness in temporal arteritis. Br J Ophthalmol 1991;75:432.
441. Postel EA, Pollock SC: Recovery of vision in a 47-year-old man with fulminant giant cell arteritis. J Clin Neuro-ophthalmol 1993;13:262–270.
442. Diamond JP: IV steroid treatment in giant cell arteritis (letter). Ophthalmology 1993;100:291–292.
443. Cornblath WT, Eggenberger ER: Progressive vision loss from giant cell arteritis despite high dose intravenous methylprednisolone. Ophthalmology 1997; 104:854–858.
444. Clearkin LG: IV steroids for central retinal artery occlusion in giant-cell arteritis (letter). Ophthalmology 1992;99:1482–1483.
445. Rubinow A, Brandt KD, Cohen AS, et al: Iatrogenic morbidity accompanying suppression of temporal arteritis by adrenal corticosteroids. Ann Ophthalmol 1984;16:258–265.
446. Diego M, Margo CE: Postural vision loss in giant cell arteritis. J Neuro-ophthalmol 1998;18:124–126.
447. Cullen JF: Temporal arteritis. Occurrence of ocular complications 7 years after diagnosis. Br J Ophthalmol 1972;56:584–588.

448. Evans JM, Batts KP, Hunder GG: Persistent giant cell arteritis despite corticosteroid treatment. Mayo Clin Proc 1994;69:1060–1061.
449. Boesen P, Dideriksen K, Stentoft J, et al: Dapsone in temporal arteritis and polymyalgia rheumatica (letter). J Rheumatol 1988;15:879–880.
450. Reinitz E, Aversa A: Long-term treatment of temporal arteritis with dapsone. Am J Med 1988;85:456–457.
451. Meadows SP: Temporal or giant cell arteritis. Proc Roy Soc Med 1966;59:329–333.
452. Birkhead NC, Wagener HP, Shick RM: Treatment of temporal arteritis with adrenal corticosteroids. Results in fifty-five cases in which lesion was proved at biopsy. JAMA 1957;163:821–827.
453. Slavin ML, Margolis AJ: Progressive anterior ischemic optic neuropathy due to giant cell arteritis despite high-dose intravenous corticosteroids (letter). Arch Ophthalmol 1988;106:1167.
454. Rauser M, Rismondo V: Ischemic optic neuropathy during corticosteroid therapy for giant cell arteritis. Arch Ophthalmol 1995;113:707–708.
455. Schneider HA, Weber AA, Ballen PH: The visual prognosis in temporal arteritis. Ann Ophthalmol 1971;3:1215–1230.
456. Soelberg Sørensen P, Lorenzen I: Giant-cell arteritis, temporal arteritis and polymyalgia rheumatica. A retrospective study of 63 patients. Acta Med Scand 1977;201:207–213.
457. Hugod C, Scheibel M: Temporal arteritis—progressive affection of vision during high-level corticosteroid therapy. A case report. Acta Med Scand 1979;205:445–446.
458. Delecoeuillerie G, Joly P, Cohen De Lara A, et al: Polymyalgia rheumatica and temporal arteritis: a retrospective analysis of prognostic features and different corticosteroid regimens (11 year survey of 210 patients). Ann Rheum Dis 1988;47:733–739.
459. Faarvang KL, Pontoppidan Thyssen E: Giant cell arteritis: loss of vision during corticosteroid therapy. J Intern Med 1989;225:215–216.
460. Myles AB, Perera T, Ridley MG: Prevention of blindness in giant cell arteritis by corticosteroid treatment. Br J Rheumatol 1992;31:103–105.
461. Harrison EQ: Complications of herpes zoster ophthalmicus. Am J Ophthalmol 1965;60:1111–1114.
462. Perlman JI, Forman S, Gonzalez ER: Retrobulbar ischemic optic neuropathy associated with sickle cell disease. J Neuro-ophthalmol 1994;14:45–48.
463. Lee AG, Brazis PW, Miller NR: Posterior ischemic optic neuropathy associated with migraine. Headache 1996;36:506–510.
464. Isayama Y, Takahashi T, Inoue M, et al: Posterior ischemic optic neuropathy. III: Clinical diagnosis. Ophthalmologica 1983;187:141–147.
465. Johnson MW, Kincaid MC, Trobe JD: Bilateral retrobulbar optic nerve infarctions after blood loss and hypotension. A clinicopathologic case study. Ophthalmology 1987;94:1577–1584.
466. Shaked G, Gavriel A, Roy-Shapira A: Anterior ischemic optic neuropathy after hemorrhagic shock. J Trauma 1998;44:923–925.
467. Drance SM, Morgan RW, Sweeney VP: Shock-induced optic neuropathy. A cause of nonprogressive glaucoma. N Engl J Med 1973;288:392–395.
468. Sweeney PJ, Breuer AC, Selhorst JB, et al: Ischemic optic neuropathy: A complication of cardiopulmonary bypass surgery. Neurology 1982;32:560–562.
469. Williams EL, Hart WM, Tempelhoff R: Postoperative ischemic optic neuropathy. Anesth Analg 1995; 80:1018–1029.
470. Katz DM, Trobe JD, Cornblath WT, et al: Ischemic optic neuropathy after lumbar spine surgery. Arch Ophthalmol 1994;112:925–931.
471. Lee AG: Ischemic optic neuropathy following lumbar spine surgery. Case report. J Neurosurg 1995; 83:348–349.
472. Rizzo JF, Lessell S: Posterior ischemic optic neuropathy during general surgery. Am J Ophthalmol 1987;103:808–811.
473. Schobel GA, Schmidbauer M, Millesi W, et al: Posterior ischemic optic neuropathy following bilateral radical neck dissection. Int J Oral Maxillofac Surg 1995;24:283–287.
474. Shapira OM, Kimmel WA, Lindsey PS, et al: Anterior ischemic optic neuropathy after open heart operations. Ann Thorac Surg 1996;61:660–666.
475. Alexandrakis G, Lam B: Bilateral posterior ischemic optic neuropathy after spinal surgery. Am J Ophthalmol 1999;127:354–355.
476. Barr CG, Glaser JS, Blankenship G: Acute disc swelling in juvenile diabetes: clinical profile and natural history in 12 cases. Arch Ophthalmol 1980;98:2185–2192.
477. Regillo CD, Brown GC, Savino PJ, et al: Diabetic papillopathy. Patient characteristics and fundus findings. Arch Ophthalmol 1995;113:889–895.
478. Skillern PG, Lokhart G: Optic neuritis and uncontrolled diabetes mellitus in 14 patients. Ann Intern Med 1959;51:468–475.
479. Ho AC, Maguire AM, Yanuzzi LA, et al: Rapidly progressive optic disc neovascularization after diabetic papillopathy. Am J Ophthalmol 1995;120: 673–675.
480. Kennedy F: Retrobulbar neuritis as an exact diagnostic sign of certain tumors and abscesses in the frontal lobes. Am J Med Sci 1911;142:355–368.
481. Wright JE, McNab AA, McDonald WI: Optic nerve glioma and the management of optic nerve tumours in the young. Br J Ophthalmol 1989;73:967–974.
482. Trobe JD, Glaser JS: Quantitative perimetry in compressive optic neuropathy and optic neuritis. Arch Ophthalmol 1978;96:1210–1216.
483. Dutton JJ: Gliomas of the anterior visual pathways. Surv Ophthalmol 1994;38:427–452.
484. Lewis RA, Gerson LP, Axelson KA, et al: von Recklinghausen neurofibromatosis. II: Incidence of optic gliomata. Ophthalmology 1984;91:929–935.
485. Haik BG, Louis LS, Bierly J, et al: Magnetic resonance imaging in the evaluation of optic nerve gliomas. Ophthalmology 1987;94:709–717.
486. Jakobiec FA, Depot MJ, Kennerdell JS, et al: Combined clinical and computed tomographic diagnosis of orbital glioma and meningioma. Ophthalmology 1984;91:137–155.
487. Alvord EC, Lofton S: Gliomas of the optic nerve or chiasm: outcome by patients' age, tumor site, and treatment. J Neurosurg 1988;68:85–98.
488. McDonnell P, Miller NR: Chiasmatic and hypothalamic extension of optic nerve glioma. Arch Ophthalmol 1983;101:1412–1415.
489. Kushner BJ: Functional amblyopia associated with abnormalities of the optic nerve. Arch Ophthalmol 1984;102:683–685.
490. Gaini SM, Tomei G, Arienta C, et al: Optic nerve and chiasmal gliomas in children. J Neurosurg Sci 1982;26:33–39.
491. Redfern RM, Scholtz CL: Long term survival with optic nerve glioma. Surg Neurol 1980;14:371–375.

492. Spoor TC, Kennerdell JS, Martinez AJ, et al: Malignant gliomas of the optic nerve pathways. Am J Ophthalmol 1980;89:284–292.
493. Hoyt WF, Meshel LG, Lessell S, et al: Malignant optic glioma of adulthood. Brain 1973;96:121–132.
494. Cunliffe IA, Moffat DA, Hardy DG, et al: Bilateral optic nerve sheath meningiomas in a patient with neurofibromatosis type 2. Br J Ophthalmol 1992; 76:310–312.
495. Bickerstaff ER, Small JM, Guest IA: The relapsing course of certain meningiomas in relation to pregnancy and menstruation. J Neurol Neurosurg Psychiatr 1958;21:89–91.
496. Sarkies NJ: Optic nerve sheath meningiomas: diagnostic features and therapeutic alternatives. Eye 1987;1:597–602.
497. Sibony PA, Krauss HR, Kennerdell JS, et al: Optic nerve sheath meningiomas: clinical manifestations. Ophthalmology 1984;91:1313–1326.
498. Wright JE, Call NB, Liaricos S: Primary optic nerve meningiomas. Br J Opthalmol 1980;64:553–558.
499. Zimmerman CF, Schatz NJ, Glaser JS: Magnetic resonance imaging of optic nerve meningiomas: enhancement with gadolinium-DTPA. Ophthalmology 1990;97:585–591.
500. Lindblom B, Truwit CL, Hoyt WF: Optic nerve sheath meningioma. Definition of intraorbital, intracanalicular, and intracranial components with magnetic resonance imaging. Ophthalmology 1992;99:560–566.
501. Mafee MF, Goodwin J, Dorodi S: Optic nerve sheath meningiomas. Role of MR imaging. Radiol Clin N Am 1999;37:37–58.
502. Smith JL, Vuksanovic MM, Yates BM, et al: Radiation therapy for primary optic nerve meningiomas. J Clin Neuro-ophthalmol 1981;1:85–99.
503. Kennerdell JS, Maroon JC, Malton M, et al: The management of optic nerve sheath meningiomas. Am J Ophthalmol 1988;106:450–457.
504. Klink DF, Miller NR, Williams J: Preservation of residual vision 2 years after stereotactic radiosurgery for a presumed optic nerve sheath meningioma. J Neuro-ophthalmol 1998;18:117–120.
505. Kupersmith MJ, Warren FA, Newell J, et al: Irradiation of meningiomas of the intracranial anterior visual pathway. Ann Neurol 1987;21:131–137.
506. Rosenstein J, Symon L: Surgical management of suprasellar meningioma. 2. Prognosis for visual function following craniotomy. J Neurosurg 1984;61: 642–648.
507. Andrews BT, Wilson CB: Suprasellar meningiomas: the effect of tumor location on postoperative visual outcome. J Neurosurg 1988;69:523–528.
508. Rosenberg LF, Miller NR: Visual results after microsurgical removal of meningiomas involving the anterior visual system. Arch Ophthalmol 1984;102:1019–1023.
509. Grisoli F, Vincentelli F, Raybaud C, et al: Intrasellar meningioma. Surg Neurol 1983;20:36–41.
510. Kline LB, Kim JY, Ceballos R: Radiation optic neuropathy. Ophthalmology 1985;92:1118–1126.
511. Wiebers DO, Whisnant JP, O'Fallon WM: The natural history of unruptured intracranial aneurysms. N Engl J Med 1981;304:696–698.
512. Farris BK, Smith JL, David NJ: The nasal junction scotoma in giant aneurysms. Ophthalmology 1986; 93:895–905.
513. Vargas ME, Kupersmith MJ, Setton A, et al: Endovascular treatment of giant aneurysms which cause visual loss. Ophthalmology 1994;101:1091–1098.
514. Ferguson GG, Drake CG: Carotid-ophthalmic aneurysms: the surgical management of those cases presenting with compression of the optic nerves and chiasm alone. Clin Neurosurg 1980;27:263–307.
515. Kupersmith MJ, Berenstein A, Choi IS, et al: Percutaneous transvascular treatment of giant carotid aneurysms: neuro-ophthalmologic findings. Neurology 1984;34:328–335.
516. Gutman I, Melamed S, Askenazi I, et al: Optic nerve compression by carotid arteries in low tension glaucoma. Graefes Arch Clin Exp Ophthalmol 1993; 231:711–717.
517. Kalenak JW, Kosmorsky GS, Hassenbusch SJ: Compression of the intracranial optic nerve mimicking unilateral normal pressure glaucoma. J Clin Neuro-ophthalmol 1992;12:230–235.
518. Jacobson DM, Warner JJ, Broste SK: Optic nerve contact and compression by the carotid artery in asymptomatic patients. Am J Ophthalmol 1997;123:677–683.
519. Grosskreutz C, Netland PA: Low-tension glaucoma. Int Ophthalmol Clin 1994;34:173–185.
520. Sommer A, Tielsch JM, Katz J, et al: Relationship between intraocular pressure and primary open angle glaucoma among white and black Americans. The Baltimore Eye Survey. Arch Ophthalmol 1991;109:1090–1095.
521. Stroman GA, Stewart WC, Golnik KC, et al: Magnetic resonance imaging in patients with low tension glaucoma. Arch Ophthalmol 1995;113:168–172.
522. Corbett JJ, Phelps CD, Eslinger P, et al: The neurologic evaluation of patients with low-tension glaucoma. Invest Ophthalmol Vis Sci 1985;26:1101–1104.
523. Bianchi-Marzoli S, Rizzo JF, Brancato R, et al: Quantitative analysis of optic disc cupping in compressive optic neuropathy. Ophthalmology 1995;102:436–440.
524. Sharma M, Volpe NJ, Dreyer EB: Methanol-induced optic nerve cupping. Arch Ophthalmol 1999;117:286.
525. Greenfield DS, Siatkowski RM, Glaser JS, et al: The cupped disc. Who needs neuroimaging? Ophthalmology 1998;105:1866–1874.
526. Wasserstrom WF, Glass JP, Posner JB: Diagnosis and treatment of leptomeningeal metastases from solid tumors: Experience with 90 patients. Cancer 1982; 49:759–769.
527. Katz J, Valsamis M, Jampel R: Ocular signs in diffuse carcinomatous meningitis. Am J Ophthalmol 1961;52: 681–690.
528. Altrocchi P, Eckman P: Meningeal carcinomatosis and blindness. J Neurol Neurosurg Psychiatry 1973;36:206–210.
529. Case Records of the MGH: N Engl J Med 1988; 318:903–916.
530. Arnold AC, Hepler RS, Foos RY: Isolated metastasis to the optic nerve. Surv Ophthalmol 1981;26:75–83.
531. Sung JU, Lam BL, Curtin VT, et al: Metastatic gastric carcinoma to the optic nerve. Arch Ophthalmol 1998;116:692–693.
532. Backhouse O, Simmons I, Frank A, et al: Optic nerve breast metastasis mimicking meningioma. Aust NZ J Ophthalmol 1998;26:247–249.
533. Mansour AM, Dinowitz K, Chaljub G, et al: Metastatic lesion of the optic nerve. J Clin Neuro-ophthalmol 1993;13:102–104.
534. Newman NJ, Grossniklaus HE, Wojno TH: Breast carcinoma metastatic to the optic nerve. Arch Ophthalmol 1996;114:102–103.
535. Kattah JC, Chrousos GC, Roberts J, et al: Metastatic prostate cancer to the optic canal. Ophthalmology 1993;100:1711–1715.

536. Strominger MB, Schatz NJ, Glaser JS: Lymphomatous optic neuropathy. Am J Ophthalmol 1993;116: 774–776.
537. Coppeto JR, Monteiro ML, Cannarozzi DB: Optic neuropathy associated with chronic lymphomatous meningitis. J Clin Neuro-ophthalmol 1988;8:39–45.
538. Donoso LA, Magargal LE, Eiferman RA: Meningeal carcinomatosis secondary to malignant lymphoma (Burkitt's pattern). J Pediatr Ophthalmol Strabis 1981;18:48–50.
539. Kline LB, Garcia JH, Harsh GR: Lymphomatous optic neuropathy. Arch Ophthalmol 1984;102:1655–1657.
540. Kay MC: Optic neuropathy secondary to lymphoma. J Clin Neuro-ophthalmol 1986;6:31–34.
541. Takahashi T, Oda Y, Isayama Y: Leukemic optic neuropathy. Ophthalmologica 1982;185:37–45.
542. Brown GC, Shields JA, Augsburger JJ, et al: Leukemic optic neuropathy. Int Ophthalmol 1981;3:111–116.
543. Currie JN, Lessell S, Lessell IM, et al: Optic neuropathy in chronic lymphocytic leukemia. Arch Ophthalmol 1988;106:654–660.
544. Norton SW, Stockman JA: Unilateral optic neuropathy following vincristine chemotherapy. J Pediatr Ophthalmol Strabis 1979;16:190–193.
545. Waterston JA, Gilligan BS: Paraneoplastic optic neuritis and external ophthalmoplegia. Aust N Z J Med 1986;16:703–704.
546. Pillay N, Gilbert JJ, Ebers GC, et al: Internuclear ophthalmoplegia and "optic neuritis": paraneoplastic effects of bronchial carcinoma. Neurology 1984;34: 788–791.
547. Boghen D, Sebag M, Michaud J: Paraneoplastic optic neuritis and encephalomyelitis. Report of a case. Arch Neurol 1988;45:353–356.
548. Malik S, Furlan AJ, Sweene PJ, et al: Optic neuropathy: a rare paraneoplastic syndrome. J Clin Neuro-ophthalmol 1992;12:137–141.
549. Luiz JE, Lee AG, Keltner JL, et al: Paraneoplastic optic neuropathy and autoantibody production in small-cell carcinoma of the lung. J Neuro-ophthalmol 1998;18:178–181.
550. de la Sayette V, Bertran F, Honnorat J, et al: Paraneoplastic cerebellar syndrome and optic neuritis with anti-CV2 antibodies: clinical response to excision of the primary tumor. Arch Neurol 1998; 55:405–408.
551. Blumenthal D, Schochet S, Jr., Gutmann L, et al: Small-cell carcinoma of the lung presenting with paraneoplastic peripheral nerve microvasculitis and optic neuropathy (letter). Muscle & Nerve 1998;21:1358–1359.
552. Schatz NJ, Lichtenstein S, Corbett JJ: Delayed radiation necrosis of the optic nerves and chiasm. In: Glaser JS, Smith JL (eds): Neuro-ophthalmology. Symposium of the University of Miami and the Bascom Palmer Eye Institute. Vol. VIII, pp 131–139. St. Louis, CV Mosby, 1975.
553. Girkin CA, Comey CH, Lunsford LD, et al: Radiation optic neuropathy after stereotactic radiosurgery. Ophthalmology 1997;104:1634–1643.
554. Leber KA, Berglöff J, Pendl G: Dose-response tolerance of the visual pathways and cranial nerves of the cavernous sinus to stereotactic radiosurgery. J Neurosurg 1998;88:43–50.
555. Zimmerman CF, Schatz NJ, Glaser GS: Magnetic resonance imaging in radiation optic neuropathy. Am J Ophthalmol 1990;110:389–394.
556. Roden D, Bosley TM, Fowble B, et al: Delayed radiation injury to the retrobulbar optic nerves and chiasm. Clinical syndrome and treatment with hyperbaric oxygen and corticosteroids. Ophthalmology 1990;97: 346–351.
557. Guy J, Schatz NJ: Hyperbaric oxygen in the treatment of radiation optic neuropathy. Ophthalmology 1986;93:1083–1090.
558. Borruat FX, Schatz NJ, Glaser JS, et al: Visual recovery from radiation induced optic neuropathy: the role of hyperbaric oxygen therapy. J Clin Neuro-ophthalmol 1993;13:98–101.
559. Glantz MJ, Burger PC, Friedman AH, et al: Treatment of radiation-induced nervous system injury with heparin and warfarin. Neurology 1994;44:2020–2027.
560. Landau K, Killer HE: Radiation damage (letter). Neurology 1996;46:889.
561. Lessell S: Toxic and deficiency optic neuropathies. In: Smith JL, Glaser JS (eds): Neuro-ophthalmology; Symposium of the University of Miami and the Bascom Palmer Eye Institute, pp 21–37. St Louis, CV Mosby, 1973.
562. Lessell S: Nutritional amblyopia. J Neuro-ophthalmol 1998;18:106–111.
563. Hamilton HE, Ellis PE, Sheets RF: Visual impairment due to optic neuropathy in pernicious anemia: Report of a case and review of the literature. Blood 1959;14:378–385.
564. Rizzo JF: Adenosine triphosphate deficiency: a genre of optic neuropathy. Neurology 1995;45:11–16.
565. Troncoso J, Mancall EL, Schatz NJ: Visual evoked responses in pernicious anemia. Arch Neurol 1979;36:168–169.
566. Lindenbaum J, Healton EB, Savage DG, et al: Neuropsychiatric disorders caused by cobalamin deficiency in the absence of anemia or macrocytosis. N Engl J Med 1988;318:1720–1728.
567. Chester EM, Agamanopolis DP, Harris JW, et al: Optic atrophy in experimental vitamin B12 deficiency in monkeys. Acta Neurol Scand 1980;61:9–26.
568. Hind VMD: Degeneration in the peripheral visual pathway of B12-deficient monkeys. Trans Ophthalmol Soc UK 1970;90:839–846.
569. Bloom SM, Merz EH, Taylor WW: Nutritional amblyopia in American prisoners of war liberated from the Japanese. Am J Ophthalmol 1946;29:1248–1257.
570. Samples JR, Younge BR: Tobacco-alcohol amblyopia. J Clin Neuro-ophthalmol 1981;1:213–218.
571. Wokes F: Tobacco amblyopia. Lancet 1958;2:526–527.
572. Rizzo JF, Lessell S: Tobacco amblyopia. Am J Ophthalmol 1993;116:84–87.
573. Heaton JM, McCormick AJA, Freeman AG: Tobacco amblyopia: clinical manifestations of vitamin B12 deficiency. Lancet 1958;2:286–290.
574. Frisén L: Fundus changes in acute malnutritional optic neuropathy. Arch Ophthalmol 1983;101:577–579.
575. Carroll FD: Nutritional amblyopia. Arch Ophthalmol 1966;76:406–411.
576. Quigley HA, Addicks EM, Green WR: Optic nerve damage in human glaucoma. III. Quantitative correlation of nerve fiber loss and visual field defect in glaucoma, ischemic neuropathy, papilledema, and toxic neuropathy. Arch Ophthalmol 1982;100: 135–146.
577. Roman GC: An epidemic in Cuba of optic neuropathy, sensorineural deafness, peripheral sensory neuropathy and dorsolateral myeloneuropathy. J Neurol Sci 1994;127:11–28.
578. Newman NJ, Torroni A, Brown MD, et al: Epidemic neuropathy in Cuba not associated with mitochondrial DNA mutations found in Leber's hereditary

optic neuropathy patients. Cuban Neuropathy Field Investigation Team. Am J Ophthalmol 1994;118: 158–168.

579. Johns DR, Neufeld MJ, Hedges TR: Mitochondrial DNA mutations in Cuban optic and peripheral neuropathy. J Neuro-ophthalmol 1994;14:135–140.
580. Johns DR, Sadun AA: Cuban epidemic optic neuropathy. Mitochondrial DNA analysis. J Neuro-ophthalmol 1994;14:130–134.
581. The Cuba Neuropathy Field Investigation Team: Epidemic optic neuropathy in Cuba—clinical characterization and risk factors. N Engl J Med 1995;333:1176–1182.
582. Sadun AA, Martone JR, Muci-Mendoza R, et al: Epidemic optic neuropathy in Cuba. Eye findings. Arch Ophthalmol 1994;112:691–699.
583. Mojon DS, Kaufmann P, Odel JG, et al: Clinical course of a cohort in the Cuban epidemic optic and peripheral neuropathy. Neurology 1997;48:19–22.
584. Hirano M, Cleary JM, Stewart AM, et al: Mitochondrial DNA mutations in an outbreak of optic neuropathy in Cuba. Neurology 1994;44:843–845.
585. Osuntokun BO, Osuntokun O: Tropical amblyopia in Nigerians. Am J Ophthalmol 1971;72:708–716.
586. Carroll FD: Jamaican optic neuropathy in immigrants to the United States. Am J Ophthalmol 1971; 71:261–265.
587. Plant GT, Mtanda AT, Arden GB, et al: An epidemic of optic neuropathy in Tanzania: characterization of the visual disorder and associated peripheral neuropathy. J Neurol Sci 1997;145:127–140.
588. Benton CD, Calhoun FP: The ocular effects of methyl alcohol poisoning. Report of a catastrophe involving three hundred and twenty persons. Trans Am Acad Ophthalmol Otolaryngol 1952;56:875–885.
589. Hayreh MS, Hayreh S, Baumbach GL, et al: Methyl alcohol poisoning. III. Ocular toxicity. Arch Ophthalmol 1977;95:1851–1858.
590. Sharpe JA, Hostovsky M, Bilbao JM, et al: Methanol optic neuropathy: a histopathological study. Neurology 1982;32:1093–1100.
591. Naeser P: Optic nerve involvement in a case of methanol poisoning. Br J Ophthalmol 1988;72:778–781.
592. McKellar MJ, Hidajat RR, Elder MJ: Acute ocular methanol toxicity: clinical and electrophysiological features. Aust N Z J Ophthalmol 1997;25:225–230.
593. Leibold JE: The ocular toxicity of ethambutol and its relation to dose. N Y Acad Sci 1966;135:904–909.
594. Barron GJ, Tepper L, Iovine G: Ocular toxicity from ethambutol. Am J Ophthalmol 1974;77:256–260.
595. DeVita EG, Miao M, Sadun AA: Optic neuropathy in ethambutol-treated renal tuberculosis. J Clin Neuro-ophthalmol 1987;7:77–86.
596. Salmon JF, Carmichael TR, Welsh NH: Use of contrast sensitivity measurement in the detection of subclinical ethambutol toxic optic neuropathy. Br J Ophthalmol 1987;71:192–196.
597. Woung LC, Jou JR, Liaw SL: Visual function in recovered ethambutol optic neuropathy. J Ocul Pharmacol Ther 1995;11:411–419.
598. Tsai RK, Lee YH: Reversibility of ethambutol optic neuropathy. J Ocul Pharmacol Ther 1997;13:473–477.
599. Garett SN, Kearney JJ, Schiffman JS: Amiodarone optic neuropathy. J Clin Neuro-ophthalmol 1988;8: 105–110.
600. Mansour AM, Puklin JE, O'Grady R: Optic nerve ultrastructure following amiodarone therapy. J Clin Neuro-ophthalmol 1988;8:231–237.
601. Nazarian SM, Jay WM: Bilateral optic neuropathy associated with amiodarone therapy. J Clin Neuro-ophthalmol 1988;8:25–28.
602. Gittinger JW, Asdourian GK: Papillopathy caused by amiodarone. Arch Ophthalmol 1987;105:349–351.
603. Feiner LA, Younge BR, Kazmier FJ, et al: Optic neuropathy and amiodarone therapy. Mayo Clin Proc 1987;62:702–717.
604. Palimar P, Cota N: Bilateral anterior ischaemic optic neuropathy following amiodarone (letter). Eye 1998;12:894–896.
605. Macaluso DC, Shults WT, Fraunfelder FT: Features of amiodarone-induced optic neuropathy. Am J Ophthalmol 1999;127:610–612.
606. Kono R: Subacute myelo-optico neuropathy, a new neurological disease prevailing in Japan. Jpn J Med Sci Biol 1971;24:195–216.
607. Khawly JA, Rubin P, Petros W, et al: Retinopathy and optic neuropathy in bone marrow transplantation for breast cancer. Ophthalmology 1996;103:87–95.
608. Fard AK, Merbs SL, Pieramici DJ: Optic nerve avulsion from a diving injury. Am J Ophthalmol 1997;124:562–564.
609. Tsopelas NV, Arvanitis PG: Avulsion of the optic nerve head after orbital trauma. Arch Ophthalmol 1998;116:394.
610. Espaillat A, To K: Optic nerve avulsion. Arch Ophthalmol 1998;116:540–541.
611. Foster BS, March GA, Lucarelli MJ, et al: Optic nerve avulsion. Arch Ophthalmol 1997;115:623–630.
612. Lessell S: Indirect optic nerve trauma. Arch Ophthalmol 1989;107:382–386.
613. Anderson RL, Panje Gross CE: Optic nerve blindness following blunt forehead trauma. Ophthalmology 1982;89:445–455.
614. Kline LB, Morawetz RB, Swaid SN: Indirect injury of the optic nerve. Neurosurgery 1984;14:756–764.
615. Joseph MP, Lessell S, Rizzo J, et al: Extracranial optic nerve decompression for traumatic optic neuropathy. Arch Ophthalmol 1990;108:1091–1093.
616. Seiff SR: High dose corticosteroids for treatment of vision loss due to indirect injury to the optic nerve. Ophthalmic Surg 1990;21:389–395.
617. Steinsapir KD, Goldberg RA: Traumatic optic neuropathy. Surv Ophthalmol 1994;38:487–518.
618. Bracken MB, Collins WF, Freeman DF, et al: A randomized, controlled trial of methylprednisolone or naloxone in the treatment of acute spinal-cord injury: results of the second national Acute Spinal Cord Injury Study. N Engl J d 1990;322:1405–1411.
619. Braughler JM, Hall ED: Current applications of "high dose" steroid therapy for CNS injury. J Neurosurg 1985;62:806–810.
620. Li KK, Teknos TN, Lai A, et al: Traumatic optic neuropathy: result in 45 consecutive surgically treated patients. Otolaryngol Head Neck Surg 1999;120:5–11.
621. Levin LA, Beck RW, Joseph MP, et al: The treatment of traumatic optic neuropathy. The international optic nerve trauma study. Ophthalmology 1999; 106:1268–1277.
622. Volpe NJ, Lessell S, Kline LB: Traumatic optic neuropathy: diagnosis and management. Int Ophthalmol Clin 1991;31:142–156.
623. Rabiah PK, Bateman JB, Demer JL, et al: Ophthalmologic findings in patients with ataxia. Am J Ophthalmol 1997;123:108–117.
624. Abe T, Abe K, Aoki M, et al: Ocular changes in patients with spinocerebellar degeneration and repeated trinucleotide expansion of spinocerebellar

ataxia type 1 gene. Am J Ophthalmol 1997;115: 231–236.
625. Landy PJ: A prospective study of the risk of developing multiple sclerosis in optic neuritis in a tropical and subtropical area. J Neurol Neurosurg Psychiatr 1983;46:659–661.
626. Sandberg-Wollheim M, Bynke H, Cronqvist S, et al: A long-term prospective study of optic neuritis: evaluation of risk factors. Ann Neurol 1990;27:386–393.
627. Slavin ML: Compression of the anterior visual pathways. In: Kline LB (ed): Optic Nerve Disorders, pp 91–137. San Francisco, American Academy of Ophthalmology and Palace Press, 1996.
628. Imperia PS, Lazarus HM, Lass JH: Ocular complications of systemic cancer chemotherapy. Surv Ophthalmol 1989;34:209–230.
629. Lessell S: Toxic and deficiency optic neuropathies. In: Walsh and Hoyt's Clinical Neuro-ophthalmology. In: Miller NR, Newman NJ (eds): 5th edition, pp. 663–680. Baltimore, Williams & Wilkins, 1998.
630. Brodsky MC, Landau K, Wilson RS, et al: Morning glory disc anomaly in neurofibromatosis type 2. Arch Ophthalmol 1999;117:839–841.
631. Bremner FD, Shallo-Hoffman J, Riordan-Eva P, et al: Comparing pupil function with visual function in patients with Leber's hereditary optic neuropathy. Invest Ophthalmol Vis Sci 1999;40:2528–2534.
632. Kerrison JB, Arnould VJ, Ferraz Sallum JM, et al: Genetic heterogeneity of dominant optic atrophy, Kjer type. Arch Ophthalmol 1999;117:805–810.
633. Jin Y-P, de Pedro-Cuesta J, Söderström M, et al: Incidence of optic neuritis in Stockholm, Sweden, 1990–1995. Arch Neurol 1999;56:975–980.
634. Rudick RA: Disease-modifying drugs for relapsing-remitting multiple sclerosis and future directions for multiple sclerosis therapeutics. Arch Neurol 1999;56:1079–1084.
635. Gonen O, Catalaa I, Babb JS, et al: Total brain N-acetylaspartate. A new measure of disease load in MS. Neurology 2000;54:15–19.
636. Li DKB, Paty DW, UBC MS/MRI Analysis Research Group, et al: Magnetic resonance imaging results of the PRISMS trial: a randomized, double-blind, placebo-controlled study of interferon-beta 1a in relapsing-remitting multiple sclerosis. Ann Neurol 1999;46:197–206.
637. Zhao GJ, Koopmans RA, Li DKB, et al: Effect of interferon beta-1b in MS. Assessment of annual accumulation of PD/T2 activity on MRI. Neurology 2000;54:200–206.
638. Trobe JD, Sieving PC, Guire KE, et al: The impact of the Optic Neuritis Treatment Trial on the practices of ophthalmologists and neurologists. Ophthalmology 1999;106:2047–2053.
639. Wingerchuk DM, Hogancamp WF, O'Brien PC, et al: The clinical course of neuromyelitis optica (Devic's syndrome). Neurology 1999;53:1107–1114.
640. Filippi M, Rocca MA, Moiola L, et al: MRI and magnetization transfer imaging changes in the brain and cervical cord of patients with Devic's neuromyelitis optica. Neurology 1999;53:1705–1710.
641. Brady KM, Brar AS, Lee AG, et al: Optic neuritis in children: clinical features and visual outcome. J AAPOS 1999;3:98–103.
642. Meadows SP: Doyne memorial lecture (1969). Retrobulbar and optic neuritis in childhood and adolescence. Trans Ophthalmol Soc U K 1970;89:603–638.
643. Maltzman JS, Lee AG, Miller NR: Optic neuropathy occurring after bee and wasp sting. Ophthalmology 2000;107:193–195.
644. Jackson TL, Farmer CKT, Kingswood C, et al: Hypotensive ischemic optic neuropathy and peritoneal dialysis. Am J Ophthalmol 1999;128:109–111.
645. Muci-Mendoza R, Arevalo JF, Ramella M, et al: Optociliary veins in optic nerve sheath meningioma. Indocyanine green videoangiography findings. Ophthalmology 1999;106:311–318.
646. Jacobson DM: Symptomatic compression of the optic nerve by the carotid artery. Ophthalmology 1999;106:1994–2004.
647. Levin LA, Gragoudas ES, Lessell S: Endothelial cell loss in irradiated optic nerves. Ophthalmology 2000;107:370–374.
648. Vaphiades MS, Newman NJ: Optic nerve enhancement on orbital magnetic resonance imaging in Leber's hereditary optic neuropathy. J Neuro-ophthalmol 1999;19:238–239.
649. Lee AG, Eggenberger ER, Kaufman DI, et al: Optic nerve enhancement on magnetic resonance imaging in anterior ischemic optic neuropathy. J Neuro-ophthalmol 1999;19:235–237.

CHAPTER 6

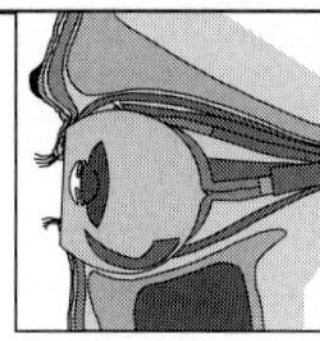

Optic Disc Swelling: Papilledema and Other Causes

The distinction between papilledema (disc swelling secondary to increased intracranial pressure), disc swelling associated with optic neuropathy, and disc elevation due to pseudopapilledema will be reviewed first. Then, the funduscopic appearance of papilledema, the associated visual loss and its mechanisms, and the differential diagnosis in and evaluation of patients with papilledema will be discussed. Conditions associated with papilledema then will be covered, with the greatest emphasis placed on diagnosis and management of a relatively common nontumor cause of papilledema, pseudotumor cerebri.

DISTINCTION OF PAPILLEDEMA FROM OPTIC NEUROPATHY, PSEUDOPAPILLEDEMA, AND OTHER CAUSES OF DISC SWELLING

Table 6–1 outlines the differential diagnosis of a swollen disc. The term *papilledema* refers to optic disc swelling due to increased intracranial pressure, and the two conditions most commonly mistaken for it are disc swelling due to optic neuropathy and pseudopapilledema (disc elevation without nerve fiber layer edema). The distinction between these three major causes of disc swelling is aided by review of the history, evaluation of visual function, ophthalmoscopic appearance of the disc, and ancillary testing. At times the diagnosis may be difficult, but there are some useful, general guidelines.[1–3]

Signs and symptoms of elevated intracranial pressure, such as headache, nausea, vomiting, and abducens paresis, should suggest the diagnosis of papilledema. However, caution should be applied in this regard, as patients may present with headache unrelated to their disc swelling. For instance, we have seen patients with migraine headaches and pseudopapilledema, and others with headache associated with optic neuritis.

Ophthalmoscopically, the disc swelling due to optic neuropathy and that due to papilledema may be identical (Fig. 6–1; see Color Plate 29). However, optic neuropathies such as optic neuritis or ischemic optic neuropathy typically lead to more severe central visual loss that is usually sudden in onset, unilateral, and associated with an afferent pupillary defect and impaired color vision.[4] Papilledema, on the other hand, is more frequently bilateral and more commonly leads to visual deficits such as enlarged blind spots and peripheral field constriction, about which the patient may not be aware. The various optic neuropathies are discussed in more detail in Chapter 5.

Pseudopapilledema

Pseudopapilledema (or pseudo-disc edema) is the term used to describe optic nerve variants or abnormalities that mimic papilledema ophthalmoscopically, including congenital anomalies,[5] tilting, hypoplasia, crowded hyperopic disc, optic disc hamartoma, myelinated nerve

TABLE 6–1. Differential Diagnosis of a Swollen Optic Disc: Causes According to Frequency

Most Common	Common	Uncommon
Papilledema	Central retinal vein occlusion	Ocular hypotony
Optic neuritis	Diabetic papillopathy	Intraocular inflammation (uveitis)
Anterior ischemic optic neuropathy		Malignant hypertension
Pseudopapilledema		Optic perineuritis
		Papillitis
		Intrinsic optic disc tumors
		Leber's hereditary optic neuropathy
		Optic nerve infiltration
		Sarcoidosis
		Lymphoma
		Leukemia
		Plasma cell dyscrasia

fibers, and optic nerve head drusen (Fig. 6–2; see Color Plates 30 to 32). Visual loss, which may occur in some cases, is long standing, painless, and frequently unnoticed by the patient. The diagnosis may be aided by serial dilated fundus examinations and review of stereo disc photographs; pseudopapilledema will be stable over time, while untreated papilledema might change. Ophthalmoscopic hallmarks of pseudopapilledema include anomalous retinal vasculature (abnormal branching pattern, for instance), absence of a central cup,

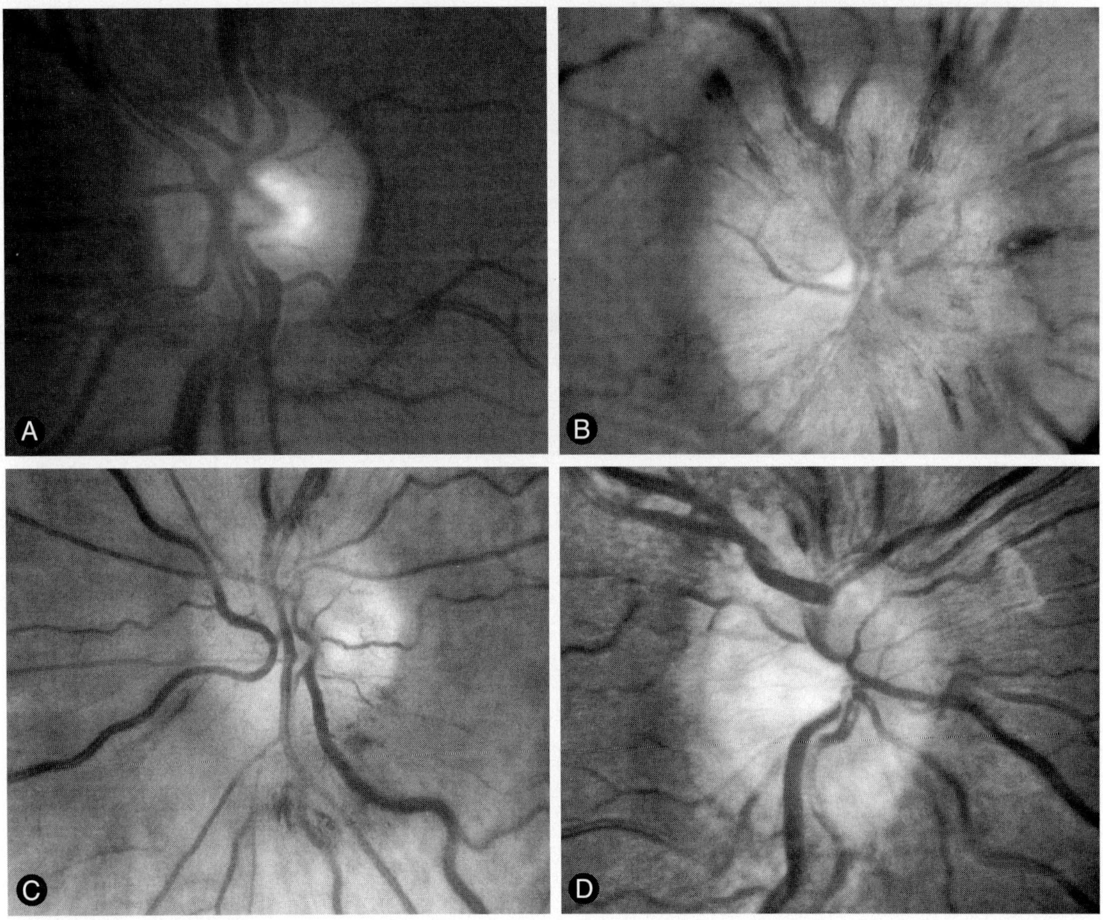

FIGURE 6–1. **A.** Normal optic disc (See Color Plate 29). Disc swelling associated with (**B**) elevated intracranial pressure (papilledema), (**C**) anterior ischemic optic neuropathy, and (**D**) optic neuritis.

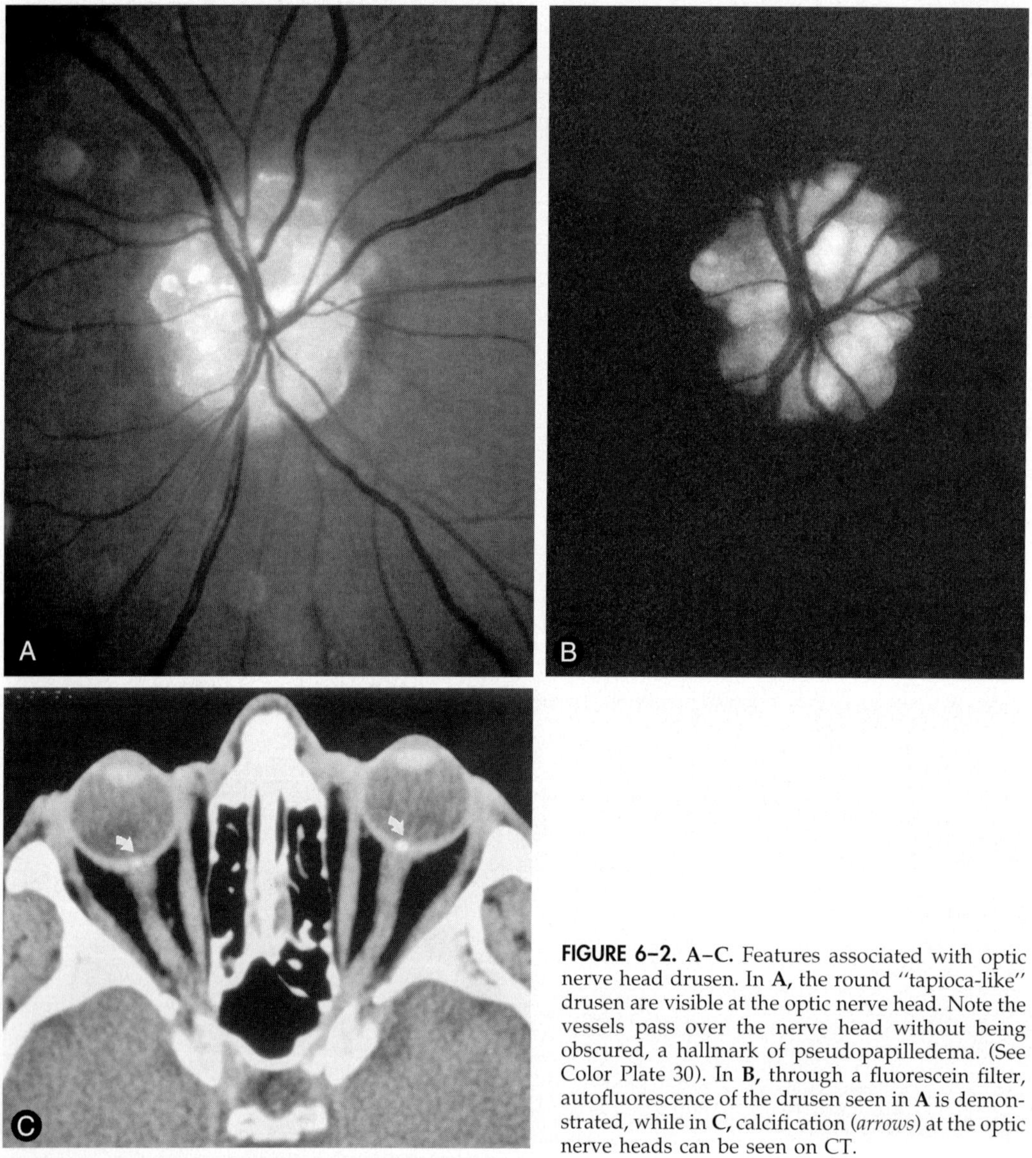

FIGURE 6–2. A–C. Features associated with optic nerve head drusen. In **A,** the round "tapioca-like" drusen are visible at the optic nerve head. Note the vessels pass over the nerve head without being obscured, a hallmark of pseudopapilledema. (See Color Plate 30). In **B,** through a fluorescein filter, autofluorescence of the drusen seen in **A** is demonstrated, while in **C,** calcification (*arrows*) at the optic nerve heads can be seen on CT.

irregular disc margins, and vessels that pass over the disc normally without being obscured by the nerve fiber layer.[6] They also tend to be less elevated without swelling of the nerve fiber layer, hemorrhages, or exudates, in contrast to discs with true disc edema. The presence of spontaneous venous pulsations favors a diagnosis of pseudopapilledema. In addition, discs with true papilledema will leak during fluorescein angiography, in contrast to those with pseudopapilledema, which tend not to leak or show only late staining.[1] Discs with pseudopapilledema often have nerve fiber-related field defects, so visual field testing cannot be used to separate pseudopapilledema from true papilledema.

Disc Drusen

Optic disc drusen (hyaline bodies) are calcium deposits within the nerve head.[7] In general, they are not visible at birth or in infancy but become more noticeable by the end of the first decade of life.[8] When on the surface of the disc, they appear as refractile, tapioca-like bodies that are easily identified ophthalmoscopically. If they are buried (between the surface and the lamina cribrosa), as they usually are in childhood, they may simply elevate the optic nerve head. Drusen are often associated with an anomalous retinal artery branching pattern, which includes a spokelike appearance secondary to trifurcations of the first-order vessels.[9, 10] The disc generally takes on a yellowish appearance.

On occasion suspected drusen can be more easily seen if the disc is retroilluminated. To perform this technique a spot or beam of light from the direct ophthalmoscope or slit lamp is focused on the nasal peripapillary retina. The disc is then observed in the darkened field next to the light. Drusen may give the disc a translucent appearance with the disc drusen highlighted.

Various types of hemorrhages can also be associated with disc drusen. The most typical is a peripapillary subretinal hemorrhage, which may ultimately cause peripapillary pigmentary disruption or hyperpigmentation. On occasion drusen-associated hemorrhages are related to a peripapillary subretinal neovascular membrane.[11]

Optic disc drusen are thought to consist of intracellular axonal debris that accumulates throughout life because of a defect in axonal metabolism.[12, 13] They are present in approximately 0.3% to 2.0% of the population, and in about two thirds of cases are bilateral.[14] Some instances are familial, inherited presumably in an autosomal dominant fashion with incomplete penetrance.[9, 324] Rarely they are associated with angioid streaks and retinitis pigmentosa,[9, 15] but there are no other established systemic associations.[7]

If optic disc drusen are suspected but cannot be definitively identified ophthalmoscopically then a diagnostic workup may confirm their presence. They may autofluoresce when photographed through a fluorescein filter (without dye injection) (Fig. 6–2).[16, 17] The most predictable way to confirm a diagnosis of disc drusen is combined A- and B-scan ultrasonography.[7, 14, 18, 325] This technique may demonstrate disc elevation secondary to highly reflective material. Computed tomography (CT) with axial sections through the nerve globe junction may also reveal calcifications secondary to drusen (Fig. 6–2).

Other Causes

Other causes of disc swelling (Fig. 6–3) that should be contrasted from papilledema include (1) central retinal vein occlusion, which is characterized additionally by dilated, tortuous veins and retinal hemorrhages; (2) ocular hypotony;[19] (3) intraocular inflammation (eg, uveitis); (4) diabetic papillopathy; (5) optic perineuritis (idiopathic or due to syphilis, for instance); (6) intrinsic optic disc tumors,[20] such as hemangiomas (in von Hippel-Lindau disease, for example), astrocytic hamartomas (in tuberous sclerosis), and optic disc gliomas; (7) Leber's hereditary optic neuropathy, (8) optic nerve infiltration by neoplasms, antibodies in plasma cell dyscrasia,[21, 326] or sarcoidosis, for instance; and (9) malignant hypertension—the associated disc swelling had been previously related to elevated cerebrospinal fluid (CSF) pressure, however, more recent experimental and clinical observations have suggested that an ischemic optic neuropathy may also be responsible.[22, 23] Disc swelling due to malignant hypertension is frequently accompanied by cotton-wool spots in the retina, and macular serous retinal detachment and lipid star formation.[24] Many of these entities are discussed in more detail in the chapters on retinal disorders and optic neuropathies (see Chapters 4 and 5).

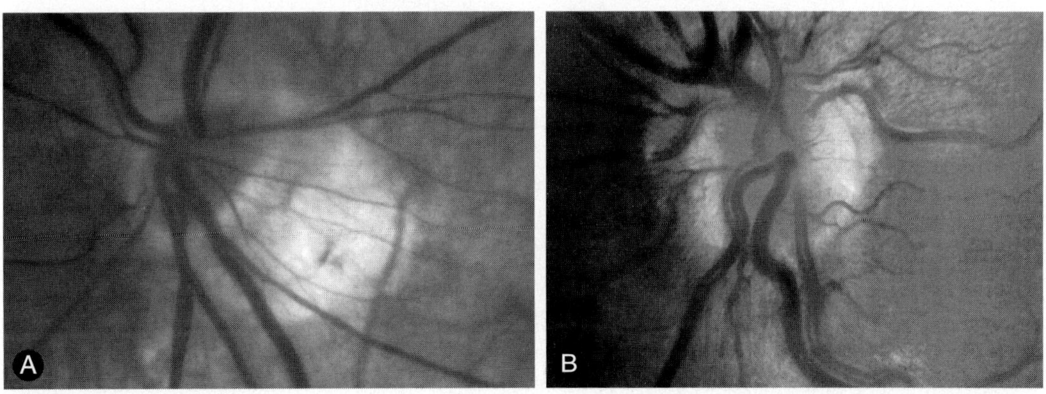

FIGURE 6–3. Other examples of pseudopapilledema include (**A**), a tilted disc, and (**B**), a congenitally small, crowded disc with anomalous vessels and absence of a central cup. (See Color Plates 31 and 32.)

FUNDUSCOPIC APPEARANCE OF PAPILLEDEMA

Mechanism

The force of elevated CSF is transmitted to tissue fluid between axons in the optic nerve head,[25] leading to axoplasmic stasis in the prelaminar portion of the optic nerve (Fig. 6–4).[26] This causes axonal swelling, which is observable ophthalmoscopically as a swollen optic disc.[27]

Early and Acute Papilledema

Early disc swelling associated with elevated intracranial pressure appears first superiorly and inferiorly, then nasally, and finally temporally (Fig. 6–5; see Color Plates 33 to 36). This pattern follows the relative thickness of the nerve fiber layer, in descending order, at different locations around the optic disc.[22] Elevation of the nerve fiber layer obscures the underlying vessels and blurs the disc margins.

Usually, the development of papilledema requires at least 1 to 5 days of persistently elevated intracranial pressure.[22] However, sudden rises in intracranial pressure, caused by an acute subarachnoid or intraparenchymal hemorrhage, for instance, occasionally may result in papilledema that develops rapidly within hours.[28] Selhorst et al[29] witnessed the development of papilledema within 1 hour in a patient with acute aneurysmal rupture. Because axoplasmic stasis could not develop so quickly, they surmised that a sudden, severe rise in intracranial pressure could force axoplasm retrogradely from the intraorbital optic nerve into the optic nerve head.

The vascular changes associated with papilledema are secondary to the nerve fiber swelling. Compression of capillaries and venules on the disc cause venous stasis and dilation, formation of microaneurysms, and disc and peripapillary radial hemorrhages. The disc becomes hyperemic because of the capillary dilation. Cotton-wool spots represent ischemic areas within the nerve fiber layer (Fig. 6–5). Compression of the central retinal vein can lead to retinal venous engorgement and tortuosity[23] and disappearance of spontaneous venous pulsations, which are pulse-related dilations and contractions of large venous branches in or overlying the disc. The best place to look for spontaneous venous pulsations is within the central cup of the disc and where the veins bend. Spontaneous venous pulsations are most evident in patients with deep and large cups. The presence of spontaneous venous pulsations implies the intracranial pressure is <180 mm H_2O at the time of viewing.[30] However, the absence of spontaneous venous pulsations does not imply elevated intracranial pressure, for as many as 10% of the normal population may not have them in either eye.[30, 31]

Grading systems for papilledema have been devised,[32] but more commonly descriptive ter-

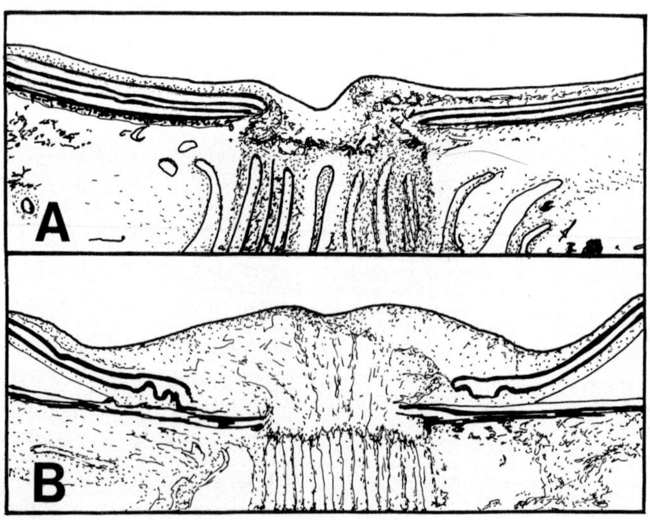

FIGURE 6–4. Drawing depicting histologic sections of normal optic nerve (**A**) and papilledema (**B**). Note the papilledema is characterized by axoplasmic stasis in the prelaminar portion of the optic nerve.

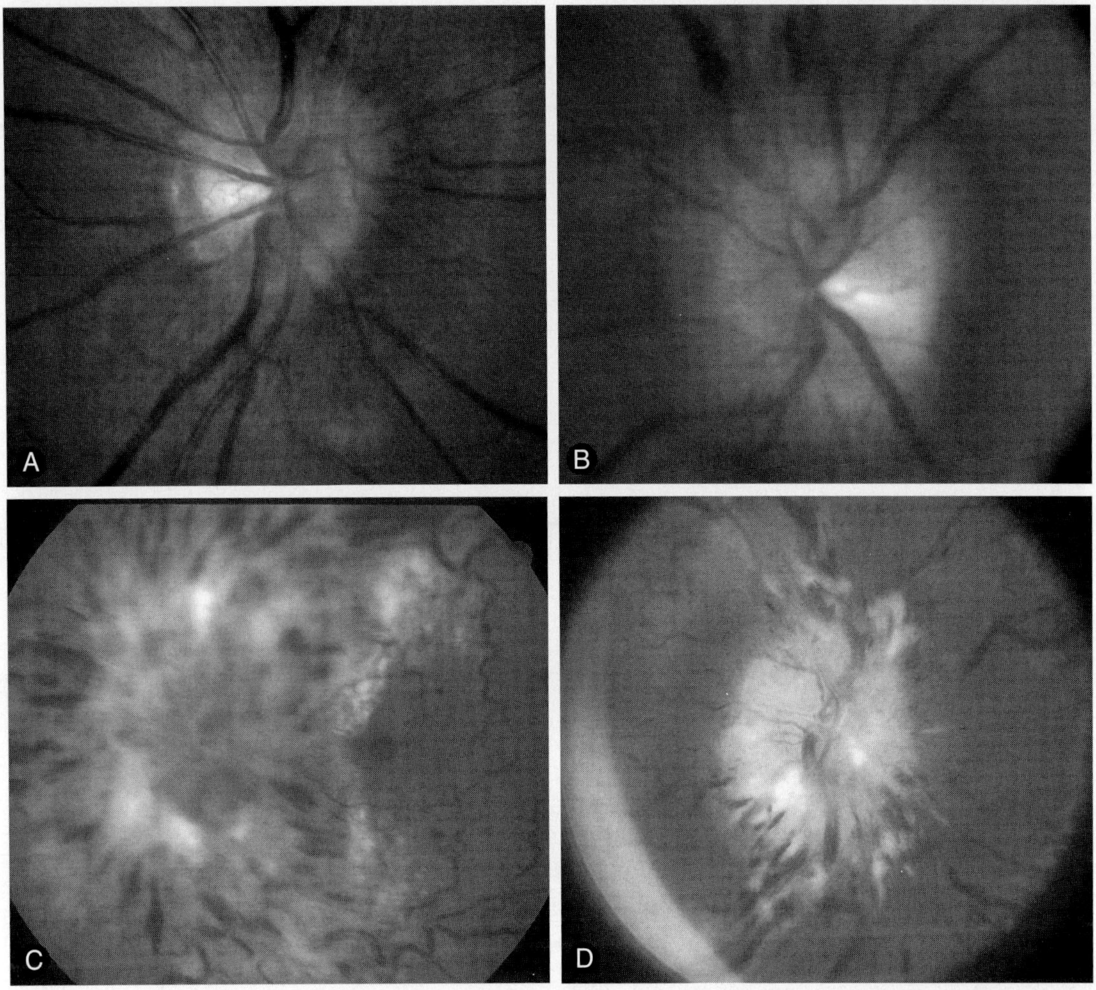

FIGURE 6–5. Various grades of early or acute papilledema. (See Color Plates 33 to 36.) In early mild papilledema of the right eye (**A**), the nerve fiber layer is slightly elevated superiorly, inferiorly, and nasally, causing mild blurring of the disc margin (horizontal lines are photographic artifact). Acute papilledema (**B**) is characterized by venous dilation, disc elevation, blurring of the disc margin, and peripapillary hemorrhages (seen superiorly in this photo). In high-grade or florid papilledema (**C**), the disc is hyperemic, the disc is so elevated that that the usual features are unrecognizable, and cotton-wool spots may indicate nerve fiber layer ischemia. Nerve fiber layer hemorrhages are also prominent. When acute papilledema is associated with multiple cotton-wool spots and disc pallor (**D**), indicative of optic nerve head ischemia, accompanying visual loss is usually moderate or severe.

minology is used.[33] The term *mild papilledema* refers to slight disc elevation with some or no peripapillary hemorrhages. *High-grade* or *florid papilledema* is characterized by severe disc elevation with cotton-wool spots, peripapillary hemorrhages, and venous engorgement (Fig. 6–5). The degree of papilledema is usually symmetric in both eyes, but asymmetric[34] and even unilateral[35–37] papilledema may occur. A subarachnoidal meshwork within the optic canal can act as an incomplete barrier to transmission of CSF pressure between the intracranial vault and anterior optic nerve.[25, 38] Anatomic differences in this meshwork may account for asymmetric papilledema as well as interpersonal variation in disc swelling with the same CSF pressure. Alternatively, Lepore[34] proposed age-related changes in the lamina cribrosa due to increased collagen and decreased elasticity might protect the optic nerve head from elevated intracranial pressure. Finally, optic atrophy (see Foster Kennedy Syndrome, below) may prevent disc swelling.

Chronic Papilledema

Table 6–2 compares the features of acute and chronic papilledema. The disc takes on a

TABLE 6–2. Funduscopic Characteristics of Acute and Chronic Papilledema

Characteristics common to both *acute* and *chronic* papilledema
Disc elevation
Venous distention and tortuosity
Obscuration of the normal disc margin and overlying retinal vessels
Absence of spontaneous venous pulsations
Characteristics typical of *acute* papilledema
Disc hyperemia
Cotton-wool spots
Peripapillary hemorrhages
Characteristics typical of *chronic* papilledema
"Champagne-cork" appearance
Overlying gliosis and extruded axoplasm (pseudodrusen)
Disc atrophy
Venous collateral vessels
Peripapillary subretinal neovascularization

"champagne-cork" appearance (Fig. 6–6; see Color Plate 37) when papilledema has been present for weeks or months. Typically, peripapillary hemorrhages are conspicuously absent. White exudates, representing extruded axoplasm, commonly overly the disc (pseudodrusen). Chronic papilledema may also be associated with venous collateral vessels (Fig. 6–7; see Color Plate 38) and peripapillary subretinal neovascularization.[39] The collateral vessels form when decreased flow through the central retinal vein causes compensatory dilation of pre-existing communications between retinal and ciliary venous circulations.[39]

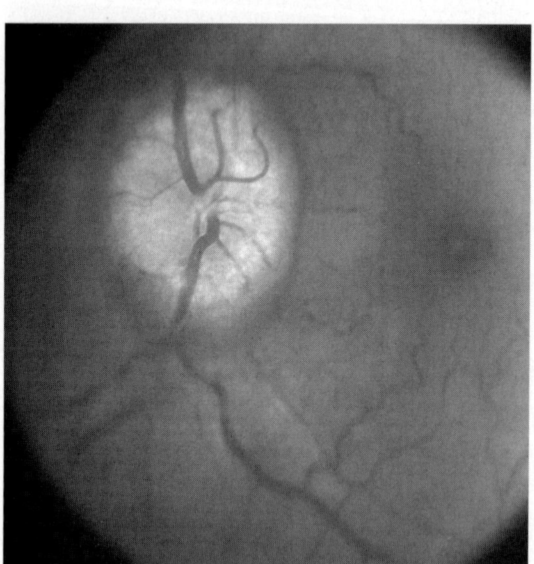

FIGURE 6–6. "Champagne-cork" appearance of chronic papilledema. The whitish, glistening areas on the optic disc head represent gliosis and extruded axoplasm. Note conspicuous absence of peripapillary hemorrhages. (See Color plate 37.)

Atrophic Papilledema

When nerve fibers die, the disc atrophies and swelling becomes pale and less prominent (Fig. 6–8; see Color Plate 39). Arterial branches, especially peripapillary, become attenuated.

Treated Papilledema

If the elevated intracranial pressure is treated prior to atrophy of nerve fibers, papilledema usually resolves completely over the ensuing weeks or months (Fig. 6–9). However, some patients are left with some residual disc elevation, especially nasally, because of gliosis (Fig. 6–10).[40]

Foster Kennedy Syndrome

Earlier this century, Foster Kennedy[41] described patients with ipsilateral disc pallor, secondary to optic nerve compression, and contralateral papilledema. Pre-existing optic atrophy precludes the development of papilledema, because there are no fibers to swell.[26] Similarly, atrophic portions of an optic nerve head cannot develop disc swelling, but intact portions can.[42] Classically, the culprit lesion in the Foster Kennedy syndrome is a subfrontal mass, typically a meningioma, which compresses the ipsilateral optic nerve, causing disc atrophy. If the lesion is large enough to cause elevated intracranial pressure, papilledema results in the contralateral eye only, owing to the ipsilateral nerve atrophy (Fig. 6–11). Bilateral optic nerve compression is another possible mechanism.[43] Nontumor causes, resulting in the pseudo-Foster Kennedy syndrome, are actually more common.[44] One example is consecutive anterior ischemic optic neuropathy, characterized by new ischemic disc swelling in one eye accompanied by long-standing disc atrophy resulting from a previous ischemic event in the other eye (see Chapter 5). Unlike the true Foster Kennedy syndrome, the eye with the disc swelling will usually have impaired visual acuity.

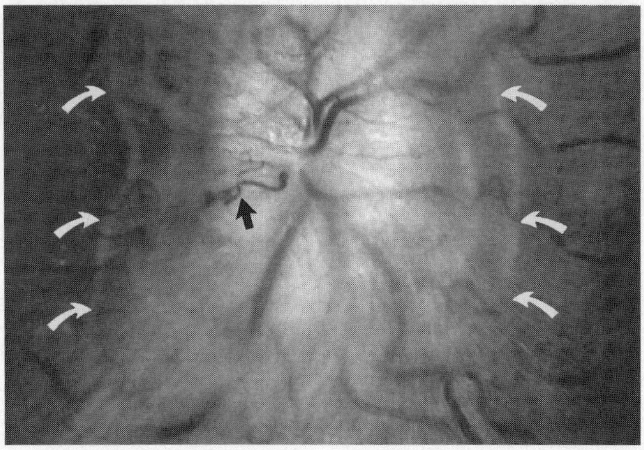

FIGURE 6–7. Peripapillary "high-water marks" (*white arrows*) indicative of previous retinal elevation associated with papilledema. Lipid exudate is visible near the white arrows on the left side of the photograph. The black arrow at 8 o'clock at the optic disc points to a venous collateral vessel. (See Color Plate 38.)

Retinal Findings Associated With Papilledema

Secondary effects on the macula are the usual causes of acute reduction in visual acuity and metamorphopsia in papilledema (Table 6–3). For instance, in severe disc swelling, fluid may extend to the macula by dissecting between the axons of the nerve fiber layer.[26, 45] Macular edema is difficult to see with a direct ophthalmoscope but is more readily visible using biomicroscopy. Retinal or choroidal folds,[46] lipid (hard exudate) stars,[47] hemorrhages,[48] and pigment epithelial and photoreceptor disturbances in the macula also may be associated with papilledema (Fig. 6–12, see Color Plates 40 to 42). Indentation of the posterior globe by a rigid optic nerve sheath is one proposed mechanism for choroidal folds in papilledema.[49] Shortening of the globe or flattening of the posterior pole may also account for the association between intracranial hypertension, papilledema, folds, and acquired hyperopia.[50, 51] Choroidal folds actually occur in Bruch's membrane.[52]

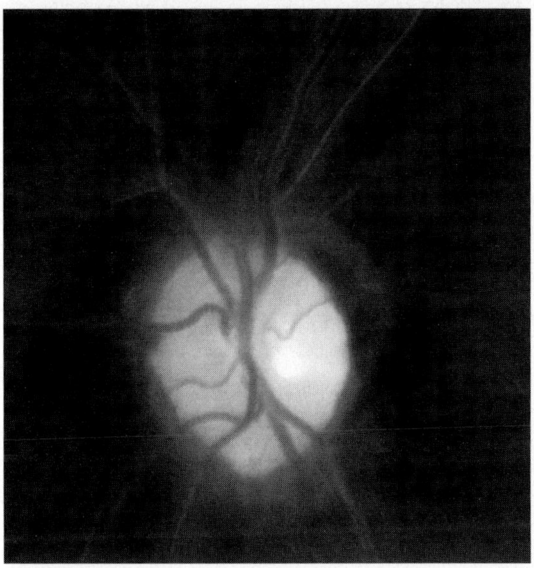

FIGURE 6–8. Chronic atrophic papilledema, characterized by disc pallor, gliosis, vessel narrowing, and resolution of disc elevation. (See Color Plate 39.)

Hemorrhages associated with papilledema are usually peripapillary and retinal (within the nerve fiber layer), but occasionally can be found more than one or two disc diameters away from the optic nerve head or in the subhyaloid and vitreous spaces.[53] Rarely, hemorrhages are due to peripapillary subretinal neovascular membranes, seen best on fluorescein angiography.[54, 55] When these membranes extend toward the fovea, photocoagulation may be indicated.[56] Venous stasis retinopathy[57] and central[58] or branch[59] retinal artery occlusion, due to compression of vascular structures in the optic nerve, are rare but have been documented.

Once the papilledema improves with the appropriate treatment, hemorrhages, folds, macular edema, and lipid stars tend to resolve as well. One may see residual macular pigment epithelial disturbances if lipid, folds, or edema had been present,[60] or circumpapillary "high-water marks" delineating the prior extent of peripapillary retinal elevation caused by disc swelling (Figs. 6–7 and 6–12C). Unfortunately, subretinal neovascular membranes and associ-

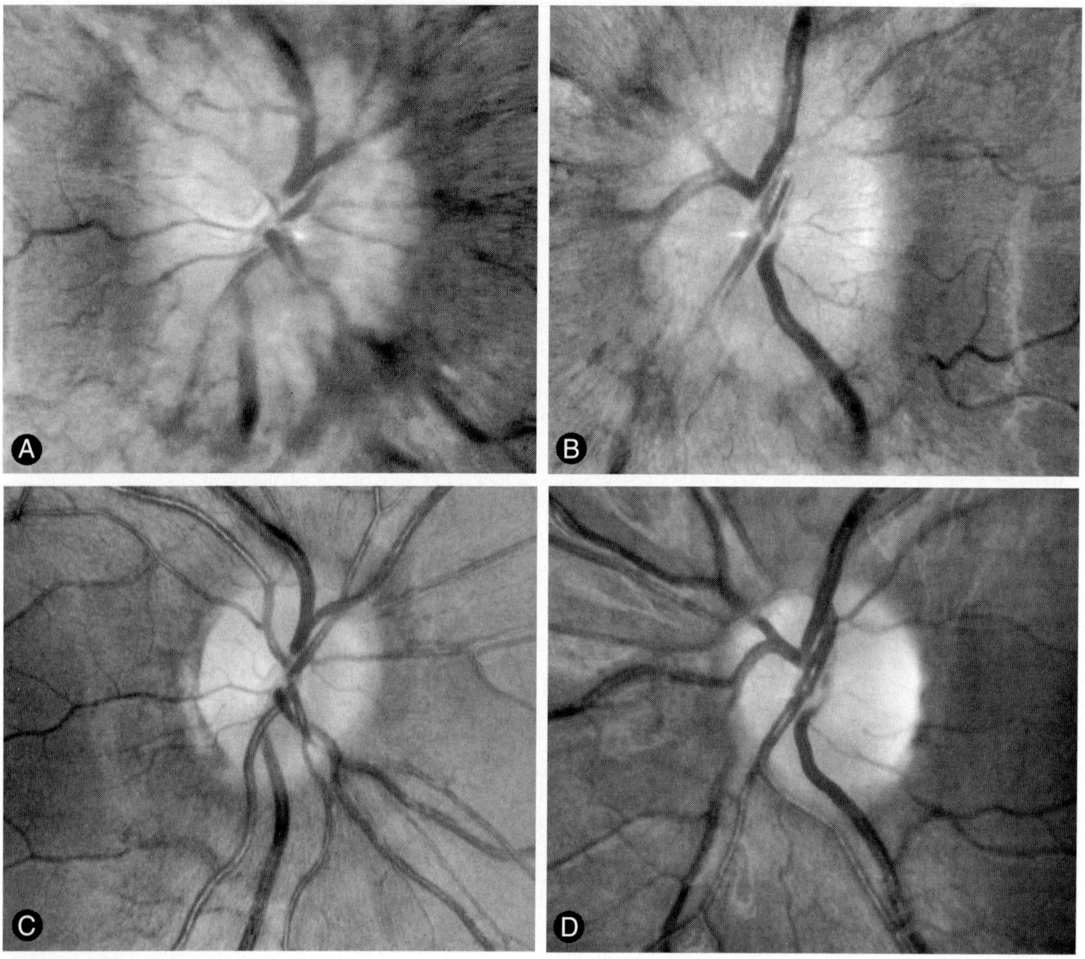

FIGURE 6–9. Papilledema associated with pseudotumor cerebri: (**A**) right eye, (**B**) left eye. Six months after medical treatment the disc swelling is completely resolved: (**C**) right eye, (**D**) left eye.

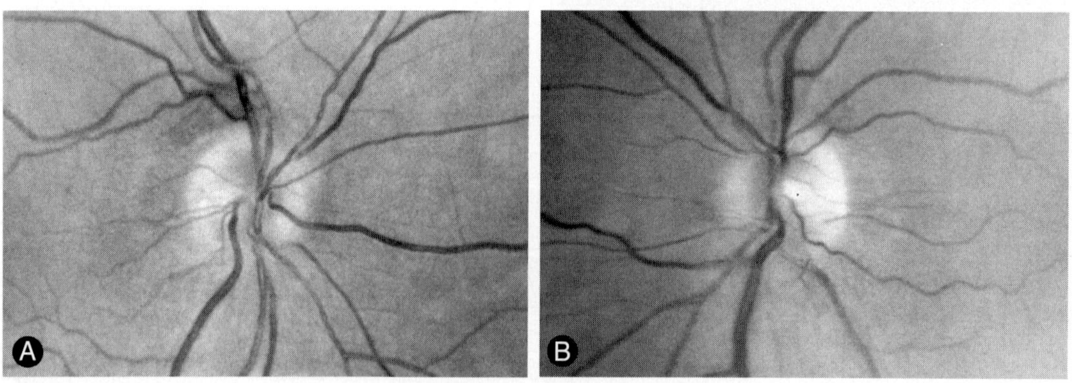

FIGURE 6–10. Resolution of papilledema with residual disc elevation associated with pseudotumor cerebri following medical and surgical therapy: (**A**) right eye, (**B**) left eye. Although the disc swelling has abated, the superior and inferior portions of both discs are still slightly elevated in a "heaped-up" fashion.

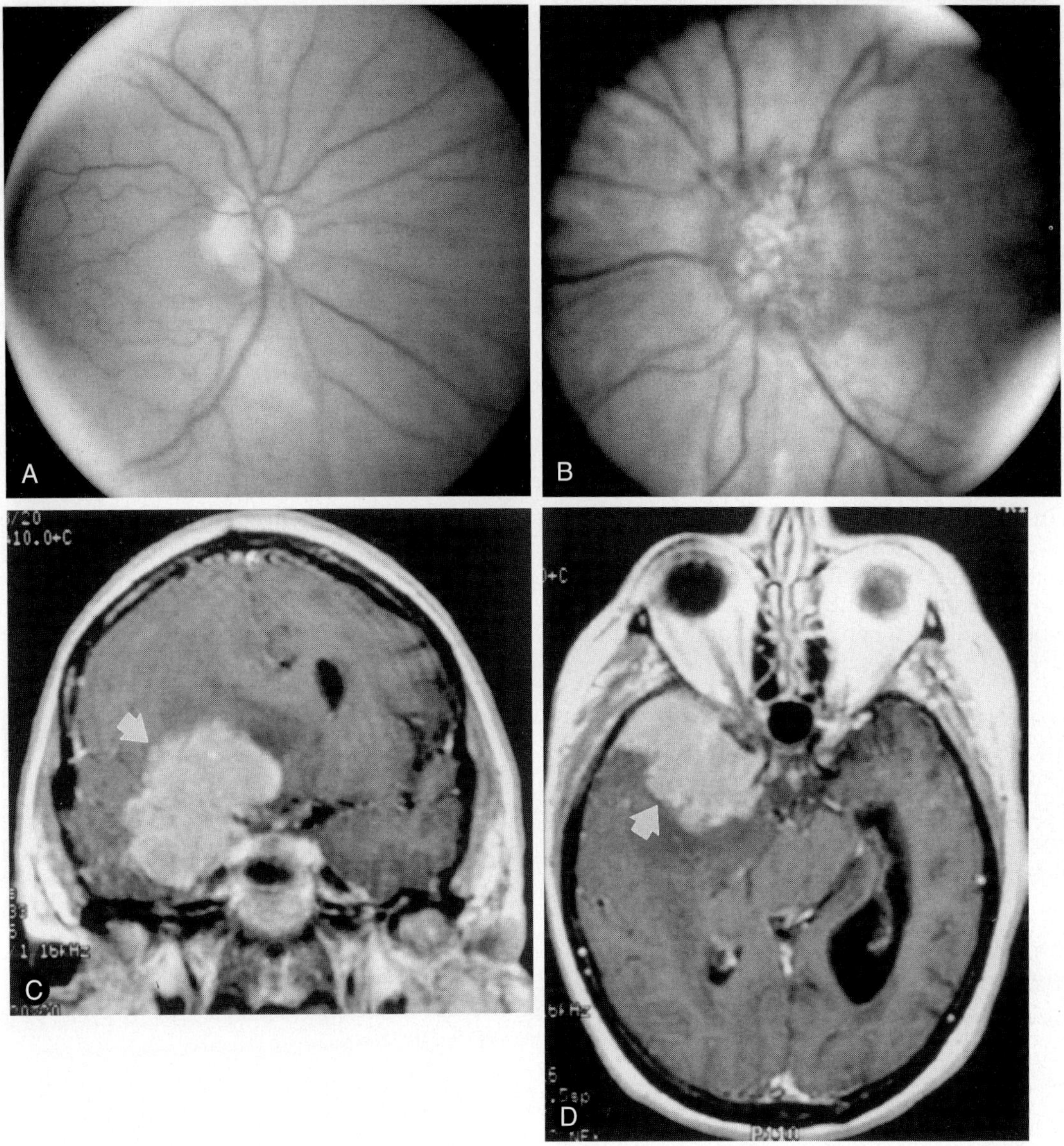

FIGURE 6–11. Foster Kennedy syndrome. This patient presented with progressive behavioral changes, headaches, and counting fingers vision in the right eye. Funduscopic examination revealed optic atrophy in the right eye (**A**) and papilledema in the left eye (**B**). Gadolinium-enhanced coronal MRI (**C**) demonstrates a large meningioma (*arrow*) compressing the right frontal and temporal lobes, right optic nerve, and third ventricle. The axial-MRI scan (**D**) shows dilation of the left lateral ventricle consistent with noncommunicating hydrocephalus.

ated subretinal hemorrhages may cause irreversible visual loss.[61]

FLUORESCEIN ANGIOGRAPHY AND ECHOGRAPHY IN PAPILLEDEMA

Hayreh[22] has detailed the typical fluorescein angiographic findings associated with papilledema. In the retinal arterial phase, fluorescence may be absent when disc swelling is severe enough to delay the prelaminar circulation. During the retinal arteriovenous phase, dilated capillaries, microaneurysms, and flame-shaped hemorrhages may be demonstrated on the surface of the disc and peripapillary retina. Fluorescein may leak from superficial dilated capillaries during the retinal

TABLE 6–3. Retinal Findings Associated with Papilledema

Common	Uncommon
Macular changes	Subretinal neovascular membrane
Edema	Venous stasis retinopathy
Lipid (hard exudate) stars	Retinal artery occlusion
Pigment epithelial disturbances	
Retinal or choroidal folds	
Hemorrhages	
Peripapillary "high-water" mark	

venous phase. During the late phase, classically there is hyperfluorescence of the superficial and deep portions of the optic disc.

In patients with papilledema, A-scan echography of the optic nerve can suggest increased subarachnoid fluid within the nerve sheath by demonstrating a reduction in nerve sheath diameter by 10% when the eye rotates laterally 30 degrees ("positive 30-degree test").[62] However, increased subarachnoid fluid is nonspecific and may be seen in optic neuritis, optic nerve trauma, and compressive optic neuropathy. Furthermore, echography is extremely operator dependent, and therefore, in general, we have not relied on its use either to diagnose or follow patients with papilledema.

VISUAL DEFICITS ASSOCIATED WITH PAPILLEDEMA AND THEIR MECHANISM

Visual loss due to papilledema is for the most part related to optic nerve head dysfunction.[63] The field deficits are similar to those in other disorders that affect the anterior optic nerve, such as glaucoma, and they do not align along the vertical meridian, as in chiasmal or retrochiasmal lesions.[64] It is less certain whether ischemia or axoplasmic stasis causes axonal

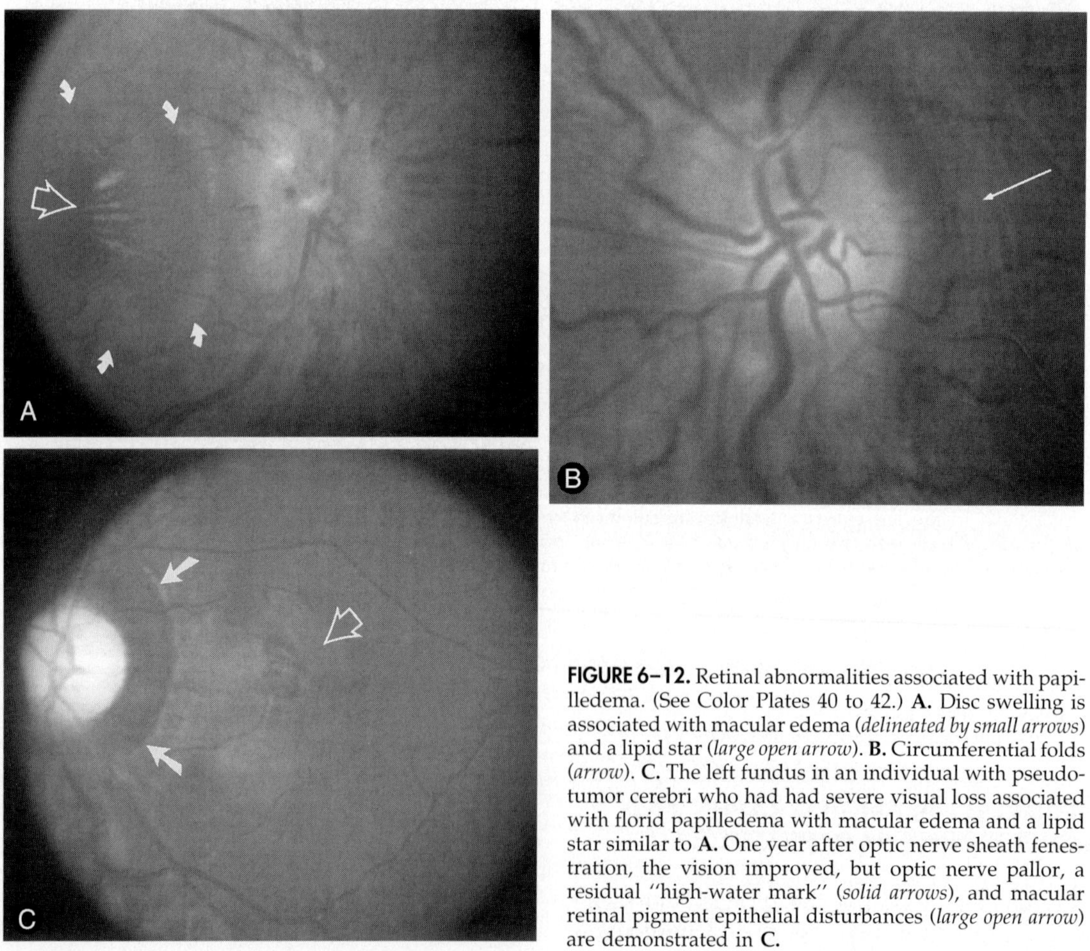

FIGURE 6–12. Retinal abnormalities associated with papilledema. (See Color Plates 40 to 42.) **A.** Disc swelling is associated with macular edema (*delineated by small arrows*) and a lipid star (*large open arrow*). **B.** Circumferential folds (*arrow*). **C.** The left fundus in an individual with pseudotumor cerebri who had had severe visual loss associated with florid papilledema with macular edema and a lipid star similar to **A.** One year after optic nerve sheath fenestration, the vision improved, but optic nerve pallor, a residual "high-water mark" (*solid arrows*), and macular retinal pigment epithelial disturbances (*large open arrow*) are demonstrated in **C.**

dysfunction. Rapid improvement in vision following optic nerve sheath decompression suggests axoplasmic stasis plays at least some part,[65] but cases with frank optic nerve ischemia have been documented as well.[66] Preexisting anemia or hypertension may be associated with more severe visual loss, perhaps by aggravating optic nerve head ischemia.[39, 67]

Blind spot enlargement is commonly associated with papilledema (Fig. 6–13). The cause is either mechanical displacement and folding of the peripapillary retina or a refractive scotoma caused by relative hyperopia due to peripapillary retinal elevation.[68] Nasal defects (especially inferiorly[69]) are also common initially, in part because the temporal arcuate bundles are densest, and hence more susceptible to axoplasmic stasis and compression.[64] Further involvement of nerve fibers leads to arcuate defects then field constriction (Fig. 6–13).[39, 70] Once sufficient nerve fiber layer loss develops, central visual acuity loss results.[39] Central visual defects and metamorphopsia in acute papilledema are uncommon, but when they occur are almost always due to retinal processes affecting the macula (see above).

Visual Field Testing[71]

Computerized threshold perimetry of the central 30 degrees of vision (stationary targets, Humphrey 30-2 program), although lengthy and tedious, in most instances is a good objective and reproducible test for patients with papilledema. Each field can be quantified using the average of all the threshold values (in decibels (dB)) for each measured area, allowing for objective, numerical comparison of serial fields. Kinetic Goldmann perimetry[72] is more appropriate for patients with significant visual loss and those who are less cooperative, such as children. However, automated perimeters are more widely available, and because of the advantages outlined above, most patients with papilledema should be tested, and if necessary, followed with serial threshold field examinations. Finger confrontation methods and tangent screen examinations are too insensitive to detect subtle visual loss.[73]

It is often difficult to correlate the severity of disc swelling with the amount of visual loss. As the papilledema becomes more chronic, nerve fibers atrophy, reducing the amount of disc swelling. Hence chronically atrophic swollen discs, likely associated with severe visual loss, tend not to be grossly elevated. However, in the acute setting it may be useful to generalize that mild disc elevation is usually associated with more minor field deficits than high-grade, florid papilledema.[39] Furthermore, at presentation, a normally shaped and colored disc without swelling should be associated with a normal visual field.

Transient Visual Obscurations

These are uni- or bilateral episodes of visual loss lasting for seconds. They can occur rarely or several times per day, and are associated with changes in posture such as standing or bending over. Likely they result from transient ischemia at the optic nerve head.[74] Transient visual obscurations do not correlate with intracranial pressure, extent of visual loss, or severity of disc edema.[75] They have also been reported in patients with other conditions causing optic nerve swelling or elevation.[74]

DIFFERENTIAL DIAGNOSIS IN PATIENTS WITH PAPILLEDEMA

Table 6–4 outlines causes of papilledema, and groups them according to frequency. A history of seizures, unilateral motor or sensory findings on examination, reflex asymmetry, or extensor plantar reflexes suggests a mass or other focal lesion. A sudden onset of severe headache, altered mentation, and neurologic deficits would be consistent with an acute intracranial hemorrhage. In a young female who is overweight or has a history or recent weight gain, and who has papilledema and a normal neurologic examination, pseudotumor cerebri is a likely possibility. Limb weakness might suggest a spinal tumor or demyelinating polyneuropathy. Hypertension should be excluded. Special considerations in children are discussed below.

EVALUATION OF THE PATIENT WITH PAPILLEDEMA

In patients with papilledema, we recommend urgent neurologic evaluation and neuroimaging (magnetic resonance imaging (MRI) or computed tomography (CT) with contrast) to rule out an intracranial mass lesion, hemorrhage, hydrocephalus, or venous thrombosis (Table 6–5). MR venography[76] should be requested as well when venous clot is suspected.

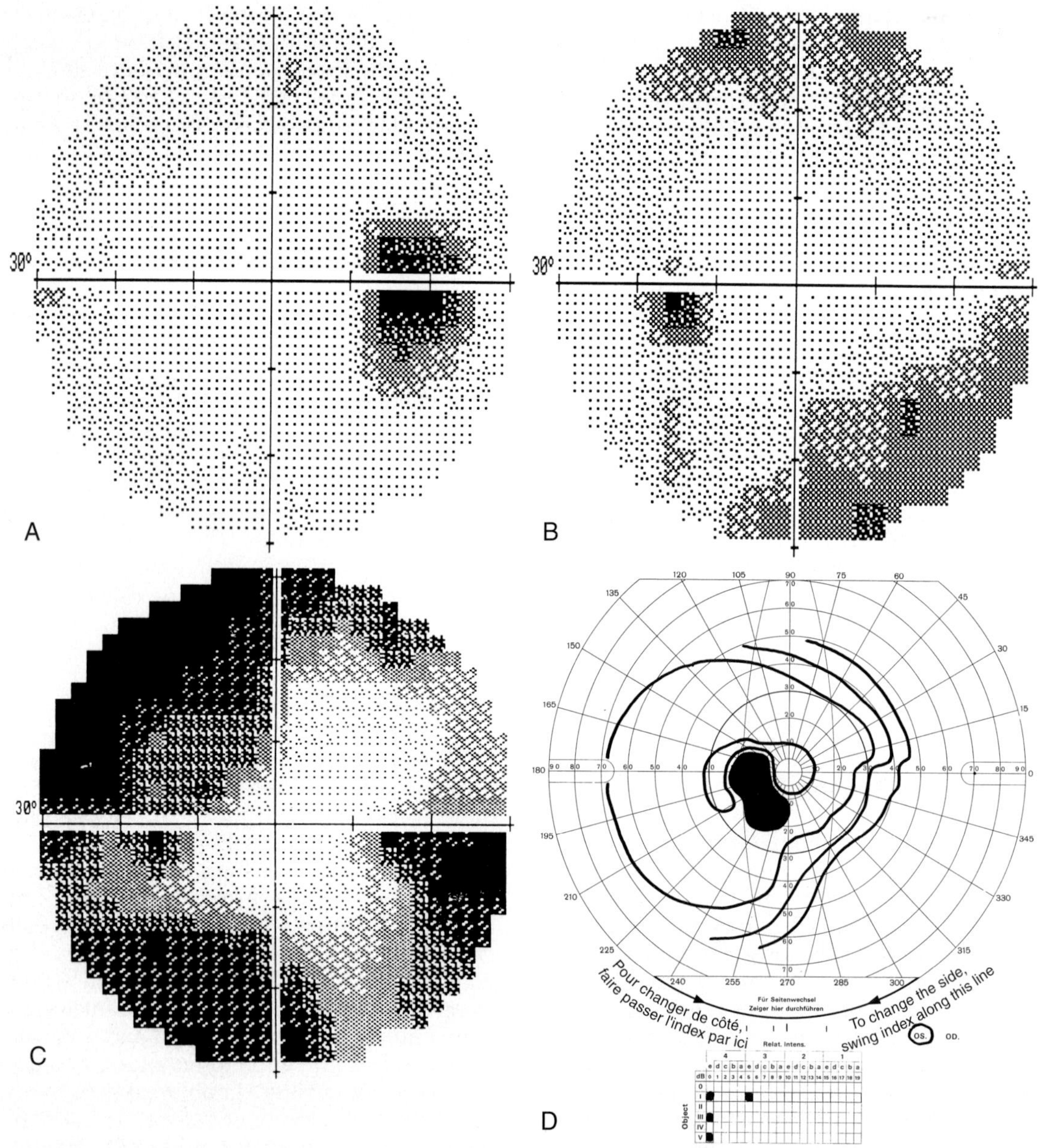

FIGURE 6–13. Examples of Humphrey (threshold) 30-2 computerized perimetry demonstrating (**A**) typical enlarged blind spot, (**B**) infranasal constriction, and (**C**) diffuse constriction due to papilledema associated with pseudotumor cerebri. The grey scale plots the central 30 degrees of vision. **D.** Goldmann (kinetic) visual field typical for visual loss associated with papilledema due to pseudotumor cerebri. Enlarged blind spot, inferior nerve fiber bundle defect, and infranasal constriction are present. (A, B, and D from Galetta SL et al. Neurol Clin 1996;14:201–222, with permission.)

MR angiography may be ordered if a dural arteriovenous malformation is considered as a possible cause of elevated intracranial pressure. If neuroimaging is normal, a lumbar puncture is necessary to rule out meningitis and to document the CSF opening pressure.[71] If neuroimaging reveals a venous thrombosis, it is still helpful to measure the opening pressure, and in these patients, as well as those with pseudotumor cerebri, the lumbar puncture often alleviates the headache. The lumbar puncture should be performed with the patient relaxed in a lateral decubitus position, with the head and spine at the same level and the neck and knees slightly flexed. Normal CSF opening pressure in an adult is <250 mm H_2O,[77] but is less in children, where the normals vary with age. CSF measurements should

TABLE 6–4. Causes of Papilledema, According to Frequency

Common	Uncommon
Intracranial mass lesion	Dural sinus arteriovenous malformation
Pseudotumor cerebri	Obstructive sleep apnea
Hydrocephalus	Guillain–Barré syndrome
Intracranial hemorrhage	Chronic inflammatory demyelinating polyneuropathy
Venous thrombosis/obstruction	Spinal cord tumors
Meningitis	Craniosynostoses
	Nonaccidental injury

also include at least those for protein, glucose, cell count and differential, Gram stain, culture, cryptococcal antigen, and India ink. Papilledema, normal neuroimaging, elevated CSF opening pressure but normal CSF constituents strongly suggests pseudotumor cerebri. CSF pleocytosis with or without elevated protein suggests meningitis. Bloody CSF or xanthochromia implies an intracranial hemorrhage, even if the neuroimaging is normal.

TABLE 6–5. Evaluation of Patients With Papilledema

I. Distinguish from other causes of disc swelling (see Table 6–1), based on clinical, funduscopic, and adjunctive laboratory features.
II. Clinical history
  - Rapidity of onset of headache and/or visual symptoms that might suggest a hemorrhage or quickly expanding mass lesion
  - Other neurologic symptoms, such as hemiparesis, sensory loss, or ataxia, to suggest a mass lesion
  - Body habitus (overweight female suggests pseudotumor cerebri)
III. Neuro-ophthalmic examination
  - Including careful visual field testing looking for field defects associated with papilledema
IV. Neurologic examination
  - Evidence of mental status abnormalities, focal neurologic abnormalities, or long tract signs suggest a mass lesion
  - Fever and stiff neck suggest meningitis
V. Neuroimaging
  - MRI or CT with contrast to exclude a mass lesion or hydrocephalus
  - MR venography, if venous sinus thrombosis suspected
VI. Lumbar puncture
  - Measurement of opening pressure when neuroimaging is unrevealing or if a venous sinus thrombosis is detected
  - CSF tests to exclude meningitis (eg, protein, glucose, cell count with differential, Gram stain, culture, cryptococcal antigen, and India ink)
  - When the clinical scenario requires the consideration of other entities: syphilis serologies, acid-fast staining, cytology for malignant cells, angiotensin converting enzyme, Lyme titers

In the emergency setting, the presence of papilledema may alter management in patients with fever, stiff neck, and altered mentation suggestive of bacterial meningitis.[78] Papilledema, indicative of elevated intracranial pressure, may reflect an abcess or hydrocephalus in these patients and a tendency to herniate. In one approach, emergent empiric intravenous (IV) antibiotics can be given, then neuroimaging performed prior to a lumbar puncture. The absence of papilledema should not be used to rule out elevated intracranial pressure.

PAPILLEDEMA IN CHILDREN

Much of the differential diagnosis of papilledema in children overlaps that of adults, but there are some special considerations in younger age groups. Of the patients seen by the neuro-ophthalmology service at the Children's Hospital of Philadelphia, by far the most common cause of papilledema is a brain neoplasm, and pseudotumor cerebri is a distant second. Other frequently seen causes are meningitis (Lyme particularly), aqueductal stenosis, venous thrombosis, craniosynostoses, and nonaccidental injury.

Papilledema may be less frequent in infants because the cranial sutures have not closed, allowing the cranial vault to expand in response to elevated intracranial pressure.[79] However, in cases where the pressure is exceedingly high or when it elevates rapidly, papilledema is still possible.[20] A bulging anterior fontanelle and enlarging head size are better indications of elevated intracranial pressure in this age group.

Craniosynostosis associated with Crouzon or Apert syndrome, for instance, refers to the premature closure of the cranial sutures. If brain growth exceeds that of the skull, elevated intracranial pressure and papilledema may result. Serial funduscopic examinations are important in the monitoring of these patients before or after craniofacial procedures.[80] The papilledema is usually chronic, and untreated cases can suffer from blindness.[81]

The most common ocular finding in nonaccidental injury (child abuse, shaken-baby syndrome, battered-child syndrome, etc[82]) is retinal hemorrhages in any layer of the retina.[83] When papilledema is seen in these cases, it usually indicates an accompanying subdural hematoma.[20] In these unfortunate instances, other evidence of nonaccidental trauma, such as ecchymoses, fractures, or burns, should be sought.[84]

MASS LESIONS

Although papilledema is an excellent sign of elevated intracranial pressure, the absence of disc swelling does not necessarily rule out an intracranial mass lesion such as a neoplasm or abcess. In a series of patients (age range 0 to 90 years) with brain tumors presenting to an emergency department,[85] only 28% had papilledema. Van Crevel[86] studied the relationship between papilledema and brain tumors, and suggested that disc swelling is less likely if the patients were older, because age-related cerebral atrophy may allow for greater tumor expansion without causing elevated intracranial pressure, and also if the tumor were located in the parietal lobe. In his study, tumor size correlated poorly with the presence of papilledema. In contrast, childhood brain tumors, which are more commonly located in the posterior fossa and frequently cause fourth-ventricular compression and noncommunicating hydrocephalus, may be more likely to present with papilledema (65% in one pediatric series[79]).

One type of cerebral neoplasm, gliomatosis cerebri, deserves particular mention, as it may mimic pseudotumor cerebri (see below). Affected patients may present initially with papilledema, elevated CSF opening pressure with normal constituents, and normal neuroimaging. However, subsequent mental status changes and neurologic deterioration are inevitable with this malignant tumor, and MRI at this point will likely demonstrate the characteristic infiltrative lesions of the cerebral hemispheres and brain stem.[87]

CEREBRAL HEMORRHAGE

Types of intracranial hemorrhages include aneurysmal or arteriovenous malformation (AVM)-related subarachnoid hemorrhage, acute subdural hematoma, and intraparenchymal hemorrhage. CT is better than MRI at identifying the presence and location of acute blood. Hemorrhagic or xanthochromic CSF can confirm a subarachnoid hemorrhage, and formal angiography should be performed when an aneurysm or AVM is suspected. MR-angiography can be used as a screening tool, but it does not have the sensitivity of conventional angiography in excluding aneurysms. Elevated intracranial pressure results from mass effect produced by a hematoma or obstructive hydrocephalus from subarachnoid blood. As discussed above, acute rises in intracranial pressure associated with intracranial hemorrhages may result in the development of papilledema within hours. However, for unclear reasons, papilledema due to subarachnoid or intraparenchymal hemorrhage occurs only in a minority, despite the presence of elevated intracranial pressure. Papilledema occurred in only 16% in one series of patients with ruptured aneurysms.[88] Therefore, normal optic nerve appearance should not be the sole criterion to exclude the presence of elevated intracranial pressure.[89]

In Terson syndrome, acute subarachnoid bleeding (more typically) or an acute subdural hematoma causes intraocular hemorrhage in the vitreous, preretinal (subhyaloid), intraretinal, or subretinal spaces (Fig. 6–14).[90] In one prospective series,[91] intraocular hemorrhages occurred in 27% of patients with subarachnoid hemorrhages, and the presence of Terson syndrome was not related to the severity of the subarachnoid hemorrhage. In another prospective study,[92, 93] ocular hemorrhages were present in 17% of patients with ruptured cerebral aneurysms. Preretinal hemorrhages usually occur between the temporal vascular arcades and can characteristically "layer out". When present, vitreous hemorrhages can prevent adequate visualization of retinal hemorrhages. Severe, sudden rises in intracranial pressure can be transmitted to the optic nerve,[94] and Garfinkel et al[91] suggested subsequent compression of both the central retinal vein and retinochoroidal anastomoses could result in an acute decrease in venous drainage from the retina and cause stasis and intraocular hemorrhage. Tracking of blood within the optic nerve sheath subarachnoid space and into the vitreous has been proposed, but similar ocular hemorrhages may be seen in patients with sudden elevations in intracranial pressure without subarachnoid hemorrhage (Fig. 6–14).

In Schultz et al's study,[90] affected eyes had visual acuities ranging from 20/20 to light perception, and the natural history was for spontaneous resorption of the blood and moderate to good spontaneous recovery of vision within 9 months. Epiretinal membranes developed commonly, but their cause was unclear. Vitrec-

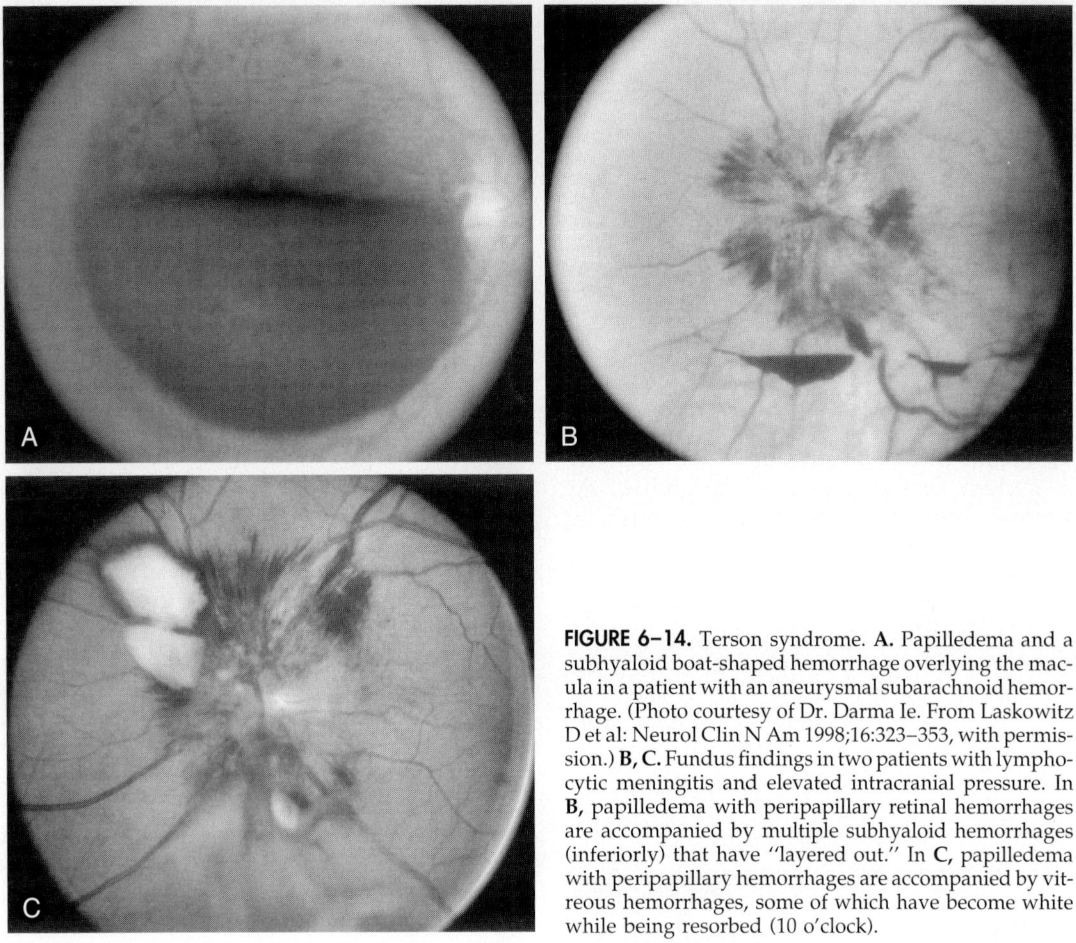

FIGURE 6–14. Terson syndrome. **A.** Papilledema and a subhyaloid boat-shaped hemorrhage overlying the macula in a patient with an aneurysmal subarachnoid hemorrhage. (Photo courtesy of Dr. Darma Ie. From Laskowitz D et al: Neurol Clin N Am 1998;16:323–353, with permission.) **B, C.** Fundus findings in two patients with lymphocytic meningitis and elevated intracranial pressure. In **B**, papilledema with peripapillary retinal hemorrhages are accompanied by multiple subhyaloid hemorrhages (inferiorly) that have "layered out." In **C**, papilledema with peripapillary hemorrhages are accompanied by vitreous hemorrhages, some of which have become white while being resorbed (10 o'clock).

tomy allowed faster recovery, but the visual prognosis was no different. Thus, vitreous surgery might be reserved for young children with immature visual systems at risk for amblyopia and adults with bilateral involvement.

TRAUMA

In one study,[29] papilledema was identified in only 3.5% of patients with acute head injury. Its presence had little correlation with the degree of elevated intracranial pressure, and its absence did not rule out increased intracranial pressure. On the other hand, papilledema is much more common (approximately 50%) in patients with chronic subdural hematomas.[29]

MENINGITIS

Patients with infectious meningitis can develop papilledema and VIth-nerve palsies associated with elevated intracranial pressure. Infectious causes include bacteria (eg, a pneumococcus), Lyme borrelia, tuberculosis,[95] and *Cryptococcus*. When basilar meningitis causes obstructive hydrocephalus, shunting is usually required.[96]

Of the patients with Lyme meningitis, papilledema and sixth nerve palsies seem more common in children affected with the disorder.[97, 98] Several authors have used the term *pseudotumor* (see below) in these cases, however, this term is inappropriate because these patients have abnormal CSF contents.[99]

Cryptococcal meningitis is notorious for causing catastrophic visual loss associated with disc swelling.[100, 101] The mechanism is either the effects of high intracranial pressure or direct invasion by the cryptococci.[102] In addition to antifungal agents,[103] acetazolamide can be used in cases with mild visual loss secondary to disc swelling.[104] However, optic nerve sheath decompression has become the treatment of choice for severe visual loss in this infection, particularly when there is elevated intracranial pressure.[105]

Papilledema due to viral or other causes of aseptic meningitis, such as chemical- or drug-induced meningitis,[106] is much less common and was seen in only 2% of patients in one series.[107] Papilledema may occur in patients with elevated intracranial pressure due to carcinomatous or sarcoid meningitis, and hydrocephalus is the usual cause in these instances.[108]

HYDROCEPHALUS

Obstructive (noncommunicating) hydrocephalus results from compression of the ventricular system or its associated foramina (eg, Monroe, Sylvian aqueduct). As outlined above, common causes include neoplasms, intraventricular or subarachnoid blood, and meningitis (Fig. 6–15). Other causes that should be considered include congenital aqueductal stenosis, myelomeningocele, and in endemic areas, cysticercosis.

In addition to treatment of the primary problem, many patients with obstructive hydrocephalus will require a shunting procedure. Papilledema, if present preoperatively, usually resolves following successful CSF diversion.[109] However, some require periodic ophthalmic or neuro-ophthalmic examinations because ocular signs may signify shunt failure even in the absence of headache, nausea, vomiting, or ventriculomegaly.[110–112] We recently treated a girl with a lumboperitoneal shunt who complained only of transient visual obscurations. Disc swelling and nerve fiber-related visual field defects had recurred, and the shunt was found to have malfunctioned.

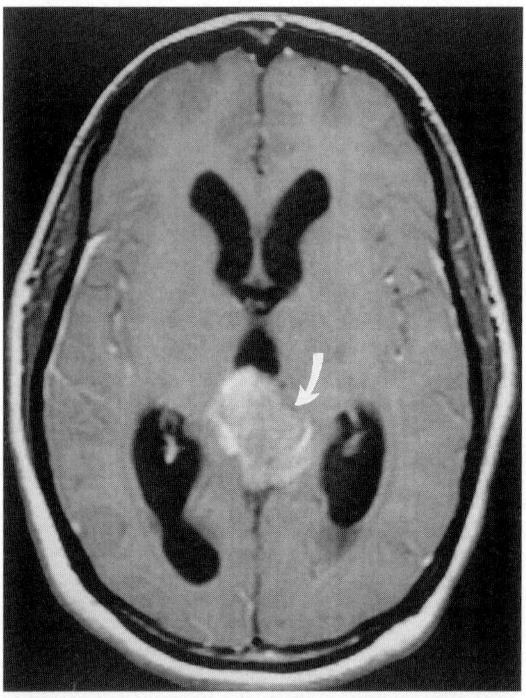

FIGURE 6–15. Noncommunicating hydrocephalus in a young woman who presented with headaches, a sixth nerve palsy, and papilledema due to a pinealblastoma (*arrow*).

A post-decompression optic neuropathy has been described, in which patients with papilledema develop acute visual loss following rapid decreases in CSF pressure due to shunting or decompressive craniotomy.[113] The postulated mechanism is hypoperfusion to the prelaminar portion of the optic nerve, and the visual prognosis is poor.[114] Fortunately, we have found this complication to be an uncommon one.

In addition, children who are shunted for hydrocephalus early in life may later develop slit-ventricle syndrome, an uncommon syndrome characterized by headaches and subnormal ventricular sizes.[115] Some of the patients we have followed for this condition developed elevated intracranial pressure and papilledema, in part due to skull noncompliance, despite normal shunt function. Treatment in these cases consisted of either acetazolamide or neurosurgical cranial vault expansion. In another subset of patients, the ventricles are normal or subnormal in size during asymptomatic periods, but when symptomatic with headaches, mild ventriculomegaly is evident. Intermittent proximal shunt malfunction is the cause in these cases, and these individuals respond to proximal shunt revision.[116]

PSEUDOTUMOR CEREBRI (IDIOPATHIC INTRACRANIAL HYPERTENSION)

Features common to all patients with pseudotumor cerebri are elevated intracranial pressure measured during a lumbar puncture, normal spinal fluid constituents, and neuroimaging that excludes a mass lesion or vascular abnormality. The diagnosis is formally established when the modified Dandy criteria[75, 117] are satisfied (Table 6–6). The greatest morbidity of the disorder is visual loss related to optic disc swelling.

TABLE 6–6. Modified Dandy Criteria for the Diagnosis of Pseudotumor Cerebri

1. Signs and symptoms of increased intracranial pressure (headache, nausea, vomiting, transient obscurations of vision, papilledema)
2. Normal neurologic exam, except for a VIth-nerve paresis
3. Elevated CSF pressure (>250 mm H_2O) with normal constituents
4. Modern neuroimaging (CT, with and without contrast, or MRI) demonstrating normal to small symmetric ventricles and excluding a mass lesion or other cause of raised intracranial pressure

Historically, another term used for this disorder was *otitic hydrocephalus,* because many cases in the preantibiotic era were associated with mastoiditis and venous thrombosis (see below). Foley[118] coined the term *benign intracranial hypertension,* which was also advocated by Weisberg[119] and even used by more recent authors.[120–122] This designation should be eschewed, however, because the condition may be associated with severe debilitating visual loss in as many as 25% of patients,[67, 123] and therefore it is not always "benign." Experts today advocate the use of the more accurate term *idiopathic intracranial hypertension.*[75, 124] However, we have found *pseudotumor cerebri* or *pseudotumor* more descriptive and easier for patients (and many physicians) to remember. Furthermore, the term *pseudotumor cerebri* is applicable in situations in which a cause is identified (ie, not idiopathic).

Demographics

In cases that are idiopathic, the patients are almost uniformly females in early adulthood and are overweight or have a history of recent weight gain. In three large series, approximately 90% were women and the mean age was 27.8 to 32.9 years.[67, 75, 125] The approximate annual incidence of pseudotumor cerebri is 0.9 to 1.7/100,000 in the general population.[126-128] However, among females 15 to 44 years of age, the incidence is 3.3 to 12.0/100,000, and among obese females in this age group, the incidence climbs to 7.9 to 21.4/100,000.[126–128] Case-control studies[125, 129] confirm that obesity and recent weight gain are more common among patients with pseudotumor cerebri than among controls. It is uncertain whether there is a racial predilection for this disorder, as the racial distribution in each reported series reflects the makeup of the local population. When men develop pseudotumor cerebri, they tend to be in a similar age distribution as affected women, they are also usually obese, and their signs and symptoms are no different than in women.[130] However, when pseudotumor cerebri in a man is suspected, the treating physician should be overly meticulous in excluding other possible causes (see below).

Although pseudotumor cerebri occurs more frequently in adults, its occurrence in pediatric patients, even infants and young children, is not uncommon.[131] Several large series have been reported,[132–142] and in contrast to the female predominance among adults, males comprise 39% to 53% of pediatric patients with pseudotumor cerebri. Affected adolescents tend to be overweight, but obesity and weight gain are not associated risk factors in patients under 11 years of age.[142] Unfortunately, children are not immune from the severe visual loss that may affect adults.[123, 133]

Associated Conditions

Table 6–7, adapted from Wall,[75] lists the conditions and drugs that are associated (purported or otherwise) with pseudotumor cerebri. The literature is replete with several disease and drug associations, but many cases must be reviewed skeptically because they fail to satisfy the modified Dandy criteria. For instance, steroid withdrawal (not steroid use) is a well-recognized, but infrequently well-documented, risk factor,[143] most commonly occurring in children on chronic corticosteroid therapy for respiratory, renal, or dermatologic disorders.[123, 136, 144] Several authors incorrectly diagnosed pseudotumor cerebri, as their patients had abnormal neurologic findings, including decreased mental status, ataxia, hemiparesis, third nerve palsy, asymmetric reflexes, and extensor plantar responses.[134, 145–147] Other reported patients lacked either CSF examinations or adequate neuroradiologic studies.[137, 148–150]

Pregnancy, menstrual irregularities, antibiotic and oral contraceptive use, and iron-deficiency anemia[151–154] have been purported risk factors, but case-control studies found their incidences to be similar among patients with pseudotumor cerebri compared with controls.[125, 129] Digre et al[155] compared pregnant patients with pseudotumor cerebri and those without, and they found that those with pseudotumor tended to be obese.

TABLE 6–7. Conditions and Drugs Associated With Pseudotumor Cerebri

Highly Likely

Decreased flow through arachnoid granulations
- Scarring from previous inflammation (eg, meningitis, sequel to subarachnoid hemorrhage)

Obstruction to venous drainage
- Venous sinus thrombosis
  - Hypercoaguable states (eg, Behçet's, ?systemic lupus erythematosus, protein C or S deficiency, antithrombin III deficiency, factor V deficiency, antiphospholipid antibody syndrome, oral contraceptive use, pregnancy, cancer, thrombocytosis, L-asparaginase, paroxysmal nocturnal hemoglobinuria)
  - Continguous infection (eg, middle-ear or mastoid—"otitic hydrocephalus")
  - Tumor related
  - Head trauma
- Bilateral radical neck dissection
- Superior vena cava syndrome
- Increased right heart pressure
- Glomus jugulare tumors

Endocrine disorders
- Addison's disease[309]
- Hypoparathyroidism
- Obesity
- Steroid withdrawal

Nutritional disorders
- Hypervitaminosis A (vitamin, liver, or isotretinoin intake)
- Hyperalimentation in deprivation dwarfism

Arteriovenous malformations
Synthetic growth hormone replacement[121, 310–313]
Tetracycline use

Probable Causes

Anabolic steroids (may cause venous sinus thrombosis)
Chlordecone (kepone)
Ketoprofen or indomethacin in Bartter syndrome
Thyroid replacement therapy in hypothyroid children[314]
Uremia

Possible Causes

Amiodarone
Diphenylhydantoin
Iron-deficiency anemia
Lithium carbonate
Nalidixic acid
Sarcoidosis
Sulfa antibiotics

Causes Frequently Cited That Are Unproven

Corticosteroid intake
Hyperthyroidism
Hypovitaminosis A[315]
Menarche
Menstrual irregularities
Multivitamin intake
Oral contraceptive use
Pregnancy

Causes Recently Cited, But Unproven

Acquired immunodeficiency syndrome (AIDS)[122, 316, 317]
Frontal sinus infection[318]
Trans-retinoic acid[319–323]
Renal transplant[329]

Cases meet the modified Dandy criteria except that a cause is found.
Adapted from Wall M: Idiopathic intracranial hypertension. Neurol Clin 1991;9:73–95, with permission.

Table 6–7 lists tetracycline as a probable risk factor, as the evidence regarding its role in pseudotumor cerebri is mounting.[327] Gardner et al[156] reviewed the literature regarding the relationship between pseudotumor and tetracycline, and its synthetic relative, minocycline. A true association was suggested in many affected patients who improved following removal of the drug and in those who experienced recurrence when the medication was restarted. The authors also suggested a combination of other factors, including genetic susceptibility. A retrospective study made similar conclusions.[157] Patients with acne often use tetracycline and vitamin A or an analog, isotretinoin, and this combination may increase the risk for pseudotumor cerebri.[158] One study[328] found serum vitamin A concentration was elevated in patients with pseudotumor cerebri.

Venous thromboses, vascular malformations, and arteriovenous fistulas are discussed in more detail in subsequent sections.

Underlying conditions that may predispose to a worse visual outcome include older age, high myopia, anemia,[39] hypertension,[67] and uremia.[159]

Mechanism

The cause of pseudotumor cerebri is unclear, but any explanation must account for elevated intracranial pressure with normal neuroimaging (without hydrocephalus), CSF constituents, and neurologic examinations. *Decreased CSF absorption by the arachnoid villi* is the most likely explanation suggested by radioisotope cisternography and other observations.[160–163] However, it is possible that decreased CSF absorption is a secondary phenomenon, resulting from compression of the arachnoid villi by elevated intracranial pressure from any cause.[164] Abnormal CSF pressure gradients caused by *increased intracranial venous pressure* may also account for decreased absorption.[120] King et al[165] performed cerebral venography and manometry in patients with pseudotumor cerebri, and they found consistently elevated venous pressures due in many cases to mural thrombi within the lateral transverse sinuses. Karahalios et al,[166] also using venography in patients with pseudotumor cerebri, discovered that in those with normal dural venous anatomy, right atrial pressures were elevated and transmitted up to the intracranial venous sinuses. They suggested elevated venous pressure as a universal mechanism for pseudotumor cerebri, even in patients without demonstrable venous outflow obstruction. *Elevated intra-abdominal pressure* secondary to obesity may increase pleural pressure and cardiac filling pressure, thereby leading to increased intracranial venous pressure and elevated intracranial pressure.[167]

Elevated brain volume secondary to cerebral edema or increased cerebral blood volume also has been proposed,[168–170] but the histologic evidence is less supportive. Sahs and Joynt,[171] reporting on brain biopsy results following subtemporal decompression, found intracellular and extracellular edema in several patients. Studies using MRI of brain water self-diffusion also suggested that increased water mobility caused interstitial and intracellular fluid accumulation.[172, 173] However, Greer found one autopsied brain and two brain biopsies to be normal.[174] Recent pathologic studies by Wall et al[175] failed to reveal cerebral edema in two patients, although the autopsies were performed 1 to 2.5 years after presentation. Wall et al[175] also reviewed three of the biopsies reported by Sahs and Joynt,[171] and the authors found no convincing evidence of cerebral edema. An *increased rate of CSF formation* is also unlikely,[176, 177] as choroid plexus papillomas tend to cause hydrocephalus.

The association between pseudotumor cerebri and female gender and obesity suggests an *endocrine basis* for the disorder.[174] Reports of pseudotumor cerebri occurring in corticosteroid-deficient states such as Addison's disease[178, 179] and adrenocorticotropic hormone (ACTH) deficiency,[156] and following removal of an ACTH-secreting pituitary adenoma,[180, 181] imply an abnormality in the adrenal–pituitary axis. Furthermore, corticosteroids in many instances effectively treat pseudotumor cerebri,[75] and corticosteroid withdrawal is associated with pseudotumor cerebri,[143] suggesting that corticosteroids have an effect on CSF dynamics. In addition, one study[182] suggested that patients with pseudotumor cerebri and orthostatic edema may have elevated vasopressin levels, leading to fluid retention. However, Soelberg Sørensen et al[183] screened a series of patients with pseudotumor cerebri and found no consistent abnormality in pituitary, gonadal, thyroid, or adrenal function.

In summary, the mechanism is likely to be decreased CSF absorption due either to dysfunction at the level of the arachnoid villi or to elevated intracranial venous pressures. The association of pseudotumor cerebri and so many other conditions suggests that these purported mechanisms may be the final common pathway, but the inciting factors may be multiple.

Presenting Signs and Symptoms

The frequency of presenting symptoms is likely underestimated in the various retrospective series,[39, 67, 118, 119, 184, 185] and the best data come from a prospective study by Wall and George.[64] Headache was the most common complaint, occurring in 94% of patients in their study. Many had related neck stiffness or retrobulbar pain, the latter sometimes exacerbated by eye movements. Seventy-two percent reported transient visual obscurations (TVOs). Photopsias (54%), diplopia (38%), and visual loss (26%) were less frequent ophthalmic complaints. Sixty percent of patients complained of a pulsatile intracranial noise, characterized either by tinnitus or a "whooshing." The bruit sounds are usually subjective (internal), but they occasionally can be auscultated or externally audible.[186] The cause of the noise is likely transmission of systolic pulsations of high-pressure CSF against the exposed walls of the dural venous sinuses, leading to turbulent blood flow through the venous sinuses.[187] Mentation and level of alertness were normal in all patients. There have also been reports of patients presenting with gaze-evoked amaurosis (see Chapter 9).[188]

Eye movement abnormalities other than abducens palsies are unusual, but third[189] and fourth nerve dysfunction,[190] internuclear ophthalmoplegia, and bilateral ophthalmoplegia[191] have been reported. Seventh nerve dysfunction is also commonly recognized.[192–194] Selky et al[195] hypothesized that facial palsies associated with elevated intracranial pressure resulted from brain stem shifts leading to stretching and compression of the extra-axial facial nerve in the bony facial canal. Cases with hemifacial spasm have also been reported.[196, 197] Technically, such patients with ophthalmoplegia and cranial nerve dysfunction other than abducens palsies do not satisfy the modified Dandy criteria, but in well-documented cases no other cause for the elevated intracranial pressure could be found.[191]

Round and Keane[198] reviewed the "minor" symptoms of elevated intracranial pressure in their patients with pseudotumor cerebri. Neck stiffness, distal extremity paresthesias, and low back pain were not uncommon. They hypothesized that these symptoms were related to nerve root irritation or spinal root pouch enlargement. Joint pain of unclear cause was another complaint described.

Neuro-ophthalmic Findings

Visual Loss. When it occurs, visual loss is typically insidious, and most patients are unaware of minor deficits because central vision is usually spared. Severe loss of visual acuity in pseudotumor cerebri is unusual[65] except when the papilledema is chronic or when there is retinal involvement,[199] such as a neurosensory retinal detachment, macular lipid exudate, or hemorrhage.[48] Most likely, the extent of visual loss does not correlate with the frequency of TVOs,[64] but conflicting opinions exist.[39] Sudden visual loss can occur although oftentimes it seems to be the result of sudden awareness, or rarely from acute optic nerve ischemia[66] or retinal artery occlusion.[55, 58, 59]

Visual field testing[71] is the most sensitive method for detecting visual loss in these patients, and the most common abnormalities are blind spot enlargement, generalized constriction of isopters, and inferior nasal field loss (see Fig. 6–13).[75] Because of reasons outlined above, we prefer to test and follow patients with computerized threshold visual fields, which tend to be more objective and reproducible. In Wall and George's prospective study,[64] 96% of patients had some abnormality detected on Goldmann perimetry, while 92% had deficits on computerized testing. As a cautionary note, we have encountered many patients with pseudotumor cerebri who have had a component of functional visual loss. In these individuals, tangent screen visual field examination may be necessary to document nonphysiologic field constriction.

Visual acuity, color vision, and pupillary reactivity are typically normal in these patients, and about one-half have abnormal contrast sensitivity,[64] in contrast to the higher incidence of visual field deficits. Sixth nerve palsies occur also in just a minority (approximately one fifth).[64] Therefore, these parameters are thought to be insensitive measures of alteration in visual function when compared to visual field testing.[75] The latency of visual evoked potentials (VEPs) were found to be correlated with CSF opening pressure by one group of investigators,[200] but others[201] found most VEPs to be normal despite the presence of visual field deficits and abnormal contrast sensitivity. Most experts, therefore, discourage using VEPs to monitor patients with pseudotumor cerebri.[75]

We do not routinely test contrast sensitivity in all patients, but some authors[202] have advocated their use. Experimental perimetric strategies[203, 204] have been investigated, but have yet to become standard practice.

Papilledema. Papilledema is uniformly present, can be asymmetric, and in uncommon instances is unilateral.[34, 35] In asymmetric cases, the vision loss is usually worse in the eye with the more severe swelling.[205] Pseudotumor cerebri without papilledema has also been reported.[206–208] The diagnosis in this last group of patients is suggested by chronic daily headache, pulsatile tinnitus, obesity, and female sex,[209] and is confirmed by lumbar puncture.

Neuroimaging.[71] Although either is acceptable, MRI of the brain without gadolinium is preferred over CT with contrast to exclude hydrocephalus or any cause of elevated intracranial pressure such as a mass lesion, venous sinus thrombosis, or dural arteriovenous malformation. Common radiographic findings in pseudotumor cerebri include an empty sella, dilation of the optic nerve sheaths,[210] and elevation of the optic disc (Fig. 6–16).[211] Occasionally on MR images the swollen optic disc will enhance.[212, 213] The empty sella is thought to result from chronically elevated intracranial pressure associated with a congenitally incompetent diaphragma sella.[214, 215] Many patients will have "slitlike" ventricles,[216] but in at least two more recent studies,[211, 217] age-matched controls had similar ventricular sizes. Some studies[218] have suggested sulci effacement on CT is a helpful radiologic sign, but we have found this to be an inconsistent feature.

Others[165, 166] have employed venography in the workup of their patients with pseudotumor cerebri. Because of the risks of the procedure, we have not done so. We prefer to use less invasive, albeit less sensitive, MR-venograms in addition to regular MR sequences as a better screen for patients suspected of having a venous sinus thrombosis (see below). Such individuals might include thin females or those with mastoiditis, for instance.

Cerebrospinal Fluid.[71] Following normal neuroimaging, a lumbar puncture is necessary to rule out meningitis, for example, and to document the CSF opening pressure. When bedside

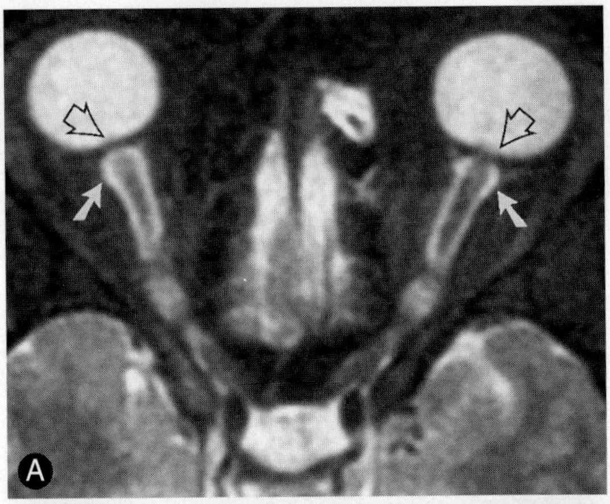

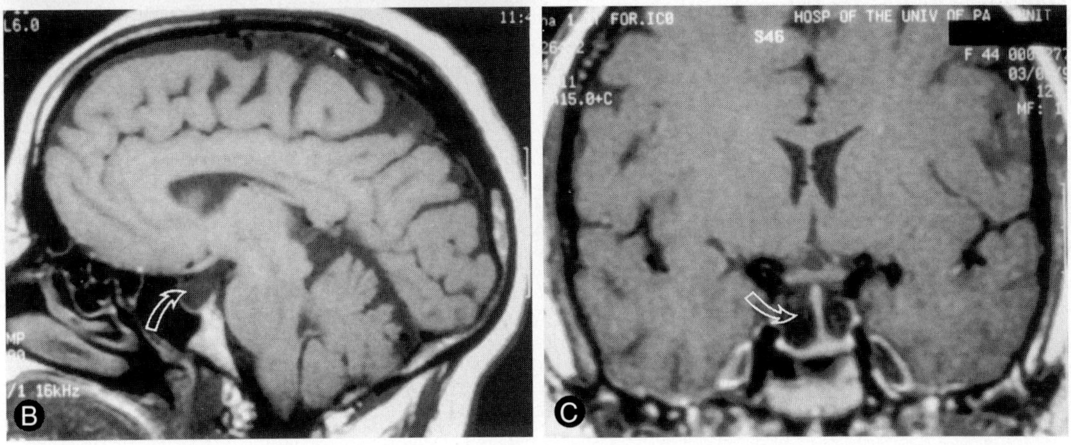

FIGURE 6–16. MRI findings associated with pseudotumor cerebri. **A.** Dilated optic nerve sheaths (*white arrows*) and indentation of the globes posteriorly (*open black arrows*) are seen (fat saturation). Empty sella (*open white arrow*) is demonstrated in (**B**) sagittal and (**C**) coronal T_1-weighted images.

lumbar punctures are difficult due to patient obesity, fluoroscopically guided lumbar punctures may be necessary. Lumbar punctures should not be performed in patients with low-lying cerebellar tonsils, because of the risk of fatal herniation.[219]

To establish the diagnosis of pseudotumor cerebri, the CSF opening pressure should exceed 250 mm H_2O, the upper limit of normal for most obese and nonobese adults.[77] Approximately 20 to 30 cc of CSF can be removed although the optimal amount has not been studied. It is not necessary to measure the closing pressure. In suspected cases with a normal CSF opening pressure, monitoring for 1 hour with an epidural transducer or subarachnoid bolt may be considered,[164] but this is rarely done in clinical practice. The cell count and glucose level should be normal, and the protein level normal or low. One study[220] found an inverse relationship between CSF opening pressure and CSF protein, while another[221] refuted this and documented CSF protein <20 mg/dl in only 26% of patients. Many patients will enjoy relief of their headache after the first lumbar puncture. Serial lumbar punctures, either to withdraw more fluid or to follow the CSF pressures, have limited role in the management of this disorder (see below).[222]

Other Imaging Modalities. Some authors have advocated the use of ultrasonography of the optic nerve[223] in the diagnosis of pseudotumor cerebri and confocal scanning laser tomography of the optic disc[224, 225] in the quantification of disc swelling and follow-up of patients with this disorder. However, we have not found these modalities to add to the clinical examination, funduscopy, neuroimaging, and CSF examination.

Management

While the diagnosis requires a neurologist, the management of patients with pseudotumor cerebri also requires the skills of an ophthalmologist or neuro-ophthalmologist.[124] The initial evaluation of a patient with suspected pseudotumor cerebri should include complete ophthalmic and neurologic examinations and computerized visual field testing. The MRI and lumbar puncture, in that order, should then be performed. Follow-up examinations should include visual fields, visual acuity, color vision, pupillary reactivity, ocular motility and alignment, and fundus appearance. Patients should be followed either weekly or biweekly initially, then, if vision stabilizes or improves, the intervals between examinations can be lengthened. To monitor disc swelling, stereo fundus photographs should be taken at presentation, then again once the papilledema resolves. The latter serves as future reference should the patient's symptoms recur. All nonpregnant obese patients are strongly encouraged to lose weight, and often they are referred to a nutritionist. Improvement in pseudotumor cerebri has been documented anecdotally following a rice/reduction diet[226] and gastric bypass surgery[227] and in retrospective studies.[228, 229] Potentially inciting risk factors, such as systemic lupus erythematosus and Addison's disease, should be treated, and offending medications, such as tetracycline and vitamin A, should be discontinued.

Treatment modalities that are no longer routinely recommended include subtemporal decompression, chronic corticosteroids, and serial lumbar punctures. The role of subtemporal or suboccipital cranial decompression (removing part of the skull to relieve elevated intracranial pressure), a treatment that causes severe side effects such as subdural hematomas and seizures, is mostly of historical interest.[230, 231] Chronic steroid treatment is complicated by elevated intraocular pressures, weight gain, and difficulty weaning off the medication.[67]

Following intracranial pressures with repeated lumbar punctures is unnecessary, impractical, invasive, and punitive.[124] They are poorly tolerated, and serial lumbar punctures are ineffective as a long-term treatment.[222] It is impossible for serial lumbar punctures alone to remove enough fluid to relieve elevated intracranial pressure, as CSF is produced at a rate of 0.35 mL/min, allowing the entire CSF circulation to be replenished in just 2 hours.[164] In fact, we believe most cases require just one (the first) spinal tap, which is both diagnostic and sometimes therapeutic, without the need of repeating the procedure. Its long-lasting effects are likely due to a persistent CSF leak at the lumbar puncture site, or to decompression of the arachnoid villi, allowing improved CSF absorption.[164] In general, there is no need for chronic monitoring of CSF pressure.[232, 233]

Corbett and Thompson have emphasized that treatment decisions should not rest on the frequency of TVOs, presence of diplopia, severity of the papilledema, abnormalities on VEPs, or CSF opening or closing pressure. Instead, the modern management of pseudotumor cerebri is based on the level of visual loss, as additional therapeutic strategies should be guided by visual fields and visual acuity (Table 6–8).[234] Thus, in addition to the measures (such as weight loss) mentioned above, treatment suggestions according to level of visual loss are as follows.

1. *For patients with no visual loss:* Patients with no visual loss, headache, or other symptoms can be observed. Those with headache may be treated with acetaminophen, nonsteroidal anti-inflammatory agents, tricyclic antidepressants, or beta-blockers, for instance (but not steroids). Acetazolamide (see below) may be used in these instances as well but may not be necessary.
2. *For patients with mild to moderate visual loss:* Most patients with pseudotumor cerebri fall into this group. Visual deficits include enlarged blind spots, arcuate defects, mild peripheral constriction, and visual acuity of 20/30 or better. Acetazolamide, a carbonic anhydrase inhibitor that decreases CSF production, is the first-line medication in these instances, although its efficacy has been documented only anecdotally[235, 236] and has

TABLE 6–8. Management of Pseudotumor Cerebri, Based on the Severity and Progression of Visual Deficits

No visual loss	Symptomatic headache (migraine) therapy Weight reduction, if necessary Acetazolamide
Mild visual loss	Acetazolamide Furosemide Weight reduction, if necessary
Severe visual loss, or progression of visual loss	Optic nerve sheath decompression (ONSD) High-dose IV steroids and acetazolamide Lumboperitoneal shunt for failed ONSD or intractable headache

not been proven by a prospective trial. We prefer acetazolamide 500-mg sequels, orally two or three times per day, as a starting dose, and will increase the total dosage to 3 g if necessary. The drug should not be given to those with sulfa allergies. Its major side effects include paresthesias of the lips, fingers, and toes (which most patients tolerate), abnormal taste, nausea, vomiting, malaise, sedation, renal calculi, and metabolic acidosis.[164, 237] The dose can be lowered in individuals not tolerating the drug.[238] Most individuals in this group will do extremely well with acetazolamide, with resolution of the field defects and papilledema within 3 to 6 months, after which the medication can be tapered. When acetazolamide is not tolerated, we switch the patient to furosemide (20 to 40 mg) and monitor the potassium level carefully. We rarely use digoxin or glycerol in these cases, but they are also reasonable alternatives.

3. *For patients with severe or progressive visual loss despite medical management:* Optic nerve sheath fenestration surgery is the primary option for these patients, which fortunately make up only a minority of those with pseudotumor cerebri. Other indications for optic nerve surgery are severe visual loss at presentation, inability to comply with medications, poor follow-up, or inability to cooperate with visual field testing.[124] As stated previously, nonorganic visual loss should be excluded since nonphysiologic tubular visual fields may be mistaken for field loss associated with papilledema.

During optic nerve sheath fenestration, windows or slits are created through the dura and arachnoid surrounding the optic nerve (Fig. 6–17), allowing CSF egress, local relief of CSF pressure, and improvement in papilledema. Although the procedure had previously been suggested for this condition,[239] three series[240–242] reported in 1988 provided the impetus for more widespread use of this technique in patients with visual loss due to pseudotumor cerebri. Acuity or fields improved in 85% to 100% of patients in these three reports. Interestingly, of the 33 patients who had only one eye operated on, 24 patients (73%) experienced improvement in disc swelling bilaterally, and of the patients who had headache, two thirds had some relief postoperatively.[124] Others[243, 244] have subsequently published similar results. The procedure may also be performed in children.[332]

When both eyes are affected by acuity or field loss, the eye with the worse vision should be operated on first. If the fellow eye does not improve and also requires surgery, that can be performed a few days later. Simultaneous bilateral surgery is ill advised. The lateral orbitotomy approach has been used,[245] but the medial approach (transconjunctival and under the medial rectus muscle) is less complicated and currently more popular. The medial approach also avoids the temporal posterior ciliary artery, and therefore makes a catastrophic vascular event involving the blood supply to the submacular choroid less likely. At the time of surgery, three longitudinal slits in the dura are made with blunt lysis of subarachnoid adhesions or alternatively a window of dura can be excised. The latter approach is more technically demanding and there has never been a study to show that it is superior to simply incising the sheath. The surgery can easily be performed with retrobulbar or sub-Tenon's local anesthesia, however, these techniques do not allow monitoring of pupil size during the surgery and or assessment of the vision immediately postoperatively.[246] While this information is not critical to the successful intraoperative or postoperative management of the patient, they do provide assurance of a good outcome to the operating surgeon. Since most of the patients are young and otherwise healthy, our preference is for general anesthesia. Admission to the hospital postoperatively affords the best management of postoperative pain and allows the staff to monitor the patient for postoperative bleeding. Some authors have suggested the use of antimetabolites[247] and drainage devices[248] in an effort to create more definitive and long-term drains. These methods are investigational without sufficient data to assess their efficiency, so at this time they are not widely employed.

Complication rates in various series are as low as 4.9%[249] and as high as 40%.[250] Minor complications include temporary motility dysfunction, usually an adduction deficit owing to the temporary disinsertion of the medial rectus muscle, and a transient tonic pupil, resulting from damage to the short ciliary nerves or their blood supply.[250] Uncommon major complications include branch and central retinal artery occlusions,[250] choroidal infarction,[251] and worsening optic neuropathy.[252, 253]

While instantaneous decompression of the optic nerve is essentially guaranteed by this procedure, whether this type of surgery pro-

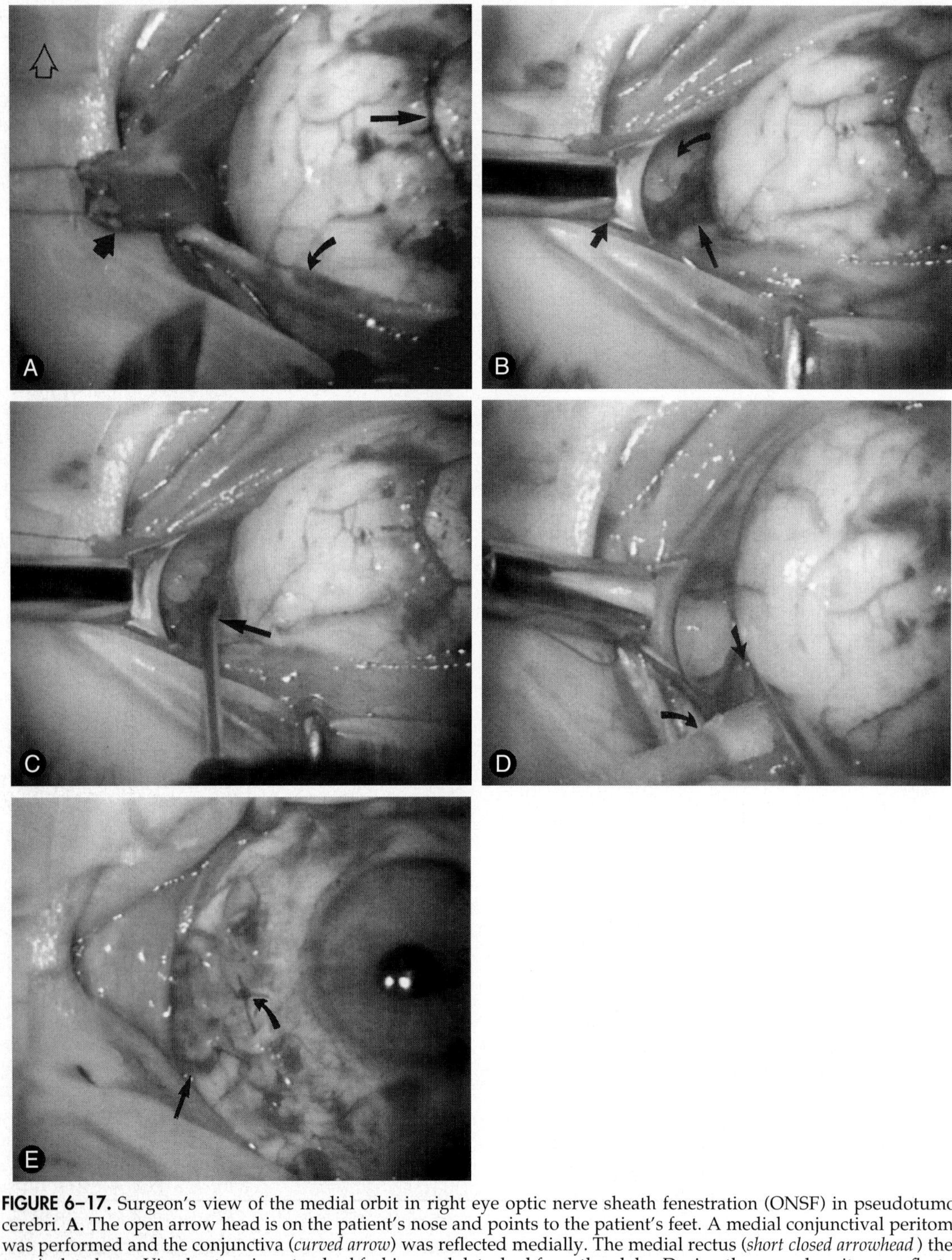

FIGURE 6–17. Surgeon's view of the medial orbit in right eye optic nerve sheath fenestration (ONSF) in pseudotumor cerebri. **A.** The open arrow head is on the patient's nose and points to the patient's feet. A medial conjunctival peritomy was performed and the conjunctiva (*curved arrow*) was reflected medially. The medial rectus (*short closed arrowhead*) then was isolated on a Vicryl suture in a standard fashion and detached from the globe. During the procedure it was reflected medially. A 5-0 Vicryl suture was then sutured into the medial rectus insertion site (*straight arrow*) in a running locking fashion. **B.** The globe was retracted upward and laterally. A medial orbital retractor (*shorter straight arrow*) was used to retract the medial rectus and medial orbital tissue toward the nose. Orbital fat (*curved arrow*) was dissected bluntly to expose the optic nerve sheath (*longer straight arrow*). Numerous ciliary vessels are visible on the optic nerve sheath. **C.** Next, an MVR blade (*arrow*) was used to create a slit (1.5 to 2 mm from the point where the sheath meets the globe) in the optic nerve sheath through which the spinal fluid egressed. The process was repeated three times. **D.** Long cotton swabs were then used to retract fat and Tenon's capsule. A curved tenotomy hook (*straight arrow*) was then passed from one previously made slit to the next within the subarachnoid space. Gentle movements were used to lyse subarachnoid adhesions. **E.** After hemostasis was achieved, the previously placed Vicryl sutures (*curved arrowhead*) were used to reattach the medial rectus muscle (*straight arrow*). The muscle was left hung back approximately 1 to 2 mm to correct for the small resection that occurred when the muscle was detached from the globe. Note the slightly irregular pupil, which is common at the end of the procedure.

vides a long-term fistula or drain is uncertain. Improvement of disc swelling in the fellow eye and resolution of headache suggests that sheath decompression acts as a filtering procedure.[254, 255] Post-operative MRI's may demonstrate a decrease in intrasheath fluid and collections of fluid within the orbit.[330] Pathologic studies of eyes following sheath decompression suggest that CSF exits either through intact open fistulas in the dura or through enclosed blebs of fibrosis.[256] Cystlike structures, contiguous to the fenestration site, have been imaged and may also act as filters.[257] However, evidence against the filtration hypothesis is (1) an inability to demonstrate extravasation of iopamidol dye into the orbit following intrathecal injection, despite its visualization in the subarachnoid space by CT, and (2) inconsistent CSF pressure measurements, both lowered and persistently elevated,[258, 259] following the procedure. Alternatively, fat and Tenon's capsule may attach to the openings or fenestrations, and extensive scarring and adhesions are almost always seen on reoperations. Chronic adhesion of the dura to the retrolaminar portion of the optic nerve may prevent the transmission of high CSF pressure to the optic nerve head.[254] Another possible mechanism for the effectiveness of sheath decompression is improved blood flow in the short posterior ciliary arteries.[209]

Optic nerve sheath decompression is more effective in reversing visual loss due to acute papilledema, in contrast to that due to chronic disc swelling.[260] In the long term, vision stabilizes or improves in the majority, but as many as 32% of operated eyes may experience deterioration following initially successful surgery.[261] A reoperation can be performed,[260] but we prefer lumboperitoneal shunting in these instances.

If the severe visual loss is sudden, if central visual loss is caused by macular edema, or if optic nerve sheath fenestration is not immediately available, then high-dose IV steroids combined with acetazolamide is another treatment option.[262] IV methylprednisolone, 250 mg qid for 5 days can be given in combination with acetazolamide sequels 500 mg tid and ranitadine. Lack of immediate improvement is an indication for optic nerve sheath decompression. The IV steroids are followed by 80 mg prednisone orally, tapered over 4 weeks in order to avoid the side effects of chronic use, and the acetazolamide is continued until the disc swelling resolves.

We reserve lumboperitoneal shunting for patients in whom headache is the major problem or in whom visual loss progresses despite optic nerve sheath fenestration.[263] Although lumboperitoneal shunting is effective in treating visual loss,[264, 265] shunt failure and low-pressure headaches are common enough in our opinion not to make it a first-line therapy.[266] Sometimes within the same patient, shunts fail several times, requiring multiple shunt revisions. Relatively small or normal ventricle sizes make ventriculoperitoneal shunting difficult.[267]

Pregnant Patients. Women who are pregnant and develop pseudotumor cerebri can be treated similarly to nonpregnant patients except for the following three caveats: (1) because of a single case report of a sacrococcygeal teratoma in an infant following the mother's use of acetazolamide in the first trimester, the drug should be reserved for use only in the last two trimesters; (2) stronger diuretics should not be used; and (3) weight reduction should not be recommended.[155, 164] Therapeutic abortions are unnecessary.

Outcome

In our experience, most patients with mild to moderate visual loss tend to recover vision following medical therapy. Papilledema usually resolves completely over weeks or months, but many patients are left with some residual disc elevation, especially nasally, macular pigment epithelial changes if lipid or edema had been present, or circumferential "high-water" marks delineating the prior extent of peripapillary retinal elevation associated with disc swelling. Thus, for future reference we obtain disc photographs following resolution of disc swelling. Recurrences in this group are relatively infrequent, so follow-up need not extend more than 6 or 12 months past tapering of medication.

Among those with severe visual loss requiring surgery, residual acuity and field deficits are not uncommon and are occasionally debilitating.[67, 123, 331] In Wall and George's series,[64] approximately 3% of eyes had visual acuity worse than 20/100. Rarely cases act in a malignant fashion and seem recalcitrant to medications, optic nerve sheath fenestration, and lumboperitoneal shunting. Furthermore, we agree with Spoor et al[261] that recurrences are more frequent in this group. Therefore, follow-up in these patients should include semiannual examinations for at least 2 to 3 years following surgery. In one series,[67] 8% of patients had return of symptoms, while in another,[185] 37% experienced recurrence. In addition to the aforementioned residual fundus changes, most patients in this group are left with some degree of optic atrophy.

VENOUS THROMBOSIS/ OBSTRUCTION

Elevated intracranial pressure and papilledema can result from thrombosis or obstruction of the cerebral dural venous sinuses, which drain blood from the brain (Fig. 6–18). The superior sagittal sinus runs along the superior portion of the falx cerebri, while the inferior sagittal sinus, which lies along the inferior portion of the falx, joins the great vein of Galen to drain into the straight sinus. The superior sagittal sinus, straight sinus, and two transverse sinues frequently join posteriorly at the confluence of sinuses (or torcular Herophili), but in many instances the superior sagittal sinus drains into the right transverse sinus and the straight sinus directly into the left transverse sinus. In turn, the transverse sinuses drain into the sigmoid sinuses, each of which empties into the internal jugular veins.[268] Impaired flow in these sinuses can cause venous hypertension and subsequently decrease CSF absorption.

The top section of Table 6–7 lists various causes. The causes of clot formation within the sinuses are multiple, but fall largely into three categories:

1. *Hypercoagulable states*. These include Behçet's disease,[269] the presence of antiphospholipid antibodies[270] or lupus anticoagulant, protein C or S deficiency,[271] antithrombin III deficiency, factor V deficiency, oral contraceptive use, pregnancy, cancer, and thrombocytosis.[272] Venous thrombosis due to hypercoagulability also is a likely mechanism for many of the pseudotumor-like presentations in patients with systemic lupus erythematosus.[273–277] L-asparaginase predisposes to clot formation by decreasing antithrombin III levels. Cerebral venous thrombosis is also a recognized complication of paroxysmal nocturnal hemoglobinuria.[278, 279]
2. *Contiguous infection*. Although antibiotics have made lateral sinus thrombosis secondary to adjoining mastoiditis or middle-ear infections uncommon,[280] such cases are still seen (Fig. 6–19).[272, 281] The mechanism is likely contiguous vessel wall inflammation and thrombophlebitis. The term *otitic hydrocephalus*[118] has been applied to these cases, but the designation is a misnomer because affected patients do not have hydrocephalus. When an abducens palsy is present, it tends to be ipsilateral to the involved ear.[118] Surgical excision of infected mastoid tissue is often required.

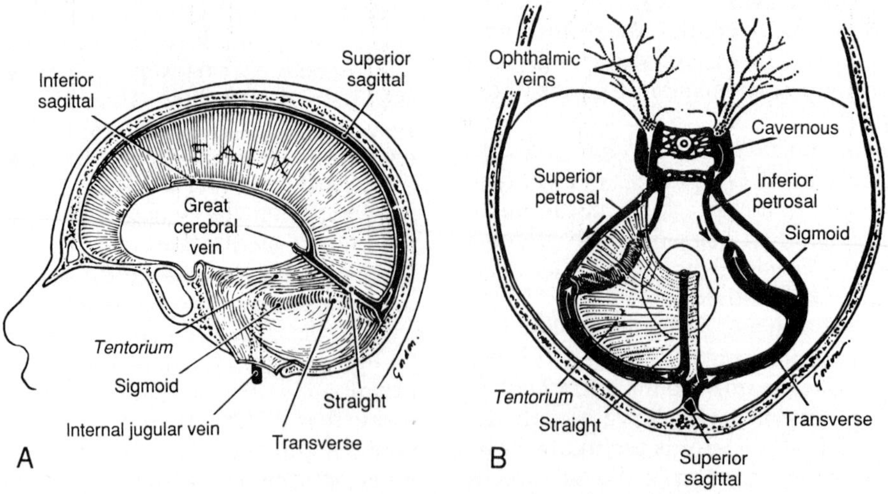

FIGURE 6–18. Major venous sinuses of the dura mater in (**A**) sagittal and (**B**) axial views. The arrows indicate the direction of blood flow. (From Moore KL: Clinically Oriented Anatomy, 3rd edition. Baltimore, Williams & Wilkins, p 688, 1992.)

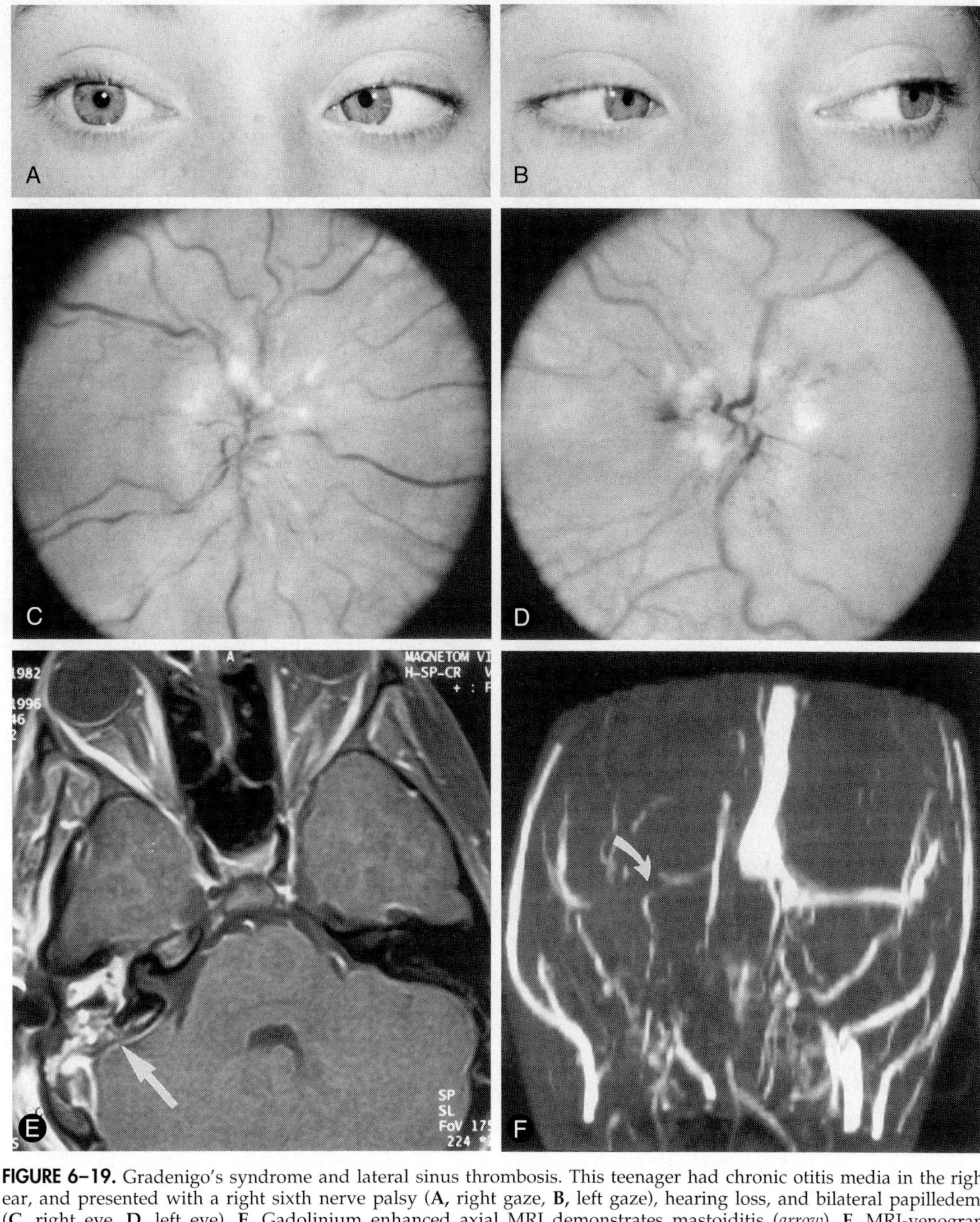

FIGURE 6–19. Gradenigo's syndrome and lateral sinus thrombosis. This teenager had chronic otitis media in the right ear, and presented with a right sixth nerve palsy (**A,** right gaze, **B,** left gaze), hearing loss, and bilateral papilledema (**C,** right eye, **D,** left eye). **E.** Gadolinium enhanced axial MRI demonstrates mastoiditis (*arrow*). **F.** MRI-venogram (TR 30, TE 9), coronal view, shows absence of flow in the transverse sinus on the right (*arrow*), consistent with venous thrombosis.

3. *Contiguous neoplasm*. Neoplasms may compress the venous sinuses, impeding venous drainage and leading to clot formation (Fig. 6–20). Reported examples include medulloblastoma, sarcoma, melanoma,[269] and meningioma.[282]

Radical neck dissection or iatrogenic ligation of one of the draining veins or sinuses can result in outflow obstruction.[272, 283] Venous catheterization (jugular or subclavian, for instance) may be associated with local clot formation and venous hypertension. Outflow ob-

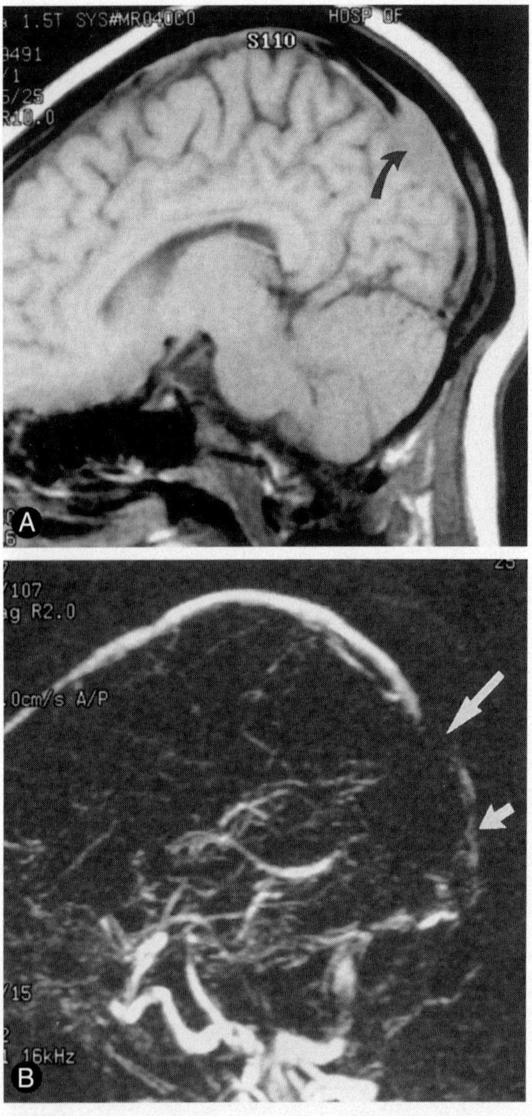

FIGURE 6–20. Venous thrombosis secondary to tumor compression by presumed lymphoma. This thin woman presented with bilateral papilledema and headaches, and the sagittal T_1-weighted MRI (**A**) demonstrated a mass (*arrow*) compressing the posterior portion of the superior sagittal sinus. **B.** The MR-venogram (TR 26, TE 9.2) shows occlusion of the sinus (*large arrow*) and poor venous flow (*small arrow*). A parotid mass was biopsied and disclosed B-cell lymphoma. The patient also had splenic and bone marrow involvement and a pleural effusion. Venous sinus compression, headaches, and disc swelling resolved following chemotherapy and whole-brain and focal radiation.

struction without clot can result from direct tumor compression by a parasagittal meningioma (superior sagittal sinus)[272, 284] or glomus jugulare[285] or other base of skull[334] tumor (jugular veins), for instance. We have also seen venous thromboses associated with epidural hematomas due to head trauma.

Presenting Signs and Symptoms

In most instances the neuro-ophthalmic features are similar to those with pseudotumor cerebri: headache, nausea and vomiting, papilledema, optic nerve-related visual loss, and sixth nerve palsies.[272, 333] However, patients may develop altered mentation, and cortical vein thrombosis and cerebral infarction can lead to hemiparesis, hemisensory loss, and seizures, for instance. Thrombosis of the transverse and sigmoid sinuses may also lead to seventh and eighth nerve dysfunction.[286]

Thromboses of the dural venous sinuses, as described above, should be distinguished from those of the deep venous drainage (internal cerebral veins, and the vein of Galen, for example). Patients with the latter tend to present more acutely with altered consciousness and long tract signs. The signs and symptoms of elevated intracranial pressure, although present, are less prominent.[287]

Neuroimaging

A safe and effective method for visualizing cerebral venous thrombosis combines MRI with gadolinium, with sagittal images especially, and MR venography.[76, 283] The clot tends to enhance on T_1-weighted enhanced MR images. Axial CT scans with contrast may demonstrate the characteristic "empty delta sign" at the intersection of the straight sinus and distal superior sagittal sinus.[283] Characteristically the ventricles are small on neuroimaging. We have found MRI and MR venography sufficient for managing these patients, without requiring the use of formal venography.

Workup

If a clot is demonstrated radiologically, prior ear infections, neck surgery, and IV catheters as a source should be excluded. Clinical evidence for Behçet's (oral and genital ulcers) or lupus (rashes or joint aches) should be investigated. The patient should be asked about oral contraceptive use or personal and family history of clotting disorders or miscarriages. In unclear cases, laboratory investigation should include screening for antiphospholipid antibodies, lupus anticoagulant, protein C or S, antithrombin III or factor V deficiency, antinuclear antibodies, and thrombocytosis. In cases without mass effect, lumbar puncture should be performed to document the opening pressure, and the vision should be assessed carefully, including visual field testing.

Treatment

If identifiable, the offending drug should be discontinued, or the underlying medical condition or mass lesion treated. Because dehydration and hypotension can aggravate cerebral thromboses, and overhydration can worsen elevated intracranial pressure, patients should be kept euvolemic with judicious use of IV fluids. We recommend anticoagulation with IV heparin for 5 to 7 days followed by warfarin, especially in cases due to primary hypercoagulable states, but not in those with evidence of hemorrhage. Selective catheterization and urokinase infusion have been used in some centers,[288] but its safety and efficacy need to be confirmed. Depending on clinical status and follow-up radiologic studies, oral anticoagulation should be continued for at least 3 months.[268]

As in pseudotumor cerebri, acetazolamide can be used to treat elevated intracranial pressure and mild field loss. Any diuretic in this setting, however, should be used with caution, with monitoring of fluid status and blood pressure because of the potential for worsening the thrombosis. Patients with progressive or severe visual loss despite medical therapy and treatment of the offending source should undergo optic nerve sheath fenestration.[284, 289] The visual outcome is favorable in most instances.[272] Lumboperitoneal shunting should be used in patients in whom headache or nausea and vomiting are refractory to acetazolamide, anticoagulation, and conservative medical therapy.

ARTERIOVENOUS MALFORMATIONS OF THE DURAL SINUSES

Prehemorrhagic dural arteriovenous malformations (AVMs) that drain into the venous sinuses (AV fistulas) can cause elevated intracranial pressure and papilledema without ventriculomegaly by increasing blood flow within the sinuses or by causing venous thrombosis.[290, 291] Both mechanisms can lead to decreased CSF absorption. Less commonly, unruptured cerebral AVMs can drain into the superior sagittal sinus and cause similar symptoms.[292] If a dural AVM drains into the transverse sinus, a cranial bruit may be audible, and the patient may complain of tinnitus.[293] The dural AVM may be evident on MRI or CT with contrast. However, formal angiography is usually required to outline the vascular anatomy.[294] Treatment options include surgical excision of the AVM or embolization. However, some larger AVMs are incurable, and elevated intracranial pressure and papilledema may require further management with acetazolamide, optic nerve sheath fenestration, or lumboperitoneal shunting.[295] Cerebral AVMs, which are much more common, are discussed in Chapter 8, while dural AVMs are reviewed in more detail in Chapter 15.

PULMONARY DISEASE

Elevated intracranial pressure and papilledema may develop in the setting of respiratory insufficiency as a result of hypercapnea-induced cerebral vasodilation.[296, 297, 335] These patients can be distinguished by their lethargy, peripheral retinal hemorrhages (due to the venous hypertension), arterial blood gas results, and high serum bicarbonate.[298]

Obese patients with the Pickwickian syndrome (sleep apnea/obesity hypoventilation syndrome) may develop papilledema,[298] and it is easy to mistakenly diagnose them with pseudotumor cerebri. Excess fat in the hypopharynx leads to obstructive sleep apnea, chronic hypoxemia and hypercapnea, pulmonary hypertension, right-sided heart failure, and venous hypertension. The papilledema tends to respond to treatment of the lung abnormalities, including oxygenation, positive airway pressure, and weight reduction, under the direction of a pulmonologist.[298] If there is mild visual field loss associated with the disc swelling, acetazolamide can be added.

GUILLAIN-BARRÉ SYNDROME AND CHRONIC INFLAMMATORY DEMYELINATING POLYNEUROPATHY

These conditions, discussed in more detail in Chapter 14, are characterized by muscle weakness and areflexia due to inflammatory demyelinating polyneuropathy. Chronic inflammatory demyelinating polyneuropathy (CIDP) has a slowly progressive or relapsing–remitting course, and rare cases with papilledema have been reported.[299, 300] In Guillain–Barré syndrome, typified by acute to subacute weakness, papilledema may be seen in approximately 1% to 3% of cases.[301] According to Ropper et al,[301] disc swelling, when it occurs, generally develops during the third week of this illness. However, papilledema may go unnoticed because daily funduscopy may not be performed in these patients, and they may be paralyzed, intubated, and unable to complain about headache or abnormal vision. We have seen one patient with Guillain–Barré syndrome[302] who received respiratory support for 3 months and upon discontinuation of ventilatory assistance, told us she had had blurry vision in the left eye for weeks. Only then was chronic papilledema detected, and the CSF pressure was measured and found to be elevated. Abducens palsies are unreliable as a sign of elevated intracranial pressure because the sixth nerves are commonly affected in Guillain–Barré syndrome.

The combination of papilledema, elevated intracranial pressure, and Guillain–Barré syndrome is generally associated with high CSF protein levels (above 200 mg/dl). Decreased CSF resorption by the arachnoid villi due to elevated protein concentrations is one proposed mechanism for the papilledema, but other possibilities include increased CSF outflow resistance, hydrocephalus,[303] and increased venous pressure.[299, 301] Several authors[301, 302, 304, 305] have used the term *pseudotumor cerebri* in these situations, however, the designation is technically incorrect if the CSF protein or neuroimaging is abnormal.

Neuro-ophthalmic management may be difficult in these instances because their poor medical condition may preclude careful assessment of visual acuity and fields. However, as in pseudotumor cerebri, acetazolamide,[299] corticosteroids,[302] and optic nerve sheath fenestration[299, 300] may be used to treat documentable visual loss, based on the level of its severity.

SPINAL CORD TUMORS

Papilledema and elevated intracranial pressure are well-established, but uncommon complications of spinal cord tumors.[306–308] Matzkin et al[306] identified 53 such cases in the literature, and approximately 40% involved spinal cord ependymomas. Elevated CSF protein causing decreased CSF absorption by the arachnoid villi has also been a purported mechanism in these instances, but abnormal CSF dynamics caused by tumor cell dissemination, tumor mucin production, recurrent subarachnoid hemorrhages, and compression of the lumbar spinal sac have been considered as well.[306]

Magnetic resonance imaging of the spine with and without gadolinium is recommended when paraparesis or quadriparesis, lumbar pain, a sensory level, hyperreflexia, extensor plantar responses, or bladder dysfunction are present. Neuroimaging of the brain in these instances may reveal associated communicating hydrocephalus. Treatment would include neurosurgical removal or biopsy of the spinal cord tumor as well as a venticulostomy or ventriculoperitoneal shunt, if necessary.

REFERENCES

1. Corbett JJ: Problems in the diagnosis and treatment of pseudotumor cerebri. Can J Neurol Sci 1983; 10:221–229.
2. Sergott RC: Diagnosis and management of vision-threatening papilledema. Semin Neurol 1986;6: 176–184.
3. Whiting AS, Johnson LN: Papilledema: clinical clues and differential diagnosis. Am Fam Physician 1992;45:1125–1134.
4. Stammen J, Unsold R, Arendt G, et al: Etiology and pathogenetic mechanisms of optic disc swelling with visual loss. An interdisciplinary prospective pilot study of 102 cases. Ophthalmologica 1999;213:40–47.
5. Brodsky MC: Congenital optic disk anomalies. Surv Ophthalmol 1994;39:89–112.
6. Hoyt WF, Pont ME: Pseudopapilledema: anomalous elevation of optic disk. JAMA 1962;181:191–196.
7. Kheterpal S, Good PA, Beale DJ, et al: Imaging of optic disc drusen: a comparative study. Eye 1995;9:67–69.
8. Hoover DL, Robb RM, Peterson RA: Optic disc drusen in childhood. J Pediatr Ophthalmol Strabismus 1988;25:191–195.
9. Lorentzen SE: Drusen of the optic disc. A clinical and genetic study. Acta Ophthalmol 1966;Suppl 90:1–180.
10. Rosenberg MA, Savino PJ, Glaser JS: A clinical analysis of pseudopapilledema. I: population, laterality, acuity, refractive error, ophthalmoscopic characteristics and coincident disease. Arch Ophthalmol 1979;97:65–70.
11. Rubinstein K, Ali M: Retinal complications of optic disc drusen. Br J Ophthalmol 1982;66:83–95.
12. Apple DJ, Rabb MF, Walsh PM: Congenital anomalies of the optic disc. Surv Ophthalmol 1982;27:3–41.
13. Tso MO: Pathology and pathogenesis of drusen of the optic nerve head. Ophthalmology 1981;88:1066–1080.
14. Boldt HC, Byrne SF, DiBernardo C: Echographic evaluation of optic disc drusen. J Clin Neuro-ophthalmol 1991;11:85–91.
15. Buys YM, Pavlin CJ: Retinitis pigmentosa, nanophthalmos, and optic disc drusen: a case report. Ophthalmology 1999;106:619–622.
16. Mustonen E, Nieminen H: Optic disc drusen—a photographic study. I: Autofluorescence pictures and

fluorescein angiography. Acta Ophthalmol 1982; 60:849–858.
17. Froula PD, Bartley GB, Garrity JA, et al: The differential diagnosis of orbital calcification as detected on computed tomography scans. Mayo Clin Proc 1993;68:256–261.
18. McNicholas MM, Power WJ, Griffin JF: Sonography in optic disk drusen: imaging findings and role in diagnosis when funduscopic findings are normal. AJR Am J Roentgenol 1994;162:161–163.
19. Kawasaki A, Purvin V: Unilateral optic disc edema following trabeculectomy. J Neuro-ophthalmol 1998; 18:121–123.
20. Brodsky MC, Baker RS, Hamed LM: The swollen optic disc in childhood. In: Pediatric Neuro-ophthalmology, pp 76–124. New York, Springer-Verlag, 1996.
21. Wong VA, Wade NK: POEMS syndrome: an unusual cause of bilateral optic disk swelling. Am J Ophthalmol 1998;126:452–454.
22. Hayreh SS: Optic disc edema in raised intracranial pressure. V. Pathogenesis. Arch Ophthalmol 1977; 95:1553–1565.
23. Hayreh SS: Pathogenesis of optic disc oedema. In: Kennard C, Rose FC (eds): Physiological Aspects of Clinical Neuro-ophthalmology, pp 431–447. Chicago, Year Book, 1988.
24. Wall M: Optic disk edema with cotton-wool spots. Surv Ophthalmol 1995;39:502–508.
25. Kardon RH: The pathogenesis of visual field loss in idiopathic intracranial hypertension. North American Neuro-ophthalmology Society meeting 1992.
26. Wirtschafter JD, Rizzo FJ, Smiley BC: Optic nerve axoplasm and papilledema. Surv Ophthalmol 1975;20:157–189.
27. Tso MOM, Hayreh SS: Optic disc edema in raised intracranial pressure. III. A pathologic study of experimental papilledema. Arch Ophthalmol 1977;95: 1448–1457.
28. Pagani LF: The rapid appearance of papilledema. J Neurosurg 1969;30:247–249.
29. Selhorst JB, Gudeman SK, Butterworth JF, et al: Papilledema after acute head injury. Neurosurg 1985; 16:357–363.
30. Levin BE: The clinical significance of spontaneous pulsations of the retinal vein. Arch Neurol 1978; 35:37–40.
31. Lorentzen SE: Incidence of spontaneous venous pulsations in the retina. Acta Ophthalmol 1970;48: 765–770.
32. Frisén L: Swelling of the optic nerve head: a staging scheme. J Neurol Neurosurg Psychiatr 1982;45:13–18.
33. Sanders M: The Bowman Lecture. Papilloedema: "The pendulum of progress." Eye 1997;11:267–294.
34. Lepore FE: Unilateral and highly asymmetric papilledema in pseudotumor cerebri. Neurology 1992; 42:676–678.
35. Strominger MB, Weiss GB, Mehler MF: Asymptomatic unilateral papilledema in pseudotumor cerebri. J Clin Neuro-ophthalmol 1992;12:238–241.
36. Yohai RA, Bullock JD, Margolis JH: Unilateral optic disk edema and a contralateral temporal fossa mass. Am J Ophthalmol 1993;115:261–262.
37. Moster ML: Unilateral disk edema in a young woman. Surv Ophthalmol 1995;39:409–416.
38. Hayreh SS: Pathogenesis of oedema of the optic disc (papilloedema). Br J Ophthalmol 1964;48:522–543.
39. Orcutt JC, Page NGR, Sanders MD: Factors affecting visual loss in benign intracranial hypertension. Ophthalmology 1984;91:1303–1312.
40. Soelberg Sørensen P, Krogsaa B, Gjerris F: Clinical course and prognosis of pseudotumor cerebri. A prospective study of 24 patients. Acta Neurol Scand 1988;77:164–172.
41. Kennedy F: A further note on the diagnostic value of retrobulbar neuritis in expanding lesions of the frontal lobes. With a report of this syndrome in a case of aneurysm of the right internal carotid artery. JAMA 1916;67:1361–1363.
42. Ing EB, Leavitt JA, Younge BR: Papilledema following bowtie optic atrophy. Arch Ophthalmol 1996; 114:356–357.
43. Watnick RL, Trobe JD: Bilateral optic nerve compression as a mechanism for the Foster Kennedy syndrome. Ophthalmology 1989;96:1793–1798.
44. Schatz NJ, Smith JL: Non-tumor causes of the Foster Kennedy syndrome. J Neurosurg 1967;27:37–44.
45. Pollock SC: Acute papilledema and visual loss in a patient with pseudotumor cerebri [letter]. Arch Ophthalmol 1987;105:752–753.
46. Mitchell DJ, Steahly LP: Pseudotumor cerebri and macular disease. Retina 1989;9:115–117.
47. Verm A, Lee AG: Bilateral optic disk edema with macular exudates as the manifesting sign of a cerebral arteriovenous malformation. Am J Ophthalmol 1997;123:422–424.
48. Talks SJ, Mossa F, Elston JS: The contribution of macular changes to visual loss in benign intracranial hypertension. Eye 1998;12:806–808.
49. Morris AT, Sanders MD: Macular changes resulting from papilloedema. Br J Ophthalmol 1980;64: 211–216.
50. Bird AC, Sanders MD: Choroidal folds in association with papilloedema. Br J Ophthalmol 1973;57:89–97.
51. Jacobson DM: Intracranial hypertension and the syndrome of acquired hyperopia with choroidal folds. J Neuro-ophthalmol 1995;15:178–185.
52. Bullock JD, Egbert PR: The origin of choroidal folds. A clinical, histopathological, and experimental study. Doc Ophthalmol 1974;37:261–293.
53. Keane JR: Papilledema with unusual ocular hemorrhages. Arch Ophthalmol 1981;99:262–263.
54. Jamison RR: Subretinal neovascularization and papilledema associated with pseudotumor cerebri. Am J Ophthalmol 1978;85:78–81.
55. Troost BT, Sufit RL, Grand MG: Sudden monocular visual loss in pseudotumor cerebri. Arch Neurol 1979;36:440–442.
56. Akova YA, Kansu T, Yazar Z, et al: Macular subretinal neovascular membrane associated with pseudotumor cerebri. J Neuro-ophthalmol 1994;14:193–195.
57. Galvin R, Sanders MD: Peripheral retinal haemorrhages with papilledema. Br J Ophthalmol 1980; 64:262–266.
58. Baker RS, Buncic JR: Sudden visual loss in pseudotumor cerebri due to central retinal artery occlusion. Arch Neurol 1984;41:1274–1276.
59. Lam BL, Siatkowski RM, Fox GM, et al: Visual loss in pseudotumor cerebri from branch retinal artery occlusion. Am J Ophthalmol 1992;113:334–336.
60. Gittinger JW, Asdourian GK: Macular abnormalities in papilledema from pseudotumor cerebri. Ophthalmology 1989;96:192–194.
61. Carter SR, Seiff SR: Macular changes in pseudotumor cerebri before and after optic nerve sheath fenestration. Ophthalmology 1995;102:937–941.
62. Galetta SL, Byrne SF, Smith JL: Echographic correlation of optic nerve sheath size and cerebrospinal fluid pressure. J Clin Neuro-ophthalmol 1989;9:79–82.

63. Hayreh SS: Optic disc edema in raised intracranial pressure. VI. Associated visual disturbances and their pathogenesis. Arch Ophthalmol 1977;95:1566–1579.
64. Wall M, George D: Idiopathic intracranial hypertension. A prospective study of 50 patients. Brain 1991;114:155–180.
65. Liu GT, Volpe NJ, Schatz NJ, et al: Severe acute visual loss caused by pseudotumor cerebri and lumboperitoneal shunt failure. Am J Ophthalmol 1996;122: 129–131.
66. Green GJ, Lessell S, Loewenstein JI: Ischemic optic neuropathy in chronic papilledema. Arch Ophthalmol 1980;98:502–504.
67. Corbett JJ, Savino PJ, Thompson HS, et al: Visual loss in pseudotumor cerebri. Follow-up of 57 patients from five to 41 years and a profile of 14 patients with permanent severe visual loss. Arch Neurol 1982; 39:461–474.
68. Corbett JJ, Jacobson DM, Mauer RC, et al: Enlargement of the blind spot caused by papilledema. Am J Ophthalmol 1988;105:261–265.
69. Hedges TR, Legge RH, Peli E, et al: Retinal nerve fiber layer changes and visual field loss in idopathic intracranial hypertension. Ophthalmology 1995;102: 1242–1247.
70. Gu XZ, Tsai JC, Wurdeman A, et al: Pattern of axonal loss in longstanding papilledema due to idiopathic intracranial hypertension. Curr Eye Res 1995;14: 173–180.
71. Galetta SL, Liu GT, Volpe NJ: Diagnostic testing in neurology. Neuro-ophthalmology. Neurol Clin 1996; 14:201–222.
72. Wall M, George D: Visual loss in pseudotumor cerebri. Incidence and defects related to visual field strategy. Arch Neurol 1987;44:170–175.
73. Wall M: Sensory visual testing in idiopathic intracranial hypertension. Measures sensitive to change. Neurology 1990;40:1859–1864.
74. Sadun AA, Currie JN, Lessell S: Transient visual obscurations with elevated optic discs. Ann Neurol 1984;16:489–494.
75. Wall M: Idiopathic intracranial hypertension. Neurol Clin 1991;9:73–95.
76. Mattle HP, Wentz KU, Edelman RR, et al: Cerebral venography with MR. Radiology 1991;178:453–458.
77. Corbett JJ, Mehta MP: Cerebrospinal fluid pressure in normal obese subjects and patients with pseudotumor cerebri. Neurology 1983;33:1386–1388.
78. Archer BD: Computed tomography before lumbar puncture in acute meningitis: a review of the risks and benefits. Can Med Assoc J 1993;148:961–965.
79. Allen ED, Byrd SE, Darling CF, et al: The clinical and radiological evaluation of primary brain tumors in children, Part I: Clinical evaluation. J Natl Med Assoc 1993;85:445–451.
80. Siddiqi SN, Posnick JC, Buncic R, et al: The detection and management of intracranial hypertension after initial suture release and decompression for craniofacial dysostosis syndromes. Neurosurg 1995;36: 703–709.
81. Billson FA, Hudson RL: Surgical treatment of chronic papilloedema in children. Br J Ophthalmol 1975; 59:92–95.
82. Wissow LS: Child abuse and neglect. N Engl J Med 1995;332:1425–1431.
83. Kaur B, Taylor D: Fundus hemorrhages in infancy. Surv Ophthalmol 1992;37:1–17.
84. Duhaime A-C, Christian CW, Rorke LB, et al: Nonaccidental head injury in infants—the "shaken-baby syndrome." N Engl J Med 1998;338:1822–1829.
85. Snyder H, Robinson K, Shah D, et al: Signs and symptoms of patients with brain tumors presenting to the emergency department. J Emerg Med 1993;11: 253–258.
86. Van Crevel H: Papilloedema, CSF pressure, and CSF flow in cerebral tumours. J Neurol Neurosurg Psychiatr 1979;42:493–500.
87. Weston P, Lear J: Gliomatosis cerebri or benign intracranial hypertension? Postgrad Med J 1995;71: 380–381.
88. Fahmy JA: Papilloedema associated with ruptured intracranial aneurysms. Acta Ophthalmol 1972;50: 793–802.
89. Steffen H, Eifert B, Aschoff A, et al: The diagnostic value of optic disc evaluation in acute elevated intracranial pressure. Ophthalmology 1996;103:1229–1232.
90. Schultz PN, Sobol WM, Weingeist TA: Long-term visual outcome in Terson syndrome. Ophthalmology 1991;98:1814–1819.
91. Garfinkle AM, Danys IR, Nicolle DA, et al: Terson's syndrome: a reversible cause of blindness following subarachnoid hemorrhage. J Neurosurg 1992;76: 766–771.
92. Frizzell RT, Kuhn F, Morris R, et al: Screening for ocular hemorrhages in patients with ruptured cerebral aneurysms: a prospective study of 99 patients. Neurosurgery 1997;41:529–534.
93. Kuhn F, Morris R, Witherspoon CD, et al: Terson syndrome. Results of vitrectomy and the significance of vitreous hemorrhage in patients with subarachnoid hemorrhage. Ophthalmology 1998;105:472–477.
94. Velikay M, Datlinger P, Stolba U, et al: Retinal detachment with severe proliferative vitreoretinopathy in Terson syndrome. Ophthalmology 1994;101:35–37.
95. Molavi A, LeFrock JL: Tuberculous meningitis. Med Clin N Am 1985;69:315–331.
96. Tang LM: Ventriculoperitoneal shunt in cryptococcal meningitis with hydrocephalus. Surg Neurol 1990; 33:314–319.
97. Lesser RL, Kornmehl EW, Pachner AR, et al: Neuro-ophthalmologic manifestations of Lyme disease. Ophthalmology 1990;97:699–706.
98. Belman AL, Iyer M, Coyle PK, et al: Neurologic manifestations in children with North American Lyme disease. Neurology 1993;43:2609–2614.
99. Balcer LJ, Winterkorn JMS, Galetta SL: The neuro-ophthalmic manifestations of Lyme disease. J Neuro-ophthalmol 1997;108:108–121.
100. Kestelyn P, Taelman H, Bogaerts J, et al: Ophthalmic manifestations of infections with Cryptococcus neoformans in patients with the acquired immunodeficiency syndrome. Am J Ophthalmol 1993;116: 721–727.
101. Rex JH, Larsen RA, Dismukes WE, et al: Catastrophic visual loss due to Cryptococcus neoformans meningitis. Medicine 1993;72:207–224.
102. Cohen DB, Glasgow BJ: Bilateral optic nerve cryptococcosis in sudden blindness in patients with acquired immune deficiency syndrome. Ophthalmology 1993;100:1689–1694.
103. van der Horst CM, Saag MS, Cloud GA, et al: Treatment of cryptococcal meningitis associated with the acquired immunodeficiency syndrome. N Engl J Med 1997;337:15–21.
104. Johnston SR, Corbett EL, Foster O, et al: Raised intracranial pressure and visual complications in AIDS patients with cryptococcal meningitis. J Infect 1992;24:185–189.

105. Garrity JA, Herman DC, Imes R, et al: Optic nerve sheath decompression for visual loss in patients with acquired immunodeficiency syndrome and cryptococcal meningitis with papilledema. Am J Ophthalmol 1993;116:472–478.
106. Strominger MB, Liu GT, Schatz NJ: Optic disk swelling and abducens palsies associated with OKT3. Am J Ophthalmol 1995;119:664–665.
107. Lamonte M, Silberstein SD, Marcelis JF: Headache associated with aseptic meningitis. Headache 1995; 35:520–526.
108. Balm M, Hammack J: Leptomeningeal carcinomatosis. Arch Neurol 1996;53:626–632.
109. Corbett JJ: Neuro-ophthalmologic complications of hydrocephalus and shunting procedures. Semin Neurol 1986;6:111–123.
110. Arroyo HA, Jan LE, McCormick AQ, et al: Permanent visual loss after shunt malfunction. Neurology 1985;35:25–29.
111. Katz DM, Trobe JD, Muraszko KM, et al: Shunt failure without ventriculomegaly proclaimed by ophthalmic findings. J Neurosurg 1994;81:721–725.
112. Lee AG: Visual loss as the manifesting symptom of ventriculoperitoneal shunt malfunction. Am J Ophthalmol 1996;122:127–129.
113. Newman NJ: Bilateral visual loss and disc edema in a 15-year-old girl. Surv Ophthalmol 1994;38:365–370.
114. Beck RW, Geenberg HS: Post-decompression optic neuropathy. J Neurosurg 1985;63:196–199.
115. Obana WG, Raskin NH, Cogen PH, et al: Antimigraine treatment for slit-ventricle syndrome. Neurosurg 1990;27:760–763.
116. Epstein F, Lapras C, Wisoff JH: 'Slit-ventricle syndrome': etiology and treatment. Pediatr Neurosci 1988;14:5–10.
117. Smith JL: Whence pseudotumor cerebri? [editorial]. J Clin Neuro-ophthalmol 1985;5:55–56.
118. Foley J: I. Benign forms of intracranial hypertension—"toxic" and "otitic" hydrocephalus. Brain 1955;78:1–13.
119. Weisberg LA: Benign intracranial hypertension. Medicine 1975;54:197–207.
120. Greitz D, Hannerz J, Rähn T, et al: MR imaging of cerebrospinal fluid dynamics in health and disease. On the vascular pathogenesis of communicating hydrocephalus and benign intracranial hypertension. Acta Radiol 1994;35:204–211.
121. Malozowski S, Tanner LA, Wysowski DK, et al: Benign intracranial hypertension in children with growth hormone deficiency treated with growth hormone. J Pediatr 1995;126:996–999.
122. Schwarz S, Husstedt IW, Georgiadis D, et al: Benign intracranial hypertension in an HIV-infected patient: headache as the only presenting sign [letter]. AIDS 1995;9:657–658.
123. Lessell S, Rosman NP: Permanent visual impairment in childhood pseudotumor cerebri. Arch Neurol 1986;43:801–804.
124. Corbett JJ, Thompson HS: The rational management of idiopathic intracranial hypertension. Arch Neurol 1989;46:1049–1051.
125. Giuseffi V, Wall M, Siegel PZ, et al: Symptoms and disease associations in idiopathic intracranial hypertension (pseudotumor cerebri): a case-control study. Neurology 1991;41:239–244.
126. Durcan FJ, Corbett JJ, Wall M: The incidence of pseudotumor cerebri. Population studies in Iowa and Louisiana. Arch Neurol 1988;45:875–877.
127. Radhakrishnan K, Ahlskog JE, Cross SA, et al: Idiopathic intracranial hypertension (pseudotumor cerebri). Descriptive epidemiology in Rochester, Minn, 1976 to 1990. Arch Neurol 1993;50:78–80.
128. Radhakrishnan K, Thacker AK, Bohlaga NH, et al: Epidemiology of idiopathic intracranial hypertension: a prospective and case-control study. J Neurol Sci 1993;116:18–28.
129. Ireland B, Corbett JJ, Wallace RB: The search for causes of idiopathic intracranial hypertension. A preliminary case-control study. Arch Neurol 1990; 47:315–320.
130. Digre KB, Corbett JJ: Pseudotumor cerebri in men. Arch Neurol 1988;45:866–872.
131. Lessell S: Pediatric pseudotumor cerebri (idiopathic intracranial hypertension). Surv Ophthalmol 1992; 37:155–166.
132. Couch R, Camfield PR, Tibbles JAR: The changing picture of pseudotumor cerebri in children. Can J Neurol Sci 1985;12:48–50.
133. Baker RS, Carter D, Hendrick EB, et al: Visual loss in pseudotumor cerebri of childhood. A follow-up study. Arch Ophthalmol 1985;103:1681–1686.
134. Grant DN: Benign intracranial hypertension. A review of 79 cases in infancy and childhood. Arch Dis Child 1971;46:651–655.
135. Hagberg B, Sillanpaa M: Benign intracranial hypertension (pseudotumor cerebri). Review and report of 18 cases. Acta Paediat Scand 1970;59:328–339.
136. Weisberg LA, Chutorian AM: Pseudotumor cerebri of childhood. Am J Dis Child 1977;131:1243–1248.
137. Rose A, Matson DD: Benign intracranial hypertension in children. Pediatrics 1967;39:227–237.
138. Babikian P, Corbett JJ, Bell W: Idiopathic intracranial hypertension in children: the Iowa experience. J Child Neurol 1994;9:144–149.
139. Gordon K: Pediatric pseudotumor cerebri: descriptive epidemiology. Can J Neurol Sci 1997;24:219–221.
140. Scott IU, Siatkowski RM, Eneyni M, et al: Idiopathic intracranial hypertension in children and adolescents. Am J Ophthalmol 1997;124:253–255.
141. Cinciripini GS, Donahue S, Borchert MS: Idiopathic intracranial hypertension in prepubertal pediatric patients: characteristics, treatment, and outcome. Am J Ophthalmol 1999;127:178–182.
142. Balcer LJ, Liu GT, Forman S, et al: Pediatric pseudotumor cerebri: relationship of age and obesity. Neurology 1999;52:870–872.
143. Liu GT, Kay MD, Bienfang DC, et al: Pseudotumor cerebri associated with corticosteroid withdrawal in inflammatory bowel disease. Am J Ophthalmol 1994;117:352–357.
144. Greer M: Benign intracranial hypertension. II. Following corticosteroid therapy. Neurology 1963;13: 439–441.
145. Dees SC, McKay HW: Occurrence of pseudotumor cerebri (benign intracranial hypertension) during treatment of children with asthma by adrenal steroids. Report of three cases. Pediatrics 1959;23:1143–1151.
146. Walker AE, Adamkiewicz JJ: Pseudotumor cerebri associated with prolonged corticosteroid therapy. Reports of four cases. JAMA 1964;188:779–784.
147. Gordon RC, Kelsey WM: Pseudotumor cerebri in congenital adrenal hyperplasia. Am J Dis Child 1967;113:727–729.
148. Neville BGR, Wilson J: Benign intracranial hypertension following corticosteroid withdrawal in childhood. Br Med J 1970;3:554–556.

149. Calcagno PL, Rubin MI: Physiologic considerations concerning corticosteroid therapy and complications in the nephrotic syndrome. J Pediatr 1961;58:686–706.
150. Cohn GA: Pseudotumor cerebri in children secondary to administration of adrenal steroids. J Neurosurg 1963;20:784–786.
151. Lubeck MJ: Papilledema caused by iron-deficiency anemia. Trans Am Acad Ophthalmol Otol 1959; 63:306–309.
152. Ikkala E, Laitinen L: Papilloedema due to iron deficiency anemia. Acta Haematol 1963;29:368–370.
153. Capriles LF: Intracranial hypertension and iron-deficiency anemia. Report of four cases. Arch Neurol 1963;9:147–153.
154. Schwaber JR, Blumberg AG: Papilledema associated with blood loss anemia. Ann Intern Med 1961; 55:1004–1007.
155. Digre KB, Varner MW, Corbett JJ: Pseudotumor cerebri and pregnancy. Neurology 1984;34:721–729.
156. Gardner K, Cox T, Digre KB: Idiopathic intracranial hypertension associated with tetracycline use in fraternal twins: case reports and review. Neurology 1995;45:6–10.
157. Chiu AM, Chuenkongkaew WL, Cornblath WT, et al: Minocycline treatment and pseudotumor cerebri syndrome. Am J Ophthalmol 1998;126:116–121.
158. Lee AG: Pseudotumor cerebri after treatment with tetracycline and isotretinoin for acne. Cutis 1995; 55:165–168.
159. Guy J, Johnston PK, Corbett JJ, et al: Treatment of visual loss in pseudotumor cerebri associated with uremia. Neurology 1990;40:28–32.
160. Johnston I: The reduced CSF absorption syndrome: a reappraisal of benign intracranial hypertension and related conditions. Lancet 1973;2:418–420.
161. Gjerris F, Sørensen PS, Vorstrup S, et al: Intracranial pressure, conductance to cerebrospinal fluid outflow and cerebral blood flow in patients with benign intracranial hypertension. Ann Neurol 1985;17:158–162.
162. Johnston I, Hawke S, Halmagyi M, et al: The pseudotumor syndrome. Disorders of cerebrospinal fluid circulation causing intracranial hypertension without ventriculomegaly. Arch Neurol 1991;48:740–747.
163. Malm J, Kristensen B, Markgren P, et al: CSF hydrodynamics in idiopathic intracranial hypertension: a long-term study. Neurology 1992;42:851–858.
164. Radhakrishnan K, Ahlskog JE, Garrity JA, et al: Idiopathic intracranial hypertension. Mayo Clin Proc 1994;69:169–180.
165. King JO, Mitchell PJ, Thomson KR, et al: Cerebral venography and manometry in idiopathic intracranial hypertension. Neurology 1995;45:2224–2228.
166. Karahalios DG, Rekate HL, Khayata MH, et al: Elevated intracranial venous pressure as a universal mechanism in pseudotumor cerebri of varying etiologies. Neurology 1996;46:198–202.
167. Sugerman HJ, DeMaria EJ, Felton WL, et al: Increased intra-abdominal pressure and cardiac filling pressures in obesity-associated pseudotumor cerebri. Neurology 1997;49:507–511.
168. Dandy WE: Intracranial pressure without brain tumor. Diagnosis and treatment. Ann Surg 1937;106:492–513.
169. Mathew NT, Meyer JS, Ott EO: Increased cerebral blood volume in benign intracranial hypertension. Neurology 1975;25:646–649.
170. Raichle ME, Grubb RL, Phelps ME, et al: Cerebral hemodynamics and metabolism in pseudotumor cerebri. Ann Neurol 1978;4:104–111.
171. Sahs AL, Joynt RJ: Brain swelling of unknown cause. Neurology 1956;6:791–803.
172. Soelberg Sørensen P, Thomsen C, Gjerris F, et al: Brain water accumulation in pseudotumor cerebri demonstrated by MR-imaging of brain water self-diffusion. Acta Neurochir (Suppl) 1990;51:363–365.
173. Gideon P, Sørensen PS, Thomsen C, et al: Increased brain water self-diffusion in patients with idiopathic intracranial hypertension. AJNR Am J Neuroradiol 1995;16:381–387.
174. Greer M: Benign intracranial hypertension. VI. Obesity. Neurology 1965;15:382–388.
175. Wall M, Dollar JD, Sadun AA, et al: Idiopathic intracranial hypertension. Lack of histologic evidence for cerebral edema. Arch Neurol 1995;52:141–145.
176. Fishman RA: Diseases of intracranial pressure: hydrocephalus, brain edema, pseudotumor, intracranial hypotension, and related disorders. In: Cerebrospinal Fluid in Diseases of the Nervous System, second ed, pp 103–155. Philadelphia, WB Saunders, 1992.
177. Gideon P, Sørensen PS, Thomsen C, et al: Assessment of CSF dynamics and venous flow in the superior sagittal sinus by MRI in idiopathic intracranial hypertension: a preliminary study. Neuroradiology 1994; 36:350–354.
178. Walsh FB: Papilledema associated with increased intracranial pressure in Addison's disease. Arch Ophthalmol 1952;47:86.
179. Alexandrakis G, Filatov V, Walsh T: Pseudotumor cerebri in a 12-year-old boy with Addison's disease. Am J Ophthalmol 1993;116:650–651.
180. Martin NA, Linfoot J, Wilson CB: Development of pseudotumor cerebri after the removal of an adrenocorticotropic hormone-secreting pituitary adenoma: case report. Neurosurgery 1981;8:699–702.
181. Weissman MN, Page LK, Bejar RL: Cushing's disease in childhood: benign intracranial hypertension after trans-sphenoidal adenomectomy. Neurosurgery 1983;13:195–197.
182. Friedman DI, Streeten DH: Idiopathic intracranial hypertension and orthostatic edema may share a common pathogenesis. Neurology 1998;50:1099–1104.
183. Soelberg Sørensen P, Gjerris F, Svenstrup B: Endocrine studies in patients with pseudotumor cerebri. Estrogen levels in blood and cerebrospinal fluid. Arch Neurol 1986;43:902–906.
184. Paterson R, DePasquale N, Mann S: Pseudotumor cerebri. Medicine 1961;40:85–99.
185. Rush JA: Pseudotumor cerebri. Clinical profile and visual outcome in 63 patients. Mayo Clin Proc 1980;55:541–546.
186. Biousse V, Newman NJ, Lessell S: Audible pulsatile tinnitus in idiopathic intracranial hypertension. Neurology 1998;50:1185–1186.
187. Lee AG: Pulsatile tinnitus as a presenting symptom of pseudotumour cerebri. J Otolaryngol 1996;25: 203–204.
188. O'Duffy D, James B, Elston J: Idiopathic intracranial hypertension presenting with gaze-evoked amaurosis. Acta Ophthalmol Scand 1998;76:119–120.
189. McCammon A, Kaufman HH, Sears ES: Transient oculomotor paralysis in pseudotumor cerebri. Neurology 1981;31:182–184.
190. Speer C, Pearlman J, Phillips PH, et al: Fourth cranial nerve palsy in pediatric patients with pseudotumor cerebri. Am J Ophthalmol 1999;127:236–237.
191. Friedman DI, Forman S, Levi L, et al: Unusual ocular motility disturbances with increased intracranial pressure. Neurology 1998;50:1893–1896.

192. Davie C, Kennedy P, Katifi HA: Seventh nerve palsy as a false localising sign [letter]. J Neurol Neurosurg Psychiatry 1992;55:510–511.
193. Davenport RJ, Will RG, Galloway PJ: Isolated intracranial hypertension presenting with trigeminal neuropathy [letter]. J Neurol Neurosurg Psychiatry 1994;57:381.
194. Dorman PJ, Campbell MJ, Maw AR: Hearing loss as a false localising sign in raised intracranial pressure [letter]. J Neurol Neurosurg Psychiatry 1995;58:516.
195. Selky AK, Dobyns WB, Yee RD: Idiopathic intracranial hypertension and facial diplegia. Neurology 1994;44:357.
196. Selky AK, Purvin VA: Hemifacial spasm. An unusual manifestation of idiopathic intracranial hypertension. J Neuro-ophthalmol 1994;14:196–198.
197. Benegas NM, Volpe NJ, Liu GT, et al: Hemifacial spasm and idiopathic intracranial hypertension [letter]. J Neuro-ophthalmol 1996;16:70.
198. Round R, Keane JR: The minor symptoms of increased intracranial pressure: 101 patients with benign intracranial hypertension. Neurology 1988;38: 1461–1464.
199. Miller NR: Walsh and Hoyt's Clinical Neuro-ophthalmology, fourth ed, pp 175–211. Baltimore, Williams & Wilkins, 1982.
200. Soelberg Sørensen P, Trojaborg W, Gjerris F, et al: Visual evoked potentials in pseudotumor cerebri. Arch Neurol 1985;42:150–153.
201. Verplanck M, Kaufman DI, Parsons T, et al: Electrophysiology versus psychophysics in the detection of visual loss in pseudotumor cerebri. Neurology 1988;38:1789–1792.
202. Wall M: Contrast sensitivity testing in pseudotumor cerebri. Ophthalmology 1986;93:4–7.
203. Keltner JL, Johnson CA: Short-wavelength automated perimetry in neuro-ophthalmic disorders. Arch Ophthalmol 1995;113:475–481.
204. Wall M, Montgomery EB: Using motion perimetry to detect visual field defects in patients with idiopathic intracranial hypertension: a comparison with conventional automated perimetry. Neurology 1995;45: 1169–1175.
205. Wall M, White WN: Asymmetric papilledema in idiopathic intracranial hypertension: prospective interocular comparison of sensory visual function. Invest Ophthalmol Vis Sci 1998;39:134–142.
206. Marcelis J, Silberstein SD: Idiopathic intracranial hypertension without papilledema. Arch Neurol 1991; 48:392–399.
207. Mathew NT, Ravishankar K, Sanin LC: Coexistence of migraine and idiopathic intracranial hypertension without papilledema. Neurology 1996;46:1226–1230.
208. Krishna R, Kosmorsky GS, Wright KW: Pseudotumor cerebri sine papilledema with unilateral sixth nerve palsy. J Neuro-ophthalmol 1998;18:53–55.
209. Wang SJ, Silberstein SD, Patterson S, et al: Idiopathic intracranial hypertension without papilledema: a case-control study in a headache center. Neurology 1998;51:245–249.
210. Mashima Y, Oshitari K, Imamura Y, et al: High-resolution magnetic resonance imaging of the intraorbital optic nerve and subarachnoid space in patients with papilledema and optic atrophy. Arch Ophthalmol 1996;114:1197–1203.
211. Gibby WA, Cohen M, Goldberg HI, et al: Pseudotumor cerebri: CT findings and correlation with vision loss. Am J Radiol 1993;160:143–146.
212. Brodsky MC, Glasier CM: Magnetic resonance visualization of the swollen optic disc in papilledema. J Neuro-ophthalmol 1995;15:122–124.
213. Brodsky MC, Vaphiades M: Magnetic resonance imaging in pseudotumor cerebri. Ophthalmology 1998;105:1686–1693.
214. Weisberg LA, Housepian EM, Saur DA: Empty sella syndrome and complication of benign intracranial hypertension. J Neurosurg 1975;43:177–180.
215. Foley KM, Posner JB: Does pseudotumor cerebri cause the empty sella syndrome? Neurology 1975;25:565–569.
216. Weisberg LA: Computerized tomography in benign intracranial hypertension. Neurology 1985;35:1075–1078.
217. Jacobson DM, Karanjia PN, Olson KA, et al: Computerized tomography ventricular size has no predictive value in diagnosing pseudotumor cerebri. Neurology 1990;40:1454–1455.
218. Rothwell PM, Gibson RJ, Sellar RJ: Computed tomographic evidence of cerebral swelling in benign intracranial hypertension. J Neurol Neurosurg Psychiatry 1994;57:1407–1409.
219. Sullivan HC: Fatal tonsillar herniation in pseudotumor cerebri. Neurology 1991;41:1142–1144.
220. Chandra V, Bellur SN, Anderson RJ: Low CSF protein concentration in idiopathic pseudotumor cerebri. Ann Neurol 1986;19:80–82.
221. Johnston PK, Corbett JJ, Maxner CE: Cerebrospinal fluid protein and opening pressure in idiopathic intracranial hypertension (pseudotumor cerebri). Neurology 1991;41:1040–1042.
222. Practice parameters: Lumbar puncture (summary statement). Neurology 1993;43:625–627.
223. Shuper A, Snir M, Barash D, et al: Ultrasonography of the optic nerves: clinical application in children with pseudotumor cerebri. J Pediatr 1997;131: 734–740.
224. Trick GL, Vesti E, Tawansy K, et al: Quantitative evaluation of papilledema in pseudotumor cerebri. Invest Ophthalmol Vis Sci 1998;39:1964–1971.
225. Mulholland DA, Craig JJ, Rankin SJ: Use of scanning laser ophthalmoscopy to monitor papilloedema in idiopathic intracranial hypertension. Br J Ophthalmol 1998;82:1301–1305.
226. Newborg B: Pseudotumor cerebri treated by rice/reduction diet. Arch Intern Med 1974;133:802–807.
227. Sugerman HJ, Felton WL, Salvant JB, et al: Effects of surgically induced weight loss on idiopathic intracranial hypertension in morbid obesity. Neurology 1995;45:1655–1659.
228. Johnson LN, Krohel GB, Madsen RW, et al: The role of weight loss and acetazolamide in the treatment of idiopathic intracranial hypertension (pseudotumor cerebri). Ophthalmology 1998;105:2313–2317.
229. Kupersmith MJ, Gamell L, Turbin R, et al: Effects of weight loss on the course of idiopathic intracranial hypertension in women. Neurology 1998;50:1094–1098.
230. Smith JL: Pseudotumor cerebri. Trans Am Acad Ophthalmol Otol 1958;62:432–440.
231. Kessler LA, Novelli PM, Reigel DH: Surgical treatment of benign intracranial hypertension—subtemporal decompression revisited. Surg Neurol 1998;50:73–76.
232. Gücer G, Viernstein L: Long-term intracranial pressure recording in the management of pseudotumor cerebri. J Neurosurg 1978;49:256–263.

233. Schoeman JF: Childhood pseudotumor cerebri: clinical and intracranial pressure response to acetazolamide and furosemide treatment in a case series. J Child Neurol 1994;9:130–134.
234. Liu GT, Volpe NJ, Galetta SL: Pseudotumor cerebri and its medical treatment. Drugs of Today 1998; 34:563–574.
235. Tomsak RL, Niffenegger AS, Remler BF: Treatment of psudotumor cerebri with Diamox (acetazolamide). J Clin Neuro-ophthalmol 1988;8:93–98.
236. Wandstrat TL, Phillips J: Pseudotumor cerebri responsive to acetazolamide [letter]. Ann Pharmacother 1995;29:318.
237. Alward WLM: Medical management of glaucoma. N Engl J Med 1998;339:1298–1307.
238. Lichter PR: Reducing side effects of carbonic anhydrase inhibitors. Ophthalmology 1981;88:266–269.
239. Smith JL, Hoyt WF, Newton TH: Optic nerve sheath decompression for relief of chronic monocular choked discs. Am J Ophthalmol 1969;68:633–639.
240. Brourman ND, Spoor TC, Ramocki JM: Optic nerve sheath decompression for pseudotumor cerebri. Arch Ophthalmol 1988;106:1378–1383.
241. Sergott RC, Savino PJ, Bosley TM: Modified optic nerve sheath decompression provides long-term visual improvement for pseudotumor cerebri. Arch Ophthalmol 1988;106:1384–1390.
242. Corbett JJ, Nerad JA, Tse DT, et al: Results of optic nerve sheath fenestration for pseudotumor cerebri. The lateral orbitotomy approach. Arch Ophthalmol 1988;106:1391–1397.
243. Pearson PA, Baker RS, Khorram R, et al: Evaluation of optic nerve sheath fenestration in pseudotumor cerebri using automated perimetry. Ophthalmology 1991;98:99–105.
244. Kelman SE, Heaps R, Wolf A, et al: Optic nerve decompression surgery improves visual function in patients with pseudotumor cerebri. Neurosurg 1992;30:391–395.
245. Tse DT, Nerad JA, Anderson RL, et al: Optic nerve sheath fenestration in pseudotumor cerebri. A lateral orbitotomy approach. Arch Ophthalmol 1988;106: 1458–1462.
246. Rizzuto PR, Spoor TC, Ramocki JM, et al: Subtenon's local anesthesia for optic nerve sheath fenestration. Am J Ophthalmol 1996;121:326–327.
247. Spoor TC, McHenry JG, Shin DH: Long-term results using adjunctive mitomycin C in optic nerve sheath decompression for pseudotumor cerebri. Ophthalmology 1995;102:2024–2028.
248. Spoor TC, McHenry JG, Shin DH: Optic nerve sheath decompression with adjunctive mitomycin and Molteno device implantation [letter]. Arch Ophthalmol 1994;112:25–26.
249. Spoor TC, McHenry JG: Complications of optic nerve sheath decompression [letter]. Ophthalmology 1993; 100:1432.
250. Plotnik JL, Kosmorsky GS: Operative complications of optic nerve sheath decompression. Ophthalmology 1993;100:683–690.
251. Rizzo JF, Lessell S: Choroidal infarction after optic nerve sheath fenestration. Ophthalmology 1994; 101:1622–1626.
252. Flynn WJ, Westfall CT, Weisman JS: Transient blindness after optic nerve sheath fenestration [letter]. Am J Ophthalmol 1994;117:678–679.
253. Brodsky MC, Rettele GA: Protracted postsurgical blindness with visual recovery following optic nerve sheath fenestration. Arch Ophthalmol 1997;115:1473–1474.
254. Keltner JL: Optic nerve sheath decompression. How does it work? Has its time come? [editorial]. Arch Ophthalmol 1988;106:1365–1369.
255. Seiff SR, Shah L: A model for the mechanism of optic nerve sheath fenestration. Arch Ophthalmol 1990; 108:1326–1329.
256. Tsai JC, Petrovich MS, Sadun AA: Histopathological and ultrastructural examination of optic nerve sheath decompression. Br J Ophthalmol 1995;79:182–185.
257. Hamed LM, Tse DT, Glaser JS, et al: Neuroimaging of the optic nerve after fenestration for management of pseudotumor cerebri. Arch Ophthalmol 1992; 110:636–639.
258. Burde RM, Karp JS, Miller RN: Reversal of visual deficit with optic nerve decompression in long-standing pseudotumor cerebri. Am J Ophthalmol 1974;77:770–772.
259. Kaye AH, Galbraith JFK, King J: Intracranial pressure following optic nerve decompression for benign intracranial hypertension. J Neurosurg 1981;55: 453–456.
260. Spoor TC, Ramocki JM, Madion MP, et al: Treatment of pseudotumor cerebri by primary and secondary optic nerve sheath decompression. Am J Ophthalmol 1991;112:177–185.
261. Spoor TC, McHenry JG: Long-term effectiveness of optic nerve sheath decompression for pseudotumor cerebri. Arch Ophthalmol 1993;111:632–635.
262. Liu GT, Glaser JS, Schatz NJ: High-dose methylprednisolone and acetazolamide for visual loss in pseudotumor cerebri. Am J Ophthalmol 1994;118:88–96.
263. Mauriello JA, Shaderowfsky P, Gizzi M, et al: Management of visual loss after optic nerve sheath decompression in patients with pseudotumor cerebri. Ophthalmology 1995;102:441–445.
264. Eggenberger ER, Miller NR, Vitale S: Lumboperitoneal shunt for the treatment of pseudotumor cerebri. Neurology 1996;46:1524–1530.
265. Burgett RA, Purvin VA, Kawasaki A: Lumboperitoneal shunting for pseudotumor cerebri. Neurology 1997;49:734–739.
266. Rosenberg ML, Corbett JJ, Smith C, et al: Cerebrospinal fluid diversion procedures in pseudotumor cerebri. Neurology 1993;43:1071–1072.
267. Tulipan N, Lavin PJ, Copeland M: Stereotactic ventriculoperitoneal shunt for idiopathic intracranial hypertension: technical note. Neurosurg 1998;43: 175–176.
268. Gordon DL: The diagnosis and management of cerebral venous thrombosis. In: Adams HP (ed): Handbook of Cerebrovascular Diseases, pp 591–612. New York, Marcel Dekker, 1993.
269. Daif A, Awada A, Al-Rajeh S, et al: Cerebral venous thrombosis in adults. A study of 40 cases from Saudi Arabia. Stroke 1995;26:1193–1195.
270. Mokri B, Jack CR, Petty GW: Pseudotumor syndrome associated with cerebral venous sinus occlusion and antiphospholipid antibodies. Stroke 1993;24:469–472.
271. Confavreux C, Brunet P, Petiot P, et al: Congenital protein C deficiency and superior sagittal sinus thrombosis causing isolated intracranial hypertension. J Neurol Neurosurg Psychiatry 1994;57:655–657.
272. Purvin VA, Trobe JD, Kosmorsky G: Neuro-ophthalmic features of cerebral venous obstruction. Arch Neurol 1995;52:880–885.
273. Silberberg DS, Laties AM: Increased intracranial pressure in disseminated lupus erythematosus. Arch Neurol 1973;29:88–90.

274. Carlow TJ, Glaser JS: Pseudotumor cerebri syndrome in systemic lupus erythematosus. JAMA 1974;228: 197–200.
275. Li EK, Ho PCP: Pseudotumor cerebri in systemic lupus erythematosus. J Rheumatol 1989;16:113–116.
276. Li EK, Chan MSY: Is pseudotumor cerebri in SLE a thrombotic event? [letter]. J Rheumatol 1990;17: 983–984.
277. Vidailhet M, Piette J-C, Wechsler B, et al: Cerebral venous thrombosis in systemic lupus erythematosus. Stroke 1990;21:1226–1231.
278. Al-Hakim M, Katirji MB, Osorio I, et al: Cerebral venous thrombosis in paroxysmal nocturnal hemoglobinuria: report of two cases. Neurology 1993; 43:742–746.
279. Hauser D, Barzilai N, Zalish M, et al: Bilateral papilledema with retinal hemorrhages in association with cerebral venous sinus thrombosis and paroxysmal nocturnal hemoglobinuria. Am J Ophthalmol 1996;122:592–593.
280. Case Records of the MGH: Case 20-1988. N Engl J Med 1988;318:1322–1328.
281. Cohen SM, Keltner JL: Thrombosis of the lateral transverse sinus with papilledema. Arch Ophthalmol 1993;111:274–275.
282. Cremer PD, Thompson EO, Johnston IH, et al: Pseudotumor cerebri and cerebral venous hypertension. Neurology 1996;47:1602–1603.
283. Lam BL, Schatz NJ, Glaser JS, et al: Pseudotumor cerebri from cranial venous obstruction. Ophthalmology 1992;99:706–712.
284. Horton JC, Seiff SR, Pitts LH, et al: Decompression of the optic nerve sheath for vision-threatening papilledema caused by dural sinus occlusion. Neurosurgery 1992;31:203–212.
285. Angeli SI, Sato Y, Gantz BJ: Glomus jugulare tumors masquerading as benign intracranial hypertension. Arch Otolaryngol Head Neck Surg 1994;120:1277–1280.
286. Kuehnen J, Schwartz A, Neff W, et al: Cranial nerve syndrome in thrombosis of the transverse/sigmoid sinuses. Brain 1998;121:381–388.
287. Crawford SC, Digre KB, Palmer CA, et al: Thrombosis of the deep venous drainage of the brain in adults. Arch Neurol 1995;52:1101–1108.
288. Horowitz M, Purdy P, Unwin H, et al: Treatment of dural sinus thrombosis using selective catheterization and urokinase. Ann Neurol 1995;38:58–67.
289. Acheson JF, Green WT, Sanders MD: Optic nerve sheath decompression for the treatment of visual failure in chronic raised intracranial pressure. J Neurol Neurosurg Psychiatry 1994;57:1426–1429.
290. Cockerell OC, Lai HM, Ross-Russell RW: Pseudotumour cerebri associated with arteriovenous malformations. Postgrad Med J 1993;69:637–640.
291. Martin TJ, Bell DA, Wilson JA: Papilledema in a man with an "occult" dural arteriovenous malformation. J Neuro-ophthalmol 1998;18:49–52.
292. Chimowitz MI, Little JR, Awad IA, et al: Intracranial hypertension associated with unruptured cerebral arteriovenous malformations. Ann Neurol 1990;27: 474–479.
293. Kühner A, Drastel A, Stoll W: Arteriovenous malformations of the transverse dural sinus. J Neurosurg 1976;45:12–19.
294. Cognard C, Gobin YP, Pierot L, et al: Cerebral dural arteriovenous fistulas: clinical and angiographic correlation with a revised classification of venous drainage. Radiology 1995;194:671–680.
295. David CA, Peerless SJ: Pseudotumor syndrome resulting from a cerebral arteriovenous malformation: case report. Neurosurg 1995;36:588–590.
296. Jozefowicz RF: Neurologic manifestations of pulmonary disease. Neurol Clin 1989;7:605–616.
297. Kirkpatrick PJ, Meyer T, Sarkies N, et al: Papilledema and visual failure in a patient with nocturnal hypoventilation [letter]. J Neurol Neurosurg Psychiatry 1994;57:1546–1547.
298. Wolin MJ, Brannon WL: Disk edema in an overweight woman. Surv Ophthalmol 1995;39:307–314.
299. Fantin A, Feist RM, Reddy CV: Intracranial hypertension and papilloedema in chronic inflammatory demyelinating polyneuropathy. Br J Ophthalmol 1993;77:193.
300. Midroni G, Dyck PJ: Chronic inflammatory demyelinating polyradiculoneuropathy: unusual clinical features and therapeutic responses. Neurology 1996;46:1206–1212.
301. Ropper AH, Wijdicks EFM, Truax BT: Papilledema and pseudotumor cerebri. Clinical features of Guillain–Barré syndrome. In: Guillain-Barré Syndrome, pp 94–95. Philadelphia, FA Davis, 1991.
302. Michaud LJ, Ried SR, Liu GT, et al: Pseudotumor cerebri with loss of vision in Guillain–Barré syndrome [abstract]. Arch Phys Med Rehabil 1994;75: 1050–1051.
303. Ersahin Y, Mutluer S, Yurtseven T: Hydrocephalus in Guillain–Barré syndrome. Clin Neurol Neurosurg 1995;97:253–255.
304. Weiss GB, Bajwa ZH, Mehler MF: Co-occurrence of pseudotumor cerebri and Guillain-Barré syndrome in an adult. Neurology 1991;41:603–604.
305. Gross FJ, Mindel JS: Pseudotumor cerebri and Guillain–Barré syndrome associated with human immunodeficiency virus infection. Neurology 1991;41: 1845–1846.
306. Matzkin DC, Slamovits TL, Genis I, et al: Disc swelling: a tall tail? Surv Ophthalmol 1992;37:130–136.
307. Oikawa S, Kyoshima K, Takemae T, et al: Multiple spinal neurinomas presenting visual disturbance as the initial symptom: case report. Surg Neurol 1992;38:309–314.
308. Breen LA: Disk edema and peripheral neuropathy. Surv Ophthalmol 1994;38:467–474.
309. Condulis N, Germain G, Charest N, et al: Pseudotumor cerebri: a presenting manifestation of Addison's disease. Clin Pediatr 1997;36:711–713.
310. Malozowski S, Tanner LA, Wysowski D, et al: Growth hormone, insulin-like growth factor I, and benign intracranial hypertension [letter]. N Engl J Med 1993;329:665–666.
311. Price DA, Clayton PE, Lloyd IC: Benign intracranial hypertension induced by growth hormone treatment [letter]. Lancet 1995;345:458–459.
312. Crock PA, McKenzie JD, Nicoll AM, et al: Benign intracranial hypertension and recombinant growth hormone therapy in Australia and New Zealand. Acta Paediatr 1998;87:381–386.
313. Rogers AH, Rogers GL, Bremer DL, et al: Pseudotumor cerebri in children receiving recombinant human growth hormone. Ophthalmology 1999;106:1186–1190.
314. Raghavan S, DiMartino-Nardi J, Saenger P, et al: Pseudotumor cerebri in an infant after L-thyroxine therapy for transient neonatal hypothyroidism. J Pediatr 1997;130:478–480.
315. Panozzo G, Babighian S, Bonora A: Association of xerophthalmia, flecked retina, and pseudotumor

cerebri caused by hypovitaminosis A. Am J Ophthalmol 1998;125:708–710.
316. Traverso F, Stagnaro R, Fazio B: Benign intracranial hypertension associated with HIV infection. Eur Neurol 1993;33:191–192.
317. Javeed N, Shaikh J, Jayaram S: Recurrent pseudotumor cerebri in an HIV-positive patient [letter]. AIDS 1995;9:817–819.
318. Keren T, Lahat E: Pseudotumor cerebri as a presenting symptom of acute sinusitis in a child. Pediatr Neurol 1998;19:153–154.
319. Mahmoud HH, Hurwitz CA, Roberts WM, et al: Tretinoin toxicity in children with acute promyelocytic leukaemia. Lancet 1993;342:1394–1395.
320. Degos L, Dombret H, Chomienne C, et al: All-*trans*-retinoic acid as a differentiating agent in the treatment of acute promyelocytic leukemia. Blood 1995;85:2643–2653.
321. Varadi G, Lossos A, Or R, et al: Successful allogeneic bone marrow transplantation in a patient with ATRA-induced pseudotumor cerebri [letter]. Am J Hematol 1995;50:147–148.
322. Colovic MD, Jankovic GM, Elezovic I, et al: Effect of all-trans-retinoic acid alone or in combination with chemotherapy in newly diagnosed acute promyelocytic leukaemia. Medical Oncology 1997;14:65–72.
323. Sano F, Tsuji K, Kunika N, et al: Pseudotumor cerebri in a patient with acute promyelocytic leukemia during treatment with all-trans-retinoic acid. Intern Med 1998;37:546–549.
324. Antcliff RJ, Spalton DJ: Are optic disc drusen inherited? Ophthalmology 1999;106:1278–1281.
325. Kurz-Levin MM, Landau K: A comparison of imaging techniques for diagnosing drusen of the optic nerve head. Arch Ophthalmol 1999;117:1045–1049.
326. Case Records of the MGH: Case 10-1987. N Engl J Med 1987;316:606–618.
327. Quinn AG, Singer SB, Buncic JR: Pediatric tetracycline-induced pseudotumor cerebri. J AAPOS 1999;3:53–57.
328. Jacobson DM, Berg R, Wall M, et al: Serum vitamin A concentration is elevated in idiopathic intracranial hypertension. Neurology 1999;53:1114–1118.
329. Obeid T, Awada A, Huraib S, et al: Pseudotumor cerebri in renal transplant recipients: a diagnostic challenge. J Nephrology 1997;10:258–260.
330. Sallomi D, Taylor H, Hibbert J, et al: The MRI appearance of the optic nerve sheath following fenestration for benign intracranial hypertension. Eur Radiol 1998;8:1193–1996.
331. Rowe FJ, Sarkis NJ: Visual outcome in a prospective study of idiopathic intracranial hypertension. Arch Ophthalmol 1999;117:1571.
332. Lee AG, patrinely JR, Edmond JC: Optic nerve sheath decompression in pediatric psuedotumor cerebri. Ophthalmic Surg Lasers 1998;29:514–517.
333. Biousse V, Ameri A, Bousser M-G: Isolated intracranial hypertension as the only sign of cerebral venous thrombosis. Neurology 1999;1537–1542.
334. Kikuchi M, Kudo S, Wada M, et al: Retropharyngeal rhabdomyosarcoma mimicking pseudotumor cerebri. Pediatr Neurol 1999;21:496–499.
335. O'Halloran HS, Berger JR, Baker RS, et al: Optic nerve edema as a consequence of respiratory disease. Neurology 1999;53:2204–2205.

CHAPTER 7

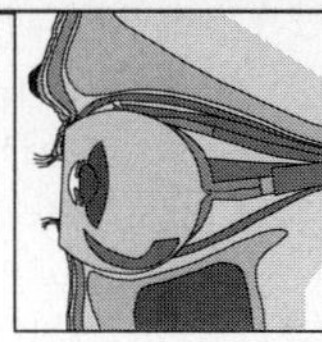

Vision Loss: Disorders of the Chiasm

Chiasmal disorders are important in the differential diagnosis of anterior visual pathway dysfunction, particularly when the visual loss is gradually progressive. Involvement of the chiasm is suggested by (1) a monocular or bitemporal hemianopia, or (2) visual loss of any type associated with endocrine dysfunction. The most common causes are compressive sellar masses, and therefore the diagnosis and management depends heavily on neuroimaging. These lesions produce visual acuity and field deficits by interfering with the optic nerves, chiasm, or optic tracts or, less often, by obstructing the third ventricle and causing chronic atrophic papilledema. Endocrinopathy is the result of pituitary, stalk, or hypothalamic dysfunction, while ocular motility abnormalities can result from lateral extension and involvement of the cavernous sinuses. Because sellar masses are so frequently associated with visual disturbances, neuro-ophthalmic evaluation often leads to their detection and is important for pretreatment assessment and subsequent follow-up.

Anatomic aspects of the chiasm and sellar and parasellar structures will be reviewed first, followed by a discussion of the neuro-ophthalmic signs and symptoms of chiasmal disease. Because of its clinical importance, pituitary and hypothalamic physiology also will be covered. The differential diagnosis of the various entities affecting the chiasm then will be discussed, in the context of the patient's age, clinical history, general physical findings, neuroimaging, and endocrine testing. Finally, the clinical features and treatment of these disorders will be detailed, with the greatest emphasis placed on the most common disorders: pituitary adenomas, craniopharyngiomas, meningiomas, aneurysms, and chiasmal–hypothalamic gliomas.

NEUROANATOMY

Intracranially, the optic nerves ascend and converge medially to join at the optic chiasm, which has the shape of the letter X when viewed from above or below. The chiasm tilts forward at an angle of 45 degrees and lies in the subarachnoid (cerebrospinal fluid (CSF) filled) space of the suprasellar cistern (Fig. 7–1). It is approximately 12 mm wide, 8 mm in anteroposterior diameter, and 4 mm thick.[1] Its posterior portion forms the anterior and inferior wall of the third ventricle. The chiasm lies inferior to the hypothalmus and anterior to the pituitary stalk (or infundibulum, which connects the hypothalamus and the pituitary) (Fig. 7–2). The pituitary gland sits 10 mm below the chiasm in a recess in the sphenoid bone called the sella turcica. The bony boundaries of the sella include the tuberculum sellae anteriorly, the dorsum sellae posteriorly, and the anterior and posterior clinoid processes superiorly (Fig. 7–3).[2] The cavernous sinuses, containing cranial nerves III, IV, V1, V2, and VI, the internal carotid arteries, and sympathetic fibers, form the lateral walls of the sella. The diaphragma sellae, penetrated only by the pituitary stalk, is a horizontal fold of dura mater that separates the pituitary gland from the suprasellar cistern (Fig. 7–3).[3] In 80% of individuals, the chiasm is located directly above the

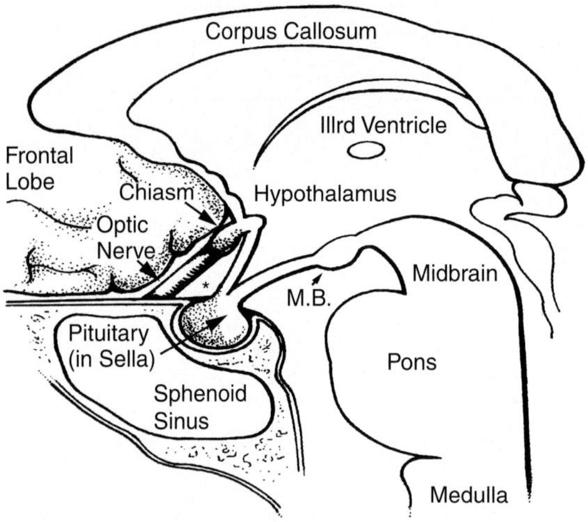

FIGURE 7–1. Sagittal view of the brain detailing the chiasm and surrounding structures. Note the optic nerves and chiasm rise at approximately 45 degrees. The chiasm lies in a CSF-filled space called the suprasellar cistern (*) bordered superiorly by the frontal lobe and inferiorly by the diaphragma sellae (which forms the roof of the sella above the pituitary gland). The chiasm is also located at the anterior and inferior part of the third ventricle, immediately inferior to the hypothalmus. M.B. = mammillary body.

pituitary gland, while in 15% it lies over the tuberculum sellae (prefixed chiasm), and in 5% it is over the dorsum sellae (postfixed chiasm) (Fig. 7–4).[4–6]

Magnetic resonance imaging (MRI) provides exquisite detail of the sellar area (Fig. 7–5). Normally on T_1-weighted MR coronal images the body of the chiasm has a dumbbell shape[460] and is located in the middle of the suprasellar cistern. More anteriorly the two optic nerves are visible, but more posteriorly the chiasm lies sandwiched between the vertically oriented third ventricle above it and the pituitary stalk below it. On coronal images within the sella the pituitary gland appears flat, and the cavernous sinuses are lateral to it. The pituitary stalk and cavernous sinuses normally enhance with gadolinium. On sagittal sections, the titled chiasm is easily identified above the pituitary. On T_1-weighted images, the anterior pituitary is isointense with the pons, but the posterior portion of pituitary is bright.[7] Details of the chiasm and sellar region are less evident with computed tomography (CT) scanning.[8]

At the chiasm, axons from the nasal retinal ganglion cells (temporal visual field) from both eyes cross, and the most ventral axons originating in the inferonasal retina bend temporarily up to 3 mm into axons of the contralateral optic nerve (Wilbrand's knee[9]) (Fig. 7–6). Recently the knee's existence has been questioned and attributed to artefact of long-term monocular enucleation.[10] Fibers from the temporal retina (containing information from the nasal field) remain ipsilateral. The ratio of crossed to uncrossed fibers is 53 : 47. The fibers transmitting visual information from the superior retina remain superior in the chiasm; those from the inferior retina remain inferiorly situated.[11,12] Approximately 90% of chiasmal fibers originate from the macula,[5] and of these, the ones that cross lie superiorly and posteriorly within the chiasm.

Most of the ganglion cell axons travelling through the optic chiasm exit posteriorly and diverge to form the left and right optic tracts. Each tract is made up of ipsilateral temporal fibers and contralateral nasal fibers. There may also exist retinal projections from the posterior chiasm to the hypothalamus, specifically the suprachiasmic nucleus or the supraoptic nucleus.[13] This pathway is thought to mediate the visual input responsible for diurnal variations of various neuroendocrine systems.

The supraclinoid portions of the carotid arteries ascend lateral to the optic chiasm. The precommunicating segments of the anterior cerebral arteries and the anterior communicating arteries are located anterior and superior (dorsal) to the chiasm. Because of the chiasm's upward tilt, the posterior portion of the circle of Willis lies behind and below it (ventral) (Fig. 7–2).[14] The chiasm derives its blood supply from an inferior and superior anastomotic group of vessels. The inferior group is made up of the superior hypophyseal arteries, which derive their blood supply from the internal carotid, posterior communicating, and posterior cerebral arteries. The superior group of vessels consists of precommunicating branches of the anterior cerebral arteries.[14] There is evidence to suggest that the body of the chiasm receives its blood supply only from the inferior group, while the lateral parts of the chiasm are fed by branches from both inferior and superior groups.[15]

NEURO-OPHTHALMIC SYMPTOMS AND SIGNS IN CHIASMAL DISORDERS

Visual Symptoms

Because most chiasmal disturbances are caused by compressive lesions, the visual loss

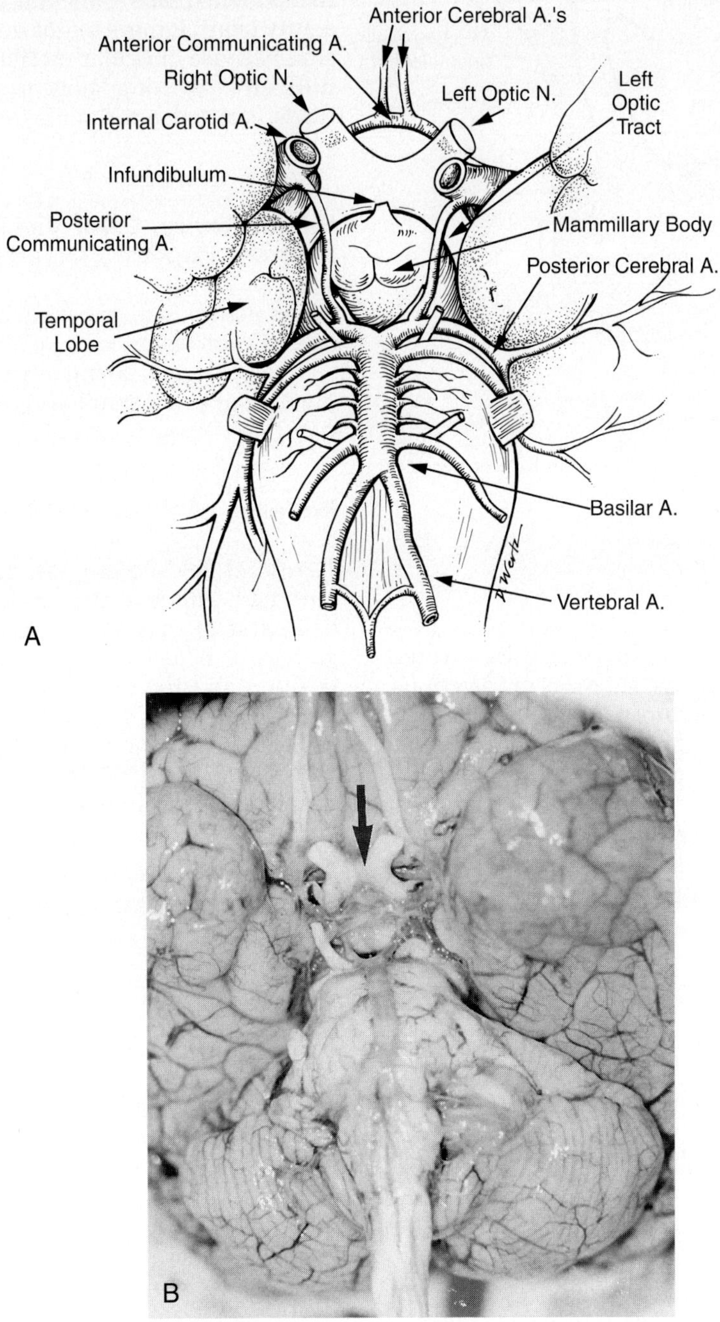

FIGURE 7–2. A. Ventral view of the brain detailing the chiasm and its relationship with the circle of Willis. Note the anterior cerebral and anterior communicating arteries lie superior (dorsal) to the optic nerves and chiasm, while the posterior communicating arteries lie inferior (ventral) to the chiasm and optic tracts. The infundibulum is immediately posterior to the body of the chiasm. A. = artery, N. = nerve. **B.** Ventral side of autopsy specimen (view corresponds roughly to the drawing in part A). The black arrow points to the chiasm.

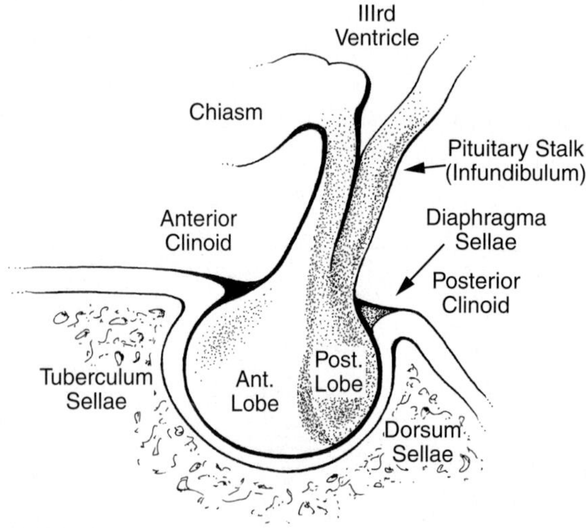

FIGURE 7–3. Drawing, sagittal view, of the chiasm, pituitary gland, and sella. Ant. Lobe = anterior lobe of the pituitary gland. Post. Lobe = posterior lobe of the pituitary gland.

is usually insidious. Acute visual loss would imply a rapidly expanding mass or infectious, vascular, or inflammatory cause, and these situations may mimic retrobulbar optic neuritis. Visual complaints are usually vague, often reflecting blurry or hazy vision or difficulty reading or focusing. Patients with slowly progressive chiasmal field loss may be without visual complaints unless acuity is abnormal,[16] and a temporal field defect may not be apparent until the patient reads only the nasal half of the acuity chart. Others might describe double vision because of ocular motility dysfunction or difficulty aligning noncorresponding nasal fields (see sensory double vision, below).

Visual Acuity, Color Vision, and Afferent Pupillary Defects

When acuity is diminished, asymmetry is the rule.[5] Color vision may be altered only in defective fields, and asymmetric lesions may produce an afferent pupillary defect.

Patterns of Visual Field Loss

Temporal field defects respecting the vertical meridian, either in one or both eyes, are the hallmarks of chiasmal dysfunction. The actual pattern of field loss depends on the chiasm's position and the exact location of the culprit lesion (Fig. 7–6). For instance, if the process affects the crossing nasal fibers in the body of the chiasm, in the case of sellar mass growing upward and impinging upon a normally situated chiasm, a classic bitemporal hemianopia

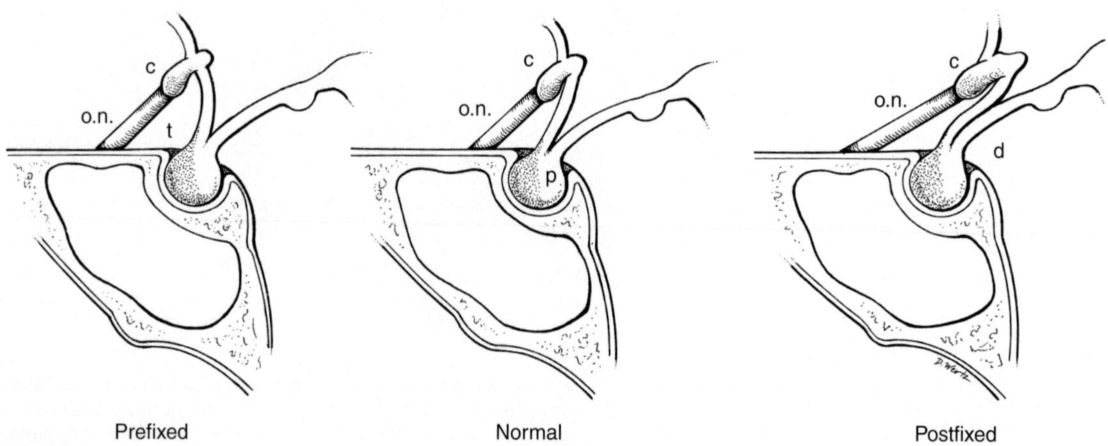

FIGURE 7–4. Relationship of the chiasm to the sella (sagittal views). Normally, in approximately 80% of individuals, the chiasm (c) is directly above the pituitary gland (p). In 15% the chiasm is prefixed and over the tuberculum sella (t), and in the remaining 5% it is postfixed and over the dorsum sella (d). o.n. = optic nerve. (Redrawn from AL Rhoton, FS Harris, WH Renn. Neuro-ophthalmology Symposium of the University of Miami and the Bascom Palmer Eye Institute, JS Glaser (ed), pp 75–105. St. Louis, C. V. Mosby, 1973, with permission.)

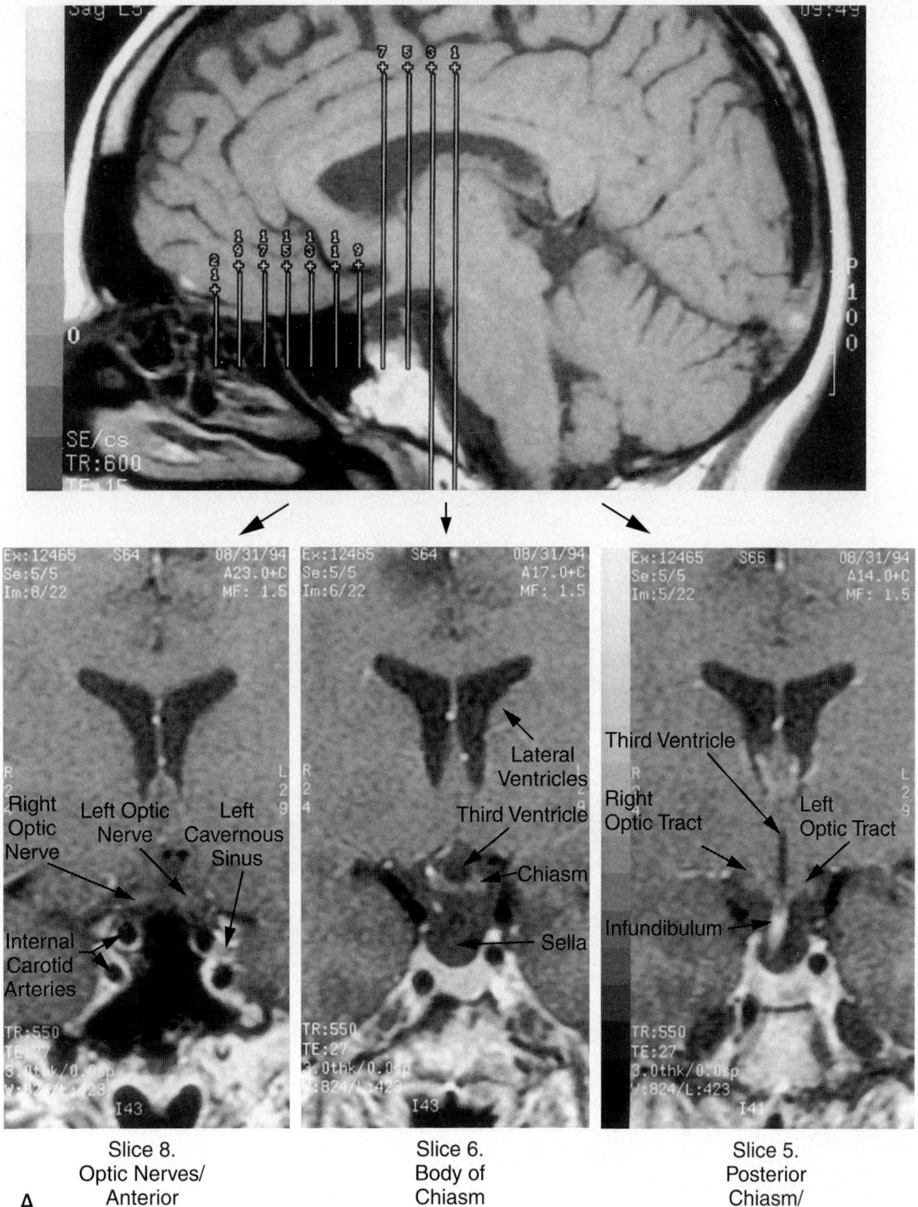

FIGURE 7–5. A. *Top:* Sagittal MRI (T_1-weighted) through the chiasm (see Fig. 7–1 for corresponding illustration and labeling of structures. *Bottom:* Corresponding coronal sections (T_1-weighted with gadolinium) through the optic nerves/anterior chiasm, body of chiasm, and posterior chiasm/optic tracts. The slice numbers are indicated in the sagittal image.

Illustration continued on following page

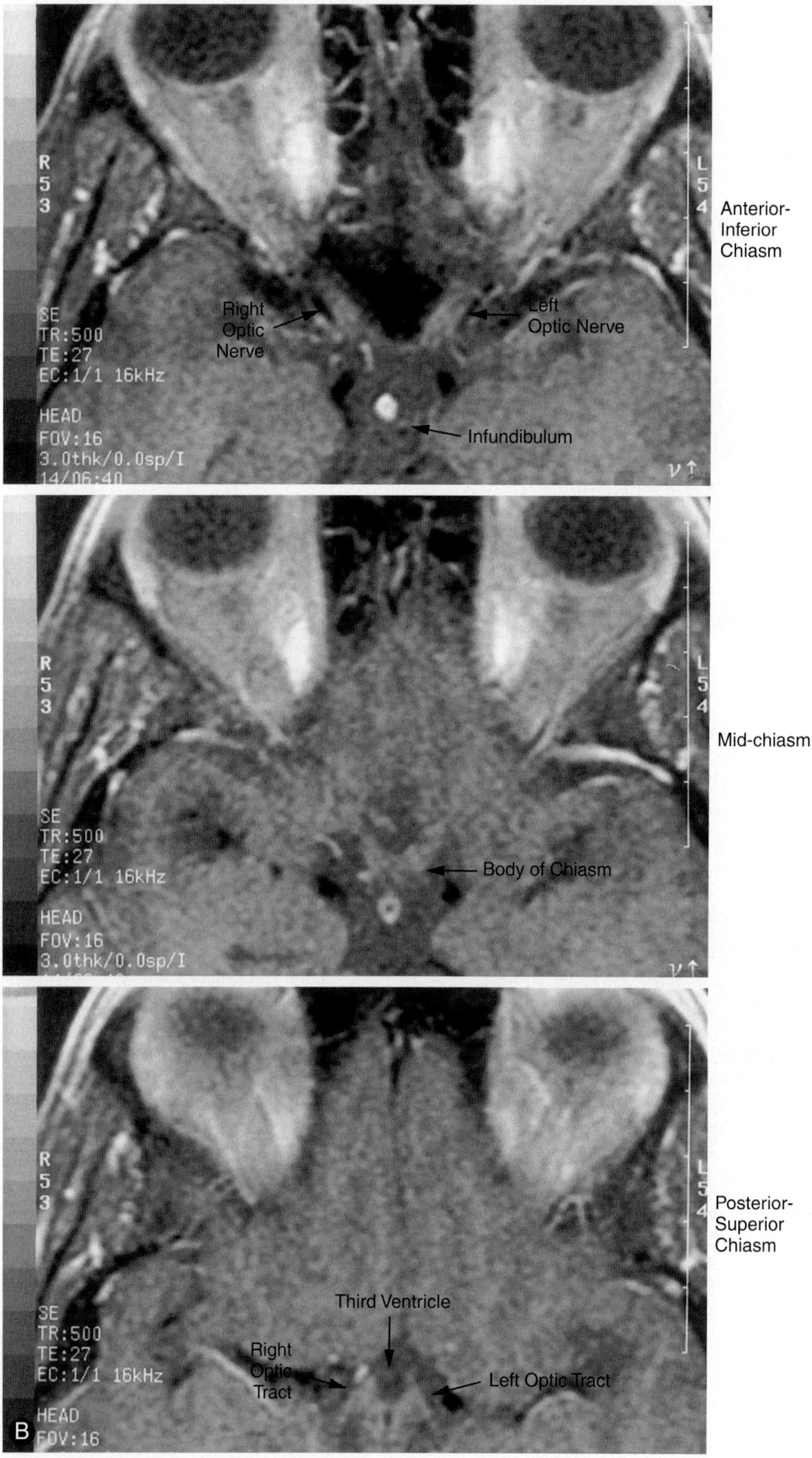

FIGURE 7–5 *Continued.* **B.** Axial MRI scans (gadolinium enhanced) through the anterior-inferior, mid-, and posterior-superior chiasm.

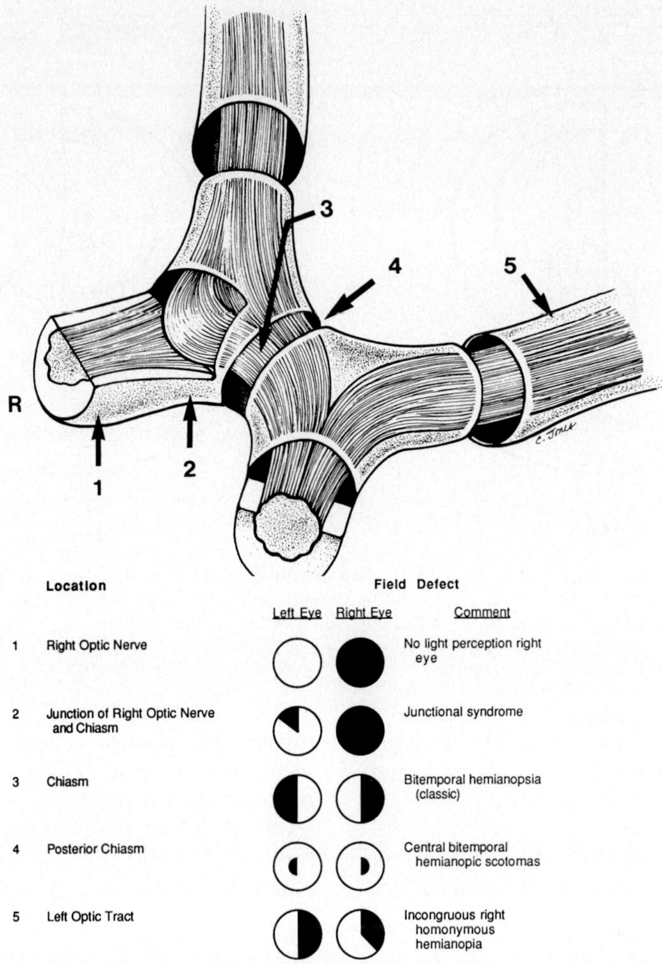

FIGURE 7–6. Optic chiasm: correlation of lesion site and field defect. Note the most ventral nasal fibers (mostly from inferior nasal retina) temporarily travel within the fellow optic nerve in Wilbrand's knee (From Liu GT: Disorders of the eyes and eyelids. In Samuels MA, Feske S (eds): The Office Practice of Neurology, p 46. New York, Churchill Livingstone, 1996, with permission. Adapted from Hoyt WF, Luis O, Arch Ophthalmol 1963;70:69–85, with permission (Copyright 1963, American Medical Association).)

is the result (Fig. 7–7). Incomplete and asymmetric bitemporal defects occur in the majority of cases (Fig. 7–8). More diffuse processes in this location can, of course, eventually cause nasal defects and acuity loss. However, it is a common observation that large sellar masses, despite compression, elevation, and flattening of the chiasm, as well as optic nerves and tracts in many instances, sometimes produce only a bitemporal hemianopia. It is unclear why the crossing fibers are so vulnerable. Mechanical distortion of nerve fiber bundles and impairment of the extrinsic vascular supply are two possible explanations, but a combination of both is likely.[9,17] An enlarging suprasellar mass might preferentially affect the inferior blood supply of the chiasm, affecting the body of the chiasm and crossing fibers,[15] and leave the more lateral and superior vascular supply of the lateral parts of the chiasm relatively spared. The relatively immediate improvement in visual fields following surgical decompression in some patients with chronic mass lesions is also enigmatic. In these instances, vascular compromise seems less likely than reversible axonal compression.

Patients with complete bitemporal hemianopias and *postfixation blindness*[18] may have trouble performing near tasks and complain of abnormal depth perception. When the eyes converge on a near target, the blind temporal fields overlap behind it (Fig. 7–9). Objects behind the fixation point are therefore not seen. Affected patients will have difficulty threading

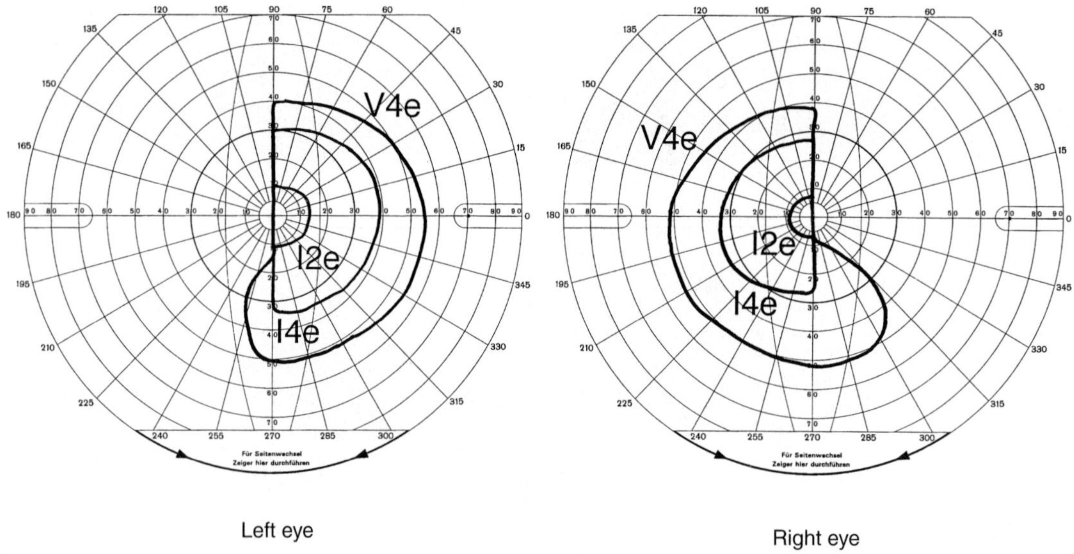

FIGURE 7–7. Bitemporal hemianopia documented on Goldmann perimetry in a patient with a craniopharyngioma compressing the chiasm from below (Fig. 7–23). Note the preservation of a small amount of temporal field in each eye inferiorly, reflecting the sparing of some fibers in the superior portion of the chiasm.

a needle, for instance. One can investigate this by having the patient fixate on a near target, then testing whether they see any objects directly behind it.

If the chiasm is postfixed (Fig. 7–4) in relationship to a sellar mass, or the lesion affects the anterior portion of the chiasm, several patterns of field loss can be seen. Patients may present with a monocular arcuate or central scotoma if the process primarily affects one optic nerve, and these instances may be difficult to separate from glaucoma or optic neuri-

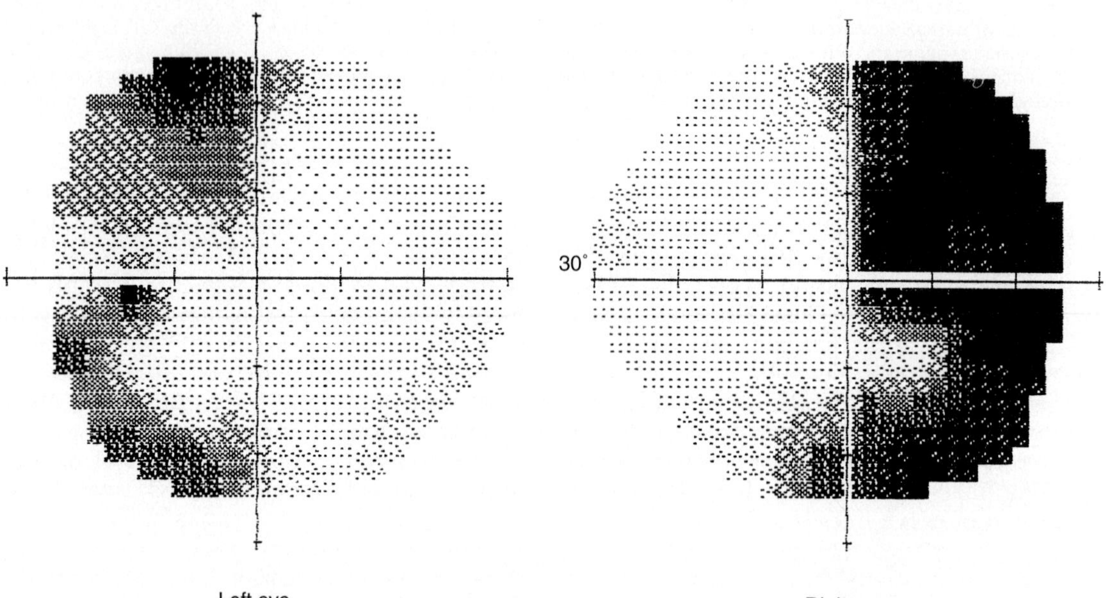

FIGURE 7–8. Incomplete, asymmetric bitemporal hemianopia documented on computerized threshold perimetry in a patient with chiasmal compression by a pituitary adenoma.

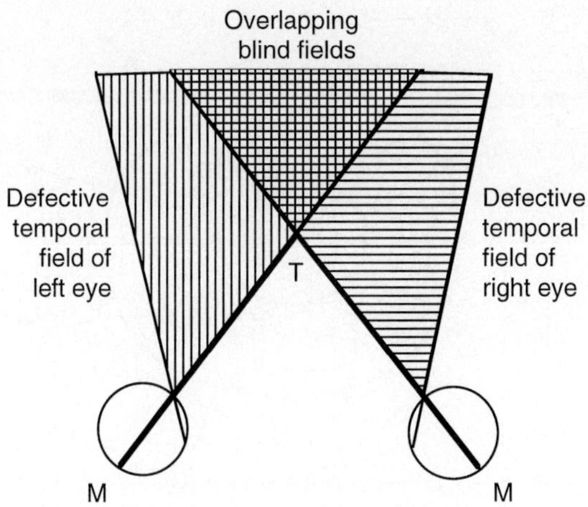

FIGURE 7–9. Postfixation blindness associated with a complete bitemporal hemianopia. When the eyes converge and fix on a near target (T), the blind temporal fields overlap behind it. Objects directly behind the target are invisible. M = macula.

tis. More characteristic of a chiasmal lesion is involvement of the ipsilateral optic nerve and Wilbrand's knee, resulting in a junctional scotoma.[19–21] This field deficit is characterized by a central scotoma or other optic nerve-related defect in the ipsilateral eye and a supratemporal defect in the other eye (Fig. 7–10). A monocular temporal field defect also localizes to the ipsilateral anterior chiasm and proximal optic nerve. Here a unilateral lesion is posterior enough to disrupt the ipsilateral crossing nasal fibers after they have segregated but is too anterior to involve the contralateral ones.[22] Since this pattern of field loss is also often functional, patients with organic monocular temporal field defects should be distinguished by an associated ipsilateral afferent pupillary defect, sometimes with optic atrophy. Less commonly, a disturbance of the crossing nerve fiber bundle anteriorly may result in an arcuate scotoma emanating from the blind spot and ending abruptly at the vertical meridian (Fig. 7–11).[23] Central bitemporal hemianopic scotomas (Fig. 7–12) or optic tract syndromes may be the product of prefixed chiasms or more posteriorly situated lesions.

The examiner should be aware of processes that produce bitemporal defects that do not respect the vertical meridian. These include tilted optic discs, sectoral (nasal) retinitis pigmentosa, and enlarged blind spots. In these cases, neuroimaging of the chiasm will obviously be unremarkable.

Binasal defects respecting the vertical meridian due to chiasmal dysfunction are extremely unusual. Theoretically this pattern can result from bilateral ectatic carotid artery compres-

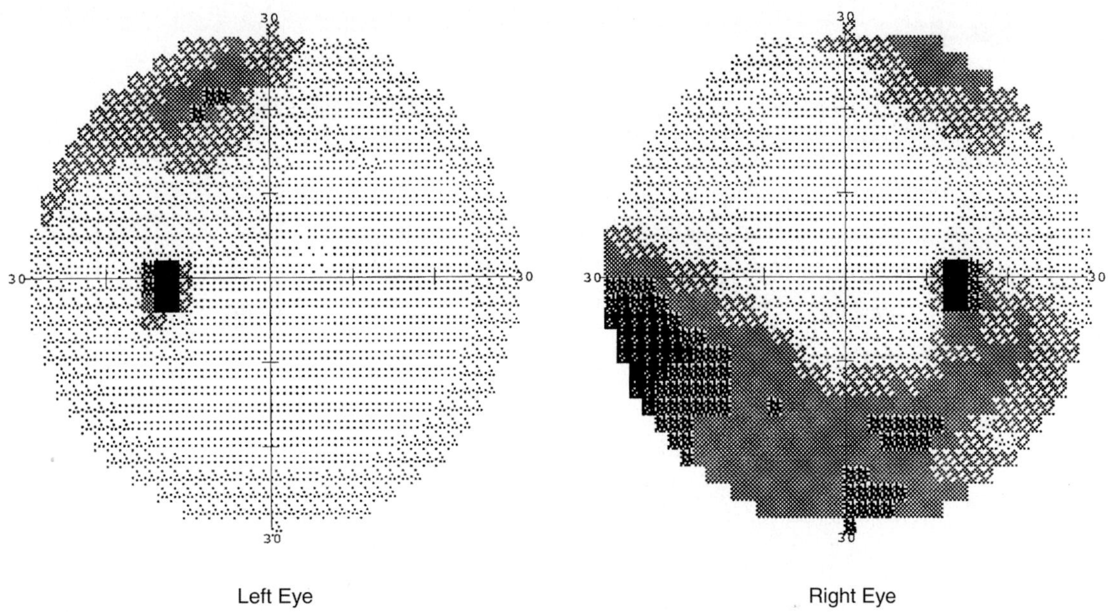

FIGURE 7–10. Junctional syndrome due to a pituitary adenoma affecting the anterior chiasm. The patient has an inferior arcuate defect in the right eye reflecting optic nerve dysfunction. The left eye has a superior temporal defect superiorly, owing to involvement of the Wilbrand's knee on the right.

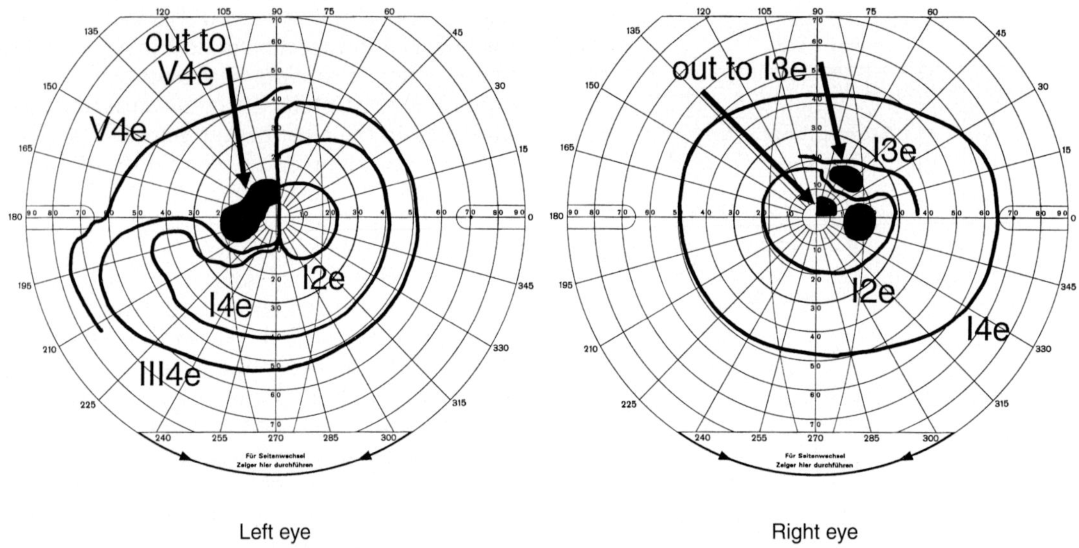

FIGURE 7–11. Goldmann visual field demonstrating a superior bitemporal hemianopia due to tumor compression. A superior arcuate scotoma in the left eye ends abruptly at the vertical meridian, a pattern that may result from a disturbance of the crossing nerve fibers from the left eye, anteriorly in the optic chiasm.

sion of the lateral portions of the chiasm, compression from a variety of chiasmal region tumors, or from third ventricular enlargement (see below). Usually binasal defects have ocular causes such as glaucoma, retinitis pigmentosa, and ischemic optic neuropathy.[24] Uncommonly, altitudinal defects can occur when crossed and uncrossed fibers are affected equally by a process involving the inferior or superior portions of the chiasm.

Optic Disc Findings

Long-standing processes can lead to optic disc pallor, but this finding is variable and does not correlate with the degree of visual loss. Nevertheless, disc pallor generally is associated with a poorer prognosis for visual improvement following treatment. Optic disc swelling in the setting of chiasmal dysfunction indicates either papilledema due to third ven-

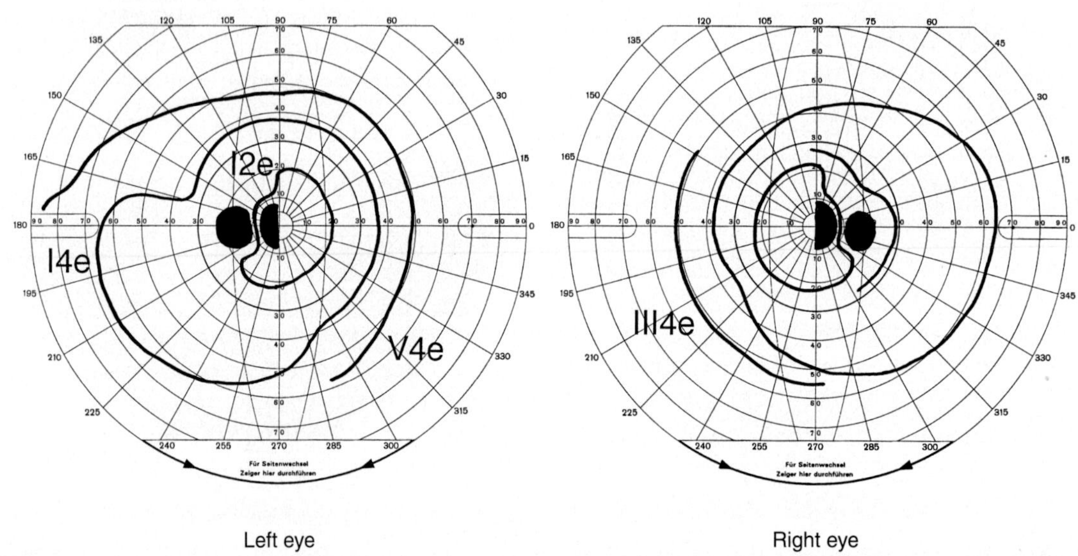

FIGURE 7–12. Goldmann visual field demonstrating central bitemporal hemianopic scotomas due to a posterior chiasmal lesion.

tricular compression by a sellar mass or an infiltrative or inflammatory process involving the anterior visual pathway.

In patients with bitemporal hemianopias, a characteristic transverse "band" optic atrophy can result from chiasmal compression of crossing nasal fibers.[25] In each eye, ganglion cells and their axons degenerate in the blind nasal hemiretina, leading to a nasal wedge of optic atrophy. Fibers from the blind nasal half of the macula are similarly affected, resulting in a temporal wedge of optic atrophy. The nerve fibers coming from "seeing" temporal macula and retina, entering the disc superiorly and inferiorly, are preserved.

Sensory Double Vision

Rarely, patients with complete bitemporal hemianopias may have odd complaints caused by an inability to align the noncorresponding nasal visual fields of each eye (hemifield slide phenomenon[18]) (Fig. 7–13). With a hypertropia, a patient may describe vertical misalignment or slippage of nasal fields. In contrast, esodeviated eyes can result in horizontal separation of nasal fields. Exodeviated eyes may cause overlap of nasal fields and so-called nonparetic diplopia.[26] One can test for these phenomena in patients with horizontal deviations by drawing a line of small dots or circles, then asking the patient to look quickly at the center of them and tell the examiner how many he sees (Fig. 7–14).

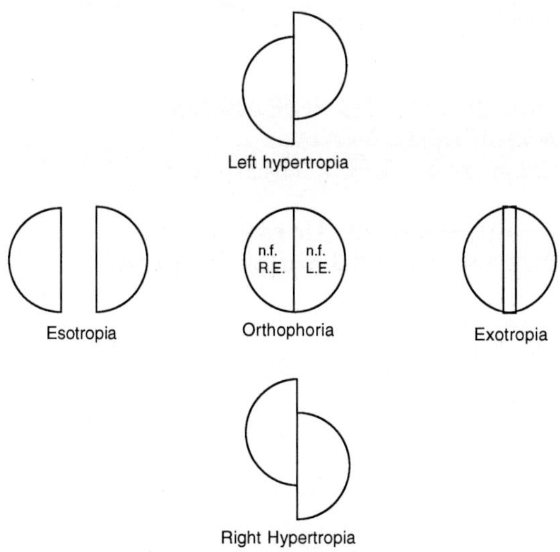

FIGURE 7–13. Hemifield slide phenomena associated with complete bitemporal hemianopia. The diagrams depict the visual fields from the patient's perspective with both eyes open (cyclopean view). If the eyes are orthophoric (no misalignment), then the nasal fields will align properly. n.f.R.E. = nasal field of the right eye, n.f.L.E. = nasal field of the left eye. However, because the nasal fields are noncorresponding, affected individuals will be unable to compensate for any tendency for ocular misalignment, and the nasal fields will drift if there is a hypertropia, esotropia, or exotropia.

Eye Movement Abnormalities

Ocular motor palsies and nystagmoid eye movements can be associated with chiasmal disorders but are uncommon. Chiasmal field loss accompanied by an ocular motor palsy implies cavernous sinus involvement, sometimes also suggested by facial pain or numbness resulting from trigeminal nerve dysfunction. The sellar process that most commonly affects both the chiasm and cavernous sinuses is pituitary apoplexy (see below).

See-saw nystagmus can be a sign of a chiasmal process, and sellar masses and trauma are the usual culprits. In this unique motility disturbance one eye elevates and intorts while the other depresses and extorts, then vice versa in a pendular fashion (Fig. 7–15).[27] The exact mechanism is unclear, but almost all patients with acquired see-saw nystagmus have either a bitemporal hemianopia or bilateral involvement of the interstitial nuclei of Cajal (INC) in the mesencephalon.[28] Most sellar masses that exhibit see-saw nystagmus are large, causing both the field defect and midbrain compression. However, each factor by itself is sufficient for the development of this motility disorder. Patients with see-saw nystagmus and chiasmal trauma, for instance, have the bitemporal hemianopia, while those with midbrain infarction or hemorrhage involving the INC have no visual loss. Proposed explanations relating the bitemporal hemianopia and see-saw nystagmus include (1) a torsional adaptive process that attempts to increase the overlap of noncorresponding nasal fields[29]; and (2) disruption of the visuovestibular connections between retina and inferior olive.[28] Rare achiasmatic and hemichiasmatic individuals, who may have normal fields, can also have see-saw nystagmus (see anomalies of the chiasm, below).[30, 31] See-saw nystagmus is also discussed in Chapter 17.

Asymmetric or Monocular Nystagmus

Young children with sellar masses such as gliomas or craniopharyngiomas in unusual

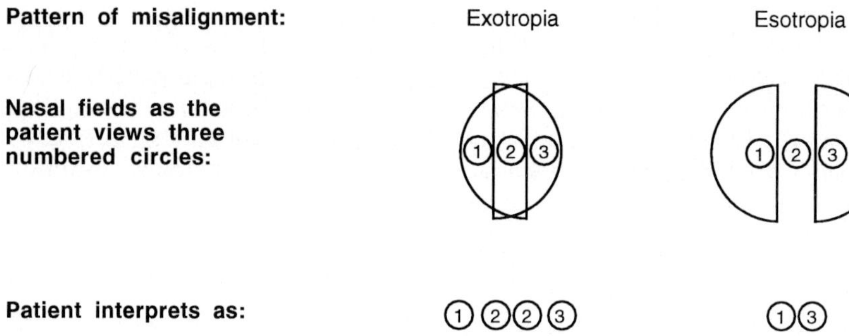

FIGURE 7–14. Sensory double vision and hemifield slide phenomena associated with complete bitemporal hemianopias. The diagrams depict the visual fields from the patient's perspective with both eyes open. As described in Figure 7–13, if a patient with a bitemporal hemianopia and an exotropia views three numbered circles, he might think he is seeing four circles. The #2 circle is contained in each nasal field and is therefore duplicated ("double vision"). A patient with an esotropia might actually see only two of the circles, because neither nasal field contains the #2 circle.

instances may present with monocular or asymmetric nystagmus when the chiasm is involved. Sometimes the full triad of nystagmus, head nodding and head tilting is present, mimicking the benign symptom complex of spasmus nutans.[32] Usually those with intracranial lesions will have reduced vision, optic atrophy, strabismus, or diencephalic syndrome,[33] and these findings will convince the examiner that neuroimaging should be performed. The mechanism by which sellar masses produce the motility disorder is not clear. For a more detailed discussion of spasmus nutans and its imitators, the reader is referred to the chapter on nystagmus and nystagmoid eye movements (Chapter 17).

Visual Field Testing

Patients with suspected chiasmal disorders should undergo careful documentation of visual fields in addition to the neuro-ophthalmic examination. Subtle superior temporal defects respecting the vertical meridian may be the first sign of a compressive sellar mass, so examiners should look carefully in these areas.[34] Goldmann kinetic perimetry may be necessary in poorly cooperative patients and those with severe visual loss. However, we prefer computerized threshold perimetry in most patients with chiasmal disturbances, as they likely will require serial field examinations to monitor disease activity. We do not advocate the use of visual evoked potentials[35] in the evaluation or follow-up of patients with chiasmal disorders.

ENDOCRINE DISTURBANCES ASSOCIATED WITH CHIASMAL DISORDERS

Pituitary Gland, Hormone Physiology, and Endocrinopathy

Traditionally, the pituitary gland is separated into the anterior (adenohypophysis) and

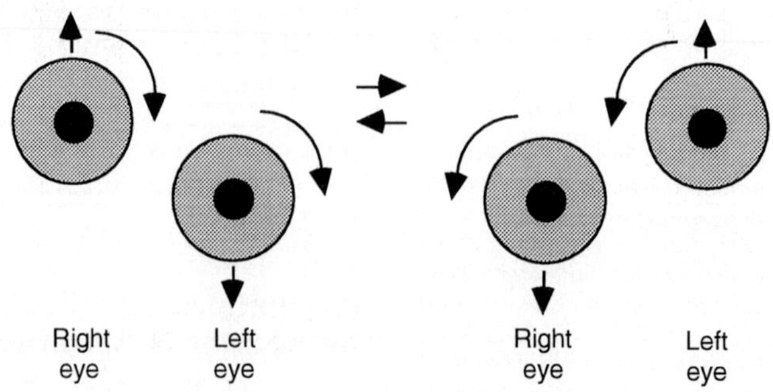

FIGURE 7–15. See-saw nystagmus. One eye depresses and extorts while the fellow eye elevates and intorts. The pattern alternates in a pendular fashion, simulating the motion of a see-saw.

posterior lobes (neurohypophysis) (see Fig. 7–3).[7] Laterally, the adenohypophysis contains cells that secrete prolactin and growth hormone (GH), while cells that produce thyroid-stimulating hormone (TSH), follicle-stimulating hormone (FSH), luteinizing hormone (LH), and adrenocorticotropic hormone (ACTH) are located medially. The hormones vasopressin (or antidiuretic hormone (ADH) and oxytocin are synthesized in the supraoptic and periventricular nuclei in the hypothalmus, then transported to the posterior lobe via long axons within the pituitary stalk.

Prolactin stimulates production of breast milk in women. GH stimulates liver production of insulin-like growth factor I (IGF-I, also called somatomedin C). Corticotropin (ACTH) causes adrenal secretion of both cortisol and androgens. TSH stimulates thyroid production of triiodothyronine (T_3) and thyroxine (T_4). In women, FSH and LH lead to estradiol and progesterone secretion, folliculogenesis, and ovulation, while in men, these two hormones stimulate testosterone secretion and spermatogenesis.[36] Hormone secretion in the adenohypophysis is regulated in part by proteins produced in the hypothalamus and brought to the pituitary via the hypophyseal portal venous system (Fig. 7–16). Dopamine tonically inhibits prolactin secretion, for example. End-organ hormone levels confer additional regulation by modulating the production of pituitary and hypothalamic releasing hormones. ADH, released in the neurohypophysis, stimulates free-water reabsortion in the collecting ducts of the kidney. Oxytocin stimulates uterine contraction and milk ejection.[36]

Because of the chiasm's proximity to the pituitary, stalk, and hypothalamus, chiasmal disorders, especially those due to mass lesions, often present concomitantly with endocrine dysfunction. In this setting, the endocrinopathies usually fall into two major categories: pituitary hormone deficiency (hypopituitarism) and hypersecretion. Hypopituitarism can be the result of compression of normal pituitary tissue, impaired blood flow of normal tissue, or interference with hypothalmic production or delivery of releasing hormones.[36] Symptoms consistent with hypopituitarism, which can vary according to sex, are outlined in Table 7–1. Of these, the most common are those associated with GH deficiency, but the most salient clinical features of hypopituitarism actually vary with age. In children, failure of normal linear growth is the dominant symptom, in adolescence it is delayed sexual maturation, and in adults it is secondary hypogonadism.[37]

On the other hand, pituitary hormone excess generally is caused either by hypersecreting pituitary adenomas or target organ failure with secondary hypersecretion. In the one exception, mild degrees of hyperprolactinemia can be associated with hypothalamic dysfunction or stalk compression, both of which result in decreased delivery of dopamine, which normally inhibits prolactin secretion, to the pituitary gland. Clinical features of pituitary hormone hypersecretion due to adenomas are highlighted in Table 7–2. When chiasmal dysfunction due to a sellar mass is present, hypopituitarism is more common than hypersecretion, but patients can have elements of one or both (for instance, when a hypersecreting adenoma compresses and compromises adjacent normal pituitary tissue).

Hypopituitarism also can be an unavoidable side effect of surgery or irradiation of sellar lesions. Thus, before and following treatment in many instances, hormone replacement will be required because cortisol and thyroxine are necessary for life, uncontrolled diabetes insipidus can be life-threatening, and gonadotropin deficiency is associated with osteoporosis and impaired reproductive and sexual functions. It is not uncommon for patients with sellar processes to require replacement regimens consisting of various combinations of corticosteroid, T_4, GH (in children), estrogen (for women), testosterone (for men), and DDAVP (desmopressin; 1-deamino-8-arginine vasopressin).

Hypothalamic Syndromes

Two childhood endocrinopathies, Russell's diencephalic syndrome[38] and precocious puberty, are the most important clinical syndromes associated with hypothalamic lesions in the pediatric age group. The diencephalic syndrome has a typical age of onset between the newborn period and 4 years of age[39] and is characterized by emaciation, hyperkinesis, and euphoria (Fig. 7–17). The weight loss is the most salient trait, and it occurs after initially normal weight gain. Children are often evaluated for failure to thrive.[40] Linear growth is unaltered. An alert appearance (due to lid retraction), vomiting, pallor, and nystagmus are other common features.[41] Optic atrophy occurs in approximately one quarter.[41] Hypothalamic chiasmal gliomas are the usual cause, and ante-

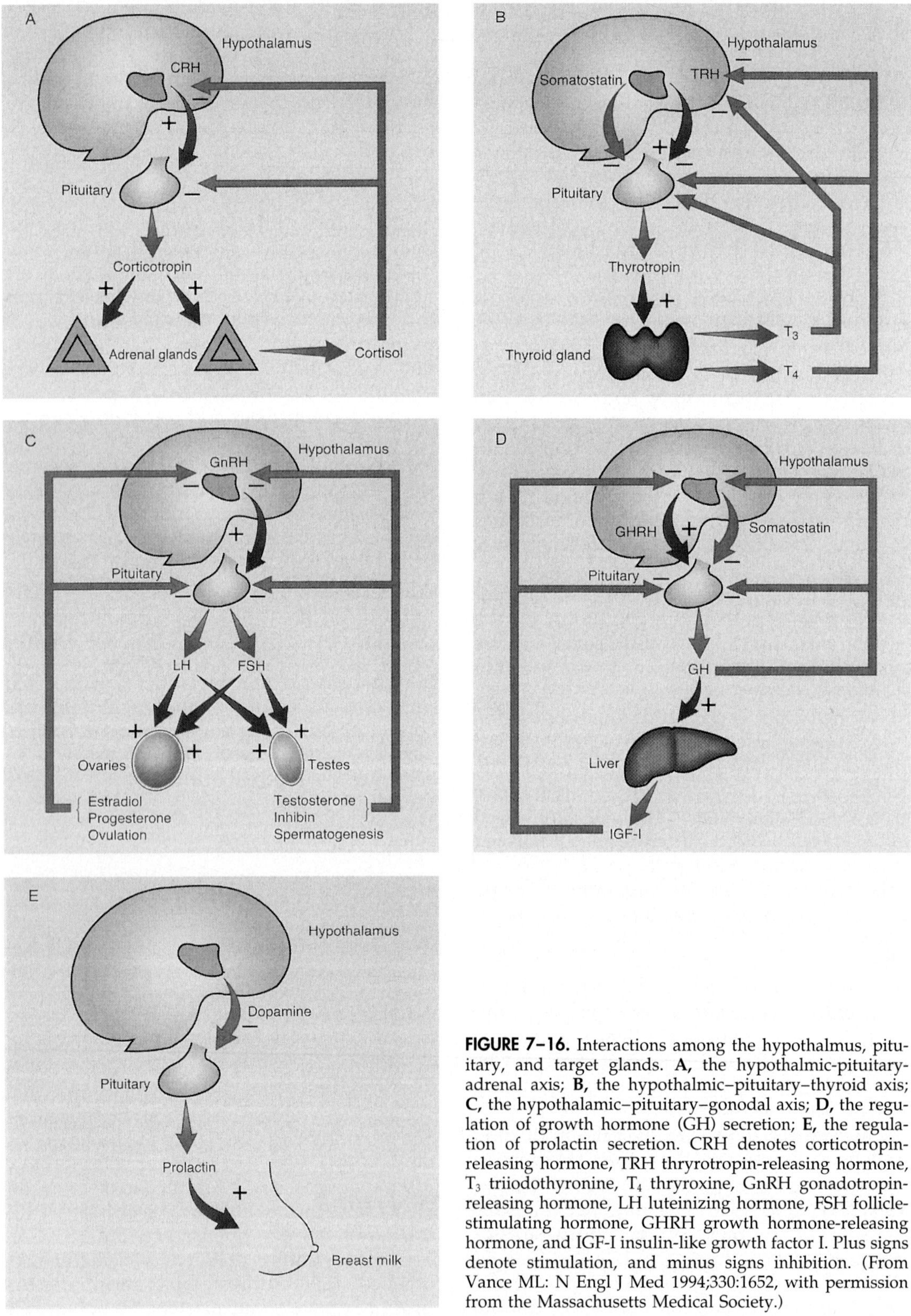

FIGURE 7–16. Interactions among the hypothalmus, pituitary, and target glands. **A,** the hypothalmic-pituitary-adrenal axis; **B,** the hypothalmic–pituitary–thyroid axis; **C,** the hypothalamic–pituitary–gonodal axis; **D,** the regulation of growth hormone (GH) secretion; **E,** the regulation of prolactin secretion. CRH denotes corticotropin-releasing hormone, TRH thryrotropin-releasing hormone, T_3 triiodothyronine, T_4 thryroxine, GnRH gonadotropin-releasing hormone, LH luteinizing hormone, FSH follicle-stimulating hormone, GHRH growth hormone-releasing hormone, and IGF-I insulin-like growth factor I. Plus signs denote stimulation, and minus signs inhibition. (From Vance ML: N Engl J Med 1994;330:1652, with permission from the Massachusetts Medical Society.)

TABLE 7–1. Typical Features of Hypopituitarism Due to Hypothalamic/Pituitary Dysfunction

	Hormones Affected	In Women	In Men	In Women and Men
Hypogonadism	↓ or nl LH ↓ or nl FSH ↓ estradiol in women ↓ testosterone in men	Oligomenorrhea or amenorrhea Dyspareunia Vaginal dryness	↓ facial and body hair Testicular atrophy Erectile dysfunction Gynecomastia	↓ libido
Hypoprolactinemia	↓ prolactin	Failure to start and maintain lactation		
Hypothyroidism	↓ or nl TSH ↓ T_3, T_4			Fatigue, weakness, inability to lose weight, puffiness, constipation, cold intolerance, memory impairment, altered mentation, bradycardia, delayed relaxation of deep tendon reflexes
Growth hormone deficiency	↓ GH, IGF-I			Short stature in children ↓ vigor, ↓ exercise tolerance ↓ body muscle:fat ratio
Hypoadrenalism	↓ or nl ACTH ↓ cortisol	Loss of axillary and pubic hair		Fatigue and malaise Postural hypotension, pallor, anorexia, and nausea
Diabetes insipidus	↓ ADH			Polyuria Polydipsia Hypernatremia
Oxytocin deficiency		↓ milk ejection during lactation		

See text for explanation of abbreviations. nl = normal.

rior hypothalmic dysfunction is one proposed mechanism for the syndrome.[41]

Precocious puberty is seen in boys more commonly than girls, and affected children are tall for age and exhibit early gonadal maturation. Responsible lesions typically lie in the floor of the third ventricle, posterior hypothalmus, tuber cinereum, or median eminence. Common causes in these areas include hamartomas of the tuber cinereum, hypothalamic gliomas, and suprasellar germ cell tumors. There may be several mechanisms, each resulting in inappropriate testosterone production. Germ cell tumors, for instance (see below), produce beta-human chorionic gonadotropin, which stimulates Leydig cells. Alternatively, hypothalamic infiltration might cause increased secretion of gonadotropin-releasing hormone.[39]

In children and adults following surgery in the hypothalmic region, for example, for treatment of craniopharyngioma, weight gain and obesity are common. This likely results from injury to satiety centers in the hypothalmus.

DIAGNOSIS/APPROACH

It is often difficult on the basis of the neuro-ophthalmic signs and symptoms alone to arrive at the specific pathologic diagnosis. The visual complaints and field patterns facilitate chiasmal localization, but are usually nondiagnositic with regards to cause. Only in rare instances, such as progressive superior bitemporal field deficits due to an expanding pituitary adenoma, does the pattern of visual loss suggest a specific entity. Rather, once a chiasmal disorder is suspected on neuro-opthalmic grounds, the diagnosis is best established by considering the patient's age, clinical history, general physical findings, neuroimaging results, and endocrine testing.

TABLE 7–2. Typical Features of Hypersecreting Syndromes Associated With Pituitary Adenomas

	Hormones Affected	In Women	In Men	In Women and Men
Hyperprolactinemia	↑ prolactin	Amenorrhea Oligomenorrhea Infertility	Impotence Gynecomastia	↓ libido Galactorrhea (rare in men)
Growth hormone excess	↑ GH, IGF-I			Acromegaly Gigantism (children)
ACTH excess (Cushing disease)	↑ or nl ACTH ↑ cortisol	Oligomenorrhea Amenorrhea	↓ libido	Sudden weight gain Moon facies Buffalo hump Hypertension Hirsuitism Acne Glucose intolerance Muscle wasting and weakness[45]
Hyperthyroidism	↑ or nl TSH ↑ T_3, T_4			Thyrotoxicosis Goiter
Excess LH/FSH	↑ or nl LH ↑ or nl FSH ↑ or nl estradiol in women ↑ testosterone in men (variable)	Amenorrhea Oligomenorrhea		Precocious puberty in childhood ↓ libido in adults

See text for details and explanation of abbreviations. nl = normal.

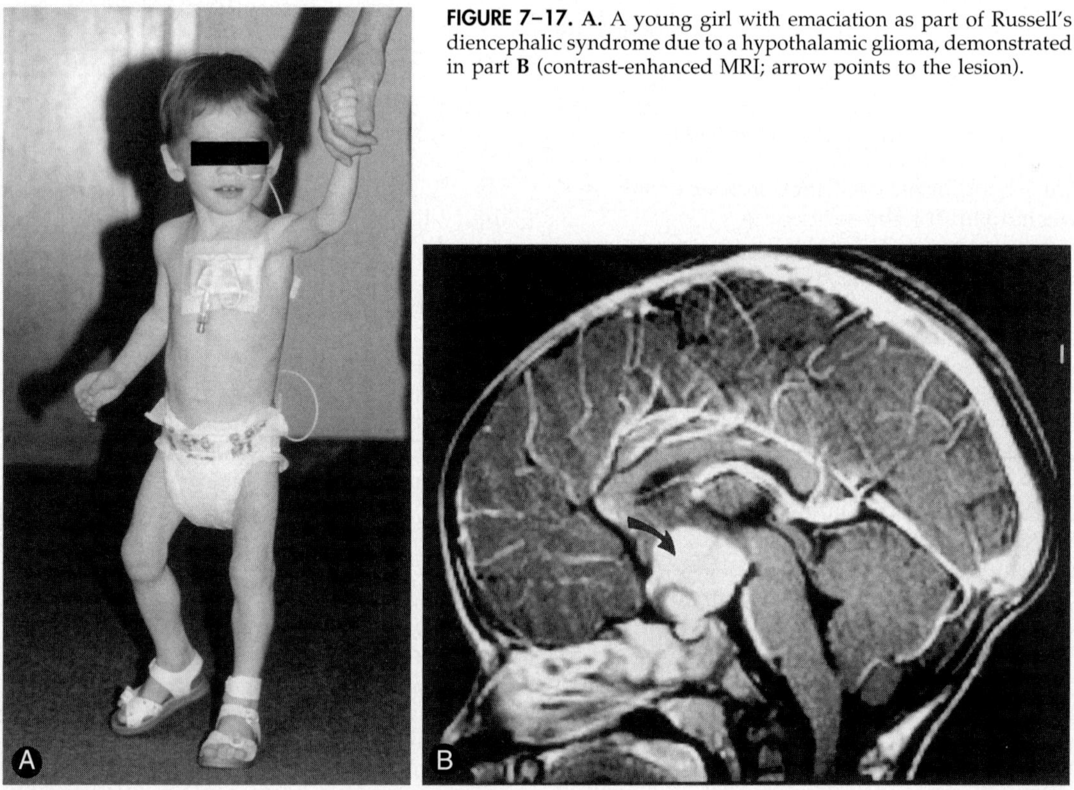

FIGURE 7–17. A. A young girl with emaciation as part of Russell's diencephalic syndrome due to a hypothalamic glioma, demonstrated in part **B** (contrast-enhanced MRI; arrow points to the lesion).

Age

Most chiasmal disorders are due to compressive lesions, many of which have a tendency to occur more frequently either in (1) children and young adults or (2) middle-aged and elderly individuals. Table 7–3 outlines the differential diagnosis of most sellar and suprasellar processes, based on age predilection and frequency. In general, tumors and masses of congenital derivation are more common in childhood, and vascular processes and metastases in late adulthood. The inflammatory, infectious, and infiltrative disorders occur at all ages.

Clinical History

Both the rate of onset of symptoms and presence and quality of endocrine features will be important. Because the most common cause is a compressive sellar mass, most visual and endocrine symptoms will be insidious. Acute chiasmal syndromes can occur when tumors enlarge suddenly, due to cyst expansion or intratumor hemorrhage, as in pituitary apoplexy. However, sudden chiasmal field loss might also suggest chiasmal neuritis, ischemia, or an instrinsic vascular malformation. Patients should also be questioned about double vision or difficulty with depth perception.

Historical features suggestive of endocrine dysfunction should be investigated. In particular, the patient should be asked about symptoms consistent either with hypopituitarism or pituitary hormone hypersecretion. While the former could be due to any sellar mass, the latter suggests a pituitary adenoma. Other types of endocrine dysfunction, such as diabetes insipidus, are characteristic of sellar sarcoidosis and germinoma, for instance. However, diabetes insipidus may be seen in many other suprasellar processes.

General Physical Findings

The examiner should look for evidence of endocrine dysfunction, and in some cases the diagnosis can be made on physical findings alone. Patients with gynecomastia, cushingoid features, or acromegaly, for example, might harbor hypersecreting pituitary adenomas. Precocious puberty suggests hypothalamic dysfunction, while growth retardation might be due to GH deficiency. Features of neurofibromatosis, such as café-au-lait spots and neu-

TABLE 7–3. Sellar and Suprasellar Processes That Can Affect the Chiasm, According to Age Group, Etiology, and Frequency

Age Group	More Common	Less Common

Pediatric–young adult	Chiasmal–hypothalamic glioma
	Craniopharyngioma
		Arteriovenous malformation
		Dermoid
		Germ cell tumors
		  Germinoma
		  Teratoma
		  Non germinoma
		Lymphocytic hypophysitis
		Pituitary adenoma
		Suprasellar arachnoid cyst

Middle age–elderly	Pituitary adenoma Meningioma Craniopharyngioma Aneurysm (internal carotid)	Choristomas Empty sella syndrome Epidermoids Infarction Malignant optic glioma Metastases to chiasm, sella, or suprasellar region Pituitary apoplexy Rathke's cleft cyst Sphenoid sinus mucocele

No particular age predilection		Histiocytosis
		Meningitis
		  Bacterial
		  Tuberculous
		Sarcoidosis

Adapted from Liu GT: In Samuels MA, Feske S (eds): The Office Practice of Neurology, pp 40–74. New York, Churchill Livingstone, 1995, with permission.

rofibromas, should also be excluded because of their association with optic pathway gliomas.

Diagnostic Studies/Neuroimaging

All patients suspected of having a chiasmal disorder should undergo enhanced and unenhanced MRI with special attention to the sellar area, including axial and 3-mm coronal and sagittal sections. If the clinical history and findings on examination suggest chronicity (long duration of symptoms and optic disc pallor, for example), neuroimaging can be performed over the next day or two. However, sudden visual loss, indicating an acute process, and optic disc swelling, a sign of possible hydrocephalus, are both indications for emergent scanning. MRI is far superior to CT in the evaluation of this region because it provides excellent anatomic detail, sagittal views, and better soft tissue imaging. The only disadvantage of MRI in this regard is its inability to demonstrate small amounts of calcification and changes in the sellar walls, which are made of cortical bone and separate the pituitary gland and cavernous sinuses. When MRI is contraindicated or intolerable, CT can still be useful, especially if contrast images and coronal views (thin 1.5-mm sections) can be obtained. In some instances CT is adjunctive to MRI by outlining bony landmarks and possibly their erosion by a sellar mass. CT can also identify calcification within suspected sellar lesions. When aneurysms are suspected because of MRI or CT findings, MRI-angiography or conventional angiography is necessary.

Intrinsic disorders of the chiasm will be suggested by radiographically demonstrated chiasmal enlargement, signal abnormality, or gadolinium enhancement. Extrinsic compression will be evident if there is a mass lesion and distortion or displacement of the chiasm.

Diagnostic Studies/Endocrine Testing

The basic outpatient endocrinologic panel should include serum prolactin, serum AM cortisol, TSH, T_4, LH, FSH, estradiol (in women), and testosterone (in men) levels. Low values, and even normal ones in some instances, are consistent with hypopituitarism (Table 7–1). High values imply hypersecretion (Table 7–2). Other tests may be ordered if a particular hypersecreting pituitary adenoma is suspected: for GH-secreting tumors, GH (after a 75-g oral glucose load) and insulin-like growth factor I (IGF-I); for Cushing syndrome, ACTH and cortisol (24-hr urine free cortisol). Some relevant details should be mentioned here:

1. As a rule, prolactin secreting macroadenomas are associated with a serum prolactin level of >150 to 200 ng/ml (normal 2 to 15 ng/ml), and elevated levels correlate with tumor size.[42] Microadenomas, hypothalmic dysfunction, pituitary stalk compression, or drugs such as neuroleptics and antidepressants lead to more modest elevations.[43] Physiologic hyperprolactinemia, also modest, occurs during pregnancy and postpartum lactation.
2. After a 75-g oral glucose load, the normal GH level is <2 ng/ml. Lack of suppression to this extent is the rule in acromegaly, and secretory spikes are frequent in this disorder. IGF-I levels are also elevated, but are more stable and correlate better with the severity of the acromegaly.[44]
3. If neuroimaging suggests a pituitary adenoma, and clinical features are consistent with ACTH hypersecretion despite normal or equivocal ACTH and cortisol levels, adjunctive testing may be required. In the overnight dexamethasone suppression test, 1 mg dexamethasone is given orally at midnight, then at 8 AM the following morning the plasma cortisol level is measured, and should be <5 μg/dl. Elevated levels suggest pituitary ACTH hypersecretion. In a more definitive suppression test, 0.5 mg dexamethasone is administered every 6 hours for 2 days and urinary cortisol is measured for 24 hours. An unchanged urine cortisol level would be consistent with inappropriate cortisol secretion. Finally, petrosal venous sinus[45] or cavernous sinus[464] ACTH sampling may be performed, but this is rarely necessary if an adenoma has already been demonstrated radiographically.

A summary of evaluation of patients with suspected chiasmal disorders is outlined in Table 7–4. The discovery of a mass lesion requires neurosurgical consultation, while the presence of endocrine dysfunction, either on clinical or laboratory grounds, should prompt a formal endocrinologic evaluation as well. The remainder of this chapter discusses the various entities leading to chiasmal dysfunction. The clinical features and the management of each are emphasized.

TABLE 7–4. Evaluation of Patients With Suspected Chiasmal Disorders

I. Consideration of patient's age
Childhood and young adulthood
Middle age and elderly

II. Clinical history
Visual symptoms
Endocrine symptoms

III. Neuro-ophthalmic examination
Including careful visual field testing

IV. General physical examination
Evidence of endocrine dysfunction
Evidence of underlying systemic disease

V. Neuroimaging
MRI, preferably, including sagittal and coronal thin cuts through the sellar region
CT, with coronal views

VI. Endocrine testing and evaluation
Serum prolactin, AM cortisol, TSH, T_4, LH, FSH, estradiol (in women), and testosterone (in men)
GH (after a 75-g oral glucose load) and IGF-I if acromegaly suspected; ACTH and dexamethasone suppression tests if inappropriate ACTH secretion suspected.

VII. Other adjunctive tests
Lumbar puncture if neuroimaging suggests an infectious, inflammatory, or infiltrative disorder

PITUITARY ADENOMAS

These tumors are the most common cause of chiasmal dysfunction in adults, and they are very common, representing about 10% to 15% of all intracranial tumors.[37] Pituitary adenomas may be found in 3.1% to 22.5% of routine autopsies, but frequently these incidental lesions are <2 mm in size.[46, 47] About 70% of pituitary adenomas occur in individuals age 30 to 50, and only 3% to 7% occur in patients less than 20.[48–50] Pituitary adenomas are uncommon but can occur in children.[51, 52]

There is disagreement whether adenomas arise from somatic mutation of a single cell or from hyperstimulation due to hypothalmic or hormonal dysregulation, or both.[50, 53] In general, they are benign epithelial neoplasms that rarely metastasize; primary pituitary carcinomas are rare. Microadenomas are adenomas <10 mm in size, and these are rarely large enough to cause chiasmal compression, while macroadenomas are those >10 mm. Pituitary adenomas are usually isolated, but they can be associated with tumors of the parathyroid gland and pancreas, and less commonly with those of the thymus, in multiple endocrine neoplasia (MEN) type I syndrome.[54, 55]

Pituitary adenomas can be classified functionally by their endocrine abnormality into two major groups: those with *nonfunctional enlargement* and those exhibiting *hormone hypersecretion*.[46] Approximately one quarter to one third of patients with clinically apparent pituitary adenomas are nonfunctioning or nonsecreting.[56, 57] On the other hand, the two most common hypersecreting adenomas are prolactinomas and GH secreting tumors, but ACTH-, TSH-, and LH/FSH-secreting tumors are also clinically important. Modern morphologic techniques have rendered the classification of pituitary adenomas based on staining characteristics, such as acidophilic, basophilic, and chromophobic, less helpful.[58]

The presentation of pituitary adenomas varies according to tumor subtype. Nonfunctioning adenomas are often asymptomatic until after they have extended beyond the sella, causing signs related to tumor enlargement and compression of surrounding structures: visual loss, headache, and hypopituitarism. Most (70%) of the large adenomas causing visual loss will be nonfunctioning.[59] In contrast, hypersecreting tumors present more commonly with characteristic endocrine symptoms, described in detail below. In all pituitary adenomas, diabetes insipidus at presentation is unusual.

Neuro-ophthalmic Symptoms and Signs

Chiasmal visual field loss is the most important neuro-ophthalmic manifestation of pituitary adenomas. Usually it is insidious and slowly progressive,[37] and often there is a delay of months or years between the onset of visual loss and diagnosis of the pituitary tumor.[16] Since the chiasm is located directly above the pituitary in most instances, the crossing inferonasal fibers are usually the first to be disturbed by upward growing adenomas, causing superotemporal defects respecting the vertical meridian. Further tumor enlargement results in more complete interruption of crossing fibers in the body of the chiasm, leading to a complete bitemporal hemianopia. Because of the distance between the diaphragm and the chiasm, only macroadenomas with significant suprasellar extension are associated with field loss. These principles are reflected in the excellent data from a review of 1000 cases by Hollenhorst and Younge.[60] Thirty percent of patients had no visual field abnormalities.

Superotemporal field defects occurred in 10%, and bitemporal hemianopias in 30%. Junctional scotomas, central scotomas, and homonymous hemianopias were less frequent, consistent with the lower incidence of postfixed and prefixed chiasms. Today, the percentage of patients presenting with field loss is probably lower, perhaps reflecting earlier tumor detection by more modern endocrinologic testing and neuroimaging.[61]

Acuity is affected less commonly (16%)[62] than visual fields. Disc pallor occurs in about 30% of patients[60] and correlates with the presence of decreased visual acuity better than with field loss or the severity of visual loss.[5] Papilledema is unusual unless the adenoma is large enough to cause hydrocephalus[63] and instead suggests other sellar processes that have a greater tendency for causing third ventricular obstruction. Formed visual hallucinations, presumable release phenomena (see Chapter 12), have been reported in association with field loss due to pituitary adenomas.[64]

Cavernous sinus invasion,[65] following lateral erosion of the thin sellar wall, may lead to ocular motor palsies (in 1% to 5% of patients[17]) or trigeminal dysfunction. However, motility disturbances are much more common with pituitary apoplexy (see below). When ocular motor palsies occur, the third nerve is the most commonly affected.[17, 60] Rarely, a third, fourth, or sixth nerve palsy is the sole presenting feature of the pituitary adenoma.[66, 67] Orbital invasion[68] and extrasellar pituitary adenomas[69] have reported but are uncommon growth patterns.

Diagnostic Studies/Neuroimaging

In 80% to 95% of microadenomas, a hypointense lesion is evident within the normal pituitary on T_1-weighted MR images.[70] A hyperintense region on T_1-weighted images usually indicates a hemorrhagic component. Most of the time (75%) the hemorrhage is not associated with clinical apoplexy (see below).[71] In about one third to one half of cases, the adenoma is hyperintense on T_2-weighted images. Contrast may be helpful if the unenhanced images are equivocal. The various types of adenomas usually can not be distinguished by MRI, although prolactinomas and GH secreting adenomas tend to be more lateral, while ACTH-, TSH-, and LH/FSH-secreting adenomas are usually more midline. This pattern reflects the normal location of the secreting cells.

Macroadenomas (Fig. 7–18) share similar MRI signal characteristics, but differ morphologically. They are characterized frequently by suprasellar extension, enlargement of the sella turcica, and a dumbbell or figure-eight shape on sagittal and coronal images (caused by the limitations of the bony sella). In some instances there is demonstrable lateral extension into the cavernous sinus. Approximately 20% of macroadenomas may exhibit radiographic

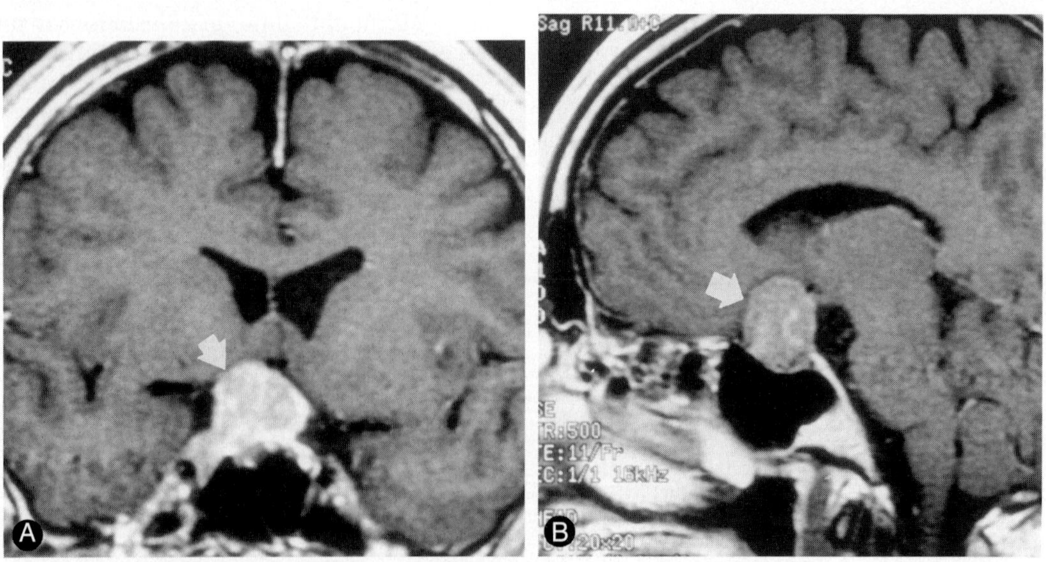

FIGURE 7–18. Enhancing, nonsecreting pituitary macroadenoma (*arrow*) seen on gadolinium enhanced MR images. **A.** Coronal view. **B.** Sagittal view.

evidence of cystic changes, necrosis, or hemorrhage, but only 1% are associated with a history of sudden clinical deterioration[70] (see pituitary apoplexy, below). MRI should be sufficient to outline vascular structures and rule out coexisting aneurysms,[72–74] so routine angiography is unnecessary in most preoperative assessments. On CT the pituitary adenomas are hypodense compared with the normal gland on both enhanced and unenhanced images.[7] Sellar erosion can be evident on CT with larger adenomas.

Diagnostic Studies/Laboratory Tests

In addition to MRI, endocrinologic studies are necessary to classify the tumor type and direct treatment (see Table 7–4). Abnormal results and their interpretation are outlined in Tables 7–1 and 7–2.

Treatment

Some generalizations regarding treatment, outcome, and management of pituitary adenomas can be made:

1. Except for prolactinomas, the first-line treatment of symptomatic adenomas is transsphenoidal neurosurgery. Advantages of this method versus a craniotomy include direct visualization of the pituitary gland and tumor, no external scars, and better tolerance of the surgery even by elderly and medically complicated individuals. Access to the sphenoid is usually via a sublabial or transnasal approach or combinations of both,[75] and tumors are removed with the aid of the operating microscope. When necessary, the sellar floor is reconstructed with a plate of nasal bone or cartilage, and the sphenoid sinus is packed with muscle, fat, or Gelfoam.[76] Postoperative diabetes insipidus (usually transient), CSF leak, visual loss, ocular motor nerve palsy, hemorrhage, and cerebral ischemia are potential complications, but the morbidity and mortality rates are usually very low.[76,77] At some institutions, the sella is exposed transnasally or transseptally using an endoscope, and the tumor removal is accomplished also endoscopically[78] or with an operating microscope.[79, 80] A pterional or transfrontal approach via craniotomy should be considered when there is extensive extrasellar tumor.[81]
2. The prognosis for visual improvement is excellent following surgical or medical decompression. Recovery to some degree may occur within days or weeks of treatment. In Trautmann and Law's large series of patients who underwent transsphenoidal surgery,[62] approximately half of those with reduced acuity experienced improvement in this parameter, while about three quarters of those with field loss had restoration or improvement in visual fields. Slightly better results were reported in smaller studies.[82, 83] Prognostic signs that are associated with lack of improvement included optic disc pallor, lengthy delay prior to diagnosis, and poor visual acuity.[5, 84] Interestingly, the degree of visual field loss has no predictive value, as patients with profound field defects still have a reasonable chance for improvement.
3. External beam radiotherapy is useful in instances of residual or recurrent tumor, but, in general, the effects are not seen for months or years.[85, 86] Patients should be informed of the possible late side effects of radiation, such as chiasmal or optic neuropathy in up to 3%,[87] hypopituitarism, brain parenchymal necrosis, and secondary neoplasms (meningiomas and sacromatous transformation of the pituitary adenoma).[85, 86, 88, 89] Stereotactic radiosurgery[90–93] allows more precise delivery of radiation to this area with less risk to surrounding tissues.
4. We recommend a neuro-ophthalmic examination, including visual field testing, within a few days of surgery if the patient is able to comply. The exam can be repeated 1 month postoperatively, and Klibanski[56] recommends follow-up MRI at this time of check for residual tumor. Serial neuroimaging and neuro-ophthalmic examinations then can be performed at 6 and 12 months postoperatively, and if stable, at yearly intervals after that. Postradiation follow-up can be similar. Follow-up of prolactinomas is slightly different because the primary treatment is medical (see below). However, if surgery or radiation becomes part of the management of a prolactinoma, the above schedule may be applied. Endocrine follow-up is also necessary.

Rarely, a delayed visual loss months or years following transsphenoidal resection without radiation can occur. The visual deficits are slowly progressive, and possible mechanisms include intrasellar herniation (empty sella) or tethering scar tissue. Some authors have advocated surgical removal of adhesions and repair of the sellar floor.[94]

Clinical Features and Treatment of Nonfunctioning and Hypersecreting Adenomas

Nonfunctioning (Nonsecreting) Pituitary Tumors. These are usually macroadenomas without clinical evidence of pituitary hormone hypersecretion.[57] In one report, visual loss occurred in 72%, hypopituitarism in 61%, headache in 36%, and cranial neuropathies in 10%.[76] Tumor compression of the normal residual pituitary gland or the stalk often leads to loss of normal LH/FSH, ACTH, and TSH secretion along with mild degrees of hyperprolactinemia.[56, 76] A minority may have panhypopituitarism.[76] In the series of Ebersold et al,[76] patients ranged from 14.5 to 78 years (median 57 years), and 74% were male and 26% female.

Although classically "nonfunctioning," immunocytochemical techniques have demonstrated that cells in the majority of these tumors are capable of producing a small amount of hormone, but not enough to elevate serum levels.[56, 57] In one surgical series,[76] 82% percent were null cell adenomas, while the rest were silent prolactinomas, gonadotropic adenomas, and corticotropic adenomas. One silent plurihormonal adenoma was encountered. Most nonfunctioning adenomas synthesize gonadotropins or their subunits.[42]

Transsphenoidal tumor removal is the treatment modality of choice. All patients with headache in the series of Ebersold et al[76] were relieved of this symptom. However, the prognosis for recovery of pituitary function following transsphenoidal surgery of nonfunctioning tumors is fair to good.[95] Because these tumors are nonfunctioning, hormone levels are unhelpful in detecting residual tumor or recurrences. In younger patients with moderate residual tumor postoperatively, local irradiation at a dose of approximately 5000 cGy, in <200-cGy fractions,[57, 96] should be considered. The ability to follow patients with small amounts of residual tumor by serial MRI may lessen the need for empiric radiation in all such patients.

In the series of Ebersold et al,[76] 6% developed symptomatic recurrences, while an additional 10% had radiographic evidence of recurrent tumor during a follow-up period of 48 to 100 months. Tumors recurred in 18% of patients who received radiotherapy and in 12% who did not. The authors were unable to draw any conclusions from this comparison because the patients with the largest tumors were the ones who underwent radiotherapy. Surgery is the preferred modality when tumors recur following radiotherapy.

Medical options are available to patients with nonfunctioning adenomas in whom surgery is contraindicated, or in whom postoperative recurrence is documented. Bromocriptine (see Prolactinomas, below), when taken long term, has been shown to decrease tumor size in a small number (16%) of patients with nonsecreting adenomas.[59, 97] Octreotide (see GH-Secreting Tumors, below) may reduce the size of some nonsecreting tumors and improve visual symptoms, occasionally within days or even hours.[57, 98, 99] The effects are often transient, and only 30% of patients have long-lasting, stable visual improvement. Thus, Sassolas et al[57] suggested using octreotide as a temporary alternative to surgery in patients with severe visual impairment. The mechanism of action of these medications in this setting is unclear. Our group has little personal experience with bromocriptine and octreotide in the treatment of nonsecreting tumors, so we would still recommend surgery when possible.

Prolactinomas. Prolactin secreting tumors are the most common hormone secreting pituitary adenomas. In women, endocrine symptoms caused by prolactinomas include galactorrhea and evidence of gonadal dysfunction such as decreased libido, amenorrhea, oligomenorrhea, and infertility (Table 7–2). In men, diminished libido, gynecomastia, and impotence are the most common manifestations, but galactorrhea is less frequent.[100] Prolactinomas have been reported in childhood and adolescence.[461]

Medical therapy with dopamine agonists, such as bromocriptine and cabergoline, which inhibit the synthesis and secretion of prolactin, are the first-line treatment of prolactinomas.[59] Bromocriptine in doses up to 2.5 to 5 mg bid or tid can afford tumor shrinkage and reduction in serum prolactin level in up to 80% of patients with prolactinomas.[101] Common side effects include nausea, vomiting, dizziness, and orthostatic hypotension, but sometimes these can be avoided by starting with lower dosages.[43] Withdrawal of bromocriptine results in tumor regrowth and recurrence of prolactinemia, so the medication must be taken indefinitely. Moster et al[102] followed 10 patients with prolactinomas treated with bromocriptine. Improvement in visual acuity and fields and reducting in tumor size occurred in 9 of 10 patients, and in general the salutary effect was sustained. Patients often noticed the visual improvement within days of starting the drug, and subsequent studies[103, 104] have confirmed the potential for rapid visual recovery (Fig. 7–19). A new longer-acting bromocriptine formulation has been developed and requires only monthly intramuscular injections.[105] Cabergoline needs to be taken only twice a week and may be better tolerated than bromocriptine.[106] Other dopamine agonists such as pergolide and quinagolide (CV 205–502)[107] have also been tried in patients with prolactionomas and visual loss.

Transsphenoidal surgery of prolactinomas is less effective,[108] as hyperprolactinemia often recurs postoperatively.[101] Radiotherapy alone may reduce tumor mass effect and prevent further growth,[85] but it is generally an ineffective treatment of hyperprolactinemia.[100] Surgery and radiotherapy should be reserved for patients who do not tolerate or who fail medical therapy.

Besser[43] recommends biweekly neuro-ophthalmic follow-up and prolactin levels initially at the start of medical therapy in individuals with compromised vision. Neuroimaging can be repeated in 6 weeks if vision and prolactin levels have improved. Alternatively, repeat neuroimaging should be performed in 2 to 3 weeks in patients who do not improve, and surgery should be recommended in such cases.

A prolactinoma in the setting of pregnancy is a special situation. During pregnancy, the normal pituitary gland increases in size by 50% to 70% due to lactotroph hyperplasia,[59] but chiasmal compression is rarely an issue. On the other hand, pregnant women with microprolactinomas have a 1% chance of developing symptomatic pituitary enlargement, but those with macroprolactinomas have a 10% to 25% chance.[100] Although bromocriptine is probably safe during pregnancy, Vance and Thorner[100] suggest stopping the medication in women with prolactinomas who become pregnant, and then monitoring visual function carefully. If visual acuity or field abnormalities develop, either continued observation or restarting bromocriptine would be a reasonable approach. Finally, transsphenoidal surgery can also be carried out successfully during pregnancy if absolutely necessary.

Growth Hormone (GH, Somatotropin)-Secreting Pituitary Tumors. According to Molitch's meta-analysis,[109] the mean age of affected patients at diagnosis is 42 years, and eapproximately half are women. Endocrine manifestations are the most common symptom, while visual field defects occurs in only 19% of patients with this type of tumor. Headaches occur in 55%, but their cause is unclear because they correlate poorly with tumor size.

Gigantism and acromegaly are the two major medical conditions that result from GH hypersecretion. Characteristic bony and soft-tissue changes occur, primarily owing to GH-induced increases in IGF-I. GH oversecretion in childhood is associated with pituitary gigantism, and in this disorder longitudinal bone growth is still possible. In acromegaly, typified by overgrowth of acral segments (hands, feet, nose, chin, and forehead),[44] epiphyseal closure has already occurred, prohibiting bone elongation.[44] The disfiguring frontal bossing and enlargement of the mandible and hands are characteristic (Fig. 7–20). Because the changes are insidious, patients may notice only a gradual increase in glove or hat size. Furthermore, because acromegaly primarily occurs in middle-aged individuals, the changes are often attributed to "normal aging." In fact, the delay between onset of symptoms and diagnosis averages 8.7 years.[109]

In addition, bony and soft-tissue overgrowth commonly results in carpal tunnel syndrome and other entrapment neuropathies.[109] Myopathy, arthropathy, and depression are also seen in association with acromegaly. Patients with acromegaly have a higher mortality rate than the normal population, due in part to greater frequencies of hypertension, diabetes, cardiovascular disease, hypertrophic cardiomyopathy, upper and lower airway restrictive pulmonary disease, and gastrointestinal malignancies (colon, especially) occurring in individuals with this endocrinopathy.[109] GH hypersecretion can also cause ocular hypertension and exophthalmos.[37] Hypogonadism occurs in 30% to 40%, likely as the result of stalk compression and hyperprolactinemia (by inhibiting gonadotropin-releasing hormone secretion).[44] Some GH-secreting adenomas cosecrete prolactin.

Definitive treatment of a GH-secreting adenomas is imperative because of their associated disfigurement and increased mortality. Transsphenoidal surgery is the primary treatment, and successful surgery results in a rapid

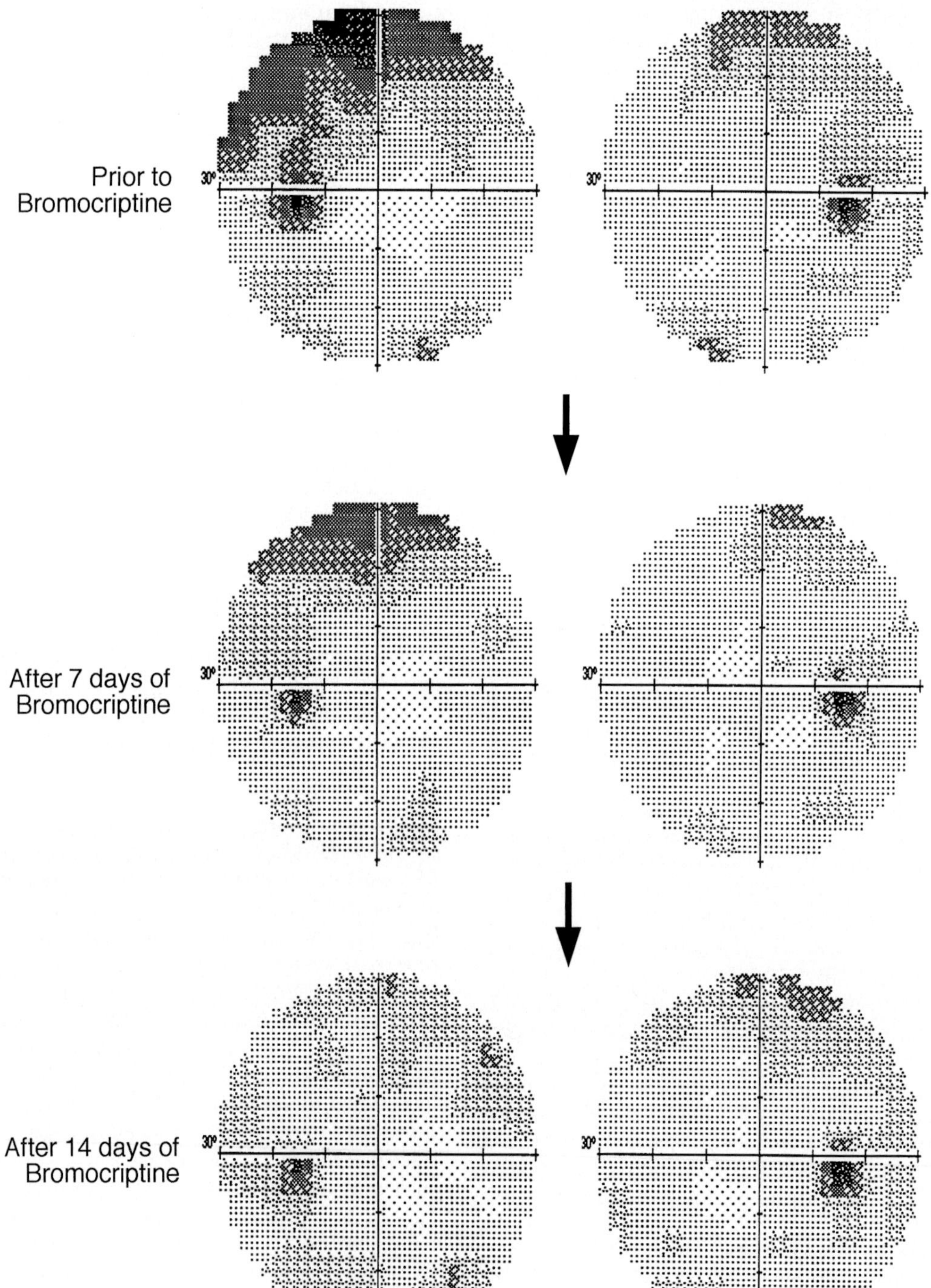

FIGURE 7–19. Rapid improvement in visual fields, especially the superior temporal defect in the left eye, in a patient with a prolactinoma and chiasmal compression treated with bromocriptine.

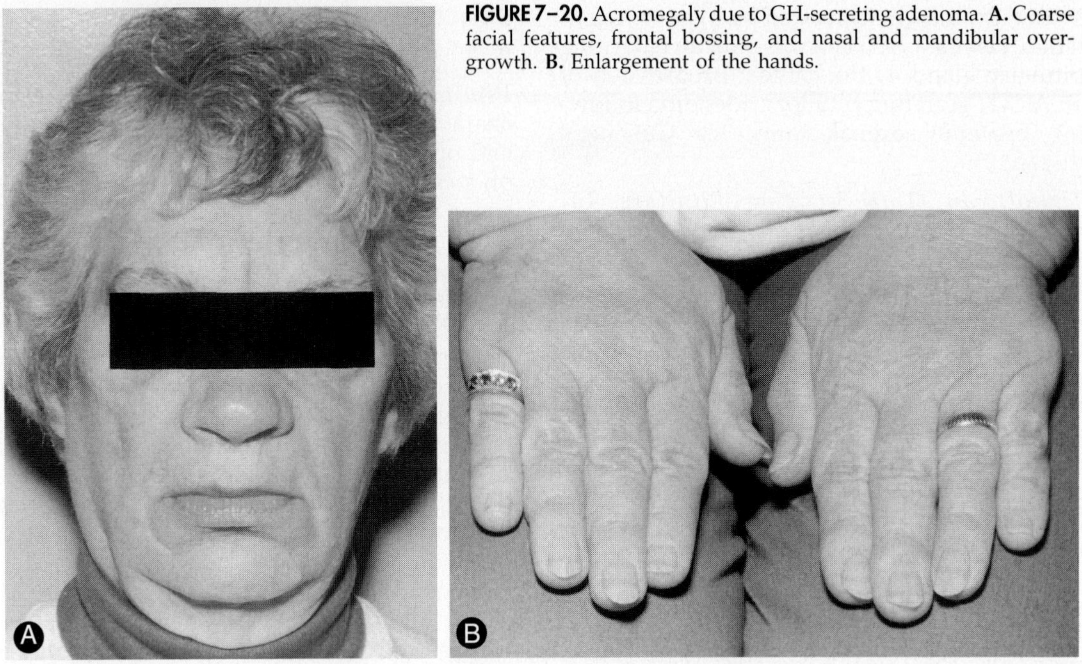

FIGURE 7–20. Acromegaly due to GH-secreting adenoma. **A.** Coarse facial features, frontal bossing, and nasal and mandibular overgrowth. **B.** Enlargement of the hands.

fall in the GH level, although usually not to normal levels.[44, 110] Unfortunately, advanced acromegalic features are rarely reversible, but mild soft-tissue enlargement can be reduced.

Surgical, medical, and radiotherapeutic treatment options can be combined in an overall approach to patients with acromegaly. In Melmed's study,[111] octreotide, a somatostatin analogue (SMS-995) administered via subcutaneous injection,[112] normalized growth hormone levels in 50%, and 37% of tumors decreased in size. Octreotide alone can lead to marked improvement in chiasmal visual field defects.[98, 99] The major side effects are transient diarrhea and nausea, and less frequent ones are gallbladder sludge and asymptomatic gallstones. Melmed's treatment algorithm[111] is a reasonable one and suggests octreotide prior to surgery to facilitate removal[113] in patients with tumors >5 mm. A cure is considered a reduction in GH levels to <2 μg/l after an oral glucose challenge. Bromocriptine and cabergoline may be used but are not as effective as octreotide.[44, 114] Cabergoline may be more efficacious than bromocriptine. Patients with persistently high GH levels in spite of these measures can be retreated with octreotide or receive radiotherapy.[85] Despite doses of 4000 to 5000 cGy, radiation can take years to lower GH levels.

Adrenocorticotropin (ACTH)-Secreting Pituitary Tumors (Cushing's disease). These adenomas occur primarily in women of childbearing age, and approximately three quarters of cases of Cushing syndrome (excess circulating cortisol) are caused by ACTH-secreting pituitary tumors (Cushing's disease).[45] Elevated ACTH levels result in adrenocortical hyperplasia and increased secretion of cortisol. Common clinical features include obesity with moon facies and a buffalo hump, hypertension, hirsutism, striae, psychiatric symptoms, gonadal dysfunction, osteopenia, and glucose intolerance.[115] Usually these tumors are microadenomas without extrasellar involvement.

Transsphenoidal removal is the procedure of choice.[116, 117] Radiotherapy can be used in patients with persistent or recurrent disease,[85, 118] but cortisol levels may not be controlled until 1 to 2 years later. In the interim, drugs such as metyrapone, ketoconazole, and aminoglutethimide, which inhibit adrenal cortisol synthesis, or cyproheptadine, sodium valproate, bromocriptine, and octreotide, which can inhibit ACTH secretion, can be used short term to control symptoms.[53] As a last resort, those individuals failing both surgery and radiation are candidates for bilateral adrenalectomy to suppress the hypercortisolism, but this procedure has no effect on pituitary size.[45] Nelson syndrome, characterized by hyperpigmentation, elevated ACTH levels, and an enlarging pituitary gland, is the clinical progression of an ACTH-secreting pituitary adenoma following bilateral adrenalectomy for Cushing's disease.[116]

Thyrotropin (TSH)-Secreting Pituitary Tumors. These are uncommon, but occur in two varieties. In the first type, which is really not a tumor per se, primary hypothyroidism leads to compensatory hyperplasia of pituitary thyrotroph cells. In Smallridge's review[119] of reported cases of this type, he found that 37% of these patients developed visual defects (types unspecified) due to pituitary enlargement and chiasmal compression. Reduction in pituitary size and improvement in visual field deficits are often successful after thyroid replacement.[120]

In contrast, the second type, a thyrotropin-secreting adenoma (thyrotropinoma), is usually associated with thyrotoxicosis due to inappropriate TSH secretion. The diagnosis is established by demonstrating high circulating levels of T_3 and T_4, normal or elevated TSH, and a pituitary lesion. Fifty-four percent of affected individuals in Smallridge's literature review[119] had abnormal visual fields (again, types unspecified). In general, patients do not develop thyroid associated orbitopathy. Transsphenoidal surgery, followed by radiation if necessary, is the treatment of choice. Thyroidectomy or radioactive iodine controls the hyperthyroidism but not the pituitary enlargement. Octreotide, which can improve chiasmal field defects in this setting, may also be considered.[98, 462, 463]

Gonadotropin (LH, FSH)-Secreting Pituitary Tumors. Patients with these adenomas are typically male and older than 40, have normal gonadal function, and typically present with visual impairment due to chiasmal compression.[121] In Snyder's series,[121] 17% of 139 men with pituitary macroadenomas had this type of tumor. In a series of 100 patients from the Mayo Clinic,[122] 43% presented with visual loss, 22% with symptoms of hypopituitarism, and 8% with headache. Hypersecretion of FSH is the most common endocrinologic abnormality. Precocious puberty results when this tumor occurs in childhood. Transsphenoidal surgery usually results in some visual improvement,[122] and octreotide may have a beneficial effect with this type of adenoma as well.[98]

Three other situations related to pituitary adenomas—pituitary apoplexy, metastases to the pituitary, and incidental pituitary adenomas—deserve special mention.

Pituitary Apoplexy. This clinical syndrome is characterized by sudden visual loss, headache, and ophthalmoplegia due to rapid expansion of a pituitary adenoma into the suprasellar space and cavernous sinuses (Fig. 7–21).[123] Defined in this way, pituitary apoplexy presents with headache in 95%, vomiting in 69%, ocular paresis in 78%, visual field deficits in 64%, and reduction in acuity in 52%.[124] Third nerve palsies are more common than fourth and sixth nerve deficits. When visual loss and headache are the primary symptoms, the condition can be confused with retrobulbar optic neuritis. Alteration in consciousness, due to diencephalic compression, hypopituitarism, facial pain or numbness, and signs of meningeal irritation (blood- or necrotic tumor tissue-induced) are common associated features. We have seen retraction nystagmus associated with pituitary apoplexy,[125] presumably due to dorsal midbrain compression, but that is rare. Diabetes insipidus is surprisingly uncommon in this setting. Most affected patients were previously unaware that they harbored a pituitary adenoma. The syndrome is uncommon, and only about 2% of pituitary adenomas will present this way.[124]

Often pituitary apoplexy is the result of extensive tumor infarction or hemorrhage. Although most cases are associated solely with a pituitary adenoma, predisposing factors may include sudden trauma, anticoagulation, alteration of pressure gradients (angiography, for example), cardiac surgery, diabetic ketoacidosis, and estrogen, bromocriptine, radiotherapy, and postpartum hemorrhage (Sheehan syndrome).

The clinical suspicion of pituitary apoplexy mandates MRI as routine CT may miss the lesion. MRI usually demonstrates a macroadenoma with heterogeneous signal characteristics due to the presence of blood, while CT can reveal an unenhancing, hyperdense sellar mass. Hemorrhage, when present, can extend in the subarachnoid space and ventricles. Lumbar puncture may demonstrate an aseptic meningitis, sometimes accompanied by red blood cells. Since the sudden headache and ocular motor palsies associated with pituitary apoplexy may mimic aneurysmal subarachnoid hemorrhage, a CSF hemorrhagic component may warrant angiographic exclusion of an aneurysm if CT and MRI are inconclusive. Transsphenoidal surgery and emergent steroid and other hormonal replacement have facilitated the management of pituitary apoplexy. Some cases improve spontaneously, either clinically[126] or radiographically, or both.[475] The prognosis for visual improvement depends more on early surgical decompression than the severity of the visual deficit. Almost all patients undergoing surgery within 1 week will experience some improvement in acuity, fields, and ocular motility.[124] A conservative approach may be appropriate for stable or improving patients without visual loss or mental status changes who have a medical contraindication for surgery.

Metastatic Tumors to the Pituitary. These can have clinical and radiographic presentions similar to those of nonsecreting pituitary adenomas, except that patients with metastases to the pituitary are more likely to have diabetes insipidus and ocular motor palsies, and a more rapidly evolving clinical course is seen.[127, 128] The most common primary sources are breast and lung. The pituitary lesion may be the first indication of malignancy, and in these instances patients may undergo transsphenoidal surgery with an incorrect preoperative diagnosis of pituitary adenoma.

Incidental Pituitary Adenomas. Incidental identification of a pituitary lesion may occur in as many as 10% of patients undergoing neuroimaging for other reasons. All such individuals require endocrinologic screening, but those with macroadenomas also need neuro-ophthalmic evaluation. If endocrine and visual function are normal, neuroradiologic and neuro-ophthalmic assessments can be repeated on a semiannual or annual basis. Surgery would be indicated if there is evidence of tumor compression or growth. Incidentally detected macroadenomas have approximately a 33% chance of enlarging, while only 15% of microadenomas will increase in size.[129–131]

CRANIOPHARYNGIOMAS

Craniopharyngiomas are cystic, calcified sellar-region tumors that constitute 1.2% to 3%

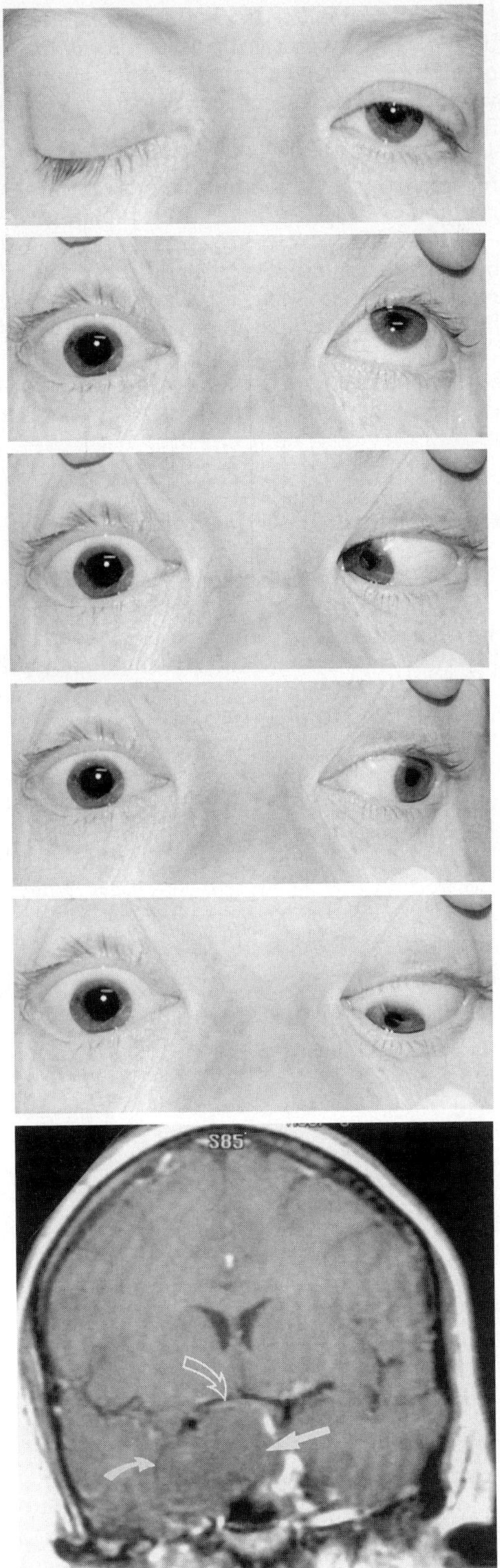

FIGURE 7–21. Pituitary apoplexy. *Top rows:* This patient developed sudden headache, complete ophthalmoplegia and mydriasis of the right eye, ptosis of the right upper eyelid, loss of sensation in the right forehead, and chiasmal field loss. *Bottom:* MRI demonstrated a heterogeneous sellar mass (*large solid arrow*) compressing the chiasm (*open arrow*) and invading the right cavernous sinus (*curved solid arrow*).

of all intracranial neoplasms.[132] They may present at any age, but in various series,[132–134] the peak age incidence occurred in either the first or second decade of life. Approximately half of all cases are seen in adults, and some present in patients in their sixth decade.[132] They are epithelial in origin and are thought to derive from remnants of Rathke's pouch, which ordinarily migrates upward from the primitive buccal cavity. Craniopharyngiomas can be found anywhere along the migratory path.[135, 136] Others have suggested that craniopharyngiomas might originate from squamous metaplasia in cells of the adenohypophysis.[136] Although benign in histology, craniopharyngiomas may act aggressively by invading local structures and by recurring despite apparent complete resection.[137]

Pathology

There are two major histologic subtypes, adamantinomatous and squamous papillary, each with different age predilections. Although seen in all age groups, adamantinomatous craniopharyngiomas most often occur in childhood.[132] The microscopic appearance is characterized by angulated columnar cells, and keratin nodules and calcification are common.[136] Cysts are present in 90% and are mixed frequently with solid components. The cyst fluid has the consistency of light machinery ("crank-case") oil and contains suspended cholesterol crystals. Although usually well defined, adamantinomatous craniopharyngiomas may adhere to surrounding brain and vascular structures.[136] Reactive gliosis and tumor islets[132] may be seen in adjacent brain tissue. These features may, in part, account for recurrences of adamantinomatous craniopharyngiomas despite "total" resection.[132]

Craniopharyngiomas in adulthood tend to be squamous papillary. Calcification, keratin nodule formation, and adamantinous epithelium are conspicuously absent in these tumors. Cysts occur in approximately 50% of cases.[132] Squamous papillary craniopharyngiomas tend to be well demarcated, and after complete resection they tend not to recur.[132, 138]

Location and Growth Characteristics

Figure 7–22 highlights the most common locations of craniopharyngiomas in relationship to the sella, suprasellar area, and third ventricle. Typically they traverse more than one of these spaces, and entirely intrasellar or intraventricular craniopharyngiomas are unusual.[139] Prechiasmatic tumors, when large, can protrude between the optic nerves and lift the A_1 segments of the anterior cerebral arteries. Retrochiasmal tumors can extend posteriorly into the third ventricle and abut the basilar artery and midbrain.[140] Their size may vary from a few millimeters to several centimeters,[70] but the majority of tumors are 2 to 4 cm in greatest

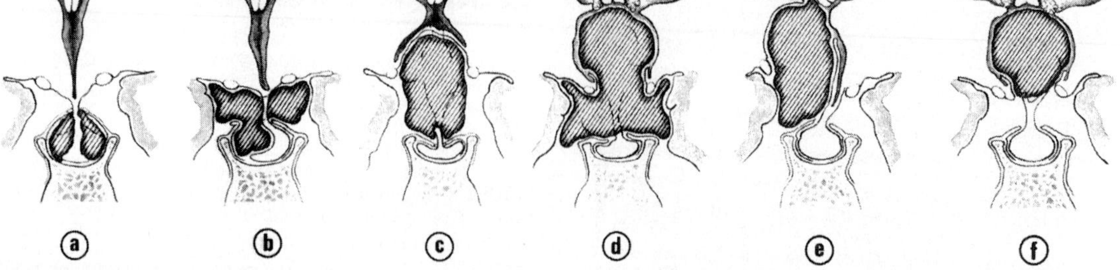

FIGURE 7–22. Diagrammatic representation of the most common locations of craniopharyngiomas. a: Purely intrasellar-infradiaphragmatic; b: intra- and suprasellar, infra- and supradiaphragmatic; c: supradiaphragmatic, parachiasmatic, extraventricular; d: intra- and extraventricular; e: paraventricular in respect to the third ventricle; and f: purely intraventricular. (From Yasargil MG, et al: J Neurosurg 1990;73:3–11, with permission.)

diameter.[138] Tumors may be densely adherent to the hypothalamus with small papillary projections.[136] Hydrocephalus, due to third ventricular compression, occurs in approximately 38% of patients.[138]

Craniopharyngiomas typically disrupt the anterior visual pathways by external compression. However, unusual instances of intrachiasmatic craniopharyngioma, causing chiasmal thickening, have been described.[141–143] Tumor extension through the optic foramen and canal into the orbit is also rare, but has been reported.[144,145] Other unusual growth patterns include spread beyond the sellar area into the anterior, middle, and posterior fossae.[146] Midbrain,[147] hemispheric,[148] and cerebellopontine angle[149] involvement has also been reported.

Fluid leakage, owing to surgical or spontaneous cyst rupture, can result in a severe chemical arachnoiditis or meningitis.[136] Spontaneous hemorrhage with subarachnoid hemorrhage is a reported but unusual complication.[150]

Symptoms

Initial manifestations can be grouped into four major categories: visual, endocrinologic, and cognitive abnormalities, and headaches.[132, 134, 138] Visual symptoms are usually the most common manifestation, occuring in 61% to 77% of patients.[132, 134, 138, 151, 152] These and endocrinologic abnormalities are discussed in more detail below. Cognitive deficits include personality changes, memory loss, depression, and confusion. Headaches are nonspecific, but are sometimes accompanied by nausea and vomiting. Some authors have touted a varied presentation according to age group, with visual loss and endocrine symptoms seen at all ages, but with headaches and papilledema occurring more frequently in childhood and mental status changes more often in adult cases.[133, 134]

Neuro-ophthalmic Signs

In Repka et al's series,[153] visual acuity was <20/40 in 41% of eyes at presentation, and approximately 15% were worse than 20/400. Bitemporal hemianopias are commonly observed field abnormalities,[133, 151] and asymmetry and incomplete defects appear to be the rule.[134, 154] Homonymous hemianopias, due to optic tract compression,[155] are less frequent.[133, 151] Usually visual impairment occurs gradually, but sudden unilateral or bilateral visual loss, mimicking retrobulbar optic neuritis, has been reported.[134, 156] The majority of patients with visual loss will have optic atrophy.[133] Sixth nerve palsies are common, and usually owe to third ventricular compression and elevated intracranial pressure, but they can also result from infiltration of the cavernous sinuses. Children may present with comitant or incomitant esotropia.[133] See-saw nystagmus may also be an associated finding.[29]

Some authors[136] have written that children with craniopharyngiomas may be less apt to report visual loss, so visual deficits at presentation may be more severe than in adults. However, not all data support this notion. In one analysis,[133] the difference was not statistically significant. In another series,[153] more children had subnormal acuities, but more adults had visual field deficits.

Endocrinologic Manifestations

Kennedy and Smith's study,[133] in which 64% of patients had endocrine abnormalities, contains excellent data regarding the frequency of these symptoms. Twenty-seven percent had complaints consistent with diabetes insipidus, 22% experienced weight gain, 20% had short stature, 36% developed various manifestations of hypogonadism, 16% had myxedema, while 24% were somnolent. Other investigators have had similar results.[145] Thomsett et al[157] found that 83% of children with craniopharyngioma had at least one hypothalamic–pituitary hormone deficiency after careful laboratory evaluation. Growth retardation is, of course, a symptom primarily of children and young adults.[105] It is uncertain whether endocrinopathy is more frequent in adults or children, because different series give conflicting results.[132, 133, 138] The syndrome of inappropriate secretion of antidiuretic hormones (SIADH) at presentation can occur but is uncommon.[465]

Diagnostic Studies/Neuroimaging

The MRI appearance of craniopharyngiomas is characteristic.[158] They are discrete intra- or suprasellar masses that can be hyperintense on T_1-weighted images. Increased amounts of cholesterol, protein, and keratin cause these tumors to be markedly hyperintense on T_2-weighted images (Fig. 7–23). Cysts appear as round masses that are hypointense on T_1-

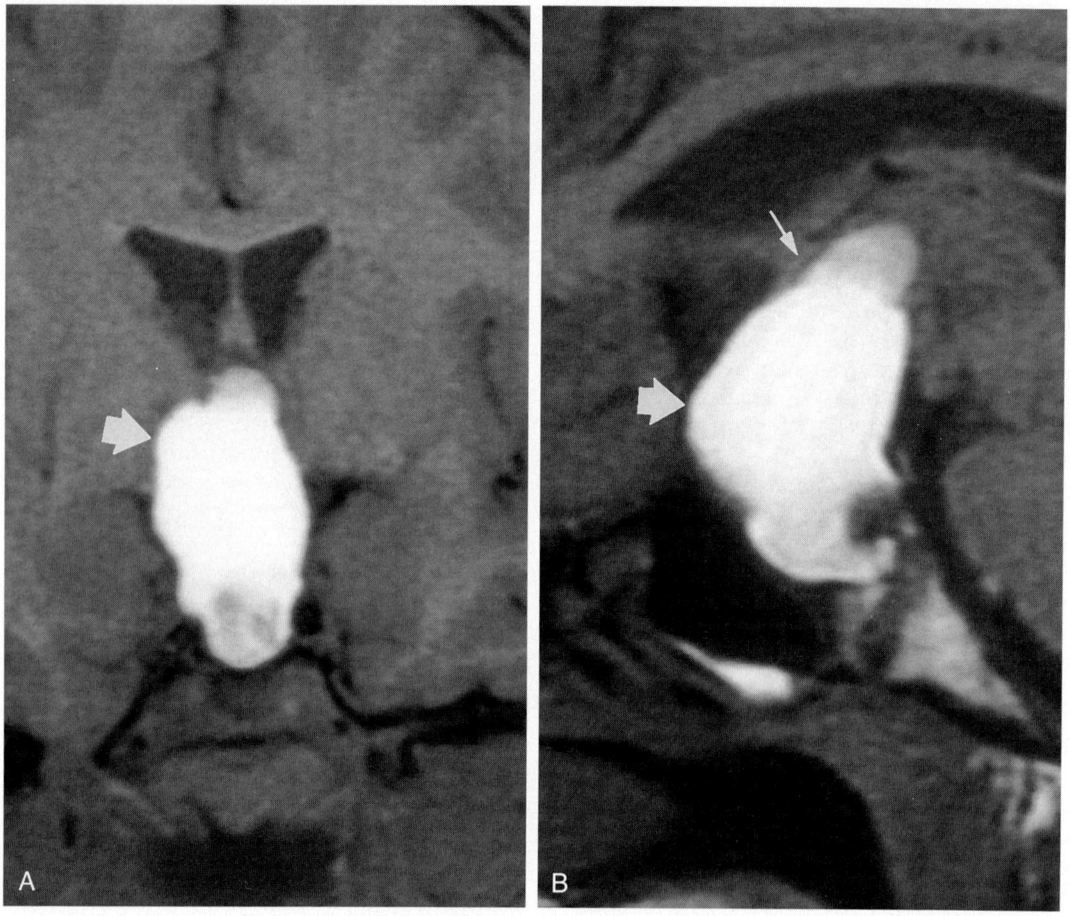

FIGURE 7–23. Large suprasellar mass (*large arrow*) that is hyperintense on MRI, T_1-weighted images, consistent with a craniopharyngioma. **A.** Coronal view. **B.** Sagittal view; the chiasm (*small arrow*) has been flattened and bowed upwards. The patient had a bitemporal hemianopia (see Fig. 7–7).

weighted images and hyperintense on T_2-weighted images. Areas of signal void within the tumor represent calcification, and on rare occasions the solid component is completely calcified. After administration of gadolinium, the solid portion may exhibit modest enhancement.[70] High signal within the optic tracts and posterior limbs of the internal capsules has been observed with MRI, producing a "moustache" appearance,[159] but resolution of this finding following tumor resection suggests perifocal edema rather than tumor invasion.[160, 161] In some instances MRI-angiography may be helpful in excluding an aneurysm[72] and defining the tumor's relationship to vascular structures within the circle of Willis, which can be either displaced or surrounded by the tumor.[148] Conventional invasive angiography, which may demonstrate absence of neovascularity or tumor staining,[162] is rarely necessary.

CT, especially with coronal views, is complementary and often diagnostic when calcification is evident (Fig. 7–24). Cysts and solid components are easily distinguishable, and the solid portions variably enhance after administration of intravenous (IV) contrast. Cysts may ring enhance. Calcification within an intra- or suprasellar mass on CT is highly characteristic of craniopharyngioms and occurs in approximately 80% of cases.[148] Thus, preoperatively many authorities would recommend MRI, with its sagittal views and emphasis on anatomic detail, as well as CT.[136]

Treatment

The primary treatment of craniopharyngiomas is neurosurgical,[163, 164] utilizing microsurgical techniques. Tumors that are primarily intrasel-

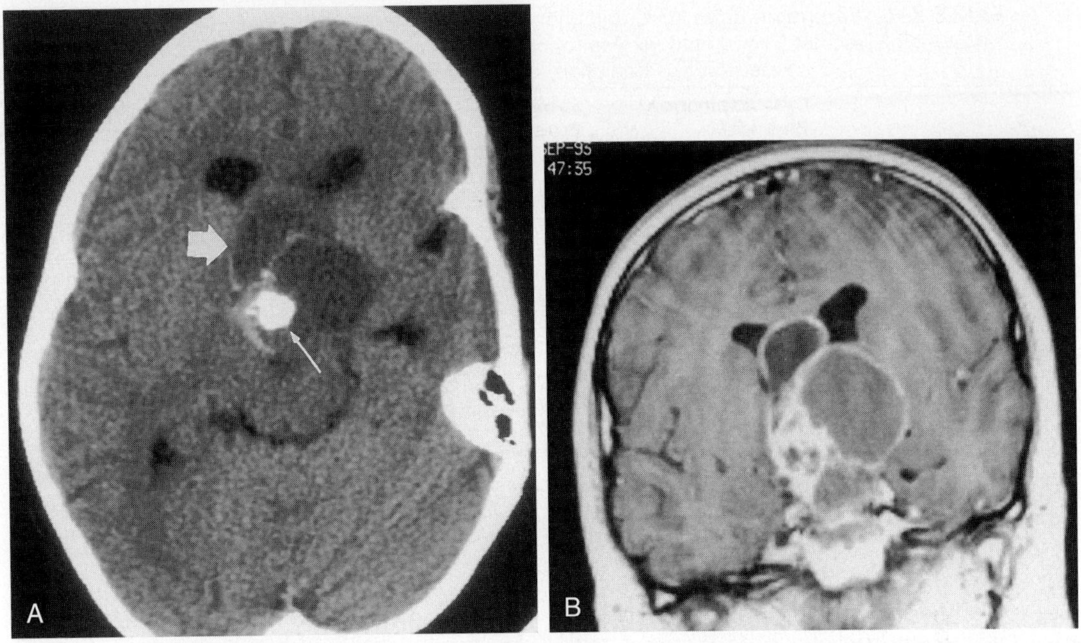

FIGURE 7–24. Multicystic craniopharyngioma. **A.** Coronal CT scan demonstrating a large, multicystic suprasellar mass (*thick white arrow*) with a hyperdensity (*long white arrow*) corresponding to an area of calcification. **B.** Corresponding gadolinium-enhanced coronal MRI scan of the same patient demonstrating large suprasellar extension and obliteration of the third ventricle.

lar or subdiaphragmatic may be amenable to transsphenoidal surgery,[62, 165–167] which offers a lower surgical morbidity. However, the two most common approaches are unilateral pterional and subfrontal[135] craniotomies, which can be combined with a transcallosal approach if the tumor involves the third ventricle,[168] or a transsphenoidal procedure when there is subdiaphragmatic extension.[145] Multiple procedures may be required for complete decompression of large and recurrent tumors.[151, 169] Shunt placement may be necessary when hydrocephalus is present.[145]

Experts disagree whether the best treatment is complete excision or subtotal resection plus radiation.[145, 151, 152] The controversy exists in part because many authors espouse just one treatment approach.[151, 170] Advocates of complete resection[140, 145, 171, 172] argue that modern neuroimaging, microsurgical techniques, and hormonal replacement therapy allow aggressive surgery, and patients are spared the side effects of radiation. However, extensive surgery can result in debilitating visual, endocrinologic, emotional, and cognitive deficits,[173, 174] and has an operative mortality of up to 11%.[136] Accidental tears in the carotid artery, leading to cerebral infarction, have been reported when complete excision was attempted.[140] Furthermore, this approach does not guarantee a cure, as recurrence rates still range from 6% to 50% despite apparent complete removal.[140, 145, 152, 171, 172]

Proponents of subtotal resection plus external beam radiation readily emphasize a lower rate of operative morbidity and mortality associated with this method of treatment.[135, 151, 175] Postoperative radiotherapy decreases the rate of recurrence and improves patient survival compared with partial removal alone.[176] Radiation doses usually range from 5000 to 5500 cGy, given in 180-cGy fractions.[152, 177] Unfortunately, dose-related radiation toxicity, manifesting as endocrinopathy, optic neuropathy, vascular events, and secondary malignancies,[178] can occur in approximately 50% of patients treated in this fashion.[170]

In order to arrive at a sensible treatment approach, several investigators[136–138, 152, 157, 177, 179, 467] compared the various treatment regimens, using retrospective analysis of patients treated at their institutions (Table 7–5). In the one study[157] that specifically addressed endocrinologic issues, hypothalamic–pituitary dysfunction occurred least commonly in patients treated with limited excision plus radiotherapy. The tumor recurrence rate was similar in children and adults.[138] In all studies, subtotal

TABLE 7–5. Recurrence Rates for Craniopharyngiomas in Series From Single Institutions and Meta-analyses That Compared Cyst Aspiration Plus Radiation, Subtotal Resection, Subtotal Resection Plus Radiation, and Total Resection Alone

	Cyst Aspiration Plus xRT	Subtotal Resection	Subtotal Resection Plus xRT	Total Resection Alone
Series/#Pts				
Shapiro (1979)/60[179]	50	78	0	23
Cabezudo (1981)/45[137]		71	6	30
Wen (1989)/52[177]		85	0	50
Weiss (1989)/31*[152]		100	20	33
Weiner (1994)/56[138]		50	63	17
Fahlbusch (1999)/148[467]				19
Meta-analysis				
Wen (1989)[177]		74	25	30
Weiss (1989)*[152]	26	75	22	26
Sanford (1991)[136]		71	21	25

Pts = patients, xRT = radiation therapy.
*Children only

resection alone had the highest rate of recurrence. Cyst aspiration plus radiation had reasonable outcomes, but was not included in most reviews. Except in one study,[138] subtotal resection combined with radiation was associated with a lower recurrence rate than total resection. Meta-analyses,[136, 152, 177] however, show that the recurrence rates for these two approaches are similar. Therefore, based on these results, the most reasonable approach seems to be to attempt complete resection if possible, especially in young children, in whom radiation is less desirable. Most tumors can be handled in this way. When involvement of visual and endocrine structures precludes complete excision, and when neuroimaging indicates residual tumor following surgery, external beam irradiation should be performed postoperatively.[137, 152, 179] This is the treatment algorithm currently practiced by the neurosurgery service at the Children's Hospital of Philadelphia.

Intracavitary brachytherapy, utilizing beta-emitting radioactive colloids, is an alternative to surgical excision when craniopharyngiomas are primarily cystic or when they recur.[180] Radiation destroys the epithelial lining, leading to cyst collapse.[181] Because the cystic components are frequently the largest part of the tumor, reduction in cyst size may result in improvement in symptoms. The most common isotopes injected stereotactically include phosphorus-32, yttrium-90, rhenium-186, and gold-198.[154] Intratumoral bleomycin, an antineoplastic antibiotic, has also been used to reduce cyst size.[182]

In the future, more craniopharyngiomas will be treated with either single-dose (gamma-knife, for example) or fractionated stereotactic radiosurgery, which deliver more concentrated radiation doses within narrower fields.[183] However, these modalities may not be suited for residual perichiasmal tumor. Ideal craniopharyngiomas for stereotactic radiosurgery are <2.5 cm and are sufficiently distant from the optic chiasm (>5 mm) to limit the chance of chiasmal radiation necrosis.[184]

Although survival in craniopharyngioma is excellent, the visual and endocrinologic complications can be devastating.[185] These are discussed separately below.

Visual Outcome. Dramatic visual recovery can occur,[186] but in general, the prognosis for visual improvement following therapy for craniopharyngiomas is modest at best[187] and less sanguine than that associated with pituitary adenomas. Repka et al[153] retrospectively compared pre- and postoperative visual examinations in 30 patients, most of whom underwent transcranial surgery for their craniopharyngiomas. The proportion of eyes with visual acuity worse than 20/40 fell from 41% preoperatively to 24% postoperatively, and those with visual field abnormalities decreased from 80% to 44%. Optic atrophy was associated with poorer postoperative visual acuities, whereas normal preoperative optic nerve appearance almost always predicted a postoperative visual acuity of 20/30 or better. Adults had a greater chance for improvement in acuity and fields compared with children, and the authors attributed this difference to longer periods of undetected visual loss in younger patients. A poorer visual prognosis in children was confirmed in another series.[188] Trautmann and Laws[62] reported 40 patients who underwent transsphenoidal surgery for craniopharyngiomas (locations not indicated). Only 2 of 13 patients with preoperative vision worse than 20/40 experienced improvement in acuity, and of 21 patients with visual field deficits, the fields returned to normal in 7. Acuity and fields worsened in two patients following surgery. Based on our personal experience, we agree with Repka and Miller[189] that "one should not be optimistic regarding postoperative visual outcome after removal of craniopharyngioma, particularly in children . . . cautious optimism may be appropriate for some adults, particularly those without ophthalmoscopic evidence of optic atrophy."

The visual outcome following intracavitary brachytherapy is similar. Van den Berge et al[154] described their results in 31 patients with cystic craniopharyngiomas, into which they stereotactically injected yttrium-90. In approximately two thirds of patients the cysts either resolved or decreased in size. However, visual acuity improved in only 29% of eyes studied, remained unchanged in 13%, and worsened in 58%. Visual field deficits improved in 28% of eyes, stabilized in 20%, and deteriorated in 52%. The authors concluded that intracavitary brachytherapy with yttrium-90 offered good radiologic results, but was not as efficacious in preserving vision. Anderson et al[181] reported more encouraging results with phosphorus-32 although in some instances multiple injections were required. Five patients were treated for recurrences following surgery and standard radiation, and all five enjoyed improvement in acuity. In three of these patients, visual fields improved (two returned to normal). Two other patients received intracavitary phosphorus-32 as primary treatment, and they also experienced improvement in acuity and visual fields.

Endocrine Outcome. Post-treatment pituitary dysfunction is the rule, usually the result of surgery but occasionally due to radiation.[157] In one series,[190] 74% of patients post-treatment had diabetes insipidus, 100% were growth hormone deficient, 72% had ACTH deficiency, 65% TSH deficiency, and 93% gonadotrophin deficiency. Results in other reports were similar.[157, 191] Thus, after treatment most patients require some combination of GH, corticosteroid, thyroid, and gonadal steroid replacement and DDAVP. Diabetes insipidus, if not present preoperatively, usually manifests 6 to 12 hours after surgery sometimes following a transient phase of SIADH. There may be slight improvement and a minority recover, but most affected patients develop permanent ADH deficiency.[39, 466] Interestingly, even without GH replacement some patients experience normal or accelerated growth post-treatment, sometimes accompanied by obesity and hyperphagia.[190, 192]

RATHKE'S CLEFT CYSTS

These lesions are similar to craniopharyngiomas in derivation, location, and symptoms, but there are some important differences. Although small incidental cysts are found commonly on neuroimaging and in the pars distalis or pars intermedia in 2% to 26% of routine autopsy cases, symptomatic Rathke's cleft cysts are unusual.[193, 194] Patients are typically older; the average age at presentation is 38 years.[193] Other dissimilarities, including a better visual prognosis, are highlighted below.

Pathology

Rathke's cleft cysts also originate from Rathke's pouch, but histopathologically are less complex than craniopharyngiomas. The cysts are lined by a single layer of cuboidal or ciliated columnar epithelium and contain a gold-colored or white serous or mucinous fluid.[195, 196] Calcification is rare.

Location and Growth Characteristics

Most cysts are intrasellar, and when symptomatic lead to headache and hypopituitarism. A prominent suprasellar component can result in chiasmal compression and hypothalamic dysfunction, and in unusual situations, obstructive hydrocephalus.[197] Rarely, symptomatic Rathke's cleft cysts are entirely suprasellar.[197, 198]

Symptoms

Voelker et al[193] reviewed the findings in 155 patients with symptomatic Rathke's cleft cyst: 8 from their institution and 147 other cases reported in the literature up to 1991. The most common presenting symptom was pituitary dysfunction, found in 69% of cases. Hypopituitarism, amenorrhea–galactorrhea, and diabetes insipidus occurred in decreasing order of frequency. Visual disturbances were present in 56% (see below), and headache in 49%. In another series,[199] the cysts were found incidentally in 14 percent of the patients.

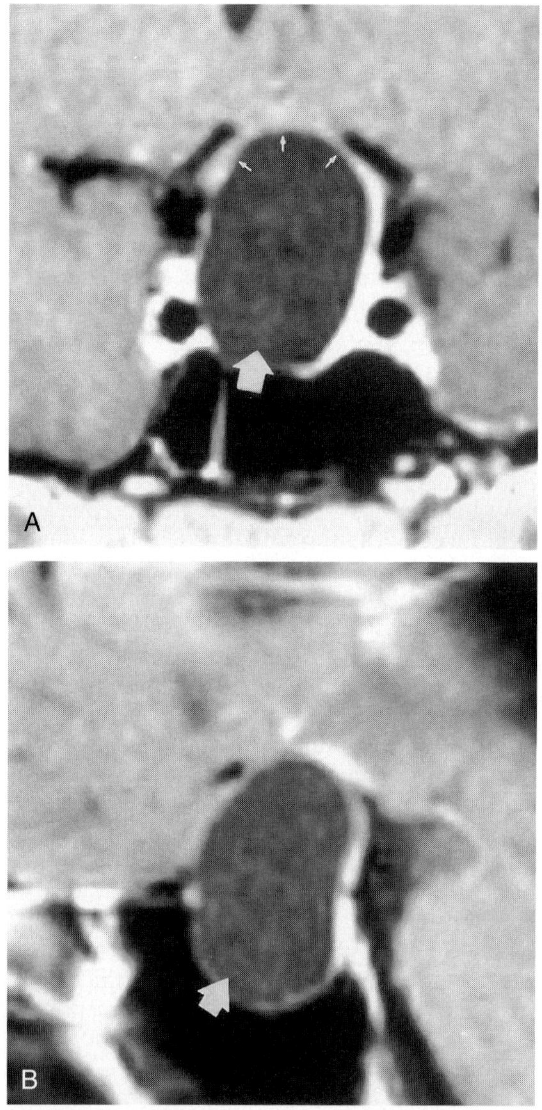

FIGURE 7–25. Symptomatic Rathke's cleft cyst (*thick arrow*), serous type, compressing the chiasm (*small arrows*). **A.** Coronal view. **B.** Sagittal view. The cyst contains fluid that is hypointense on these postcontrast T_1-weighted MR images, and the cyst wall enhances. Like CSF, the cyst fluid was bright on T_2-weighted images (not shown). The patient had a bitemporal hemianopia. (Courtesy of Lawrence Gray, OD.)

Neuro-ophthalmic Signs

Approximately one half of patients have visual field deficits, and about one quarter will have visual acuity loss.[193, 200] In the series of Rao et al,[196] 9 of 11 patients had field defects. In all instances the deficit indicated a chiasmal disturbance: five of these nine were bitemporal, while the other four had monocular temporal field abnormalities.

Diagnostic Studies/Neuroimaging

There are two characteristic patterns. Serous lesions are hypodense on CT, and on MRI they are hypointense in T_1-weighted images and hyperintense on T_2-weighted images, like CSF (Fig. 7–25).[201] On the other hand, mucoid cysts on CT are either isodense or hyperdense, compared with brain. On MRI they are hyperintense on T_1-weighted images and iso- or hypointense on T_2-weighted images.[202] The cyst wall (rim) may enhance, and blood or hemosiderin can also be evident.[203, 204]

Treatment

Neurosurgical decompression is curative and often affords symptomatic improvement. Because Rathke's cleft cysts are primarily intrasellar, transsphenoidal drainage and biopsy of the cyst wall is the favored surgical approach.[165, 199, 200, 205] Associated morbidity and mortality is limited to diabetes insipidus. In one series,[205] headache was cured in all cases in which it was present preoperatively, but endocrine outcomes were variable. Hypopituitarism and diabetes insipidus frequently persist.[193] Large suprasellar components may require removal via craniotomy.[199] Recurrences requiring repeat drainage can occur[206, 207] but are uncommon, and adjunctive radiation or chemotherapy is unnecessary.

Visual Outcome

In contrast to visual loss associated with craniopharyngiomas, the visual prognosis associated with Rathke's pouch cysts is excellent following decompression. Voelker et al[193] found resolution or improvement of visual field deficits in 89% of affected patients, and 81% of those with subnormal visual acuity also enjoyed some improvement. Seventy-five percent of the patients of Rao et al[196] experienced postoperative improvement in visual function. Following transsphenoidal surgery, El-Mahdy et al[200] found 66.6% of eyes had improvement in visual acuity, and 68% in the visual field.

SUPRASELLAR ARACHNOID CYSTS

These are uncommon lesions, and they are thought to derive from an anomaly in Liliequist's membrane, either as a diverticulum or as a cleavage within the membrane and CSF secretion into the cavity.[208] On CT and MRI, suprasellar arachnoid cysts contain fluid with neuroimaging characteristics of CSF, and the cyst wall does not enhance. The cysts are usually noncommunicating, but in some instances may connect with the basal cisterns. Rare instances of intraluminal hemorrhage may give a cyst a "blue-domed" appearance.[209] Half of cases present before 6 years of age.[208] Common clinical features include signs and symptoms of slowly progressive obstructive hydrocephalus, visual impairment, endocrine dysfunction, spasticity and gait disturbances.[210] Approximately 10% of patients will have a peculiar to-and-fro head bobbing.[210, 211]

Asymptomatic suprasellar arachnoid cysts can be observed, but in symptomatic cases the treatment is neurosurgical.[212] Endoscopic ventriculocystosomy seems to be the safest and most effective technique.[210] Removal or fenestration via subfrontal craniotomy or fenestration of the cyst into the lateral ventricle and shunt insertion are other options.[208, 210]

MENINGIOMAS OF THE SKULL BASE

Meningiomas can affect the chiasm when they arise from the tuberculum sellae, anterior clinoid processes, or diaphragma sellae (see Fig. 7–3). Dorsum sellae meningiomas are rare.[213] When they become large enough, juxta- and parasellar meningiomas can also cause chiasmal compression, but these are discussed in the chapters dealing with their primary neuro-ophthalmic disturbance: planum sphenoidale, olfactory groove, and optic sheath meningiomas in Chapter 5, and middle and lateral sphenoid wing and cavernous sinus meningiomas in Chapter 15. This section will concentrate on the meningiomas that occur primarily in the suprasellar region, which account for approximately 8% of all intracranial meningiomas.[214]

Pathology

Meningiomas arise from the arachnoid mater,[214] and in particular suprasellar meningiomas derive from the meninges covering the medial portion of the sphenoid bone, tuberculum, and anterior clinoid processes. They tend to be vascular and firm in consistency.[215] Histologically they are usually of the "classic" variety, characterized by whorls and psammoma bodies.[216] "Classic" subtypes include meningotheliomatous, fibroblastic, transitional, psammomatous, and angiomatous.[217] Other classes of meningiomas, such as angioblastic,[217] are much less common in the sellar region. For the most part meningiomas grow slowly, are benign, and cause dysfunction by compressing adjacent structures. They generally do not invade brain. They can grow exclusively along a dural surface (en plaque meningioma) or a similar flat dural component can be attached to a more clearly defined soft tissue mass (dural tail).

Associations

Progesterone and sometimes estrogen receptors can be found in meningiomas. The functional significance of these receptors is not clear, except meningiomas are more common in women than in men, can enlarge during pregnancy and during hormonal replacement, and are associated with breast carcinoma. They are found frequently in patients with neurofibromatosis type 2 and prior intracranial irradiation. They generally present in middle and older age. Metastases from distant systemic cancers are recognized to spread to meningiomas.[218]

Neuro-ophthalmic Symptoms and Signs

Painless, progressive visual loss is a feature of almost all symptomatic suprasellar meningiomas, and often it is the only manifestation.[215] The pattern of the visual deficit depends on the exact location of the meningioma in relationship to the optic nerve, chiasm, and tract (see below). Because meningiomas take years to enlarge, visual loss is usually accompanied by optic atrophy. Disc pallor correlates better with loss of visual acuity rather than with field loss.[219] Third ventricular obstruction and papilledema can occur in association with large meningiomas, but big asymmetric tumors involving the optic foramen may instead present with ipsilateral optic disc pallor and contralateral disc swelling (Foster Kennedy syndrome, see Chapter 6). Optociliary shunt vessels would be more characteristic of intraorbital optic nerve sheath meningiomas, but in some rare instances they can occur with suprasellar meningiomas.[214] Ocular motility deficits, proptosis, and eye pain can result when there is more lateral involvement of the superior orbital fissure or cavernous sinus.

Other Symptoms and Signs

Headache, usually frontal, occurs in about half of patients.[215] Much less frequent symptoms include changes in personality or mentation (due to frontal lobe dysfunction), anosmia, and seizures. Endocrine dysfunction is also uncommon, but when it occurs the symptoms are consistent with hypopituitarism.[215]

Diagnostic Studies/Neuroimaging

On CT meningiomas are round and isodense compared with brain on unenhanced scans, may be partially calcified, and enhance uniformly with contrast (Fig. 7–26)[216] Surrounding cerebral edema may be evident.[220] Hyperostosis, bony erosion, and calcification are best demonstrated by CT. On T_1-weighted MR images, meningiomas are usually isointense to grey matter (Fig. 7–27), and less commonly are hypointense. Half the time on T_2-weighted images, they remain isointense, while in remaining instances they are hyperintense. Thickening of the dura, a wide dural base, a dural tail, and homogeneous gadolinium enhancement are also characteristic features.[70] MRI-angiography or conventional angiography may be necessary to outline the tumor's relationship to vascular structures.[221] Angiography may be necessary in the preoperative evaluation of these meningiomas because large tumors commonly elevate and encase the proximal anterior cerebral arteries. Conventional angiography also may add more information regarding arterial supply and venous drainage, especially if embolization is considered.[222]

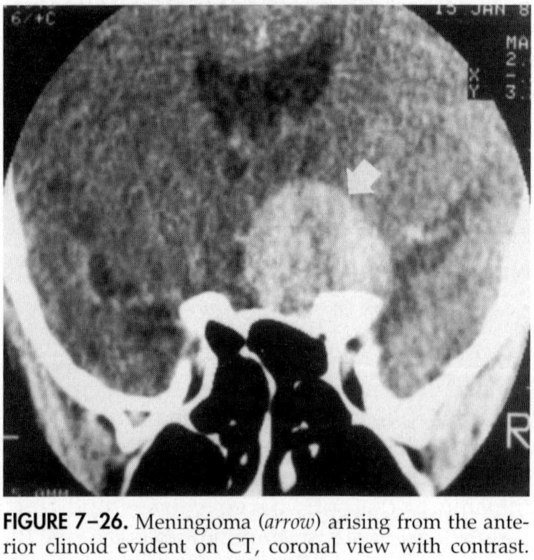

FIGURE 7–26. Meningioma (*arrow*) arising from the anterior clinoid evident on CT, coronal view with contrast. (Courtesy of Lawrence Gray, OD.)

Treatment

Visual loss is the best indication for intervention, which is primarily neurosurgical. Most patients are treated preoperatively with dexamethasone and phenytoin. In some instances preoperative embolization facilitates removal, given the hypervascularity of these lesions.[223] Pterional or subfrontal craniotomies are the most popular surgical approaches.[224] When the tumor is densely adherent to the internal carotid or anterior cerebral arteries or the anterior visual pathway, a subtotal resection is recommended.[222, 225] External beam radiation (5000 to 5500 cGy)[226] or gamma-knife stereotactic radiosurgery[227, 228] should be considered when there is residual or recurrent tumor, or when surgery is contraindicated. Experience with stereotactic brachytherapy with iodine-125 seeds is too limited to allow serious consideration of this modality as either a primary or an adjuvant therapy.[229, 230]

Alternatively, observation may be the best approach in some cases. Elderly patients or poor operative candidates with mild to minimal visual loss, for instance, may be better off with conservative management. Hormonal therapy may be another option when tumors recur despite surgery or radiation, when they become unresectable because of location, or when these traditional approaches are contraindicated.[231] Experience with suprasellar meningiomas, however, is limited,[232] and some

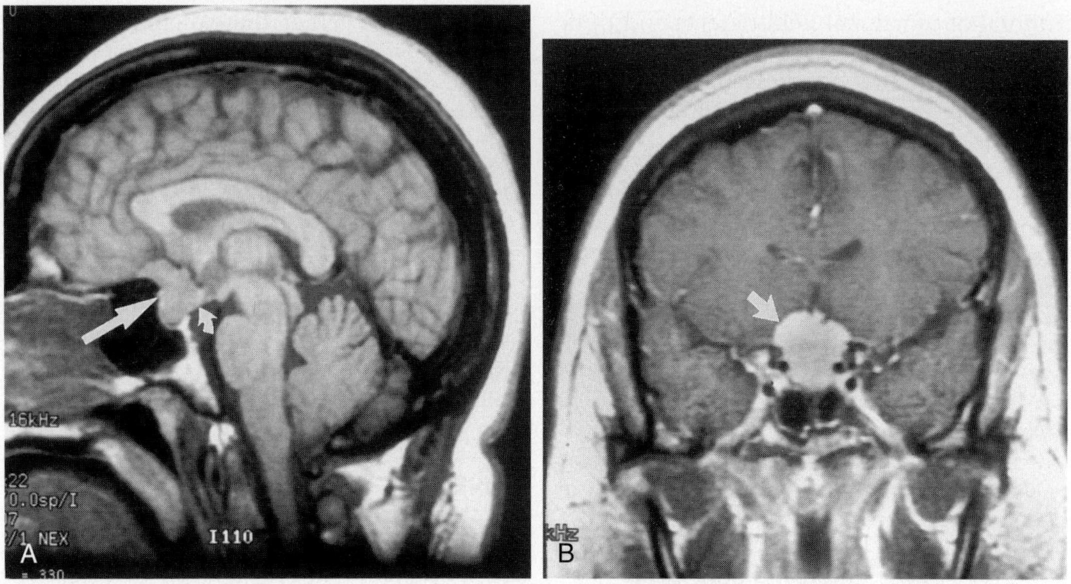

FIGURE 7–27. A. Tuberculum sella meningioma (*larger arrow*) visible on unenhanced T_1-weighted sagittal MRI. The mass extends anteriorly along the planum sphenoidale and posteroinferiorly into the sella turcica. Posterior and inferior displacement of the chiasm (*smaller arrow*) caused a bitemporal hemianopia. **B.** Coronal enhanced MR image of the same tuberculum sella meningioma (*arrow*) as in part A.

hormonal treatments such as RU-486 are poorly tolerated because of a flulike side effect.

Outcome

The chance for visual improvement following neurosurgical decompression is good and only slightly less than that of treated pituitary adenomas. However, this is tempered by the fact that suprasellar meningiomas have higher risk of recurrence, and their surgical removal is associated with much higher rates of visual loss, morbidity, and mortality. In a large series by Symon and Rosenstein,[215, 233] 64% experienced some improvement in visual acuity or fields, while visual function remained unchanged in 12% and worsened in 24%. Other authors[219, 224, 234, 235] have described similar results. Patients with large tumor size and longstanding or severe visual deficits tend to have the poorest visual prognosis,[233] but those factors do not preclude the chance for some visual recovery following surgery.[219, 224] Radiation alone in some instances can afford visual improvement as well.[226] Symon and Rosenstein[215] found that one third of partially resected tumors recurred, compared with only 1.4% of completely resected ones. Recurrences typically occurred years (average 3.7 years) after initial therapy, and were treated either with radiation or repeat craniotomy.

Suprasellar Meningiomas

The three major types of suprasellar meningiomas, tuberculum sellae, anterior clinoidal, and diaphragma sellae, are considered separately below, as they differ slightly in presentation and treatment. They are named after the bony or meningeal structure from which they arise. There is considerable overlap, and when the tumors are large sometimes the distinction is artificial. The classification, however, is most useful regarding outcome. In general, meningiomas restricted to the tuberculum sellae have a more favorable visual prognosis following surgical decompression. On the other hand, those involving the anterior clinoid and diaphragma sellae are more difficult to remove completely and are associated with higher rates of operative visual loss, postoperative visual deterioration,[224] and surgical morbidity.

Tuberculum Sellae Meningiomas. The tuberculum sellae lies midline in the sphenoid bone, and is anterior and inferior to the chiasm. Classically tuberculum sella meningiomas present in middle age, and interfere with the anterior portion of the chiasm, causing asymmetric bitemporal or junctional field defects and optic atrophy (Fig. 7–27). Loss of vision is usually insidious and progressive. Grant and Hedges[236] observed a characteristic pattern: the visual loss was "invariably asymmetric in its progression and accompanied initially by central hemianopic temporal visual field defects. Slowly developing blindness in one eye with diminution of acuity is then accompanied by a temporal field defect in the opposite eye." This temporal sequence of progressive monocular visual loss followed months later by fellow eye involvement was confirmed by Gregorius et al.[219] In some instances the visual loss may mimic retrobulbar optic neuritis or fluctuate.[234, 237] Ocular motor palsies and proptosis are very unusual, reflecting the midline origin of the tumor.[236]

Because of their location, sometimes radical resection of tumor, dura, and bone is possible. Surgical morbidity consists of further visual impairment and hypopituitarism, including diabetes insipidus. Operative visual loss usually is the result of interruption of the blood supply of the chiasm or optic nerve. The small surgical mortality is in part due to the risk of pulmonary embolism.[237]

Anterior Clinoidal Meningiomas. The two anterior clinoid processes lie on the medial ridge of the lesser wings of the sphenoid bone. They look like two triangles pointing toward the back of the head. On each side of midline, the intracranial and canalicular portions of the optic nerve, and the internal carotid artery, exiting from the cavernous sinus just below the nerve, lie just inferomedial to the anterior clinoid process. Meningiomas of the anterior clinoid can cause either an optic neuropathy or chiasmal disturbance. Foster Kennedy syndrome and superior orbital fissure or cavernous sinus involvement are more common with this type, given its more lateral location.[238] Complete neurosurgical removal may be impossible when the tumor encases either the optic nerve or internal carotid artery, and adjuvant radiotherapy is required in these instances. Surgical mortality, related to injury of the internal carotid or middle cerebral arteries, can be as high as 42%.[238] Visual recovery in general is poor.

Diaghragma Sella Meningiomas. A less common type of meningioma in this area arises from the diaphragma sellae. Kinjo et al[239] presented their personal experience with 12 such patients and reviewed 27 other reported cases. Visual field disturbances are still frequent with this variation. When these meningiomas originate from the diaphragm's upper leaf, they grow upward into the suprasellar cistern, so their presentation and management are similar to those of other suprasellar meningiomas. Those originating from the lower leaf, when they grow large enough, expand the sella, and can mimic a nonsecreting pituitary adenoma clinically and radiographically.[240] Some of the latter type may be amenable to a combined transsphenoidal–transcranial resection. In either type, however, complete resection may be limited when the tumor encases the chiasm or pituitary stalk.

ANEURYSMS

Because of the intimate relationship of the circle of Willis to the chiasm and sella (Fig. 7–2), large saccular aneurysms in this area can cause chiasmal visual loss and endocrinopathy.[241, 242] In some instances, their presentation may be indistinguishable from a pituitary adenoma or craniopharyngioma.[243] Prior to angiography and modern neuroimaging, transsphenoidal surgery for a presumed pituitary tumor had the potential for disastrous blood loss if in fact an aneurysm eroding the sella was present.[244]

Pathology/Demographics

Aneurysms most likely develop from congential defects in arterial walls, and pathologically they are characterized by disruption of the media and fibrinoid changes.[245] In addition, hypertension, hemodynamic stress, and atherosclerosis likely play a role in their development.[246] Affected patients tend to be female and middle aged.

Location and Growth Characteristics

Any aneurysm arising from the anterior circle of Willis may compress the chiasm (Fig. 7–28), but chiasmal syndromes are most characteristic of those of the supraclinoid internal carotid artery. These tend to be large (several centimeters in diameter) with upward and medial growth, resulting in compression of the anterolateral portion of the chiasm.

Carotid–ophthalmic artery aneurysms are also frequently associated with chiasmal disturbances. This type of aneurysm arises in the first 2 mm of the internal carotid artery above

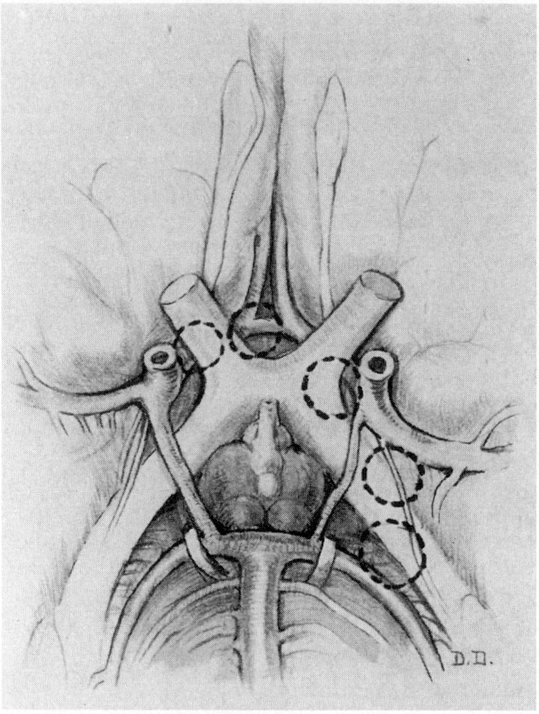

FIGURE 7–28. Common sites of aneurysms and where they might compress the optic nerves, chiasm, or tract. (From Jefferson G: Compression of the chiasma, optic nerves, and optic tracts by intracranial aneurysms. Brain 1937;60:444–497, with permission from Oxford University Press.)

the cavernous sinus. The overwhelming majority of individuals presenting with visual loss are women. There is up to a 20% incidence of bilateral carotid–ophthalmic aneurysms and many affected individuals have multiple aneurysms elsewhere.[245] When they enlarge superiorly, they can erode the ipsilateral anterior clinoid process, then grow upward toward the chiasm. Anterior chiasmal compression is the likely cause of visual loss in these instances, and these aneuryms are similar to anterior clinoidal meningiomas in location and associated field defects.

When cavernous or anterior communicating artery aneurysms cause visual loss, the mechanism is usually optic nerve compression.[247] However, less commonly these two types can cause chiasmal disturbances, depending on their growth pattern.[247] For instance, cavernous aneurysms can extend medially to invade the pituitary fossa, then superiorly to compress the chiasm. Anterior communicating aneurysms with downward extension (because the anterior communicating artery is above the chiasm) rarely can encroach upon the chiasm.[248]

Pregnancy may be associated with a higher risk of aneurysmal rupture, with subsequent high rates of morbidity and mortality for both the mother and the fetus. Thus, in their review of the management of a pregnant patient with aneurysmal visual loss, Shutter et al[249] emphasized that pregnancy should not alter the neurosurgical management of symptomatic ruptured or unruptured aneurysms.

Symptoms

Some individuals have headache, although most patients with visually symptomatic aneurysms in this area will not.[250] Retro-orbital pain is also an occasional accompanying feature. Visual loss and endocrinopathy have already been alluded to, and will be discussed in more detail below. Although many patients will be present with neuro-ophthalmic symptoms, others may present following aneurysmal rupture, and the visual loss is detected at that time. The ocular features of aneurysmal rupture and subarachnoid hemorrhage are discussed in the chapter on disc swelling (Chapter 6).

Neuro-ophthalmic Signs

Their visual presentation is usually similar to that of other sellar masses, with chronic visual acuity and field loss and optic atrophy. However, the examiner should be alerted to the possibility of an aneurysm if the visual loss fluctuates. Sudden worsening or improvement can result from aneurysmal thrombosis or dilation, and acute visual loss might be the result of hemorrhage into the chiasm.[245] In addition, aneurysmal chiasmal disturbances tend to produce very asymmetric field loss. A symmetric bitemporal hemianopia caused by an aneurysm would be unusual and more suggestive of a pituitary adenoma.

Because of their varying location and growth patterns described above, the different aneurysmal subtypes are purported to have characteristic patterns of chiasmal visual loss:

1. *Supraclinoid carotid artery aneurysms.* These arise from the supraclinoid portion of the internal caroid artery. Visual loss is typically highly asymmetric and sequential, beginning in the ipsilateral eye.[251] Because the aneurysm is lateral to the chiasm, the visual loss in the ipsilateral eye is first nasal, then central and temporal. Vision is usually se-

verely reduced in this eye, then as the aneurysm enlarges, the crossing nasal fibers of the other eye are affected. The end result is a blind ipsilateral eye and a temporal defect in the fellow eye.[247] Uncommonly the aneurysms compress the chiasm from above rather than from the side. In these cases the patients can develop an asymmetric bitemporal hemianopia.

2. *Carotid-ophthalmic aneurysms.* In Ferguson and Drake's series[250] of 100 patients with carotid–ophthalmic aneurysms, which arise from the origin of the ophthalmic artery, 32 (25 of 61 with intact aneurysms, 7 of 39 with ruptured aneurysms) had visual abnormalities. Twenty-eight of the 32 patients harbored giant aneurysms (>2.5 cm in diameter). Sixteen of the 32 patients had evidence of chiasmal compression, based on the pattern of field loss (3 of the 16 had bilateral aneurysms). The chiasmal field defects fell roughly into two groups: asymmetric bitemporal hemianopias and junctional field loss characterized by severe visual loss in the ipsilateral eye and a temporal field defect in the fellow eye. Carotid–ophthalmic aneurysms are discussed further in the chapter on optic neuropathies (Chapter 5).
3. *Cavernous carotid aneurysms.* The diagnosis is suggested by signs of cavernous sinus involvement: third, fourth, or sixth nerve palsies, ipsilateral facial pain or dysesthesias, or Horner syndrome. In the late stages of aneurysmal expansion, optic nerve and pituitary dysfunction may occur. These aneurysms receive more attention in Chapter 15.
4. *Anterior communicating aneurysms.* An aneurysm of the anterior communicating artery or of its junction with an anterior cerebral artery more commonly ruptures before becoming large enough to compress the optic apparatus.[247] When visual loss occurs, monocular or binocular inferior altitudinal defects can be observed because of the aneurysm's location above the anterior visual pathway. Chiasmal compression and bitemporal hemianopias are rare but can result from an aneurysm of this type growing downward between the optic nerves, then enlarging and forcing the chiasm upward and backward.[247, 248, 252]
5. *Posterior communicating aneurysms.* The most common neuro-ophthalmic presentation associated with an aneurysm at the junction of the internal carotid and posterior communicating artery is a pupil-involving third nerve palsy. Visual loss is unusual because the aneurysm usually points away from the optic pathways. However, when a giant posterior communicating aneurysm projects into the suprasellar region, the optic tract can be involved. Rarely, medial chiasmal compression and a bitemporal hemianopia can be observed.[253] These aneurysms also receive more attention in Chapters 13 and 15.

Endocrinologic Manifestations

The frequency of endocrinopathy has not been well studied, but it is clear that hypopituitarism of varying degrees can occur as a result of pituitary or stalk compression by an adjacent suprasellar aneurysm.[244] Following treatment, it is interesting that few patients require endocrine replacement, in contrast to those with other types of sellar lesions.[245]

Diagnostic Studies/Neuroimaging

On MRI suprasellar aneurysms will appear as round lesions in this area (Fig. 7–29A). The signal characteristics depend on the presence of clot. Nonthrombosed aneurysms have a telltale internal signal void (hypointense on T_1-weighted images) produced by rapid blood flow and disappearance of protons before they have a chance to emit a signal.[254] Aneurysmal blood flow can also cause a characteristic phase-encoded artifact that runs through the aneurysm and across the image.[70] Partially thrombosed aneurysms contain clot that can appear laminated and bright on T_1- and T_2-weighted images, mixed with areas of signal void. Hemosiderin, evident as dark areas on T_2-weighted images, may be visible outside of the aneurysm in adjacent tissues. Gradient-echo images may be helpful in demonstrating intraluminal flow in equivocal cases.[255]

On CT aneurysmal calcification may be evident, and aneurysms contrast enhance. CT is better than MRI in detecting the presence of subarachnoid hemorrhage (when that is an issue) and in delineating the relationship of the aneurysm to bony structures.

When aneurysms are suspected, MRI-angiography should be performed. Since most of the suprasellar aneurysms that cause visual loss are giant ones, MRI-angiography should

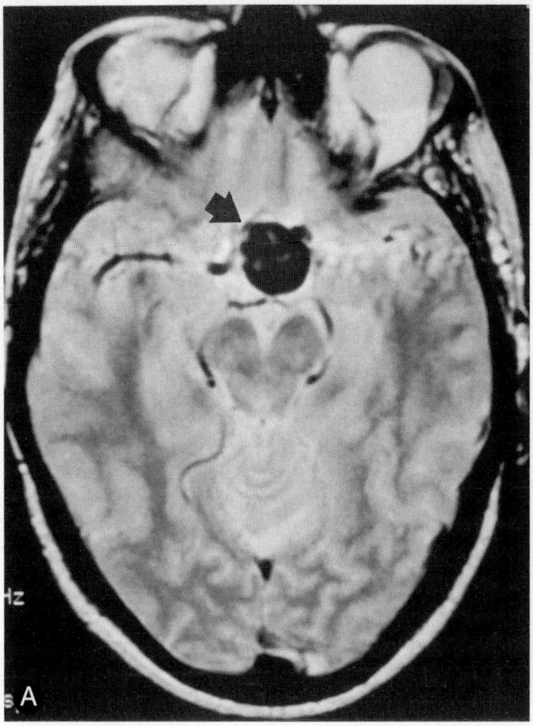

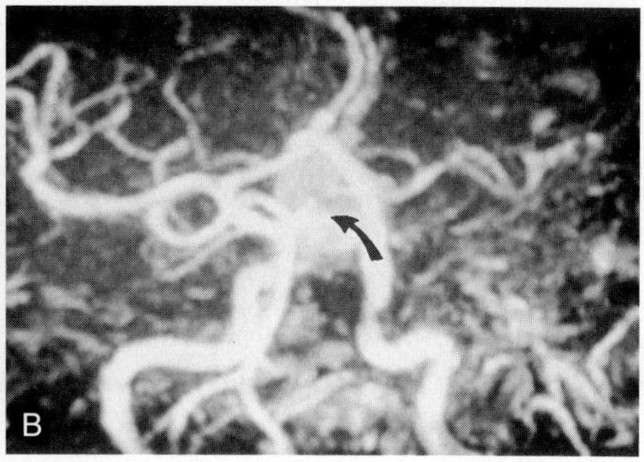

FIGURE 7–29. Internal carotid artery aneurysm that presented with an incomplete bitemporal hemianopia. **A.** T_2-weighted MRI revealed a round flow-void (*arrow*). **B.** MR-angiography confirmed a large internal carotid aneurysm (*curved arrow*).

provide a reasonable screening tool (Fig. 7–29B). Treatment decisions will almost always require conventional angiography to locate the neck of the aneurysm and to delineate the aneurysm's exact blood supply and its relationship to surrounding vessels. Angiography also screens for the presence of other intracranial aneurysms. An aneurysm detected on MRI may appear smaller on angiography if it is partially thrombosed with a small lumen.[245]

Treatment

In general, aneurysms that cause compressive chiasmal syndromes should be treated. A nonruptured aneurysm needs to be occluded to prevent symptom progression or subarachnoid hemorrhage, which is associated with a 8% to 60% mortality rate even before an affected individual reaches the hospital.[246] Even after admission to the hospital, the mortality rate following subarachnoid hemorrhage is 37%.[246] Patients whose aneurysms have ruptured, and who are salvageable, require definitive treatment to prevent rebleeding. The treatment modality depends on the location and size of the aneurysm, as well as the age and medical condition of the patient, and institutional preference. One large study[256] suggested that the morbidity and mortality associated with surgery greatly exceeded the risk of bleeding in unruptured aneurysms <1 cm in patients without any previous history of subarachnoid hemorrhage.

Neurosurgical clipping of the aneurysm remains the most popular approach.[257, 258, 474] When feasible, a metal clip with a spring closure is placed around the aneurysmal neck to isolate it from the parent vessel. When small perforating arteries arise from the aneurysms, clipping may be undesirable. Percutaneous intra-arterial (endovascular) embolization of the aneurysm with balloons or metallic coils, and balloon occlusion of the parent artery, are two alternatives in patients with inoperable aneurysms.[259, 260]

Visual Outcome

In Ferguson and Drake's series,[250] of those with visual deficits who survived and were treated, approximately half had some improvement in visual acuity or field, one third remained unchanged, and about 15% worsened.

VASCULAR MALFORMATIONS INTRINSIC TO THE CHIASM

Maitland et al[261] used the term *chiasmal apoplexy* to describe sudden visual loss due to an intrachiasmal hematoma. Vascular malformations are the usual cause although in one of Maitland et al's cases,[261] the hemorrhage was associated with an optic glioma. Characteristically, acute visual loss is accompanied by headache, and the usual age of onset is in the third or fourth decade.[262] Because the hematomas distend but are usually confined to the chiasm, endocrine symptoms, meningismus, and focal neurologic signs are conspicuously absent. The various subtypes of vascular malformations instrinsic to the chiasm are discussed below.

Cavernous Angiomas (Cavernous Hemangiomas, Cavernomas)

Kupersmith[263] describes these histologically as "irregular sinusoids of vascular channels" without interposed neuronal tissue and without a major arterial supply or venous drainage. Usually they are sporadic, but in rare instances familial cavernous hemangiomas can present in the chiasm.[264] Symptoms in the chiasm are due to hemorrhage and are frequently sudden.[265] On MRI the chiasm is enlarged (Fig. 7–30), and the cavernous angioma is usually heterogenous on T_1-weighted MR images and contains dark areas on T_2-weighted images indicative of hemosiderin.[266] On CT a calcified or enhancing suprasellar mass can be detected. Not infrequently, angiography fails to demonstrate these lesions because of their slow flow characteristics.

The best management of symptomatic cavernous angiomas in the chiasm is unclear.[267] Several authors[262, 268] have advocated microsurgical removal of these lesions to prevent further hemorrhages. On the other hand, we have managed two patients with recurrent hemorrhages and visual loss that have resolved spontaneously over weeks following the ictus. It would seem unwise to subject all individuals with a chiasmal cavernous angioma to a craniotomy and unnecessary surgery involving the optic apparatus when some display a benign course.

Arteriovenous Malformations (AVMs)

Rarely, AVMs, composed of direct arterial communication with veins, occur in the chiasm

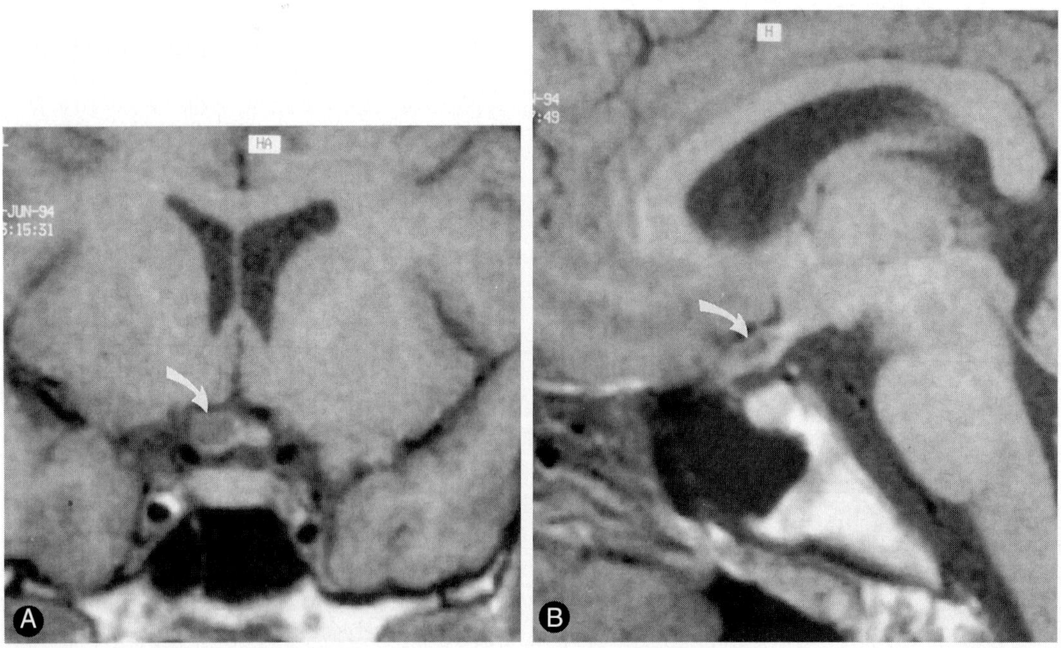

FIGURE 7–30. Cavernous hemangioma (*curved arrow*) of the chiasm demonstrated on T_1-weighted coronal (**A**) and sagittal (**B**) MR images. This patient presented with servere headache and sudden visual loss, which resolved spontaneously.

and cause a bitemporal hemianopia when they bleed. Lavin et al[269] reported two patients in whom formal angiography failed to demonstrate any vessel abnormalities, but chiasmal cryptic AVMs were confirmed histopathologically. The first presented with repeated episodes of visual loss that resolved either spontaneously or following surgical decompression of the hematomas. The second patient had just one acute episode of visual loss prior to surgery. CT in both patients revealed high-density suprasellar masses. Surgical removal of these AVMs should be considered. External compression of the chiasm by AVMs is discussed below. AVMs of the cerebral hemispheres, which are much more common, are discussed in Chapter 8.

Venous Angiomas

These represent developmental anomalies of the venous system and are usually asymptomatic.[263] One rare case of a chiasmal venous angioma presenting apoplectically has been described.[270]

Other Vascular Malformations

Balcer et al[271] reported the rare occurrence of a hemangioblastoma of the chiasm in a patient with von Hippel–Lindau disease. The chiasmal lesion was accompanied by retinal capillary hemangiomas and cervicomedullary hemangioblastomas.

OTHER VASCULAR PROCESSES AFFECTING THE CHIASM

Ischemic Chiasmal Syndrome

Patients with vasculopathic risk factors may develop small-vessel infarction of the chiasm.[272] However, for unclear reasons this is unusual. This diagnosis might be entertained in an elderly patient with diabetes or hypertension, with or without a previous history of small-vessel strokes, who develops a sudden bitemporal hemianopia or bilateral visual loss. Neuroimaging fails to reveal a sellar mass, but typical small-vessel-related white matter and basal ganglia lesions may be evident.

Like posterior ischemic optic neuropathy, atherosclerotic ischemic chiasmal syndrome must be a diagnosis of exclusion. Vasculitidies such as giant cell arteritis can all cause infarction of the chiasm.[272] MRI may reveal chiasmal T_2 high signal or enhancement. When vasculitis is suspected, appropriate studies should be obtained (see descriptions of atypical optic neuritis and giant cell arteritis in Chapter 5, and vasculitides in Chapter 8) and high-dose IV steroids should be considered.

Compression by Atherosclerotic Anterior Cerebral and Internal Carotid Arteries

In our opinion, this is even more uncommon. Dolichoectatic sclerotic anterior cerebral arteries can cause bitemporal field loss either by direct chiasmal compression[272, 273] or by impairing the blood supply of the chiasm.[274] Previous cases were documented with formal angiography, but today MRI and MRI-angiography should be sufficient to confirm the diagnosis. It is unclear whether surgical decompression is the best treatment approach.

In one case report,[275] atherosclerotic internal carotid artery compression of the optic nerves mimicked a sellar mass. The patient presented with a bitemporal hemianopia, and unroofing of the optic canals resulted in improvement in visual fields. The close anatomic relationship of the internal carotid artery and the optic nerves and chiasm predisposes to compressive neuropathy, even when the carotid artery is normal.[276]

Optic neuropathy due to these causes is discussed in Chapter 5.

Compression by an Arteriovenous Malformation (AVM)

In contrast to the smaller cryptic chiasmal AVMs that present acutely, extrinsic compression by larger AVMs is more insidious. Sibony et al[277] described two patients with large, angiographically evident AVMs affecting the chiasm. One was suprasellar and fed by the right ophthalmic artery, while the other was a large frontal AVM. Both patients had long-standing evidence of decreasing vision. We have seen a similar case in which the AVM's draining vein compressed the chiasm.[278] Endocrine disturbances, mimicking those associated with a pituitary macroadenoma, may occur when the AVM is intrasellar.[279]

CHIASMAL/HYPOTHALAMIC GLIOMAS

Chiasmal/hypothalamic gliomas, along with craniopharyngiomas, constitute the two most common sellar masses in children. In general, optic gliomas or optic pathway tumors are intrinsic, sometimes hamartoma-like tumors of the anterior visual pathways (optic nerve, chiasm, and tracts) and hypothalamus. These tumors are rare, but they comprise 5% of all childhood brain tumors and 30% of all brain tumors in children less than 5 years old at The Children's Hospital of Philadelphia.[280] Between 59% and 70% present before age 10, and another 20% to 22% by age 20.[281, 282]

Optic nerve gliomas, which involve only the optic nerve, are reviewed in the chapter on optic neuropathies (Chapter 5). In general the greatest morbidity of optic nerve gliomas is visual loss, and the mortality rate is extremely low.[281] On the other hand, optic pathway tumors involving the chiasm and/or hypothalamus, given their location, often present with endocrine dysfunction and are associated with higher morbidity and mortality rates. Therefore, they must be managed differently. Chiasmal/hypothalamic gliomas comprise approximately 75% of all optic pathway gliomas.[282]

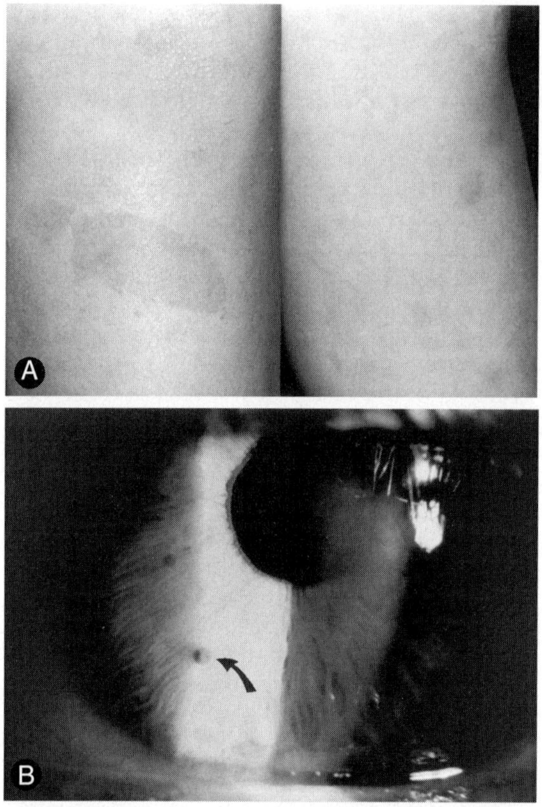

FIGURE 7–31. Neurofibromatosis type 1. **A.** Typical café-au-lait spots on the skin. **B.** Iris Lisch nodules (*arrow*), in an individual with a dark iris, evident on slit-lamp examination.

Association With Neurofibromatosis Type 1 (NF-1)

The incidence of neurofibromatosis type 1 (NF-1, von Recklinghausen's disease) among patients with optic gliomas is 10% to 70% (average 29%).[282] Because of the strong association, all patients with newly discovered optic gliomas should be screened for NF-1. Diagnostic criteria for NF-1 include two or more of the following: (1) café-au-lait spots on the skin (Fig. 7–31A), (2) cutaneous neurofibromas, (3) axillary or inguinal freckling, (4) optic gliomas, (5) iris hamartomas (Lisch nodules) (Fig. 7–31B), (6) bony lesion such as sphenoid wing dysplasia, and (7) family history of NF-1.[283] Thus, in a patient with an optic glioma, the presence of any other feature of NF-1 establishes the diagnosis. Although there have been a few reported individuals with neurofibromatosis type 2 (bilateral acoustic neuromas) and optic pathway tumors,[284] an association has not been confirmed.

In one study by Lewis et al,[285] 15% of patients with NF-1 were found to have optic pathway gliomas when screened with brain CT. Importantly, Lewis et al found that only one third of these patients with radiographically demonstrated gliomas were symptomatic with either subnormal vision or optic atrophy. Listernick et al[286] found 19% of their NF-1 patients had optic gliomas. This slightly higher proportion in this study may have resulted from the fact that patients were screened with both CT and MRI, the latter of which may be more sensitive in detecting optic pathway involvement. All symptomatic optic pathway tumors in Listernick et al's study were diagnosed before 6 years of age. A newly symptomatic optic pathway glioma would be very unusual in adulthood.[468]

There is considerable debate whether all children with NF-1 should undergo routine neuroimaging[287, 288] or visual evoked potentials[289, 290] to screen for optic pathway tumors. Currently at The Children's Hospital of Philadelphia, the decision to perform MRI is made on an individual basis. MRI scans are obtained in NF-1 patients with an abnormal neurologic exam or learning disability, attentional deficit, endocrinopathy, or developmental delay. Every patient with NF-1 receives at least an annual neuro-ophthalmologic examination, and unexplained acuity, color, or field loss, afferent pupillary defect, proptosis, or optic atrophy would also mandate neuroimaging.[291] Because there is no evidence that treating an asymptomatic optic glioma in patients with NF-1 prevents subsequent visual loss, in general there is no advantage in detecting these lesions at an early stage with screening neuroimaging. Even after a normal MRI scan, the neuro-ophthalmologic status of a young patient with NF-1 is still closely monitored, because optic gliomas may still develop despite the unremarkable initial neuroimaging.[292, 293] Our NF-1 patients do not undergo visual evoked potentials, because the testing is associated with unacceptable false positive[290] and false negative rates[294] regarding tumor detection. The neuro-ophthalmic examination is a more reliable screen, even in young children.[295]

Pathology

Optic gliomas, like cystic cerebellar astrocytomas, are juvenile pilocytic astrocytomas.[296] In general, these are benign, low-grade glial tumors, which are grade 1 in the World Health Organization classification of gliomas.[297] Other pathologic features include eosinophilic Rosenthal fibers and the absence of mitotic figures. Extracellular accumulation of acid mucopolysaccharide may account for some instances of tumor enlargement,[298, 299] and resorption of this mucosubstance may explain spontaneous shrinkage of some optic nerve and chiasmal gliomas. Other possible mechanisms for tumor growth include proliferation of neoplastic cells and reactive arachnoidal proliferation.[282] Optic gliomas should be distinguished from cerebral gliomas and malignant optic gliomas of adulthood, which are discussed in the subsequent section.

Location and Growth Characteristics

Gliomas involving the chiasm and the optic nerves are termed *anterior chiasmal gliomas,* while those with extension into the optic tracts or hypothalamus are classified as *posterior chiasmal gliomas.*

For decades, the growth potential of these optic gliomas has been a controversial issue. Hoyt and Baghdassarian[300] advocated the notion that they are benign hamartomas: "optic gliomata are clinically indolent tumours that tend to enlarge, cause symptoms early in life, and remain static thereafter. Unlike the rare glioblastomata that arise in the adult optic nerve, childhood gliomata do no undergo malignant degeneration. They have features of congenital hamartomata." On the other hand, more recent histopathologic studies have suggested that optic gliomas are true neoplasms.[301]

It has been our personal experience that chiasmal/hypothalamic gliomas behave unpredictably, and their growth rates span a wide spectrum. Some do behave like hamartomas,[302] but some grow over years, then stop, while others continue to enlarge and cause progressive symptoms despite all interventions. In rare instances, spontaneous improvement in vision and radiographic appearance can also occur.[303–309] Central nervous system and abdominal (via ventriculoperitoneal shunting) metastases also have been documented.[310–314] In general, the morbidity and mortality of anterior chiasmal gliomas are much less compared to those with posterior extension.[281, 315, 316]

In neurofibromatosis, there is a relatively high rate of second intracranial tumors such as cerebral gliomas.[470]

Symptoms

Because they are slow growing, chiasmal/hypothalamic gliomas tend to present insidiously with visual loss with optic atrophy and/or endocrine dysfunction. Headache can be a common complaint, especially when the third ventricle is obstructed by a large hypothalamic component.

Neuro-ophthalmic Signs

Visual acuity varies at presentation, but profound acuity loss (worse than 20/200) is not uncommon.[282] Monocular or bitemporal field defects occur in about 40% of cases, and other patterns of field loss include unilateral or bilateral optic nerve-related deficits, homonymous defects due to optic tract involvement, or diffuse visual loss.[302] In general, it is difficult to correlate an optic glioma's location with the field defect, as dysfunction of anatomically involved structures does not always occur. Despite diffuse infiltration of the anterior visual pathway, an optic glioma may present solely with bitemporal hemianopia or a unilateral central scotoma. In the extreme case of some patients with neurofibromatosis with large radiographically demonstrated lesions, there may be no visual field defect. In addition, optic gliomas may progress radiographically without change in visual function, and vision can worsen without any change in size of the lesion.[317]

Visual loss rarely can occur apoplectically,[318] and in some instances this behavior may reflect sudden cyst enlargement rather than tumor growth per se. Young children, who might not complain of visual loss, may present with strabismus owing to poor vision in one eye. Other presentations include monocular[319] or asymmetric nystagmus or the full triad of head nodding, head tilting, and nystagmus, mimicking spasmus nutans.[33, 320] Optic atrophy is the rule, but optic nerve infiltration or third ventricular obstruction with hydrocephalus may be associated with disc swelling (Fig. 7–32). A large optic nerve component might also lead to proptosis. Cranial neuropathies in general are not associated with chiasmal/hypothalamic gliomas.

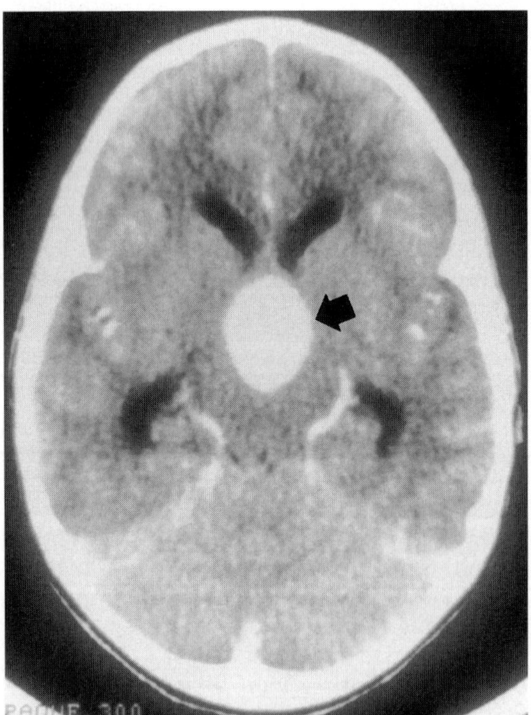

FIGURE 7–32. Axial CT scan showing contrast-enhancing globular chiasmal/hypothalamic glioma (*arrow*) obstructing the third ventricle and causing hydrocephalus.

Endocrinologic Manifestations

Endocrine signs and symptoms can be a prominent feature when the glioma either originates or extends into the hypothalmus.[321, 469] Russell's diencephalic syndrome and precocious puberty are the two most common endocrinopathies at presentation,[40, 314] while diabetes insipidus and hypopituitarism are uncommon initial symptoms.

Diagnostic Studies/Neuroimaging

MRI is preferable to CT in the evaluation of these tumors because of the availability of coronal images and its superior ability in imaging the optic tract/hypothalamic extent of the lesion.[322, 323] Chiasmal gliomas are seen best on coronal images, and they appear as instrinsic enlargement of the chiasm,[324] occasionally with a cystic component (Fig. 7–33).[325] When the optic nerves are also involved and enlarged, the anterior chiasm looks like a upside-down pair of pants on axial images. Chiasmal/hypothalamic gliomas are usually round suprasellar masses, and often it is difficult to tell whether the growth arises from the chiasm or hypothalamus (Fig. 7–34A, B). The lesions are isointense or hypointense on T_1-weighted images, hyperintense on T_2-weighted images, and may enhance with gadolinium.[70] Optic tract involvement can be evident when the tracts are bright on T_2 and enhanced images (Fig. 7–34C).[326]

When there is instrinsic enlargement of visual pathways in any child or an individual of any age with NF-1, the MRI appearance is almost pathognomonic. Masqueraders include gangliogliomas, germ cell tumors, sarcoidosis, and intrachiasmal craniopharyngiomas. Although chiasmal neuritis may have a similar neuroradiologic appearance, its sudden visual loss should easily distinguish that entity from a chiasmal glioma. Malignant optic gliomas can be distinguished clinically by rapidly progressive visual loss and onset in adulthood.

Fletcher et al[317] outlined three characteristics of chiasmal gliomas evident on CT: tubular thickening of the optic nerve and chiasm, a suprasellar tumor with contiguous optic nerve expansion, and a suprasellar tumor with optic tract involvement. The diagnosis can not be made with certainty in the case of a globular suprasellar mass without optic nerve or tract extension.

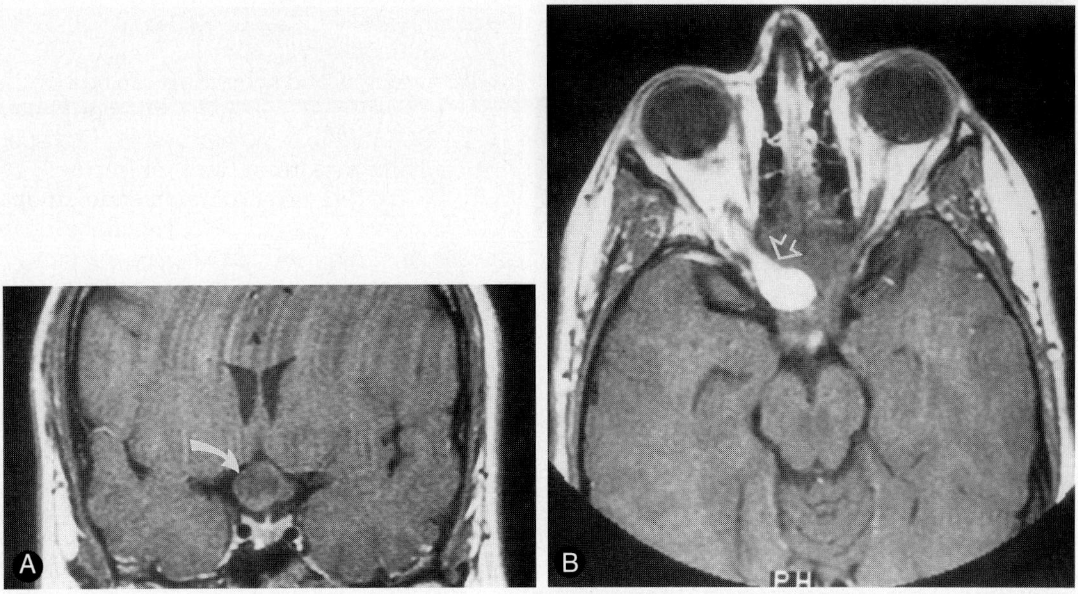

FIGURE 7–33. Anterior chiasmal glioma. **A.** Unenhanced coronal T_1-weighted MRI scan demonstrating intrinsic chiasmal enlargement (*arrow*) with a cystic (hypointense) component. **B.** In the same patient, axial MR image with gadolinium shows anterior extension of the tumor, reflected by enlargement and enhancement of the right optic nerve (*arrow*).

Findings on plain skull roentgenograms include enlargement or J-shaped excavation of the sella.[282] Concomitant optic nerve involvement may lead to enlargement of the optic foramen or canal. Roentgenograms are rarely necessary when CT or MRI are available.

Treatment

Despite the myriad of retrospective series and reviews by authorities on the subject,[281, 282, 300, 302, 315, 316, 327–346] the best treatment of chiasmal/hypothalamic gliomas is unfortunately still unclear. The controversy exists in part because the tumors are heterogeneous in terms of clinical presentation, location, and natural history, and each institution has its own bias with regard to treatment approach. Many studies failed to include complete neuro-ophthalmic data, and older studies were performed prior to the availability of MRI, which has greatly improved tumor localization. A prospective, controlled trial is necessary to resolve these issues, but such a study would have to account for tumor heterogeneity and include long follow-up. The tumors grow slowly, and in some instances many years may pass following treatment before they progress again.

The neuro-oncology service at The Children's Hospital of Philadelphia[343, 344] currently maintains an individualized approach to chiasmal/hypothalmic gliomas based on (1) location of the tumor on MRI, (2) tumor size, (3) neuro-ophthalmic status, (4) endocrine status, and (5) the presence of NF-1. *Anterior chiasmal gliomas,* especially in patients with NF-1, do not require a biopsy, and without evidence of radiographic or clinical (visual or endocrine) progression, can be observed.[315] The MRI and neuro-ophthalmic examination, including visual fields, should be repeated in 6 to 18 weeks, then semiannually if stable. If the lesion is confined to the optic nerves and chiasm, biopsy or surgery carries the chance of causing further visual loss, and therefore should be avoided in such instances.

Evidence of progression on two successive neuro-ophthalmologic or radiologic examinations would be an indication for external beam radiation (approximately 4500 to 5000 cGy in divided doses[347]). In many instances radiation can halt tumor growth and the progression of visual loss.[336, 337, 348–351] Less commonly, vision improves.[352] The major side effects of cranial irradiation for optic gliomas, which include mental retardation, endocrinopathies, and cerebrovascular disease,[353, 354] must be considered, particularly in smaller children who are most vulnerable to these complications. Radionecrosis of the chiasm also has been reported.[355]

If the patient is less than 6 years of age, chemotherapy may be used to halt progression

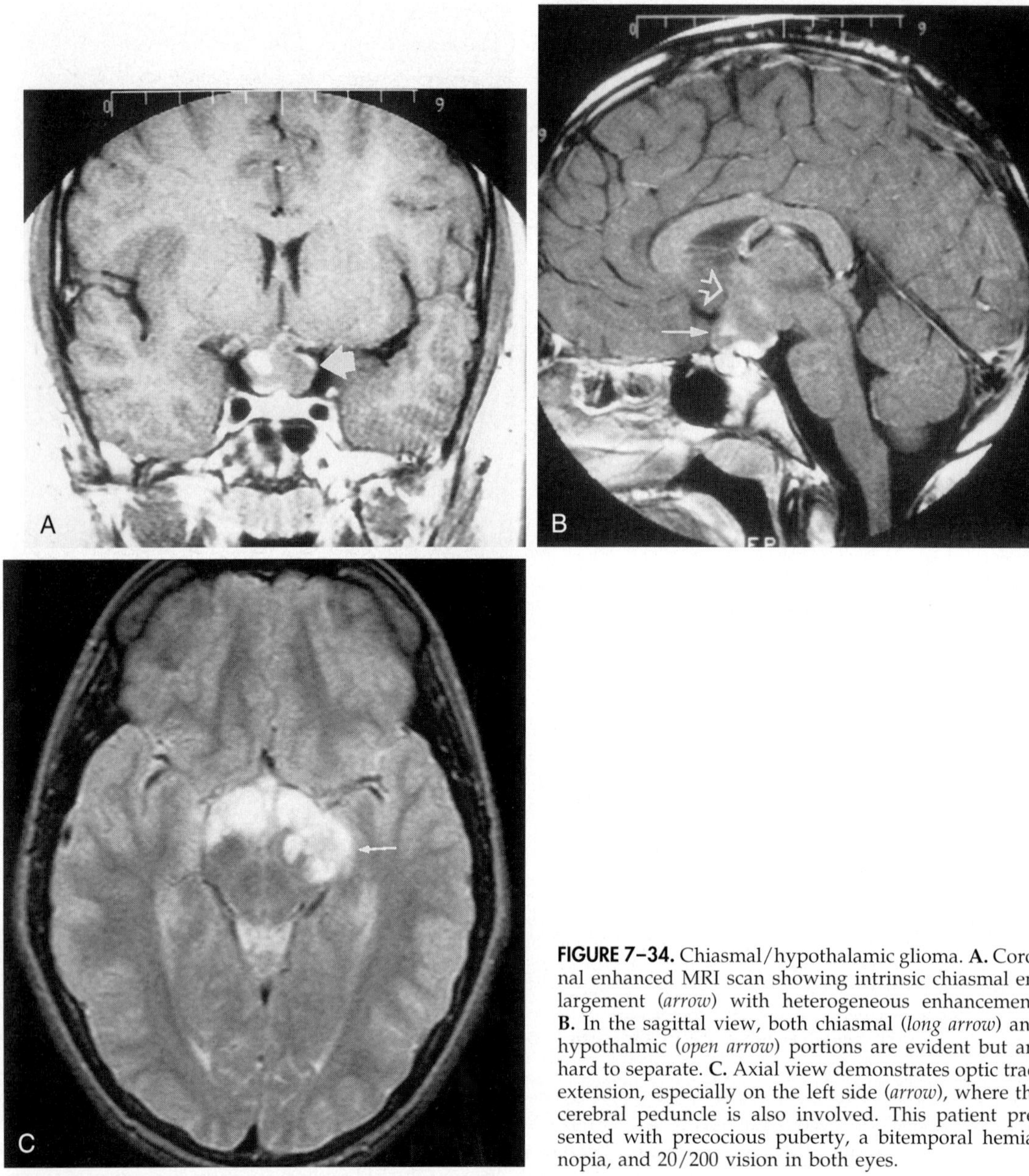

FIGURE 7–34. Chiasmal/hypothalamic glioma. **A.** Coronal enhanced MRI scan showing intrinsic chiasmal enlargement (*arrow*) with heterogeneous enhancement. **B.** In the sagittal view, both chiasmal (*long arrow*) and hypothalmic (*open arrow*) portions are evident but are hard to separate. **C.** Axial view demonstrates optic tract extension, especially on the left side (*arrow*), where the cerebral peduncle is also involved. This patient presented with precocious puberty, a bitemporal hemianopia, and 20/200 vision in both eyes.

for a few years, allowing radiation treatment to be delayed or avoided in such instances.[280, 356, 357] Currently vincristine and carboplatin (preferred now over actinomycin D) are first-line agents[358]; topotecan and oral etoposide (VP-16) are other alternatives, especially when the tumors recur.[359] *Cis*-retinoic acid, alpha-2a interferon and VP-16 have been used in patients with neurofibromatosis. Chemotherapy may be utilized when radiation fails. Furthermore, in the case of a very young child with a chiasmal/hypothalamic glioma and profound visual loss, it is reasonable to initiate chemotherapy without evidence of progression, as the child's age may preclude detection of small changes in vision. In young children with grossly asymmetric visual loss, part-time monocular patching of the better eye should also be considered when superimposed amblyopia may be present (see Chapter 5).

Posterior chiasmal gliomas in patients with NF-1 may be observed, particularly when their neuro-ophthalmic examination is normal. In those without NF-1 and with hypothalamic involvement, a biopsy of that part should be performed because the differential diagnosis, which includes craniopharyngiomas or germinomas, for instance, can be broad. Since these posterior gliomas have a poorer prognosis, it may be prudent in some cases then to institute radiation or chemotherapy right away, without requiring documentation of radiographic or clinical progression. It has been debated whether partial or radical resection of a globular hypothalamic component, in cases without extensive optic nerve or tract involvement, enhances the prognosis.[339, 341, 342, 344] Large tumors, obstruction of the foramina of Monro, and cysts associated with visual progression are other reasonable indications for neurosurgical intervention.[360] However, it is unclear whether aggressive surgery, which can be associated with vascular occlusion, endocrinopathy, and further visual loss, is necessary in every instance.

Outcome

In Dutton's meta-analysis of reported cases,[282] there seemed to be little long-term (10-year) difference between chiasmal gliomas treated with radiation and those which were observed with regards to rate of visual stabilization/improvement (69.3% vs 76.8%), visual worsening (30.7% vs 23.2%), tumor recurrence/progression (41.5% vs 41.9%), and mortality (27.6% vs 28.6%). However, it is our experience, as well as that of others,[316, 348] that radiation is associated with good short-term stabilization in vision and tumor size, and in many instances tumor bulk decreases. Contrary to series reporting high rates of visual improvement following radiotherapy, in one instance 43%,[348] we have found visual improvement is uncommon. We inform patients that stabilization in vision and tumor size is considered successful treatment. Unfortunately, we agree that eventual tumor progression following years of stability after radiation is not uncommon.[334] Persistent endocrine dysfunction is very common.[345]

Also in Dutton's meta-analysis,[282] anterior chiasmal gliomas had a lower rate of recurrence or progression following radiation compared with posterior chiasmal gliomas (41.2% vs 51.1%) and a lower mortality rate (23.2% vs 43.2%). It has been our impression that children who present at a very young age in general have a poor prognosis, but that those with NF-1 have a better prognosis. While some authors have agreed with our observations,[333, 341, 471] analyses of larger numbers of patients have not arrived at the same conclusions regarding the protective effect of NF-1.[281, 282, 346]

MALIGNANT OPTIC CHIASMAL GLIOMAS OF ADULTHOOD

These uncommon tumors also primarily involve the anterior visual pathway, and occur primarily in middle-age and elderly individuals. In contrast to the aforementioned pediatric optic gliomas, however, malignant optic chiasmal gliomas of adulthood cause rapidly progressive bilateral visual loss, and are uniformly lethal. Some cases have been associated with prior intracranial irradiation.[361] Only a handful of unusual cases in children have been reported.[362]

Pathology, Location, and Growth Characteristics

These tumors should be considered glioblastomas of the anterior visual pathway, although some would also include anaplastic astrocytomas in this location. Hoyt et al[363] called these lesions a "common type of brain tumour in an uncommon location." Initially malignant optic gliomas affect just one optic nerve, then within several weeks spread to the chiasm and other optic nerve before reaching the optic tracts, hypothalamus, internal capsules, and basal ganglia.

Symptoms and Signs

Initially, patients appear to have optic neuritis in one eye, with monocular visual loss occurring over a few weeks, and the optic disc is either normal or exhibits only mild disc swelling.[363] They may also complain of ocular pain exacerbated by eye movements. Within the ensuing weeks or months, visual loss progresses, often accompanied by funduscopic evidence of a central retinal artery or venous occlusion due to tumor infiltration of the proximal optic nerve. Later, vision in the other eye becomes involved, and eventually each eye suffers from severe visual loss. Cerebral extension is manifested by hypothalamic disturbances, hemiparesis, and altered mental status.

Diagnostic Studies/Neuroimaging

Typically on MRI, the chiasm is enlarged and enhances with gadolinium. As the lesion progresses, radiographic involvement of the optic tracts, hypothalamus, and other cerebral structures becomes evident (Fig. 7–35).[364, 365] On CT, adult chiasmal gliomas may appear cystic with ring enhancement and mimic other suprasellar masses.[366] Since the neuroimaging features are nonspecific, the diagnosis relies more on the patient's age and rapidly progressive symptoms.

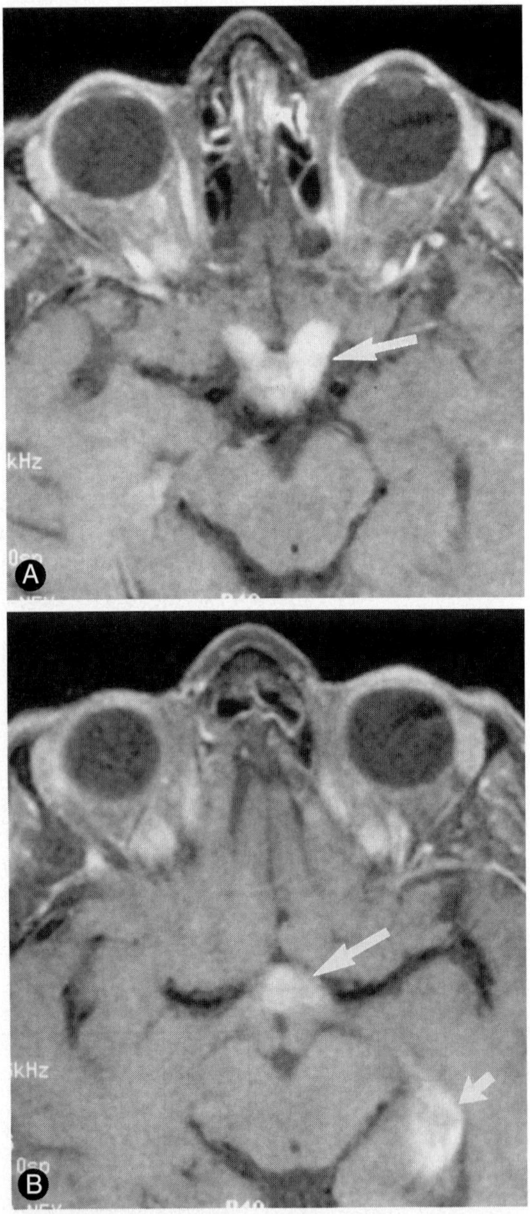

FIGURE 7–35. Malignant chiasmal glioma, which presented with rapidly progressive visual loss and was biopsy proven. **A.** Axial MRI scan with gadolinium demonstates chiasmal enlargement and enhancement (*arrow*). **B.** Axial MRI scan with gadolinium, dorsal to the view in part A, revealing tumor involvement of the left optic tract (*larger arrow*) and lateral geniculate nucleus (*smaller arrow*).

Treatment

The results of most treatment modalities in this disorder are disappointing. Steroids usually have only some transient benefit. In exceptional instances, combined radiation and chemotherapy may prolong survival.[367]

HYPOTHALAMIC (TUBER CINEREUM) HAMARTOMAS

These lesions present primarily with precocious puberty because they release luteinizing hormone releasing hormone (LHRH), and other common clinical features can include gelastic seizures, mental retardation and behavioral disturbances. However, when they grow large enough, they can compress the chiasm. Hypothalamic hamartomas are noninvasive, rarely grow in size, and microscopically are composed of neurons and glia. Radiographically, they appear as round sessile or pedunculated masses ("collar buttons") attached to the posterior hypothalamus between the infundibulum and mamillary bodies.[368] They are isointense relative to grey matter on T_1-weighted MR images and are homogeneous and hyperintense on T_2-weighted images.

When the clinical, radiographic, and endocrinologic (LHRH levels, for example) features are consistent with a hypothalamic hamartoma, observation with serial biannual or annual neuroimaging and examinations may be sufficient. Treatment of the precocious puberty consists of hormonal suppression therapy. Surgical management should be reserved for chiasmal compression, atypical lesions, progressive enlargement, and instances where medical management fails to control endocrine dysfunction.[368, 369]

GANGLIOGLIOMAS

Gangliogliomas are central nervous system neoplasms that contain neuronal and glial elements. These tumors may arise anywhere in the neuroaxis but are more common in the cerebral hemispheres and spinal cord.[370] Patients usually present with intellectual and behavioral abnormalities, seizures, or focal neurologic deficits.[371] Ganglioneuromas are histologically similar tumors found in the peripheral nervous system although previous authors have used the terms interchangeably.[372]

Gangliogliomas involving the anterior visual pathways are uncommon,[373] but we have had experience with three patients with chiasmal syndromes, each with distinct mechanisms.[374] One had unique tumor invasion of optic nerves and chiasm by medial extension of a temporal lobe ganglioglioma into the suprasellar area. Subarachnoid dissemination was also present. The ganglioglioma in the second patient was intrinsic to the hypothalamus and chiasm (Fig. 7–36), while the tumor in the third invaded both optic tracts with lateral compression of the chiasm by a cyst. The second patient had a bitemporal hemianopia, while the other two had severe bilateral visual loss. All had optic atrophy.

Gangliogliomas intrinsic to the chiasm are unusual. Chilton et al[373] reported a 33-year-old man with a ganglioglioma of the optic chiasm and right optic tract, and they found only a few other well-documented cases with clinicopathologic correlation. Since the optic nerve and chiasm do not contain neuronal cell bodies, these gangliogliomas may have arisen from ectopic neural tissue or more primitive neurons, or spread from the floor of the third ventricle. Because of their indolent visual loss

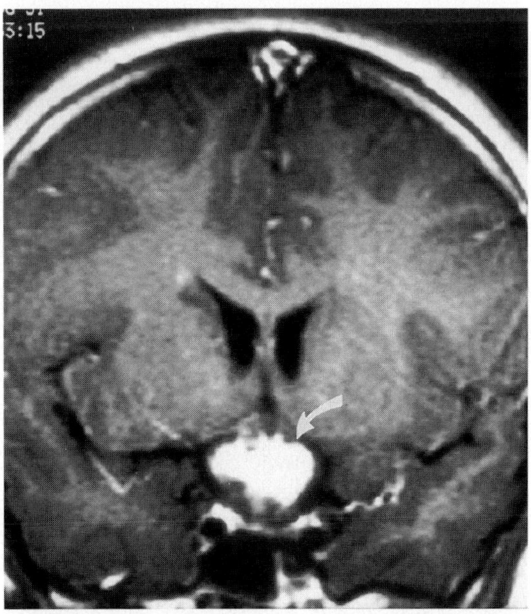

FIGURE 7–36. Ganglioglioma of the chiasm. Coronal MRI demonstrating intrinsic chiasmal enlargement and enhancement (*arrow*) (From Liu GT, Galetta SL, Rorke LB, et al: Gangliogliomas of the optic chiasm. Neurology 1996;46:1669–1673, with permission.)

associated with optic nerve or chiasmal enlargement, gangliogliomas intrinsic to the anterior visual pathway may mimic optic gliomas clinically and radiologically.[375]

When gangliogliomas arise from the floor of the third ventricle,[376] extrinsic chiasmal compression by these tumors can occur. Pituitary or hypothalmic dysfunction sometimes accompanied by visual loss due to obstructive hydrocephalus and chronic papilledema, is the more common presentation of gangliogliomas in this region.

Gangliogliomas are usually slowly growing neoplasms, and occasionally behave like hamartomas. When surgically accessible, complete resection is usually curative, with radiation and chemotherapy reserved for cases with progression or recurrence.[377, 378] However, when the chiasm and hypothalamus are involved, complete surgical resection is impossible. In these instances, patients should undergo subtotal removal followed by radiotherapy, but the visual prognosis is varied.

GERM CELL TUMORS

Intracranially, these tumors arise in midline structures, particularly the suprasellar and pineal regions. The reason for the predilection for those areas is not clear, but these may be sites of primordial germ cell migration during ontogeny.[379] Most are diagnosed between 10 and 21 years of age,[369] and there is no sex preponderance for suprasellar lesions.[380] Actually, extracranial sites are more common and include the gonads (testicular seminomas and ovarian dysgerminomas, for example), retroperitonium, and mediastinum.[369]

There are three major groups of intracranial germ cell neoplasms: germinomas, teratomas, and nongerminoma germ cell tumors.[379] Suprasellar germinomas include tumors previously termed ectopic pinealomas,[381] atypical teratomas,[382] or dysgerminomas. They are composed of primordial, polygonal germ cells with lymphocytic infiltration, and these tend to have the best prognosis because of their radiosensitivity. Teratomas, on the other hand, consist of differentiated tissue of all three germ layers. Pure teratomas are benign and also have a good prognosis. The nongerminoma germ cell tumors include embryonal carcinomas, yolk sac or endodermal sinus tumors, choriocarcinomas, and immature teratomas.[369] As these are nonradiosensitive, they have the worst prognosis.

Location and Growth Characteristics

Suprasellar germ cell tumors tend to be located inferior and posterior to the chiasm. Frequently they infiltrate the hypothalamus, infundibulum, and optic nerves. Subarachnoid, intra-axial, and subependymal (ventricular) seeding unfortunately is not uncommon.[382] Germinomas can secrete human chorionic gonadotropin (HCG), alpha-fetoprotein, and carcinoembryonic antigen (CEA). In a minority of cases there is concomitant involvement of both the suprasellar region and the pineal gland, a presentation known as *multiple midline germinomas*[347] (Fig. 7–37).

Symptom and Signs

The symptom triad of diabetes insipidus, visual loss, and hypopituitarism is present in the majority of patients with suprasellar germ cell tumors.[380, 381] Of these, diabetes insipidus is the most common, occurring in almost all patients in some series.[382, 383] It is usually the initial symptom and can be present for years prior to diagnosis. Visual deficits result either from tumor compression or infiltration of the chiasm.[383] Thus bitemporal hemianopias as well as nondescript field loss can be observed,[382, 384] and optic atrophy is very common. Papilledema due to elevated intracranial pressure and ocular motor palsies occur in only a very small minority.[385] Hypothalamic and pituitary dysfunction manifests as, in decreasing order of frequency, hypogonadism, panhypopituitarism, hypothyroidism, dwarfism, hypocortisolism, central hyperthermia, cachexia, and precocious puberty.[381] Tumor beta-HCG production stimulates Leydig cells to secrete testosterone, leading to precocious puberty in males.

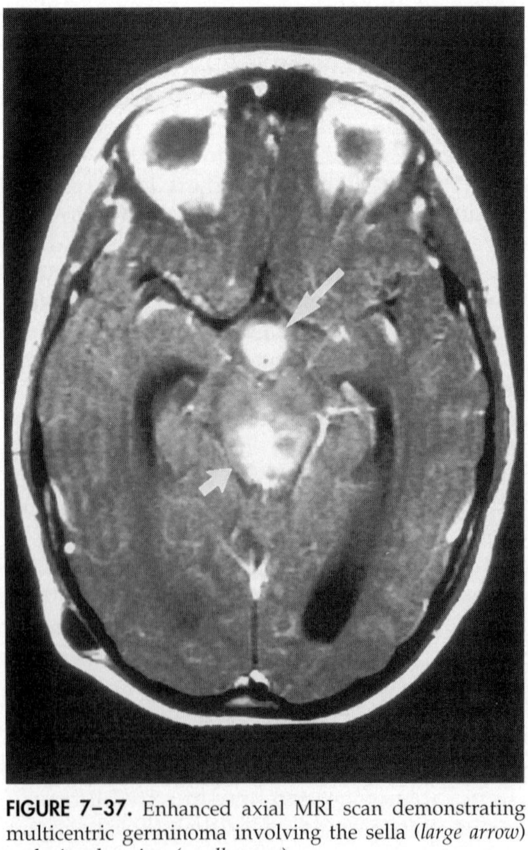

FIGURE 7–37. Enhanced axial MRI scan demonstrating multicentric germinoma involving the sella (*large arrow*) and pineal region (*small arrow*).

Diagnostic Studies/Neuroimaging

By the time they present, suprasellar germinomas are usually already large. They are homogeneous and only rarely have cystic components. On MRI they are mildly hypointense on T_1-weighted images and hyperintense on T_2-weighted images, and enhance with contrast. Teratomas tend to be more heterogeneous with evidence of fat or calcification.[70] On CT the lesions are iso- or high density, and they also contrast enhance.[384]

Diagnostic Studies/Laboratory Tests

Along with the standard endocrinologic screening, serum and CSF beta-HCG and alpha-fetoprotein levels should be evaluated. These tumor markers are helpful in monitoring treatment. High beta-HCG levels suggest choriocarcinoma. CSF also should be sent for cytologic examination, which can reveal abnormal cells when there is a germ cell tumor.

Treatment

Previously, germinomas were empirically irradiated, sometimes supported by an abnormal CSF cytology.[384] However, modern neurosurgical techniques, a preference for histologic confirmation,[379] and the observation that decompression of the anterior visual pathways can result in visual improvement have made subtotal resection the preferable approach.[385] Benign teratomas require no further therapy, and pure germinomas respond well to postoperative radiation. Younger children may undergo chemotherapy to delay radiation. Recurrent disease may necessitate chemotherapy.[386] The more aggressive nongerminoma germ cell tumors require both craniospinal irradiation and adjuvant chemotherapy.[347]

Outcome

Recurrence and survival rates depend heavily on tumor histology. In one series,[385] patients with intracranial germinomas had a 85% long-term survival rate, while those with intracranial nongerminoma germ cell tumors had only a 45% survival rate.

MISCELLANEOUS GROWTHS

Epidermoids and Dermoids

Epidemoids and dermoids are congenital inclusions of germ layers that occur at the time of neural tube closure.[387] Epidermoids consist of ectodermal germ cells, while dermoids contain both ectodermal and mesodermal germ layers. Visual disturbances, and less commonly hypopituitarism, diabetes insipidus, and cranial neuropathies, can occur when these lesions are in the suprasellar region.[70] On MRI suprasellar epidermoids and dermoids appear as round homogeneous masses that are hyperintense on T_1- and T_2-weighted images. Their signal characteristics are similar to subcutaneous fat, reflecting the presence of glandular tissue from hair follicles and sebaceous and apocrine glands.

Chiasmal Metastases

Cohen and Lessell[388] described three such cases, each presenting with acuity loss and bitemporal hemianopia. Breast and lung cancer were the primary malignancies in two of the patients, while in the third no primary was found. Dexamethasone and radiation, with chemotherapy in one case, offered some visual recovery.

Sellar and Chiasmal Lymphoma

Primary B-cell central nervous system lymphoma should be considered when there is a sellar mass in any immunocompromised individual, especially one with acquired immunodeficiency syndrome. In addition, cases in immunocompetent individuals have been described. In one, lymphoma intrinsic to the chiasm was discovered, and the lesion was steroid responsive.[389] Another reported patient presented with visual loss, impotence, decreased libido, diabetes insipidus, and hearing loss.[390] MRI revealed an enhancing suprasellar mass involving the infundibulum, mammillary bodies, chiasm, and fornix. Biopsy revealed lymphoma, and the patient was treated with high-dose methotrexate followed by radiation.

Choristomas (Gangliocytomas, Granular Cell Tumors, Myoblastomas, and Infundibulomas)

Choristomas are very rare tumors that can occur in the sellar area and cause visual loss.[391, 392] Choristomas are composed of histologically normal tissue in an abnormal location (heterotopias). In one report of a patient with slowly progressive visual loss owing to a chiasmal choristoma, fibrous tissue and smooth muscle were found in the optic nerve and chiasm.[393] Surgical removal seems to be the most reasonable approach.

Chordomas and Chondrosarcomas

These skull base tumors more commonly present with ocular motor palsies so are discussed in more detail in Chapter 15. However, rarely chordomas and chondrosarcomas involving the central skull base can present with chiasmal interference and bitemporal hemianopias.[394]

CHIASMAL NEURITIS

Autopsy studies of patients with multiple sclerosis commonly reveal demyelinating lesions in the chiasm. In addition, occasionally patients with optic neuritis with complaints in just one eye are found to have a bitemporal field defects on formal perimetry.[395, 396] However, clinically evident chiasmal neuritis occurs much less frequently than ordinary optic neuritis. Newman et al[397] described five such patients and reviewed the reported cases with clinical correlation up to 1991. Most affected individuals were young adult or middle-aged females. The rate of onset of the visual loss was variable, and chiasmal field defects were often accompanied by evidence of optic nerve involvement. MRI typically showed chiasmal enlargement and enhancement, along with instrinsic bright T_2 signal. Although most individuals improved with or without corticosteroids, for unclear reasons patients took longer (months) to recover than those with ordinary optic neuritis.

In an individual with a history of multiple sclerosis, no further workup is required. In other cases, systemic lupus erythematosus, sarcoidosis, and other systemic disorders should be excluded by appropriate testing (antinuclear antibodies, angiotensin converting enzyme (ACE), erythrocyte sedimentation rate, Lyme antibodies, CSF ACE, and chest roentgenography and/or gallium scan). Optic gliomas appear similar radiographically, but they can be distinguished clinically by their more insidious visual loss.

In the Optic Neuritis Treatment Trial,[398] patients with optic neuritis who were given corticosteroids recovered more quickly, but their visual outcomes at 1 year were similar to those given placebo. However, we think chiasmal neuritis is a different situation because of the bilateral nature of the visual loss. If the field defects are subtle, then it might be reasonable to observe. On the other hand, we would treat those patients with dense bitemporal defects or severe acuity loss with 3 to 5 days of high-dose (1 g) IV methylprednisolone, followed by a short taper of oral prednisone over 5 to 10 days.

INFLAMMATORY MASSES

Inflammatory suprasellar masses include sarcoidosis, histiocytosis X, lymphocytic adenohypophysitis, idiopathic granulomatous hypophysitis, and optochiasmatic arachnoiditis. The first two are much more common than the others. In unusual cases, these disorders can present with isolated sellar lesions without systemic involvement, thereby mimicking pituitary tumors or craniopharyngiomas. In such instances, a transsphenoidal or stereotactic biopsy is required to establish the diagnosis.

Sarcoidosis

Because of its tendency to involve the basal meninges, it is not uncommon for sarcoidosis to affect the chiasm, hypothalamus, or pituitary gland.[399, 400, 472] The typical scenario is a bitemporal hemianopia or some other pattern of bilateral visual loss, diabetes insipidus, obesity, and hypopituitarism—with or without systemic involvement.[401, 402] Chronic cases usually present with optic atrophy, but concomitant optic nerve involvement may be associated with disc swelling. Concurrent uveitis or facial nerve or ocular motor palsies are highly suggestive of sarcoid. On MRI, suprasellar sarcoid appears as an irregular, infiltrative mass that is isointense to brain on T_1-weighted images and hyperintense on T_2-weighted images.[403] On CT the suprasellar lesions contrast enhance.[404] Sarcoid also can be intrinsic to the chiasm and optic nerves, causing radiographic enlargement and gadolinium enhancement of the anterior visual pathway.[405] In one series of chiasmal sarcoid,[406] four of four patients had elevated CSF protein. Gelwan et al[407] treated four patients with chiasmal sarcoid and visual loss with high-dose IV corticosteroids. Visual improvement was usually temporary, and subsequent deteriorations necessitated radiation, then immunosuppressive medications such as azathioprine or chlorambucil. Other steroid sparing agents such as cyclophosphamide, methotrexate,[408] and cyclosporine[400] have been used in sarcoidosis in this region.

Further details regarding the histopathology, diagnosis, and treatment of sarcoidosis involving the anterior visual pathway are discussed in Chapter 5.

Langerhans' Cell Histiocytosis (Histiocytosis X)

Pathologically, this disorder is typified by distinctive granulomas resulting from idiopathic proliferation of histiocytes, plasma cells, and eosinophilic inflammatory cells.[409] Other terms for Langerhans' cell histiocytosis have been used, depending on its focality and severity. Eosinophilic granuloma is the preferred designation when the process is unifocal. Hand–Schüller–Christian disease, the multifocal type, has a classic triad of exophthalmos, diabetes insipidus and skull lesions. The cells are well-differentiated in these two types. In contrast, Letterer–Siwe disease is a more aggressive form characterized by poorly differentiated histiocytes and multiorgan involvment.

Intracranial Langerhans' cell histiocytosis occurs more commonly in children and males and has a predilection for the hypothalmus.[409]

Endocrine disturbances are the most common manifestation, and the most frequent of these are diabetes insipidus, GH deficiency, and delayed puberty.[369] Visual loss due to compression of the anterior visual pathway can occur.[410, 411] Previous or concurrent skin, bone, or reticuloendothelial involvement should suggest the diagnosis, but cases can be isolated to the central nervous system (CNS). Surgical removal, chemotherapy, immunosuppression, and radiation therapy are all reasonable treatment options, depending on the extent of CNS and systemic involvement.[412]

Lymphocytic Adenohypophysitis

This entity occurs predominantly in younger women and is most common during pregnancy or in the postpartum period.[413] It is a presumed autoimmune disease,[37] as other associated conditions include Sjögren's disease, thyroiditis, pernicious anemia, rheumatoid arthritis, and insulin dependent diabetes.[414] The disorder is characterized histopathologically by plasma cell and lymphocyte infiltration of the pituitary, and clinically by headaches and hyperprolactinemia or hypopituitarism out of proportion to the degree of radiographic pituitary enlargement.[415] Bitemporal field defects may occur when extrasellar extension involves the chiasm.[415–417] On MRI, lymphocytic adenohypophysitis appears as a symmetric, solid sellar mass that is isotense with grey matter on T_1- and T_2-weighted images and that gadolinium enhances.[415, 418] The lesions are homogeneous and contrast enhancing on CT. Because the clinical and radiographic features can be confused with those of a pituitary adenoma,[419] a definitive diagnosis requires a biopsy. Chiasmal compression is an indication for partial resection, but complete removal, often resulting in unwarranted panhypopituitarism, should be avoided.[417] Corticosteroids may be used adjunctively.

Idiopathic Granulomatous Hypophysitis (Giant Cell Granuloma)

This related disorder can involve the pituitary, infundibulum, and potentially the chiasm.[420] Granulomatous hypophysitis typically presents in middle-aged or older women with hypopituitarism and diabetes insipidus. The older age predilection, diabetes insipidus, MRI evidence of infundibular thickening, and granulomatous inflammation distinguish this disorder from lymphocytic adenohypophysitis. Lack of systemic involvement separates it from the aforementioned granulomatous processes. Transsphenoidal biopsy is usualy necessary to establish the diagnosis, and corticosteroids are the treatment of choice. Rarely, granulomatous hypophysitis caused by a ruptured intrasellar Rathke's cleft cyst can be identified.[421]

Optochiasmatic Arachnoiditis

An inflammatory response in the suprasellar space may occur idiopathically or in association with head trauma or infections such as tuberculosis and cysticercosis (see below). In addition, optochiasmatic arachnoiditis may be induced by muslin wrapping of intracranial aneurysms in this region.[422]

INFECTIONS

Because the chiasm is surrounded by CSF, it is particularly vulnerable to any of the infectious meningitidies. In addition to tuberculous meningitis, which is discussed in more detail below, purulent meningitis due to *Streptococcus pneumoniae, Staphylococcus, Pseudomonas aeruginosa, Cryptococcus,* and syphilis infrequently can involve the chiasm. Other types of infections in this area are discussed below as well.

Tuberculosis

Pathologically, tuberculous meningitis is characterized by a thick greyish, gelatinous exudate at the base of brain and cisterns, consisting of polymorphonuclear cell infiltration, fibrin, endarteritis, and caseous necrosis.[423] With modern multidrug therapy, anterior visual pathway involvement in tuberculous meningitis has become exceedingly rare in developed nations.[424] However, we treated a previously healthy, immunocompetent 11-year-old boy who developed blindness, optic atrophy, and bilateral partial third nerve palsies as early sequelae of tuberculous meningitis. MRI revealed perichiasmal and basal cistern enhancement (Fig. 7–38).[425] Some authors have termed this process *tuberculous optochiasmatic arachnoiditis.*[426] When this occurs, visual field defects may be scotomatous or hemianopic, but more typically concentric contraction is present.[426] The diagnosis is supported by MRI

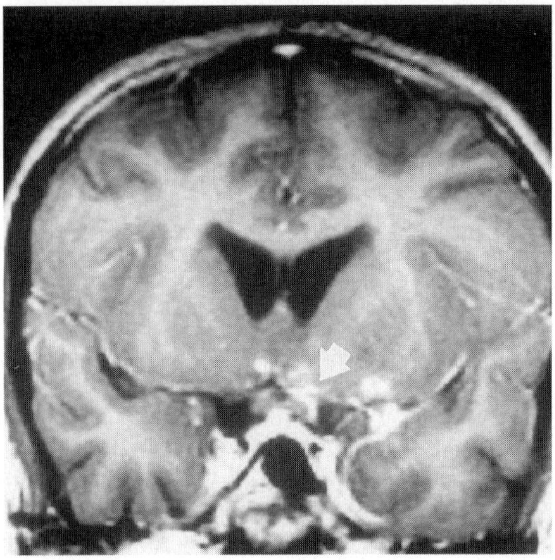

FIGURE 7–38. This patient with tuberculous meningitis presented with blindness, third nerve palsies, and altered mental status. The coronal MRI scan with gadolinium demonstrated perichiasmal enhancement (*arrow*), presumably due to arachnoiditis. (From Silverman IE, Liu GT, Bilaniuk LT, et al: Tuberculous meningitis with blindness and peri-chiasmal involvement on MRI. Pediatr Neurol 1995;12:65–67, with permission.)

evidence of perichiasmal enhancement. CSF analysis should be consistent with tuberculous meningitis (low glucose, lymphocytic or polymorphonuclear pleocytosis, and elevated protein).[427] Unfortunately, CSF acid-fast bacilli smears are often negative, and tubercle bacilli cultures takes days or weeks. For those reasons, polymerase chain reaction (PCR) for rapid detection of *Mycobacterium tuberculosis* in the CSF is gaining in popularity as a diagnostic tool.[428, 429] Antituberculous medication is the primary therapy in this disorder, at times in combination with neurosurgical lysis of adhesions.[426] Tuberculomas of the chiasm also have been described, but are even more uncommon.

Pituitary Abscesses

These are rare. Typically patients present with visual field loss and meningitis, or they appear as if they have a pituitary tumor: headache, bitemporal hemianopia, and hypopituitarism.[430, 431] The etiology of primary pituitary abscesses includes contiguous sphenoid sinus or cavernous sinus infection, meningitis, bacteremia, and CSF leaks. They may also occur secondarily when existing lesions such as pituitary adenomas, craniopharyngiomas, or Rathke's cleft become infected.[391] Pituitary abscesses are typically iso- or hypointense on T_1-weighted MRI and rim enhance.[432] Antibiotics should be administered, and if there is no response, the abscess can be drained transsphenoidally.[431]

Cysticercosis

In unusual instances cysticerci may infect the suprasellar cistern or sella and imitate a pituitary tumor.[433] On MRI or CT, calcified cysts may be evident, and if large enough the cysts can cause hydrocephalus. Proximity to the meninges or ventricular system can result in lymphocytic or eosinophilic meningitis. The diagnosis should be suspected when the neuroradiologic findings are suggestive in an individual from an endemic area (Central America, for example) or in a person who might have had direct contact with someone else who is infected with the parasite. Serum serologic testing for antibodies directed against the responsible tapeworm, *Taenia solium,* is the most sensitive and specific test for cysticercosis. Corticosteroids and anticysticercal drugs such as praziquantel or albendazole should be administered, and the presence of hydrocephalus may require a shunting procedure. Surgical removal is sometimes necessary for large lesions. Cisternal cysticercosis may have a poor prognosis despite treatment. Chronic inflammation of cysts and meninges can cause fibrosis and adhesions, leading to impairment of CSF flow and vasculitis with subsequent brain infarction.[433]

SIDE EFFECTS OF RADIATION

In the previous sections on pituitary adenomas and craniopharyngiomas, we alluded to the hazards of radiotherapy near the sellar area. This section will discuss in greater detail those that can cause chiasmal visual loss: radionecrosis of the chiasm and secondary neoplasms.

Chiasmal Radionecrosis

This complication has been most frequently reported following radiation treatment of pituitary adenomas, craniopharyngiomas, meningiomas, and other tumors near the skull base. Risk factors include radiation dose exceeding 4800 cGy, fractional dosage >200 cGy, overlapping treatment fields, and concurrent chemotherapy.[434] In one study, the time between completion of radiation therapy and onset of visual symptoms ranged from 4 to 35 months.[435] Visual loss is painless and can be either acute or gradual. Both eyes may be involved simultaneously or sequentially, with fellow eye involvement separated by weeks or months. Acutely the fundus appearance is normal, but eventually optic atrophy ensues.

Neuroimaging is required to confirm the diagnosis and exclude recurrent or secondary tumor. Typically, radionecrosis of the chiasm causes intrinsic enlargement and gadolinium enhancement on MRI.[436, 437] In general there are no visible signal changes within the chiasm on T_1- and T_2-weighted images.[438] Involvement of surrounding structures, such as the hypothalamus, frontal lobes, or pons, is often evident due to contrast enhancement.[439] With a history of previous radiation, the MRI findings are virtually diagnostic and obviate the need for further testing or biopsy.[440] CT, with or without enhancement, can be insensitive to subtle changes. In equivocal cases, positron emission tomography (PET) with 18-fluorine-deoxyglucose may be helpful in distinguishing radiation necrosis from tumor. The former is hypometabolic on PET, while recurrent or secondary tumors are hypermetabolic.

The pathophysiology and relative merits of treatment with corticosteroids, hyperbaric oxygen, and heparin are discussed under radiation optic neuropathy in Chapter 5.

Secondary Tumors

Radiation-induced tumors of the chiasm are unusual but have been reported. Hufnagel et al[441] reported a 41-year-old man who developed rapidly progressive visual loss due to a malignant optic chiasmal glioma 8 years following radiotherapy for a prolactinoma.

THIRD VENTRICULAR ENLARGEMENT

The neuro-ophthalmologic complications of third ventricular enlargement are described in an excellent review by Osher et al.[442] Rarely, third ventricle dilation causes downward chiasmal compression and a bitemporal hemianopia, owing to the intimate relationship of those two structures. Optic tract and optic nerve disturbances can also occur if the chiasm is pre- or postfixed, respectively. Proptosis, ocular motor palsies due to cavernous sinus compression, and Parinaud syndrome can be other complications. Posterior fossa tumors are the most common cause of the hydrocephalus in these instances, while aqueductal stenosis and postmeningitic adhesions are less frequent causes. Shunting procedures can improve visual field deficits and other symptoms.

Theoretically, binasal hemianopias may result from third ventricular enlargement if the chiasm and optic nerves are pushed downward and laterally against the carotid arteries. We agree with Osher et al[442] that binasal defects in the setting of hydrocephalus are much more commonly caused by papilledema.

CHIASMAL TRAUMA

In the setting of blunt head trauma, vision loss much less commonly localizes to the chiasm compared to the optic nerve. Nonetheless, a traumatic chiasmal syndrome is well recognized. Blunt frontal head trauma is the usual cause, and patients wake up with a nonprogressive bitemporal hemianopia, often complete.[443] Common associated findings include ocular motility deficits, anosmia, deafness, CSF rhinorrhea and otorrhea, and diabetes insipidus due to trauma to the pituitary stalk.[444] In a few instances see-saw nystagmus is related to chiasmal trauma.[28] Neuroimaging may reveal longitudinal disruption of the chiasm.[445] The mechanism of the bitemporal hemianopia is unclear, and proposed theories include stretching of the body of the chiasm,[444] a vascular insult, or contusion hemorrhage, necrosis, or tears.[446] Two patients with traumatic chiasmal syndrome were found to have midline basilar skull fractures through the midclivus, sella turcica floor, dorsum sellae, and sphenoid sinus, suggesting the chiasm was torn.[443]

EMPTY SELLA SYNDROME

In this condition, the sella is enlarged and the pituitary flattened against the sellar floor because of arachnoid herniation through a defect in the diaphragm (see Figure 6–16).[36] In primary empty sella, the defect is presumably congenital, while in secondary cases it results from surgery, radiation, infarction of a pituitary adenoma, or elevated intracranial pressure. In most instances when the sella is empty, it is CSF filled. However, occasionally the suprasellar portions of the optic nerves, chiasm, and tracts and anterioinferior third ventricle herniate into the space.[447] Bitemporal field deficits can occur in primary empty sellae,[448] but they are uncommon and seem unrelated to the amount of herniation.[447] Visual loss is usually nonprogressive, so surgical intervention is for the most part unnecessary. In primary cases endocrine function is usually preserved. Visual acuity and field loss in secondary empty sella is multifactorial and more likely the result of the original process. An empty sella is commonly observed in patients with pseudotumor cerebri,[449] but generally does not contribute to visual loss or endocrine dysfunction because herniation of suprasellar structures does not occur.

SPHENOID SINUS MUCOCELES

These can be considered retention cysts of the sinus, in many instances owing to inflammatory blockage of the draining ostium.[450] They consist of a sterile creamy fluid that is sometimes purulent.[391] Enlargement usually causes headache and orbital apex interference, however, chiasmal syndromes have been reported.[451] Surgical drainage of these mucoceles is best achieved via transnasal or transoral routes by an otolaryngologist.

DEVELOPMENTAL ANOMALIES OF THE CHIASM

These are rare and include chiasms that are either malformed or miswired.[473] Transsphenoidal encephaloceles, for instance, are characterized by congenital downward herniation of the optic nerves, chiasm, tract, and hypothalamus through the sphenoid bone.[452] Hypopituitarism, agenesis of the corpus callosum, and other cranial midline defects, such as hypertelorism, cleft lip, and cleft palate, are frequent accompanying features. Bitemporal hemianopias are the most common visual field defect. Disc atrophy is the usual fundus finding, but many patients instead have optic nerve colobomas or morning-glory disc anomalies (see Chapter 5). Indications for surgical intervention include progressive visual loss (uncommon), epipharyngeal respiratory obstruction, and CSF rhinorrhea. The surgeon is always careful to reduce rather than amputate the sac containing neural and endocrine structures.

Chiasmal aplasia or asymmetry can be associated with anophthalmia, which results from faulty development of one or both optic vesicles.[453] Chiasmal dysplasia can accompany optic nerve hypoplasia, absence of the septum pellucidum, and pituitary ectopia (de Morsier's septo-optic dysplasia) (Fig. 7–39).[9] A hereditary chiasmal optic neuropathy, without any major abnormalities on neuroimaging, has also been described.[454]

Miswiring of retinal fibers in the chiasm occurs almost exclusively in albinos, in whom some temporal ganglion cell axons can cross and project to the contralateral lateral geniculate nucleus. Greater activation of the contralateral occipital lobe following monocular stimulation has been demonstrated using visual evoked potentials[455] and functional MRI.[456] The appearance of the chiasm on MRI seems to be unaffected.[457] Two unusual nonalbino patients without chiasms were described by Apkarian et al.[458] These individuals had optic nerves that projected solely ipsilaterally to the optic tracts. Their visual fields were normal, but they had reduced acuity, esotropia, torticollis, and head tremor. Eye movement recordings demonstrated congenital nystagmus waveforms in the horizontal plane and seesaw nystagmus in the vertical and torsional planes.

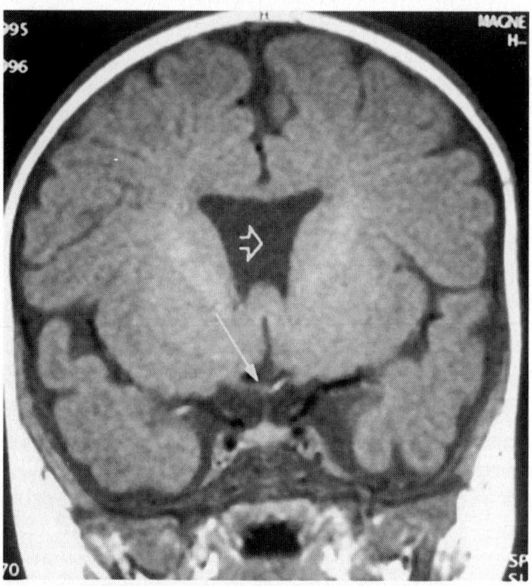

FIGURE 7–39. de Morsier syndrome. The coronal T_1-weighted MRI scan shows a thin chiasm (*thin arrow*) and absence of the septum pellucidum (*open arrow*) in a child with bilateral optic nerve hypoplasia.

REFERENCES

1. Hupp SL, Kline LB: Magnetic resonance imaging of the optic chiasm. Surv Ophthalmol 1991;36:207–216.
2. Lechan RM: Neuroendocrinology of pituitary hormone regulation. Endocrinol Metab Clin North Am 1987;16:475–501.
3. Ciric I: Pituitary tumors. Neurol Clin 1985;3:751–768.
4. Bergland RM, Ray BS, Torack RM: Anatomical variations in the pituitary gland and adjacent structures in 225 human autopsy cases. J Neurosurg 1968;28:93–99.
5. Melen O: Neuro-ophthalmologic features of pituitary tumors. Endocrinol Metab Clin North Am 1987;16: 585–608.
6. Doyle AJ: Optic chiasm position on MR images. AJNR 1990;11:553–555.
7. Elster AD: Modern imaging of the pituitary. Radiology 1993;187:1–14.
8. Kline LB, Vitek JJ, Acker JD: Computed tomography in the evaluation of the optic chiasm. Surv Ophthalmol 1983;27:387–396.
9. Hoyt WF: Correlative functional anatomy of the optic chiasm. 1969. Clin Neurosurg 1970;17:189–208.
10. Horton JC: Wilbrand's knee of the primate optic chiasm is an artefact of monocular enucleation. Trans Am Ophthalmol Soc 1997;95:579–609.
11. Liu GT: Disorders of the eyes and eyelids. In: Samuels MA, Feske S (eds): The Office Practice of Neurology, pp 40–74. New York, Churchill Livingstone, 1995.
12. Newman NM: The visual afferent pathways. Anatomic considerations. In: Neuro-ophthalmology: A Practical Text, pp 3–26. East Norwalk, Conn, Appleton & Lange, 1992.
13. Glaser JS, Sadun AA: Anatomy of the visual sensory system. In: Glaser JS (ed): Neuro-ophthalmology, second ed., pp 61–82. Philadelphia, JB Lippincott., 1990.
14. Kupersmith MJ: Circulation of the eye, orbit, cranial nerves, and brain. In: Neurovascular Neuro-ophthalmology, pp 1–67. Berlin, Springer-Verlag, 1993.
15. Bergland R, Ray BS: The arterial supply of the human optic chiasm. J Neurosurg 1969;31:327–334.
16. Elkington SG: Pituitary adenoma: preoperative symptomatology in a series of 260 patients. Br J Ophthalmol 1968;52:322–328.
17. Wary SH: Neuro-ophthalmic manifestations of pituitary and parasellar lesions. Clin Neurosurg 1977;24: 86–117.
18. Kirkham TH: The ocular symptomatology of pituitary tumours. Proc R Soc Med 1972;65:1–2 (517–518).
19. Bird AC: Field loss due to lesions at the anterior angle of the chiasm. Proc R Soc Med 1972;65:3–4 (519–520).
20. Mojon DS, Odel JG, Rios RJ, et al: Pituitary adenoma revealed by paracentral junctional scotoma of Traquair. Ophthalmologica 1997;211:104–108.
21. Karanjia N, Jacobson DM: Compression of the prechiasmatic optic nerve produces a junctional scotoma. Am J Ophthalmol 1999;128:256–258.
22. Hershenfeld SA, Sharpe JA: Monocular temporal hemianopia. Br J Ophthalmol 1993;77:424–427.
23. Trobe JD: Chromophobe adenoma presenting with a hemianopic temporal arcuate scotoma. Am J Ophthalmol 1974;77:388–392.
24. Salinas-Garcia RF, Smith JL: Binasal hemianopia. Surg Neurol 1978;10:187–194.
25. Unsold R, Hoyt WF: Band atrophy of the optic nerve. Arch Ophthalmol 1980;98:1637–1638.
26. Lyle TK, Clover P: Ocular symptoms and signs in pituitary tumours. Proc R Soc Med 1961;54:611–619.
27. Daroff RB: See-saw nystagmus. Neurology 1965;15: 874–877.
28. Nakada T, Kwee IL: Seesaw nystagmus. Role of visuovestibular interaction in its pathogenesis. J Clin Neuro-ophthalmol 1988;8:171–177.
29. Arnott EJ, Miller SJH: See saw nystagmus. Trans Ophthalmol Soc UK 1970;90:491–496.
30. Dell'Osso LF: See-saw nystagmus in dogs and humans. Neurology 1996;47:1372–1374.
31. Dell'Osso LF, Daroff RB: Two additional scenarios for see-saw nystagmus: achiasma and hemichiasma. J Neuro-ophthalmol 1998;18:112–113.
32. Gottlob I, Zubcov A, Catalano RA, et al: Signs distinguishing spasmus nutans (with and without central nervous system lesions) from infantile nystagmus. Ophthalmology 1990;97:1166–1175.
33. Lavery MA, O'Neill JF, Chu FC, et al: Acquired nystagmus in early childhood: A presenting sign of intracranial tumor. Ophthalmology 1984;91:425–435.
34. Trobe JD, Acosta PC, Krischer JP: A screening method for chiasmal visual-field defects. Arch Ophthalmol 1981;99:264–271.
35. Kooi KA, Yamada T, Marshall RE: Field studies of monocularly evoked cerebral potentials in bitemporal hemianopsia. Neurology 1973;23:1217–1225.
36. Vance ML: Hypopituitarism. N Engl J Med 1994;330: 1651–1661.
37. Abboud CF, Laws EJ: Diagnosis of pituitary tumors. Endocrinol Metab Clin North Am 1988;17:241–280.
38. Russell A: A diencephalic syndrome of emaciation in infancy and childhood. Arch Dis Child 1951;26:274.
39. Costin G: Endocrine disorders associated with tumors of the pituitary and hypothalamus. Pediatr Clin North Am 1979;26:15–31.
40. Poussaint TY, Barnes PD, Nichols K, et al: Diencephalic syndrome: clinical features and imaging findings. AJNR 1997;18:1499–1505.
41. Burr IM, Slonim AE, Danish RK, et al: Diencephalic syndrome revisited. J Pediatr 1976;88:439–444.
42. Aron DC, Tyrrell JB, Wilson CB: Pituitary tumors. Current concepts in diagnosis and management. West J Med 1995;162:340–352.
43. Besser M: Criteria for medical as opposed to surgical treatment of prolactinomas. Acta Endocrinol (Copenh) 1993;129 (Suppl 1):27–30.
44. Baumann G: Acromegaly. Endocrinol Metab Clin North Am 1987;16:685–703.
45. Orth DN: Cushing's syndrome. N Engl J Med 1995;332:791–803.
46. Post KD, Muraszko K: Management of pituitary tumors. Neurol Clin 1986;4:801–831.
47. Teramoto A, Hirakawa K, Sanno N, et al: Incidental pituitary lesions in 1,000 unselected autopsy specimens. Radiology 1994;193:161–164.
48. Di Rocco C, Maira G, Borelli P: Pituitary microadenomas in children. Childs Brain 1982;9:165–178.
49. Shalet SM: Pituitary adenomas in childhood. Acta Endocrinol Suppl (Copenh) 1986;279:434–439.
50. Faglia G: Epidemiology and pathogenesis of pituitary adenomas. Acta Endocrinol (Copenh) 1993;1:1–5.
51. Lee AG, Sforza PD, Fard AK, et al: Pituitary adenoma in children. J Neuro-ophthalmol 1998;18:102–105.
52. Abe T, Lüdecke DK, Saeger W: Clinically nonsecreting pituitary adenomas in childhood and adolescence. Neurosurgery 1998;42:744–750.
53. Alford FP, Arnott R: Medical management of pituitary tumours. Med J Aust 1992;157:57–60.
54. Keltner JI, Gittinger JW, Burde RM, et al: Endocrinological associations of pituitary tumors. Surv Ophthalmol 1980;25:31–36.

55. Simcic KJ, Moreno AJ: Tumors of the pituitary, pancreas, and parathyroid glands in a patient with multiple endocrine neoplasia Type 1. N Engl J Med 1998;339:1602.
56. Klibanski A: Nonsecreting pituitary tumors. Endocrinol Metab Clin North Am 1987;16:793–804.
57. Sassolas G, Trouillas J, Treluyer C, et al: Management of nonfunctioning pituitary adenomas. Acta Endocrinol (Copenh) 1993;129 (Suppl 1):21–26.
58. Kovacs K, Horvath E: Pathology of pituitary tumors. Endocrinol Metab Clin North Am 1987;16:529–551.
59. Bevan JS, Webster J, Burke CW, et al: Dopamine agonists and pituitary tumor shrinkage. Endocrine Rev 1992;13:220–240.
60. Hollenhorst RW, Younge BR: Ocular manifestations produced by adenomas of the pituitary gland: analysis of 1,000 cases. In: Kohler PO, Ross GT (eds): Diagnosis and Treatment of Pituitary Tumors, pp 53–64. Amsterdam, Excepta Medica-American Elsevier, 1973.
61. Anderson D, Faber P, Marcovitz S, et al: Pituitary tumors and the ophthalmologist. Ophthalmology 1983;90:1265–1270.
62. Trautmann JC, Laws ER: Visual status after transsphenoidal surgery at the Mayo Clinic, 1971–1982. Am J Ophthalmol 1983;96:200–208.
63. Zikel OM, Atkinson JL, Hurley DL: Prolactinoma manifesting with symptomatic hydrocephalus. Mayo Clin Proc 1999;74:475–477.
64. Dawson DJ, Enoch BA, Shepherd DI: Formed visual hallucinations with pituitary adenomas. BMJ 1984; 289:414.
65. Knosp E, Steiner E, Kitz K, et al: Pituitary adenomas with invasion of the cavernous sinus space: a magnetic resonance imaging classification compared with surgical findings. Neurosurgery 1993;33:610–617.
66. Saul RF, Hilliker JK: Third nerve palsy: the presenting sign of a pituitary adenoma in five patients and the only neurological sign in four patients. J Clin Neuro-ophthalmol 1985;5:185–193.
67. Petermann SH, Newman NJ: Pituitary macroadenoma manifesting as an isolated fourth nerve palsy. Am J Ophthalmol 1999;127:235–236.
68. Spiegel PH, Karcioglu ZA: Orbital invasion by pituitary adenoma. Am J Ophthalmol 1994;270–271.
69. Matsumura A, Meguro K, Doi M, et al: Suprasellar ectopic pituitary adenoma: case report and review of the literature. Neurosurgery 1990;26:681–685.
70. Kucharczyk W, Montanera WJ: The sella and parasellar region. In: Atlas SW (ed): Magnetic Resonance Imaging of the Brain and Spine, pp 625–667. New York, Raven Press, 1991.
71. Ostrov SG, Quencer RM, Hoffman JC, et al: Hemorrhage within pituitary adenomas: how often associated with pituitary apoplexy syndrome? AJNR 1989;10:503–510.
72. Jakubowski J, Kendall B: Coincidental aneurysms with tumours of pituitary origin. J Neurol Neurosurg Psychiatry 1978;41:972–979.
73. Weir B: Pituitary tumors and aneurysms: case report and review of the literature. Neurosurgery 1992;30: 585–591.
74. Pant B, Arita K, Kurisu K, et al: Incidence of intracranial aneurysm associated with pituitary adenoma. Neurosurg Rev 1997;20:13–17.
75. Laws ER: Pituitary surgery. Endocrinol Metab Clin North Am 1987;16:647–665.
76. Ebersold MJ, Quast LM, Laws ER, et al: Long-term results in transsphenoidal removal of nonfunctioning pituitary adenomas. J Neurosurg 1986;64:713–719.
77. Ciric I, Ragin A, Baumgartner C, et al: Complications of transsphenoidal surgery: results of a national survey, review of the literature, and personal experience. Neurosurgery 1997;40:225–236.
78. Jho HD, Carrau RL, Ko Y, et al: Endoscopic pituitary surgery: an early experience. Surg Neurol 1997;47: 213–222.
79. Yaniv E, Rappaport ZH: Endoscopic transseptal transsphenoidal surgery for pituitary tumors. Neurosurgery 1997;40:944–946.
80. Sheehan MT, Atkinson JLD, Kasperbauer JL: Preliminary comparison of the endoscopic transnasal vs. the sublabial approach for clinically nonfunctioning pituitary macroadenomas. Mayo Clin Proc 1999;74: 661–670.
81. Adams CB, Burke CW: Current modes of treatment of pituitary tumours [editorial]. Br J Neurosurg 1993;7:123–127.
82. Lennestand G: Visual recovery after treatment for pituitary adenoma. Acta Ophthalmol 1983;61:1104–1117.
83. Cohen AR, Cooper PR, Kupersmith MJ, et al: Visual recovery after transsphenoidal removal of pituitary adenomas. Neurosurgery 1985;17:446–452.
84. Klauber A, Rasmussen P, Lindholm J: Pituitary adenoma and visual function. The prognostic value of clinical, ophthalmological and neuroradiological findings in 51 patients subjected to operation. Acta Ophthalmol 1978;56:252–263.
85. Halberg FE, Sheline GE: Radiotherapy of pituitary tumors. Endocrinol Metab Clin North Am 1987;16: 667–684.
86. Capo H, Kupersmith MJ: Efficacy and complications of radiotherapy of anterior visual pathway tumors. Neurol Clin 1991;9:179–203.
87. Wen PY, Loeffler JS: Advances in the diagnosis and management of pituitary tumors. Curr Opin Oncol 1995;7:56–62.
88. Al-Mefty O, Kersh JE, Routh A, et al: The long-term side effects of radiation therapy for benign brain tumors in adults. J Neurosurg 1990;73:502–512.
89. Alexander MJ, DeSalles AA, Tomiyasu U: Multiple radiation-induced intracranial lesions after treatment for pituitary adenoma. Case report. J Neurosurg 1998;88:111–115.
90. Kondziolka D, Lunsford LD, Flickinger JC: Gamma knife radiosurgery for pituitary tumors: imaging, visual, and endocrine results [abstract]. Acta Neurochir (Wien) 1993;122:148.
91. Pollock BE, Gorman DA, Schomberg PJ, et al: The Mayo Clinic gamma knife experience: indications and initial results. Mayo Clin Proc 1999;74:5–13.
92. Mitsumori M, Shrieve DC, Alexander E, et al: Initial clinical results of LINAC-based stereotactic radiosurgery and stereotactic radiotherapy for pituitary adenomas. Int J Radiat Oncol Biol Phys 1998;42:573–580.
93. Jackson IM, Noren G: Role of gamma knife therapy in the management of pituitary tumors. Endocrinol Metab Clin North Am 1999;28:133–142.
94. Czech T, Wolfsberger S, Reitner A, et al: Delayed visual deterioration after surgery for pituitary adenoma. Acta Neurochirurg 1999;141:45–51.
95. Arafah BM, Brodkey JS, Manni A, et al: Recovery of pituitary function following surgical removal of large nonfunctioning pituitary adenomas. Clin Endocrinol 1982;17:213–222.
96. Breen P, Flickinger JC, Kondziolka D, et al: Radiotherapy for nonfunctional pituitary adenoma: analysis

of long-term tumor control. J Neurosurg 1998;89: 933–938.
97. Van Schaardenburg D, Roelfsema F, Van Seters AP, et al: Bromocriptine therapy for non-functioning pituitary adenomas. Clin Endocrinol 1989;30:475–484.
98. Warnet A, Timsit J, Chanson P, et al: The effect of somatostatin analogue on chiasmal dysfunction from pituitary macroadenomas. J Neurosurg 1989;71: 687–691.
99. Warnet A, Harris AG, Renard E, et al: A prospective multicenter trial of octreotide in 24 patients with visual field defects caused by nonfunctioning and gonadotropin-secreting pituitary adenomas. Neurosurgery 1997;41:786–797.
100. Vance ML, Thorner MO: Prolactinomas. Endocrinol Metab Clin North Am 1987;16:731–753.
101. Serri O: Progress in the management of hyperprolactinemia [editorial]. N Engl J Med 1994;331:942–944.
102. Moster ML, Savino PJ, Schatz NJ, et al: Visual function in prolactinoma patients treated with bromocriptine. Ophthalmology 1985;92:1332–1341.
103. Lesser RL, Zheutlin JD, Boghen D, et al: Visual function improvement in patients with macroprolactinomas treated with bromocriptine. Am J Ophthalmol 1990;109:535–543.
104. Mbanya J-CN, Mendelow AD, Crawford PJ, et al: Rapid resolution of visual abnormalities with medical therapy alone in patients with large prolactinomas. Br J Neurosurg 1993;7:519–527.
105. Jaquet P: Medical therapy of prolactinomas. Acta Endocrinol (Copenh) 1993;129 (Suppl 1):31–33.
106. Webster J, Piscitelli G, Polli A, et al: A comparison of cabergoline and bromocriptine in the treatment of hyperprolactinemic amenorrhea. N Engl J Med 1994;331:904–909.
107. Grochowicki M, Khafallah Y, Vighetto A, et al: Ophthalmic results in patients with macroprolactinomas treated with a new prolactin inhibitor CV 205–502. Br J Ophthalmol 1993;77:785–788.
108. van't Verlaat JW: The use of surgery for the treatment of prolactinomas. Acta Endocrinol (Copenh) 1993;129 (Suppl 1):34–37.
109. Molitch ME: Clinical manifestations of acromegaly. Endocrinol Metab Clin North Am 1992;21:597–614.
110. Davis DH, Laws ER, Ilstrup DM, et al: Results of surgical treatment for growth hormone-secreting pituitary adenomas. J Neurosurg 1993;79:70–75.
111. Melmed S: Medical management of acromegaly—what and when? Acta Endocrinol (Copenh) 1993;129 (Suppl 1):13–17.
112. Lamberts SWJ, van der Lely A-J, de Herder WW, et al: Octreotide. N Engl J Med 1996;334:246–254.
113. Stevenaert A: Presurgical octreotide treatment in acromegaly. Acta Endocrinol (Copenh) 1993;129 (Suppl 1):18–20.
114. Abs R, Verhelst J, Maiter D, et al: Cabergoline in the treatment of acromegaly: a study in 64 patients. J Clin Endocrinol Metabol 1998;83:374–378.
115. Aron DC, Findling JW, Tyrell JB: Cushing's disease. Endocrinol Metab Clin North Am 1987;16:705–730.
116. Tyrell JB, Wilson CB: Cushing's disease. Therapy of pituitary adenomas. Endocrinol Metab Clin North Am 1994;23:925–938.
117. Utiger RD: Treatment, and retreatment of Cushing's disease [editorial]. N Engl J Med 1997;336:215–217.
118. Estrada J, Boronat M, Mielgo M, et al: The long-term outcome of pituitary irradiation after unsuccessful transsphenoidal surgery in Cushing's disease. N Engl J Med 1997;336:172–177.
119. Smallridge RC: Thyrotropin-secreting pituitary tumors. Endocrinol Metab Clin North Am 1987;16: 765–792.
120. Yamamoto K, Saito K, Takai T, et al: Visual field defects and pituitary enlargement in primary hypothyroidism. J Clin Endocrinol Metab 1983;57:283–287.
121. Snyder PJ: Gonadotroph cell pituitary adenomas. Endocrinol Metab Clin North Am 1987;16:755–764.
122. Young WF, Scheithauer BW, Kovacs KT, et al: Gonadotroph adenoma of the pituitary gland: a clinicopathologic analysis of 100 cases. Mayo Clin Proc 1996;71: 649–656.
123. Cardoso ER, Peterson EW: Pituitary apoplexy: a review. Neurosurgery 1984;14:363–373.
124. Bills DC, Meyer FB, Laws ER, et al: A retrospective analysis of pituitary apoplexy. Neurosurgery 1993;33: 602–608.
125. Poisson M, Van Effentere R, Mashaly R: Pituitary apoplexy with retraction nystagmus. Ann Neurol 1980;7:286.
126. David NJ, Gargano FP, Glaser JS: Pituitary apoplexy in clinical perspective. In: Glaser JS, Smith JL (eds): Neuro-ophthalmology. Symposium of the University of Miami and the Bascom Palmer Eye Institute. Vol. VIII, pp 140–165. St. Louis, CV Mosby, 1975.
127. Juneau P, Schoene WC, Black P: Malignant tumors in the pituitary gland. Arch Neurol 1992;49:555–558.
128. Aaberg TM, Kay M, Sternau L: Metastatic tumors to the pituitary. Am J Ophthalmol 1995;119:779–785.
129. Molitch ME: Incidental pituitary adenomas. Am J Med Sci 1993;306:262–264.
130. Molitch ME: Evaluation and treatment of the patient with a pituitary incidentaloma. J Clin Endocrinol Metab 1995;80:3–6.
131. Molitch ME: Approach to the incidentally discovered pituitary mass. Cancer Treatment & Research 1997;89:73–90.
132. Adamson TE, Wiestler OD, Kleihues P, et al: Correlation of clinical and pathological features in surgically treated craniopharyngiomas. J Neurosurg 1990;73: 12–17.
133. Kennedy HB, Smith RJ: Eye signs in craniopharyngioma. Br J Ophthalmol 1975;59:689–695.
134. Crane TB, Yee RD, Hepler RS, et al: Clinical manifestations and radiologic findings in craniopharyngiomas in adults. Am J Ophthalmol 1982;94:220–228.
135. Shillito JJ: Craniopharyngiomas: the subfrontal approach, or none at all? Clin Neurosurg 1980;27: 188–205.
136. Sanford RA, Muhlbauer MS: Craniopharyngioma in children. Neurol Clin 1991;9:453–465.
137. Cabezudo JM, Vaquero J, Areitio E, et al: Craniopharyngiomas: a critical approach to treatment. J Neurosurg 1981;55:371–375.
138. Weiner HL, Wisoff JH, Rosenberg ME, et al: Craniopharyngiomas: a clinicopathological analysis of factors predictive of recurrence and functional outcome. Neurosurgery 1994;35:1001–1010.
139. McLone DG, Raimondi AJ, Naidich TP: Craniopharyngiomas. Child's Brain 1982;9:188–200.
140. Hoffman HJ, De Silva M, Humphreys RP, et al: Aggressive surgical management of craniopharyngiomas in children. J Neurosurg 1992;76:47–52.
141. Duff TA, Levine R: Intrachiasmatic craniopharyngioma. Case report. J Neurosurg 1983;59:176–178.
142. Brodsky MC, Hoyt WF, Barnwell SL, et al: Intrachiasmatic craniopharyngioma: a rare cause of chiasmal thickening. Case report. J Neurosurg 1988;68: 300–302.

143. Brummitt ML, Kline LB, Wilson ER: Craniopharyngioma: pitfalls in diagnosis. J Clin Neuro-ophthalmol 1992;12:77–81.
144. Block MA, Goree JA, Jimenez JP: Craniopharyngioma with optic canal enlargement simulating glioma of the optic chiasm. Case report. J Neurosurg 1973;39: 523–527.
145. Yasargil MG, Curcic M, Kis M, et al: Total removal of craniopharyngiomas. Approaches and long-term results in 144 patients. J Neurosurg 1990;73:3–11.
146. Petito CK, DeGirolami U, Earle KM: Craniopharyngiomas: a clinical and pathological review. Cancer 1976;37:1944–1952.
147. Waga S, Morikawa A, Sakakura M: Craniopharyngioma with midbrain involvement. Arch Neurol 1979;36:319–320.
148. Young SC, Zimmerman RA, Nowell MA, et al: Giant cystic craniopharyngiomas. Neuroradiology 1987;29: 468–473.
149. Altinors N, Senveli E, Erdogan A, et al: Craniopharyngioma of the cerebellopontine angle. Case report. J Neurosurg 1984;60:842–844.
150. Yamamoto T, Yoneda S, Funatsu N: Spontaneous haemorrhage in craniopharyngioma [letter]. J Neurol Neurosurg Psychiatry 1989;52:803–804.
151. Baskin DS, Wilson CB: Surgical management of craniopharyngiomas. A review of 74 cases. J Neurosurg 1986;65:22–27.
152. Weiss M, Sutton L, Marcial V, et al: The role of radiation therapy in the management of childhood craniopharyngioma. Int J Radiat Oncol Biol Phys 1989;17: 1313–1321.
153. Repka MX, Miller NR, Miller M: Visual outcome after surgical removal of craniopharyngiomas. Ophthalmology 1989;96:195–199.
154. van den Berge JH, Blaauw G, Breeman WAP, et al: Intracavitary brachytherapy of cystic craniopharyngiomas. J Neurosurg 1992;77:545–550.
155. Savino PJ, Paris M, Schatz NJ, et al: Optic tract syndrome. A review of 21 patients. Arch Ophthalmol 1978;96:656–663.
156. Cappaert WE, Kiprov RV: Craniopharyngioma presenting as unilateral central visual loss. Ann Ophthalmol 1981;13:703–704.
157. Thomsett MJ, Conte FA, Kaplan SL, et al: Endocrine and neurologic outcome in childhood craniopharyngioma. J Pediatr 1980;97:728–735.
158. Johnson LN, Hepler RS, Yee RD, et al: Magnetic resonance imaging of craniopharyngioma. Am J Ophthalmol 1986;102:242–244.
159. Nagahata M, Hosoya T, Kayama T, et al: Edema along the optic tract: a useful MR finding for the diagnosis of craniopharyngiomas. AJNR 1998;19:1753–1757.
160. Higashi S, Yamashita J, Fujisawa H, et al: "Moustache" appearance in craniopharyngiomas: unique magnetic resonance imaging and computed tomographic findings of perifocal edema. Neurosurgery 1990;27:993–996.
161. Youl BD, Plant GT, Stevens JM, et al: Three cases of craniopharyngioma showing optic tract hypersignal on MRI. Neurology 1990;40:1416–1419.
162. Numaguchi Y, Kishikawa T, Ikeda J, et al: Neuroradiological manifestations of suprasellar pituitary adenomas, meningiomas and craniopharyngiomas. Neuroradiology 1981;21:67–74.
163. Pierre-Kahn A, Sainte-Rose C, Renier D: Surgical approach to children with craniopharyngiomas and severly impaired vision: special considerations. Pediatr Neurosurg 1994;21 (Suppl 1):50–56.
164. Allen MB, Yaghmai F: Diagnosis and treatment of pituitary tumors and craniopharyngiomas. In: Allen MB, Miller RH (eds): Essential of Neurosurgery. A Guide to Clinical Practice, pp 211–228. New York, McGraw-Hill, 1995.
165. Landolt AM, Zachmann M: Results of transphenoidal extirpation of craniopharyngiomas and Rathke's cysts. Neurosurgery 1991;28:410–415.
166. Honegger J, Buchfelder M, Fahlbusch R, et al: Transsphenoidal microsurgery for craniopharyngioma. Surg Neurol 1992;37:189–196.
167. Norris JS, Pavaresh M, Afshar F: Primary transsphenoidal microsurgery in the treatment of craniopharyngiomas. Br J Neurosurg 1998;12:305–312.
168. Long DM, Leibrock L: The transcallosal approach to the anterior ventricular system and its application in the therapy of craniopharyngioma. Clin Neurosurg 1980;27:160–168.
169. Caldarelli M, di Rocco C, Papacci F, et al: Management of recurrent craniopharyngioma. Acta Neurochir 1998;140:447–454.
170. Regine WF, Mohiuddin M, Kramer S: Long-term results of pediatric and adult craniopharyngiomas treated with combined surgery and radiation. Radiother Oncol 1993;27:13–21.
171. Symon L, Sprich W: Radical excision of craniopharyngioma. Results in 20 patients. J Neurosurg 1985;62:174–181.
172. Symon L, Pell MF, Habib AH: Radical excision of craniopharyngioma by the temporal route: a review of 50 patients. Br J Neurosurg 1991;5:539–549.
173. Cavazzuti V, Fischer EG, Welch K, et al: Neurological and psychophysiological sequelae following different treatments of craniopharyngioma in children. J Neurosurg 1983;59:409–417.
174. De Vile CJ, Grant DB, Kendall BE, et al: Management of childhood craniopharyngioma: can the morbidity of radical surgery be predicted? J Neurosurg 1996;85:73–81.
175. Fischer EG, Welch K, Shillito J, et al: Craniopharyngiomas in children. Long-term effects of conservative surgical procedures combined with radiation therapy. J Neurosurg 1990;73:534–540.
176. Manaka S, Teramoto A, Takakura K: The efficacy of radiotherapy for craniopharyngioma. J Neurosurg 1985;62:648–656.
177. Wen BC, Hussey DH, Staples J, et al: A comparison of the roles of surgery and radiation therapy in the management of craniopharyngiomas. Int J Radiat Oncol Biol Phys 1989;16:17–24.
178. Sogg RL, Donaldson SS, Yorke CN: Malignant astrocytoma following radiotherapy of a craniopharyngioma. J Neurosurg 1978;48:622–627.
179. Shapiro K, Till K, Grant DN: Craniopharyngiomas in childhood. A rational approach to treatment. J Neurosurg 1979;50:617–623.
180. Voges J, Sturm V, Lehrke R, et al: Cystic craniopharyngioma: long-term results after intracavitary irradiation with stereotactically applied colloidal beta-emitting radioactive sources. J Neurosurg 1997;40: 263–269.
181. Anderson DR, Trobe JD, Taren JA, et al: Visual outcome in cystic craniopharyngiomas treated with intracavitary phosphorus-32. Ophthalmology 1989;96: 1786–1792.
182. Cavalheiro S, Sparapani FV, Franco JO, et al: Use of bleomycin in intratumoral chemotherapy for cystic craniopharyngioma. Case report. J Neurosurg 1996;84:124–126.

183. Kobayashi T, Tanaka T, Kida Y: Stereotactic gamma radiosurgery of craniopharyngiomas. Pediatr Neurosurg 1994;21 (Suppl 1):69–74.
184. Stephanian E, Lunsford LD, Coffey RJ, et al: Stereotactic radiosurgery. Neurosurg Clin North Am 1992;3:207–218.
185. Fisher PG, Jenab J, Goldthwaite PT, et al: Outcomes and failure patterns in childhood craniopharyngiomas. Childs Nerv Syst 1998;14:558–563.
186. Mutlukan E, Cullen JF: Visual outcome after craniopharyngioma [letter]. Ophthalmology 1990;97:539–540.
187. Sorva R, Heiskanen O, Perheentupa J: Craniopharyngioma surgery in children: endocrine and visual outcome. Childs Nerv Syst 1988;4:97–99.
188. Abrams LS, Repka MX: Visual outcome of craniopharyngioma in children. J Pediatr Ophthalmol Strabismus 1997;34:223–228.
189. Repka MX, Miller NR: Visual outcome after craniopharyngioma [comment]. Ophthalmology 1990;97: 539–540.
190. Lyen KR, Grant DB: Endocrine function, morbidity, and mortality after surgery for craniopharyngioma. Arch Dis Child 1982;57:837–841.
191. Newman CB, Levine LS, New MI: Endocrine function in children with intrasellar and suprasellar neoplasms: before and after therapy. Am J Dis Child 1981;135:259–266.
192. Tiulpakov AN, Mazerkina NA, Brook CG, et al: Growth in children with craniopharyngioma following surgery. Clin Endocrinol 1998;49:733–738.
193. Voelker JL, Campbell RL, Muller J: Clinical, radiographic, and pathological features of symptomatic Rathke's cleft cysts. J Neurosurg 1991;74:535–544.
194. Oka H, Kawano N, Suwa T, et al: Radiological study of symptomatic Rathke's cleft cysts. Neurosurgery 1994;35:632–636.
195. Kucharczyk W, Peck WW, Kelly WM, et al: Rathke cleft cysts: CT, MR imaging, and pathologic features. Radiology 1987;165:491–495.
196. Rao GP, Blyth CP, Jeffreys RV: Ophthalmic manifestations of Rathke's cleft cysts. Am J Ophthalmol 1995;119:86–91.
197. Barrow DL, Spector RH, Takei Y, et al: Symptomatic Rathke's cleft cysts located entirely in the suprasellar region: review of diagnosis, management, and pathogenesis. Neurosurgery 1985;16:766–772.
198. Itoh J, Usui K: An entirely suprasellar symptomatic Rathke's cleft cyst: case report. Neurosurgery 1992; 30:581–584.
199. Ross DA, Norman D, Wilson CB: Radiologic characteristics and results of surgical management of Rathke's cysts in 43 patients. Neurosurgery 1992;30: 173–178.
200. el-Mahdy W, Powell M: Transsphenoidal management of 28 symptomatic Rathke's cleft cysts, with special reference to visual and hormonal recovery. Neurosurgery 1998;42:7–16.
201. Maggio WW, Cail WS, Brookeman JR, et al: Rathke's cleft cyst: computed tomographic and magnetic resonance imaging appearances. Neurosurgery 1987;21: 60–62.
202. Hayashi Y, Tachibana O, Muramatsu N, et al: Rathke cleft cyst: MR and biomedical analysis of cyst content. J Comput Assist Tomogr 1999;23:34–38.
203. Crenshaw WB, Chew FS: Rathke's cleft cyst. AJR 1992;158:1312.
204. Kurisaka M, Fukui N, Sakamoto T, et al: A case of Rathke's cleft cyst with apoplexy. Child's Nerv Syst 1998;14:343–347.
205. Midha R, Jay V, Smyth HS: Transsphenoidal management of Rathke's cleft cysts. A clinicopathological review of 10 cases. Surg Neurol 1991;35:446–454.
206. Iraci G, Giordano R, Gerosa M, et al: Ocular involvement in recurrent cyst of Rathke's cleft: Case report. Ann Ophthalmol 1979;11:94–98.
207. Mukherjee JJ, Islam N, Kaltsas G, et al: Clinical, radiological and pathological features of patients with Rathke's cleft cysts: tumors that may recur. J Clin Endocrinol Metabol 1997;82:2357–2362.
208. Rappaport ZH: Suprasellar arachnoid cysts: options in operative management. Acta Neurochir (Wien) 1993;122:71–75.
209. Burnbaum MD, Harbison JW, Selhorst JB, et al: Blue-domed cyst with optic nerve compression. J Neurol Neurosurg Psychiatry 1978;41:987–991.
210. Pierre KA, Capelle L, Brauner R, et al: Presentation and management of suprasellar arachnoid cysts. Review of 20 cases. J Neurosurg 1990;73:355–359.
211. Benton JW, Nellhaus G, Huttenlocher PR, et al: The bobble-head doll syndrome. Report of unique truncal tremor associated with third ventricular cyst and hydrocephalus in children. Neurology 1966;16:725–729.
212. Chun BB, Lee AG, Coughlin WF, et al: Unusual presentations of sellar arachnoid cyst. J Neuro-ophthalmol 1998;18:246–249.
213. Abe T, Matsumoto K, Homma H, et al: Dorsum sellae meningioma mimicking pituitary macroadenoma: case report. Surg Neurol 1999;51:543–546.
214. Wilson WB: Meningiomas of the anterior visual system. Surv Ophthalmol 1981;26:109–127.
215. Symon L, Rosenstein J: Surgical management of suprasellar meningioma. Part 1: The influence of tumor size, duration of symptoms, and microsurgery on surgical outcome in 101 consecutive cases. J Neurosurg 1984;61:633–641.
216. Black PM: Meningiomas. Neurosurgery 1993;32: 643–657.
217. Chou SM, Miles JM: The pathology of meningiomas. In: A1-Mefty O (ed): Meningiomas, pp 37–57. New York, Raven Press, 1991.
218. Lee A, Wallace C, Rewcastle B, et al: Metastases to meningioma. AJNR 1998;19:1120–1122.
219. Gregorius FK, Hepler RS, Stern WE: Loss and recovery of vision with suprasellar meningiomas. J Neurosurg 1975;42:69–75.
220. Brihaye J, Brihaye-van Geertruyden M: Management and surgical outcome of suprasellar meningiomas. Acta Neurochir (Wein) [Suppl] 1988;42:124–129.
221. Yeakley JW, Kulkarni MV, McArdle CB, et al: High-resolution MR imaging of juxtasellar meningiomas with CT and angiographic correlation. AJNR 1988; 9:279–285.
222. Ojemann RG: Management of cranial and spinal meningiomas (honored guest presentation). Clin Neurosurg 1993;40:321–383.
223. Rodesch G, Lasjaunias P: Embolization and meningiomas. In: A1-Mefty O (ed): Meningiomas, pp 285–297. New York, Raven Press, 1991.
224. Andrews BT, Wilson CB: Suprasellar meningiomas: the effect of tumor location on postoperative visual outcome. J Neurosurg 1988;69:523–528.
225. Probst C: Possibilities and limitations of microsurgery in patients with meningiomas of the sellar region. Acta Neurochir (Wien) 1987;84:99–102.
226. Kupersmith MJ, Warren FA, Newall J, et al: Irradiation of meningiomas of the intracranial anterior visual pathway. Ann Neurol 1987;21:131–137.

227. Kondziolka D, Lunsford LD, Coffey RJ, et al: Stereotactic radiosurgery of meningiomas. J Neurosurg 1991;74:552–559.
228. Hakim R, Alexander E, Loeffler JS, et al: Results of linear accelerator-based radiosurgery for intracranial meningiomas. Neurosurgery 1998;42:446–453.
229. Gutin PH, Leibel SA, Hosobuchi Y, et al: Brachytherapy of recurrent tumors of the skull base and spine with iodine-125 sources. Neurosurgery 1987;20:938–945.
230. Kumar PP, Patil AA, Leibrock LG, et al: Continuous low-dose rate brachytherapy with high activity iodine-125 seeds in the management of meningiomas. Int J Radiat Oncology Biol Phys 1993;25:325–328.
231. Schrell UMH, Fahlbusch R: Hormonal manipulation of cerebral meningiomas. In: A1-Mefty O (ed): Meningiomas, pp 273–283. New York, Raven Press, 1991.
232. Grunberg SM, Weiss MH, Spitz IM, et al: Treatment of unresectable meningiomas with the antiprogesterone agent mifepristone. J Neurosurg 1991;74:861–866.
233. Rosenstein J, Symon L: Surgical management of suprasellar meningioma. Part 2: Prognosis for visual function following craniotomy. J Neurosurg 1984;61:642–648.
234. Finn JE, Mount LA: Meningiomas of tuberculum sellae and planum sphenoidale: a review of 83 cases. Arch Ophthalmol 1974;92:23–27.
235. Rosenberg L, Miller NR: Visual results after microsurgical removal of meningioma involving the anterior visual system. Arch Ophthalmol 1984;102:1019–1023.
236. Grant FC, Hedges TR: Ocular findings in meningiomas of the tuberculum sellae. Arch Ophthalmol 1956;56:163–170.
237. Al-Mefty O, Smith RR: Tuberculum sellae meningiomas. In: Al-Mefty O (ed): Meningiomas, pp 395–411. New York, Raven Press, 1991.
238. Al-Mefty O: Clinoidal meningiomas. In: Al-Mefty O (ed): Meningiomas, pp 427–443. New York, Raven Press, 1991.
239. Kinjo T, Al-Mefty O, Ciric I: Diaphragma sellae meningiomas. Neurosurgery 1995;36:1082–1092.
240. Cappabianca P, Cirillo S, Alfieri A, et al: Pituitary macroadenoma and diaphragma sellae meningioma: differential diagnosis on MRI. Neuroradiology 1999;41:22–26.
241. Kasner SE, Liu GT, Galetta SL: Neuro-ophthalmologic aspects of aneurysms. Neuroimag Clin North Am 1997;7:679–692.
242. Date I, Asari S, Ohmoto T: Cerebral aneurysms causing visual symptoms: their features and surgical outcome. Clin Neurol Neurosurg 1998;100:259–267.
243. Walsh FB: Visual field defect due to aneurysms at the circle of Willis. Arch Ophthalmol 1964;71:15–27.
244. White JC, Ballantine HT: Intrasellar aneurysms simulating hypophyseal tumors. J Neurosurg 1961;18:34–50.
245. Kupersmith MJ: Aneurysms involving the motor and sensory visual pathways. In: Neurovascular Neuro-ophthalmology, pp 239–300. Berlin, Springer-Verlag, 1993.
246. Meyer FB, Morita A, Puumala MR, et al: Medical and surgical management of intracranial aneurysms. Mayo Clin Proc 1995;70:153–172.
247. Peiris JB, Ross Russell RW: Giant aneurysms of the carotid system presenting as visual field defect. J Neurol Neurosurg Psychiatr 1980;43:1053–1064.
248. Højer-Pedersen E, Haase J: Giant anterior communicating artery aneurysm with bitemporal hemianopsia: case report. Neurosurgery 1981;8:703–706.
249. Shutter LA, Kline LB, Fisher WS: Visual loss and a suprasellar mass complicated by pregnancy. Surv Ophthalmol 1993;38:63–69.
250. Ferguson G, Drake CG: Carotid-ophthalmic aneurysms: visual abnormalities in 32 patients and the results of treatment. Surg Neurol 1981;16:1–8.
251. Bird AC, Nolan B, Gargano FP, et al: Unruptured aneurysm of the supraclinoid carotid artery. Neurology 1970;20:445–454.
252. Date I, Akioka T, Ohmoto T: Penetration of the optic chiasm by a ruptured anterior communicating artery aneurysm. Case report. J Neurosurg 1997;87:324–326.
253. Raymond LA, Tew J: Large suprasellar aneurysms imitating pituitary tumor. J Neurol Neurosurg Psychiatr 1978;41:83–87.
254. Biondi A, Scialfa G, Scotti G: Intracranial aneurysms: MR imaging. Neuroradiology 1988;30:214–218.
255. Atlas SW, Mark AS, Fram EK, et al: Vascular intracranial lesions: applications of gradient-echo MR imaging. Radiology 1988;169:455–461.
256. The International Study of Unruptured Intracranial Aneurysms Investigators: Unruptured intracranial aneurysms-risk of rupture and risks of surgical intervention. N Engl J Med 1998;339:1725–1733.
257. Schievink WI: Intracranial aneurysms. N Engl J Med 1997;336:28–40.
258. De Jesús O, Sekhar LN, Riedel CJ: Clinoid and paraclinoid aneurysms: surgical anatomy, operative techniques, and outcome. Surg Neurol 1999;51:477–487.
259. Guterman LR, Hopkins LN: Endovascular treatment of cerebral aneurysms. Diagnosis and treatment. Clin Neurosurg 1993;40:56–83.
260. Nichols DA, Meyer FB, Piepgras DG, et al: Endovascular treatment of intracranial aneurysms. Mayo Clin Proc 1994;69:272–285.
261. Maitland CG, Abiko S, Hoyt WF, et al.: Chiasm apoplexy: report of four cases. J Neurosurg 1982;56:118–122.
262. Hwang J-F, Yau C-W, Huang J-K, et al: Apoplectic optochiasmal syndrome due to intrinsic cavernous hemangioma. Case report. J Clin Neuro-ophthalmol 1993;13:232–236.
263. Kupersmith MJ: Vascular malformations of the brain. In: Neurovascular Neuro-ophthalmology, pp 301–351, Berlin, Springer-Verlag, 1993.
264. Corboy JR, Galetta SL: Familial cavernous angiomas manifesting with an acute chiasmal syndrome. Am J Ophthalmol 1989;108:245–250.
265. Mohr G, Hardy J, Gauvin P: Chiasmal apoplexy due to ruptured cavernous hemangioma of the optic chiasm. Surg Neurol 1985;24:636–640.
266. Tien R, Dillon WP: MR imaging of cavernous hemangioma of the optic chiasm. J Comput Assist Tomogr 1989;13:1087–1088.
267. Warner JEA, Rizzo JF, Brown EW, et al: Recurrent chiasmal apoplexy due to cavernous malformation. J Neuro-ophthalmol 1996;16:99–106.
268. Hassler W, Zentner J, Wilhelm H: Cavernous angiomas of the anterior visual pathways. J Clin Neuro-ophthalmol 1989;9:160–164.
269. Lavin PJM, McCrary JA, Roessmann U, et al: Chiasmal apoplexy: hemorrhage from a cryptic vascular malformation in the optic chiasm. Neurology 1984;34:1007–1011.
270. Fermaglich J, Kattah J, Manz H: Venous angioma of the optic chiasm. Ann Neurol 1978;4:470–471.
271. Balcer LJ, Galetta SL, Curtis M, et al: von Hippel-Lindau disease manifesting as a chiasmal syndrome. Surv Ophthalmol 1995;39:302–306.

272. Lee KF, Schatz NJ, Savino PJ: Ischemic chiasmal syndrome. In: Glaser JS, Smith JL, (eds): Neuro-ophthalmology. Symposium of the University of Miami and the Bascom Palmer Eye Institute. Vol. VIII, pp 115–130. St. Louis, CV Mosby, 1975.
273. Jacobson DM: Symptomatic compression of the optic nerve by the carotid artery. Clinical profile of 18 patients with 24 affected eyes identified by magnetic resonance imaging. Ophthalmology 1999;106:1994–2004.
274. Hilton GF, Hoyt WF: An arteriosclerotic chiasmal syndrome. Bitemporal hemianopia associated with fusiform dilatation of the anterior cerebral arteries. JAMA 1966;196:1018–1020.
275. Matsuo K, Kobayashi S, Sugita K: Bitemporal hemianopsia associated with sclerosis of the intracranial internal carotid arteries. J Neurosurg 1980;53: 566–569.
276. Golnik KC, Hund PW, Stroman GA, et al: Magnetic resonance imaging in patients with unexplained optic neuropathy. Ophthalmology 1996;103:515–530.
277. Sibony PA, Lessell S, Wray S: Chiasmal syndrome caused by arteriovenous malformations. Arch Ophthalmol 1982;100:438–442.
278. Volpe NJ, Sharma MC, Galetta SL, et al: Orbital drainage from cerebral arteriovenous malformations. Neurosurgery 2000;46:820–824.
279. Gould TJ, Johnson LN, Colapinto EV, et al: Intrasellar vascular malformation mimicking a pituitary macroadenoma. J Neuro-ophthalmol 1996;16:199–203.
280. Packer RJ: Treatment of chiasmatic/hypothalamic gliomas of childhood with chemotherapy. In: Smith JL, Katz RS (eds): Neuro-ophthalmology Enters the Nineties, pp 145–151. Hialeah, Dutton, 1988.
281. Alvord EC, Lofton S: Gliomas of the optic nerve or chiasm: outcome by patients' age, tumor site, and treatment. J Neurosurg 1988;68:85–98.
282. Dutton JJ: Gliomas of the anterior visual pathways. Surv Ophthalmol 1994;38:427–452.
283. Ragge NK: Clinical and genetic patterns of neurofibromatosis 1 and 2. Br J Ophthalmol 1993;77:662–672.
284. Bouzas EA, Parry DM, Eldridge R, et al: Visual impairment in patients with neurofibromatosis 2. Neurology 1993;43:622–623.
285. Lewis RA, Gerson LP, Axelson KA, et al: von Recklinghausen neurofibromatosis. II. Incidence of optic gliomata. Ophthalmology 1984;91:929–935.
286. Listernick R, Charrow J, Greenwald M, et al: Natural history of optic pathway tumors in children with neurofibromatosis type 1: a longitudinal study. J Pediatr 1994;125:63–66.
287. Champion MP, Robinson RO: Screening for optic gliomas in neurofibromatosis type 1: the role of neuroimaging [letter]. J Pediatr 1995;127:507–508.
288. Listernick R, Louis DN, Packer RJ, et al: Optic pathway gliomas in children with neurofibromatosis 1: consensus statement from the NF1 optic pathway glioma task force. Ann Neurol 1997;41:143–149.
289. Jabbari B, Maitland CG, Morris LM, et al: The value of visual evoked potential as a screening test in neurofibromatosis. Arch Neurol 1985;42:1072–1074.
290. North K, Cochineas C, Tang E, et al: Optic gliomas in neurofibromatosis type 1: role of visual evoked potentials. Pediatr Neurol 1994;10:117–123.
291. Listernick R, Charrow J: Screening for optic gliomas in neurofibromatosis type 1: the role of neuroimaging [reply]. J Pediatr 1995;127:507–508.
292. Listernick R, Charrow J, Greenwald M: Emergence of optic pathway gliomas in children with neurofibromatosis type 1 after normal neuroimaging results. J Pediatr 1992;121:584–587.
293. Massry GG, Morgan CF, Chung SM: Evidence of optic pathway gliomas after previously negative neuroimaging. Ophthalmology 1997;104:930–935.
294. Rossi LN, Pastorino G, Scotti G, et al: Early diagnosis of optic glioma in children with neurofibromatosis type 1. Childs Nerv Syst 1994;10:426–429.
295. Liu GT, Molloy PT, Needle M, et al: Optic gliomas in neurofibromatosis type 1: role of visual evoked potentials [letter]. Pediatr Neurol 1995;12:89–90.
296. Borit A, Richardson EP: The biological and clinical behaviour of pilocytic astrocytomas of the optic pathways. Brain 1982;105:161–187.
297. Coakley KJ, Huston J, Scheithauer BW, et al: Pilocytic astrocytomas: well-demarcated magnetic resonance appearance despite frequent infiltration histologically. Mayo Clin Proc 1995;70:747–751.
298. Anderson DR, Spencer WH: Ultrastructural and histochemical observations of optic nerve gliomas. Arch Ophthalmol 1970;83:324–335.
299. Bilgiç S, Erbengi A, Tinaztepe B, et al: Optic glioma of childhood: clinical, histopathological, and histochemical observations. Br J Ophthalmol 1989;73: 832–837.
300. Hoyt WF, Baghdassarian SA: Optic glioma of childhood: natural history and rationale for conservative management. Br J Ophthalmol 1969;53:793–798.
301. Burnstine MA, Levin LA, Louis DN, et al: Nucleolar organizer regions in optic gliomas. Brain 1993;116: 1465–1476.
302. Glaser JS, Hoyt WF, Corbett J: Visual morbidity with chiasmal glioma. Arch Ophthalmol 1971;85:3–12.
303. Tym R: Piloid gliomas of the anterior optic pathways. Br J Surg 1961;49:322–331.
304. Venes JL, Latack J, Kandt RS: Postoperative regression of opticochiasmatic astrocytoma: a case for expectant therapy. Neurosurgery 1984;15:421–423.
305. Kanamori M, Shibuya M, Yoshida J, et al: Long-term follow-up of patients with optic glioma. Childs Nerv Syst 1985;1:272–278.
306. Brzowski A, Bazan C, Mumma J, et al: Spontaneous regression of optic glioma in a patient with neurofibromatosis. Neurology 1992;42:679–681.
307. Liu GT, Lessell S: Spontaneous visual improvement in chiasmal gliomas. Am J Ophthalmol 1992;114: 193–201.
308. Takeuchi H, Kabuto M, Sato K, et al: Chiasmal gliomas with spontaneous regression: proliferation and apoptosis. Childs Nerv Syst 1997;13:229–233.
309. Gottschalk S, Tavakolian R, Buske A, et al: Spontaneous remission of chiasmatic/hypothalamic masses in neurofibromatosis type 1: report of two cases. Neuroradiology 1999;41:199–201.
310. Trigg ME, Swanson JD, Letellier MA: Metastasis of an optic glioma through a ventriculoperitoneal shunt. Cancer 1983;52:599–601.
311. Civitello LA, Packer RJ, Rorke LB, et al: Leptomeningeal dissemination of low-grade gliomas in childhood. Neurology 1988;38:562–566.
312. de Keizer RJW, de Wolff-Rouendaal D, Bots GTAM, et al: Optic glioma with intraocular tumor and seeding in a child with neurofibromatosis. Am J Ophthalmol 1989;108:717–725.
313. Bruggers CS, Friedman HS, Phillips PC, et al: Leptomeningeal dissemination of optic pathway gliomas in three children. Am J Ophthalmol 1991;111:719–723.
314. Perilongo G, Carollo C, Salviati L, et al: Diencephalic syndrome and disseminated juvenile pilocytic astro-

cytomas of the hypothalamic-optic chiasm region. Cancer 1997;80:142–146.
315. Miller NR, Iliff WJ, Green WR: Evaluation and management of gliomas of the anterior visual pathways. Brain 1974;97:743–754.
316. Jenkin D, Angyalfi S, Becker L, et al: Optic glioma in children: surveillance, resection, or irradiation? Int J Radiat Oncol Biol Phys 1993;25:215–225.
317. Fletcher WA, Imes RK, Hoyt WF: Chiasmal gliomas: appearance and long-term changes demonstrated by computerized tomography. J Neurosurg 1986;65: 154–159.
318. Pfaffenbach DD, Kearns TP, Hollenhorst RW: An unusual case of optic nerve-chiasmal glioma. Am J Ophthalmol 1972;74:523–525.
319. Schulman JA, Shults WT, Jones JM: Monocular vertical nystagmus as an initial sign of chiasmal glioma. Am J Ophthalmol 1979;87:87–90.
320. Kelly TW: Optic glioma presenting as spasmus nutans. Pediatrics 1970;45:295–296.
321. Brauner R, Malandry F, Rappaport R, et al: Growth and endocrine disorders in optic glioma. Eur J Pediatr 1990;149:825–828.
322. Holman RE, Grimson BS, Drayer BP, et al: Magnetic resonance imaging of optic gliomas. Am J Ophthalmol 1985;100:596–601.
323. Haik BG, Saint Louis L, Bierly J, et al: Magnetic resonance imaging in the evaluation of optic nerve gliomas. Ophthalmology 1987;94:709–717.
324. Hollander MD, FitzPatrick M, O'Connor SG, et al: Optic gliomas. Radiol Clin North Am 1999;37:59–71.
325. Wilson WB, Finkel RS, McCleary L, et al: Large cystic optic glioma. Neurology 1990;40:1898–1900.
326. Brown EW, Riccardi VM, Mawad M, et al: MR imaging of optic pathways in patients with neurofibromatosis. AJNR 1987;8:1031–1036.
327. Wong IG, Lubow M: Management of optic glioma of childhood: a review of 42 cases. In: Smith JL (ed): Neuro-ophthalmology. Symposium of the University of Miami and the Bascom Palmer Eye Institute. Vol. VI, pp 51–60. St. Louis, CV Mosby, 1972.
328. Glaser JS: Gliomas of the anterior visual pathway in childhood: rationale for conservative management. In: Brockhurst RJ, Boruchoff SA, Hutchinson BT, Lessell S (eds): Controversy in Ophthalmology, pp 897–906. Philadelphia, WB Saunders, 1977.
329. Oxenhandler DC, Sayers MP: The dilemma of childhood optic gliomas. J Neurosurg 1978;48:34–41.
330. Heiskanen O, Raitta C, Torsti R: The management and prognosis of gliomas of the optic pathways in children. Acta Neurochirurg 1978;43:193–199.
331. DeSousa AL, Kalsbeck JE, Mealey J, et al: Optic chiasmatic glioma in children. Am J Ophthalmol 1979;87: 376–381.
332. Sung DI: Suprasellar tumors in children: a review of clinical manifestations and managements. Cancer 1982;50:1420–1425.
333. Rush JA, Younge BR, Campbell RJ, et al: Optic glioma: long-term follow-up of 85 histopathologically verified cases. Ophthalmology 1982;89:1213–1219.
334. Packer RJ, Savino PJ, Bilaniuk LT, et al: Chiasmatic gliomas of childhood. A reappraisal of natural history and effectiveness of cranial irradiation. Childs Brain 1983;10:393–403.
335. Imes RK, Hoyt WF: Childhood chiasmal gliomas: update on the fate of patients in the 1969 San Francisco study. Br J Ophthalmol 1986;70:179–182.
336. Wong JYC, Uhl V, Wara WM, et al: Optic gliomas: a reanalysis of the University of California, San Francisco experience. Cancer 1987;60:1847–1855.
337. Flickinger JC, Torres C, Deutsch M: Management of low-grade gliomas of the optic nerve and chiasm. Cancer 1988;61:635–642.
338. Gittinger JW: To image or not to image. Surv Ophthalmol 1988;32:350–356.
339. Rodriguez LA, Edwards MSB, Levin VA: Management of hypothalamic gliomas in children: an analysis of 33 cases. Neurosurgery 1990;26:242–247.
340. Cohen ME, Duffner PK: Optic pathway tumors. Neurol Clin 1991;9:467–477.
341. Hoffman HJ, Humphreys RP, Drake JM, et al: Optic pathway/hypothalamic gliomas: a dilemma in management. Pediatr Neurosurg 1993;19:186–195.
342. Nishio S, Takeshita I, Fujiwara S, et al: Opticohypothalamic glioma: an analysis of 16 cases. Childs Nerv Syst 1993;9:334–338.
343. Janss AJ, Grundy R, Cnaan A, et al: Optic pathway and hypothalamic chiasmatic gliomas in children younger than age 5 years with a 6-year follow-up. Cancer 1995;75:1051–1059.
344. Sutton LN, Molloy PT, Sernyak H, et al: Long-term outcome of hypothalamic/chiasmatic astrocytomas in children treated with conservative surgery. J Neurosurg 1995;83:583–589.
345. Medlock MD, Madsen JR, Barnes PD, et al: Optic chiasm astrocytomas of childhood. 1. Long-term follow-up. Pediatr Neurosurg 1997;27:121–128.
346. Chan MY, Foong AP, Heisey DM, et al: Potential prognostic factors of relapse-free survival in childhood optic pathway glioma: a multivariate analysis. Pediatr Neurosurg 1998;29:23–28.
347. Halperin EC, Constine LS, Tarbell NJ, et al: Supratentorial brain tumors except ependymoma; brain tumors in babies and very young children. In: Pediatric Radiation Oncology, second ed., pp 40–89. New York, Raven Press, 1994.
348. Horwich A, Bloom HJG: Optic gliomas: radiation therapy and prognosis. Int J Radiat Oncol Biol Phys 1985;11:1067–1079.
349. Kovalic JJ, Grigsby PW, Shepard MJ, et al: Radiation therapy for gliomas of the optic nerve and chiasm. Int J Radiat Oncol Biol Phys 1990;18:927–932.
350. Tao ML, Barnes PD, Billett AL, et al: Childhood optic chiasm gliomas: radiographic response following radiotherapy and long-term clinical outcome. Int J Radiat Oncol Biol Phys 1997;39:579–587.
351. Cappelli C, Grill J, Raquin M, et al: Long-term follow up of 69 patients treated for optic pathway tumours before the chemotherapy era. Arch Dis Child 1998;79:334–338.
352. Adams C, Fletcher WA, Myles ST: Chiasmal glioma in neurofibromatosis type 1 with severe visual loss regained with radiation. Pediatr Neurol 1997;17: 80–82.
353. Hirata Y, Matsukado Y, Mihara Y, et al: Occlusion of the internal carotid artery after radiation therapy for the chiasmal lesion. Acta Neurochirurg 1985;74: 141–147.
354. Grill J, Couanet D, Cappelli C, et al: Radiation-induced cerebral vasculopathy in children with neurofibromatosis and optic pathway glioma. Ann Neurol 1999;45:393–396.
355. Warman R, Glaser JS, Quencer RM: Radionecrosis of optico-hypothalamic glioma. Neuro-ophthalmol 1989;9:219–226.
356. Packer RJ, Sutton LN, Bilaniuk LT, et al: Treatment of chiasmatic/hypothalamic gliomas of childhood with chemotherapy: an update. Ann Neurol 1988;23: 79–85.

357. Moghrabi A, Friedman HS, Burger PC, et al: Carboplatin treatment of progressive optic pathway gliomas to delay radiation. J Neurosurg 1993;79:223–227.
358. Packer RJ, Ater J, Allen J, et al: Carboplatin and vincristine chemotherapy for children with newly diagnosed progressive low-grade gliomas. J Neurosurg 1997;86:747–754.
359. Chamberlain MC: Recurrent chiasmatic-hypothalmic glioma treated with oral etoposide. Arch Neurol 1995;52:509–513.
360. Medlock MD, Scott RM: Optic chiasm astrocytomas of childhood. 2. Surgical management. Pediatr Neurosurg 1997;27:129–136.
361. Wilson WB, Feinsod M, Hoyt WF, et al: Malignant evolution of childhood chiasmal pilocytic astrocytoma. Neurology 1976;26:322–325.
362. Safneck JR, Napier LB, Halliday WC: Malignant astrocytoma of the optic nerve in a child. Can J Neurol Sci 1992;19:498–503.
363. Hoyt WF, Meshel LG, Lessell S, et al: Malignant optic glioma of adulthood. Brain 1973;96:121–132.
364. Millar WS, Tartaglino LM, Sergott RC, et al: MR of malignant optic glioma of adulthood. AJNR 1995;16:1673–1676.
365. Woiciechowsky C, Vogel S, Meyer R, et al: Magnetic resonance imaging of a glioblastoma of the optic chiasm. Case report. J Neurosurg 1995;83:923–925.
366. Barbaro NM, Rosenblum ML, Maitland CG, et al: Malignant optic glioma presenting radiologically as a "cystic" suprasellar mass: case report and review of the literature. Neurosurgery 1982;11:787–789.
367. Albers GW, Hoyt WF, Forno LS, et al: Treatment response in malignant optic glioma of adulthood. Neurology 1988;38:1071–1074.
368. Burton EM, Ball WS, Crane K, et al: Hamartomas of tuber cinereum: comparison of MR and CT findings in 4 cases. AJNR 1989;10:497–502.
369. Styne DM: The therapy for hypothalamic-pituitary tumors. Endocrinol Metab Clin North Am 1993;22: 631–648.
370. Miller DC, Lang FF, Epstein FJ: Central nervous system gangliogliomas. Part 1: Pathology. J Neurosurg 1993;79:859–866.
371. Sutton LN, Packer RJ, Rorke LB, et al: Cerebral gangliogliomas during childhood. Neurosurgery 1983;13: 124–128.
372. Cogan DG, Poppen JL, Hicks SP: Ganglioneuroma of chiasm and optic nerves. Arch Ophthalmol 1961;65:481–482.
373. Chilton J, Caughron MR, Kepes JJ: Ganglioglioma of the optic chiasm: case report and review of the literature. Neurosurgery 1990;26:1042–1045.
374. Liu GT, Galetta SL, Rorke LB, et al: Gangliogliomas of the optic chiasm. Neurology 1996;46:1669–1673.
375. Sugiyama K, Goishi J, Sogabe T, et al: Ganglioglioma of the optic pathway. Surg Neurol 1992;37:22–25.
376. Courville CB, Anderson FM: Neuro-gliogenic tumors of the central nervous system. Report of two additional cases of ganglioglioma of the brain. Bull Los Ang Neurol Soc 1941;6:154–176.
377. Johannsson JH, Rekate HL, Roessmann U: Gangliogliomas: pathological and clinical correlation. J Neurosurg 1981;54:58–63.
378. Lang FF, Epstein FJ, Ransohoff J, et al: Central nervous system gangliogliomas. Part 2: Clinical outcome. J Neurosurg 1993;79:867–873.
379. Allen JC: Controversies in management of intracranial germ cell tumors. Neurol Clin 1991;9:441–452.
380. Bowman CB, Farris BK: Primary chiasmal germinoma. J Clin Neuro-ophthalmol 1990;10:9–17.
381. Izquierdo JM, Rougerie J, Lapras C, et al: The so-called ectopic pinealomas. A cooperative study of 15 cases. Childs Brain 1979; 5:505–512.
382. Camins MB, Mount LA: Primary suprasellar atypical teratoma. Brain 1974;97:447–456.
383. Kageyama N, Belsky R: Ectopic pinealoma in the chiasmal region. Neurology 1961;11:318–327.
384. Takeuchi J, Handa H, Nagata I: Suprasellar germinoma. J Neurosurg 1978;49:41–48.
385. Hoffman HJ, Otsubo H, Hendrick EB, et al: Intracranial germ-cell tumors in children. J Neurosurg 1991;74:545–551.
386. Neuwelt EA, Frenkel EP, Smith RG: Suprasellar germinomas (ectopic pinealomas): aspects of immunological characterization and successful chemotherapeutic responses in recurrent disease. Neurosurgery 1980;7:352–358.
387. Houston LW, Hinke ML: Neuroradiology case of the day: suprasellar epidermoid. AJR 1986;146:1094–1095.
388. Cohen MM, Lessell S: Chiasmal syndrome due to metastases. Arch Neurol 1979;36:565–567.
389. Gray RS, Abrahams JJ, Hufnagel TJ, et al: Ghost-cell tumor of the optic chiasm. Primary CNS lymphoma. J Clin Neuro-ophthalmol 1989;9:98–104.
390. Case Records of the MGH: N Engl J Med 1994;331: 861–868.
391. Post KD, McCormick PC, Bello JA: Differential diagnosis of pituitary tumors. Endocrinol Metab Clin North Am 1987;16:609–645.
392. Cone L, Srinivasan M, Romanul FC: Granular cell tumor (choristoma) of the neurohypophysis: two cases and a review of the literature. AJNR 1990;11: 403–406.
393. Kazim M, Kennerdell JS, Maroon J, et al: Choristoma of the optic nerve and chiasm. Arch Ophthalmol 1992;110:236–238.
394. Volpe NJ, Liebsch NJ, Munzenrider JE, et al: Neuro-ophthalmologic findings in chordoma and chondrosarcoma of the skull base. Am J Ophthalmol 1993;115: 97–104.
395. Keltner JL, Johnson CA, Spurr JO, et al: Baseline visual field profile of optic neuritis. The experience of the optic neuritis treatment trial. Optic Neuritis Study Group. Arch Ophthalmol 1993;111:231–234.
396. Beck RW, Kupersmith MJ, Cleary PA, et al: Fellow eye abnormalities in acute unilateral optic neuritis. Experience of the optic neuritis treatment trial. Ophthalmology 1993;100:691–697.
397. Newman NJ, Lessell S, Winterkorn JMS: Optic chiasmal neuritis. Neurology 1991;41:1203–1210.
398. Beck RW, Cleary PA, the Optic Neuritis Study Group: Optic neuritis treatment trial. One year follow-up results. Arch Ophthalmol 1993;111:773–775.
399. Case Records of the MGH: N Engl J Med 1996;335: 1668–1674.
400. Zajicek JP, Scolding NJ, Foster O, et al: Central nervous system sarcoidosis-diagnosis and management. Q J Med 1999;92:103–117.
401. Shealy CN, Kahana L, Engel FL, et al: Hypothalamic pituitary sarcoidosis. Am J Med 1961;30:46–55.
402. Walsh TJ, Smith JL: Sarcoidosis and suprasellar mass. In: Smith JL (ed): Neuroophthalmology. Symposium of the University of Miami and the Bascom Palmer Eye Institute. Vol. IV, pp 167–177. St. Louis, CV Mosby, 1968.

403. Hayes WS, Sherman JL, Stern BJ, et al: MR and CT evaluation of intracranial sarcoidosis. AJR 1987;149: 1043–1049.
404. Case Records of the MGH: N Engl J Med 1991;324: 677–687.
405. Beck AD, Newman NJ, Grossniklaus HE, et al: Optic nerve enlargement and chronic visual loss. Surv Ophthalmol 1994;38:555–566.
406. Tang RA, Grotta JC, Lee KF, et al: Chiasmal syndrome in sarcoidosis. Arch Ophthalmol 1983;101:1069–1073.
407. Gelwan MJ, Kellen RI, Burde RM, et al: Sarcoidosis of the anterior visual pathway: successes and failures. J Neurol Neurosurg Psychiatr 1988;51:1473–1480.
408. Lower EE, Broderick JP, Brott TG, et al: Diagnosis and management of neurological sarcoidosis. Arch Intern Med 1997;157:1864–1868.
409. Tibbs PA, Challa V, Mortara RH: Isolated histiocytosis X of the hypothalamus. J Neurosurg 1978;49:929–934.
410. Goodman RH, Post KD, Molitsch ME, et al: Eosinophilic granuloma mimicking a pituitary tumor. Neurosurgery 1979;5:723–725.
411. Job OM, Schatz NJ, Glaser JS: Visual loss with Langerhans cell histiocytosis: multifocal central nervous system involvement. J Neuro-ophthalmol 1999;19:49–53.
412. Halperin EC, Constine LS, Tarbell NJ, et al: Langerhans' cell histiocytosis. In: Pediatric Radiation Oncology, second ed, pp 446–472. New York, Raven Press, 1994.
413. Kerrison JB, Lee AG: Acute loss of vision during pregnancy due to a suprasellar mass. Surv Ophthalmol 1997;41:402–408.
414. Li J-Y, Lai P-H, Lam H-C, et al: Hypertrophic cranial pachymeningitis and lymphocytic hypophysitis in Sjögren's syndrome. Neurology 1999;52:420–423.
415. Case Records of the MGH: N Engl J Med 1995;333: 441–447.
416. Baskin DS, Townsend JJ, Wilson CB: Lymphocytic adenohypophysitis of pregnancy simulating a pituitary adenoma: a distinct pathological entity. J Neurosurg 1982;56:148–153.
417. Levine SN, Benzel EC, Fowler MR, et al: Lymphocytic hypophysitis: clinical, radiological, and magnetic resonance imaging characterization. Neurosurgery 1988;22:937–941.
418. Saiwai S, Inoue Y, Ishihara T, et al: Lymphocytic adenohypophysitis: skull radiographs and MRI. Neuroradiology 1998;40:114–120.
419. Hungerford GD, Biggs PJ, Levine JH, et al: Lymphoid adenohypophysitis with radiologic and clinical findings resembling a pituitary tumor. AJNR 1982;3: 444–446.
420. Case Records of the MGH: N Engl J Med 1985; 312:297–305.
421. Roncaroli F, Bacci A, Frank G, et al: Granulomatous hypophysitis caused by a ruptured intrasellar Rathke's cleft cyst: report of a case and review of the literature. Neurosurgery 1998;43:146–149.
422. Lee AG, Cech DA, Rose JE, et al: Recurrent visual loss due to muslin-induced optochiasmatic arachnoiditis. Neuro-ophthalmology 1997;18:199–204.
423. Okazaki H: Infectious disease. In: Fundamentals of Neuropathology, second ed, pp, 115–147. New York, Igaku-Shoin, 1989.
424. Hepler RS: Miscellaneous optic neuropathies. In: Albert DM, Jakobiec FA (eds): Principles and Practice of Ophthalmology, pp 2604–2615. Philadelphia, WB Saunders, 1993.
425. Silverman IE, Liu GT, Bilaniuk LT, et al: Tuberculous meningitis with blindness and peri-chiasmal involvement on MRI. Pediatr Neurol 1995;12:65–67.
426. Navarro IM, Peralta VHR, Leon JAM, et al: Tuberculous optochiasmatic arachnoiditis. Neurosurgery 1981;9:654–660.
427. Fishman RA: CSF findings in diseases of the nervous system. In: Cerebrospinal Fluid in Diseases of the Nervous System, second ed, pp, 253–343. Philadelphia, WB Saunders, 1992.
428. Kox LFF, Kuijper S, Kolk AHJ: Early diagnosis of tuberculous meningitis by polymerase chain reaction. Neurology 1995;45:2228–2232.
429. Nguyen LN, Kox LFF, Pham LD, et al: The potential contribution of the polymerase chain reaction to the diagnosis of tuberculous meningitis. Arch Neurol 1996;53:771–776.
430. Lindholm J, Rasmussen P, Korsgaard O: Intrasellar or pituitary abscess. J Neurosurg 1973;38:616–619.
431. Domingue JN, Wilson CB: Pituitary abscess. Report of seven cases and review of the literature. J Neurosurg 1977;46:601–608.
432. Wolansky LJ, Gallagher JD, Heary RF, et al: MRI of pituitary abscess: two cases and review of the literature. Neuroradiology 1997;39:499–503.
433. Case Records of the MGH: N Engl J Med 1993;328: 566–573.
434. Ebner R, Slamovits TL, Friedland S, et al: Visual loss following treatment of sphenoid sinus carcinoma. Surv Ophthalmol 1995;40:62–68.
435. Roden D, Bosley TM, Fowble B, et al: Delayed radiation injury to the retrobulbar optic nerves and chiasm. Ophthalmology 1990;97:346–351.
436. Zimmerman CF, Schatz NJ, Glaser JS: Magnetic resonance imaging of radiation optic neuropathy. Am J Ophthalmol 1990;110:389–394.
437. Piquemal R, Cottier JP, Arsène S, et al: Radiation-induced optic neuropathy 4 years after radiation: report of a case followed up with MRI. Neuroradiology 1998;40:439–441.
438. Guy J, Mancuso A, Beck R, et al: Radiation-induced optic neuropathy: a magnetic resonance imaging study. J Neurosurg 1991;74:426–432.
439. Tachibana O, Yamaguchi N, Yamashima T, et al: Radiation necrosis of the optic chiasm, optic tract, hypothalamus, and upper pons after radiotherapy for pituitary adenomas, detected by gadolinium-enhanced T1-weighted magnetic resonance imaging: case report. Neurosurgery 1990;27:640–643.
440. Hudgins PA, Newman NJ, Dillon WP, et al: Radiation-induced optic neuropathy: characteristic appearances on gadolinium-enhanced MR. AJNR 1992;13:235–238.
441. Hufnagel TJ, Kim JH, Lesser R, et al: Malignant glioma of the optic chiasm eight years after radiotherapy for prolactinoma. Am J Ophthalmol 1988;106:1701–1705.
442. Osher RH, Corbett JJ, Schatz NJ, et al: Neuro-ophthalmological complications of enlargement of the third ventricle. Br J Ophthalmol 1978;62:536–542.
443. Heinz GW, Nunery WR, Grossman CB: Traumatic chiasmal syndrome associated with midline basilar skull fractures. Am J Ophthalmol 1994;117:90–96.
444. Savino PJ, Glaser JS, Schatz NJ: Traumatic chiasmal syndrome. Neurology 1980;30:963–970.
445. Sharma R, Goyal M, Sharma A, et al: Traumatic transection of the optic chiasm: magnetic resonance evaluation. Australas Radiol 1998;42:80–82.

446. Lindenberg R, Walsh FB, Sacks JG: The chiasm. In: Neuropathology of Vision: An Atlas, pp, 197–313. Philadelphia, Lea & Febiger, 1973.
447. Kaufman B, Tomsak RL, Kaufman BA, et al: Herniation of suprasellar visual system and third ventricle into empty sellae: morphologic and clinical considerations. AJNR 1989;10:65–76.
448. Buckman MT, Husain M, Carlow TJ, et al: Primary empty sella syndrome with visual field defects. Am J Med 1976;61:124–128.
449. Weisberg LA, Housepian EM, Saur DA: Empty sella syndrome and complication of benign intracranial hypertension. J Neurosurg 1975;43:177–180.
450. Nugent GR, Sprinkle P, Bloor BM: Sphenoid sinus mucoceles. J Neurosurg 1970;32:443–451.
451. Goodwin JA, Glaser JS: Chiasmal syndrome in sphenoid sinus mucocele. Ann Neurol 1978;4:440–444.
452. Smith DE, Murphy MJ, Hitchon PW, et al: Transsphenoidal encephaloceles. Surg Neurol 1983;20:471–480.
453. Brodsky MC, Frindik JP: Hypothalmic-hypophyseal dysgenesis as a neuroimaging correlate of pituitary hormone deficiency in anophthalmia. Am J Ophthalmol 1996;122:747–748.
454. Pomeranz HD, Lessell S: A hereditary chiasmal optic neuropathy. Arch Ophthalmol 1999;117:128–131.
455. Bouzas EA, Caruso RC, Drews-Bankiewicz MA, et al: Evoked potential analysis of visual pathways in human albinism. Ophthalmology 1994;101:309–314.
456. Hedera P, Lai S, Haacke EM, et al: Abnormal connectivity of the visual pathway in human albinos demonstrated by susceptibility-sensitized MRI. Neurology 1994;44:1921–1926.
457. Brodsky MC, Glasier CM, Creel DJ: Magnetic resonance imaging of the visual pathways in human albinos. J Pediatr Ophthalmol Strabismus 1993;30:382–385.
458. Apkarian P, Bour LJ, Barth PG, et al: Non-decussating retinal-fugal fibre syndrome. An inborn achiasmatic malformation associated with visuotopic misrouting, visual evoked potential ipsilateral asymmetry and nystagmus. Brain 1995;118:1195–1216.
459. Levy A, Lightman SL: Diagnosis and management of pituitary tumours. BMJ 1994;308:1087–1091.
460. Wagner AL, Murtagh FR, Hazlett KS, et al: Measurement of the normal optic chiasm on coronal MR images. AJNR: Am J Neuroradiol 1997;18:723–726.
461. Colao A, Loche S, Cappa M, et al: Prolactinomas in children and adolescents. Clinical presentation and long-term follow-up. J Clin Endocrinol Metabol 1998;83:2777–2780.
462. Fukuda T, Yokoyama N, Tamai M, et al: Thyrotropin secreting pituitary adenoma effectively treated with octreotide. Intern Med 1998;37:1027–1030.
463. Iglesias P, Diez JJ: Long-term preoperative management of thyrotropin-secreting pituitary adenoma with octreotide. J Endocrinol Invest 1998;21:775–778.
464. Teramoto A, Yoshida Y, Sanno N, et al: Cavernous sinus sampling in patients with adrenocorticotrophic hormone-dependent Cushing's syndrome with emphasis on inter- and intracavernous adrenocorticotrophic hormone gradients. J Neurosurg 1998;89:762–768.
465. Gonzales-Portillo G, Tomita T: The syndrome of inappropriate secretion of antidiuretic hormone: an unusual presentation for childhood craniopharyngioma: report of three cases. Neurosurgery 1998; 42:917–921.
466. Honegger J, Buchfelder M, Fahlbusch R: Surgical treatment of craniopharyngiomas: endocrinological results. J Neurosurg 1999;90:251–257.
467. Fahlbusch R, Honegger J, Paulus W, et al: Surgical treatment of craniopharyngiomas: experience with 168 patients. J Neurosurg 1999;90:237–250.
468. Créange A, Zeller J, Rostaing-Rigattieri S, et al: Neurological complications of neurofibromatosis type 1 in adulthood. Brain 1999;122:473–481.
469. Cnossen MH, Stam EN, Cooiman LC, et al: Endocrinologic disorders and optic pathway gliomas in children with neurofibromatosis type 1. Pediatrics 1997;100:667–670.
470. Friedman JM, Birch P: An association between optic glioma and other tumours of the central nervous system in neurofibromatosis type 1. Neuropediatrics 1997;28:131–132.
471. Chan MY, Foong AP, Heisey DM, et al: Potential prognostic factors of relapse-free survival in childhood optic pathway glioma: a multivariate analysis. Pediatr Neurosurg 1998;29:23–28.
472. Guoth MS, Kim J, de Lotbiniere AC, et al: Neurosarcoidosis presenting as hypopituitarism and a cystic pituitary mass. Am J Med Sci 1998;315:220–224.
473. Thompson DA, Kriss A, Chong K, et al: Visual-evoked potential evidence of chiasmal hypoplasia. Ophthalmology 1999;106:2354–2361.
474. Cawley CM, Zipfel GJ, Day AL: Surgical treatment of paraclinoid and ophthalmic aneurysms. Neurosurg Clin N Am 1998;9:765–783.
475. Schatz NJ, Job OM, Glaser JS: Spontaneous resolution of pituitary adenoma after apoplexy. J Neuroophthalmol 2000;20:42–44.

CHAPTER 8

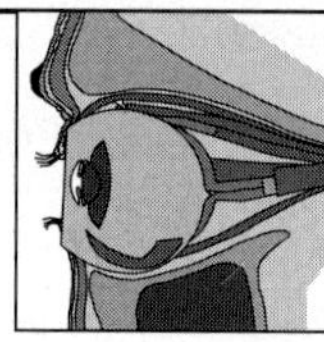

Retrochiasmal Disorders

The retrochiasmal afferent visual pathways include the optic tract, lateral geniculate nucleus, optic radiations, and striate cortex. The most common neuro-ophthalmic presentation of a unilateral retrochiasmal disturbance is a homonymous hemianopic field defect with normal acuity.

In adults, the most common cause of unilateral retrochiasmal visual loss is a stroke (Table 8–1).[1, 2] In Smith's study[3] of isolated and nonisolated hemianopias in adults, 42% were caused by stroke, while in the report of Trobe et al,[4] isolated homonymous hemianopias in adults were due to a stroke in 89% of cases. In contrast, in a pediatric series[5] from the Children's Hospital of Philadelphia, brain neoplasms involving the visual pathways or their associated biopsy or removal were the most common cause (Table 8–2). Cerebrovascular disease, cerebral hemorrhages, and trauma are also causes in children, but are seen less commonly.

The beginning of this chapter will be subdivided by localization, with neuroanatomy, clinical presentation, and common causes described in each section. The subsequent section details the diagnosis and management of lesions in the optic radiations and occipital lobe. Emphasis will be placed on cerebrovascular disease, since it is seen most frequently.

LESIONS OF THE RETROCHIASMAL PATHWAYS

OPTIC TRACT

In adults, optic tract lesions are relatively uncommon and accounted for only 3% of hemianopias in Smith's series.[3] The higher frequency of tract involvement in children (8/36 (22%), Table 8–2) may in part relate to the higher incidence of sellar masses and the lower incidence of strokes in the pediatric age group.

Neuroanatomy

The afferent visual fibers (ganglion cell axons) exit the chiasm posteriorly and diverge to form the left and right optic tracts, each of which is made up of ipsilateral temporal retinal fibers and contralateral nasal fibers (see Figs. 3–1, 3–3, and 7–6). The optic tracts sweep around and above the infundibulum, below the third ventricle, and superomedially to the uncal gyri (see Figs. 7–2 and 7–5). They then turn posterolaterally to the interpenduncular cistern, just ventral to the rostral midbrain and cerebral peduncles.

Most of the tract fibers synapse within the ipsilateral lateral geniculate nucleus, however, some axons depart from the optic tract to complete the afferent limb of the pupillary light reflex. These pupillary fibers pass ventral to the medial geniculate nucleus, then continue through the brachium of the superior colliculi before reaching the pretectal nuclei, where they synapse. In turn, these nuclei connect bilaterally to the Edinger–Westphal nuclei in the oculomotor complex (see Fig. 13–2).

The blood supply of the optic tract is variable but typically comes from an anastamotic network of branches from the posterior communicating and anterior choroidal arteries (from the internal carotid artery (ICA)) (Fig. 8–1).[6]

TABLE 8–1. Frequency of Causes (by Category and Primary Location) of Hemifield Loss in Inpatient and Outpatient Adults Seen by One of the Authors (G.T.L.) From 7/93 to 10/96

	Optic Tract	Optic Radiations	Occipital Lobe	Total
Vascular (68%)				
Stroke (infarction)		6	17	23 (52%)
Hemorrhage		1	5	6 (14%)
Aneurysm	1			1 (2%)
Neoplasm (18%)				
Preoperative or following neurosurgical removal of neoplasm involving the visual pathways		7	1	8 (18%)
Trauma (4%)		1	1	2 (4%)
Other (9%)		3	1	4 (9%)
Total				44

All patients had CT or MRI confirmation of the lesion and localization.

Symptoms and Signs

Visual Field Defects. Incomplete optic tract lesions characteristically result in highly incongruous homonymous hemianopias of variable density and with sloping margins (Fig. 8–2).[7] The explanation for the incongruity observed in optic tract lesions is anatomic. Since the optic tract is the first structure in the anterior visual pathway where uncrossed and crossed axons combine, fibers carrying information from corresponding areas within the contralateral homonymous hemifield may still be widely separated.[7] Thus a partial tract lesion may affect the visual field in each eye asymmetrically. If the lesion progresses to involve the entire optic tract, the result is a complete macular-splitting contralateral hemianopia.

TABLE 8–2. Frequency of Causes (by Category and Primary Location) of Hemifield Loss in Pediatric Patients Seen at the Children's Hospital of Philadelphia from 7/93 to 2/97

	Optic Tract	Optic Radiations	Occipital Lobe	Total
Neoplasm (39%)				
Preoperative	5		1	6 (17%)
Following neurosurgical removal of neoplasm involving the visual pathways	2	4	2	8 (22%)
Vascular (25%)				
Stroke (Infarction)		2	2	4 (11%)
Hemorrhage	1	1	2	4 (11%)
Following neurosurgical removal of hematoma involving anterior visual pathway			1	1 (3%)
Trauma (19%)				
Nonsurgical		4	1	5 (14%)
Neurosurgical—during operations that did not involve tumors in the visual pathways			2	2 (6%)
Other (17%)				
Congenital		2		2 (6%)
Other		3	1	4 (11%)
Total				36

(From Liu GT, Galetta SL. Neurology 1997;49:1748–1749, with permission.)

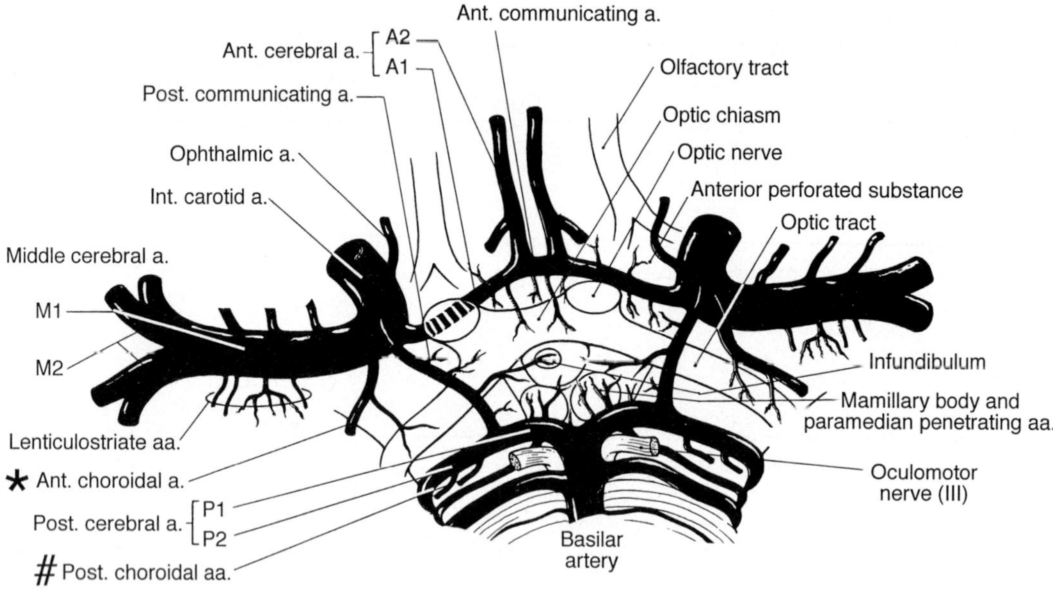

FIGURE 8–1. Relationship of the anterior choroidal artery (*) and the posterior choroidal arteries (#) to the circle of Willis. The anterior choroidal artery is a branch of the internal carotid/middle cerebral artery complex, and the posterior choroidal artery is a branch of the posterior cerebral artery. a. = artery, aa. = arteries. (Adapted from Haines DE: Neuroanatomy. An Atlas of Structures, Sections, and Systems, p 24. Baltimore, Williams & Wilkins, 1995, with permission.)

Other Neuro-ophthalmic Signs. Acuity is preserved in an isolated tract lesion, but a relative afferent pupillary defect in the contralateral eye may be observed. In fact, a homonymous hemianopia accompanied by normal visual acuities but a relative afferent pupillary defect ipsilateral to the field defect is highly suggestive of an optic tract disturbance. If the chiasm or optic nerves are also involved, by a large sellar mass, for instance, acuity may be reduced, and an afferent pupillary defect may be evident in the eye with the greater visual

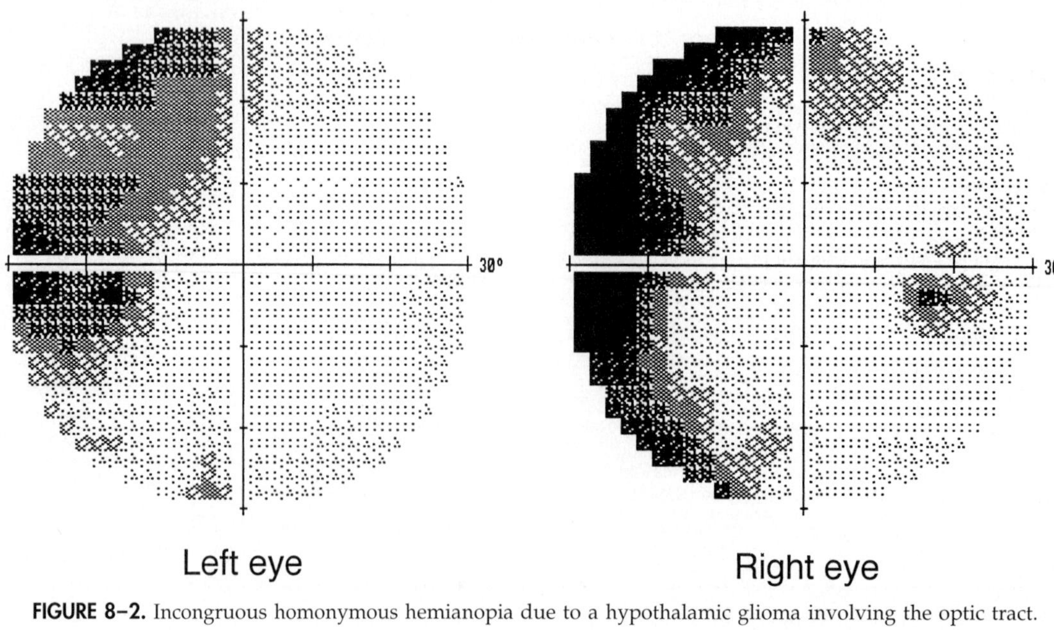

FIGURE 8–2. Incongruous homonymous hemianopia due to a hypothalamic glioma involving the optic tract.

field loss. In most cases, the afferent pupillary defect is observed in the eye contralateral to the optic tract lesion as the temporal field loss is usually larger than the nasal field loss (also see Chapter 13), reflecting the disturbance of more crossed then uncrossed fibers. Other described pupillary abnormalities include contralateral mydriasis (Behr's pupil), and hemianopic pupillary reactivity (Wernicke's pupil). However, both of these pupillary abnormalities are of uncertain clinical significance, and their existence is debated.[8]

Because presynaptic ganglion cell axons are interrupted, patients with isolated tract lesions may have bilateral optic atrophy with ipsilateral temporal pallor and contralateral "bow-tie" or "band" atrophy (Fig. 8–3; see Color Plate 43) Larger lesions also affecting the chiasm or optic nerves may produce diffuse bilateral optic atrophy. A homonymous hemianopia accompanied by optic atrophy would be consistent with a disturbance of either the optic tract or lateral geniculate nucleus.

Other Symptoms and Signs. Because of its proximity to the optic tract, the cerebral peduncle can be simultaneously affected by compressive mass lesions, leading to a hemiparesis on the same side as the hemianopia. Endocrine disturbances, owing to involvement of the pituitary, stalk, or hypothalamus, may also be seen. In Bender and Bodis-Wollner's series of patients with optic tract lesions,[9] 5 of their 12 patients had memory problems, and 3 of these had visual hallucinations, and the authors attributed these symptoms to temporal lobe involvement.

Etiology

Because of the anatomic relationship between the two, any process that can involve the optic chiasm (see Table 7-3) may also affect the optic tract, and therefore the differential diagnosis is similar. If the chiasm is prefixed (short intracranial optic nerves), an enlarging sellar mass is likely to cause posterior chiasmal or optic tract interference. Sellar disturbances are discussed in detail in Chapter 7. In addition, temporal lobe masses may cause optic tract disturbances, but in these instances it may be difficult to distinguish pressure on the optic tract from involvement of the optic radiations.

Among 21 patients with optic tract syndromes in one series,[8] the most common causes were craniopharyngiomas (8/21 (38%)), aneurysms (3/21 (14%)) (Fig. 8–4), and pituitary adenomas (3/21 (14%)). Other less frequent causes seen were trauma, temporal lobe tumor, demyelination, meningioma, pinealoma, and malignant astrocytoma. In another series,[9] suprasellar masses were also the most common cause. Because of the rich anastomotic blood supply from the anterior choroidal and posterior cerebral arteries, ischemic tract lesions were not seen in either study and are therefore considered unusual.[10] With the use of modern neuroimaging, more patients with multiple sclerosis and symptomatic demyelination of the optic tract have been recognized (Fig. 8–5).[11] In addition, individuals with homonymous hemianopias due to arteriovascular malformations[12] and metastases[13] involving the optic tract and congenital absence of the optic tract[14] have been described. Overall, these studies together serve to emphasize that an optic tract lesion is more often caused by a mass lesion.

LATERAL GENICULATE NUCLEUS

Ganglion cell axons traveling in the optic tract end in the lateral geniculate nucleus (LGN), where they synapse with neurons that form the optic radiations. Isolated disturbances of the lateral geniculate are even less common than those of the optic tract. However, when they occur, they are sometimes recognized by the characteristic patterns of sectorial hemianopic field loss.

Neuroanatomy

The LGN, situated within the lateral recess of the choroidal fissure, above the ambient cistern,[15] is considered part of the thalamus (Fig. 8–6). Coronally, the LGN has six neuronal layers, and the input into each is monocular and retinotopically organized (Fig. 8–7). Visual information from the ipsilateral eye synapses within layers 2, 3, and 5, while that from the contralateral eye synapses within laminae 1, 4, and 6. Furthermore, macular vision is subserved by the middle wedge (hilum), while the medial and lateral horns carry information from the inferior and superior quadrants, respectively (Fig. 8–8).

Layers 1 and 2 contain large neurons (magnocellular LGN layers), while layers 3 through 6 contain smaller neurons (parvocellular LGN layers). Studies suggest the existence of at least

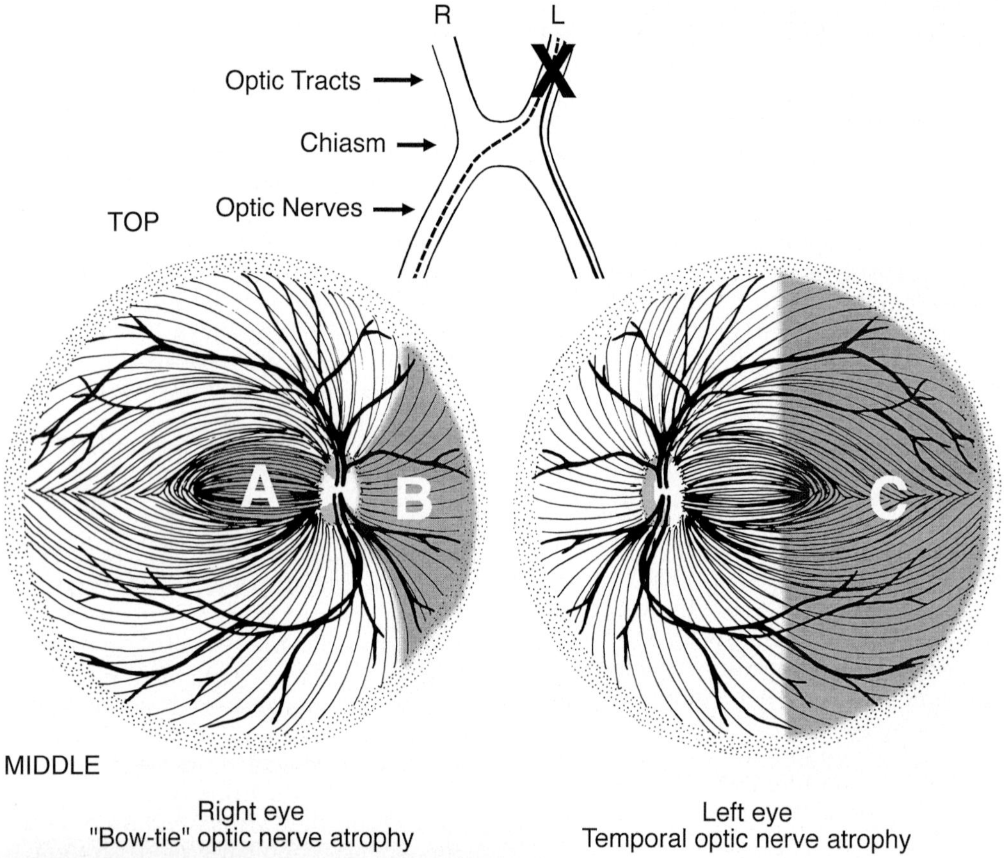

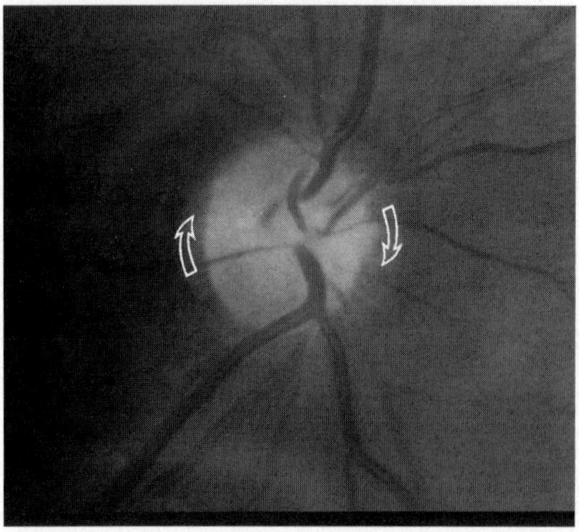

BOTTOM

FIGURE 8–3. "Bow-tie" atrophy due to an optic tract lesion. TOP: Following a chronic lesion ("X") in the left optic tract, three groups of retinal ganglion cell fibers atrophy: MIDDLE: A, those from the nasal half of the macula in the right eye; B, those from the nasal retina in the right eye; and C, those from the temporal retina of the left eye. A and B result in a bow-tie or band pattern of optic atrophy (*white areas*) in the right disc, and C results in temporal atrophy of the left disc (*white area*). BOTTOM: This pattern of optic atrophy is similar to that seen in homonymous hemioptic atrophy due to a congenital lesion of the geniculocalcarine pathway (see Color Plate 43).

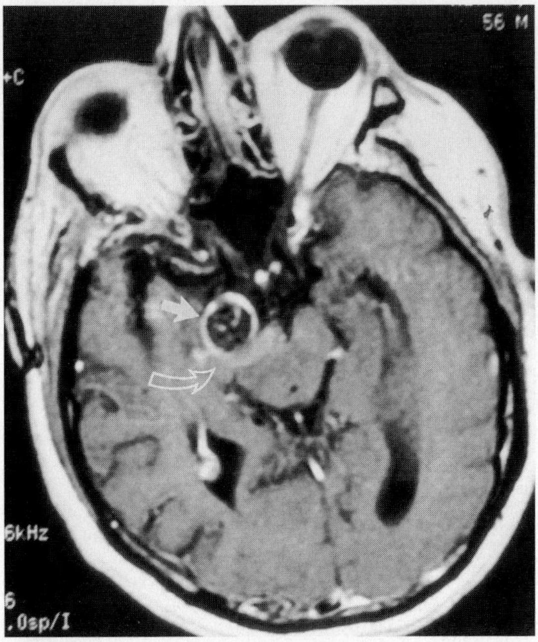

FIGURE 8–4. Supraclinoid aneurym (*solid arrow*) compressing the optic tract (*open arrow*).

two types of retinal ganglion cells (M and P, respectively) that project preferentially to each group, and that each layer may have distinct projections within the striate cortex as well. The M-group of retinal ganglion cells are important in motion detection while P-cells serve form and color vision (see Chapters 4, 5, and 8 for further discussion).

The LGN also has a rich anastomotic blood supply made up of the anterior and posterior choroidal arteries. While the anterior choroidal artery derives from the ICA, the posterior choroidal arteries, consisting of one medial and two lateral arteries, are branches of the posterior cerebral artery (PCA) and arise distal to the thalamogeniculate arteries.[16] The medial and lateral horns of the LGN are supplied by the anterior choroidal artery, and the hilum by the posterior choroidal artery and its branches (Figs. 8–1 and 8–8).[17] In about 50% of cases, small portions of the LGN receive blood from other small posterior cerebral artery branches. Ischemic lesions to the posterior portion of the optic tract and the LGN are considered rare due to their rich anastomotic blood supply.[6, 18]

Symptoms and Signs

Visual Field Defects. Compressive or infiltrative lesions of the LGN typically cause an incongruous contralateral homonymous hemianopia. When the disturbance involves the LGN completely, the result is a complete hemianopia.

Two patterns of field loss, although rare, are highly suggestive of LGN involvement and owe to its blood supply pattern and retinotopic organization[19]:

1. A *horizontal homonymous sectoranopia* is the hallmark of posterior choroidal artery territory infarction (Fig. 8–9).[17] The field defect, which characteristically points inward toward and involves fixation, results from involvement of the central hilum of the LGN.[20] Several authors, however, have cautioned that horizontal homonymous sectoranopias are nonspecific, and similar visual field abnormalities may result from lesions in the optic radiations[21, 22] or occipital cortex.[23]
2. Also uncommon, but highly localizable is the "mirror image" field defect: an *upper and lower homonymous sectoranopia* (Fig. 8–10). Sometimes, this field defect is referred to as a "quadruple sectoranopia." This pattern of field loss results from anterior choroidal artery infarction, affecting the medial and lateral horns of the LGN.[24]

Other Neuro-ophthalmic Signs. Like optic tract lesions, acuity should be normal in processes involving only the LGN, and hemianopic patterns of optic atrophy may be evident.[24, 25] However, because ganglion cell axons subserving the pupillary light reflex leave the anterior visual pathway prior to the LGN (see Fig. 13–2), lesions of the LGN only should have

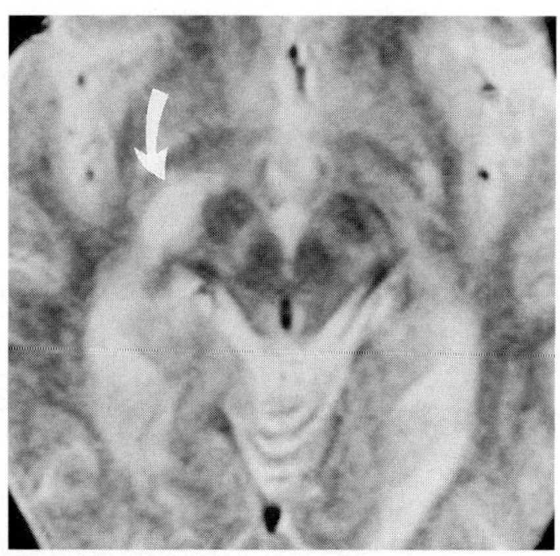

FIGURE 8–5. Optic tract demyelination (*solid arrow*) in multiple sclerosis associated with an incongruous left homonymous hemianopia.

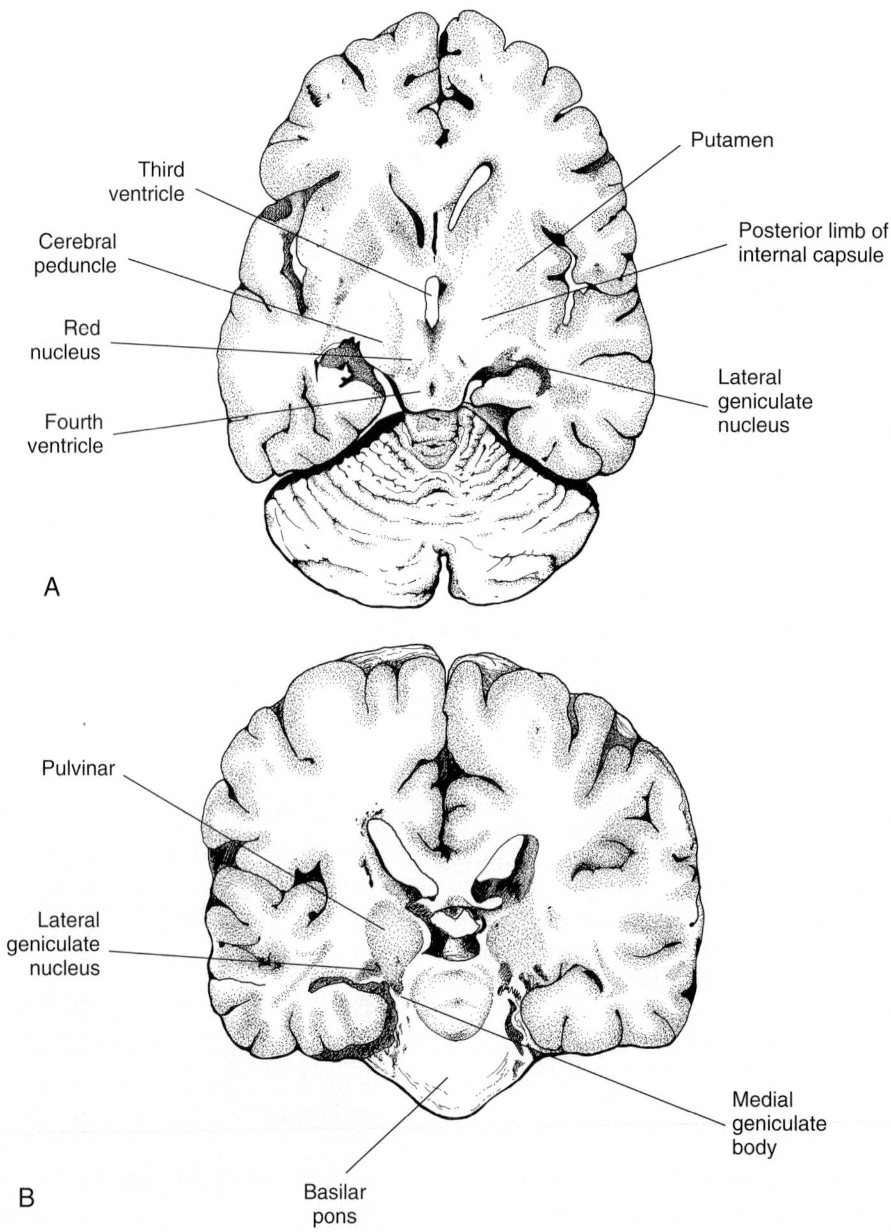

FIGURE 8–6. Location of the lateral geniculate nucleus. **A.** Axial view at the level of the midbrain. **B.** Coronal view through the pulvinar and basilar pons. (Adapted from Haines DE: Neuroanatomy. An Atlas of Structures, Sections, and Systems. Baltimore, Williams & Wilkins, 1995, with permission.)

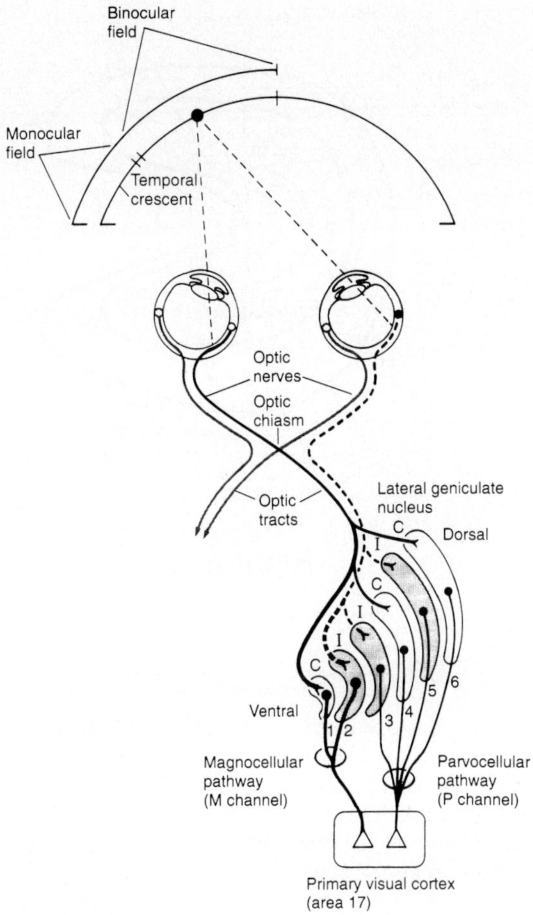

FIGURE 8–7. Inputs into and outputs from layers of the lateral geniculate nucleus (LGN). Inputs from the right hemiretina of each eye project to different layers of the right LGN to create a complete representation of the left visual hemifield. Similarly, fibers from the left hemiretina of each eye project to the left LGN (not shown). The temporal crescent is not represented in contralateral inputs. Layers 1 and 2 are the magnocellular layers; layers 4 through 6 are the parvocellular layers. All of these project to area 17, the primary visual cortex. (From Mason C, Kandel ER: Central Visual Pathways, p 425. Norwalk, Conn, Appleton & Lange, 1991, with permission.)

no influence on pupillary reactivity or size and should not cause a relative afferent pupillary defect.

Other Signs and Symptoms. Thalamic involvement due to posterior choroidal artery territory infarction may lead to contralateral sensory loss and language and memory disturbances.[17] Anterior choroidal artery infarction is typically also associated with hemiparesis and hemisensory loss ipsila'eral to the hemianopia, and these symptoms are likely due to involvement of the motor and sensory pathways in the posterior limb of the internal capsule.[26]

Etiology

Small-vessel occlusion in the territories of the anterior and posterior choroidal arteries may cause LGN-related field disturbances.[27] Recognizing these visual field defects not only suggests the cause of the lesion, but also predicts the circulation involved. Vascular accidents in these distributions have also been reported following intentional and inadvertent neurosurgical ligation.[24, 26] In addition, LGN damage due to trauma[28, 29] and bilateral quadruple sectoranopias from bilateral LGN involvement in central myelinolysis[30] have been described.

OPTIC RADIATIONS

Postsynaptic fibers from the LGN form the optic radiations, which are destined for the calcarine cortex.

Neuroanatomy

The optic radiations (geniculocalcarine fibers) exit dorsally from the LGN, then spread into

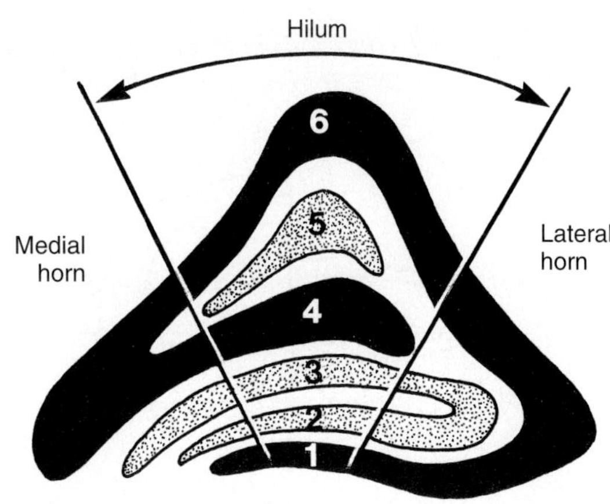

FIGURE 8–8. Coronal view of the lateral geniculate nucleus: layers, retinotopic organization, and vascular supply. Visual information from the ipsilateral eye synapses within layers 2, 3, and 5, while that from the contralateral eye synapses within layers 1, 4, and 6. Macular vision is subserved by the middle wedge (hilum), which is supplied by the posterior choroidal artery. The medial and lateral horns carry information from the inferior and superior quadrants, respectively, and are fed by anterior choroidal artery.

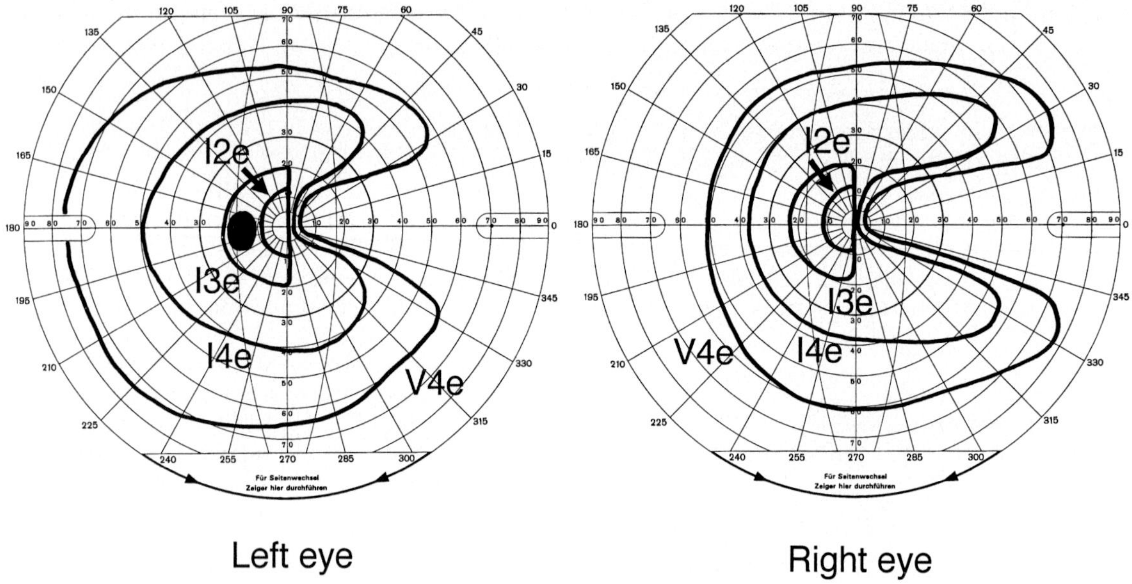

FIGURE 8–9. Wedge-shaped sectoranopia typical of left posterior choroidal infarction and involvement of the hilum of the left lateral geniculate nucleus.

two major bundles (see Fig. 3-1). The group of fibers containing contralateral superior quadrant visual information (inferior fascicle) curves in an anteroinferior direction into the anterior pole of the temporal lobe, forming Meyer's loop. Since the fibers dedicated to the macula do not extend anteriorly, they may be spared in anterior temporal lobe lesions that involve the optic radiations. The superior fascicle lies deep within the parietal lobe and subserves visual information from the contralateral inferior quadrant. The temporal and parietal fascicles project in a retinotopic fashion to the lower and upper banks of calcarine cortex, respectively.

The temporal portion of the optic radiations receives its blood supply from the anterior choroidal artery and other middle cerebral artery

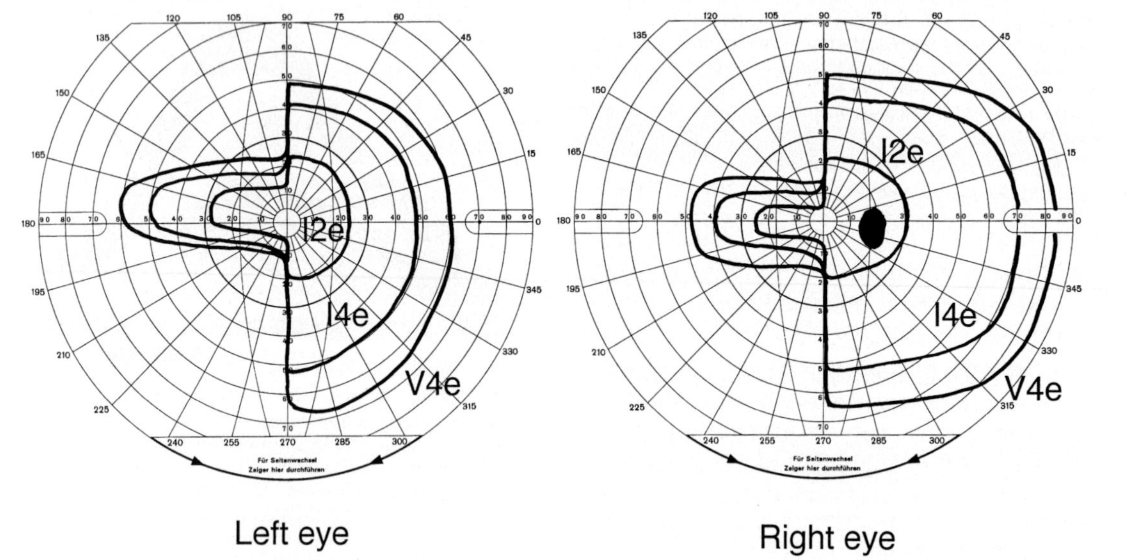

FIGURE 8–10. Upper and lower (quadruple) sectoranopia, characteristic of anterior choroidal infraction and involvement of the medial and lateral portions of the right lateral geniculate nucleus.

(MCA) branches within the sylvian fissure (Fig. 8–11), including the lenticulostriate and inferior temporo-occipital artery. The distal branches of the MCA, including the angular and posterior temporal arteries, supply the more superiorly situated parietal fascicles.[31] The most posterior portions of the optic radiations, just before their entry into the occipital lobe, are supplied by the superior temporo-occipital sylvian artery branch of the MCA, and the anterior temporal and calcarine arteries of the PCA.[6, 18]

Symptoms and Signs

Visual Field Defects. An isolated lesion of Meyer's loop will typically lead to an incongruous contralateral homonymous hemianopia denser superiorly ("pie in the sky" defect) (Fig. 8–12).[350] In contrast, lesions of the parietal lobe characteristically will lead to incongruous defects more prominent inferiorly (Fig. 8–13), and rarely quadrantanopias respecting the horizontal meridian can be seen.[32, 33] In clinical practice, there is significant variation in these findings, especially with regard to congruity. Complete interruption of the optic radiations will cause a dense homonymous hemianopia (Fig. 8–14). Bilateral lesions of the optic radiations will cause *cerebral blindness*.

Other Neuro-ophthalmic Signs. Visual acuity is spared in unilateral lesions, but can be impaired if bilateral lesions are present. Pupillary responses are normal in disturbances limited to the optic radiations. The optic discs are also normal unless the lesion is large enough to cause mass effect or obstruction of the ventricular system and lead to papilledema. In addition, long-standing or congenital optic radiation lesions may be associated with optic atrophy as a result of transsynaptic degeneration.

A homonymous hemianopia or quadrantanopia due to deep parietal lobe lesions may be associated with a defective optokinetic response when the targets are drawn toward the side of the lesion (see Chapter 17). Similarly, slow pursuit will be defective in the direction ipsilateral to the lesion (see Chapter 16). The combination of the hemianopia, defective optokinetic response, and poor tracking result from co-involvement of the optic radiations and adjacent descending corticobulbar fibers from the parieto-occipitotemporal pursuit area. In contrast, normal optokinetic responses would be expected in a hemianopia due to a lesion solely within the occipital lobe. Patients

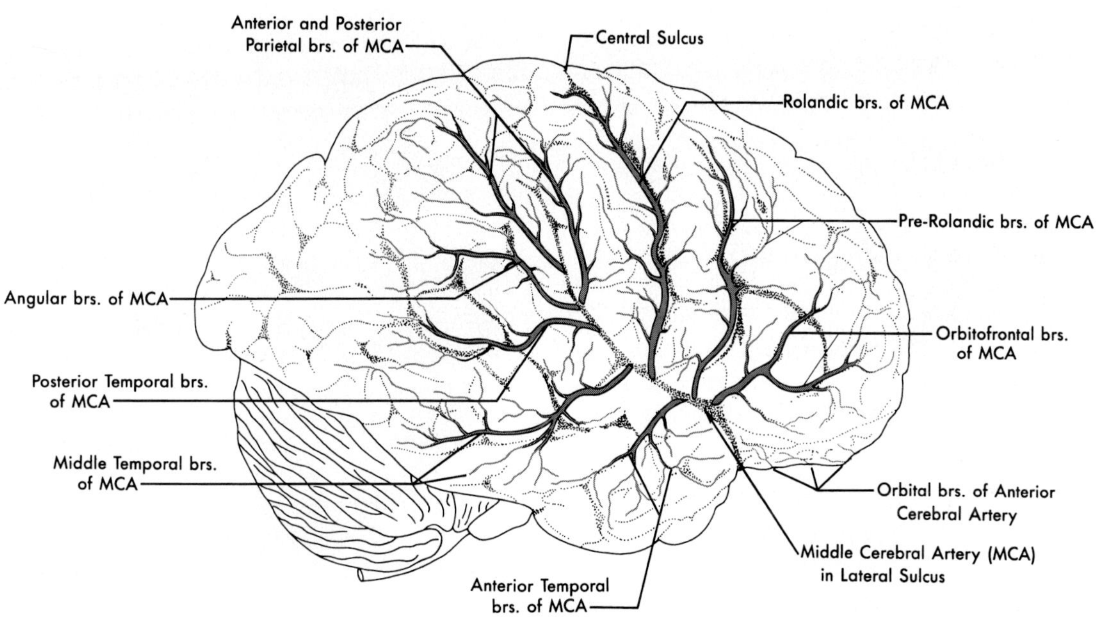

FIGURE 8–11. Branches of the middle cerebral artery (MCA). Lateral view of the right cerebral hemisphere showing the location and general branching pattern of the middle cerebral artery. The middle cerebral artery branches in the depths of the lateral sulcus. brs. = branches. (From Haines DE: Neuroanatomy. An Atlas of Structures, Sections, and Systems, p 17. Baltimore, Williams & Wilkins, 1995, with permission.)

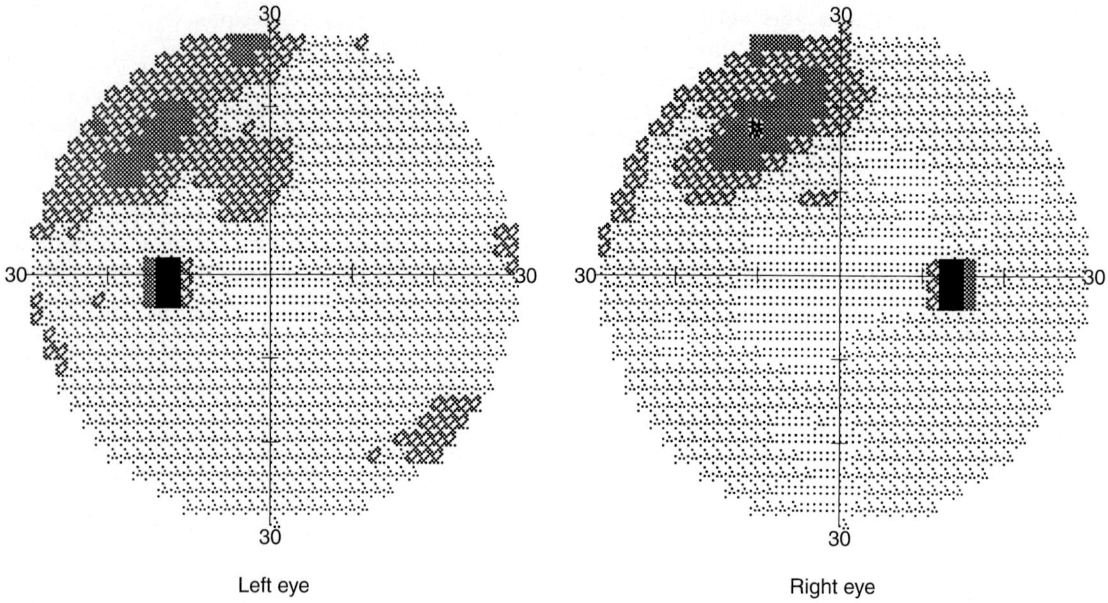

FIGURE 8–12. Upper left visual field ("pie in the sky") defect due to a right temporal lobe glioma.

with a hemianopia or neglect may also have a gaze preference away from the visual deficit.

During attempted eye closure, normally each eye has an upward and outward trajectory (Bell's phenomenon). However, in the majority of hemispheric lesions, both eyes will deviate up and away from the side of the lesion. This phenomenon, known as *Cogan's spasticity of conjugate gaze,*[34, 35] has been attributed to an increased tone in contralateral gaze

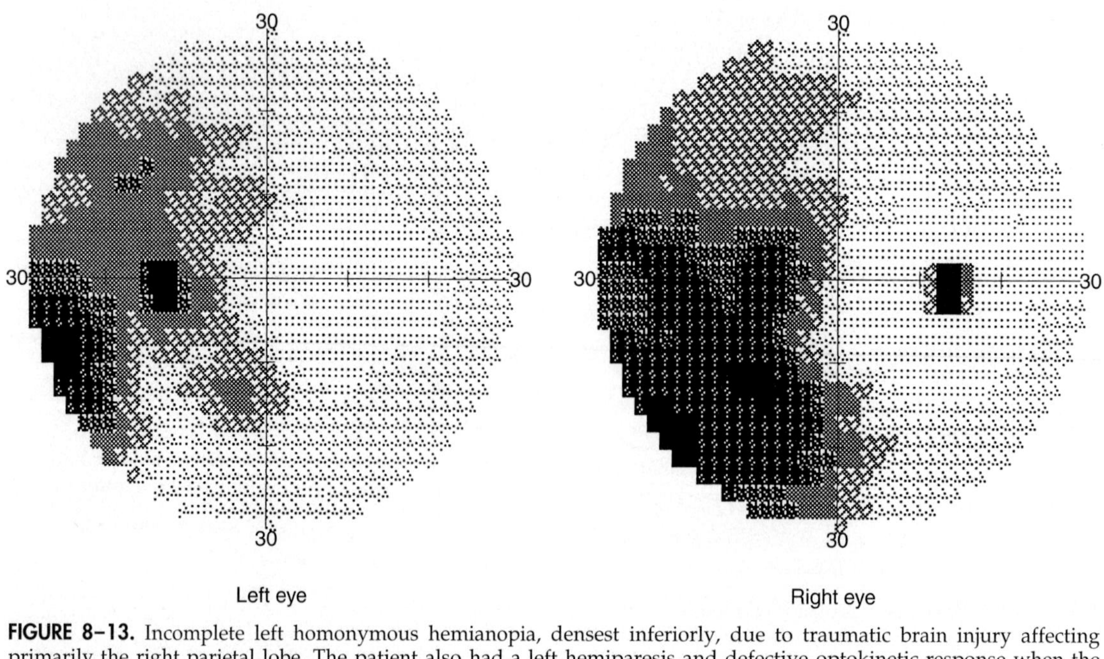

FIGURE 8–13. Incomplete left homonymous hemianopia, densest inferiorly, due to traumatic brain injury affecting primarily the right parietal lobe. The patient also had a left hemiparesis and defective optokinetic response when the targets were drawn to his right.

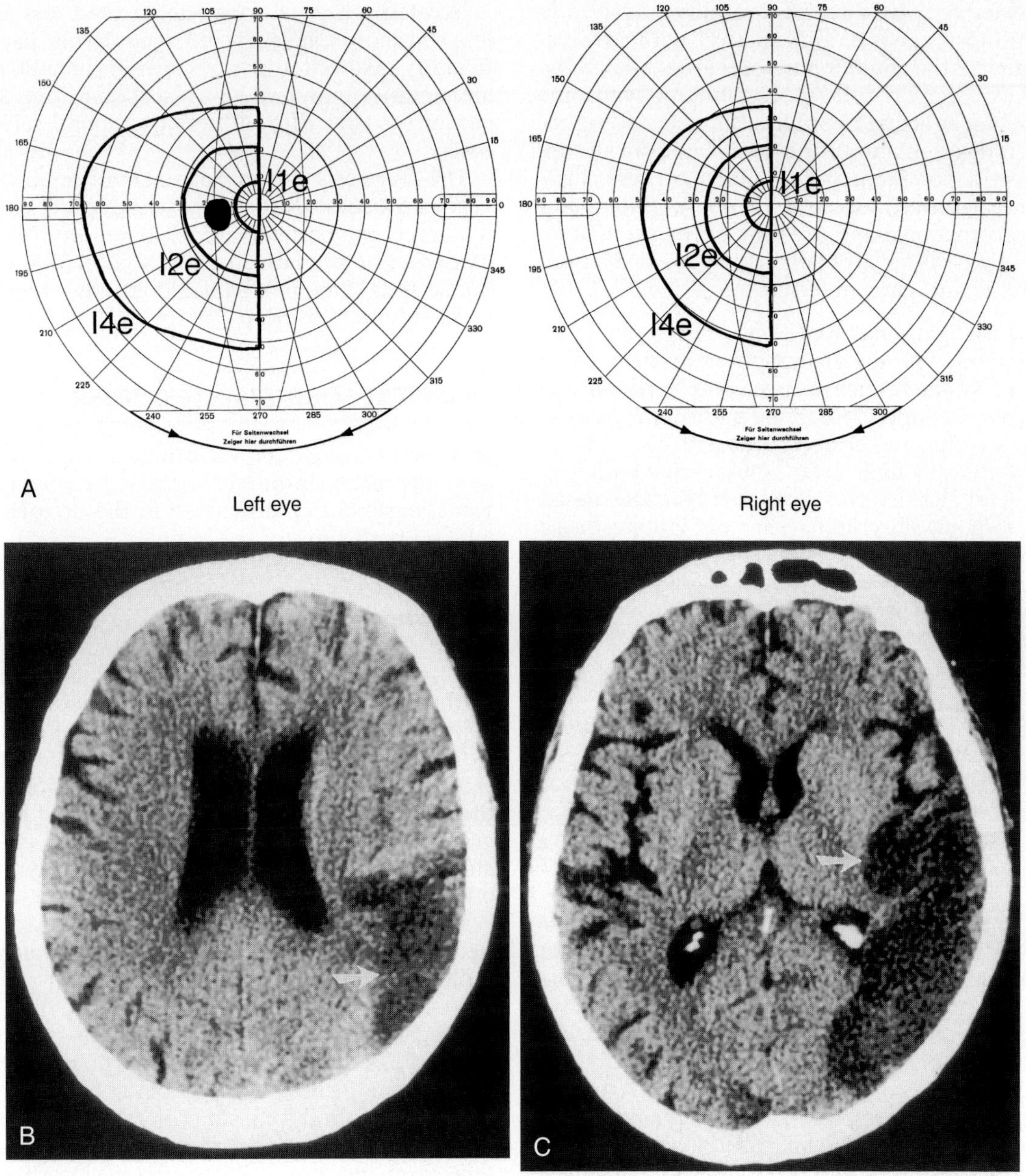

FIGURE 8–14. A. Complete, macular splitting right homonymous hemianopia due to large left middle cerebral artery infraction depicted in the axial CT scans in **B** and **C. B.** The hypodense area (*arrow*) in the left parietal region. **C.** A more ventral slice depicting the hypodense infraction (*arrow*) in the left temporal lobe. The patient was also aphasic.

deviation or a decreased ability to suppress attention to the contralateral hemispace.[36] Overall, we find this sign to be relatively unreliable since such lateral gaze deviations with eye closure may be seen with normal patients. Furthermore, patients with established parietal optic radiation lesions may have a normal Bell's phenomenon.

Other Cortical Symptoms and Signs. Hemianopias that result from lesions of the optic radiations are often associated with other "cortically based" neurologic findings. Temporal lobe lesions may be accompanied by personality changes, complex partial seizures, memory deficits, fluent aphasia (if the dominant side is involved), or Klüver–Bucy syndrome (hypersexuality, placidity, hyperorality, visual and auditory agnosia, and apathy) with involvement of the anterior temporal lobes bilaterally. A conduction aphasia, Gerstmann syndrome (finger agnosia, agraphia, acalculia, and right–left disorientation), and tactile agnosia all suggest a dominant parietal lobe process. Left-sided neglect, topographic memory loss, and constructional and dressing apraxias, in association with a left hemianopia, suggest a nondominant, parietal lesion.

Other Symptoms and Signs. Hemispheric lesions may produce a homonymous field defect and ipsilateral hemiparesis and hyperreflexia when the optic radiations and motor strip or descending motor fibers are disrupted. A homonymous field defect in combination with ipsilateral sensory loss, astereognosis, decreased two-point discrimination, or graphesthesia suggests a parietal lesion. A process within the nondominant (usually right) parietal lobe can also produce a contralateral neglect syndrome or hemianopia, accompanied by contralateral sensory inattention. Pain, hemianesthesia, or choreoathetoid movements and an ipsilateral homonymous field deficit implies co-involvement of the thalamus and optic radiations.

Etiology

Strokes in the MCA distribution (Fig. 8–14) and neoplasms are the most common causes of optic radiation hemianopias in adults (Table 8–1). Hemorrhages, trauma, infections, and degenerative diseases are also seen but are less common.

An occlusion of the proximal MCA would cause a contralateral hemianopia, a contralateral hemiparesis due to disturbance of the motor cortex or descending corticospinal tracts, and sensory loss resulting from involvement of the postcentral gyrus or ascending fibers from the thalamus. Aphasia or neglect may be observed in MCA occlusion, depending on whether the stroke affects the dominant or nondominant hemisphere, respectively. Anterior division MCA strokes can be recognized by the predominantly motor findings and nonfluent (Broca's) aphasia, while posterior division MCA strokes have more salient sensory and fluent (Wernicke's) language deficits. MCA strokes associated with hemianopias are either fronto-parietal, parietal, or parieto-temporal.

Isolated temporal lobe-related field loss is less common. Causes include neoplasms, particularly glial cell tumors, herpes encephalitis, and anterior temporal lobe resection for recalcitrant seizures due to mesial temporal sclerosis.[37]

The diagnosis and management of cerebrovascular disease, tumors, and other processes that affect the parietal and temporal lobes are discussed in more detail in the section following occipital lobe-related field loss, since there is considerable overlap.

OCCIPITAL LOBE/STRIATE CORTEX

Brodmann area 17 (or V1, primary, calcarine, or striate cortex) is the end organ of the afferent visual system and is situated in the occipital lobe on both sides of the brain.

Neuroanatomy

The upper bank of striate cortex lies superior to the calcarine fissure, and the lower bank below the fissure (see Figs. 3–1 and 8–15). Other boundaries of striate cortex include the splenium of the corpus callosum anteriorly, the interhemispheric fissure medially, and the occipital pole posteriorly. Laterally, some striate cortex may be visible on the posteriolateral outer surface of the occipital lobes.

Neuronal input arrives in a retinotopic fashion from fibers of the LGN and synapses within striate cortex, which is divided into six layers. Entry is primarily into the thick, light-colored layer 4, which is visible to the naked eye and has been termed the *stria of Gennari*.[38] Fibers from the medial aspect of the LGN, carrying information from superior retina, project to the upper bank of the calcarine cortex, while those from the lateral aspect, carrying information from the inferior retina, project to the lower bank. The inferior visual fields are thus represented within the upper bank, and the superior visual fields within the lower bank. Left and right visual fields are represented within right and left occipital lobes, respectively.

Macular projections from the central 10 degrees of vision synapse in the occipital pole and occupy 55% to 60% of the entire surface area of striate cortex.[39–41] The occipital tip is devoted to foveal vision. The anterior striate cortex, comprising approximately 8% to 10% of striate cortex,[42] is monocularly innervated

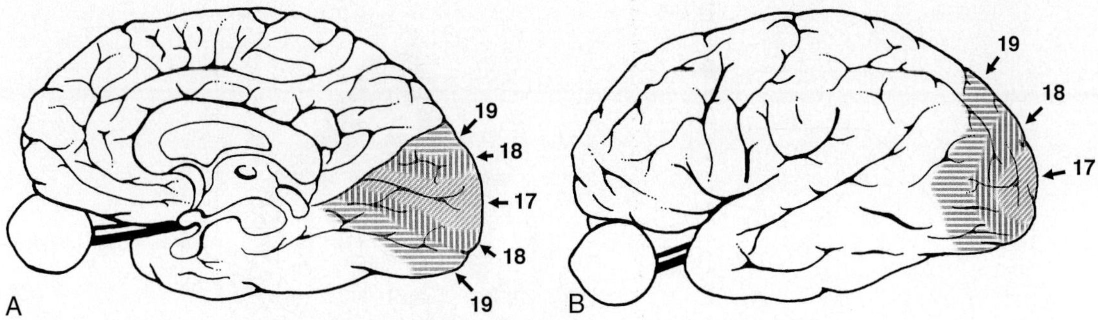

FIGURE 8–15. Medial (**A**) and lateral (**B**) views of the occipital lobe in relationship to the rest of the brain. Areas 17, 18, and 19 are highlighted.

and subserves the temporal 30 degrees of the visual field of the contralateral eye (Fig. 8–16). The horizontal meridian of the visual field lies deep within the calcarine fissure at the calcarine bank, while the vertical meridian lies along the calcarine lips (Fig. 8–17).[43]

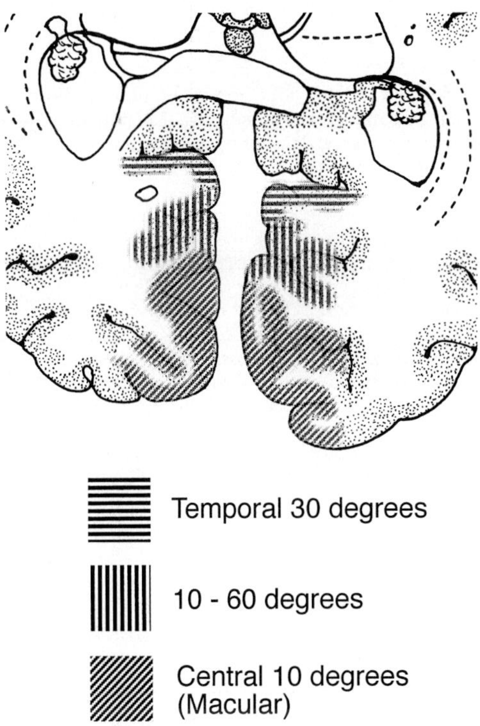

FIGURE 8–16. Retinotopic organization of the striate of cortex (axial section at the level of the calcarine fissures, viewed inferiorly; the lower bank of the occipital lobe is cut away). Approximately 55% to 60% of the surface area of striate cortex, located posteriorly, is responsible for the central 10 degrees of vision. The anterior striate cortex subserves the temporal 30 degrees of the visual field of the contralateral eye.

The majority of the blood supply to striate cortex derives from branches of the PCA (Fig. 8–18): the calcarine artery, mostly, with lesser contributions from the posterior temporal and parieto-occipital arteries.[44] In most cases, small penetrating branches from the calcarine artery supply both the upper and lower banks of calcarine cortex. In up to one third of cases, one major branch to each bank may be seen. At the occipital pole, there is an anastomosis between PCA vessels and the superior temporo-occipital sylvian artery from the MCA. This dual blood supply to the area responsible for central vision is one vascular explanation for macular sparing in the setting of PCA occlusion.

The PCAs are normally considered part of the posterior circulation of the brain, as usually both PCAs arise from the distal bifurcation of the basilar artery (Fig. 8–1). In some anomalous cases, however, a PCA may derive its blood supply from the anterior portion of the circle of Willis. These variations include (1) a persistent trigeminal artery,[45] and (2) persistence of the fetal origin of the PCA from the ICA.[46]

Symptoms and Signs

Visual Field Defects. Unilateral occipital lobe lesions may cause a contralateral congruous homonymous hemianopia respecting the vertical meridian. The following visual field features, when present, are specific to occipital lobe disturbances. These features are often better identified with Goldmann or tangent screen perimetry compared with automated perimetry.[351]

1. *Macular sparing.* PCA infarction may produce a hemianopia with macular sparing

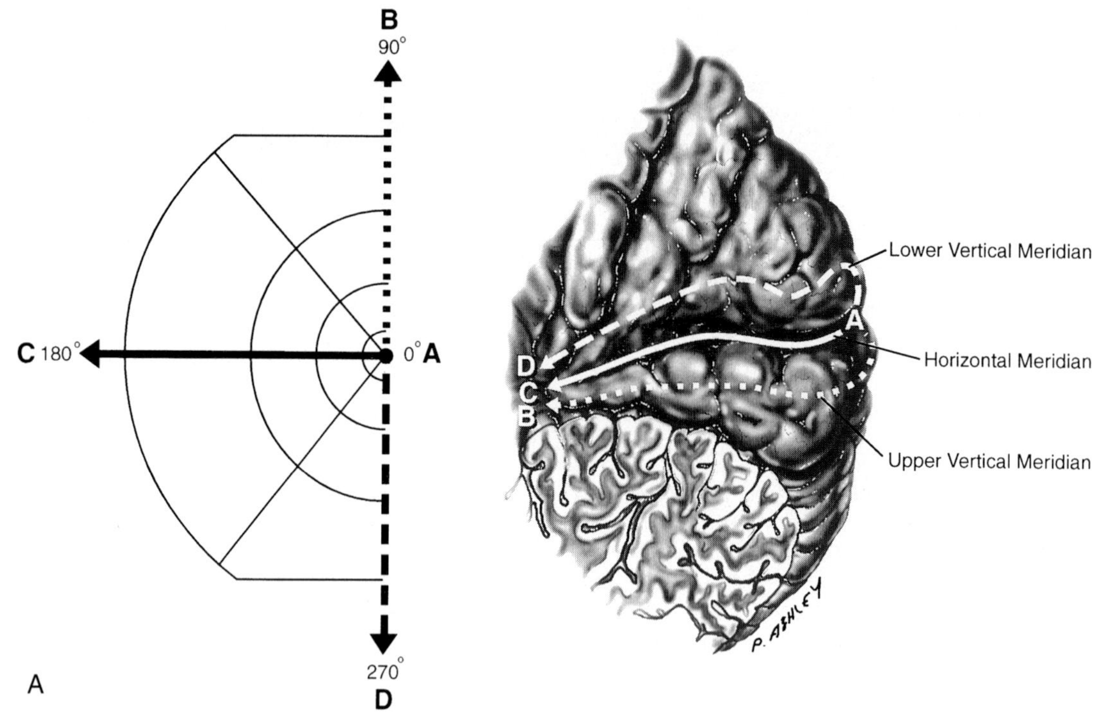

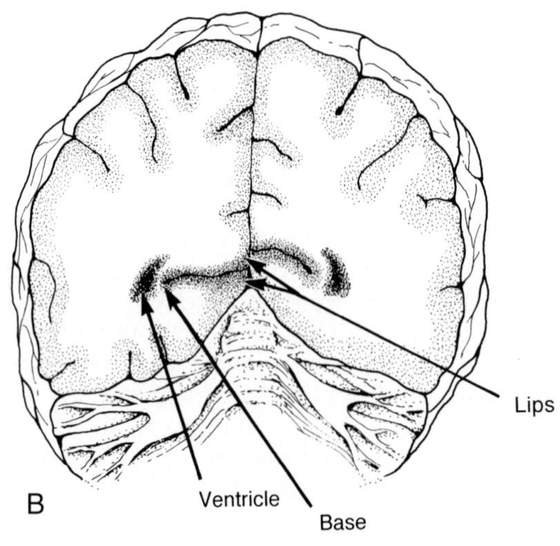

FIGURE 8–17. Occipital lobe representation of the vertical horizontal meridians. **A.** The left visual hemifield is demonstrated with the corresponding right calcarine fissure opened to reveal the fissure base and calcarine banks. The vertical hemianopic meridian is represented along the borders of the calcarine lips. The lower vertical meridian of the visual field, line AD, is represented along the perimeter of upper striate cortex (ie, the margin of the upper calcarine lip). The upper vertical meridian of the visual field, line AB, is similarly represented along the border of the lower calcarine lip. The horizontal meridian of the visual field, line AC, follows the contour of the base of the calcarine fissure. **B.** This coronal section through the occipital region shows the relationship of the calcarine lips to the base of the calcarine sulcus that flanks the medial wall of the posterior ventricular horn. (From Gray LG, Galetta SL, Schatz NJ: Neurology 1998;50:1170–1173, with permission.)

(Fig. 8–19) (as opposed to macular splitting), and this feature is characteristic of occipital lobe-related hemianopias. Proposed mechanisms include the dual vascular supply of the occipital poles, bilateral representation of the maculae, and test artifact due to poor central fixation by the patient.[47] However, a recent clinicoradiologic study[48] provided evidence for unilateral macular representation. In addition, a study

FIGURE 8–18. Posterior cerebral artery. **A.** Ventral view of the cerebral hemispheres with brainstem removed showing the branching pattern of the posterior cerebral artery (PCA) and some branches of the anterior (ACA) and middle cerebral arteries (MCA). **B.** Midsagittal view of the cerebral hemisphere and diencephalon showing the locations and branching patterns of the ACA and PCA. br. = branch, brs. = branches, LS = lenticulostriate. (From Haines DE: Neuroanatomy. An Atlas of Structures, Sections, and Systems, p 27. Baltimore, Williams & Wilkins, 1995, with permission.)

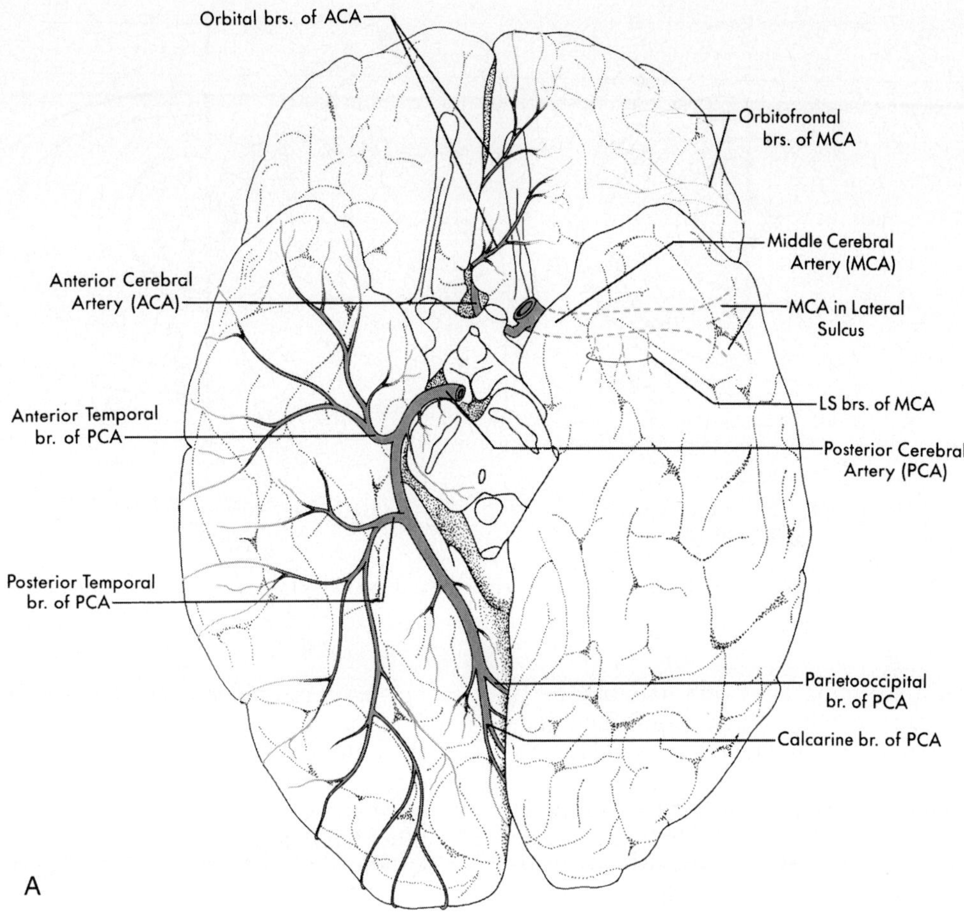

A

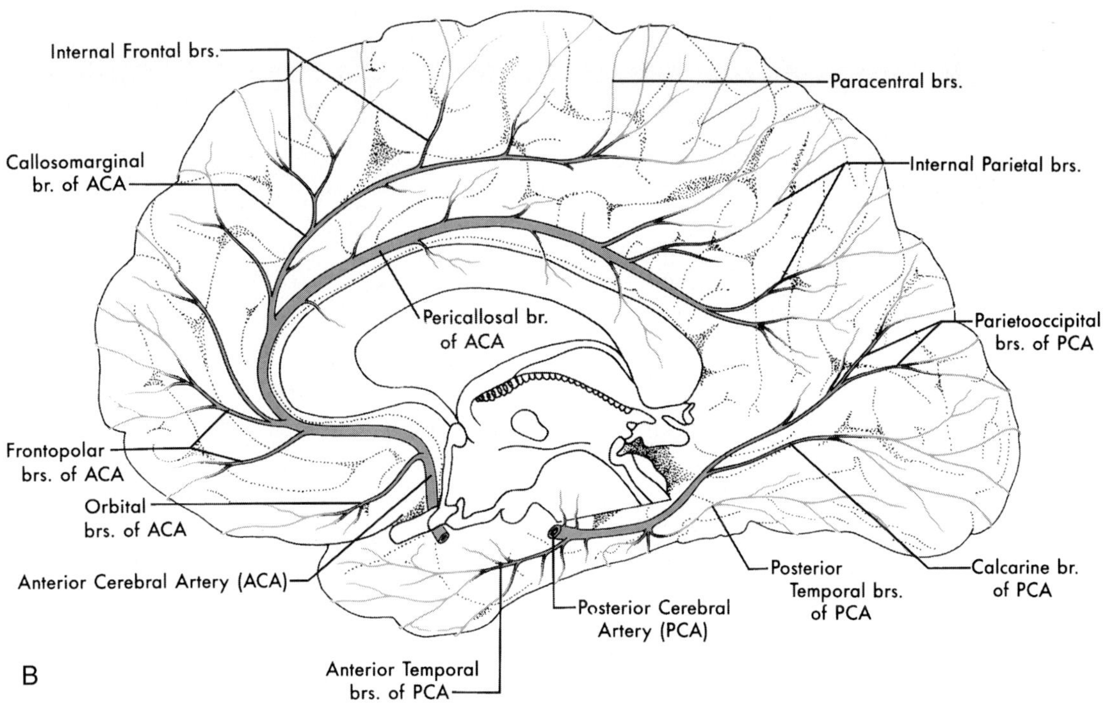

B

(See legend on page 310.)

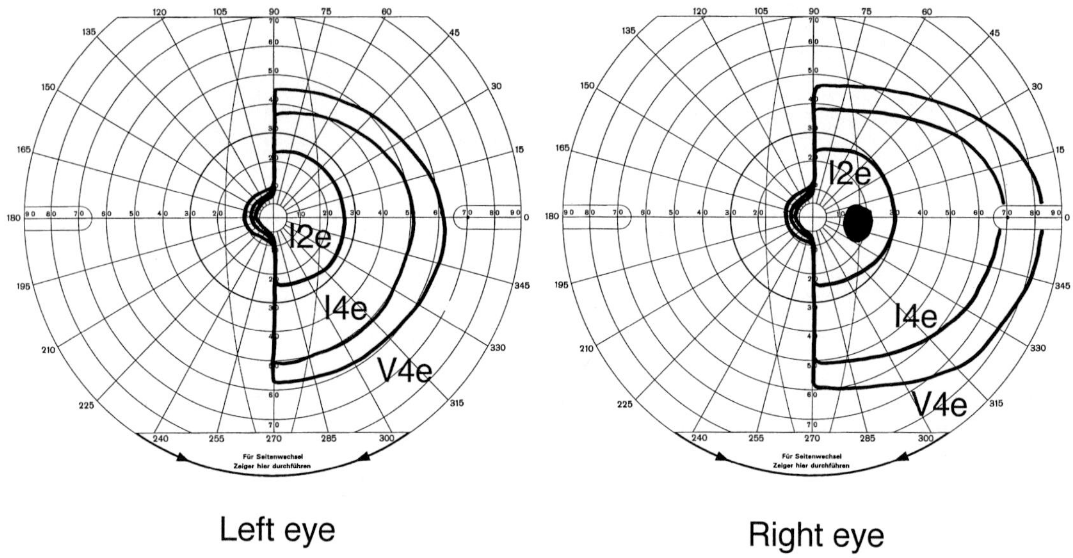

FIGURE 8–19. Macular-sparing left homonymous hemianopia due to a right posterior cerebral artery stroke.

using a scanning laser ophthalmoscope to stimulate the retina directly confirmed macular sparing in occipital lobe-related hemianopias.[49]

2. *Homonymous hemianopic central scotomas.* These scotomas also a telltale sign of a unilateral occipital lobe tip disturbance (Fig. 8–20). On rare occasions they are paracentral.[50]
3. *Sparing or involvement of the temporal crescent.* If an occipital lobe lesion does not involve the anterior striate cortex, the temporal 30 degrees of the visual field of the contralateral eye may be spared (Fig. 8–21).[51] On the other hand, lesions restricted to the anterior striate cortex may selectively affect the temporal 30 degrees of vision of the contralateral eye.[52, 53]

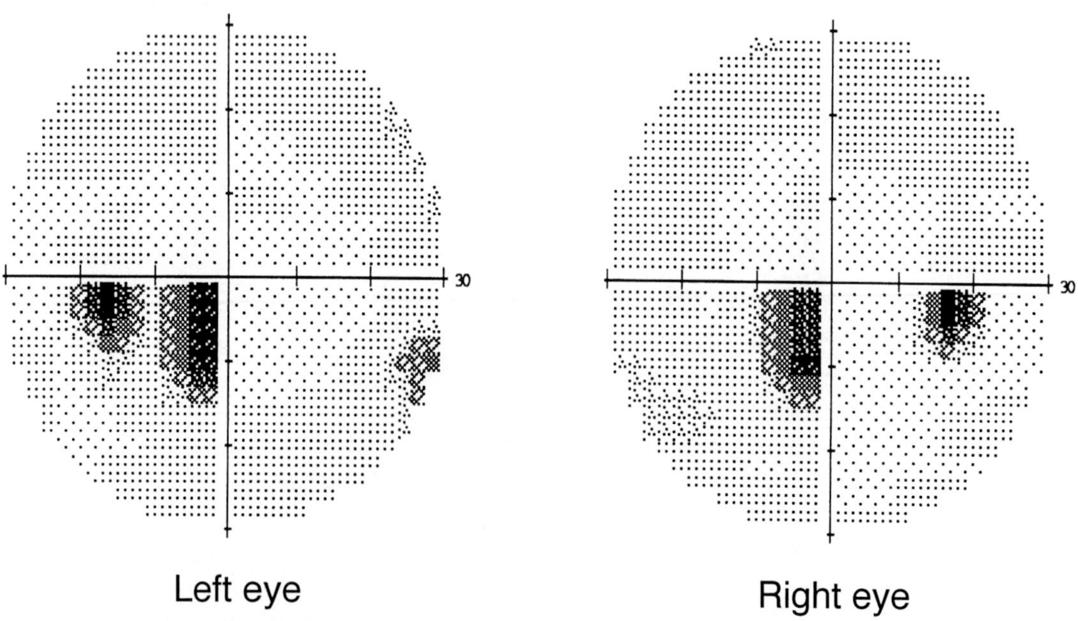

FIGURE 8–20. Left homonymous inferior quadrantic central scotomas due to a neoplasm of the right occipital tip.

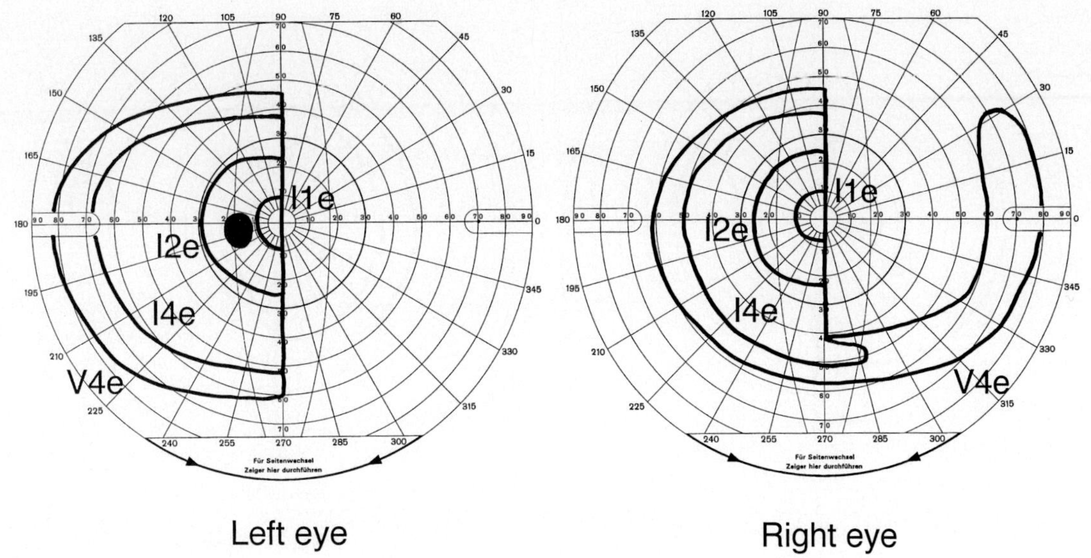

FIGURE 8–21. Right homonymous hemianopia with sparing of the temporal crescent in the right eye. This resulted from a left posterior cerebral artery infarction that spared the anterior striate cortex on that side.

Bilateral posterior cerebral artery infarction may lead to bilateral macular-sparing hemianopias, with a characteristic "keyhole" visual field (Fig. 8–22). Patients are left with residual vision in the central 5 to 10 degrees. The preserved tunnel is often asymmetric with a vertical step-off that helps to distinguish this field defect from ocular causes of field constriction.

Restricted lesions of the upper or lower bank of the calcarine cortex may cause quadrantic field defects (Fig. 8–23).[33] It has been suggested that occipital lobe quadrantanopias with strict horizontal meridian sparing are more likely the result of an extrastriate lesion involving V2 (area 18) and V3 (area 19) (see Fig. 8–15 and Chapter 9).[54] However, either a striate or extrastriate lesion can be responsible.[55]

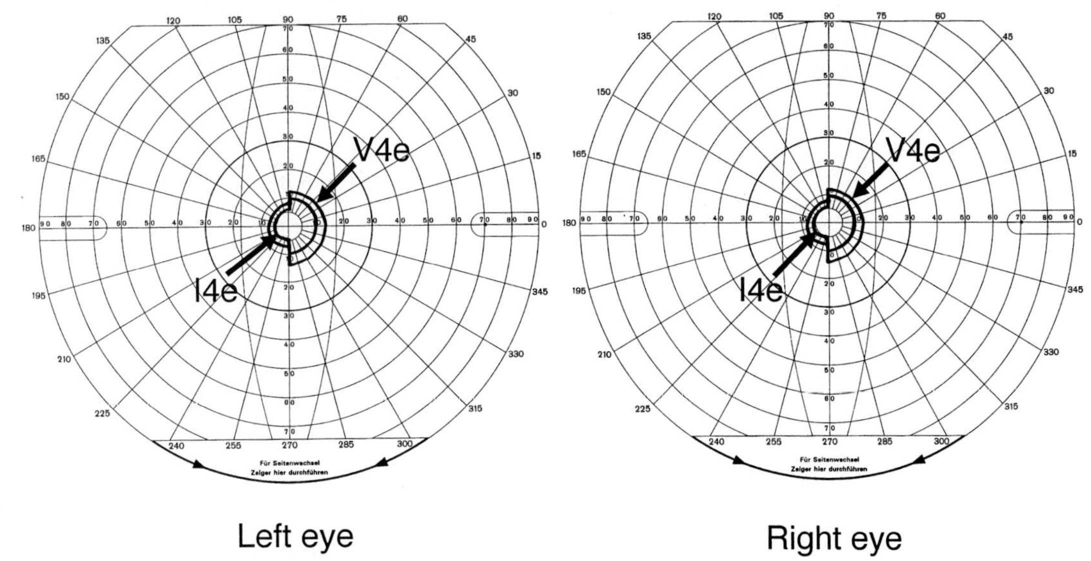

FIGURE 8–22. "Keyhole" visual field defect due to bilateral posterior cerebral artery infarctions. Sparing of central vision is greater in the right visual field than the left, and the demarcation (step-off) between the two respects the vertical meridian.

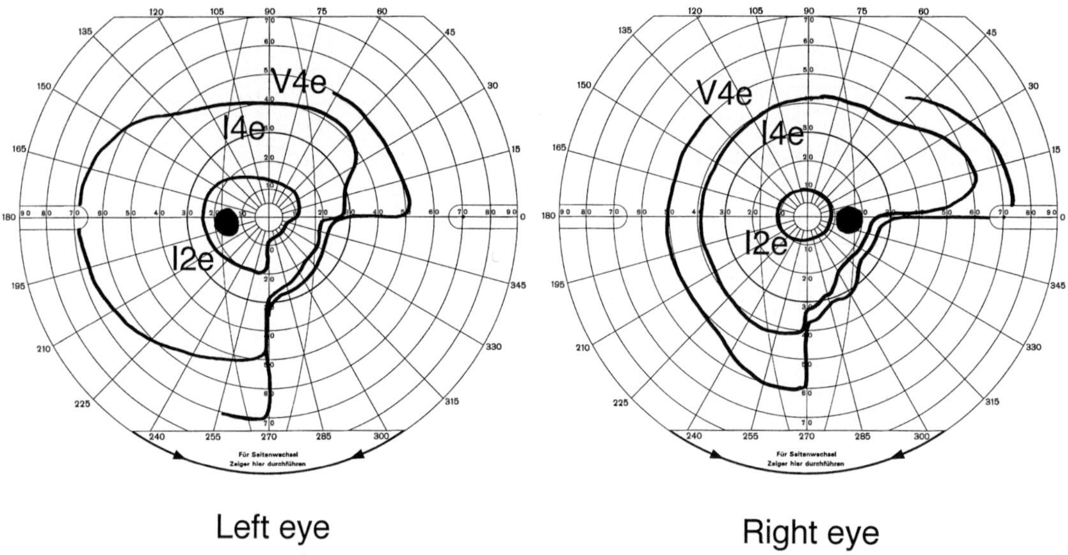

FIGURE 8–23. Right homonymous inferior quadrantanopia from left upper bank infarction of the occipital lobe. Note there is a suggestion of macular sparing.

Crossed quadrantanopias may result from a lesion of one lower bank and the contralateral upper ban This has been called the *checkerboard visual field*.[56]

Bilateral upper or lower bank disturbances produce altitudinal hemianopias respecting the horizontal meridian (Fig. 8–24).[57] This pattern may be mistaken for similar visual field deficits caused by bilateral optic neuropathies. The vertical meridian can be spared if the calcarine lips are not involved, while horizontal meridian sparing may be seen if the base of the calcarine banks deep within the calcarine fissure is uninvolved.[43]

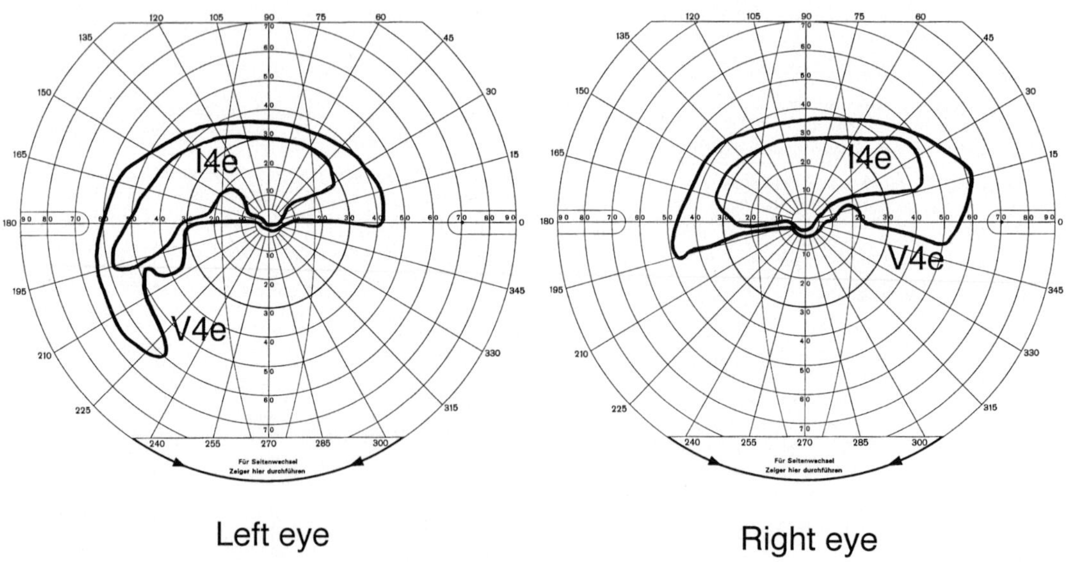

FIGURE 8–24. Bilateral inferior altitudinal hemianopia from bilateral parietal–occipital hemorrhages. The patient also had Balint syndrome (see Chapter 9).

Cerebral Blindness. This condition, characterized by blindness, absent blink to threat[58] and optokinetic responses, normal pupillary reactivity, and normal fundi, results from bilateral retrogeniculate dysfunction. When lesions to both occipital lobes are responsible, as opposed to bilateral involvement of the optic radiations, the term *cortical blindness* may be applied (Fig. 8–25). Clinically, patients with cerebral blindness can be distinguished from those with pregeniculate lesions by the presence of intact pupillary light responses. Cerebral blind patients may confabulate visual perceptions or deny their blindness (*Anton syndrome*). Some of these patients have additional, contributory frontal or temporal lobe lesions that alter recognition, memory, and behavior.

The Riddoch Phenomenon and Blindsight. Riddoch[59] and Holmes[60] observed that individuals recovering from occipital lobe injuries first perceive moving objects but not stationary ones. The Riddoch phenomenon can be observed during confrontation field testing by comparing the patient's responses to moving and still targets. More recently it has been shown that rare patients with uni- or bilateral occipital lesions lose object recognition but in some instances may have "blindsight," an unconscious ability to locate light sources and detect moving targets in affected fields.[61–67, 352, 353] Some have argued that patients with blindsight have some residual visual function in this apparent blind field, and it is merely conscious vision that is impaired. Extrageniculostriate vision resulting from a "second" more primitive, secondary visual pathway consisting of retino-tectal-pulvinar connections with parietal lobe[68] and with V5, the putative motion detection area (see Chapter 9 for further discussion of the role of V5), have been invoked to explain the Riddoch phenomenon and blindsight.[62–66, 69–72] Recent evidence,[73, 74] however, has suggested that residual subcortical connections with V5 are not necessary for these phenomena to occur. Alternative mechanisms[75] include small residual islands of vision not detectable by routine perimetry,[76] direct connections from the lateral geniculate nucleus to extrastriate areas V2 and V4[77] (see Chapter 9) and, less likely, light scatter in the retina.[78] It should be noted that the Riddoch phenomenon is not specific for lesions of the striate cortex and may be observed with lesions of the anterior visual pathway as well.[79]

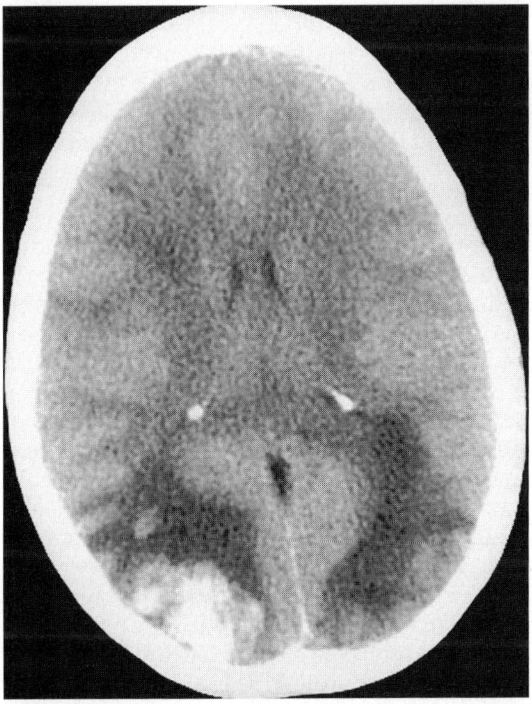

FIGURE 8–25. CT-demonstrated bilateral occipital lobe hemorrhagic lesions and edema, presumably due to aspergillosis, in a patient with leukemia and cortical blindness.

Other Neuro-ophthalmic Signs. Visual acuity is affected only if bilateral lesions are present. Any level of visual acuity is possible with bilateral retrochiasmal lesions, but the acuities should be symmetric unless there is superimposed anterior visual pathway disease.

Occipital lobe hemianopias that are stroke related are often isolated, unless a proximal PCA occlusion leads to a third nerve palsy. We have also seen several individuals with acute PCA strokes who complained of pain in the distribution of the ophthalmic division of the trigeminal nerve, ipsilateral to the vascular occlusion. One proposed mechanism is referred pain due to trigeminal innervation of the circle of Willis.[80]

A patient with a unilateral hemianopia due to occipital lobe infarction will have a normal optokinetic response. In contrast, one with a hemianopia owing to an occipital lobe mass with edema extending into the parietal lobe might have an abnormal optokinetic response when the targets are drawn ipsilaterally to the lesion (Cogan's rule).

Upper bank occipital lobe lesions may be associated with Balint syndrome. Lower bank lesions may be accompanied by hemiachromatopsia, prosopagnosia, and object agnosias.

Alexia without agraphia may follow a left occipital lesion with involvement of the splenium of the corpus callosum. These higher cortical disorders are discussed in Chapter 9.

Other unusual visual phenomena observed following occipital lobe injury include palinopsia (persistence of visual images) and optic allesthesia (abnormal object orientation in space). These symptoms are discussed in more detail in Chapter 12.

Other Symptoms and Signs. As alluded to above, a proximal PCA occlusion may cause a midbrain and occipital lobe infarction.[81, 82] Resulting signs might include an ipsilateral third nerve palsy, contralateral ataxia or hemiparesis, and contralateral hemianopia.[354] PCA occlusion may also lead to memory or personality changes from mesial-temporal or thalamic involvement.[83] Thalamic lesions may also lead to sensory loss.[355] The "top of the basilar syndrome"[84] (discussed in more detail in Chapters 15 and 16) often includes signs and symptoms of unilateral or bilateral PCA occlusion. Hemianopias related to occipital lobe infarction also may be associated with brain stem signs and other types of ocular motor dysfunction such as nystagmus, skew deviation, or gaze palsies, if the cause is vertebrobasilar occlusion. Insidious field loss accompanied by language or cognitive decline suggests a mass lesion or dementing illness.

Etiology

In adults, the most common cause of a occipital lobe hemianopia is a PCA stroke (Table 8–1 and Fig. 8–26) A homonymous hemianopia, with or without macular sparing, unaccompanied by any other neurologic signs or symptoms, would be the most common presentation of a PCA stroke.

In elderly patients, the differential diagnosis of occipital lobe dysfunction also includes lobar hemorrhage due to amyloid angiopathy. Infectious causes include abscesses, progressive multifocal leukoencephalopathy, and Creutzfeldt–Jakob disease. In children, adrenoleukodystrophy and MELAS (mitochondrial myopathy, encephalopathy, lactic acidosis, and strokelike episodes) may be responsible for hemianopias. Ictal or postictal hemianopias, and complicated migraine leading to occipital lube infarction are uncommon.

Important acquired and congenital causes of cortical blindness[85] are listed in Table 8–3.

DIAGNOSIS AND MANAGEMENT OF DISTURBANCES OF THE OPTIC RADIATIONS AND OCCIPITAL LOBE

Because processes that affect the optic radiations and occipital lobe are very similar, they are discussed together in the following sections.

CEREBROVASCULAR DISEASE (ISCHEMIC STROKE)

Occlusion of the middle or posterior cerebral arteries is suggested by the sudden onset of neurologic symptoms in an elderly individual with cerebrovascular risk factors such as atrial fibrillation, hypertension,[86] diabetes, smoking,[87, 88] and hypercholesterolemia.[89] Loosely defined, a transient ischemic attack (TIA) is a cerebrovascular event that lasts for a few minutes or hours, and a stroke is one that produces a fixed deficit that lasts for more than a day. TIAs are discussed in more detail in Chapter 10.

MCA strokes are associated with cardiogenic emboli, internal carotid occlusion, and ICA dissection.[90] Common causes of PCA infarction include embolism from the heart and a more proximal vascular lesion in the vertebral or basilar arteries.[91, 92] Posterior division MCA strokes, leading to Wernicke's aphasia and hemianopia, and isolated PCA infarcts are frequently cardioembolic.[93] Less commonly, MCA and PCA infarction can result from local atherostenosis,[94] migraine, or a hypercoagulable state.[91]

Neuroimaging. CT, which is fast and readily available, can be performed in the emergency setting to differentiate between an ischemic and a hemorrhagic stroke. Small strokes may be more visible with MRI, especially on T_2-weighted and fluid level attenuated inversion recovery (FLAIR) images (Fig. 8–26). Neither CT or conventional MRI may show any abnormality within the first 6 hours after the stroke ictus. New MRI techniques such as diffusion-weighted imaging (Fig. 8–26),[95, 356] which detects changes in the random motion of water molecules, and perfusion-weighted imaging, which may identify ischemic areas with low blood volume, may delineate brain ischemia before CT or routine MRI is able. MRI-angiography of the carotid system and circle of Willis is frequently helpful when establishing the stroke mechanism.

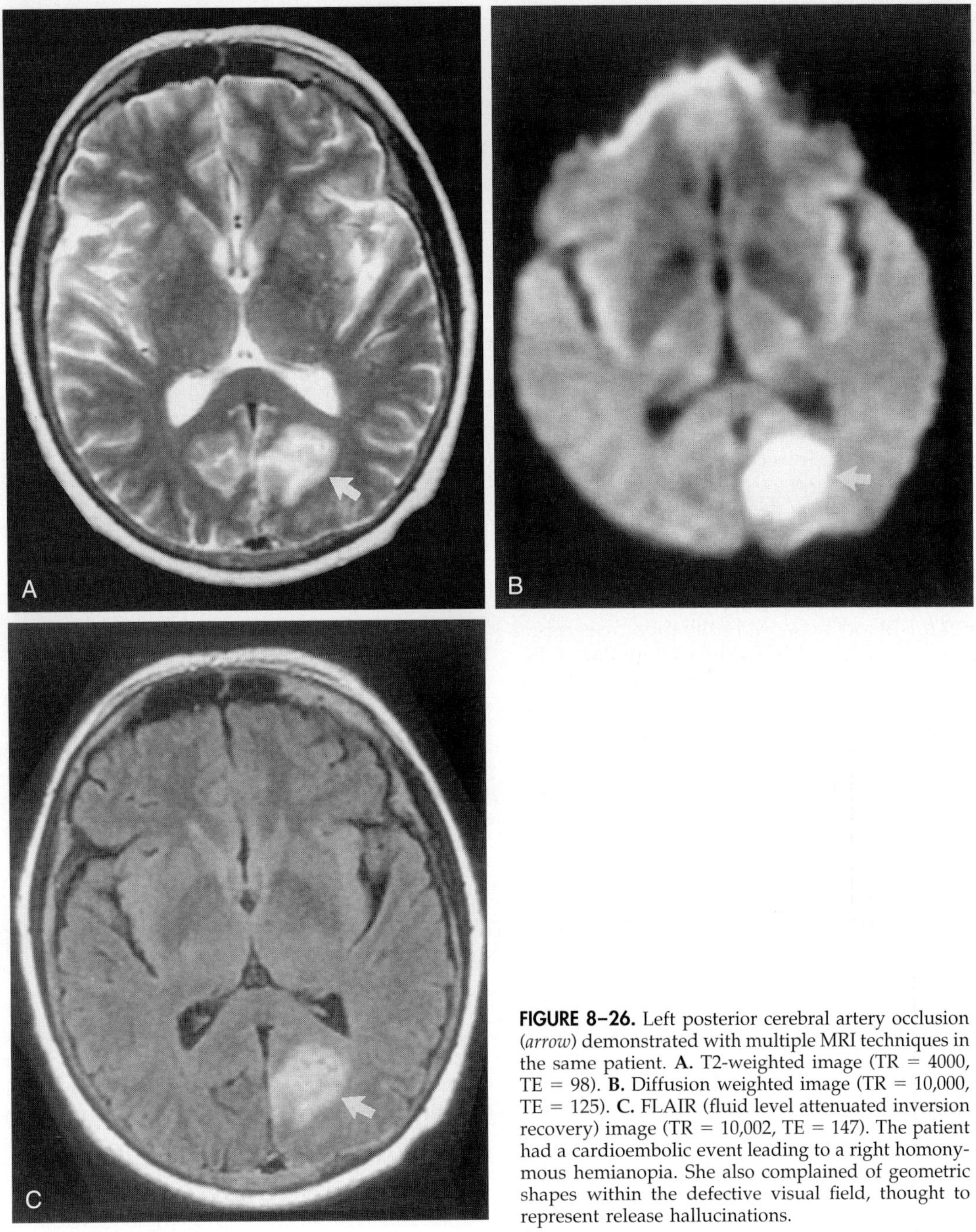

FIGURE 8–26. Left posterior cerebral artery occlusion (*arrow*) demonstrated with multiple MRI techniques in the same patient. **A.** T2-weighted image (TR = 4000, TE = 98). **B.** Diffusion weighted image (TR = 10,000, TE = 125). **C.** FLAIR (fluid level attenuated inversion recovery) image (TR = 10,002, TE = 147). The patient had a cardioembolic event leading to a right homonymous hemianopia. She also complained of geometric shapes within the defective visual field, thought to represent release hallucinations.

Treatment. The best treatment for stroke is primary prevention according to the underlying medical or vascular condition.[96, 97] Control of hypertension, lowering serum cholesterol, cessation of smoking, and exercise may reduce the risk of stroke.[98, 99] Reducing glucose, dietary modification, and avoidance of obesity are also recommended, but to date these measures have not been proven to reduce the risk of cerebrovascular events.[98] Considerations regarding asymptomatic carotid stenosis are reviewed in Chapter 10. Treatment of underlying cardiac and hypercoagulable states and secondary prevention are discussed separately in more detail below.

While the details of the management of acute stroke patients are beyond the scope of this book, it is helpful to mention some basic

TABLE 8–3. Important Causes of Cortical Blindness

Acquired
Vascular
Bilateral posterior cerebral artery infarction
Cardiac surgery
Cerebral angiography
Hypoxia
Reversible leukoencephalopathies
Hypertensive encephalopathy
Peripartum state
FK-501
Cyclosporine
Carbon monoxide poisoning
Creutzfeldt–Jakob disease
Trauma
Progressive multifocal leukoencephalopathy
Alzheimer's disease
Congenital
Hypoxemic–ischemic encephalopathy
Periventricular leukomalacia
Cortical dysplasia

points. Acute stroke therapy is aimed at either limiting neuronal damage or re-establishing cerebral blood flow. Maintenance of cerebral perfusion pressure, lying the patient flat, delivering oxygen, and normalization of serum glucose, body temperature, and intravascular volume are recommended.[100, 101]

At many centers, thrombolytic therapy in selected patients with acute ischemic stroke is given to allow rapid recanalization of occluded vessels,[102, 103, 357] but its use is controversial.[104] Two large randomized studies[105, 106] evaluated intravenous (IV) recombinant tissue plasminogen activator (rt-PA) in patients with acute ischemic stroke and a clinically significant neurologic defect. Patients with small-vessel occlusive, large-vessel occlusive, and cardioembolic strokes were enrolled.[107] They had to have been evaluated within 3 to 6 hours of onset of symptoms, and CT had to demonstrate the absence of early infarction or hemorrhage.[107, 108] Functional neurologic outcomes were improved and disability reduced in treated patients.[109] Enthusiasm for thrombolytic agents, however, has been tempered by the high risk of associated cerebral hemorrhage. IV streptokinase[110] has been shown to be unsafe, although selective intra-arterial thrombolysis with urokinase has been used in some settings.[111] The use of heparin and antiplatelet agents such as aspirin is discussed in more detail below in the sections on cardioembolic stroke and ischemic stroke, respectively.

Neuroprotective agents have also been studied in stroke therapy.[112] Cerebral ischemia causes excessive release of the neurotransmitter glutamate, which in turn worsens ischemic injury by acting on N-methyl-D-aspartate (NMDA) receptors, which allows excessive intracellular entry of calcium and sodium. Agents that are NMDA receptor antagonists or competitive antagonists of the glutamate or glycine recognition sites of the NMDA receptor are currently being investigated. However, many such drugs have been hampered by unacceptable side effects such as hypotension, and several have failed to show any benefit in drug trials. Methods for modifying the immune response to stroke have also been proposed.[113, 114]

In elderly patients, field deficits from cerebral infarction that persist for more than 48 hours have a relatively poor prognosis for recovery.[115] However, in children and young adults the prognosis is much better, as visual field improvement sometimes can be observed days or weeks following the ictus.

Cardioembolism

Frequent cardioembolic causes of cerebral infarction include atrial fibrillation, regional or global wall hypokinesis, valvular disease, and patent foramen ovale.[93] Less common causes include atrial myxoma and endocarditis.

Atrial Fibrillation. Stroke occurs in 4.5% of untreated patients with atrial fibrillation per year.[116] In nonrheumatic atrial fibrillation, the risk of stroke is approximately five times that of the normal population, and in atrial fibrillation associated with rheumatic valvular disease, there is a 17-fold increase in risk.[117]

Although treatment should be individualized under the direction of a cardiologist, in general patients with atrial fibrillation should receive prophylaxis for thromboembolism. Warfarin, adjusted to maintain an international normalized ratio (INR) of 2.0 to 3.0,[118] has been proven to reduce the risk of stroke and secondary cerebrovascular events.[119–124] Cerebral hemorrhage is the most feared complication, but the risk is low at the aforementioned INRs. In patients with contraindications such as poorly controlled hypertension, inability to comply, gait instability, and history of bleeding, aspirin may be used.[125] Cardiac rate can be controlled by digoxin, beta-blockers, or calcium channel blockers.[116]

In acute stroke due to atrial fibrillation, when the infarct is nonhemorrhagic and mild to moderate in size, emergent anticoagulation with IV heparin,[358] followed by warfarin, should be instituted to reduce the risk of reembolus. Larger embolic infarctions have a greater tendency for spontaneous hemorrhagic transformation.[126] Nevertheless, some authors suggest IV heparin even in large[127] and hemorrhagic[128] embolic infarcts if the patient is relatively intact neurologically and at continued high risk for recurrent cardiac source emboli.

Hypokinetic Wall Motion Abnormalities. Especially within the first 2 weeks following a myocardial infarction, focal areas of left ventricular akinesia or dyskinesia may predispose to the development of mural thrombi with resultant cerebral and systemic emboli. The risk may extend for several years following myocardial infarction, and a decreased ejection fraction and older age were found to be independent predictors of an increased risk of stroke in one study.[129] Long-term anticoagulation, usually warfarin, is generally given to at-risk patients without contraindications. However, to our knowledge warfarin and aspirin have not been compared in this setting. Treatment is similar in patients with low ejection fraction from dilated cardiomyopathy from myocarditis and amyloid, for example. In patients with acute ischemic events (see atrial fibrillation above) who are not already anticoagulated, emergent IV heparin followed by warfarin is recommended.

Patent Foramen Ovale. In younger patients without other stroke risk factors and in those whose neurologic deficit followed Valsalva or cough, this mechanism should be considered.[130] Asymptomatic deep venous thromboses may result in paradoxic emboli if clot material passes through a patent foramen ovale. The diagnosis may be established with a transesophageal echocardiogram bubble study, during which a small amount of air mixed in saline is injected into an antecubital vein. Excessive microbubbles detected in the left atrium in resting states or after Valsalva may indicate a right-to-left interatrial shunt. However, because patent foramen ovales are overrepresented in patients with cerebral infarcts of uncertain cause,[131] it is often difficult to correlate them with cerebrovascular events. Therefore, treatment, consisting of anticoagulation with warfarin or antiplatelet agents, or transcatheter or surgical closure of the defect,[132] should be determined on a case by case basis.[133]

Valvular Disease. Mitral valve prolapse and mitral annulus calcification are also associated with higher risk of TIA and stroke.[93] However, like patent foramen ovale, they are such common echocardiographic findings that it is sometimes hard to assign any clinical significance to them in a patient with a cerebrovascular event.[359] Nevertheless, antiplatelet therapy is frequently recommended. Prosthetic heart valves, because of their inherent thrombogenicity, require long-term warfarin anticoagulation.

Atrial Myxoma. Although histologically benign, these primary tumors of the heart may produce devastating effects when pieces detach and embolize to the brain or systemically. They are usually located within the left atrium, and are generally polypoid, pedunculated, round, or oval, with a smooth or lobulated surface.[134] Myxomas typically present either with embolism or intracardiac obstruction. Transesophageal echocardiography, CT, or MRI of the chest may demonstrate these lesions, and surgical removal is the treatment of choice.

Endocarditis. Stroke due to septic emboli may complicate infective endocarditis in approximately 21% of cases.[135] Typical organisms include *Staphylococcus aureus* and *Streptococcus*. Intracranial hemorrhages may also develop, some related to mycotic aneurysms.[136] The diagnosis of infective endocarditis is established on the basis of a valvular vegetation seen on transthoracic or transesophageal echocardiography and positive blood cultures. Other systemic emboli, such as ocular Roth spots, often aid in the diagnosis. Other neurologic complications of infective endocarditis include encephalopathy, meningitis, brain abscess, seizures, and headache.[137, 138] Most cerebral embolic phenomena occur early in the patient's course before the control of infection, so treatment is primarily antibiotics without anticoagulation.[135] Valve replacement may take place once the infection is controlled.

Other Causes of Ischemic Stroke

Carotid Artery Disease. In the absence of cardioembolic phenomena, signs and symptoms of retinal or hemispheric ischemia demand exclusion of carotid artery stenosis. Infarction may result from carotid artery occlusion or emboli from an ulcerated atheromatous plaque. The evaluation and management of carotid stenosis is discussed in more detail in Chapter 10. Carotid artery dissection, which can produce ipsilateral Horner syndrome, carotidynia (pain), dysgeusia (abnormal taste), and cortical ischemia or stroke, is discussed in more detail in Chapter 13.

Vertebrobasilar Disease. Ischemia in the posterior cerebral artery distribution may result from *vertebral* or *basilar artery stenosis*. Usually field defects due vertebrobasilar insufficiency are accompanied by other indications of brain stem or cerebellar ischemia such as diplopia, dysarthria, or ataxia.[92] *Vertebral artery dissection*,[139] due to trauma or chiropractic manipulation, for instance, may also result in upstream posterior cerebral artery ischemia. Alternatively, *vertebral artery origin occlusive disease*, similar to carotid atheromatous plaques, may produce basilar or posterior cerebral artery strokes by intracranial intra-arterial embolism.[140] Not readily surgical amenable, in situ vertebrobasilar disease generally is best treated with antiplatelet agents, but vertebral artery dissection, stroke in evolution, and crescendo TIAs may require more aggressive anticoagulation with heparin and warfarin. Some authors have also used thrombolysis successfully in basilar artery stroke.[141, 142]

Thromobosis in the Circle of Willis (in Situ Thrombosis). Atherosclerosis of the middle and posterior cerebral arteries may be detected noninvasively using MRI-angiography, and symptomatic stenosis is is usually treated medically with antiplatelet agents such as aspirin. In those failing or not tolerating aspirin, platelet antiaggregants such as clopidrogrel and ticlopidine can be used. Diarrhea and rash are common with ticlopidine, and because of potential neutropenia, use of the drug requires hematologic monitoring.[143–145] Clopidrogrel, which is preferable because it is safer than ticlopidine, in one study was slightly more effective than aspirin in reducing vascular events.[146] However, we have observed a patient who developed neutropenia on ticlopidine as well as clopidrogrel.

Dipyridamole in combination with aspirin may have some benefit over aspirin alone in the prevention of TIA or stroke.[147, 360] Extracranial–intracranial arterial bypass operations failed to reduce the risk of stroke in patients with symptomatic atherosclerotic disease of the internal carotid or middle cerebral artery.[148]

Hypercoagulable States. These conditions account for approximately 1% of ischemic strokes but up to 4% of strokes in young adults.[149] These include hematologic disorders such as protein C or S, factor V, or antithrombin III deficiency,[150] which are treated with chronic warfarin anticoagulation, and abnormalities of formed blood elements such as polycythemia vera, sickle cell anemia, sickle-C disease, and essential thrombocythemia.[151] Prothombotic states such as oral contraceptive use,[152, 153] pregnancy,[154] and cancer (Trousseau syndrome) should also be considered.[155]

Autoantibody syndromes, due to antiphospholipid (anticardiolipin, for example) antibodies and lupus anticoagulants, are also associated with hypercoagulability.[151] Several reports[156, 157] have described the presence of these antibodies in patients with cerebral ischemia, even in those without systemic lupus erythematosus. However, their exact relationship to stroke is uncertain,[158, 159] and the mechanism for the predisposition to thrombosis is unclear.[160] Furthermore, the best treatment, either aspirin or warfarin, is controversial,[161, 162] but warfarin is preferred in patients with recurrent ischemic events.

Cardiac Surgery. Open heart surgery remains the most common iatrogenic cause of stroke.[163] Perioperative mechanisms include (1) macroemboli from trauma to diseased brittle, atherosclerotic blood vessels or from intracardiac entrapment of air or particles; (2) microemboli produced by the cardiopulmonary bypass machinery; (3) alterations in blood pressure and oxygenation, and (4) pre-existing cerebrovascular or carotid disease.[164–166]

Aortic Arch Emboli. This is likely an underrecognized source of cerebral embolism.[167, 168] In patients studied with transesophageal echocardiography, atherosclerotic plaques >4 mm thick in the aortic arch were found to be associated with ischemic stroke[169] and to be predictors of recurrent brain infarction and other vascular events.[170] Aspirin may be recommended when these lesions are detected, however, the best treatment of aortic arch atherosclerosis is currently uncertain.[133]

Transtentorial Herniation. Large neoplastic or hemorrhagic lesions causing downward transtentorial herniation may cause compression of the posterior cerebral arteries at the edge of the tentorium. Both unilateral hemianopias and cortical blindness may be produced.[171]

Migraine. Homonymous hemianopic field defects in migraine are usually transient and are therefore discussed in more detail in Chapter

10. However, if the deficit lasts for more than 7 days, or if a parietal or occipital lobe infarction is demonstrated on neuroimaging, the International Headache Society diagnosis of "migrainous cerebral infarction" is suggested.[172] The rest of the diagnostic criteria are (1) the patient has previously fulfilled the criteria for migraine with aura; (2) the attack is typical of previous attacks; and (3) other causes of infarction have been excluded.[172, 173]

Epidemiologic studies have now confirmed migraine as an independent risk factor for stroke.[174, 175] We strongly discourage our migraine patients from smoking or using oral contraception, in order to reduce the chance of stroke. Any combination of risk factors may be synergistic.

In patients with migraine-related occipital infarction, basilar artery or PCA stenosis or spasm may be evident on MRI-angiography. However, in some instances the stroke does not respect the usual MCA or PCA territories (see example in Chapter 19), suggesting that a strictly vascular mechanism is insufficient to explain all migraine-related stroke phenomena. The exact pathogenesis of migraine-related stroke is unclear, but a combination of coagulation, hemodynamic factors, and neuronal factors is likely to be responsible.[176]

The best treatment of patients with migraine-related stroke is unknown. Use of aspirin, exclusion of other causes of stroke, and migraine prophylaxis is one recommended approach. Migraine treatment is discussed in more detail in Chapter 19.

Stroke in Young Adults and Children

Strokes in patients less than 40 years old are relatively uncommon. In young adults, cardiogenic emboli and atherosclerotic occlusive disease are the two most common identifiable causes of stroke.[177] Other causes that should be considered in this age group include hypercoagulable states, nonatherosclerotic vascular disease (dissection or moyamoya vessels, for instance), illicit drug use, and migraine. One study found that a cause may not be found in approximately one third of patients despite an exhaustive search.[178] In children, cyanotic heart disease and sickle cell disease are seen more often as causes of stroke, and atherosclerosis is rarely considered.[179]

HEMORRHAGE

Table 8–4 highlights some of the more important causes of intracerebral hemorrhages.

TABLE 8–4. Important Causes of Intracerebral Hemorrhage

Hypertension
Amyloid angiopathy
Vascular malformations
Arteriovenous malformations
Cavernous angiomas
Saccular or mycotic aneurysms
Trauma
Hemorrhagic infarction
Anticoagulant treatment and bleeding diathesis
Hemorrhage into intracranial tumors
Drug related

Evaluation of patients with suspected intracerebral hemorrhage begins with unenhanced CT.[180] A CT scan is easily obtained and makes it possible to determine the size of the hemorrhage, the extent of mass effect, and whether the ventricular system is compromised. Follow-up MRI is often helpful to ensure that the hemorrhage is not from an underlying arteriovenous malformation or brain tumor. In addition, MRI-angiography provides a useful noninvasive way to screen for aneurysms. Because MRI-angiography may miss some aneurysms,[181] conventional angiography is indicated when the cause of the intracerebral hemorrhage remains uncertain. In most instances patients with intracerebral hemorrhages will be managed in a neurointensive care unit setting, with attention directed toward managing blood pressure and intracranial pressure. Depending on the nature of the hemorrhage, neurosurgical evacuation may be considered if the patient's condition deteriorates or if shunting is required.[182]

Hypertensive Hemorrhage

In order of decreasing frequency, hemorrhages associated with long-standing hypertension arise in the putamen, thalamus, pons, cerebellum, and cerebral white matter. When large enough, thalamic hemorrhages may cause hemianopias by involving the LGN (Fig. 8–27), while putaminal and lobar hemorrhages may disrupt the optic radiations.[183] When the hemorrhages are limited to brain parenchyma, treatment is usually supportive. Intraventricular blood may lead to hydrocephalus and thus may require shunting.

Amyloid Angiopathy

This entity should be considered highly in any elderly individual with posteriorly situated lo-

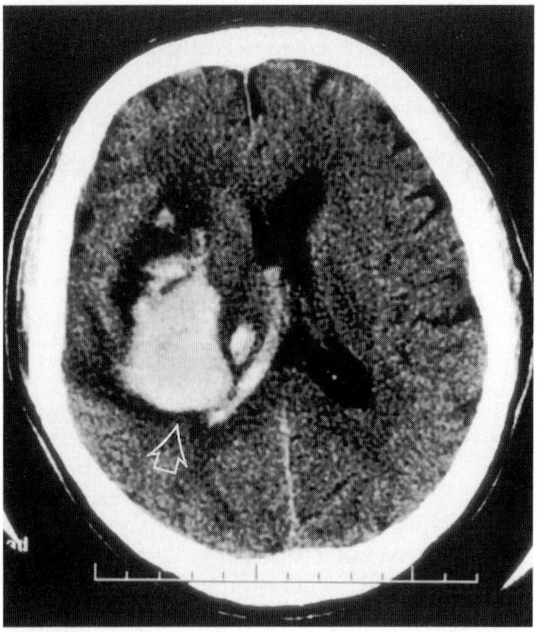

FIGURE 8–27. Hypertensive thalamic hemorrhage (*arrow*) on axial CT. The patient had a left homonymous hemianopia and left hemiplegia.

bar hemorrhages. In contrast to hypertensive hemorrhages, cerebral amyloid angiopathy tends to produce one or more episodes of lobar hemorrhage (Fig. 8–28), with a propensity to to affect the parieto-occipital regions.[184] The lobar distribution of hemorrhage in cerebral amyloid angiopathy reflects the preferential deposition of amyloid in the superficial and leptomeningeal arteries.[184] Pathologically, vessel walls contain congophilic material, which exhibits apple-green birefringence when viewed with polarized light, and fibrinoid necrosis is often seen (Fig. 8–28).[185] It has been suggested that the amyloid in this vascular disorder is the same as the amyloid found in senile plaques in Alzheimer's disease.[186]

Autopsy studies have found a greater frequency of cerebral amyloid angiopathy with increasing age. Approximately 5% of individuals from 60 to 69 years of age have cerebral amyloid angiopathy, compared with more than 50% of patients in their 90s.[187] Despite this high frequency of vessel involvement, the reason hemorrhage is still relatively infrequent in the affected population remains unclear. Predisposition to hemorrhage may be related to the severity of amyloid deposition, the presence of fibrinoid necrosis,[188] and possession of the apolipoprotein E ∈2 and ∈4 alleles.[189, 190, 361]

Although a definitive diagnosis requires a pathologic analysis of brain tissue, biopsy of the brain is rarely performed given the availability of neuroimaging to exclude other causes, the absence of effective therapy, and the advanced age of most patients with cerebral amyloid angiopathy. Most diagnoses are made postmortem. The clinical diagnosis of "probable cerebral amyloid angiopathy" can be made in a patient older than 60 years of age with multiple lobar hemorrhages with no other cause of bleeding.[191] Because of increased fragility of vessels affected by amyloid deposition, conservative management is preferred over surgical evacuation of the hematoma.[192] Antiplatelet agents or anticoagulants should be withdrawn.[191]

Arteriovascular Malformations

Arteriovenous malformations (AVMs) are dysplastic vascular lesions in which the normal capillary bed is replaced by a convolution of abnormally connected arterial and venous channels.[193] Intracranial AVMs are thought to form secondary to developmental arrest during cerebrovascular development. Usually intraparenchymal cerebral AVMs are supplied by large branches of the circle of Willis. Dural AVMs, which tend to be more superficially located, result from communications between the arteries that supply the dura mater and the intracranial venous sinuses. The afferent and efferent vessels of AVMs may vary considerably in their course, size, and number. In some instances, the entire lesion may be only a few millimeters in size, while in others, a whole cerebral lobe may be involved. The intervening cerebral tissue is often gliotic, and the surrounding neural tissue characteristically shows some degree of atrophy. Neurologic abnormalities and visual field defects are caused most commonly by compression of local structures, ischemia, or hemorrhage.

The majority of AVMs are sporadic although familial cases have been documented.[194] Men are affected slightly more often than women (1.4:1),[195] and the majority of individuals do not present until their second or third decade. Malformations often become symptomatic during times of hormonal fluctuation, accelerating growth, or accentuated intravascular volume such as puberty or pregnancy.[196] Neurocutaneous syndromes linked with intracranial AVMs include the Wyburn–Mason, Osler–Weber–Rendu, Sturge–Weber (see congenital conditions, below), and Klippel–Theraunay–Weber syndromes.[196]

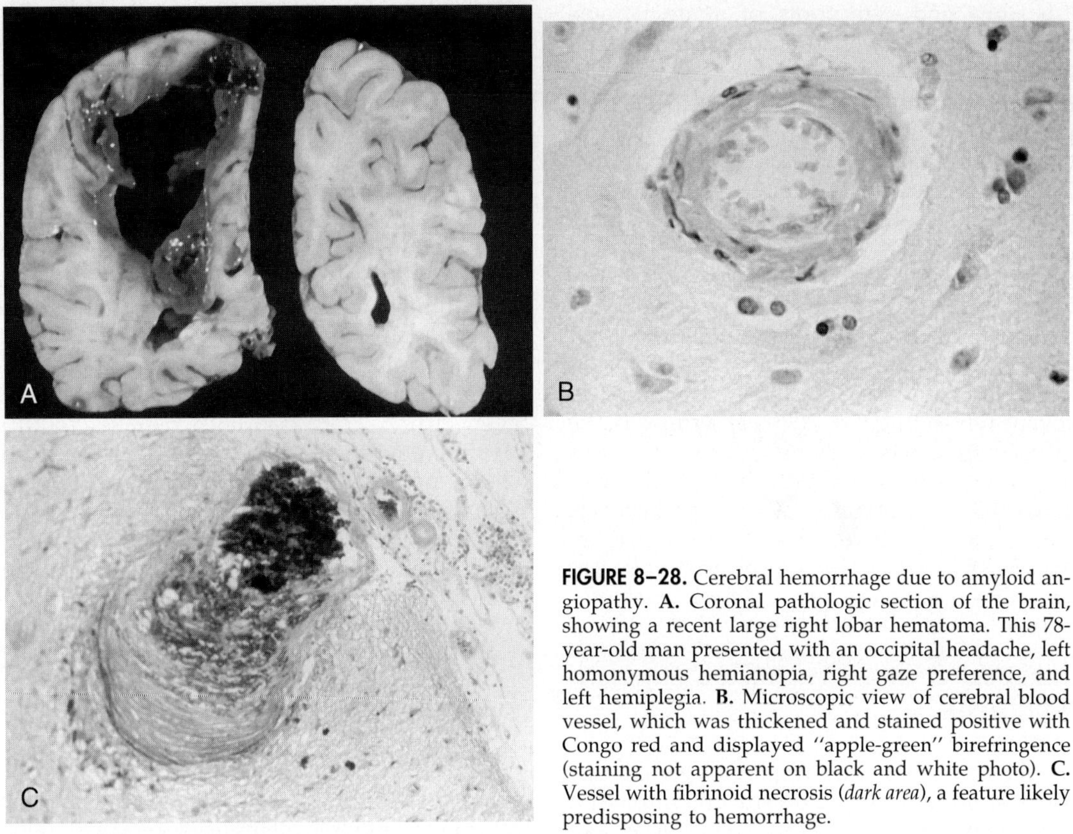

FIGURE 8–28. Cerebral hemorrhage due to amyloid angiopathy. **A.** Coronal pathologic section of the brain, showing a recent large right lobar hematoma. This 78-year-old man presented with an occipital headache, left homonymous hemianopia, right gaze preference, and left hemiplegia. **B.** Microscopic view of cerebral blood vessel, which was thickened and stained positive with Congo red and displayed "apple-green" birefringence (staining not apparent on black and white photo). **C.** Vessel with fibrinoid necrosis (*dark area*), a feature likely predisposing to hemorrhage.

The most common presentation of an intracranial AVM is intraparenchymal or subarachnoid hemorrhage, often with a focal neurologic deficit. Seizures and headaches are the next most frequent presentations. Subjective bruits are more common with extracranial AVMs, and only sometimes is the bruit audible. Dural AVMs can cause cortical disturbances but also present with venous sinus congestion from obstruction or arterialization. Many individuals with unruptured occipital lobe AVMs present with transient visual field defects or positive visual phenomena (scintillating scotomas, fortification spectra, or spots, for example) followed by headache, mimicking migraine.[197] Usually in these cases the distinguishing feature is an overwhelming headache or a residual field deficit, but sometimes differentiating between migraine and AVM is dificult on clinical grounds alone.

Radiographically, cerebral AVMs are usually identified by their serpiginous flow voids on T_1- and T_2-weighted images.[198] When patients present with large hemorrhages, AVMs may be masked and may not be evident on routine neuroimaging. MRI-angiography is often helpful in demonstrating the feeding arteries and abnormal tangle of vessels. Formal angiography is required for proper definition of the vascular anatomy.

Definitive treatment is neurosurgical removal of the AVM, especially when superficially located.[199] In some instances endovascular embolization of feeding vessels may reduce the size of the lesion, making it more surgically amenable. When they involve the optic radiations or occipital lobe with partial hemifield loss, unfortunately following embolization or surgical extirpation the field defects can worsen or become complete.[197, 200] Smaller AVMs are now treatable with stereotactic radiation therapy.[201] The treatment of large AVMs in neurologically eloquent areas is still unsatisfactory.[202]

Cavernous Angiomas (Cavernomas)

Although these small vascular malformations often occur in the cortex and cerebral white matter, associated retrochiasmal field defects are relatively uncommon. They may present with signs and symptoms of acute hemorrhage.[203] Alternatively, asymptomatic cavernous angiomas may be detected on neuroimaging done for other reasons. They consist of dilated spaces filled with blood without intervening neural tissue, separated by fibrous collagenous bands.[204] Their histopathologic and radiographic features are discussed in more detail in the section on cavernous angiomas of the chiasm (Chapter 7).

Treatment of cavernous angiomas depends on their location and symptomatology. For symptomatic superficial lesions, surgery is effective and safe, and should be considered to prevent rebleeding.[205, 206] Deeper symptomatic lesions may also be remove, but in such cases observation is often a better option because of the morbidity associated with such surgery. Unfortunately recurrent bleeding often mandates surgical removal. Asymptomatic cavernous angiomas should be treated conservatively.

VASCULITIS

Vasculitis is the broad term used to characterize those disorders associated with inflammation of blood vessels. Some of these conditions, like giant cell arteritis, purely affect vessels, while others, like systemic lupus erthematosus, produce inflammation of connective tissue, including blood vessels. It is helpful to divide central nervous system (CNS) vasculitis into two categories based on whether there is evidence of systemic disease. *Primary CNS vasculitis* is the term used to describe those entities in which the vasculitis process is limited to the CNS and eyes. Typically those patients with *systemic vasculitis,* such as temporal arteritis or systemic lupus erythematosus, will demonstrate signs and symptoms suggesting a more widespread angiitic process before the CNS is involved.

Primary CNS Vasculitis (Angiitis)

This idiopathic disorder is characterized by vasculitis restricted to the blood vessels of the brain and spinal cord.[207–216] Typically, there are multiple bilateral infarcts involving the cortex and subcortical white matter,[217, 218] often in a young individual. Scattered punctate enhancing lesions have also been observed.[219] Like conventional angiography,[217, 220] MRI-angiography may show cut-off of vessels, aneurysms, and beading but may be particularly limited in cases where a small-vessel vasculitis like granulomatous angiitis (GANS) is suspected. Biopsy of the leptomeninges is the only definitive method to establish the diagnosis of primary angiitis of the CNS.[209, 221] Pathologically, this disorder affects small- and medium-size vessels. The cellular infiltrate is composed of lymphocytes, macrophages, and giant cells in all layers of the vessel wall.

Without treatment, patients usually suffer recurrent strokes and die within several years. The administration of prednisone and cyclophosphamide may produce remission and even cure.[209, 210, 212, 214] Many patients require treatment for years. When repeat angiography shows normal findings, the immunosuppressive agent may be tapered.[220]

Other primary CNS vasculitides, such as Susac and Cogan syndrome, and Eales disease, which are typified more by their retinal manifestations, are discussed in Chapter 4.

Systemic Vasculitis

Giant Cell (Temporal) Arteritis. The pathology, systemic associations, diagnosis, and treatment of giant cell arteritis, especially with regard to arteritic ischemic optic neuropathy, are reviewed in greater detail in Chapter 5.

Transient ischemic attacks and cerebaral infarcts in giant cell arteritis may occur in any vascular distribution, but there is a tendency for involvement of the posterior circulation.[222–225, 364] Thus, from a neuro-ophthalmic prospective, hemifield defects and cortical blindness may ensue as the result of an occipital lobe infarction.[222, 226, 227] The preponderance of posterior circulation ischemia in giant cell arteritis reflects the predilection for arteritic involvement of the extracranial vertebral arteries.[228] The pathologic changes of ischemic brain injury related to giant cell arteritis include (1) inflammatory obstruction of vessels with a striking propensity for the arteritic involvement to cease as the vessel penetrates the dura intracranially; (2) embolism distal from an inflamed artery; and (3) a propagating thrombosis.[229]

Treatment of giant cell arteritis associated with brain ischemia has no established regimen. We advocate pulsed high-dose IV methylprednisolone but this regimen may also fail.[230] Since the mechanism of the brain ischemia may be inflammatory occlusive disease, consideration should be given to administration of heparin and overhydration to help evolving low flow or thromboembolic states.

Systemic Lupus Erythematosus (SLE). Permanent homonymous visual field defects may occur, either evolving acutely or over several days.[231–234] Occasionally, a homonymous field defect may herald the diagnosis of SLE.[235]

Potential causes of cortical ischemia in SLE include emboli from Libman–Sachs endocarditis, thrombotic infarction associated with antiphospholipid antibodies, vasospasm, and true vasculitis. Most pathologic studies of patients with ischemic visual or neurologic deficits have not demonstrated inflammation of the intracranial arteries. In the classic clinicopathologic study of 24 patients with SLE (18 with CNS manifestations), Johnson and Richardson[236] found true vasculitis in only 12.5%. Vascular necrosis was noted in 23%, fibrin thrombi in 12.5% and microinfarction in 70%.[236] Similar findings have been found in more contemporary neuropathologic studies.[237, 238]

Pulsed IV methylprednisolone for 3 days followed by oral prednisone 1–2 mg/kg per day for at least 1 month, along with IV heparin with plans to convert to warfarin, are recommended in patients with SLE and cortical ischemia. It is also particularly important to look for a source of emboli and the presence of antiphospholipid antibodies. Finding antiphospholipid antibodies in this setting usually requires the patient to undergo long-term anticoagulation.

The optic neuropathy associated with SLE is discussed in Chapter 5.

REVERSIBLE POSTERIOR LEUKOENCEPHALOPATHIES

A reversible posterior leukoencephalopathy syndrome, characterized by transient headache, seizures, hemianopia or cortical blindness, visual neglect, and mental status changes, is now well recognized.[239] The condition occurs in adults as well as children.[240] Causes usually fall into two groups. In the first group, consisting of malignant hypertension and eclampsia, the common feature is elevation in blood pressure. The second group is composed of patients treated with the immunosuppressive agents cyclosporine and FK-506 (tacrolimus),[241] and blood pressure is abnormal in only some of these cases. Neuroimaging in this syndrome typically demonstrates extensive bilateral white matter edema and lesions that are hypodense on CT and high signal on T_2-weighted MR images.[242, 243] The lesions can be diffuse, but they predominate in the posterior hemispheres. Both the clinical symptoms and radiographic abnormalities usually resolve within days to weeks following treatment of the hypertension or lowering of the dosage or cessation of the offending drug.

Malignant Hypertension and Eclampsia

The mechanism in malignant hypertension and eclampsia is likely defective autoregulation of the brain vasculature caused by sudden elevations in blood pressure.[239] Resulting vasodilation and vasoconstriction cause breakdown of the blood–brain barrier, with fluid transudation and petechial hemorrhages. Malignant hypertension with reversible leukoencephalopathy typically occurs in patients with a history of renal insufficiency.[244] In one report[245] erythropoietin, given to patients with chronic anemia related to end-stage renal disease, was an aggravating factor. Reversible leukoencephalopathy in eclampsia typically develops before delivery but has been reported up to 9 days postpartum.[246] One child with acquired immunodeficiency syndrome has been reported with this condition.[247]

Drugs

Cyclosporine produces the reversible posterior leukoencephalopathy typically at toxic levels.[248, 249] Aggravating factors appear to be cranial irradiation, hypomagnesemia, hypercholesterolemia, high-dose steriods, hypertension, and uremia.[249] The mechanism of this complication is unclear, but may reflect either direct neurotoxicity or a vasculopathy.[239] FK-506 (tacrolimus) is similar to cyclosporine in its action and toxic side effects. Similiar reversible cortical blindness and white matter lesions have been observed.[250] Interferon alpha has also been associated with this disorder.

NEOPLASMS OF THE CEREBRAL HEMISPHERES

In adults, the cerebral hemispheres are the most common location of brain tumors. Patients with neoplastic mass lesions of the parietal, temporal, or occipital lobes can present subacutely (days) or chronically (weeks) with altered mentation, focal neurologic findings, seizures, or symptoms of elevated intracranial pressure such as headache, nausea, or vomiting.[251] Visual field defects caused by such tumors are insidious, and worsen slowly as the tumor enlarges. Acute neurologic sysmptoms are suggestive of hemorrhage within the tumor. Visual field loss may also result as a complication of tumor treatment as in neurosurgical removal or cranial irradiation.[252]

Tumor types can be subdivided by whether they arose from primary brain tissue or metastasized from a systemic neoplasm. In children, most brain tumors are primary (Fig. 8–29), and brain metastases are much less common.

Tumors in Adults

Primary Tumors. Common supratentorial primary tumors of the brain include those that are intrinsic and those that are extrinsic to the brain. Primary intraparenchymal tumors of the brain on MRI or CT typically are heterogeneously enhancing masses with surrounding edema.

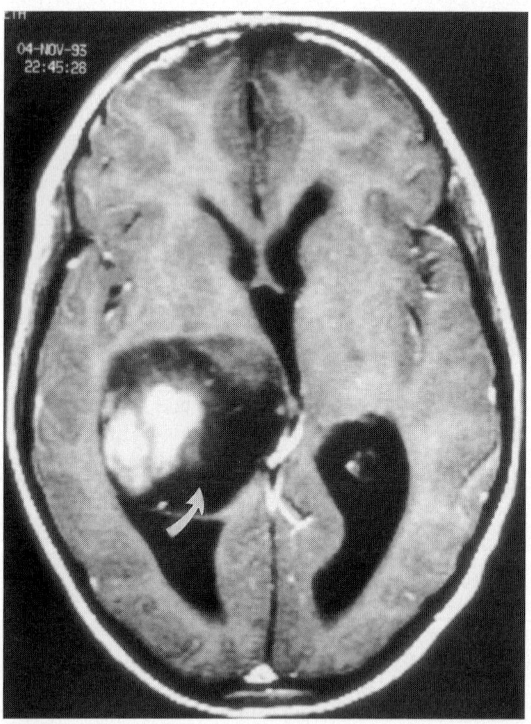

FIGURE 8–29. MRI demonstrating gadolinium-enhancing anaplatic astrocytoma of the thalamus (*arrow*) and hydrocephalus in child who presented with headaches and a left homonymous hemianopia.

Gliomas are the most common primary intraparenchymal brain tumors.[253] They are subdivided into astroglial neoplasms, oligodendrogliomas, gangliogliomas, and ependymomas. The astroglial neoplasms are further categorized, in order of increasing malignancy, into astrocytomas, anaplastic astrocytomas, and glioblastoma multiformes.[254] Generally, astrocytomas in the cerebral hemispheres are treated with complete resection, then observed without further treatment, but that is controversial.[255] Anaplastic astrocytomas and glioblastomas are treated with surgery, followed by radiation and chemotherapy. The prognosis in malignant gliomas is dismal, but age dependent: patients younger than 40 have an approximately 64% chance of survival at 18 months, while those over 60 have an 8% survival rate.[254]

Intraventricular tumors, such as choroid plexus papillomas and meningiomas, can cause hemifield defects if they involve the posterior horn of the lateral ventricle. Extraparenchymal meningiomas may lead to hemianopias if they grow large enough and are located along the hemispheric convexities.

Primary CNS lymphoma should be considered in any patient infected with human immunodeficiency virus (HIV). However, large-cell CNS lymphomas of B-cell origin have become well recognized in immunocompetent individuals as well.[256] Cerebrospinal fluid (CSF) cytology is only sometimes helpful, and often biopsy is necessary for a definitive diagnosis. A minority of individuals may develop intraocular spread and uveitis, and in these patients intravitreal sampling may be helpful. A combination of chemotherapy and radiotherapy was the most effective treatment in one report.[257]

Metastatic Tumors. The most common metastatic tumors to the brain originate from the lung and breast, but melanomas and genitourinary, gastrointestinal, and gynecologic tumors should also be considered.[258, 259] Only rarely do sarcomas, thyroid cancers, and head and neck tumors spread to the brain. MRI or CT typically demonstrates solitary or multiple ring-enhancing lesions at the grey–white matter junction with surrounding edema.

When metastases are suspected, but a systemic cancer is unknown, workup to detect a source would include at least chest roentgenography, chest and abdominal CT, carcinoembryonic antigen levels, stool guaiac study, bone scanning, and mammography.[259] Brain biopsy is required when no source can be identified. When a systemic cancer is known, treatment may be presumptive. Treatment with corticosteroids is almost always beneficial, and seizure prophylaxis in many instances is also recommended. Whole-brain radiation is usually given, but there is evidence to suggest that patients with a solitary metastasis benefit from surgical resection plus radiation rather than radiation alone.[260] The overall prognosis for patients with brain metastasis is still poor, but they tend to die of their systemic disease rather than from neurologic complications.[259]

Childhood Tumors

In contrast to adults, only 25% to 40% of childhood brain tumors arise in the cerebral hemispheres. The tumor types are similar, except meningiomas are less common, and supratentorial primitive neuroectodermal tumors, gangliogliomas, and ependymomas are more frequently seen.

INFECTIONS

Progressive Multifocal Leukoencephalopathy

Progressive multifocal leukoencephalopathy (PML) is a demyelinating viral infection caused by reactivation of a human papovavirus, JC virus (the initials stand for the first patient in whom the virus was isolated). The virus causes demyelination by lysing oligodendrocytes.[261] PML is characterized pathologically by a triad of multifocal demyelination, hyperchromatic, enlarged oligodendroglial nuclei, and enlarged bizarre astrocytes with lobulated hyperchromatic nuclei.[262, 263]

PML occurs primarily in immunocompromised individuals. Although originally described in patients with leukemia and lymphoma,[262] today most cases are seen in those infected with HIV,[264] in whom 5% are likely to develop PML.[263] Other predisposing conditions include sarcoidosis, SLE, macroglobulinemia, and immunosuppressive treatment following organ transplantation.[265]

PML presents insidiously with homonymous hemianopia, cortical blindness,[266] language disturbances, motor weakness, sensory loss, incoordination, and dementia.[267] Posterior fossa involvement, which is less common, can lead to ataxia, dysarthria, and cranial nerve palsies.[266] While most patients suffer from an inexorably progressive decline followed by death within months of their diagnosis, occasionally some experience a spontaneously relapsing–remitting or static course.[267, 268]

CT usually reveals diffuse white matter hypodensities in the posterior optic radiations (Fig. 8–30). MRI is best at demonstrating the extent and confluence of white matter involvement (see Chapter 9). The lesions are hypointense on T_1-weighted MR images and hyperintense on T_2-weighted images, and mass effect is typically absent. The lack of gadolinium enhancement usually distinguishes PML radiographically from CNS lymphoma.[269] However, a small number of cases of PML exhibit gadolinium enhancement, particularly around the lesion border. Magnetization transfer imaging, which is sensitive to demyelination, may aid in the radiologic diagnosis.[270] Routine CSF ex-

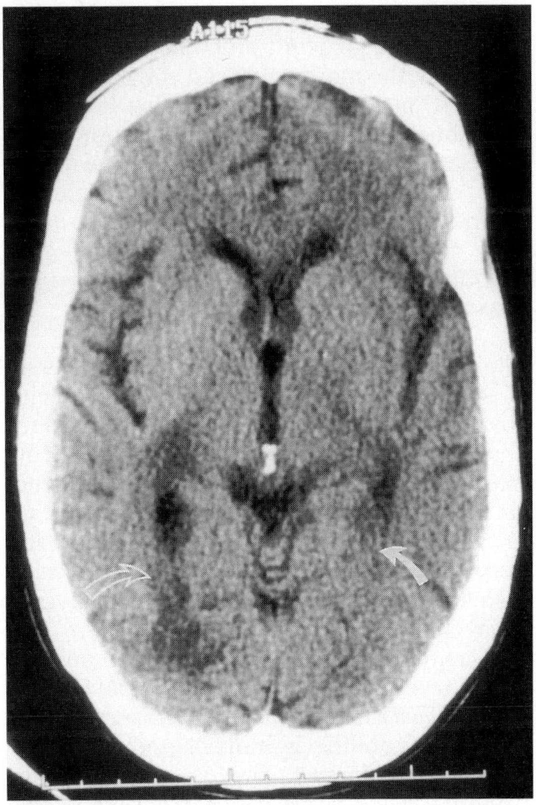

FIGURE 8–30. Progressive multifocal leukoencephalopathy in a patient with AIDS and a left homonymous hemianopia. The nonenhanced CT scan demonstrates hypodensity of the optic radiations, affecting the right hemisphere (*open arrow*) more than the left (*closed arrow*).

amination is generally unhelpful, although polymerase chain reaction testing for the JC virus in the CSF is highly sensitive and specific for PML.[271, 272] If necessary, the diagnosis may be confirmed by stereotactic biopsy.

No direct treatment has been proven to be effective. Despite supportive anectodal reports,[273] larger studies have demonstrated that neither IV nor intrathecal cytarabine improves survival in patients with PML.[274] However, the use of highly active antiretroviral therapy aimed at reducing HIV load seems also to improve the prognosis of PML.[275] This regimen is sometimes combined with cidofovir, another antiviral agent.[365]

Creutzfeldt–Jakob Disease

Uncommonly, hemianopias may be the initial presentation of Creutzfeldt–Jakob disease (CJD), and the neuroimaging, neurologic examination, and electroencephalography may be inconclusive in the early stages of the disease. However, usually by the time visual field loss is evident in patients with CJD, they are too demented for acuity and formal visual field testing. In the more advanced stages, patients with CJD often exhibit cortical blindness. Like Alzheimer's disease, CJD more commonly is associated with higher cortical visual disorders, so CJD is discussed in more detail in Chapter 9.

Abscesses

The presence of infectious cerebral abscesses is suggested by fever, seizures, headache, acute or subacute focal neurologic signs and symptoms, and multiple rim-enhancing masses on MRI or CT. The differential diagnosis includes bacterial, fungal, and parasitic infections.[276] Although contiguous infection and penetrating trauma are two recognized mechanisms, hematogenous spread is the most common cause.

Causitive bacterial agents include aerobes (eg, *Streptococcus viridans* and *Staphylococcus aureus*), anaerobes (eg, *Peptostreptococcus*), treponemes (syphilitic gummas), and mycobacteria (tuberculomas). The usual settings for bacterial abscesses are endocarditis, sinus disease, trauma, and sepsis.[277] Fungal infections include aspergillosis, cryptococcosis, histoplasmosis, coccidioidomycosis, and blastomycosis. These infections, especially aspergillosis, are well recognized in immunocompromised patients following bone marrow or liver transplantation.[278] Common parasitic abscesses include toxoplasmosis, which should be considered in any patients infected with HIV,[279] and cysticercosis, which should be suspected in individuals from endemic areas or with a history of travel to Central America or southeast Asia.

The diagnosis of a cerebral abscess usually can be established based on blood cultures or serum serologies, but occasionally needle or open biopsy is required. The appropriate antibacterial, antifungal, or antiparasitic drug can then be administered.

TRAUMA

Hemianopias and other types of retrochiasmal field loss can result from intra-axial and extra-axial disturbances related to head trauma. The most common setting is a motor vehicle accident, and one mechanism is diffuse and focal axonal injury affecting the optic radiations. Diffuse axonal injury, characterized by axonal stretching or tearing in the corpus callosum, subcortical white matter, cerebellar peduncles, and brain stem, results from shearing forces due to rotational acceleration and decelaration.[280, 281] Radiographically, punctate hemorrhages and edema are frequently evident acutely, but later atrophy and encephalomalacia often supervene.

Occasionally, conventional neuroimaging studies may be normal despite the presence of traumatically induced homonymous hemianopia. In such situations functional neuroimaging such as positron emission tomography (PET) or single photon emission computed tomography (SPECT) may confirm the localization of the suspected injury.[282]

If large enough, subdural and epidural hematomas overlying the cerebral convexities may compress the optic radiations. Intra-axial hematomas may also occur. Downward herniation in these settings may lead to impingement of the posterior cerebral artery and occipital lobe stroke. Other causes of injury include penetration by sharp objects and gun shots. In children, transient cortical visual loss may occur following minor or apparently trivial trauma. Blindness usually resolves within 24 hours, and neuroimaging is typically normal. Purported mechanisms include migrainous visual loss or vasospasm.[283]

ALZHEIMER'S DISEASE

Rarely, patients with Alzheimer's disease may present with a hemianopia.[284] However, more commonly the visual deficits in Alzheimer's disease are visuo-spatial due to involvement of the visual association cortices, and the geniculocalcarine pathways are spared.[285, 286] Thus this disorder is discussed in more detail in Chapter 9.

DEMYELINATION

Uncommonly a large demyelinating lesion in the optic radiations may cause a homonymous hemianopia.[11, 32, 287] This may occur in the setting of idiopathic demyelination, multiple sclerosis, or acute disseminated encephalomyelitis. Similar to optic neuritis, the prognosis for spontaneous visual recovery is good, with or without corticosteroids.[11] Small lesions in the optic radiations, which are very common radiographically, are usually clinically silent.[288] More destructive demyelinating lesions in the optic radiations may be seen in acute multiple sclerosis or acute hemorrhagic leukoencephalitis.

CONGENITAL/INFANTILE DISTURBANCES

Causes discussed here included those that occur in utero or during birth. Children with unilateral hemianopias since birth are often without visual complaints and may escape detection.[289, 290] On the other hand, if the visual loss is bilateral, children usually present with poor fixation, nystagmus, or strabismus. Visual acuity may be severely affected in the bilateral cases, sometimes as poor as no light perception in both eyes.[291] The terms *cortical blindness* and *cortical* or *cerebral visual impairment* have been used to describe the impairment in such patients.[292]

Because of the congenital nature of the retrochiasmal visual dysfunction, many affected patients develop an abnormal optic disc appearance resulting from transsynaptic degeneration. Commonly recognized subtypes of associated disc abnormalities in this setting include homonymous hemianopic hypoplasia, associated with unilateral hemispheric injury (see Chapter 5),[293] optic nerve hypoplasia, dysplasia, or atrophy, and enlarged cupping.[294] Nystagmus is usually not a feature of isolated, congenital retrochiasmal lesions unless these secondary optic disc abnormalities are also present.[295]

In one study[296] of 70 children with cortical visual impairment, periventricular leukomalacia was the most common cause in preterm infants, while hypoxic ischemic encephalopathy was the most common cause in term infants. Because these two disorders are usually bilateral, they are less common causes in children with unilateral hemianopias, in whom neoplasms are more frequent.[5]

Periventricular Leukomalacia

In premature and low birthweight infants, there is a predilection for ischemic injury to the periventricular white matter. Immature vascular development, watershed ischemia, and disturbances of myelinogenesis have been suggested mechanisms to account for the prenatal vulnerability of the white matter in these locales.[297–299] CT and MRI frequently demonstrate reduced amounts of periventricular white matter and ventricular dilation, particularly where the optic radiations course around the occipital horn of the lateral ventricle. Affected areas are often hyperintense on T_2-weighted MR images (Fig. 8–31),[300] but these changes may not be evident until the child is several months to a year old, once myelination has occurred. Usually the process is bilateral, but for unclear reasons occasionally one hemisphere can be involved much more than the other.[301] More severe cases, frequently resulting in cerebral visual impairment,[302] may be associated with cystic leukomalacia or a history of intraventricular hemorrhage and hydrocephalus.

Stroke in Utero

Occasionally a child with a hemianopia is found to have a porencephalic (filled with CSF) lesion, which respects the MCA or PCA vascular territories.[303] An in utero vascular insult is presumed to have caused the cortical abnormality. In addition to the visual field defect, children with in utero MCA strokes usually have a hemiparesis and hemibody atrophy.[304] Often the cause of the stroke is not found, but both the child and the mother should be evaluated for hypercoagulable disorders.[305]

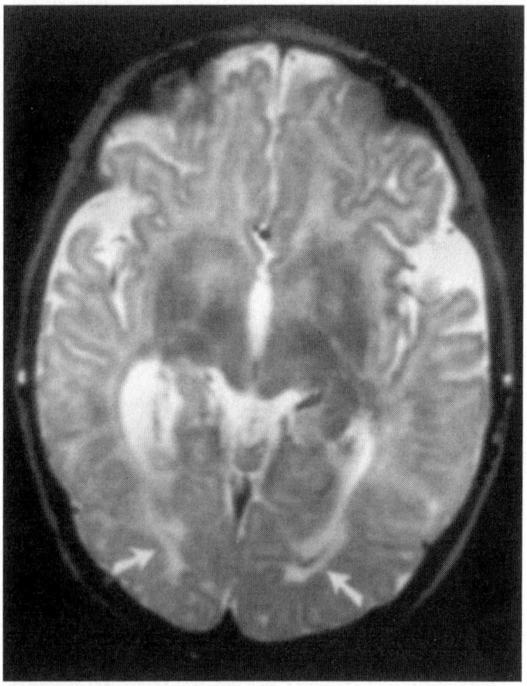

FIGURE 8–31. Periventricular leukomalacia, most apparent as the bright areas posteriorly (*arrows*), in this T_2-weighted axial MR image.

Cortical Dysplasia

Congenital retrochiasmal field loss may also be caused by cerebral cortex that is malformed and dysfunctional.[303,306] Dysplastic cortex, usually a disorder of cortical migration, is characterized radiographycally by the absence of the normal gyral and sulcal pattern, seen best on MRI. Generalized developmental disorders of cerebral cortex include lissencephaly (agyria), pachygyria, band heterotopia, subependymal heterotopias, and hemimegalancephaly.[307] In addition to focal cortical dysplasias, other focal processes include polymicrogyria, focal subcortical heterotopias, schizencephaly, which is characterized by cerebral clefts,[308] and tuberous sclerosis (see Chapter 4).[307] The most common presentation of a cortical dysplasia is epilepsy.[309]

Hypoxic Ischemic Encephalopathy

In contrast to the aforementioned prenatal disorders, hypoxic ischemic encephalopathy is more typically associated with perinatal birth asphyxia.[310, 311] Neuroimaging typically demonstrates diffuse tissue loss involving white and grey matter structures with compensatory ventricular dilation (Fig. 8–32) The changes may be severe, resulting in cystic encephalomalacia. The children may exhibit microcephaly, developmental delay, cortical visual loss, quadriparesis, spasticity, and seizures. Visual function may be as poor as "tunnel" vision, light perception only, and even no light perception.[312] The severity of visual dysfunction typically correlates with the amount of radiographically evident damage to the optic radiations and striate and parastriate cortices.[292, 313, 314]

Mitochondrial Myopathy, Encephalopathy, Lactic Acidosis, and Strokelike Episodes (MELAS)

MELAS, first characterized by Pavlakis et al,[315] is a mitochondrial disorder typified clinically by recurrent migraine or strokelike episodes in children and young adults. Attacks usually consist of headache, nausea, vomiting, focal and generalized seizures, followed by transient hemianopia, cortical blindness, or hemiparesis.[316, 317] Other less commonly associated ophthalmologic features include bilateral ptosis, chronic external ophthalmoplegia, diffuse choroidal atrophy, atypical pigmentary retinopathy with macular involvement,

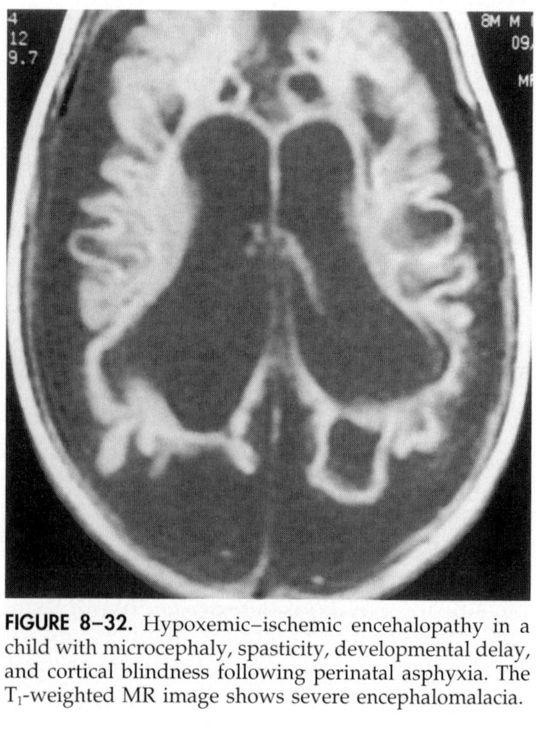

FIGURE 8–32. Hypoxemic–ischemic encehalopathy in a child with microcephaly, spasticity, developmental delay, and cortical blindness following perinatal asphyxia. The T_1-weighted MR image shows severe encephalomalacia.

optic atrophy, and patchy atrophy of the iris stroma.[318, 319, 366] However, the ocular findings are usually absent.

MELAS is a relatively uncommon disorder, and was not included in a childhood series of hemifield loss that spanned 3.5 years.[5] In a study of 38 patients between 18 and 45 years of age with an occipital lobe stroke, MELAS was diagnosed in one.[320]

Onset is usually in childhood, and cases after age 40 are exceptional.[321, 322, 367] There is usually a history of normal early development, short stature, and exercise intolerance due to muscle weakness, some patients may have sensorineural hearing loss. Eventually, however, progressive neurologic decline, dementia, and eventually death is the typical course. An earlier onset of symptoms (occurring before age 2) is associated with more rapid progression.[323]

Pathology. Affected cortical areas are characterized pathologically by spongy degeneration most prominent at the crests of gyri, and on electron microscopy the blood vessels contain abnormal mitochondria within the vascular smooth muscle and in endothelial cells.[324] Muscle biopsies may reveal ragged red fibers and other evidence of defective mitochondria.[325]

Diagnostic Studies. Eighty to ninety percent of patients with MELAS have an associated point mutation in the mitochondrial DNA at nucleotide 3243 of $tRNA^{Leu(UUR)}$.[321] Less common mutations are seen at nucleotide 3271 of $tRNA^{Leu(UUR)}$, in the subunit 4 of complex I (ND4),[321] and at nucleotide 1642 of $tRNA^{Val}$.[326] Serum and CSF lactate are typically elevated. MELAS, along with Kearn–Sayre syndrome, chronic external ophthalmoplegia (see Chapter 15), and MERRF (myoclonic epilepsy with ragged red fibers), are the mitochondrial myopathies associated with ragged red fibers on muscle biopsy. During strokelike episodes, T_2-weighted MRI usually reveals hyperintensities in the temporal, parietal, and occipital cortices, not respecting the usual MCA or PCA vascular territories.[324] MR spectroscopy may reveal increased lactate in the occipital and temporal lobes,[324] and on CT basal ganglia calcification may be seen.

Treatment. Vitamins, coenzymes (Q10, for example), riboflavin, nicotinamide,[327] and dichloroacetate[326] have been associated either with anectodal improvement in clinical symptoms and signs or decrease in serum lactate. However, most current treatments are unable to alter the ultimate progression of the disease.

Other Childhood Disorders

Adrenoleukodystrophy. In this rare X-linked childhood disorder of young boys, CNS demyelination is caused by a defect in peroxisomal long-chain fatty acid metabolism.[328, 329] Long-chain fatty acids accumulate in the brain white matter and adrenal glands, leading to abnormal behavior and cognition, visual loss, gait disturbances, skin hyperpigmentation, and hypoadrenalism.[330] The neurologic and systemic abnormalities usually precede the visual manifestations by several years. Visual disturbances, which are either retrochiasmal or due to optic nerve demyelination with associated optic atrophy, are typically relentlessly progressive in untreated cases.[331, 332] The diagnosis is suggested when elevated levels of serum very long-chain fatty acids are detected. Treatments include Lorenzo oil or bone marrow transplantation. An adult form[333] and an adrenomyeloneuropathic variant[334, 335] have also been described.

Sturge–Weber (Encephalotrigeminal Angiomatosis). This phakomatosis is characterized by a facial capillary hemangioma, often accompanied by a leptomeningeal vascular malformation (Fig. 8–33).[336] The inheritance pattern is sporadic.[337] The facial lesion has a port-wine color and is usually unilateral. Commonly associated ocular findings include glaucoma and a "tomato ketchup" fundus due to choroidal involvement by the hemangioma. The intracranial vascular disturbance is usually located in the posterior half of the brain and can often cause a homonymous hemianopia, seizures, developmental delay, or hemiparesis.[338–340] On neuroimaging, cortical atrophy, leptomeningeal enhancement, and gyriform cortical calcification are pathognomonic. Transient field defects may be the result of seizures or ischemia.

Meningitis. Cortical damage associated with bacterial meningitis may be caused by arterial occlusion or venous thrombosis. More severely affected children can develop encephalomalacia with loculated cysts.

Delayed Visual Maturation. This well-recognized condition is characterized by abnormal visual function in the first year of life despite apparently normal and intact visual pathways.[341] Pupillary reactivity, funduscopic appearance, and neuroimaging are normal. Uniformly, vision improves spontaneously. Delayed myelination of the posterior visual pathways or delayed dendrite and synapse

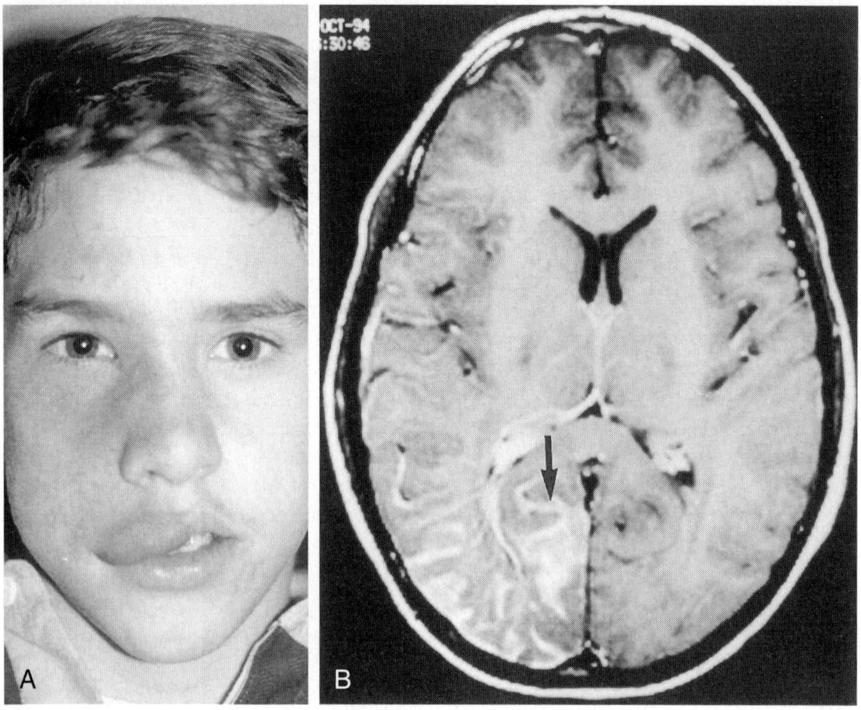

FIGURE 8–33. Sturge–Weber syndrome. **A.** This teenage boy with a right facial angioma had a transient left homonymous hemianopia. **B.** Gyral enhancement (*arrow*) of the right occipital lobe was demonstrated by MRI.

formation in the striate cortex have been implicated. Masqueraders, such as Leber's congenital amaurosis and congenital ocular motor apraxia (see Chapter 16), must be excluded.

ICTAL

Both ictal homonymous hemianopias and ictal cortical blindness are well recognized but infrequent. Postictal hemifield loss and cortical blindness are even less common and suggest an underlying, irritative structural lesion. Visual loss associated with seizures is discussed in more detail in Chapter 10.

FUNCTIONAL

Functional homonymous hemifield loss is unusual and is discussed in Chapter 11.

DIAGNOSTIC EVALUATION IN PATIENTS WITH SUSPECTED RETROCHIASMAL LESIONS

Neuroimaging

All patients with homonymous hemianopias require neuroimaging, preferably MRI. Attention to the sella and optic tract is required when the field defect is associated with optic atrophy or an afferent pupillary defect. When a stroke is suspected, because of the sudden onset of visual loss in a middle-aged or an elderly patient with vasculopathic risk factors, diffusion-weighted and FLAIR images can be obtained in addition to routine T_1- and T_2-weighted and gadolinium-enhanced scans. When MRI is contraindicated, due to claustrophobia, cardiac pacemaker, or aneurysm clips, for example, CT with and without contrast can be performed.

Vascular anatomy may be assessed with MRI-angiography of the circle of Willis, carotid arteries, and vertebral arteries. Cerebral angiography may be necessary for more definitive evaluation, such as prior to endarterectomy.

Some experimental functional neuroimaging techniques may be helpful in cases where MRI or CT is inconclusive. Using PET or SPECT techniques, hypoperfusion in visual cortex areas may be demonstrated in patients with unexplained visual field loss.[282, 342, 362] Functional MRI can highlight areas of cortical activation by detecting small changes in local blood flow.[363] This technique may be more helpful for localization of normally functioning areas of brain.

Other Diagnostic Studies

Blood studies are indicated when specific pathologic processes are suspected. Vascular events may require evaluation of the erythrocyte sedimentation rate (ESR), rapid plasmin reagin (RPR), antinuclear antibody (ANA), and coagulation indices such as prothrombin time, partial thromboplastin time (PT and PTT), and platelet count. The ESR and C-reactive protein are particularly important in the evaluation of transient or permanent visual loss in the elderly to rule out giant cell arteritis. In young individuals without an obvious risk factor for stroke, protein C, protein S, antithrombin III, factor V, antiphospholipid antibody, and anticardiolipin antibody levels should be obtained. Cardiac source emboli can be excluded by an electrocardiogram, cardiac monitoring (telemetry or Holter), and transthoracic echocardiography (TTE). If the TTE is unrevealing, and a patent foramen ovale or valvular abnormality is still highly suspected, then transesophageal echocardiography (TEE) can be ordered.

Other noninvasive vascular techniques may complement MRI-angiography in the patient with a suspected stroke. These include carotid doppler studies, which are most helpful in the evaluation of extracranial carotid artery disease, and transcranial doppler studies, which may aid in the detection of intracranial stenosis, collateral flow, and vasospasm.

A toxicology screen is necessary if drug use is suspected. Most intracranial mass lesions require either at least brain biopsy if a primary neoplasm is suspected, or a metastatic evaluation if multiple metastases are more likely. In many cases of demyelinating disease, other autoimmune, inflammatory, a infectious disorders should be excluded by evaluating the ANA, angiotensin converting enzyme (ACE), Lyme titre, and ESR, for instance.

Visual evoked potentials (VEPs) may have a useful role in children with cortical visual impairment, as a normal study may be associated with a favorable visual outcome.[341] However, abnormal VEPs do not preclude visual improvement.[343] VEPs probably have no clinical utility in adults with retrochiasmal field loss.

PRACTICAL ADVICE, HEMIANOPIC PRISMS, AND VISUAL REHABILITATION

Initially, patients with acquired homonymous hemianopias may not notice their field defect, especially if a right hemispheric lesion is responsible. Eventually, however, most adult patients become aware of their defective peripheral vision.

Those with dense field deficits may bump into objects in their blind hemifield. We caution affected patients that they have to turn their head to see into the defective field, but most learn to do that anyway. We also instruct family members to approach the patient from within the intact hemifield, and keep food, utensils, and beverages within the patient's intact hemifield when eating. At least initially, patients with dense hemianopias should not be allowed to cross the street independently. Furthermore, their defective vision prohibits them from driving.

Many have difficulty reading, because a left hemianopia may hamper their ability to find the beginning of the next line, and a right hemianopia may not allow them to appreciate the entire line of words. Macular splitting and paracentral defects may make seeing individual words difficult. A colored piece of paper placed vertically along the left or right side of the page is often helpful when the margins are a source of difficulty. It can also be used horizontally and moved down the lines of the page. Other strategies include teaching patients with left hemianopias to shift their gaze to the left side of every line and to the first letter of every word, and instructing those with right hemianopias to reach the end of a word before going to the next.[115]

Hemianopic Prisms

Patients with chronic, dense homonymous hemianopias can be offered prism therapy,[344, 345] but only a minority of them will find it beneficial. Base-out prism therapy should be attempted only in individuals who have normal mentation and in whom the hemianopia is isolated. A 15- to 45- (usually 30-) diopter base-out Fresnel press-on prism can be placed on the temporal half of an eyeglass ipsilateral to the hemianopia (Fig. 8–34). This optically displaces images in the blind half of vision into the good hemifield. A central area can be trimmed from the Fresnel prism to reduce double vision. The patients who like the prism therapy are those who use the prism to notice novel objects in their blind field; they then turn their head in that direction to use their good field to see the objects more clearly. Unfortunately, most individuals find this too

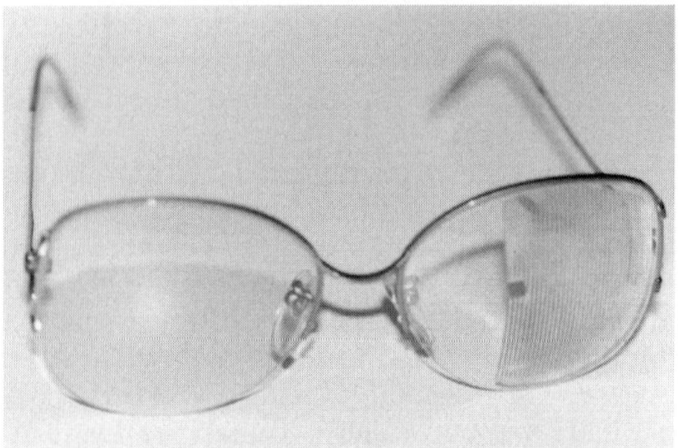

FIGURE 8–34. Hemianopic prism for an individual with a left homonymous visual field defect. A 30-diopter base-out Fresnel prism is placed over the temporal half of the left lens. A notch was cut out over the optical center to reduce double vision.

confusing and suboptimal and only 20% to 30% continue to use it. It certainly does not improve their vision to the point where they can drive or read normally. In the only controlled study, no functional benefit in activities of daily living was demonstrated.[346] Wide-angle lenses or mirror devices attached to the spectacle frame have also been used with limited success.

Visual Rehabilitation

We have found that visual occupational therapy and rehabilitation is relatively unhelpful. Compensatory oculomotor strategies, designed to enhance visual saccades into and exploration within the defective hemifield, may be tried.[115] Training of blindsight and recovering some lost visual field have also been attempted.[115,347,348] Although study parameters, such as search times and saccadic accuracy, may be improved,[349] proof is scant from any comparative study that visual training after injury makes any difference in the speed or amount of functional visual recovery.

REFERENCES

1. Huber A: Homonymous hemianopia (editorial). Neuro-ophthalmol 1992;12:351–366.
2. Fujino T, Kigazawa K, Yamada R: Homonymous hemianopia. A retrospective study of 140 cases. Neuro-ophthalmol 1986;6:17–21.
3. Smith JL: Homonymous hemianopia. A review of 100 cases. Am J Ophthalmol 1962;54:616–622.
4. Trobe JD, Lorber ML, Schlezinger NS: Isolated homonymous hemianopia. A review of 104 cases. Arch Ophthalmol 1973;89:377–381.
5. Liu GT, Galetta SL: Homonymous hemifield loss in children. Neurology 1997;49:1748–1749.
6. Kupersmith MJ: Circulation of the eye, orbit, cranial nerves, and brain. In: Neurovascular Neuro-ophthalmology, pp 1–67. Berlin, Springer-Verlag, 1993.
7. Harrington DO, Drake MV: Postchiasmal visual pathway. In: The Visual Fields. Text and Atlas of Clinical Perimetry, 6th edition, pp 311–361. St. Louis, CV Mosby, 1990.
8. Savino PJ, Paris M, Schatz NJ, et al: Optic tract syndrome. A review of 21 patients. Arch Ophthalmol 1978;96:656–663.
9. Bender MB, Bodis-Wollner I: Visual dysfunctions in optic tract lesions. Ann Neurol 1978;3:187–193.
10. Archer JS, Gracies J-M, Tohver E, et al: Bilateral optic disk pallor after unilateral internal carotid artery occlusion. Neurology 1998;50:809–811.
11. Plant GT, Kermode AG, Turano G, et al: Symptomatic retrochiasmal lesions in multiple sclerosis: clinical features, visual evoked potentials, and magnetic resonance imaging. Neurology 1992;42:68–76.
12. Kupersmith MJ, Vargas M, Hoyt WF, et al: Optic tract atrophy with cerebral arteriovenous malformations. Direct and transsynaptic degeneration. Neurology 1994;44:80–83.
13. Groom M, Kay MD, Vicinanza-Adami C, et al: Optic tract syndrome secondary to metastatic breast cancer. Am J Ophthalmol 1998;125:115–118.
14. Margo CE, Hamed LM, McCarty J: Congenital optic tract syndrome. Arch Ophthalmol 1991;109:1120–1122.
15. Horton JC, Landau K, Maeder P, et al: Magnetic resonance imaging of the human lateral geniculate body. Arch Neurol 1990;47:1201–1206.
16. Carpenter MB: Blood supply of the central nervous system. In: Core Text of Neuroanatomy, 4th edition, pp 391–416. Baltimore, Williams & Wilkins, 1991.
17. Neau J-P, Bogousslavsky J: The syndrome of posterior choroidal artery territory infarction. Ann Neurol 1996;39:779–788.
18. Glaser JS, Sadun AA: Anatomy of the visual sensory system. In: Glaser JS (ed): Neuro-ophthalmology, 2nd edition, pp 61–82. Philadelphia, JB Lippincott, 1990.
19. Gunderson CH, Hoyt WF: Geniculate hemianopia: incongruous homonymous field defects in two patients with partial lesions of the lateral geniculate nucleus. J Neurol Neurosurg Psychiatr 1971;34:1–6.
20. Schaklett DE, O'Connor PS, Dorwart RH, et al: Congruous and incongruous sectorial visual field defects with lesions of the lateral geniculate nucleus. Am J Ophthalmol 1984;98:283–290.
21. Carter JE, O'Connor P, Shacklett D, et al: Lesions of the optic radiations mimicking lateral geniculate nucleus visual field defects. J Neurol Neurosurg Psychiatry 1985;48:982–988.
22. Grochowicki M, Vighetto A: Homonymous horizontal sectoranopia: report of four cases. Br J Ophthalmol 1991;75:624–628.
23. Grossman M, Galetta SL, Nichols CW, et al: Horizontal homonymous sectoral field defect after ischemic infarction of the occipital cortex. Am J Ophthalmol 1990;109:234–236.
24. Frisén L: Quadruple sectoranopsia and sectorial optic atrophy: a syndrome of the distal anterior choroidal artery. J Neurol Neurosurg Psychiatry 1979;42: 590–594.
25. Frisén L, Homegaard L, Rosencrantz M: Sectorial optic atrophy and homonymous, horizontal sectoranop-

sia: a lateral choroidal artery syndrome. J Neurol Neurosurg Psychiatry 1978;41:374–380.

26. Suzuki H, Fujita K, Ehara K, et al: Anterior choroidal artery syndrome after surgery for internal carotid artery aneurysms. Neurosurgery 1992;31:132–136.
27. Luco C, Hoppe A, Schweitzer M, et al: Visual field defects in vascular lesions of the lateral geniculate body. J Neurol Neurosurg Psychiatry 1992;55:12–15.
28. Borruat F-X, Maeder P: Sectoranopia after head trauma: evidence of lateral geniculate body lesion on MRI. Neurology 1995;45:590–592.
29. Kosmorsky G, Lancione RR: When fighting makes you see black holes instead of stars. J Neuro-ophthalmol 1998;18:255–257.
30. Donahue SP, Kardon RH, Thompson HS: Hourglass-shaped visual fields as a sign of bilateral lateral geniculate myelinolysis. Am J Ophthalmol 1995;119: 378–380.
31. Tatu L, Moulin T, Bogousslavsky J, et al: Arterial territories of the human brain. Cerebral hemispheres. Neurology 1998;50:1699–1708.
32. Borruat F-X, Siatkowski RM, Schatz NJ, et al: Congruous quadrantanopia and optic radiation lesion. Neurology 1993;43:1430–1432.
33. Jacobson DM: The localizing value of a quadrantanopia. Arch Neurol 1997;54:401–404.
34. Cogan DG: Neurologic significance of lateral conjugate deviation of the eyes on forced closure of the lids. Arch Ophthalmol 1948;39:37–42.
35. Smith JL, Gay AJ, Cogan DG: The spasticity of conjugate gaze phenomenon. Arch Ophthalmol 1959;62: 694–696.
36. Sullivan HC, Kaminski HJ, Mass EF, et al: Lateral deviation of the eyes on forced lid closure in patients with cerebral lesions. Arch Ophthalmol 1991;48: 310–311.
37. Tecoma ES, Laxer KD, Barbaro NM, et al: Frequency and characteristics of visual field deficits after surgery for mesial temporal sclerosis. Neurology 1993;43: 1235–1238.
38. Zeki S: The P and M pathways and 'what and where' doctrine. In: A Vision of the Brain, pp 186–196. Oxford, Blackwell Scientific, 1993.
39. Horton JC, Hoyt WF: The representation of the visual field in human striate cortex. A revision of the classic Holmes map. Arch Ophthalmol 1991;109:816–824.
40. McFadzean R, Brosnahan D, Hadley D, et al: Representation of the visual field in the occipital striate cortex. Br J Ophthalmol 1994;78:185–190.
41. Wong AMF, Sharpe JA: Representation of the visual field in human occipital cortex. Arch Ophthalmol 1999;117:208–217.
42. Horton JC: Arrangement of ocular dominance columns in human visual cortex. Arch Ophthalmol 1990;108:1025–1031.
43. Gray LG, Galetta SL, Schatz NJ: Vertical and horizontal meridian sparing in occipital lobe homonymous hemianopia. Neurology 1998;50:1170–1173.
44. Smith CG, Richardson WFG: The course and distribution of the arteries supplying the visual (striate) cortex. Am J Ophthalmol 1966;61:1391–1396.
45. Gasecki AP, Fox AJ, Daneault N: Bilateral occipital infarctions associated with carotid stenosis in a patient with persistent trigeminal artery. Stroke 1994;25:1520–1523.
46. Balcer LJ, Galetta SL, Hurst RW, et al: Occipital lobe infarction from a carotid artery embolic source. J Neuro-ophthalmol 1996;16:33–35.
47. Bischoff P, Lang J, Huber A: Macular sparing as a perimetric artifact. Am J Ophthalmol 1995;119:72–80.
48. Gray LG, Galetta SL, Siegal T, et al: The central visual field in homonymous hemianopia. Arch Neurol 1997;54:312–317.
49. Trauzettel-Klosinski S, Reinhard J: The vertical field border in hemianopia and its significance for fixation and reading. Invest Ophthalmol Vis Sci 1998;39:2177–2186.
50. Kölmel HW: Homonymous paracentral scotomas. J Neurol 1987;235:22–25.
51. Benton S, Levy I, Swash M: Vision in the temporal crescent in occipital infarction. Brain 1980;103:83–97.
52. Landau K, Wichmann W, Valavanis A: The missing temporal crescent. Am J Ophthalmol 1995;119: 345–349.
53. Chavis PS, Al-Hazmi A, Clunie D, et al: Temporal crescent syndrome with magnetic resonance correlation. J Neuro-ophthalmol 1997;17:151–155.
54. Horton JC, Hoyt WF: Quadrantic visual field defects. A hallmark of lesions in extrastriate (V2/V3) cortex. Brain 1991;114:1703–1718.
55. McFadzean RM, Hadley DM: Homonymous quadrantanopia specting the horizontal meridian. A feature of striate and extrastriate cortical disease. Neurology 1997;49:1741–1746.
56. Cross SA, Smith JL: Crossed-quadrant homonymous hemianopsia. The "checkerboard" field defect. J Clin Neuro-ophthalmol 1982;2:149–158.
57. Newman RP, Kinkel WR, Jacobs L: Altitudinal hemianopia caused by occipital infarctions. Clinical and computerized tomographic correlations. Arch Neurol 1984;41:413–418.
58. Liu GT, Ronthal M: Reflex blink to visual threat. J Clin Neuro-ophthalmol 1992;12:47–56.
59. Riddoch G: Dissociation of visual perceptions due to occipital injuries, with especial reference to appreciation of movement. Brain 1917;40:15–57.
60. Holmes G: Disturbances of vision by cerebral lesions. Br J Ophthalmol 1918;2:353–384.
61. Pöppel E, Held R, Frost D: Residual visual function after brain wounds involving the central visual pathways in man. Nature 1973;243:295–296.
62. Sanders MD, Warrington EK, Marshall J, et al: "Blindsight" vision in a field defect. Lancet 1974;1:707–708.
63. Damasio AR, Damasio H, Ferro JM, et al: Recovery from hemianopia in man: evidence for collicular vision? Lancet 1974;2:110.
64. Weiskrantz L, Warrington EK, Sanders MD, et al: Visual capacity in the hemianopic field following a restricted occipital ablation. Brain 1974;97:709–728.
65. Barbur JL, Ruddock KH, Waterfield VA: Human visual responses in the absence of the geniculo-calcarine projection. Brain 1980;103:905–928.
66. Blythe IM, Kennard C, Ruddock KH: Residual vision in patients with retrogeniculate lesions of the visual pathways. Brain 1987;110:887–905.
67. Stoerig P, Cowey A: Blindsight in man and monkey. Brain 1997;120:535–559.
68. Zihl J, Von Cramon D: The contribution of the 'second' visual system to directed visual attention in man. Brain 1979;102:835–856.
69. Schneider GE: Two visual systems. Brain mechanisms for localization and discrimination are dissociated by tectal and cortical lesions. Science 1969;163: 895–902.
70. Rafal R, Smith J, Krantz J, et al: Extrageniculate vision in hemianopic humans: saccade inhibition by signals in the blind field. Science 1990;250:118–120.

71. Zeki S, ffytche DH: The Riddoch syndrome: insights into the neurobiology of conscious vision. Brain 1998;121:25–45.
72. Stoerig P, Kleinschmidt A, Frahm J: No visual responses in denervated VI: high-resolution functional magnetic resonance imaging of a blindsight patient. Neuroreport 1998;9:21–25.
73. Barton JJ, Sharpe JA: Smooth pursuit and saccades to moving targets in blind hemifields. A comparison of medial occipital, lateral occipital and optic radiation lesions. Brain 1997;120:681–699.
74. Barton JJ, Sharpe JA: Motion direction discrimination in blind hemifields. Ann Neurol 1997;41:255–264.
75. Farah M, Feinberg TE: Perception and awareness. In: Feinberg TE, Farah MJ (eds): Behavirol Neurology and Neuropsychology, pp 357–368. New York, McGraw–Hill, 1997.
76. Fendrich R, Wessinger CM, Gazzaniga MS: Residual vision in a scotoma: implications for blindsight. Science 1992;258:1489–1491.
77. Cowey A, Stoerig P: The neurobiology of blindsight. Trends Neurosci 1991;14:140–145.
78. Campion J, Latto R, Smith YM: Is blindsight an effect of scattered light, spared cortex, and near-threshold vision? Behav Brain Sci 1983;6:423–486.
79. Safran AB, Glaser JS: Statokinetic dissociation in lesions of the anterior visual pathways. A reappraisal of the Riddoch phenomenon. Arch Ophthalmol 1980;98:291–295.
80. Liu GT: Anatomy and physiology of the trigeminal nerve. In: Miller NR, Newman NJ (eds): Walsh and Hoyt's Clinical Neuro-ophthalmology, 4th edition, pp 1595–1648. Baltimore, Williams & Wilkins, 1998.
81. Hommel M, Besson G, Pollak P, et al: Hemiplegia in posterior cerebral artery occulsion. Neurology 1990; 40:1496–1499.
82. Hommel M, Moreaud O, Besson G, et al: Site of arterial occlusion in the hemiplegic posterior cerebral artery syndrome. Neurology 1991;41:604–605.
83. Chambers BR, Brooder RJ, Donnan GA: Proximal posterior cerebral artery occlusion simulating middle cerebral artery occlusion. Neurology 1991;41: 385–390.
84. Caplan LR: "Top of the basilar syndrome." Neurology 1980;30:72–79.
85. Aldrich MS, Alessi AG, Beck RW, et al: Cortical blindness: etiology, diagnosis, and prognosis. Ann Neurol 1987;21:149–158.
86. Dyken ML, Wolf PA, Barnett HJM, et al: Risk factors in stroke. Stroke 1984;15:1105–1111.
87. Colditz GA, Bonita R, Stampfer MJ, et al: Cigarette smoking and risk of stroke in middle-aged women. N Engl J Med 1988;318:937–941.
88. Wolf PA, D'Agostino RB, Kannel WB, et al: Cigarette smoking as a risk factor for stroke. The Framingham study. JAMA 1988;259:1025–1029.
89. Iso H, Jacobs DR, Wentworth D, et al: Serum cholesterol levels and six-year mortality from stroke in 350,977 men screened for the multiple risk factor intervention trial. N Engl J Med 1989;320:904–910.
90. Heinsius T, Bogousslavsky J, Melle GV: Large infarcts in the middle cerebral artery territory. Etiology and outcome patterns. Neurology 1998;50:341–350.
91. Pessin MS, Lathi ES, Cohen MB, et al: Clinical features and mechanism of occipital infarction. Ann Neurol 1987;21:290–299.
92. Bogousslavsky J, Regli F, Maeder P, et al: The etiology of posterior circulation infarcts: a prospective study using magnetic resonance imaging and magnetic resonance angiography. Neurology 1993;43:1528–1533.
93. Cerebral embolism task force: Cardiogenic brain embolism. The second report of the cerebral embolism task force. Arch Neurol 1989;46:727–743.
94. Pessin MS, Kwan ES, DeWitt LD, et al: Posterior cerebral artery stenosis. Ann Neurol 1987;21:85–89.
95. Lutsep HL, Albers GW, DeCrespigny A, et al: Clinical utility of diffusion-weighted magnetic resonance imaging in the assessment of ischemic stroke. Ann Neurol 1997;41:574–580.
96. Sacco RL: Risk factors, outcomes, and stroke subtypes for ischemic stroke. Neurology 1997;49(Suppl 4): S39–S44.
97. Sacco RL: Identifying patient populations at high risk for stroke. Neurology 1998;51(Suppl 3):S27–S30.
98. Bronner LL, Kanter DS, Manson JE: Primary prevention of stroke. N Engl J Med 1995;333:1392–1400.
99. Hebert PR, Gaziano JM, Chan KS, et al: Cholesterol lowering with statin drugs, risk of stroke, and total mortality: an overview of randomized trials. JAMA 1997;278:313–321.
100. Raps EC: Acute treatment of ischemic stroke. New horizons in stroke prevention: raising the standard of care. Philadelphia, October 25, 1997:31–39.
101. Saver JL, Starkman S: State of the art medical management of acute ischemic stroke. J Stroke Cerebrovasc Dis 1997;6:189–194.
102. Adams HP, Brott TG, Furlan AJ, et al: Guidelines for thrombolytic therapy for acute stroke: a supplement to the guidelines for the management of patients with acute ischemic stroke. A statement for healthcare professionals from a special writing group of the Stroke Council, American Heart Association. Circulation 1996;94:1167–1174.
103. Lyden PD, Grotta JC, Levine SR, et al: Intravenous thrombolysis for acute stroke. Neurology 1997;49: 14–29.
104. Caplan LR, Mohr JP, Kistler JP, et al: Should thrombolytic therapy be the first-line treatment for acute stroke? N Engl J Med 1997;337:1309–1313.
105. Hacke W, Kaste M, Fieschi C, et al: Intravenous thrombolysis with recombinant tissue plasminogen activator for acute hemispheric stroke: the European Cooperative Acute Stroke Study (ECASS). JAMA 1995;274:1017–1025.
106. The National Institute of Neurological Disorders and Stroke rt-PA Stroke Study Group: Tissue plasminogen activator for acute ischemic stroke. N Engl J Med 1995;333:1581–1587.
107. Morgenstern LB: rtPA in acute ischemic stroke: the North American perspective. Neurology 1997;49 (Suppl 4):S63–S65.
108. Hacke W: rtPA in acute ischemic stroke: European perspective. Neurology 1997;49(Suppl 4):S60–S62.
109. Kwiatkowski TG, Libman RB, Frankel M, et al: Effects of tissue plasminogen activator for acute ischemic stroke at one year. N Engl J Med 1999;340:1781–1787.
110. The Multicenter Acute Stroke Trial–Europe Study Group: Thrombolytic therapy with streptokinase in acute ischemic stroke. N Engl J Med 1996;335: 145–150.
111. Hurst RW, Raps EC, Zager E, et al: Selective intraarterial thrombolysis in acute stroke: implications for emergency management. J Stroke Cerebrovasc Dis 1994;4:30–35.
112. Lees KR: Cerestat and other NMDA antagonists in ischemic stroke. Neurology 1997;49(Suppl 4):S66–S69.

113. Rothlein R: Overview of leukocyte adhesion. Neurology 1997;49(Suppl 4):S3–S4.
114. Hallenbeck JM: Cytokines, macrophages, and leukocytes in brain ischemia. Neurology 1997;49(Suppl 4):S5–S9.
115. Pambakian AL, Kennard C: Can visual function be restored in patients with homonymous hemianopia? Br J Ophthalmol 1997;81:324–328.
116. Blackshear JL, Kopecky SL, Litin SC, et al: Management of atrial fibrillation in adults: prevention of thromboembolism and symptomatic treatment. Mayo Clin Proc 1996;71:150–160.
117. Wolf PA, Dawber TR, Thomas HE, et al: Epidemiologic assessment of chronic atrial fibrillation and risk of stroke. Neurology 1978;28:973–977.
118. Hylek EM, Skates SJ, Sheehan MA, et al: An analysis of the lowest effective intensity of prophylactic anticoagulation for patients with nonrheumatic atrial fibrillation. N Engl J Med 1996;335:540–546.
119. Peterson P, Boysen G, Godtfredson J, et al: Placebo-controlled, randomised trial of warfarin and aspirin for prevention of thromboembolic complications in chromic atrial fibrillation. The Copenhagen AFASAK study. Lancet 1989;1:175–179.
120. The Boston Area Anticoagulation Trial for Atrial Fibrillation investigators: The effect of low-dose warfarin on the risk of stroke in patients with nonrheumatic atrial fibrillation. N Engl J Med 1990;323:1505–1511.
121. Stroke Prevention in Atrial Fibrillation investigators: Stroke Prevention in Atrial Fibrillation Study: final results. Circulation 1991;84:527–539.
122. Ezelkowitz MD, Bridgers SL, James KE, et al: Warfarin in the prevention of stroke associated with nonrheumatic atrial fibrillation. N Engl J Med 1992; 327:1406–1412.
123. EAFT (European Atrial Fibrillation Trial) study group: Secondary prevention in non-rheumatic atrial fibrillation after transient ischaemic attack or minor stroke. Lancet 1993;342:1255–1262.
124. Stroke Prevention in Atrial Fibrillation investigators: Warfarin versus aspirin for prevention of thromboembolism in atrial fibrillation. Lancet 1994;343: 687–691.
125. Hart RG, Sherman DG, Easton JD, et al: Prevention of stroke in patients with nonvalvular atrial fibrillation. Neurology 1998;51:674–681.
126. Hart RG, Easton JD: Hemorrhagic infarcts. Stroke 1986;17:586–589.
127. Chamorro A, Vila N, Saiz A, et al: Early anticoagulation after large cerebral embolic infarction: a safety study. Neurology 1995;45:861–865.
128. Pessin MS, Estol CJ, Lafranchise F, et al: Safety of anticoagulation after hemorrhagic infarction. Neurology 1993;43:1298–1303.
129. Loh E, St. John Sutton M, Wun C-CC, et al: Ventricular dysfunction and the risk of stroke after myocardial infarction. N Engl J Med 1997;336:251–257.
130. Lechat P, Mass JL, Lascault G, et al: Prevalence of patent foramen ovale in patients with stroke. N Engl J Med 1988;318:1148–1152.
131. Petty GW, Khandheria BK, Chu CP, et al: Patent foramen ovale in patients with cerebral infarction. A transesophageal echocardiographic study. Arch Neurol 1997;54:819–822.
132. Devuyst G, Bogousslavsky J, Ruchat P, et al: Prognosis after stroke followed by surgical closure of patent foramen ovale: a prospective follow-up study with brain MRI and simultaneous transesophageal and transcranial Doppler ultrasound. Neurology 1996;47: 1162–1166.
133. Saver JL: Emerging risk factors for stroke: patent foramen ovale, proximal aortic atherosclerosis, antiphospholipid antibodies, and activated protein C resistance. J Stroke Cerebrovasc Dis 1997;6:167–172.
134. Reynen K: Cardiac myxomas. N Engl J Med 1995; 333:1610–1617.
135. Hart RG, Foster JW, Luther MF, et al: Stroke in infective endocarditis. Stroke 1990;21:695–700.
136. Brust JCM, Dickinson PCT, Hughes JEO, et al: The diagnosis and treatment of cerebral mycotic aneurysms. Ann Neurol 1990;27:238–246.
137. Pruitt AA, Rubin RH, Karchmer AW, et al: Neurologic complications of bacterial endocarditis. Medicine 1978;57:329–343.
138. Kanter MC, Hart RG: Neurologic complications of infective endocarditis. Neurology 1991;41:1015–1020.
139. Hicks PA, Leavitt JA, Mokri B: Ophthalmic manifestations of vertebral artery dissection. Patients seen at the Mayo Clinic from 1976 to 1992. Ophthalmology 1994;101:1786–1792.
140. Caplan LR, Amarenco P, Rosengart A, et al: Embolism from vertebral artery origin occlusive disease. Neurology 1992;42:1505–1512.
141. Wijdicks EFM, Nichols DA, Thielen KR, et al: Intra-arterial thrombolysis in acute basilar artery thromboembolism: the initial Mayo Clinic experience. Mayo Clin Proc 1997;72:1005–1013.
142. Grond M, Rudolf J, Schmülling S, et al: Early intravenous thrombolysis with recombinant tissue-type plasminogen activator in vertebrobasilar ischemic stroke. Arch Neurol 1998;55:466–469.
143. Hass WK, Easton JD, Adams HP, et al: A randomized trial comparing ticlopidine hydrochloride with aspirin for the prevention of stroke in high-risk patients. N Engl J Med 1989;321:501–507.
144. Gent M, Blakely JA, Easton JD, et al: The Canadian American Ticlopidine Study (CATS) in thromboembolic stroke. Lancet 1989;1:1215–1220.
145. Weisberg LA, the Ticlopidine Aspirin Stroke Study Group: The efficacy and safety of ticlopidine ans aspirin in non-whites: analysis of a patient subgroup from the Ticlopidine Aspirin Stroke Study. Neurology 1993;43:27–31.
146. CAPRIE Steering Committee: A randomised, blinded trial of clopidogrel versus aspirin in patients at risk of ischaemic events (CAPRIE). Lancet 1996;348:1329–1339.
147. Diener HC, Cunha L, Forbes C, et al: European Stroke Prevention Study 2: dipyridamole and acetylsalicylic acid in the secondary prevention of stroke. J Neurol Sci 1996;143:1–13.
148. The EC/IC bypass study group: Failure of extracranial-intracranial arterial bypass to reduce the risk of ischemic stroke. Results of an international randomized trial. N Engl J Med 1985;313:1191–1200.
149. Samuels MA, Thalinger K: Cerebrovascular manifestations of selected hematologic diseases. Semin Neurol 1991;11:411–418.
150. High KA: Antithrombin III, protein C, and protein S. Naturally occurring anticoagulant proteins. Arch Pathol Lab Med 1988;112:28–36.
151. Hart RG, Kanter MC: Hematologic disorders and ischemic stroke. Stroke 1990;21:1111–1121.
152. Irey NS, McAllister HA, Henry JM: Oral contraceptives and stroke in young women: a clinicopathologic correlation. Neurology 1978;28:1216–1219.

153. Longstreth WT, Swanson PD: Oral contraceptives and stroke. Stroke 1984;15:747–750.
154. Kittner SJ, Stern BJ, Feeser BR, et al: Pregnancy and the risk of stroke. N Engl J Med 1996;335:768–774.
155. Schafer AI: The hypercoagulable states. Ann Intern Med 1985;102:814–828.
156. Levine SR, Deegan MJ, Futrell N, et al: Cerebrovascular and neurologic disease associated with antiphospholipid antibodies: 48 cases. Neurology 1990;40: 1181–1189.
157. Brey RL, Hart RG, Sherman DG, et al: Antiphospholipid antibodies and cerebral ischemia in young people. Neurology 1990;40:1190–1196.
158. The Antiphospholipid Antibodies and Stroke Study Group (APASS): Anticardiolipin antibodies and the risk of recurrent thrombo-occlusive events and death. Neurology 1997;48:91–94.
159. Tanne D, D'Olhaberriague L, Schultz LR, et al: Anticardiolipin antibodies and their associations with cerebrovascular risk factors. Neurology 1999;52: 1368–1373.
160. Coull BM, Goodnight SH: Antiphospholipid antibodies, prethrombotic states, and stroke. Stroke 1990; 21:1370–1374.
161. Khamashta MA, Cuadrado MJ, Mujic F, et al: The management of thrombosis in the antiphospholipid-antibody syndrome. N Engl J Med 1995;332:993–997.
162. Lockshin MD: Answers to the antiphospholipid-antibody syndrome? (editorial). N Engl J Med 1995; 332:1025–1027.
163. Roach GW, Kanchuger M, Mangano CM, et al: Adverse cerebral outcomes after coronary bypass surgery. N Engl J Med 1996;335:1857–1863.
164. Furlan AJ, Breuer AC: Central nervous system complications of open heart surgery. Stroke 1984;15: 912–915.
165. Gilman S: Neurological complications of open heart surgery. Ann Neurol 1990;28:475–476.
166. Swain JA: Cardiac surgery and the brain (editorial). N Engl J Med 1993;329:1119–1120.
167. Horowitz DR, Tuhrim S, Budd J, et al: Aortic plaque in patients with brain ischemia: diagnosis by transesophageal echocardiography. Neurology 1992;42: 1602–1604.
168. Amarenco P, Duyckaerts C, Tzourio C, et al: The prevalence of ulcerated plaques in the aortic arch in patients with stroke. N Engl J Med 1992;326:221–225.
169. Amarenco P, Cohen A, Tzourio C, et al: Atherosclerotic disease of the aortic arch and the risk of ischemic stroke. N Engl J Med 1994;331:1474–1479.
170. The French Study of Aortic Plaques in Stroke Group: Atherosclerotic disease of the aortic arch as a risk factor for recurrent ischemic stroke. N Engl J Med 1996;334:1216–1221.
171. Keane JR: Blindness following tentorial herniation. Ann Neurol 1980;8:186–190.
172. Headache classification committee of the International Headache Society: classification and diagnostic criteria for headache disorders, cranial neuralgias and facial pain. Cephalgia 1988;8(Suppl 7):1–96.
173. Welch KMA: Relationship of stroke and migraine. Neurology 1994;44(suppl 7):S33–S36.
174. Buring JE, Hebert P, Romero J, et al: Migraine and subsequent risk of stroke in the physicians' health study. Arch Neurol 1995;52:129–134.
175. Merikangas KR, Fenton BT, Cheng SH, et al: Association between migraine and stroke in a large-scale epidemiological study of the United States. Arch Neurol 1997;54:362–368.
176. Welch KMA, Levine SR: Migraine-related stroke in the context of the International Headache Society classification of head pain. Arch Neurol 1990;47: 458–462.
177. Bevan H, Sharma K, Bradley W: Stroke in young adults. Stroke 1990;21:382–386.
178. Kittner SJ, Stern BJ, Wozniak M, et al: Cerebral infarction in young adults. The Baltimore–Washington cooperative young stroke study. Neurology 1998;50: 890–894.
179. Williams LS, Garg BP, Cohen M, et al: Subtypes of ischemic stroke in children and young adults. Neurology 1997;49:1541–1545.
180. Javeed N, Khan Z, Jayaram S, et al: Cerebral amyloid angiopathy. Res Staff Phys 1995;41:21–28.
181. Korogi Y, Takahashi M, Mabuchi M: Intracranial aneurysms: diagnostic accuracy of three-dimensional time of flight MR angiography. Radiology 1994;193: 181–186.
182. Kotapka MJ, Flamm ES: Surgical management of spontaneous intracerebral hemorrhage. In: Adams HP (ed): Handbook of Cerebrovascular Diseases, pp 451–466. New York, Marcel Dekker, 1993.
183. Hier DB, Davis KR, Richardson EP, et al: Hypertensive putaminal hemorrhage. Ann Neurol 1977; 1:152–159.
184. Kase CS: Intracerebral hemorrhage: nonhypertensive causes. Stroke 1986;17:590–595.
185. Case records of the Massachusetts General Hospital: Case 27-1991. N Engl J Med 1991;325:42–54.
186. Case records of the Massachusetts General Hospital: Case 22-1996. N Engl J Med 1996;335:189–196.
187. Vinters HV, Gilbert JJ: Cerebral amyloid angiopathy: incidence and complications in the aging brain. II: The distribution of amyloid vascular changes. Stroke 1983;14:924–928.
188. Vonsattel JPG, Myers RH, Hedley-Whyte ET, et al: Cerebral amyloid angiopathy without and with cerebral hemorrhages: a comparative histological study. Ann Neurol 1991;30:637–649.
189. Nicoll JAR, Burnett C, Leth S, et al: High frequency of apolipoprotein E $\epsilon 2$ allele in hemorrhage due to cerebral amyloid angiopathy. Ann Neurol 1997;41: 716–721.
190. Greenberg SM, Hyman BT: Cerebral amyloid angiopathy and apolipoprotein E: bad news for the good allele? (editorial). Ann Neurol 1997;41:701–702.
191. Greenberg SM: Cerebral amyloid angiopathy. Prospects for clinical diagnosis and treatment. Neurology 1998;51:690–694.
192. Greene GM, Godersky JC, Biller J, et al: Surgical experience with cerebral amyloid angiopathy. Stroke 1990;21:1545–1549.
193. Bennett J, Volpe NJ, Liu GT, et al: Neurovascular neuro-ophthalmology. In: Jakobiec FA, Albert D (eds): Principles of Ophthalmology, 2nd edition, vol 5, pp 4238–4274. Philadelphia, WB Saunders, 1999.
194. Yokoyama K, Asano Y, Murakawa T, et al: Familial occurence of arteriovenous malformation of the brain. J Neurosurg 1991;74:585–589.
195. Mingrino S: Supratentorial arteriovenous malformations of the brain. Adv Tech Stand Neurosurg 1978;5:93–123.
196. Kupersmith MJ: Vascular malformations of the brain. In: Neurovascular neuro-ophthalmology, pp 301–351. Berlin, Springer-Verlag, 1993.
197. Kupersmith MJ, Vargas ME, Yashar A, et al: Occipital arteriovenous malformations. Visual disturbances and presentation. Neurology 1996;46:953–957.

198. Lee K, Holman BL: Images in clinical medicine. Cerebral arteriovenous malformation. N Engl J Med 1995;332:923.
199. The Arteriovenous Malformation Study Group: Arteriovenous malformations of the brain in adults. N Engl J Med 1999;340:1812–1818.
200. Bartolomei J, Wecht DA, Chaloupka J, et al: Occipital lobe vascular malformations: prevalence of visual field deficits and prognosis after therapeutic intervention. Neurosurgery 1998;43:415–421.
201. Steinberg GK, Fabrikant JI, Marks MP, et al: Stereotactic heavy-charged-particle Bragg-peak radiation for intracranial arteriovenous malformations. N Engl J Med 1990;323:96–101.
202. Heros RC, Korosue K: Radiation treatment of cerebral arteriovenous malformations (editorial). N Engl J Med 1990;323:127–129.
203. Tagle P, Huete I, Méndez J, et al: Intracranial cavernous angioma: presentation and management. J Neurosurg 1986;64:720–723.
204. Bartlett JE, Kishore PRS: Intracranial cavernous hemangioma. Am J Roentgenol 1977;128:653–656.
205. Acciarri N, Padovani R, Giulioni M, et al: Intracranial and orbital cavernous angiomas: a review of 74 surgical cases. Br J Neurosurg 1993;7:529–539.
206. Tomlinson FH, Houser OW, Scheithauer BW, et al: Angiographically occult vascular malformations: a correlative study of features on magnetic resonance imaging and histological examination. Neurosurgery 1994;34:792–799.
207. Moore PM, Cupps TR: Neurological complications of vasculitis. Ann Neurol 1983;14:155–167.
208. Kattah JC, Cupps TR, Di Chiro G, et al: An unusual case of central nervous system vasculitis. J Neurol 1987;234:344–347.
209. Sigal LH: The neurologic presenation of vasculitic and rheumatologic syndromes: a review. Medicine 1987;66:157–180.
210. Moore PM: Diagnosis and management of isolated angiitis of the central nervous system. Neurology 1989;39:167–173.
211. Levin JR, Awerbuch G, Nigro MA, et al: Isolated angiitis of the central nervous system in children. Ann Neurol 1989;26:478.
212. Zimmerman RS, Young HG, Hadfield MG: Granulomatous angiitis of the nervous system. Surg Neurol 1990;33:206–212.
213. Calabrese LH, Furlan AJ, Gragg, LA, et al: Primary angiitis of the central nervous system: diagnostic criteria and clinical approach. Cleve Clin J Med 1992;59:293–306.
214. Calabrese LH, Gragg LA, Furlan AJ: Benign angiopathy: a distinct subset of angiographically defined primary angiitis of the central nervous system. J Rheumatol 1993;20:2046–2050.
215. Rhodes RH, Madelaire NC, Petrelli M, et al: Primary angiitis and angiopathy of the central nervous system and their relationship to systemic giant cell arteritis. Arch Pathol lab Med 1995;119:334–349.
216. Ozawa T, Sasaki O, Sorimachi T, et al: Primary angiitis of the central nervous system: report of two cases and review of the literature. Neurosurgery 1995;36: 173–179.
217. Vollmer TL, Guarnaccia J, Harrington W, et al: Idiopathic angiitis of the central nervous system. Diagnostic challenges. Arch Neurol 1993;50:925–930.
218. Ehsan T, Hasan S, Powers JM, et al: Serial magnetic resonance imaging in isolated angiitis of the central nervous system. Neurology 1995;45:1462–1465.
219. Shoemaker E, Lin ZS, Rae Grant AD, et al: Primary angiitis of the central nervous system: unusual MR appearance. AJNR Am J Neuroradiol 1994;15: 331–334.
220. Alhalabi M, Moore PM: Serial angiography in isolated angiitis of the CNS. Neurology 1994;44:1221–1226.
221. Younger DS, Hays AP, Brust JCM, et al: Granulomatous angiitis of the brain: an inflammatory reaction of diverse etiology. Arch Neurol 1988;45:514–518.
222. Caselli RJ, Hunder GG, Whisnant JP: Neurologic disease in biopsy proven giant cell (temporal) arteritis. Neurology 1988;38:352–359.
223. Caselli RJ, Daube JR, Hunder GG, et al: Peripheral neuropathic syndromes in giant cell (temporal) arteritis. Neurology 1988;38:685–689.
224. Hunder GG: Polymyalgia rheumatica and giant cell arteritis. In: Cecil Textbook of Medicine, pp 1498–1500. Philadelphia, WB Saunders, 1996.
225. Caselli RJ, Hunder GG: Neurologic aspects of giant cell (temporal) arteritis. Rheum Dis Clin North Am 1990;19:941–953.
226. Chisholm IH: Cortical blindness in cranial arteritis. Br J Ophthalmol 1975;59:332–333.
227. Nevyas JY, Nevyas HJ: Giant cell arteritis with normal erythrocyte sedimentation rate: a management dilemma. Metab Pediatr Syst Ophthalmol 1987;10: 18–21.
228. Wilkinson IMS, Russell RWR: Arteries of the head and neck in giant cell arteritis. A pathological study to show the pattern of arterial involvement. Arch Neurol 1972;27:378–391.
229. Cullen JF, Coleiro JA: Ophthalmic complications of giant cell arteritis. Surv Ophthalmol 1976;20:247–260.
230. Galetta SL, Balcer LJ, Liu GT: Giant cell arteritis with unusual flow related neuro-ophthalmologic manifestations. Neurology 1997;49:1463–1465.
231. Trevor RP, Sondheimer FK, Fessel WJ, et al: Angiographic demonstration of major cerebral vessel occlusion in systemic lupus erythematosus. Neuroradiology 1972;4:202–207.
232. Brandt KD, Lessell S, Cohen AS: Cerebral disorders of vision in systemic lupus erythematosus. Ann Interm Med 1975;83:163–169.
233. Lessell S: The neuro-ophthalmology of systemic lupus erythematosus. Doc Ophthalmol 1979;47:13–42.
234. Honda Y: Scintillating scotoma as the first symptom of systemic lupus erythematosus. Am J Ophthalmol 1985;99:607.
235. Rubin BR, De Horatius RJ: Acute visual loss in systemic lupus erythematosus. J Am Optom Assoc 1989;89:73–77.
236. Johnson RT, Richardson EP: The neurological manifestations of systemic lupus erythematosus. A clinical-pathological study of 24 cases and review of the literature. Medicine 1968;47:337–369.
237. Ellis SG, Verity MA: Central nervous system involvement in systemic lupus erythematosus: a review of neuropathologic findings in 57 cases, 1955–1977. Semin Arthritis Rheum 1979;8:212–221.
238. Devinsky O, Petito CK, Alonso DR: Clinical and neuropathological findings in systemic lupus erythematosus: the role of vasculitis, heart emboli, and thrombotic thrombocytopenic purpura. Ann Neurol 1988;23:380–384.
239. Hinchey J, Chaves C, Appignani B, et al: A reversible posterior leukoencephalopathy syndrome. N Engl J Med 1996;334:494–500.

240. Pavlakis SG, Frank Y, Kalina P, et al: Occipital-parietal encephalopathy: a new name for an old syndrome. Pediatr Neurol 1997;16:145–148.
241. Torocsik HV, Curless RG, Post J, et al: FK506-induced leukoencephalopathy in children with organ transplants. Neurology 1999;52:1497–1500.
242. Sanders TG, Clayman DA, Sanchez-Ramos L, et al: Brain in eclampsia: MR imaging with clinical correlation. Radiology 1991;180:475–478.
243. Ay H, Buonanno FS, Schaefer PW, et al: Posterior leukoencephalopathy without severe hypertension. Utility of diffusion-weighted MRI. Neurology 1998; 51:1369–1376.
244. Beutler JJ, Koomans HA: Malignant hypertension: still a challenge. Nephrol Dial Transplant 1997;12: 2019–2023.
245. Delanty N, Vaughn C, Frucht S, et al: Erythropoietin-associated hypertensive posterior leukoencephalopathy. Neurology 1997;49:686–689.
246. Raps EC, Galetta SL, Broderick M, et al: Delayed peripartum vasculopathy: cerebral eclampsia revisited. Ann Neurol 1993;33:222–225.
247. Frank Y, Pavlakis S, Black K, et al: Reversible occipital-parietal encephalopathy syndrome in an HIV-infected child. Neurology 1998;51:915–916.
248. Rubin Am, Kang H: Cerebral blindness and encephalopathy with cyclosporin A toxicity. Neurology 1987;37:1072–1076.
249. Patchell RA: Neurological complications of organ transplantation. Ann Neurol 1994;36:688–703.
250. Shutter LA, Green JP, Newman NJ, et al: Cortical blindness and white matter lesions in a patient receiving FK506 after liver transplantation. Neurology 1993;43:2417–2418.
251. Synder H, Robinson K, Shah D, et al: Signs and symptoms of patients with brain tumors presenting to the emergency department. J Emerg Med 1993;11: 253–258.
252. Pomeranz HD, Henson JW, Lessell S: Radiation-associated cerebral blindness. Am J Ophthalmol 1998;126:609–611.
253. Radhakrishnan K, Mokri B, Parisi PE, et al: The trends in incidence of primary brain tumors in the population of Rochester, Minnesota. Ann Neurol 1995;37: 67–73.
254. Black PM: Brain tumors. N Engl J Med 1991;324:1471–1476 (part one), 1555–1564 (part two).
255. Shaw EG: Low-grade glioma: to treat or not to treat? A radiation oncologist's viewpoint. Arch Neurol 1990;47:1138–1139.
256. Case records of the Massachusetts General Hospital: Case 33-1988. N Engl J Med 1988;319:426–436.
257. DeAngelis LM, Yahalom J, Heinemann MH, et al: Primary CNS lymphoma: combined treatment with chemotherapy and radiotherapy. Neurology 1990;40: 80–86.
258. Cairncross JG, Kim J-H, Posner JB: Radiation therapy for brain metastases. Ann Neurol 1980;7:529–541.
259. Posner JB: Intracranial metastases. In: Neurologic Complications of Cancer, pp 77–110. Philadelphia, FA Davis, 1995.
260. Patchell RA, Tibbs PA, Walsh JW, et al: A randomized trial of surgery in the treatment of single metastases to the brain. N Engl J Med 1990;322:494–500.
261. Greenlee JE: Progressive multifocal leukoencephalopathy—progress made and lessons relearned (editorial). N Engl J Med 1998;338:1378–1380.
262. Richardson EP: Progressive multifocal leukoencephalopathy 30 years later (editorial). N Engl J Med 1988;318:315–317.
263. Berger JR, Concha M: Progressive multifocal leukoencephalopathy: the evolution of a disease once considered rare. J Neurovirol 1995;1:5–18.
264. Gillespie SM, Chang Y, Lemp G, et al: Progressive multifocal leukoencephalopathy in persons infected with human immunodeficiency virus, San Francisco, 1981–1989. Ann Neurol 1991;30:597–604.
265. Case records of the Massachusetts General Hospital: Case 20-1995. N Engl J Med 1995;332:1773–1780.
266. Ormerod LD, Rhodes RH, Gross SA, et al: Ophthalmologic manifestations of acquired immune deficiency syndrome-associated progressive multifocal leukoencephalopathy. Ophthalmology 1996;103: 899–906.
267. Berger JR, Levy RM: The neurologic complications of human immunodeficiency virus infection. Med Clin North Am 1993;77:1–23.
268. Berger JR, Levy RM, Flomenhoft D, et al: Predictive factors for prolonged survival in acquired immunodeficiency syndrome-associated progressive multifocal leukoencephalopathy. Ann Neurol 1998;44: 341–349.
269. Weiss PJ, DeMarco JK: Images in clinical medicine. Progressive multifocal leukoencephalopathy. N Engl J Med 1994;330:1197.
270. Kasner S, Galetta SL, McGowan JC, et al: Magnetization transfer imaging in progressive multifocal leukoencephalopathy. Neurology 1997;48:534–536.
271. Major EO, Ault GS: Progressive multifocal leukoencephalopathy: clinical and laboratory observations on a viral induced demyelinating disease in the immunodeficient patient. Curr Opin Neurol 1995;8: 184–190.
272. Koralnik IJ, Boden D, Mai VX, et al: JC virus DNA load in patients with and without progressive multifocal leukoencephalopathy. Neurology 1999;52: 253–260.
273. Garrels K, Kucharczyk W, Wortzman G, et al: Progressive multifocal leukoencephalopathy: clinical and MR response to treatment. AJNR Am J Neuroradiol 1996;17:597–600.
274. Hall CD, Dafni U, Simpson D, et al: Failure of cytarabine in progressive multifocal leukoencephalopathy associated with human immunodeficiency virus infection. N Engl J Med 1998;338:1345–1351.
275. Clifford DB, Yiannoutsos C, Glicksman M, et al: HAART improves prognosis in HIV-associated progressive multifocal leukoencephalopathy. Neurology 1999;52:623–625.
276. Case records of the Massachusetts General Hospital: Case 39-1996. N Engl J Med 1996;335:1906–1914.
277. Case records of the Massachusetts General Hospital: Case 31-1991. N Engl J Med 1991;325:341–350.
278. Boes B, Bashir R, Boes C, et al: Central nervous system aspergillosis. J Neuroimaging 1994;4:123–129.
279. Evaluation and management of intracranial mass lesions in AIDS. Report of the quality standards subcommittee of the Americans Academy of Neurology. Neurology 1998;50:21–26.
280. Adelson PD, Kochanek PM: Head injury in children. J Child Neurol 1998;13:2–15.
281. Gennarelli TA, Thibault LE, Graham DI: Diffuse axonal injury: an important form of traumatic brain damage. Neuroscientist 1998;4:202–215.
282. Silverman IE, Grossman M, Galetta SL, et al: Understanding human visual cortex: the role of functional imaging. Neuropsychiatr Neuropsych Behav Neurol 1995;8:241–254.

283. Brodsky MC, Baker RS, Hamed LM: The apparently blind infant. In: Pediatric Neuro-ophthalmology, pp 1–41. New York, Springer-Verlag, 1996.
284. Mendez MF, Tomsak RL, Remler B: Disorders of the visual system in Alzheimer's disease. J Clin Neuro-ophthalmol 1990;10:62–69.
285. Katz B, Rimmer S: Ophthalmologic manifestations of Alzheimer's disease. Surv Ophthalmol 1989;34: 31–43.
286. Rizzo JF, Cronin-Golomb A, Growdon JH, et al: Retinocalcarine function in Alzheimer's disease. A clinical and electrophysiologic study. Arch Neurol 1992;49:93–101.
287. Cesareo M, Pozzilli C, Ristori G, et al: Crossed quadrant homonymous hemianopsia in a case of multiple sclerosis. Clin Neurol Neurosurg 1995;97:324–327.
288. Hornabrook RS, Miller DH, Newton MR, et al: Frequent involvement of the optic radiation in patients with acute isolated optic neuritis. Neurology 1992;42:77–79.
289. Bajandas FJ, McBeath JB, Smith JL: Congenital homonymous hemianopia. Am J Ophthalmol 1976;82: 498–500.
290. Bosley TM, Kiyosawa M, Moster M, et al: Neuroimaging and positron emission tomography of congenital homonymous hemianopsia. Am J Ophthalmol 1991;111:413–418.
291. Eken P, de Vries LS, van Nieuwenhuizen O, et al: Early predictors of cerebral visual impairment in infants with cystic leukomalacia. Neuropediatrics 1996; 27:16–25.
292. Cioni G, Fazzi B, Ipata AE, et al: Correlation between cerebral visual impairment and magnetic resonance imaging in children with neonatal encephalopathy. Dev Med Child Neurol 1996;38:120–132.
293. Hoyt WF, Rios-Montenegro EN, Behrens MM, et al: Homonymous hemioptic hypoplasia. Fundoscopic features in standard and red-free illustration in three patients with congenital hemiplegia. Br J Ophthalmol 1972;56:537–545.
294. Jacobson L, Hellström A, Flodmark O: Large cups in normal-sized optic discs. A variant of optic nerve hypoplasia in children with periventricular leukomalacia. Arch Ophthalmol 1997;115:1263–1269.
295. Jacobson L, Ygge J, Flodmark O: Nystagmus in periventricular leucomalacia. Br J Ophthalmol 1998;82: 1026–1032.
296. Flodmark O, Jan JE, Wong PKH: Computed tomography of the brains of children with cortical visual impairment. Dev Med Child Neurol 1990;32:611–620.
297. Takashima S, Iida K, Deguchi K: Periventricular leukomalacia, glial development and myelination. Early Hum Dev 1995;43:177–184.
298. Leviton A, Gilles F: Ventriculomegaly, delayed myelination, white matter hypoplasia, and "periventricular" leukomalacia: how are they related? Pediatr Neurol 1996;15:127–136.
299. Volpe JJ: Neurologic outcome of prematurity. Arch Neurol 1998;55:297–300.
300. Uggetti C, Egitto MG, Fazzi E, et al: Cerebral visual impairment in periventricular leukomalacia: MR correlation. AJNR Am J Neuroradial 1996;17:979–985.
301. Ragge NK, Barkovich AJ, Hoyt WF, et al: Isolated congenital hemianopia caused by prenatal injury to the optic radiation. Arch Neurol 1991;48:1088–1091.
302. Cioni G, Fazzi B, Coluccini M, et al.: Cerebral visual impairment in preterm infants with periventricular leukomalacia. Pediatr Neurol 1997;17:331–338.
303. Lambert SR, Kriss A, Taylor D: Detection of isolated occipital lobe anomalies during early childhood. Dev Med Child Neurol 1990;32:451–455.
304. Mercuri E, Spano M, Bruccini G, et al: Visual outcome in children with congenital hemiplegia: correlation with MRI findings. Neuropediatrics 1996;27:184–188.
305. Thorarensen O, Ryan S, Hunter J, et al: Factor V Leiden mutation: an unrecognized cause of hemiplegic cerebral palsy, neonatal stroke, and placental thrombosis. Ann Neurol 1997;42:372–375.
306. Tychsen L, Hoyt WF: Occipital lobe dysplasia. Magnetic resonance findings in two cases of isolated congenital hemianopsia. Arch Ophthalmol 1985;103: 680–682.
307. Kuzniecky RI: Magnetic resonance imaging in developmental disorders of the cerebral cortex. Epilepsia 1994;35:S44–56.
308. Barkovich AJ, Kjos BO: Schizencephaly: correlation of clinical findings with MR characteristics. AJNR Am J Neuroradiol 1992;13:85–94.
309. Raymond AA, Fish DR, Sisodiya SM, et al: Abnormalities of gyration, heterotopias, tuberous sclerosis, focal cortical dysplasia, microdysgenesis, dysembryoplastic neuroepithelial tumour and dysgenesis of the archicortex in epilepsy. Clinical, EEG and neuroimaging features in 100 adult patients. Brain 1995;118:629–660.
310. Hill A, Volpe JJ: Perinatal asphyxia: clinical aspects. Clin Perinatol 1989;16:435–457.
311. Volpe JJ: Hypoxic-ischemic encephalopathy. In: Neurology of the Newborn, 3rd edition, pp 211–369. Philadelphia, WB Saunders, 1995.
312. van Hof-van Duin J, Mohn G: Visual defects in children after cerebral hypoxia. Behav Brain Res 1984; 14:147–155.
313. Lambert SR, Hoyt CS, Jan JE, et al: Visual recovery from hypoxic cortical blindness during childhood. Computed tomographic and magnetic resonance imaging predictors. Arch Ophthalmol 1987;105:1371–1377.
314. Casteels I, Demaerel P, Spileers W, et al: Cortical visual impairment following perinatal hypoxia: clinicoradiologic correlation using magnetic resonance imaging. J Pediatr Ophthalmol Strabismus 1997;34: 297–305.
315. Pavlakis SG, Phillips PC, DiMauro S, et al: Mitochondrial myopathy, encephalopathy, lactic acidosis, and strokelike episodes: a distinctive clinical syndrome. Ann Neurol 1984;16:481–488.
316. Newman NJ: Neuro-ophthalmology of mitochondrial disorders in children. Pediatric Neuro-ophthalmology course. American Academy of Neurology, 1998; Minneapolis.
317. DiMauro S, Schon EA: Mitochondrial DNA and diseases of the nervous system: the spectrum. Neuroscientist 1998;4:53–63.
318. Rummelt V, Folberg R, Ionasescu V, et al: Ocular pathology of MELAS syndrome with mitochondrial DNA nucleotide 3243 point mutation. Ophthalmology 1993;100:1757–1766.
319. Sue CM, Mitchell P, Crimmins DS, et al: Pigmentary retinopathy associated with the mitochondrial DNA 3243 point mutation. Neurology 1997;49:1013–1017.
320. Majamaa K, Turkka J, Kärppä M, et al: The common MELAS mutation A3243G in mithondrial DNA among young patients with an occipital brain infarct. Neurology 1997;49:1331–1334.
321. Hirano M, Pavlakis SG: Mitochondrial myopathy, encephalopathy, lactic acidosis, and strokelike epi-

sodes (MELAS): current concepts. J Child Neurol 1994;9:4–13.
322. Kimata KG, Gordan L, Ajax, et al: A case of late-onset MELAS. Arch Neurol 1998;55:722–725.
323. Koo B, Becker LE, Chuang S, et al: Mitochondrial encephalomyopathy, lactic acidosis, stroke-like episodes (MELAS): clinical, radiological, pathological, and genetic observations. Ann Neurol 1993;34:25–32.
324. Clark JM, Marks MP, Adalsteinsson E, et al: MELAS: clinical and pathologic correlations with MRI, xenon/CT, and MR spectroscopy. Neurology 1996;46:223–227.
325. Case records of the Massachusetts General Hospital: Case 39-1998. N Engl J Med 1998;339:1914–1923.
326. Saitoh S, Momoi MY, Yamagata T, et al: Effects of dichloroacetate in three patients with MELAS. Neurology 1998;50:531–534.
327. Penn AMW, Lee JWK, Thuillier P, et al: MELAS syndrome with mitochondrial $tRNA^{Leu\,(UUR)}$ mutation: correlation of clinical state, nerve conduction, and muscle ^{31}P magnetic resonance spectroscopy during treatment with nicotinamide and riboflavin. Neurology 1992;42:2147–2152.
328. Moser HW: Adrenoleukodystrophy: survey of 303 cases: biochemistry, diagnosis, and therapy. Ann Neurol 1984;16:628–641.
329. Moser HW: Adrenoleukodystrophy: phenotype, genetics, pathogenesis and therapy. Brain 1997;120:1485–1508.
330. Schaumberg HH, Powers JM, Raine CS, et al: Adrenoleukodystrophy: a clinical and pathological study of 17 cases. Arch Neurol 1975;32:577–591.
331. Wray SH, Cogan DG, Kuwabara T, et al: Adrenoleukodystrophy with disease of the eye and optic nerve. Am J Ophthalmol 1976;82:480–485.
332. Traboulsi EI, Maumenee IH: Ophthalmologic manifestations of X-linked childhood adrenoleukodystrophy. Ophthalmology 1987;94:47–52.
333. Farrell DF, Hamilton SR, Knauss TA, et al: X-linked adrenoleukodystrophy: adult cerebral variant. Neurology 1993;43:1518–1522.
334. Griffin JW, Goren E, Schaumburg H, et al: Adrenomyeloneuropathy: a probable variant of adrenoleukodystrophy. Neurology 1977;27:1107–1113.
335. Kaplan PW, Kruse B, Tusa RJ, et al: Visual system abnormalities in adrenomyeloneuropathy. Ann Neurol 1995;37:550–552.
336. Brodsky MC, Baker RS, Hamed LM: Neuro-ophthalmologic manifestations of systemic and intracranial disease. In: Pediatric Neuro-ophthalmology, pp 399–465. New York, Springer-Verlag, 1996.
337. Richard JM: The phacomatoses: neurocutaneous disorders. In: Wright KW (ed): Pediatric Ophthalmology and Strabismus, pp 673–687. St. Louis, CV Mosby, 1995.
338. Pascual-Castroviejo I, Diaz-Gonzalez C, Garcia-Melian RM, et al: Sturge–Weber syndrome: study of 40 patients. Pediatr Neurol 1993;9:283–288.
339. Maria BL, Neufeld JA, Rosainz LC, et al: High prevalence of bihemispheric structural and functional defects in Sturge–Weber syndrome. J Child Neurol 1998;13:595–605.
340. Maria BL, Neufeld JA, Rosainz LC, et al: Central nervous system structure and function in Sturge-Weber syndrome: evidence of neurologic and radiologic progression. J Child Neurol 1998;13:606–618.
341. Good WV, Jan JE, DeSa L, et al: Cortical visual impairment in children. Surv Ophthalmol 1994;38:351–364.
342. Moster MM, Galetta SL, Schatz NJ: Physiologic functional imaging in "functional" visual loss. Surv Ophthalmol 1996;40:395–399.
343. Granet DB, Hertle RW, Quinn GE, et al: The visual-evoked response in infants with cerebral visual impairment. Am J Ophthalmol 1993;116:437–443.
344. Smith JL, Weiner IG, Lucero AJ: Hemianopic Fresnel prisms. J Clin Neuro-ophthalmol 1982;2:19–22.
345. Perlin RR, Dziadul J: Fresnel prisms for field enhancement of patients with constricted or hemianopic visual fields. J Am Optom Assoc 1991;62:58–64.
346. Rossi PW, Kheyfets S, Reding MJ: Fresnel prisms improve visual perception in stroke patients with homonymous hemianopia or unilateral visual neglect. Neurology 1990;40:1597–1599.
347. Zihl J, Von Cramen D: Restitution of visual function in patients with cerebral blindness. J Neurol Neurosurg Psychiatry 1979; 42:312–322.
348. Zihl J, Von Cramen D: Visual field recovery from scotoma in patients with postgeniculate damage. A review of 55 cases. Brain 1985;108:335–365.
349. Kerkhoff G, Münßinger U, Meier EK: Neurovisual rehabilitation in cerebral blindness. Arch Neurol 1994;51:474–481.
350. Hughes TS, Abou-Khalil B, Lavin PJM, et al: Visual field defects after temporal lobe resection. A prospective quantitative analysis. Neurology 1999;53:167–172.
351. Wong AMF, Sharpe JA: A comparison of tangent screen, Goldmann, and Humphrey perimetry in the detection and localization of occipital lesions. Ophthalmology 2000;107:527–544.
352. Weiskrantz L, Cowey A, Barbur JL: Differential pupillary constriction and awareness in the absence of striate cortex. Brain 1999;122:1533–1538.
353. Morland AB, Jones SR, Finlay AL, et al: Visual perception of motion, luminance and colour in a human hemianope. Brain 1999;122:1183–1198.
354. Yamamoto Y, Georgiadis AL, Chang H-M, et al: Posterior cerebral artery territory infarcts in the New England Medical Center posterior circulation registry. Arch Neurol 1999;56:824–832.
355. Georgiadis AL, Yamamoto Y, Kwan ES, et al: Anatomy of sensory findings in patients with posterior cerebral artery territory infarction. Arch Neurol 1999;56:835–838.
356. Fisher M, Albers GW: Applications of diffusion-perfusion magnetic resonance imaging in acute ischemic stroke. Neurology 1999;52:1750–1756.
357. Tanne D, Bates VE, Verro P, et al: Initial clinical experience with tissue plasminogen activator for acute ischemic stroke: a multicenter survey. Neurology 1999;53:424–427.
358. Chamorro A, Vila N, Ascaso C, et al: Heparin in acute stroke with atrial fibrillation. Clinical relevance of very early treatment. Arch Neurol 1999;56:1098–1102.
359. Gilon D, Buonanno FS, Joffe MM, et al: Lack of evidence of an association between mitral-valve prolapse and stroke in young patients. N Engl J Med 1999;341:8–13.
360. Wilterdink JL, Easton JD: Dipyridamole plus aspirin in cerebrovascular disease. Arch Neurol 1999;56:1087–1092.
361. O'Donnell HC, Rosano J, Knudsen KA, et al: Apolipoprotein E genotype and the risk of recurrent lobar intracerebral hemorrhage. N Engl J Med 2000;342:240–245.

362. Wang A-G, Liu R-S, Liu J-H, et al: Positron emission tomography scan in cortical visual loss in patients with organophosphate intoxication. Ophthalmology 1999;106:1287–1291.
363. Miki A, Nakajima T, Abe A, et al: Occipital lobe dysfunction revealed by functional brain imaging in a patient with traumatic visual field loss. Neuro-Ophthalmology 1999;22:127–132.
364. Thielen KR, Wijdicks EFM, Nichols DA: Giant cell (temporal) arteritis: involvement of the vertebral and internal carotid arteries. Mayo Clin Proc 1998;73: 444–446.
365. De Luca A, Fantoni M, Tartaglione T, et al: Response to cidofovir after failure of antiretroviral therapy alone in AIDS-associated progressive multifocal leukoencephalopathy. Neurology 1999;52:891–892.
366. Latkany P, Ciulla TA, Cacchillo PF, et al: Mitochondrial maculopathy: geographic atrophy of the macula in the MELAS associated A to G 3243 mitochondrial DNA point mutation. Am J Ophthalmol 1999;128: 112–114.
367. Sharfstein SR, Gordon MF, Libman RB, et al: Adult-onset MELAS presenting as herpes encephalitis. Arch Neurol 1999;56:241–243.

CHAPTER 9

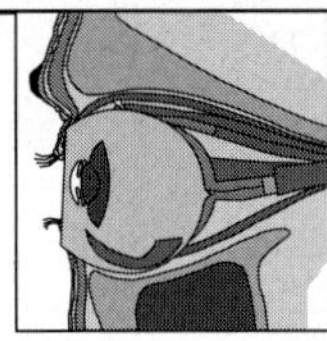

Disorders of Higher Cortical Visual Function

While the anterior visual and geniculocalcarine pathways deliver the elemental visual data from the eyes to striate cortex, the higher cortical visual (or association) areas perform the more complex interpretation of this visual information.[1] Deficits caused by damage to these areas are characterized by abnormalities in visual processing or attention often despite otherwise relatively normal visual acuity and fields. This chapter will detail the important higher cortical visual disorders (Table 9–1), then highlight some of the neurologic diseases that commonly cause them.

NEUROANATOMIC ORGANIZATION OF HIGHER CORTICAL AREAS

Areas V_1 and V_2 to V_5 designate striate cortex (Brodmann area 17) and higher cortical (or association) visual areas, respectively. The higher cortical visual areas are divided anatomically and functionally into ventral and dorsal pathways (Fig. 9–1, middle). In general, the ventral stream (occipitotemporal) is more concerned with object recognition ("what") and represents the continuation of the parvocellular pathway (Fig. 9–1, bottom).[2] Area V_4, situated in the fusiform and lingual gyri, is responsible for color perception within the contralateral hemifield.[3] Bilateral mesial occipitotemporal regions are necessary for object and facial recognition.[4–6] On the other hand, the dorsal stream carries out functions related to spatial orientation[7] (the "where" pathway) and is the extension of the magnocellular pathway (Fig. 9–1, top). The parietal lobe is devoted to directed attention. Recent studies suggest that area V_5, within the lateral occipitotemporal region, is important for motion perception. Areas V_2 and V_3 correspond roughly to Brodmann areas 18 and 19, respectively.

IMPORTANT CONCEPTS IN HIGHER CORTICAL VISUAL DISORDERS

The various higher cortical visual disorders will be discussed below by cerebral localization. However, two concepts, disconnection and simultaneous occurrence, should be considered in any review of these conditions.

Disconnection

While some of the higher cortical disorders result from damage to vital cortical areas, such as the color center in the inferior occipitotemporal lobe, others result from disconnecting the occipital lobe from visual association areas. This disconnection concept was popularized by Geschwind.[8, 9] Examples would include a lesion involving white matter pathways connecting striate cortex and facial recognition centers or another connecting to language areas. Table 9–1 indicates which higher cortical visual disorders are thought to be disconnection syndromes and which are due to direct damage to cortical structures.

Simultaneous Occurrence

The higher cortical visual disorders are not mutually exclusive. Rather, because of the

TABLE 9–1. Important Higher Cortical Visual Disturbances, Their Main and Associated Clinical Features, and Their Most Common Localization

Syndrome	Main Clinical Features	Commonly Associated Clinical Features	Most Common Localization	Disconnection?
Alexia without agraphia	Ability to write but not read	Right homonymous hemianopia	Left occipital lobe and splenium of corpus callosum	Yes
Hemiachromatopsia	Loss of color vision in one hemifield	Ipsilateral homonymous upper quadrantanopia	Contralateral occipitotemporal lobe in the fusiform (and lingual) gyri (V_4)	No
Visual object agnosia	Inability to recognize visualized objects	Alexia without agraphia Prosopagnosia	Bilateral occipitotemporal lobes involving the inferior longitudinal fasciculi	Yes
Prosopagnosia	Inability to recognize faces	Alexia without agraphia Visual object agnosia	Bilateral occipitotemporal lobes involving the midfusiform gyri	Sometimes
Akinetopsia	Defective motion perception	None	Bilateral lateral occipitotemporal lobes (V_5)	No
Visual hemi-inattention	Neglect of visual stimuli in left hemispace	Inattention Left-sided sensory loss and weakness	Right inferior parietal lobule	No
Balint syndrome	Simultanagnosia Ocular apraxia Optic ataxia	Bilateral inferior altitudinal visual field defects	Bilateral parietooccipital lobes	Yes for some features

proximity of many of the important cortical areas and white matter tracts in the parietal, occipital, and temporal lobes, many syndromes occur simultaneously. For instance, a combination of visual field defects, visual recognition, and reading disorders often results from concomitant involvement of the occipital and occipitotemporal lobes (Table 9–1).

SYMPTOMS AND SIGNS

Neuro-ophthalmic Symptoms

Most subjective complaints due to involvement of visual association areas are usually vague, such as "I have blurry vision" or "I'm having trouble seeing." Rarely, patients will complain of difficulty seeing colors or recognizing faces. Many such patients have seen numerous eye specialists and reportedly have normal examinations. Some individuals with inattention or dementia are unaware of their visual deficits, and the family members are the ones who bring them to medical attention. Another group of patients are seen after a stroke or neurosurgical intervention. Visual field loss may cause the dominant symptoms but careful examination reveals that complaints of "trouble reading and seeing" may be the result of higher cortical dysfunction.

Neurologic Symptoms

Higher cortical visual disturbances should be suspected when patients complain of loss of memory, confusion, disorientation, or behavioral changes suggestive of a dementing illness or hemispheric lesion. Their families may report that the patients seem no longer able to take care of themselves or that they get lost frequently.

Signs on Examination

Visual acuity is usually normal. Visual fields in each quadrant and with double simultaneous

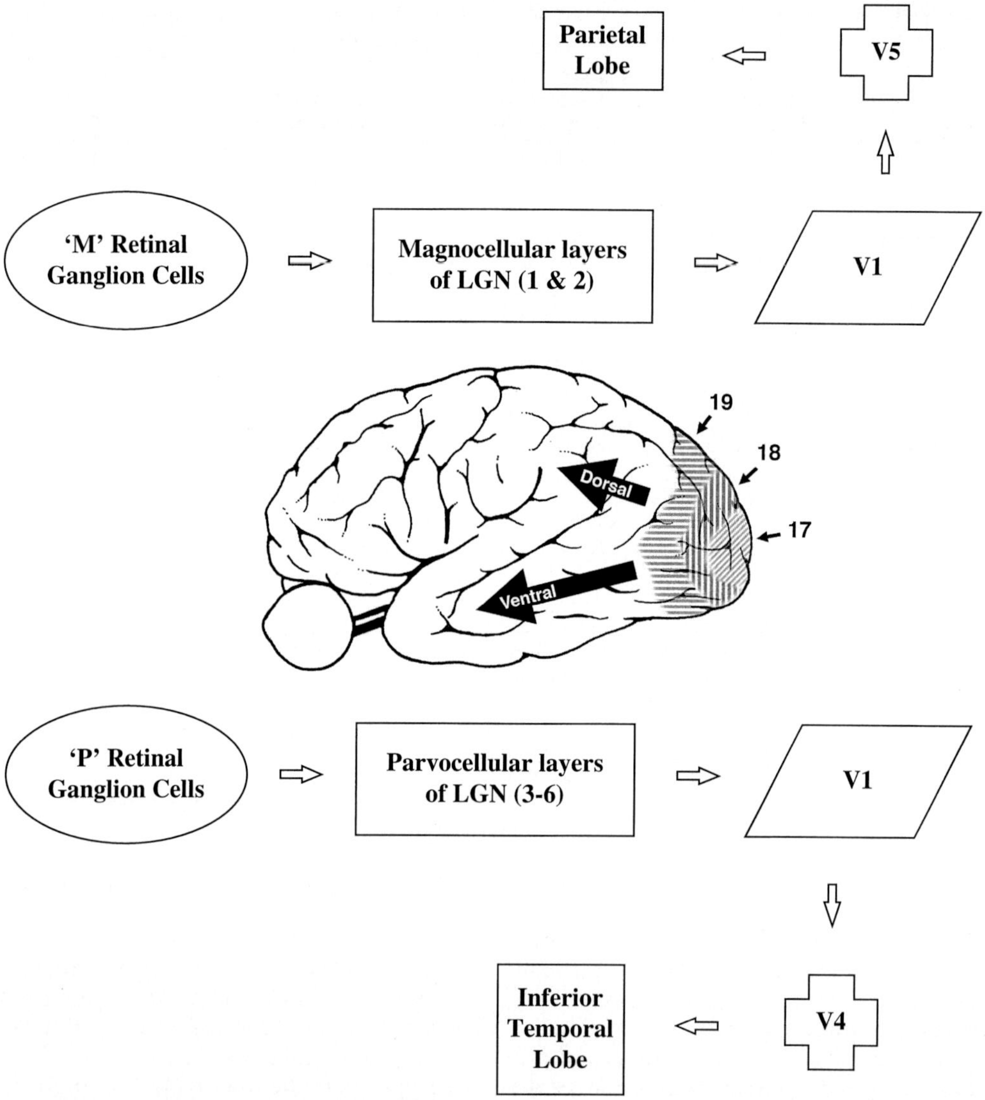

FIGURE 9–1. Middle. Diagram of dorsal and ventral higher cortical visual streams. Lateral view of the brain. In an oversimplification, after reaching area 17, visual information passes through areas 18 and 19, then dorsally for spatial analysis and ventrally for object analysis (see Figs. 9–2 and 9–3). Schematic diagrams of dorsal stream (magnocellular pathway) for spatial relations and "where" analysis (**Top**) and ventral stream (parvocellular pathway) for color and "what" analysis (**Bottom**), from retina to higher cortical visual areas. LGN = lateral geniculate nucleus.

stimulation should be tested to exclude visual inattention. Color vision, reading, and writing should also be examined. In addition, magazine pictures with familiar faces and pictures with complex scenery can be used to screen for higher cortical dysfunction. Sometimes figure and clock drawings are also helpful. Table 9–2 highlights the various examination techniques helpful in patients with suspected higher cortical visual disorders, and these methods are also reviewed in detail in Chapter 2.

OCCIPITAL LOBE DISTURBANCES

Disorders of V_1 are described in Chapter 8. Areas V_2 and V_3 surround V_1 above and below the calcarine sulcus (see Fig. 8–15). Isolated and clinically apparent lesions of V_2 and V_3 are unusual, but a combined lesion of V_2 and V_3 restricted to the upper or lower bank typically causes a homonymous quadrantic visual field defect.[10]

TABLE 9–2. Examination Techniques Helpful in Patients With Suspected Higher Cortical Visual Disorders

Test	Result	Higher Cortical Disorder to Suspect
Reading and writing	Able to write but not read	Alexia without agraphia
Ishihara color plates	Can see colors but not the numbers	Simultanaganosia
Ishihara color plates	Misses all the digits on one side	Hemiachromatopsia
Magazine pictures	Identifies only part and not the whole scene	Simultanaganosia
Famous faces in pictures and familiar ones in identification cards	Can not identify familiar faces	Prosopagnosia
Name objects presented visually	Unable to identify objects by sight but can with verbal description	Visual object agnosia
Clock drawing	Draws only the right half	Hemineglect

See Chapter 2 for a detailed description of each test.

Another condition, alexia without agraphia, is a more commonly recognized occipital lobe syndrome and is detailed below.

Alexia Without Agraphia

Often aphasic patients who have difficulty reading also have difficulty writing. However, patients with a left occipital lesion and ipsilateral coinvolvement of the splenium of the corpus callosum or adjacent periventricular white matter may develop *alexia without agraphia* (or *pure alexia* or *"word blindness"*). First characterized by Dejerine,[11] this is a disconnection syndrome characterized by a right homonymous field deficit and sparing of key language areas, but an inability to access lexical visual information processed in the right occipital lobe (Fig. 9–2). Geschwind[8, 9] emphasized that reading is impossible if the left angular gyrus, which is responsible for converting written to spoken language, is deprived of visual information. Affected patients are therefore unable to read words, but they are able to write, speak, comprehend, and repeat normally. Ironically, then, they are unable to read what they write. Patients have a common compensatory strategy, called letter-by-letter reading, during which they sequentially name each letter of a word.[12–14] Alexia and agraphia together would be caused by an angular gyrus lesion.

Many variations on the classic description of alexia without agraphia have been described:

1. *Other lesions.* Alexia without agraphia due to infarction of the left lateral geniculate body and splenium of the corpus callosum has been reported.[15]
2. *No hemianopia.* Less commonly patients have been described with alexia without agraphia but with normal visual fields.[16–20] It is possible that periventricular white matter lesions in the left occipital lobe alone may spare striate cortex but interfere with the transfer of visual information from both ipsilateral and contralateral striate cortex to the language areas by undercutting the angular gyrus.[21]
3. *Left hemiparalexia.* Patients with isolated lesions of the splenium of the corpus callosum

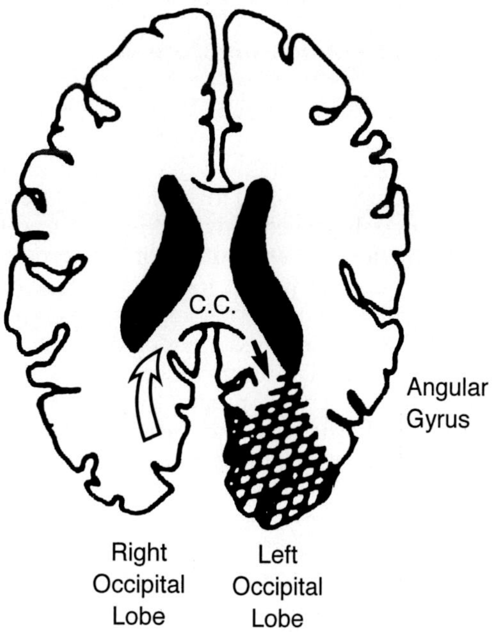

FIGURE 9–2. Localization of lesion in patients with alexia without agraphia and right homonymous hemianopia. Because of the left lateral and mesial occipital lobe involvement, visual information can come only from the right occipital lobe. However, owing to disruption of the paraventricular white matter and the outflow of the corpus callosum (C.C.), this visual information cannot access the angular gyrus in the language areas. (Adapted from Damasio AR, Damasio H: The anatomic basis of pure alexia. Neurology 1983;33:1573–1583, with permission.)

may have intact visual fields, but are unable to transfer visual information from the right occipital lobe to the left angular gyrus.[22] This may cause an inability to read the left side of words despite the absence of a hemianopia.

4. *Other associated higher cortical visual disturbances.* Several cases have been reported where alexia without agraphia occurs together with various combinations of apperceptive visual agnosia, prosopagnosia,[23, 24] visuospatial disorientation, optic ataxia, and hemiachromatopsia (these are all discussed below).[21] The condition has also been associated with color-naming deficits (see below).[25]

While the most common cause of alexia without agraphia is a posterior cerebral artery (PCA) distribution stroke,[26] it has also been reported in association with intracerebral hemorrhages,[27] arteriovenous malformations, tumors, abscesses, migraine, herpes encephalitis,[28] and multiple sclerosis.[29]

OCCIPITOTEMPORAL DISTURBANCES

Cerebral Hemiachromatopsia

More than a century ago, Verrey[30] described hemiachromatopsia, the loss of color vision in one hemifield, and claimed that a functionally separate cortex existed for color processing. However, it has been only in the past two to three decades that the notion of a neuroanatomically distinct region for color vision has been accepted.[31] Lesion studies in primates and humans have designated a region of the visual association cortex known as V_4 to be critical for color processing.[32] In humans the V_4 homolog resides in the lingual and fusiform gyri, located in the ventromedial occipitotemporal cortex (Fig. 9–3).[33] There is an area V_4 on both sides of the brain, and each mediates color vision in the opposite hemifield.

Functional neuroimaging has helped to confirm the specialization of V_4. Positron emission tomography (PET) studies of individuals viewing a multicolored abstract display show increased blood flow to V_1/V_2 and the lingual and fusiform gyri.[34] Studies using functional magnetic resonance imaging (MRI), comparing brain activation during colored versus black-and-white stimulus conditions, found the most significant changes in brain oxygenation occurred in the fusiform gyrus.[35, 36] Likewise, electrical cortical stimulation studies in epilepsy patients confirm the presence of a specialized color center in humans.[319, 320]

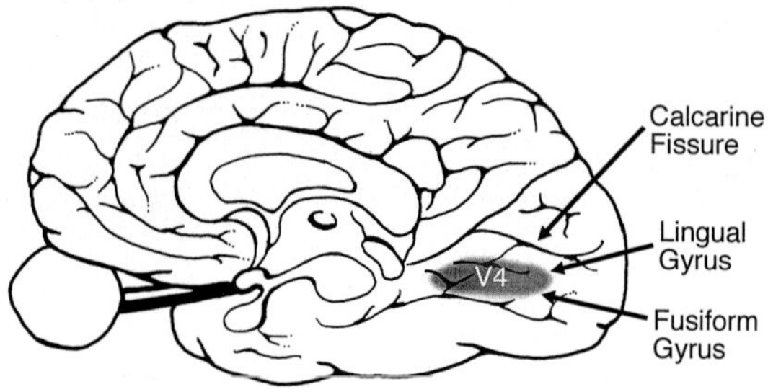

FIGURE 9–3. Medial view of the brain demonstrating the location of V_4, human color center, which lies primarily in the posterior fusiform gyrus, with a lesser contribution from the lingual gyrus.

Symptoms. Many patients with hemiachromatopsia are unaware of their color deficit, perhaps because the other hemifield has intact color vision, or because they ignore their deficit (*anosognosia*). Hemiachromatopsia can occur in the left or right hemifield. When bilateral V_4 lesions occur, patients may develop central achromatopsia, or defective color vision in both hemifields. In comparison to those with hemiachromatopsia, bilaterally affected patients may be more likely to describe their color deficit, which may differ from a loss of brightness to a complete inability to perceive colors. This variation may reflect a range of color processing impairment with different psychophysical correlates.[37] For instance, patients with partial color deficits, or *dyschromatopsia,* may perceive longer-wavelength colors, such as reds and oranges, relatively well. They may find blues and greens more difficult to discriminate. This dissociation may in part owe to the fewer number, and therefore greater vulnerability, of shorter-wavelength-selective cells in V_4.[31] Hue discrimination often becomes extremely difficult, and the described effect is a "greying" or "washing-out" of vision.[38] Some liken the impact to a switch from a color television to a black-and-white one.[39]

Signs. Since acquired cerebral color deficits tend to occur in quadrants or hemifields, they are best detected during confrontation field testing using colored swatches, sticks, or threads. Color plate testing may also reveal a hemidefect in color vision if the patient consistently misses the left-sided digits, for instance. However, color plate identification may be normal as may be more formal color testing, such as D-15 or Farnsworth–Munsell 100-hue tests, if color vision is normal within central fixation. These and other techniques of color testing are reviewed in detail in Chapter 2.

Associated Signs. Cerebral hemiachromatopsia is rarely an isolated finding. More commonly a contralateral homonymous upper quadrantanopia and defective color vision in the inferior quadrant is observed clinically (Fig. 9–4).[33] This combination is likely the result of the proximity between the lingual and fusiform gyri and the inferior optic radiations, inferior striate cortex, and inferior extrastriate cor-

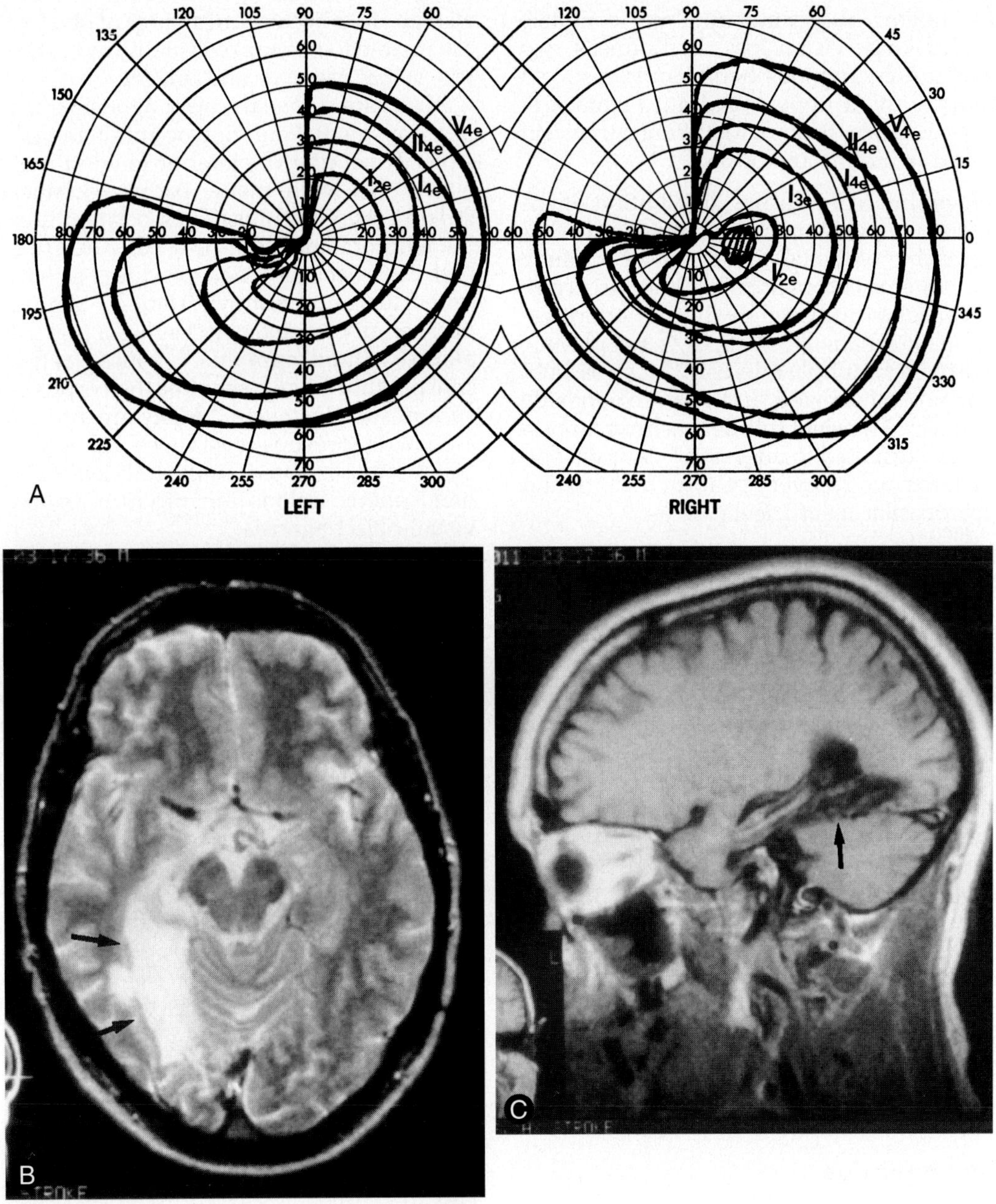

FIGURE 9–4. Visual field and neuroimaging in a patient with cerebral hemiachromatopsia of the left hemifield. **A.** Goldmann perimetry demonstrates a left homonymous superior quadrantanopia with an intact inferior quadrant. Axial (**B**) and Sagittal (**C**) MRI images reveal an infarction involving the right occipito-temporal gyri (*arrows*). (From Paulson HL, Galetta SL, Grossman M, et al: Hemiachromatopsia of unilateral occipitotemporal infarcts. Am J Ophthalmol 1994;118:518–523, with permission from Elsevier Science.)

tex (V_2/V_3).[10] Visual acuity is normal when the lesions are unilateral. Hemiachromatopsia may also be associated with alexia without agraphia (see above) when the lesion is left sided,[40] or prosopagnosia (see below).[3, 41, 42]

When isolated cerebral full-field hemiachromatopsia occurs, it is often in the setting of a developing or receding hemianopia.[42] Albert et al[43] described a monocular man who suffered cortical blindness only to recover with a partial right superor quadrantanopia yet complete left-sided color vision loss. In Kölmel's two cases,[44] a homonymous hemianopia resolved eventually to an upper quadrant hemiachromatopsia, in one instance following a transient full-field hemiachromatopsia.

Etiology. Infarction in the distribution of the posterior temporal or common temporal arteries, branches of the PCA, is the most common cause of hemiachromatopsia. Other less common causes include removal of an arteriovenous malformation,[45] trauma,[46] neoplasm,[42] hemorrhage, multiple sclerosis,[47] abscess, subarachnoid hemorrhage, and carbon monoxide poisoning.[48] Transient full-field achromatopsia has been attributed to migraine,[49] occipital epilepsy (after the recovery of form vision), and vertebrobasilar insufficiency.[50]

Other Cortical Color Processing Deficits. Patients with *color anomia,* or *color name aphasia,* have an inability to name colors despite normal color perception, as evidenced by their intact ability to match colors and identify pseudoisochromatic color plates. They also have difficulty pointing to named colors. This disorder can be associated with alexia without agraphia (see above),[25] and patients commonly have a right homonymous hemianopia.[39] The usual cause is a left PCA stroke involving the mesial occipitotemporal region.[51] Those with *color agnosia,* or *color amnesia,* have trouble naming the specific color of common objects, such as blood or a stop sign, despite normal color perception and language function. In one published case,[52] color agnosia was caused by bilateral medical temporal and left inferotemporo-occipital infarctions. Both color anomia and color agnosia are rare.[53]

Visual Agnosias

A *visual object agnosia* is an inability to recognize visualized objects despite relatively normal vision, memory, language, and intellectual function.[54] In this condition, naming function is intact, as patients are able to identify objects by touching and feeling them or by listening to a verbal description.[55] Sometimes a distinction between associative and apperceptive agnosias is made.

Patients with associative visual object agnosia have relatively normal vision within intact visual fields. They are able to draw or copy what they see, indicating their perception is relatively normal.[23] Upon request, they can also produce accurate drawings of objects they are unable to recognize visually, indicating intact visual memory and imagery.[23]

Associative visual object agnosia suggests bilateral medial inferior occipitotemporal lesions disrupting the inferior longitudinal fasculus,[56, 57] a white matter pathway connecting striate cortex with visual association areas in the temporal lobe. This is usually due to bilateral PCA occlusion and produces a "visual–verbal disconnection syndrome."[58] Many cases of associative visual object agnosia also exhibit alexia without agraphia,[23, 59] likely reflecting concomitant involvement of the corpus callosum in such instances.[56] Many are also associated with prosopagnosia (see below).[23] Less commonly, isolated unilateral left or right hemispheric lesions can produce associative visual object agnosia.[59]

In apperceptive visual object agnosia, patients have confounding deficits in shape and form perception although elemental acuity and fields are still relatively normal.[54] For instance, patients with apperceptive visual agnosia have difficulty copying geometric figures. In one study,[60] patients also had difficulty recognizing and naming line drawings, recognizing complex shapes, and mentally manipulating objects by rotation, for instance. The exact anatomic substrate is unclear, but some neuroimaging and PET studies have demonstrated lesions or hypoperfusion in bilateral temporo-occipital cortices.[61–63] A number of cases of apperceptive visual agnosia have been reported following carbon monoxide toxicity,[24, 64, 65] which has a predilection for causing occipital lobe damage.

Prosopagnosia

This section will review facial recognition and its related disorder, prosopagnosia, which is a dramatic visual agnosia for faces.

Facial Recognition. Physiologic studies have established that occipitotemporal structures bilaterally are involved in human facial recognition (Fig. 9–5). In one study,[66] electrodes on the surfaces of the striate and extrastriate cortex of epilepsy patients were used. The authors found areas bilaterally in the fusiform and lingual gyri in which electrical potentials were evoked in reponse to seeing faces, but not scrambled faces, cars, or butterflies. Depth electrode studies have also suggested that the medial occipitotemporal lobe and limbic structures such as the amygdala and hippocampus participate in facial recognition.[67, 68] In PET studies,[69–71] bilateral fusiform gyrus, lingual gyri, anterior temporal cortex, and right parahippocampal gyrus were activated while subjects identified faces. Using functional MRI, Puce et al[72]. found that bilaterally the mid-fusiform, inferior temporal gyri, and occipital temporal sulci activated during a viewing task consisting of unfamiliar faces but not during viewing of scrambled faces. Kanwisher[73] also used functional MRI to demonstrate the specificity of the right fusiform gyrus in facial recognition and perception. This area activated more strongly during viewing of faces when compared with common objects, scrambled faces, houses, and human hands.

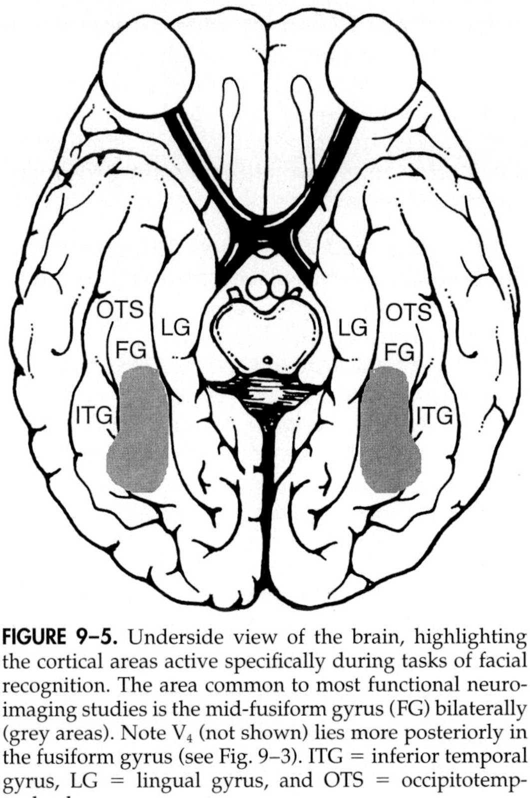

FIGURE 9–5. Underside view of the brain, highlighting the cortical areas active specifically during tasks of facial recognition. The area common to most functional neuroimaging studies is the mid-fusiform gyrus (FG) bilaterally (grey areas). Note V_4 (not shown) lies more posteriorly in the fusiform gyrus (see Fig. 9–3). ITG = inferior temporal gyrus, LG = lingual gyrus, and OTS = occipitotemporal sulcus.

Signs and Symptoms in Prosopagnosia. Patients with prosopagnosia initially are often aware of their condition, commonly reporting the inability to recognize the faces of friends and family.[74] A typical complaint is that the patients finds their own face in the mirror as unfamiliar, but know that the image must be theirs.[75] Likewise, prosopagnosics usually report knowing that they are looking at faces, and often they can identify the gender, race, and approximate age of the persons.[74] Often patients use contextual clues such as posture, body movement,[75] and especially voices to identify familiar faces.[76] Most patients exhibit both a retrograde and anterograde defect, as they often can not recognize old faces or learn new ones.[39] Sometimes the disorder is so striking and odd that affected patients may be mistakenly diagnosed with a psychiatric disease.[74]

Associated Signs. Prosopagnosia may be isolated but more commonly is associated with elemental visual or other higher cortical deficits. Unilateral homonymous hemianopias are typically present, but because the responsible lesions are typically occipitotemporal (see below), superior altitudinal or upper quadrantanopias are also seen.[4] Occasionally bilateral visual field deficits and related visual acuity loss are observed. Associated higher cortical abnormalities include achromatopsia,[77] alexia without agraphia,[78] left hemispatial neglect,[79] visual memory deficits,[6] visual object agnosia (see below),[80] visuospatial disorientation, impaired visual imagery,[24] color agnosia,[56] and anosognosia.[81]

Neuropsychological Aspects. Because prosopagnosia is a type of visual agnosia, there are probably also varying degrees of associative and apperceptive components in prosopagnosia.[82] Patients with a more apperceptive type would be expected to have more difficulty with a face-matching task than those with an associative type. This ability is most commonly examined using the Benton–Van Allen test for facial recognition.[83] This task evaluates a subject's ability to match photographs of unfamiliar faces in the front and three-quarter angle views, and under different lighting conditions. Many patients, probably with a greater apperceptive component, are impaired at face-matching.[84, 85] Some prosopagnosics perform within normal limits when completing this type of task.[83, 84] They either have a larger associative component or may employ a different matching strategy, perhaps with left hemispheric compensation (see laterality discussion below).[86] Further evidence for an associative component in some patients with prosopagnosia can be seen in patients who can correctly draw generic faces,[87] scan faces,[88, 89] estimate a person's age[83] and gender,[87] and interpret and imitate facial expressions.[90, 91] Evidence of an apperceptive component can be seen in patients with prosopagnosia who have difficulty discerning curved stimuli,[92] face-related features such as eye gaze,[93] and gender.[90]

Similar to patients with blindsight (see Chapter 8), some patients with prosopagnosia report an inability to remember or distinguish faces, but careful testing may reveal some unconscious or covert ability to do so.[87, 94–98] Access to faces stored in memory must be intact. For instance, some patients perform better than chance at deciding which of two names corresponds to a famous face, despite reporting no recognition throughout the trials and claiming to be guessing.[96] One patient correctly matched 86% (within standard deviation of controls) on a forced-choice face-to-name matching task, despite reporting familiarity with only 6% of the stimuli.[99] However, covert recognition is an inconsistent finding in patients with prosopagnosia.[90, 100, 101]

Relationship of Prosopagnosia to Other Visual Agnosias. In some patients with prosopagnosia, problems with recognition are restricted to faces only.[102] However, more commonly, there is also some degree of visual object agnosia although the facial deficits are usually more salient and severe than with other objects. One study reported a patient with recognition of 92% of objects versus only 62% of facial stimuli.[103] One prosopagnosic was unimpaired at naming real objects but was not able to discern articles belonging to her from similar objects.[104] One possible explanation is that prosopagnosia, and the visual object agnosia that is often associated with it, results from a defect in discriminating visually ambiguous stimuli from within a category.[5, 6, 105, 106]

Patients with prosopagnosia may also have difficulty recognizing familiar animals. One former bird watcher lost the ability to identify birds with the onset of her prosopagnosia.[107] Likewise, a farmer reported the inability to recognize his cattle, although he was able to do so before the onset of prosopagnosia.[107] However, another patient who began acquiring sheep after developing prosopagnosia was more successful on identification tasks involving his sheep than on identical tasks with human faces.[108]

Etiology and Associations. The most common cause of prosopagnosia is a PCA stroke, although any process that can damage the occipitotemporal lobes may be responsible. Thus other causes include carbon monoxide poisoning,[24] temporal lobectomy, encephalitis,[88, 109, 110] neoplasms,[80] right temporal lobe atrophy,[111] trauma,[6] and Alzheimer's disease.[112] More diffuse processes include alcohol intoxication,[113] Asperger syndrome (a form of autism),[114] and psychosis due to schizophrenia and mescaline.[115] One epidemiologic study found that prosopagnosia occurred significantly more frequently in males than in females,[116] which might be a reflection of either a higher incidence of stroke or a different lateralization of facial recognition in males.

Capgras Syndrome. Prosopagnosia is similar in its presentation to Capgras syndrome, a delusional disorder. A patient with Capgras syndrome feels that a friend or relative has been replaced by an impostor.[117, 118] There are some authors who believe that some patients with Capgras syndrome have prosopagnosia.[117] Evidence for this was found in one patient who began experiencing Capgras delusions at age 19 and reported having prosopagnosic symptoms as a child; she accidentally grabbed the hands of other women when shopping with her mother. MRI revealed bilateral occipitotemporal lesions similar to those often found in patients with prosopagnosia (see below).[119]

Localization and Uni-versus Bilaterality of the Lesions. Most cases of prosopagnosia that have come to autopsy show bilateral lesions in the occipitotemporal region.[4, 5, 56, 120] Usually the damage was due to bilateral infarcts in the territories of the PCAs.[121] Based on necropsy data alone, the question of whether bilateral lesions were necessary for prosopagnosia remained controversial because the autopsies in many instances were performed years after the onset of symptoms. Therefore, other lesions may have occurred between symptom onset and death. A more definitive study was published by Landis et al,[122] who presented necropsy findings of a woman who died 10 days after developing prosopagnosia. A single infarct in the territory of the right PCA was discovered.

Many authors have reported patients with prosopagnosia and bilateral posterior lesions documented with CT[6, 78, 84, 123] or MRI.[79] In contrast to necropsy data, however, multiple cases have been reported of prosopagnosics with only right-sided lesions as uncovered by CT[124, 125] or MRI.[111, 126, 127] Thus it appears that bilateral lesions are often seen in patients with prosopagnosia, but in several instances a unilateral right-sided lesion was sufficient to cause the deficit.

There is in fact evidence for a right-sided cerebral dominance for facial recognition in humans. One study compared the performance of right-lesioned to left-lesioned patients (both groups classified using CT data) on a facial identification task. Patients with right-sided lesions performed significantly worse than left-lesioned patients and controls.[128] Prosopagnosia was also observed in a patient who had undergone a right hemispherectomy.[129]

Lesion Location. Most of the reported lesions are localized within the right occipitotemporal region.[130] However, the critical structure involved in this area can vary between the inferior occipitotemporal cortex, the fusiform gyrus, and the hippocampal region.[131] A larger study correlated two separate extrastriate lesion positions to two cognitive deficits. Damage to the fusiform gyri, when accompanied with right-sided infacts in the occipitotemporal or ventromedial regions, led to problems in perceiving facial detail. Patients with damage to the right parahippocampal gyrus, and the accompanying occipitotemporal or ventromedial damage in the right hemisphere, exhibited a deficit in connecting faces to memory stores.[70]

Outcome. Although it may be an enduring condition, patients may eventually recover from prosopagnosia, especially if damage is confined to the right hemisphere.[84, 132] One study tracked the progress of 18 patients who developed prosopagnosia as a result of a right hemisphere stroke. The median time required for 50% of the patients to recover from the prosopagnosic symptoms was 9 weeks.[132] Another prosopagnosic with a right-sided lesion, as observed with MRI, regained the ability to recognize famous faces as well as friends and family 2 months after the onset of his symptoms. However, he remained unable to identify the faces of people whom he met after the onset of symptoms.[127] Bilateral damage may be necessary in order for the prosopagnosic symptoms to endure past the acute period.[39]

Optic Aphasia

In contrast, patients with optic aphasia, which is a condition closely related to visual object agnosia, are unable to name visually presented material or point to named objects although they may recognize them. They are able to name and recognize what they may hear or feel. The responsible lesion is usually unilateral and involves the left posterior cerebral hemisphere. This disorder likely is another visuoverbal disconnection syndrome.[8] However, patients with optic aphasia may have better recognizing capabilities than those with object agnosia because of relatively preserved access to right hemispheric perceptual/semantic systems.[133]

Visual Memory Disturbances

The ability to remember visual information requires storing then retrieving it.[134] Ross[135] reported two patients with bilateral posterior temporal lobe infarctions and loss of visual recent memory. Tactile, verbal, and nonverbal auditory memory functions were normal, but they could not recognize faces. Attributing the visual memory deficit to a disconnection syndrome, he hypothesized that the bilateral lesions disrupted tracts between primary visual cortex and structures important for memory, such as the medial temporal lobe. Other patients with similar bilateral temporal lobe lesions and prosopagnosia have been described,[5, 6] suggesting that recognition of faces and visual memory share similar mechanisms.

Evidence for lateralization and the role of the right temporal lobe in visual memory is provided by studies of patients who, following right temporal lobectomy, exhibit defective recognition of visual material[136] and of a patient with damage to the right frontotemporal region following middle cerebral artery aneurysm rupture who had defective memory of new visual objects and faces[137]; and by PCA amobarbital tests, which suggest that the right temporal lobe is important for remembering visual aspects of an object, while the left temporal lobe is more critical for recalling the object's verbal representation.[138] Functional MRI studies have demonstrated that the ventrolateral prefrontal cortex mediates human visual working memory, which is the process of retaining visual information for a brief period so that it is available for immediate use.[139]

Other similar patients with impaired visual memory have been described following infarction of the right dorsomedial thalamic nucleus[140] and damage to the anterior commissure and right fornix,[141] structures also important in the formation and retrieval of visual information.

Akinetopsia

Recent evidence has demonstrated that lateral occipitotemporal lesions affecting area V_5 (Fig. 9–6), which lies in the posterior bank of the superior temporal sulcus, may result in defective motion perception, or *akinetopsia*.[142] Animal experiments first suggested that the comparable location in monkeys, area MT, contains cells that receive direct connections from striate cortex and are highly motion selective.[143] Lesions to area MT impair motion perception in the contralateral hemifield.[144] Zihl et al[145] described a seminal patient with defective motion perception due to bilateral cortical venous infarctions involving the temporoparietal and occipital periventricular and subcortical white matter, posterior portion of the middle temporal gyrus, and lateral occipital gyri. Striate cortex was spared. When the patient poured tea or coffee into a cup the fluid "appeared to be frozen, like a glacier." She was unable to judge the speed of a moving car, but could identify the car without difficulty. Follow-up studies[146, 147] reported the patient's MRI scans, which confirmed the bilateral lesions involving the upper part of the occipital gyri and the adjacent portion of the middle temporal gyri, with the main focus of damage in the upper banks of the anterior occipital sulcus. Thus both the animal and clinical literature suggested the existence of a cortical area, separate from striate cortex, which mediates visual motion perception.

Other experimental evidence in normal humans has continued to support this notion. PET studies of individuals viewing moving black-and-white random-square patterns show increased blood flow to the temporo-parieto-occipital junction.[34] Functional MRI studies demonstrate increased activation of lateral occipitotemporal cortex in association with viewing moving stimuli.[148, 149] Likewise, electrical cortical stimulation in epilepsy patients has confirmed the presence of a specialized motion area in humans concentrated at the occipitotemporol parietal junction.[319, 320]

Some drugs have been reported to cause akinetopsia. Two cases of akinetopsia related to use of nefazodone, an antidepressant that blocks serotonin (5-HT_2) receptors and the reuptake of 5-HT, have been reported.[156]

Riddoch Phenomena, Blindsight, and V_5. One explanation for the Riddoch phenomenon and

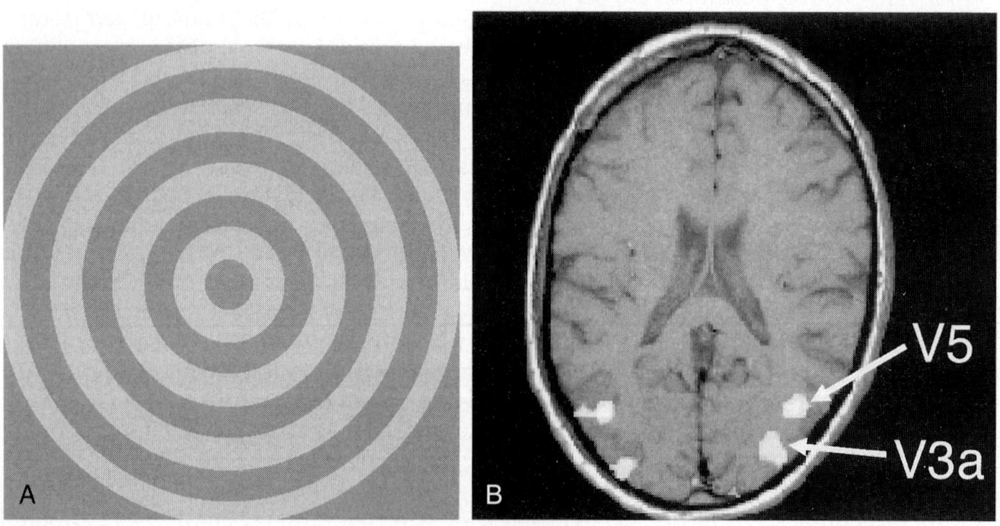

FIGURE 9–6. Functional magnetic resonance imaging (fMRI) demonstration of motion sensitive areas of the brain. **A.** Stimulus consisting of concentric rings, one cycle per degree of visual angle, which expanded and contracted at a speed of 1 degree of visual angle per second. The gray and light gray ring contrast is 22%. The stimulus paradigm alternated eight cycles of 30 seconds of moving rings then 30 seconds of stationary rings. **B.** Areas (V5 and V3a) activated by the moving rings but not the stationary ones are superimposed on the subject's corresponding T1-weighted image. The height threshold of the activation map was set at $p < 0.001$ (uncorrected). (G. R. Bonhomme, A. Miki, and G. T. Liu).

for blindsight, in which individuals with field loss due to striate cortex damage are able to perceive motion or have unconscious vision, respectively (for further discussion of these phenomena see Chapter 8), is the preservation of parallel retino-tecto-pulvinar connections with V_5. In one study,[150] a patient with a left occipital lesion who was able perceive fast- but not slow-moving stimuli within an otherwise blind hemifield underwent visual evoked potential testing. This demonstrated that V_5 was activated despite the destruction of V_1 (striate cortex), suggesting that in addition to the main pathway from V_1 to V_5, there existed another pathway to V_5 that bypassed V_1. Another study[151] suggested that in patients with visual field loss due to cerebral hemispheric lesions, those with preserved motion detection tended to have sparing of lateral temporo-occipital cortex, while those without motion detection usually had involvement of this area. In PET and functional MRI studies of patients with unilateral occipital lobe infarction, ipsilateral lateral temporo-occipital cortex is still activated during optokinetic stimulation[152] and when moving stimuli are presented in the blind hemifield.[153–155]

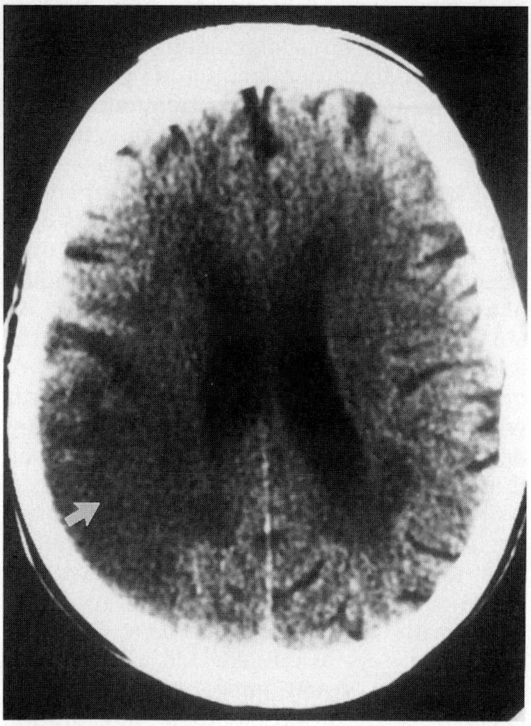

FIGURE 9–7. Axial CT scan showing a right parietal hypodensity (*arrow*), consistent with infarction, in a patient with left hemineglect.

PARIETAL DISTURBANCES

Right parietal lesions (Fig. 9–7) may result in *sensory neglect* of visual, tactile, and auditory stimuli in left hemispace.[132] *Motor neglect*, a defect in exploration of and responding to stimuli in contralateral hemispace, may also occur. Affected patients sometimes also display visual or spatial disorientation, a difficulty in localizing objects visually, to their left.[157–159] However, visual disorientation occurs more commonly in bilateral lesions (see Balint syndrome, below). Other symptoms of right parietal injury include dressing and constructional apraxia, failure to recognize one side of the body (*asomatognosia*), and a denial of neurologic impairment (*anosognosia*). These deficits are unaccounted for by visual field loss, other primary sensory deficits, or motor weakness.[160, 161]

Parietal areas involved likely include the superior parietal lobule (human area 7) or inferior parietal lobule (human areas 39 and 40) or both.[162, 163] In addition, left neglect syndromes resulting from right-sided lesions are more common because the right hemisphere is dominant for the distribution of attention.[164] In other words, the left hemisphere attends to the right side of space, while the right hemisphere attends to both sides. Thus a left-sided lesion tends not to cause neglect because the intact right hemisphere is still able to attend to the right side.

The majority of this section will review sensory neglect of visual stimuli.

Visual Neglect (Hemi-inattention)

The term *unilateral visual hemi-inattention* describes the neglect of visual stimuli in a homonymous half-field despite an intact geniculostriate system. Patients with this phenomenon clinically may be difficult to distinguish from those with a homonymous hemianopia, but unlike the latter, those with hemi-inattention will be more likely to detect the stimulus if their attention is directed to the neglected side (assuming central fixation is maintained).[165] In more subtle cases the visual fields will be normal to confrontation, but if comparable visual stimuli are presented simultaneously in right and left hemifields (double simultaneous stimulation), the one contralateral to the lesion will be ignored. When the neglect is dense, however, the absence of a hemianopia is frequently difficult to prove. If the parietal lesion is large enough, often both the neglect and a hemianopia are present.

Bedside tests for hemi-inattention, such as line or letter cancellation, line bisection, or figure and clock drawing, are reviewed in Chapter 2. In line or letter cancellation, patients with left neglect tend to identify targets only in their right hemispace. During line bisection, when patients are asked to identify the middle of a horizontal line, those with left neglect often pick a point that is on the right side of the line. The numbers of a clock may be drawn only on the right side of a clockface. Patients with both left hemi-inattention and hemianopia tend to do more poorly on these tests than those with hemi-inattention alone.[166]

Several theories have attempted to explain neglect. Bisiach et al[167] attributed unilateral neglect to a defect in the internal mental representation of the external world, as some patients with left hemineglect have defective mental imagery of the left side of space (see discussion of visual imagery, below). Others[165, 168–170] have proposed that an interruption in the corticolimbic–reticular loop causes a defect in the orienting response toward stimuli in the contralateral hemispace. Mesulam[171–173] hypothesized that a cortical network involving posterior parietal lobe, frontal lobe, and cingulate gyrus mediates directed attention. Damage to any one or more components could lead to a neglect syndrome (see discussion of frontal lobe lesions, below).[174] In Mesulam's scheme, the posterior parietal component provides an internal sensory map of extrapersonal space, the frontal component a mechanism for scanning and exploring, and the cingulate a spatial map for motivation. Because these proposed mechanisms are not mutually exclusive, a combination of them may also apply.[175–177]

Subcortical Lesions. Unilateral neglect behavior less commonly may result from subcortical lesions. Examples include damage to the thalamus,[178, 179] striatum (putamen and head of caudate) and adjacent deep white matter,[180–182] and callosal infarction.[183] These lesions may cause neglect by indirect effects on the parietal lobe by, for example, disrupting subcortical–cortical connections. Diaschisis, a poorly understood transient depression of function elsewhere in the brain due to a focal cerebral lesion, may be another explanation.[184]

Treatment. Patients with severe left-sided neglect can be some of the most difficult to rehabilitate, and their functional disability and prognosis for recovery is often poorer than that for individuals with global aphasia or hemiplegia.[185, 186] Many patients with neglect are difficult to help because they are unaware of or deny their deficit. One study found that those with larger right-sided lesions and with preexisting cortical atrophy had a poorer prognosis for recovery.[187]

The treatment of visual hemi-inattention is largely adaptive. Like in patients with hemianopias, those with hemi-inattention should have their bed within their room arranged to face their non-neglected side. Similarly, family and friends should be instructed to approach the patient from the *intact side.* Visual hemi-inattention precludes driving, cooking, crossing the street unaided, or working with heavy machinery. A vertical colored strip of paper can be placed along the left margin of text to facilitate reading, with instructions given to the patient to find the paper when moving down to the next line.

Other treatment options, although touted because of their positive effects during neuropsychological testing, are either unsatisfactory or unproven when improvement in activities of daily living is the goal.[185] We have found hemianopic prisms[188] (see Chapter 8) relatively unhelpful in patients with left-sided neglect, particularly because of the confusion they cause in patients who likely also have visual disorientation. Prism adaptation of both eyes leads to only a transient improvement.[189] The use of hemispatial sunglasses, which shade the non-neglected side of each eye and force viewing into the neglected side, has been reported anectodally as effective.[190] Another technique involves the use of visual imagery and trains patients to pretend their eyes are like the light of a lighthouse, sweeping far to the left and right.[191] An alternative strategy, which trains patients to turn their heads to the left, utilizes the intact right visual field for scanning. Phasic alerting, which uses a warning sound, can correct visual awareness[192] but is impractical outside of the experimental setting.

In addition, vestibular stimulation by cold water, for instance, may have some efficacy in patients with visual neglect.[193] This maneuver may train patients to orient toward the affected hemispatial field. We have no personal experience with this technique, which in any case is only temporary. Lastly, dopamine agonists have been shown anecdotally to improve neglect.[194] However, this therapy has not been evaluated in a controlled fashion, and in one

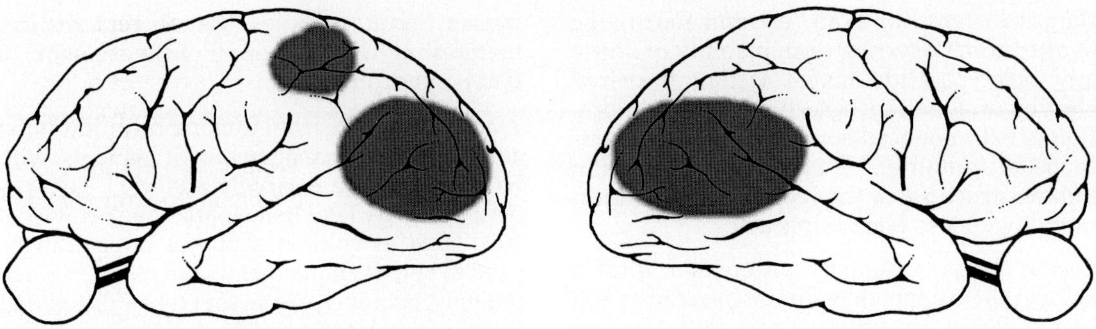

FIGURE 9–8. Location of lesions in Balint's original patient. The two largest areas of damage were in the parietal lobes bilaterally, but there was also a lesion near the left central sulcus.

study bromocriptine actually worsened some aspects of hemispatial neglect.[195]

PARIETO-OCCIPITAL DISTURBANCES

Balint Syndrome

Balint[196, 197] first analyzed this symptom complex, and Holmes[198] later elaborated his description. It results most frequently from bilateral symmetric parieto-occipital cortical or white matter injury (Figs. 9–8 and 9–9). In the minority of cases there is additional frontal lobe involvement.[199] In its most severe form, patients with Balint syndrome appear disabled and almost completely blind except for macular sparing: they bump into objects and often require assistance while walking in the room, they do not refixate on novel stimuli in their visual periphery and they do not blink to threat, but they become tremendously visually fixated on single objects.[200] The full syndrome consists of *simultanagnosia* (or simultaneous agnosia), *ocular apraxia* (a deficit in shifting gaze), and *optic ataxia* (a defect in reaching under visual guidance).[199, 201] Each of these elements, which may be seen alone or in combination, will be briefly considered below.

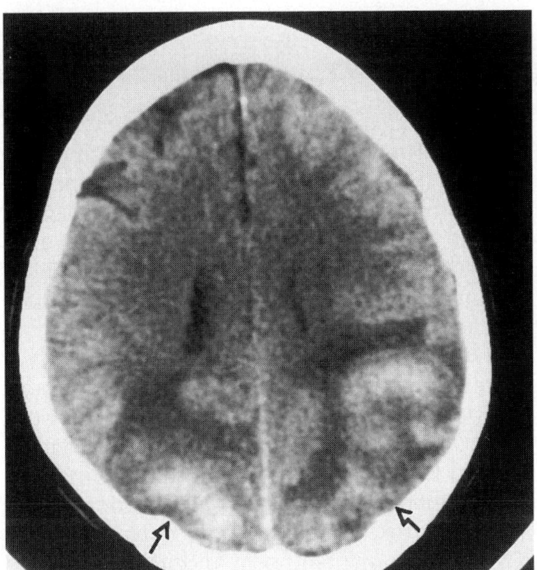

FIGURE 9–9. Axial CT scan of a patient with bilateral parieto-occipital hemorrhages and Balint syndrome. The patient had an inferior altitudinal visual field deficit in both eyes (see Fig. 8–24), simultanagnosia, optic ataxia, and ocular apraxia.

Simultanagnosia. Simultanagnosia, a striking deficit in Balint syndrome, is the element seen most often in isolation. It is defined as an inability to grasp the entire meaning of a picture despite an intact capacity to recognize the picture's individual constituent elements.[39] Thus, affected patients may be unable to identify a picture of a landscape but are able to recognize a small tree within it. Such patients may be able to read single 20/20 letters but can read words only by spelling them out loud. Despite normal color vision, patients with simultanagnosia may also have difficulty with the Ishihara color plate examination (see Chapter 2),[202] which requires them to identify colored numbers created by small dots. Chapter 2 reviews other tests for simultanagnosia.

Simultanagnosia may reflect bilaterally defective visual attention,[203, 204] as the lesions in Balint syndrome typically involve Brodmann areas 7 (superior parietal lobule), 19 (dorsorostral occipital lobe), and sometimes 39 (inferior parietal lobule).[205] These are areas important for visual attention. Several authors have offered the absent blink to visual threat response as evidence for decreased visual attention in this disorder.[206, 207] One authority[7] attributed the visual behavior to an "extreme narrowing of attention," referring to an inability to notice any object outside foveal vision. Impaired shifting of attention, defective visual exploration of extrapersonal space, leading to deficits in visual scanning,[208–210] and an impairment in linking structural descriptions and object location[211] have also been implicated.

Ocular Apraxia. Patients with ocular apraxia are unable to generate voluntary saccades, but their involuntary reflexive saccades are normal. The terms *psychic gaze paralysis* and *spasm of fixation* have also been used. Possible mechanisms include a disconnection of the occipital lobe from the frontal eye fields or uncertainty about the target's location.[200] In its purest form, ocular apraxia is associated with normal pursuit eye movements, but in fact many patients have defective pursuit as well. Other clinical features and mechanisms of ocular apraxia, which is also seen in other disorders, are reviewed in Chapter 16.

Optic Ataxia. Although patients with optic ataxia may be able to see an object of regard, they may reach for it inaccurately. Optic ataxia is also known as *visuomotor ataxia.* The deficit is unassociated with any cerebellar dysfunction or motor weakness. Instead, optic ataxia may result from a disconnection of the occipital lobe from motor centers more anteriorly in the frontal lobe, where the reaching is programmed.[7, 205, 212, 213] A defect in the internal representation of extrapersonal space, and damage to areas responsible for integrating panoramic visual information with proprioceptive information relating to the upper extremity,[205, 214] are alternative explanations.

Other Neuro-ophthalmic Signs. As alluded to earlier, the blink to threat response may be absent even within intact visual fields.[215] Spatial or visual disorientation, a difficulty in localizing and finding objects in extrapersonal space by sight alone, is another prominent feature in a number of cases.[198, 199, 216] Although the visual fields may be normal,[39] often bilateral inferior altitudinal defects are present[216, 217] owing to the frequent involvement of the superior banks of the occipital lobes.

Etiology. The usual cause is watershed infarction in the setting of hypoperfusion following cardiac or respiratory arrest, but patients with cardiogenic emboli, Alzheimer's disease,[218] Creutzfeldt–Jakob disease, adrenoleukodystrophy,[219] or progressive multifocal leukoencephalopathy[220] (see Chapter 8) may also present with complex visual disturbances manifesting with any or all of the elements of Balint syndrome.

Treatment. Aside from treating the underlying condition, the management of patients with Balint syndrome is largely adaptive. Like patients with parietal hemispatial neglect, visual cues such as colored strips of paper can be used to help them read and scan pages.[221] Some patients, however, are so severely affected that they are rendered visually disabled.

Posterior Cortical Atrophy

The syndrome of "posterior cortical atrophy" has been applied to a progressive illness characterized by some combination of alexia with or without agraphia, visual agnosia, components of Balint syndrome, Gerstmann syndrome (left–right confusion, finger agnosia, acalculia, and agraphia), and transcortical sensory aphasia (fluent aphasia with intact ability to repeat).[222–224] Memory, insight, and judgment are affected later in the course of the disease. Neuroimaging reveals cerebral atrophy, more severe posteriorly. Etiologic considerations include Alzheimer's, Pick's, and Creutzfeldt–Jakob diseases. Posterior cortical atrophy is thought to be a unique presentation of these conditions.[225]

Visual Imagery

Although visual imagery is not solely a parietal lobe function, lesions in this area may affect this cognitive function. Numerous neuropsychological and functional neuroimaging studies have suggested that many of the same areas of the brain that are responsible for viewing and interpreting an object are also important for imagining it.[226–230] For instance, patients with occipital lobe lesions and a contralateral hemianopia or quadrantanopia can have defective visual imagery ipsilateral to the field defect.[231] In addition, PET studies have demonstrated that patients with acquired blindness due to anterior visual pathway lesions activate visual cortex during mental imagery.[232] Patients with prosopagnosia and achromatopsia may have an imagery disorder involving faces and colors of objects.[233] Individuals with visual agnosias for particular objects, living versus nonliving, for example, may have selective loss of visual imagery for the same types of items.[234]

Furthermore, imagining an object or scene requires the ability to generate an internal representation of objects and scenes in extrapersonal space. This is one of the tasks of the inferior parietal lobule. Thus patients with right parietal lobe lesions may neglect the left side of visual images. For instance, Bisiach and Luzzatti[235] asked patients with left hemineglect to imagine they were looking at the Piazza del Duomo in Milan. When they were asked to describe the view from the side of the square opposite the cathedral, they described fewer landmarks on the left side of their imagined scene. Then they were asked to recall the view of the square from the other side on the cathedral steps. Again they neglected more details on their left, but they described correctly objects on the right they had previously ignored from the other side! Other patients with visual disorientation and defective visuospatial imagery have been described.[233]

However, there are notable exceptions to this concept that perception, higher cortical function, and imagery are highly correlated, implying the mechanism for imagery may be much more complicated. In fact, several cases have shown that perception and imagery can be dissociated. For instance, patients with hemianopias and cortical blindness have been reported with intact visual imagery.[236, 237] Some patients with cerebral achromatopsia have preserved color imagery.[238, 239] In addition, a patient with a right parietal lesion and left-sided representational neglect without visual perceptual neglect,[240] and others with visual agnosia but intact visual imagery,[61, 241] have been reported.

FRONTAL LOBE DISTURBANCES

Frontal lobe neglect is well recognized in humans.[242, 243] It can be denser than parietal neglect and mimic a homonymous hemianopia.[162] Cogan[244] in fact used the term *pseudohemianopsia* to refer to patients with this disorder. In contrast to those with a hemianopia from parietal or occipital injury, however, the frontal defect is usually transient. Furthermore, frontal neglect may preferentially affect exploratory–motor rather than perceptual–sensory tasks.[245] Many patients will have a hemiparesis and mild difficulty with contraversive lateral gaze, consistent with adjacent involvement of the motor strip as well as the more anterior frontal eye fields. In one study[246] of patients with frontal neglect of the left hemispace, all lesions involved the inferior frontal gyrus (Brodmann's area 44) and the underlying white matter. Part of premotor cortex, this area is the homologue of Broca's area in the right hemisphere.

DISEASES COMMONLY ASSOCIATED WITH HIGHER CORTICAL VISUAL DISTURBANCES

The most common cause of a higher cortical visual disturbance is a vaso-occlusive stroke. Typically the PCA or one of its branches is involved unilaterally or bilaterally, affecting the occipital, occipitotemporal, and occipitoparietal areas. Middle cerebral artery strokes may cause parietal or frontal lobe syndromes. Other causes include neoplasms, hemorrhages, multiple sclerosis, abscesses, trauma, progressive multifocal leukoencephalopathy, and carbon monoxide poisoning. The differential diagnosis is similar to that of retrochiasmal disturbances (see Chapter 8).

However, two dementing illnesses, Alzheimer's disease and Creutzfeldt–Jakob disease, have a predilection for visual association cortices. Thus each condition will be reviewed here. In each section, the neurologic, neuro-ophthalmic, laboratory, and pathologic features will be discussed, followed by treatment issues.

Alzheimer's Disease

Alzheimer's disease, a degenerative condition, is highlighted by gradually progressive dementia, which in turn is characterized by (i) a loss of intellect sufficient enough to interfere with social or occupational functions, (ii) memory loss, and (iii) a clear sensorium. The disease is considered probable if these features are present, the age of onset is between 40 and 90, and other neurologic diseases that could account for the deficits are absent.[247] The terms *presenile* and *senile dementia* refer to dementia that occurs either before or after age 65, respectively.

Alzheimer's disease is the most common cause of dementia in North America and Europe,[248] accounting for at least half of cases.[249] Its prevalence increases with age. In one population study,[250] of individuals 65 to 74 years of age, 3.0% had probable Alzheimer's disease, while 18.7% of persons 75 to 84 years old and 47.2% of those over 85 had the disorder. Thus, as the general population ages in the future, this disease is likely to become more prevalent. Besides advanced age, other risk factors for the disease include small head size, a history of head trauma, and low intelligence.[251]

Neurologic Symptoms and Signs. Aside from the insidious memory loss that defines this condition, patients with Alzheimer's disease may develop language deficits, particularly word-finding difficulties. Personality changes, problems with concentration, and a change in affect may also occur, and some patients become psychotic and agitated. In later stages deterioration in social skills and motor impairment may also become evident. In general, though, the cranial nerves, motor strength, sensation, gait, and reflexes are all normal. Extrapyramidal signs such as bradykinesia and tremor may be observed, as some patients have co-existing Parkinson's disease. Job loss, home care, nursing home placement, and eventual demise comprise the inevitable progression in most instances. Patient survival is usually between 5 to 12 years following disease onset.[248]

Differential Diagnosis. Depression, multi-infarct dementia, extrapyramidal disorders, hypothyroidism, and toxic–metabolic disorders (for instance, drug toxicity) are the most common conditions mistaken for Alzheimer's disease. The reader is referred to recently published reviews[248, 252, 253] for lists and discussions of the less common disorders to be considered in the differential diagnosis of dementia.

Neuro-ophthalmic Symptoms and Signs. The visual disturbances in Alzheimer's disease tend to be higher cortical in nature.[254] In one study[255] of community-based patients with Alzheimer's disease, approximately one half had a visual object agnosia, while one fifth had Balint syndrome. Prosopagnosia, visual hallucinations (see Chapter 12), defective visual motion discrimination,[256, 257] abnormal form perception,[258] poor performance on visuospatial tasks,[259, 260] right-sided neglect, alexia without agraphia, and diminished curiosity of novel or unusual visual stimuli[261] may also occur. Because patients with Alzheimer's disease and higher cortical visual disturbances usually have normal visual acuity, relatively clear ocular media, and a normal funduscopic appearance, many such patients have persistent visual complaints despite visits to several ophthalmologists and numerous changes in eyeglass prescriptions.

In contrast, some studies have suggested patients with Alzheimer's disease may also have more elementary visual deficits involving the primary visual pathways. Deficits in visual acuity,[262] visual fields,[254] contrast sensitivity,[263] stereoacuity,[264, 265] and color vision,[266] and abnormal visual evoked potentials[267] and electroretinograms[268, 269] have been reported. However, these results are only inconsistently observed, and some studies are hampered by limitations in patient testing. For instance, some authors[270, 271] were unable to demonstrate any clinical or electrophysiologic abnormalities in primary visual function that were not also observed in age-matched controls. In addition, in one study[272] of patients with Alzheimer's disease who underwent computerized perimetry, many had nonspecific visual field constriction. However, the numbers of fixation losses and false-negative and -positive responses for each patient were very high, making any conclusions difficult.

Diagnostic Studies. The results of neuroradiologic studies, both anatomic and functional, tend to be nonspecific in patients with Alzheimer's disease. CT and MRI, although helpful in excluding a mass lesion, multiple infarcts, or normal-pressure hydrocephalus, are usually either normal or reveal diffuse cortical atrophy. PET and other blood flow studies may demonstrate decreased rates of glucose metabolism in the posterior cingulate, parietal, parieto-occipital, temporal, and prefrontal regions.[273, 274] Lumbar puncture, which is often performed to exclude cryptococcal or carcinomatous meningitis or tertiary syphilis, is generally unremarkable. However, spinal fluid levels of tau may be elevated and those of beta-amyloid protein (see pathology, below) may be decreased in patients with Alzheimer's disease.[275, 321] Sometimes an electroencephalogram, which is either normal or shows diffuse slowing in Alzheimer's disease, is obtained when Creutzfeldt–Jakob disease is also considered.

The apolipoprotein E ∈4 allele is associated with the sporadic and late-onset forms of Alzheimer's disease. However, the presence of the ∈4 allele does not predict the future onset of Alzheimer's disease, and not all patients with Alzheimer's disease have the ∈4 allele. Therefore testing for the ∈4 allele is not routinely performed.[276] In the much less common early-onset familial cases, amyloid precursor protein, presenilin 1, and presenilin 2 genes may be identified.[277–279]

Although skin and olfactory epithelium biopsies, along with fibroblast and platelet analysis, have been previously suggested, their utility has not been established.[276] Pupillary supersensitivity to dilute tropicamide is also unhelpful, and this topic is reviewed in Chapter 13.

Pathology. The diagnosis of Alzheimer's disease can be confirmed only histologically, by either biopsy or postmortem examination. The diagnostic pathologic features include neurofibrillary tangles, which are characterized by paired helical fibers composed of altered forms of the microtubule-associated protein tau, and senile plaques, consisting of insoluable beta-amyloid protein.[280–283] Also seen are granulovacuolar degeneration, amyloid (congophilic) deposition in vessel walls, and Hirano bodies, which are eosinophilic filaments. Cell loss in the basal forebrain cholinergic complex and decreased choline acetyltranferase activity suggest that defective cholinergic transmission may be associated with the disease.[284]

The visual deficits in Alzheimer's disease are usually attributed to neurofibrillary tangles in visual association areas with relative less involvement of the retino-geniculo-calcarine pathways, including striate cortex.[285–287] Levine et al[288] described a patient with Alzheimer's, visual object agnosia, visual field constriction, and impaired contrast sensitivity. The postmortem examination revealed the density of tangles was highest in the occipitoparietal areas and lowest in the frontal lobes. A similar distribution of lesions was found in a group of Alzheimer's patients presenting with Balint syndrome.[289] Alzheimer's patients who are visually symptomatic are more likely to demonstrate tangles in the occipitoparietal regions than those who have normal visual function.[290]

Pathologic findings in the primary visual pathways have also been found,[267] but like analogous clinical observations, the results are inconsistent. The density of retinal ganglion cells subserving the central 11 degrees of vision is reduced in patients with Alzheimer's disease as well as in age-matched control patients.[291]

Treatment. A detailed overview of the various pharmacologic agents that may be used in Alzheimer's disease is beyond the scope of this section, so the reader is referred to reviews on this topic.[292–294, 322] However, some principles will be discussed here. Based on notion that enhancing central cholinergic neurotransmission might improve the cognitive and behavioral aspects of Alzheimer's disease, cholinesterase inhibitors such as physostigmine, tacrine (tetrahydroaminoacridine),[295] and donepezil have been used. Although proven to be mildly effective, their use is limited by gastrointestinal side effects and risk of hepatotoxicity, especially with tacrine. Medications or vitamins, such as selegiline or vitamin E (alpha-tocopherol), that increase the levels of brain catecholamines and protect against oxidative damage to neurons have also been used.[296] In general, these medications are only mildly effective. Patients may also require medical treatment of agitation, depression, and psychosis, which may include visual hallucinations (see Chapter 12).

Creutzfeldt–Jakob Disease

Creutzfeldt–Jakob disease, a relatively uncommon neurodegenerative disorder in adults, is characterized by rapidly progressive dementia and myoclonus. In contrast to patients with Alzheimer's disease, who deteriorate slowly over years, individuals with Creutzfeldt–Jakob disease tend to worsen quickly over weeks to months. In one large study,[297] the range of onset was 16 to 82 years of age, and the most frequent age group affected was the 60 to 64 age bracket.

Creutzfeldt–Jakob disease, along with kuru, Gerstmann–Sträussler syndrome, and fatal familial insomnia, make up a group of dementing illnesses known as *human transmissible spongiform encephalopathies.*[298] Clinically, kuru and Gerstmann–Sträussler syndrome present primarily with cerebellar syndromes, and dementia occurs at later stages. Scrapie and bovine spongiform encephalopathy (mad cow disease) are related neurodegenerative diseases seen more commonly in animals. The likely infectious agents in these conditions are proteinaceous particles called prions (PrP = prion protein), which are devoid of nucleic acids.[299]

Although most cases of Creutzfeldt–Jakob disease are sporadic, some are iatrogenic, due to growth hormone derived from human cadaveric pituitary glands, reuse of stereotactic electroencephalography electrodes, and corneal[300] or cadavaric dural transplantation. Rarely, cases are familial.

Neurologic Symptoms and Signs. The disorder usually starts with gradual memory loss and behavioral abnormalities. Some patients present with additional sleep disturbances, depression, weight loss, anorexia, or anxiety. Cerebellar dysfunction, typified by ataxia and dysarthria, may also be evident. Usually within a few weeks or months of onset, mental and motor functions deteriorate rapidly. Global dementia, cerebellar incoordination, rigidity, and startle-induced or spontaneous myoclonic jerk typify the later stages of the illness.[297]

Neuro-ophthalmic Symptoms and Signs. Patients with the Heidenhain (occipitoparietal) variant may have visual field defects such as homonymous hemianopia or quadrantanopia.[301] Cortical blindness, visual hallucinations, visual agnosia, palinopsia,[302] and Balint syndrome may also occur.[303] Usually the fundus is normal, but rare patients with optic atrophy have been reported.[304] Ocular motor disturbances, including supranuclear (eg, Parinaud's syndrome) and infranuclear gaze palsies, nystagmus, and slow saccades,[305] and eyelid abnormalities such as ptosis and apraxia of eyelid opening may also be observed.

Visual abnormalities may predate dementia or behavioral changes. However, frequently by the time visual signs and symptoms develop, patients with Creutzfeldt–Jakob disease are too confused and uncooperative for careful documentation and accurate testing of their visual function.

Pathology. Creutzfeldt–Jakob disease is characterized neuropathologically by neuronal loss, prominent gliosis, and spongiosis in cortex, thalamus, basal ganglia, and cerebellum.[297] Occasionally fine, radiating eosinophilic kuru amyloid plaques may be observed.[306] Immunohistochemistry with antibodies against the prion protein can provide additional confirmation of the disease.[307] In the Heidenhain variant, the neuropathologic abnormalities are most pronounced in the parietal and occipital lobes.[308] Although tissue damage is usually confined to the central nervous system, some reports have documented involvement of the optic nerve head[309] and retina.[310]

Diagnostic Studies. One of the most useful tests in this disorder is electroencephalography. In moderately to severely affected patients, the electroencephalogram may contain 1- to 2-Hz rhythmic periodic sharp-wave complexes or a slow-wave burst–suppression pattern.[311] Some patients may have an abnormal electroretinogram with a B1-wave decrease and relative preservation of the A wave.[310]

The definitive diagnosis of Creutzfeldt–Jakob disease can be made only with a biopsy or autopsy. However, spinal fluid analysis for the 14-3-3 brain protein is a highly sensitive and specific (96% for both) laboratory test for the sporadic form of this disorder.[312, 313] Caution in its use should be applied, because autopsy-proven false negatives can occur, and false-positive 14-3-3 assay results have been reported in patients with herpes simplex encephalitis, hypoxic brain injury, and intracerebral metastases.[313] The 14-3-3 spinal fluid analysis is therefore recommended for use only in patients for whom the clinical suspicion of Creutzfeldt–Jakob disease is high.

Conventional T_1- and T_2-weighted MR images are frequently normal in patients with Creutzfeldt–Jakob disease. However, diffusion-weighted MR sequences may demonstrate otherwise undetectable signal abnormalities in the cortex or basal ganglia.[314–316, 323, 324] This modality may be useful in the detection of brain abnormalities in patients with early signs and symptoms. Single photon emission computed tomography may also show hypoperfusion in the occipital lobes in patients with the Heidenhain variant of Creutzfeldt–Jakob disease.[317]

Treatment. Unfortunately, Creutzfeldt–Jakob disease is uniformly fatal, usually within 1 year of onset,[318] and there is no effective treatment.

REFERENCES

1. Zeki S: The visual association cortex. Curr Opin Neurobiol 1993;3:155–159.
2. Zeki S: The P and M pathways and the 'what and where' doctrine. In: A Vision of the Brain, pp 186–196. Oxford, Blackwell Scientific, 1993.
3. Damasio A, Yamada T, Damasio H, et al: Central achromatopsia: behavioral, anatomic, and physiologic aspects. Neurology 1980;30:1064–1071.
4. Meadows JC: The anatomical basis of prosopagnosia. J Neurol Neurosurg Psychiatry 1974;37:489–501.
5. Damasio AR, Damasio H, Van Hoesen GW: Prosopagnosia: anatomic basis and behavioral mechanisms. Neurology 1982;32:331–341.
6. Bauer RM, Trobe JD: Visual memory and perceptual impairments in prosopagnosia. J Clin Neuro-ophthalmol 1984;4:39–46.
7. De Renzi E: Disorders of spatial orientation. In: Vinken PJ, Bruyn GW, Klawans HL (eds): Handbook of Clinical Neurology. Neuropsychology, pp 405–422. Amsterdam, Elsevier, 1985.
8. Geschwind N: Disconnection syndromes in animal and man. Brain 1965;88:237–294, 585–644.
9. Absher JR, Benson DF: Disconnection syndromes: an overview of Geschwind's contributions. Neurology 1993;43:862–867.

10. Horton JC, Hoyt WF: Quadrantic visual field defects. A hallmark of lesions in extrastriate (V2/V3) cortex. Brain 1991;114:1703–1718.
11. Dejerine J: Contribution à l'étude anatomopathologique et clinique des differentes variétés de cécité verbale. Mem Soc Biol 1892;4:61–90.
12. Coslett HB, Saffran EM, Greenbaum S, et al: Reading in pure alexia. The effect of strategy. Brain 1993; 116:21–37.
13. Arguin M, Bub DN: Pure alexia: attempted rehabilitation and its implications for interpretation of the deficit. Brain Lang 1994;47:233–268.
14. Coslett HB: Acquired dyslexia. In: Feinberg TE, Farah MJ (eds): Behavioral Neurology and Neuropsychology, pp 197–208. New York, McGraw–Hill, 1997.
15. Stommel EW, Friedman RJ, Reeves AG: Alexia without agraphia associated with spleniogeniculate infarction. Neurology 1991;41:587–588.
16. Greenblatt SH: Alexia without agraphia or hemianopsia: anatomical analysis of an autopsied case. Brain 1973;96:307.
17. Greenblatt SH: Subangular alexia without agraphia or hemianopsia. Brain Lang 1976;3:229–245.
18. Vincent FM, Sadowsky CH, Saunders RL, et al: Alexia without agraphia, hemianopia or color-naming defect: a disconnection syndrome. Neurology 1977;27: 689–691.
19. Henderson VW, Friedman RB, Teng EL, et al: Left hemisphere pathways in reading: inferences from pure alexia without hemianopia. Neurology 1985; 35:962–968.
20. Iragui VJ, Kritchevsky M: Alexia without agraphia or hemianopia in parietal infarction (letter). J Neurol Neurosurg Psychiatry 1991;54:841–842.
21. Damasio AR, Damasio H: The anatomic basis of pure alexia. Neurology 1983;33:1573–1583.
22. Binder JR, Lazar RM, Tatemichi TK, et al: Left hemiparalexia. Neurology 1992;42:562–569.
23. Rubens AB, Benson DF: Associative visual agnosia. Arch Neurol 1971;24:305–316.
24. Sparr SA, Jay M, Drislane FW, et al: A historic case of visual agnosia revisited after 40 years. Brain 1991;114:789–800.
25. Geschwind N, Fusillo M: Color naming defects in association with alexia. Arch Neurol 1966;15:137–146.
26. Quint DJ, Gilmore JL: Alexia without agraphia. Neuroradiology 1992;34:210–214.
27. Weisberg LA, Wall M: Alexia without agraphia: clinical-computed tomographic correlations. Neuroradiology 1987;29:283–286.
28. Erdem S, Kansu T: Alexia without either agraphia or hemianopia in temporal lobe lesion due to herpes simplex encephalitis. J Neuro-ophthalmol 1995;15: 102–104.
29. Dogulu CF, Kansu T, Karabudak R: Alexia without agraphia in multiple sclerosis [letter]. J Neurol Neurosurg Psychiatry 1996;61:528.
30. Verrey D: Hémiachromatopsie droite absolue. Arch Ophthal (Paris) 1888;8:289–301.
31. Zeki S: A century of cerebral achromatopsia. Brain 1990;113:1721–1777.
32. Rizzo M, Nawrot M, Blake R, et al: A human visual disorder resembling area V4 dysfunction in the monkey. Neurology 1992;42:1175–1180.
33. Paulson HL, Galetta SL, Grossman M, et al: Hemiachromatopsia of unilateral occipitotemporal infarcts. Am J Ophthalmol 1994;118:518–523.
34. Zeki S, Watson JDG, Lueck CJ, et al: A direct demonstration of functional specialization in human visual cortex. J Neurosci 1991;11:641–649.
35. Sakai K, Watanabe E, Onodera Y, et al: Functional mapping of the human colour centre with echo-planar magnetic resonance imaging. Proc R Soc Lond [Biol] 1995;261:89–98.
36. McKeefry DJ, Zeki S: The position and topography of the human colour centre as revealed by functional magnetic resonance imaging. Brain 1997;120:2229–2242.
37. Rizzo M, Smith V, Pokorny J, et al: Color perception profiles in central achromatopsia. Neurology 1993; 43:995–1001.
38. Meadows JC: Disturbed perception of colours associated with localized cerebral lesions. Brain 1974;97: 615–632.
39. Damasio AR: Disorders of complex visual processing: agnosias, achromatopsia, Balint's syndrome, and related difficulties of orientation and construction. In: Mesulam M-M (ed): Principles of Behavioral Neurology, pp 259–288. Philadelphia, FA Davis, 1985.
40. Freedman L, Costa L: Pure alexia and right hemiachromatopsia in posterior dementia. J Neurol Neurosurg Psychiatry 1992;55:500–502.
41. Brazis PW, Biller J, Fine M: Central achromatopsia (letter). Neurology 1981;31:920–921.
42. Green GJ, Lessell S: Acquired cerebral dyschromatopsia. Arch Ophthalmol 1977;95:121–128.
43. Albert ML, Reches A, Silverberg R: Hemianopic colour blindness. J Neurol Neurosurg Psychiatry 1975; 38:546–549.
44. Kölmel HW: Pure homonymous hemiachromatopsia: findings with neuro-ophthalmologic examination and imaging procedures. Eur Arch Psychiatry Neurol Sci 1988;237:237–243.
45. Silverman IE, Galetta SL: Partial color loss in hemiachromatopsia. Neuro-ophthalmology 1995;15:127–134.
46. Heywood CA, Wilson B, Cowey A: A case study of cortical colour 'blindness' with relatively intact achromatic discrimination. J Neurol Neurosurg Psychiatry 1987;50:22–29.
47. Müller T, Büttner T, Kuhn W, et al: Achromatopsia as a symptom of multiple sclerosis. Neuro-ophthalmology 1994;14:277–278.
48. Fine RD, Parker GD: Disturbance of central vision after carbon monoxide poisoning. Aust NZ J Ophthalmol 1996;24:137–141.
49. Lawden MC, Cleland PG: Achromatopsia in the aura of migraine. J Neurol Neurosurg Psychiatry 1993;56: 708–709.
50. Lapresle J, Metreau R, Annabi A: Transient achromatopsia in vertebrobasilar insufficiency. J Neurol 1977; 215:155–158.
51. Mohr JP, Leicester J, Stoddard LT, et al: Right hemianopia with memory and color deficits in circumscribed left posterior cerebral artery territory infarction. Neurology 1971;21:1104–1113.
52. Schnider A, Landis T, Regard M, et al: Dissociation of color from object in amnesia. Arch Neurol 1992;49:982–985.
53. Tranel D: Disorders of color processing (perception, imagery, recognition, and naming). In: Feinberg TE, Farah MJ (eds): Behavioral Neurology and Neuropsychology, pp 257–265. New York, McGraw–Hill, 1997.
54. Farah MJ, Feinberg TE: Visual object agnosia. In: Feinberg TE, Farah MJ (eds): Behavioral Neurology and Neuropsychology, pp 239–255. New York, McGraw–Hill, 1997.
55. Bender MB, Feldman M: The so-called "visual agnosias." Brain 1972;95:173–186.

56. Benson DF, Segarra J, Albert ML: Visual agnosia-prosopagnosia. A clinicopathologic correlation. Arch Neurol 1974;30:307–310.
57. Albert ML, Soffer D, Silverberg R, et al: The anatomic basis of visual agnosia. Neurology 1979;29:876–879.
58. Albert ML, Reches A, Silverberg R: Associative visual agnosia without alexia. Neurology 1975;25:322–326.
59. Feinberg TE, Schindler RJ, Ochoa E, et al: Associative visual agnosia and alexia without prosopagnosia. Cortex 1994;30:395–411.
60. Grossman M, Galetta S, D'Esposito M: Object recognition difficulty in visual apperceptive agnosia. Brain Cogn 1997;33:306–342.
61. Shelton PA, Bowers D, Duara R, et al: Apperceptive visual agnosia: a case study. Brain Cogn 1994;25:1–23.
62. Grossman M, Galetta S, Ding X-S, et al: Clinical and positron emission tomography studies of visual apperceptive agnosia. Neuropsychiatr Neuropsychol Behav Neurol 1996;9:70–77.
63. Ferreira CT, Ceccaldi M, Giusiano B, et al: Separate visual pathways for perception of actions and objects: evidence from a case of apperceptive agnosia. J Neurol Neurosurg Psychiatry 1998;65:382–385.
64. Benson DF, Greenberg JP: Visual form agnosia: a specific defect in visual discrimination. Arch Neurol 1969;20:82–89.
65. Campion J, Latto R: Apperceptive agnosia due to carbon monoxide poisoning. An interpretation based on critical band masking from disseminated lesions. Behav Brain Res 1985;15:227–240.
66. Allison T, McCarthy G, Nobre A, et al: Human extrastriate visual cortex and the perception of faces, words, numbers, and colors. Cereb Cortex 1994; 4:544–554.
67. Seeck M, Mainwaring N, Ives J, et al: Differential neural activity in the human temporal lobe evoked by faces of family members and friends. Ann Neurol 1993;34:369–372.
68. Seeck M, Schomer D, Mainwaring N, et al: Selectively distributed processing of visual object recognition in the temporal and frontal lobes of the human brain. Ann Neurol 1995;37:538–545.
69. Sergent J, Ohta S, MacDonald B: Functional neuroanatomy of face and object processing. Brain 1992; 115:15–36.
70. Sergent J, Signoret JL: Functional and anatomical decomposition of face processing: evidence from prosopagnosia and PET study of normal subjects. Philos Trans R Soc Lond Biol 1992;335:55–61.
71. Andreasen NC, O'Leary DS, Arndt S, et al.: Neural substrates of facial recognition. J Neuropsychiatry Clin Neurosci 1996;8:139–146.
72. Puce A, Allison T, Gore JC, et al: Face-sensitive regions in human extrastriate cortex studied by functional MRI. J Neurophysiol 1995;74:1192–1199.
73. Kanwisher N, McDermott J, Chun MM: The fusiform face area: a module in human extrastriate cortex specialized for the perception of faces. J Neurosci 1997; 17:4302–4311.
74. De Renzi E: Prosopagnosia. In: Feinberg TE, Farah MJ (eds): Behavioral Neurology and Neuropsychology, pp 245–255. New York, McGraw–Hill, 1997.
75. Damasio AR, Tranel D, Damasio H: Face agnosia and the neural substrates of memory. Annu Rev Neurosci 1990;13:89–109.
76. Farah MJ, Rabinowitz C, Quinn GE, et al: Early commitment of neural substrates for face recognition. Cogn Neuropsychol (in press).
77. Adachi-Usami E, Tsukamoto M, Shimada Y: Color vision and color pattern visual evoked cortical potentials in a patient with acquired cerebral dyschromatopsia. Doc Ophthalmol 1995;90:259–269.
78. Aptman M, Levin H, Senelick RC: Alexia without agraphia in a left-handed patient with prosopagnosia. Neurology 1977;27:533–536.
79. Takahashi N, Kawamura M, Hirayama K, et al: Prosopagnosia: a clinical and anatomical study of four patients. Cortex 1995;31:317–329.
80. Levine DN: Prosopagnosia and visual object agnosia: a behavioral study. Brain Lang 1978;5:341–365.
81. Jacome DE: Subcortical prosopagnosia and anosognosia. Am J Med Sci 1986;292:386–388.
82. De Renzi E, Faglioni P, Grossi D, et al: Apperceptive and associative forms of prosopagnosia. Cortex 1991;27:213–221.
83. Benton AL, Van Allen MW: Prosopagnosia and facial discrimination. J Neurol Sci 1972;15:167–172.
84. Malone DR, Morris HH, Kay MC, et al: Prosopagnosia: a double dissociation between the recognition of familiar and unfamiliar faces. J Neurol Neurosurg Psychiatry 1982;45:820–822.
85. Davidoff J, Landis T: Recognition of unfamiliar faces in prosopagnosia. Neuropsychologia 1990;28:1143–1161.
86. Christen L, Landis T, Regard M: Left hemispheric functional compensation in prosopagnosia? A tachistoscopic study with unilaterally lesioned patients. Hum Neurobiol 1985;4:9–14.
87. Bruyer R, Laterre C, Seron X, et al: A case of prosopagnosia with some preserved covert remembrance of familiar faces. Brain Cogn 1983;2:257–284.
88. Rizzo M, Corbett JJ, Thompson HS, et al: Spatial contrast sensitivity in facial recognition. Neurology 1986;36:1254–1256.
89. Rizzo M, Hurtig R, Damasio AR: The role of scanpaths in facial recognition and learning. Ann Neurol 1987;22:41–45.
90. Young AW, Ellis HD: Childhood prosopagnosia. Brain Cogn 1989;9:16–47.
91. Roudier M, Marcie P, Grancher AS, et al: Discrimination of facial identity and of emotions in Alzheimer's disease. J Neurol Sci 1998;154:151–158.
92. Kosslyn SM, Hamilton SE, Bernstein JH: The perception of curvature can be selectively disrupted in prosopagnosia. Brain Cogn 1995;27:36–58.
93. Campbell R, Heywood CA, Cowey A, et al: Sensitivity to eye gaze in prosopagnosic patients and monkeys with superior temporal sulcus ablation. Neuropsychologia 1990;28:1123–1142.
94. Sergent J, Poncet M: From covert to overt recognition of faces in a prosopagnosic patient. Brain 1990;113: 989–1004.
95. De Haan EHF, Young AW, Newcombe F: Covert and overt recognition in prosopagnosia. Brain 1991;11: 2575–2591.
96. Sergent J, Signoret JL: Implicit access to knowledge derived from unrecognized faces in prosopagnosia. Cereb Cortex 1992;2:389–400.
97. Farah MJ, O'Reilly RC, Vecera SP: Dissociated overt and covert recognition as an emergent property of a lesioned neural network. Psychol Rev 1993;100:571–588.
98. Farah MJ, Feinberg TE: Consciousness of perception after brain damage. Semin Neurol 1997;17:145–152.
99. Diamond BJ, Valentine T, Mayes AR, et al: Evidence of covert recognition in a prosopagnosic patient. Cortex 1994;30:377–393.

100. Newcombe F, Young AW, De Haan EH: Prosopagnosia and object agnosia without covert recognition. Neuropsychologia 1989;27:179–191.
101. Bruyer R: Covert face recognition in prosopagnosia: a review. Brain Cogn 1991;15:223–235.
102. De Renzi E, di Pellegrino G: Prosopagnosia and alexia without object agnosia. Cortex 1998;34:403–415.
103. Farah MJ, Levinson KL, Klein KL: Face perception and within-category discrimination in prosopagnosia. Neuropsychologia 1995;33:661–674.
104. Habib M: Visual hypoemotionality and prosopagnosia associated with right temporal lobe isolation. Neuropsychologia 1986;24:577–582.
105. Henke K, Schweinberger SR, Grigo A, et al: Specificity of face recognition: recognition of exemplars of non-face objects in prosopagnosia. Cortex 1998;34:289–296.
106. Dixon MJ, Bub DN, Arguin M: Semantic and visual determinants of face recognition in a prosopagnosic patient. J Cog Neurosci 1998;10:362–376.
107. Bornstein B, Sroka H, Munitz H: Prosopagnosia with animal face agnosia. Cortex 1969;5:164–169.
108. McNeil JE, Warrington EK: Prosopagnosia: a face-specific disorder. Q J Exp Psychol [A] 1993;46:1–10.
109. McCarthy RA, Evans JJ, Hodges JR: Topographic amnesia: spatial memory disorder, perceptual dysfunction, or category specific semantic memory impairment? J Neurol Neurosurg Psychiatry 1996;60: 318–325.
110. Carlesimo GA, Sabbadini M, Loasses A, et al: Analysis of the memory impairment in a post-encephalitic patient with focal retrograde amnesia. Cortex 1998; 34:449–460.
111. Evans JJ, Heggs AJ, Antoun N, et al: Progressive prosopagnosia associated with selective right temporal lobe atrophy. A new syndrome? Brain 1995; 118:1–13.
112. Mendez MF, Martin RJ, Smyth KA, et al: Disturbances of person identification in Alzheimer's disease. A retrospective study. J Nerv Ment Dis 1992;180:94–96.
113. Werth R, Steinbach T: Symptoms of prosopagnosia in intoxicated subjects. Percept Mot Skills 1991; 73:399–412.
114. Kracke I: Developmental prosopagnosia in Asperger syndrome: presentation and discussion of an individual case. Dev Med Child Neurol 1994;36:873–886.
115. Harrington A, Oepen G, Spitzer M: Disordered recognition and perception of human faces in acute schizophrenia and experimental psychosis. Compr Psychiatry 1989;30:376–384.
116. Mazzucchi A, Biber C: Is prosopagnosia more frequent in males than in females? Cortex 1983;19: 509–516.
117. Shraberg D, Weitzel WD: Prosopagnosia and the Capgras syndrome. J Clin Psychiatry 1979;40:313–316.
118. Gibbs A, Andrewes D: Capgras' syndrome or prosopagnosia? (letter). Br J Psychiatry 1988;153:853.
119. Lewis SW: Brain imaging in a case of Capgras' syndrome. Br J Psychiatry 1987;150:117–121.
120. Cohn R, Neumann MA, Wood DH: Prosopagnosia: a clinicopathological study. Ann Neurol 1977;1: 177–182.
121. Gloning I, Gloning K, Jellinger K, et al: A case of "prosopagnosia" with necropsy findings. Neuropsychologia 1970;8:199–204.
122. Landis T, Regard M, Bliestle A, et al: Prosopagnosia and agnosia for noncanonical views. An autopsied case. Brain 1988;111:1287–1297.
123. Kay MC, Levin HS: Prosopagnosia. Am J Ophthalmol 1982;94:75–80.
124. Landis T, Cummings JL, Christen L, et al: Are unilateral right posterior cerebral lesions sufficient to cause prosopagnosia? Clinical and radiological findings in six additional patients. Cortex 1986;22:243–252.
125. De Renzi E: Prosopagnosia in two patients with CT scan evidence of damage confined to the right hemisphere. Neuropsychologia 1986;24:385–389.
126. De Renzi E, Perani D, Carlesimo GA, et al: Prosopagnosia can be associated with damage confined to the right hemisphere—an MRI and PET study and a review of the literature. Neuropsychologia 1994;32: 893–902.
127. Tohgi H, Watanabe K, Takahashi H, et al: Prosopagnosia without topographagnosia and object agnosia associated with a lesion confined to the right occipitotemporal region. J Neurol 1994;241:470–474.
128. Rösler A, Lanquillon S, Dippel O, et al: Impairment of facial recognition in patients with right cerebral infarcts quantified by computer aided "morphing." J Neurol Neurosurg Psychiatry 1997;62:261–264.
129. Sergent J, Villemure JG: Prosopagnosia in a right hemispherectomized patient. Brain 1989;112:975–995.
130. Whiteley AM, Warrington EK: Prosopagnosia: a clinical, psychological, and anatomical study of three patients. J Neurol Neurosurg Psychiatry 1977;40:395–403.
131. Clarke S, Lindemann A, Maeder P, et al: Face recognition and postero-inferior hemispheric lesions. Neuropsychologia 1997;35:1555–1563.
132. Hier DB, Mondlock J, Caplan LR: Recovery of behavioral abnormalities after right hemisphere stroke. Neurology 1983;33:337–344.
133. Schnider A, Benson DF, Scharre DW: Visual agnosia and optic aphasia: are they anatomically distinct? Cortex 1994;30:445–457.
134. Rubin DC, Greenberg DL: Visual memory-deficit amnesia: a distinct amnesic presentation and etiology. Proc Natl Acad Sci USA 1998;95:5413–5416.
135. Ross ED: Sensory-specific and fractional disorders of recent memory in man. I. Isolated loss of visual recent memory. Arch Neurol 1980;37:193–200.
136. Kimura D: Right temporal-lobe damage. Arch Neurol 1963;8:48–55.
137. Hanley JR, Pearson NA, Young AW: Impaired memory for new visual forms. Brain 1990;113:1131–1148.
138. Kaplan RF, Meadows M-E, Verfaellie M, et al: Lateralization of memory for the visual attributes of objects: evidence from the posterior cerebral artery amobarbital test. Neurology 1994;44:1069–1073.
139. Ungerleider LG, Courtney SM, Haxby JV: A neural system for human visual working memory. Proc Natl Acad Sci USA 1998;95:883–890.
140. Speedie LJ, Heilman KM: Anterograde memory deficits for visuospatial material after infarction of the right thalamus. Arch Neurol 1983;40:183–186.
141. Botez-Marquard T, Botez MI: Visual memory deficits after damage to the anterior commissure and right fornix. Arch Neurol 1992;49:321–324.
142. Zeki S: Cerebral akinetopsia (visual motion blindness). A review. Brain 1991;114:811–824.
143. Zeki SM: Functional organization of a visual area in the posterior bank of the superior temporal sulcus of the rhesus monkey. J Physiol 1974;236:549–573.
144. Newsome WT, Paré EB: A selective impairment of motion perception following lesions of the middle

temporal visual area (MT). J Neurosci 1988;8:2201–2211.
145. Zihl J, Von Cramon D, Mai N, et al: Selective disturbance of movement vision after bilateral brain damage. Brain 1983;106:313–340.
146. Zihl J, Von Cramon D, Mai N, et al: Disturbance of movement vision after bilateral posterior brain damage. Further evidence and follow up observations. Brain 1991;114:2235–2252.
147. Shipp S, de Jong BM, Frackowiak RSJ, et al: The brain activity related to residual motion vision in a patient with bilateral lesions of V5. Brain 1994;117:1023–1038.
148. Tootell RB, Reppas JB, Kwong KK, et al: Functional analysis of human MT and related visual cortical areas using magnetic resonance imaging. J Neurosci 1995;15:3215–3230.
149. Barton JJS, Simpson T, Diriakopoulos E, et al: Functional MRI of lateral occipitotemporal cortex during pursuit and motion perception. Ann Neurol 1996; 40:387–398.
150. Ffytch DH, Guy CN, Zeki S: Motion specific responses from a blind hemifield. Brain 1996;119:1971–1982.
151. Barton JJS, Sharpe JA, Raymond JE: Retinotopic and directional defects in motion discrimination in humans with cerebral lesions. Ann Neurol 1995;37: 665–675.
152. Brandt T, Bucher SF, Seelos KC, et al: Bilateral functional MRI activation of the basal ganglia and middle temporal/medial superior temporal motion-sensitive areas. Arch Neurol 1998;55:1126–1131.
153. Barbur J, Watson JDG, Frackowiak RSJ, et al: Conscious visual perception without V1. Brain 1993; 116:1293–1302.
154. Zeki S, Ffytche DH: The Riddoch syndrome: insights into the neurobiology of conscious vision. Brain 1998;121:25–45.
155. Stoerig P, Kleinschmidt A, Frahm J: No visual responses in denervated V1: high resolution functional magnetic resonance imaging of a blindsight patient. Neuroreport 1998;9:21–25.
156. Horton JC, Trobe JD: Akinetopsia from nefazodone toxicity. Am J Ophthalmol 1999;128:530–531.
157. Riddoch G: Visual disorientation in homonymous half-fields. Brain 1935;5:376–382.
158. Brain WR: Visual disorientation with special reference to lesions of the right cerebral hemisphere. Brain 1941;64:244–272.
159. Cole M, Schutta HS, Warrington EK. Visual disorientation in homonymous half-fields. Neurology 1962; 12:257–263.
160. Baynes K, Holtzman JD, Volpe BT: Components of visual attention. Alterations in response pattern to visual stimuli following parietal lobe infarction. Brain 1986;109:99–114.
161. Vallar G, Sandroni P, Rusconi ML, et al: Hemianopia, hemianesthesia, and spatial neglect: a study with visual evoked potentials. Neuropsychologia 1991;24: 609–622.
162. Mesulam M-M: Attention, confusional states, and neglect. In: Mesulam M-M (ed): Principles of Behavioral Neurology, pp 125–168. Philadelphia, FA Davis, 1985.
163. Vallar G, Perani D: The anatomy of unilateral neglect after right-hemisphere stroke lesions. A clinical/CT-scan correlation study in man. Neuropsychologia 1986;24:609–622.
164. Weintraub S, Mesulam M-M: Right cerebral dominance in spatial attention. Further evidence based on ipsilateral neglect. Arch Neurol 1987;44:621–625.
165. Heilman KM, Valenstein E, Watson RT: The neglect syndrome. In: Vinken PJ, Bruyn GW, Klawans HL (eds): Handbook of Clinical Neurology, Vol. 1(45), Clinical Neuropsychology, pp 153–183. Amsterdam, Elsevier, 1985.
166. Doricchi F, Angelelli P: Misrepresentation of horizontal space in left unilateral neglect. Role of hemianopia. Neurology 1999;52:1845–1852.
167. Bisiach E, Luzzatti C, Perani D: Unilateral neglect, representational schema and consciousness. Brain 1979;102:609–618.
168. Heilman KM, Valenstein E: Mechanisms underlying hemispatial neglect. Ann Neurol 1979;5:166–170.
169. Heilman KM, Bowers D, Coslett HB, et al: Directional hypokinesia: prolonged reaction times for leftward movements in patients with right hemisphere lesions and neglect. Neurology 1985;35:855–859.
170. Meador KJ, Watxon RT, Bowers D, et al: Hypometria with hemispatial and limb motor neglect. Brain 1986;109:293–305.
171. Mesulam M-M: A cortical network for directed attention and unilateral neglect. Ann Neurol 1981;10: 309–325.
172. Daffner KR, Ahern GL, Weintraub S, et al: Dissociated neglect behavior following sequential strokes in the right hemisphere. Ann Neurol 1990;28:97–101.
173. Mesulam M-M: Large-scale neurocognitive networks and distributed processing for attention, language, and memory. Ann Neurol 1990;28:597–613.
174. Watson RT, Heilman KM, Cauthen JC, et al: Neglect after cingulectomy. Neurology 1973;23:1003–1007.
175. Coslett HB, Bowers D, Fitzpatrick E, et al: Directional hypokinesia and hemispatial inattention in neglect. Brain 1990;113:475–486.
176. D'Esposito M, McGlinchey-Berroth M, Alexander MP, et al: Dissociable cognitive and neural mechanisms of unilateral visual neglect. Neurology 1993; 43:2638–2644.
177. Bartolomeo P, D'Erme P, Perri R, et al: Perception and action in hemispatial neglect. Neuropsychologia 1998;36:227–237.
178. Watson RT, Heilman KM: Thalamic neglect. Neurology 1979;29:690–694.
179. Watson RT, Valenstein E, Heilman KM: Thalamic neglect. Possible role of the medial thalamus and nucleus reticularis in behavior. Arch Neurol 1981; 38:501–506.
180. Healton EB, Navarro C, Bressman S, et al: Subcortical neglect. Neurology 1982;32:776–778.
181. Chamorro A, Sacco RL, Ciecierski K, et al: Visual hemineglect and hemihallucinations in a patient with a subcortical infarction. Neurology 1990;40:1463–1464.
182. Sakashita Y: Visual attentional disturbance with unilateral lesions in the basal ganglia and deep white matter. Ann Neurol 1991;30:673–677.
183. Kashiwagi A, Kashiwagi T, Nishikawa T, et al: Hemispatial neglect in a patient with callosal infarction. Brain 1990;113:1005–1023.
184. Perani D, Vallar G, Cappa S, et al: Aphasia and neglect after subcortical stroke. A clinical/cerebral perfusion correlation study. Brain 1987;110:1211–1229.
185. D'Esposito M: Specific stroke syndromes. In: Mills VM, Cassidy JW, Katz DI (eds): Neurologic Rehabilitation: a Guide to Diagnosis, Prognosis, and Treatment Planning, pp 59–103. Malden, Blackwell Science, 1997.
186. Kalra L, Perez I, Gupta S, et al: The influence of visual neglect on stroke rehabilitation. Stroke 1997;28:1386–1391.

187. Levine D, Warach JD, Benowitz L, et al: Left spatial neglect: effects of lesion size and premorbid brain atrophy on severity and recovery following right cerebral infarction. Neurology 1986;36:362–366.
188. Rossi PW, Kheyfets S, Reding MJ: Fresnel prisms improve visual perception in stroke patients with homonymous hemianopia or unilateral visual neglect. Neurology 1990;40:1597–1599.
189. Rossetti Y, Rode G, Pisella L, et al: Prism adaptation to a rightward optical deviation rehabilitates left hemispatial neglect. Nature 1998;395:166–169.
190. Arai T, Ohi H, Sasaki H, et al: Hemispatial sunglasses: effect on unilateral spatial neglect. Arch Phys Med Rehab 1997;78:230–232.
191. Niemeier JP: The Lighthouse Strategy: use of a visual imagery technique to treat visual inattention in stroke patients. Brain Injury 1998;12:399–406.
192. Robertson IH, Mattingley JB, Rorden C, et al: Phasic alerting of neglect patients overcomes their spatial deficit in visual awareness. Nature 1998;395:169–172.
193. Rubens AB: Caloric stimulation and unilateral visual neglect. Neurology 1985;35:1019–1024.
194. Fleet WS, Valenstein E, Watson RT, et al: Dopamine agonist therapy for neglect in humans. Neurology 1987;37:1765–1771.
195. Grujic Z, Mapstone M, Gitelman DR, et al: Dopamine agonists reorient visual exploration away from the neglected hemispace. Neurology 1998;51:1395–1398.
196. Bálint R: Seelenlähmung des "Schauens," optische Ataxie, räumliche Störung der Aufmerksamkeit. Monatsschr Psychiatr Neurol 1909;25:51–81.
197. Husain M, Stein J: Rezsö Balint and his most celebrated case. Arch Neurol 1988;45:89–93.
198. Holmes G: Disturbances of visual orientation. Br J Ophthalmol 1918;2:449–486, 506–518.
199. Hausser CO, Robert F, Giard N: Balint's syndrome. Can J Neurol Sci 1980;7:157–161.
200. Rafal RD: Balint syndrome. In: Feinberg TE, Farah MJ (eds): Behavioral Neurology and Neuropsychology, pp 337–356. New York, McGraw–Hill, 1997.
201. Rizzo M: "Balint's syndrome" and associated visuospatial disorders. Baillières Clin Neurol 1993;2: 415–437.
202. Brazis PW, Graff-Radford NR, Newman NJ, et al: Ishihara color plates as a test for simultanagnosia. Am J Ophthalmol 1998;126:850–851.
203. Rizzo M, Hurtig R: Looking but not seeing: attention, perception, and eye movements in simultanagnosia. Neurology 1987;37:1642–1648.
204. Rizzo M, Robin DA: Simultanagnosia: a defect of sustained attention yields insights on visual information processing. Neurology 1990;40:447–455.
205. Damasio AR, Benton AL: Impairment of hand movements under visual guidance. Neurology 1979;29: 170–178.
206. Pierrot-Deseilligny C, Gray F, Brunet P: Infarcts of both inferior parietal lobules with impairment of visually guided eye movements, peripheral visual inattention and optic ataxia. Brain 1986;109:81–97.
207. Watson RT, Rapcsak SZ: Loss of spontaneous blinking in a patient with Balint's syndrome. Arch Neurol 1989;46:567–570.
208. Tyler HR: Abnormalities of perception with defective eye movements (Bálint's syndrome). Cortex 1968;4: 154–171.
209. De Renzi E: Disorders of Space Exploration and Cognition, pp 57–137. Chichester, John Wiley & Sons, 1982.
210. Verfaellie M, Rapcsak SZ, Heilman KM: Impaired shifting of attention in Balint's syndrome. Brain Cogn 1990;12:195–204.
211. Coslett HB, Saffran E: Simultanagnosia: to see but not two see. Brain 1991;113:1523–1545.
212. Rondot P, De Recondo J, Ribadeau Dumas JL: Visuomotor ataxia. Brain 1977;100:355–376.
213. Nagaratnam N, Grice D, Kalouche H: Optic ataxia following unilateral stroke. J Neurol Sci 1998;155: 204–207.
214. Levine DN, Kaufman KJ, Mohr JP: Inaccurate reaching associated with a superior parietal lobe tumor. Neurology 1978;28:556–561.
215. Liu GT, Ronthal M: Reflex blink to visual threat. J Clin Neuro-ophthalmol 1992;12:47–56.
216. Holmes G, Horrax G: Disturbances of spatial orientation and visual attention with loss of stereoscopic vision. Arch Neurol Psychiatr 1919;1:385–407.
217. Godwin-Austen RB: A case of visual disorientation. J Neurol Neurosurg Psychiatry 1965;28:453–458.
218. Graff-Radford NR, Bolling JP, Earnest F, et al: Simultanagnosia as the initial sign of degenerative dementia. Mayo Clin Proc 1993;68:955–964.
219. Uyama E, Iwagoe H, Maeda J, et al: Presenile-onset cerebral adrenoleukodystrophy presenting as Balint's syndrome and dementia. Neurology 1993;43:1249–1251.
220. Moulingnier A, de Saint Martin L, Mahieux F, et al: Balint's syndrome (letter). Neurology 1995;45:1030–1031.
221. Perez FM, Tunkel RS, Lachmann EA, et al: Balint's syndrome arising from bilateral posterior cortical atrophy or infarction: rehabilitation strategies and their limitation. Disabil Rehabil 1996;18:300–304.
222. Benson DF, Davis RJ, Snyder BD: Posterior cortical atrophy. Arch Neurol 1988;45:789–793.
223. Ardila A, Rosselli M, Arvizu L, et al: Alexia and agraphia in posterior cortical atrophy. Neuropsychiatry Neuropsychol Behav Neurol 1997;10:52–59.
224. Mendez MF, Cherrier MM: The evolution of alexia and simultanagnosia in posterior cortical atrophy. Neuropsychiatry Neuropsychol Behav Neurol 1998; 11:76–82.
225. Freedman L, Selchen DH, Black SE, et al: Posterior cortical dementia with alexia: neurobehavioural, MRI, and PET findings. J Neurol Neurosurg Psychiatry 1991;54:443–448.
226. Farah MJ: The neurologic basis of mental imagery: a componential analysis. Cognition 1984;18:245–272.
227. Farah MJ, Peronnet F, Gonon MA, et al: Electrophysiological evidence for a shared representational medium for visual images and visual percepts. J Exp Psychol Gen 1988;117:248–257.
228. Farah MJ: Is visual imagery really visual? Overlooked evidence from neuropsychology. Psychol Rev 1988; 95:307–317.
229. Kosslyn SM, Alpert NM, Thompson WL, et al: Visual mental imagery activates topographically organized visual cortex: PET investigations. J Cogn Neurosci 1993;5:263–287.
230. Kosslyn SM, Thompson WL, Alpert NM: Neural systems shared by visual imagery and visual perception: a positron emission tomography study. Neuroimage 1997;6:320–334.
231. Butter CM, Kosslyn S, Mijovic-Prelec D, et al: Field-specific deficits in visual imagery following hemianopia due to unilateral occipital infarcts. Brain 1997;120:217–228.

232. Büchel C, Price C, Frackowiak RSJ, et al: Different activation patterns in the visual cortex of late and congenitally blind subjects. Brain 1998;121: 409–419.
233. Levine DN, Warach J, Farah M: Two visual systems in mental imagery: dissociation of 'what' and 'where' in imagery disorders due to bilateral posterior cerebral lesions. Neurology 1985;35:1010–1018.
234. Mehta Z, Newcombe F, De Haan E: Selective loss of imagery in a case of visual agnosia. Neuropsychologia 1992;30:645–655.
235. Bisiach E, Luzzatti C: Unilateral neglect of representational space. Cortex 1978;14:129–133.
236. Chatterjee A, Southwood MH: Cortical blindness and visual imagery. Neurology 1995;45:2189–2195.
237. Goldenberg G, Müllbacher W, Nowak A: Imagery without perception—a case study of anosognosia for cortical blindness. Neuropsychologia 1995;33:1373–1382.
238. Shuren JE, Brott TG, Schefft BK, et al: Preserved color imagery in an achromatopsic. Neuropsychologia 1996;34:485–489.
239. Bartolomeo P, Bachoud-Lévi A–C, Denes G: Preserved imagery for colours in a patient with cerebral achromatopsia. Cortex 1997;33:369–378.
240. Beschin N, Cocchini G, Della Sala S, et al: What the eyes perceive, the brain ignores: a case of pure unilateral representational neglect. Cortex 1997;33:3–26.
241. Behrmann M, Moscovitch M, Winocur G: Intact visual imagery and impaired visual perception in a patient with visual agnosia. J Exp Psychol Hum Percept Perform 1994;20:1068–1087.
242. Heilman KM, Valenstein E: Frontal lobe neglect in man. Neurology 1972;22:660–664.
243. Stein S, Volpe BT: Classical "parietal" neglect syndrome after subcortical right frontal lobe infarction. Neurology 1983;33:797–799.
244. Cogan DG: Neurology of the Ocular Muscles, pp 104–105. Springfield Ill, Charles C Thomas, 1956.
245. Liu GT, Bolton AK, Price BH, et al: Dissociated perceptual-sensory and exploratory-motor neglect. J Neurol Neurosurg Psychiatry 1992;55:701–726.
246. Husain M, Kennard C: Visual neglect associated with frontal lobe infarction. J Neurol 1996;243:652–657.
247. McKhann G, Drachman D, Folstein M, et al: Clinical diagnosis of Alzheimer's disease: Report of the NINCDS-ADRDA Work Group under the auspices of the Department of Health and Human Services Task Force on Alzheimer's disease. Neurology 1984;34:939–944.
248. Friedland RP: Alzheimer's disease: clinical features and differential diagnosis. Neurology 1993;43(Suppl 4):S45–S51.
249. Skoog I, Nilsson L, Palmertz B, et al: A population-based study of dementia in 85-year olds. N Engl J Med 1993;328:153–158.
250. Evans DE, Funkenstein HH, Albert MS, et al: Prevalence of Alzheimer's disease in a community population of older persons. Higher than previously reported. JAMA 1989;262:2551–2556.
251. Cummings JL, Vinters HV, Cole GM, et al: Alzheimer's disease. Etiologies, pathophysiology, cognitive reserve, and treatment opportunities. Neurology 1998;51(Suppl 1):S2–S17.
252. Fleming KC, Adams AC, Petersen RC: Dementia: diagnosis and evaluation. Mayo Clin Proc 1995;70: 1093–1107.
253. Geldmacher DS, Whitehouse PJ: Evaluation of dementia. N Engl J Med 1996;335:330–336.
254. Mendez MF, Tomsak RL, Remler B: Disorders of the visual system in Alzheimer's disease. J Clin Neuro-ophthalmol 1990;10:62–69.
255. Mendez MF, Mendez MA, Martin R, et al: Complex visual disturbances in Alzheimer's disease. Neurology 1990;40:439–443.
256. Trick GL, Silverman SE: Visual sensitivity to motion: age-related changes and deficits in senile dementia of the Alzheimer type. Neurology 1991;41:1437–1440.
257. Silverman SE, Tran DB, Zimmerman KM, et al: Dissociation between the detection and perception of motion in Alzheimer's disease. Neurology 1994;44:1814–1818.
258. Rizzo M, Nawrot M: Perception of movement and shape in Alzheimer's disease. Brain 1998;121:2259–2270.
259. Trobe JD, Butter CM: A screening test for integrative visual dysfunction in Alzheimer's disease. Arch Ophthalmol 1993;111:815–818.
260. Butter CM, Trobe JD, Foster NL, et al: Visual-spatial deficits explain visual symptoms in Alzheimer's disease. Am J Ophthalmol 1996;122:97–105.
261. Daffner KR, Scinto LFM, Weintraub S, et al: Diminished curiosity in patients with probable Alzheimer's disease as measured by exploratory eye movements. Neurology 1992;42:320–328.
262. Sadun AA, Borchert M, De Vita E, et al: Assessment of visual impairment in patients with Alzheimer's disease. Am J Ophthalmol 1987;104:113–120.
263. Hutton JT, Morris JL, Elias JW, et al: Contrast sensitivity dysfunction in Alzheimer's disease. Neurology 1993;43:2328–2330.
264. Mendola JD, Cronin-Golomb A, Corkin S, et al: Prevalence of visual deficits in Alzheimer's disease. Optom Vis Sci 1995;72:155–167.
265. Cronin-Golomb A: Vision in Alzheimer's disease. Gerontologist 1995;3:370–376.
266. Cronin-Golomb A, Sugiura R, Corkin S, et al: Incomplete achromatopsia in Alzheimer's disease. Neurobiol Aging 1993;14:471–477.
267. Katz B, Rimmer S: Ophthalmologic manifestations of Alzheimer's disease. Surv Ophthalmol 1989;34: 31–43.
268. Katz B, Rimmer S, Iragui V, et al: Abnormal pattern electroretinogram in Alzheimer's disease: evidence for retinal ganglion cell degeneration? Ann Neurol 1989;26:221–225.
269. Trick GL, Barris MC, Bickler-Bluth M: Abnormal pattern electroretinograms in patients with senile dementia of the Alzheimer type. Ann Neurol 1989; 26:226–231.
270. Cronin-Golomb A, Corkin S, Rizzo JF, et al: Visual dysfunction in Alzheimer's disease. relation to normal aging. Ann Neurol 1991;29:41–52.
271. Rizzo JF, Cronin-Golomb A, Growdon JH, et al: Retinocalcarine function in Alzheimer's disease. A clinical and electrophysiologic study. Arch Neurol 1992;49:93–101.
272. Trick GL, Trick LR, Morris P, et al: Visual field loss in senile dementia of the Alzheimer's type. Neurology 1995;45:68–74.
273. Reiman EM, Caselli RJ, Yun LS, et al: Preclinical evidence of Alzheimer's disease in persons homozygous for the ε4 allele for apolipoprotein E. N Engl J Med 1996;334:752–758.

274. Sandson TA, O'Connor M, Sperling RA, et al: Noninvasive perfusion MRI in Alzheimer's disease. Neurology 1996;47:1339–1342.
275. Galasko D, Chang L, Motter R, et al: High cerebrospinal fluid tau and low amyloid β42 levels in the clinical diagnosis of Alzheimer disease and relation to apolipoprotein E genotype. Arch Neurol 1998;55: 937–945.
276. The Ronald and Nancy Reagan Research Institute of the Alzheimer's Association and the National Institute on Aging Working Group: Consensus report of the working group on: "Molecular and biochemical markers of Alzheimer's disease." Neurobiol Aging 1998;19:109–116.
277. Roses AD: Genetic testing for Alzheimer disease. Arch Neurol 1997;54:1226–1229.
278. Blacker D, Tanzi RE: The genetics of Alzheimer disease. Current status and future prospects. Arch Neurol 1998;55: 294–296.
279. Martin JB: Molecular basis of the neurodegenerative disorders. N Engl J Med 1999;340:1970–1980.
280. Rumble B, Retallack R, Hilbich C, et al: Amyloid A4 protein and its precursor in Down's syndrome and Alzheimer's disease. N Engl J Med 1989;320:1446–1452.
281. Selkoe DJ: Aging, amyloid, and Alzheimer's disease (editorial). N Engl J Med 1989;320:1484–1487.
282. Yankner BA, Mesulam M-M: β-amyloid and the pathogenesis of Alzheimer's disease. N Engl J Med 1991;325:1849–1857.
283. Masters CL, Beyreuther K: Alzheimer's disease. BMJ 1998;316:446–448.
284. Mayeux R: Therapeutic strategies in Alzheimer's disease. Neurology 1990;40:175–180.
285. Lewis DA, Campbell MJ, Terry RD, et al: Laminar and regional distribution of neurofibrillary tangles and neuritic plaques in Alzheimer's disease: a quantitative study of visual and auditory cortices. J Neurosci 1987;7:1799–1808.
286. Arnold SE, Hyman BT, Flory J, et al: The topographical and neuroanatomical distribution of neurofibrillary tangles and neuritic plaques in the cerebral cortex of patients with Alzheimer's disease. Cereb Cortex 1991;1:103–116.
287. Giannakopoulos P, Gold G, Duc M, et al: Neuroanatomical correlates of visual agnosia in Alzheimer's disease. A clinicopathological study. Neurology 1999;52:71–77.
288. Levine DN, Lee JM, Fisher CM: The visual variant of Alzheimer's disease. Neurology 1993;43:305–313.
289. Hof PR, Bouras C, Constantinidis J, et al: Balint's syndrome in Alzheimer's disease: specific disruption of the occipito-parietal visual pathway. Brain Res 1989;493:368–375.
290. Hof PR, Bouras C, Constantinidis J, et al: Selective disconnection of specific visual association pathways in cases of Alzheimer's disease presenting with Balint's syndrome. J Neuropathol Exp Neurol 1990; 49:168–184.
291. Curcio CA, Drucker DN: Retinal ganglion cells in Alzheimer's and aging. Ann Neurol 1993;33:248–257.
292. Borson S, Raskind MA: Clinical features and pharmacologic treatment of behavioral symptoms of Alzheimer's disease. Neurology 1997;48 (Suppl 6):S17–S24.
293. Aisen PS, Davis KL: The search for disease-modifying treatment for Alzheimer's disease. Neurology 1997; 48 (Suppl 6):S35–S41.
294. Farlow MR, Evans RM: Pharmacologic treatment of cognition in Alzheimer's dementia. Neurology 1998; 51 (Suppl 1):S36–S44.
295. Gautheir S, Bouchard R, Lamontagne A, et al: Tetrahydroaminoacridine-lecithin combination treatment in patients with intermediate-stage Alzheimer's disease. N Engl J Med 1990;322:1272–1276.
296. Sano M, Ernesto C, Thomas RG, et al: A controlled trial of selegiline, alpha-tocopherol, or both as treatment for Alzheimer's disease. N Engl J Med 1997; 336:1216–1222.
297. Brown P, Gibbs CJ, Rodgers-Johnson P, et al: Human spongiform encephalopathy: the National Institutes of Health series of 300 cases of experimentally transmitted disease. Ann Neurol 1994;35:513–529.
298. Haywood AM: Transmissible spongiform encephalopathies. N Engl J Med 1997;337:1821–1828.
299. Prusiner SB, Hsiao KK: Human prion diseases. Ann Neurol 1994;35:385–395.
300. Heckmann JG, Lang CJG, Petruch F, et al: Transmission of Creutzfeldt–Jakob disease via a corneal transplant. J Neurol Neurosurg Psychiatry 1997;63: 388–390.
301. Vargas ME, Kupersmith MJ, Savino PJ, et al: Homonymous field defect as the first manifestation of Creutzfeldt-Jakob disease. Am J Ophthalmol 1995; 119:497–504.
302. Purvin V, Bonnin J, Goodman J: Palinopsia as a presenting manifestation of Creutzfeldt–Jakob disease. J Clin Neuro-ophthalmol 1989;9:242–246.
303. Neetens A, Martin JJ: Neuro-ophthalmologic aspects of prion diseases. Neuro-ophthalmology 1998;19: 137–144.
304. Lesser RL, Albert DM, Bobowick AR, et al: Creutzfeldt–Jakob disease and optic atrophy. Am J Ophthalmol 1979;87:317–321.
305. Grant MP, Cohen M, Peterson RB, et al: Abnormal eye movements in Creutzfeldt–Jakob disease. Ann Neurol 1993;34:192–197.
306. Case Records of the MGH: Case 17-1993. N Engl J Med 1993;328:1259–1266.
307. Kretzschmar HA, Ironside JW, DeArmond SJ, et al: Diagnostic criteria for sporadic Creutzfeldt–Jakob disease. Arch Neurol 1996;53:913–920.
308. Furlan AJ, Henry CE, Sweeney PJ, et al: Focal EEG abnormalities in Heidenhain's variant of Jakob–Creutzfeldt disease. Arch Neurol 1981;38:312–314.
309. Roth AM, Keltner JL, Ellis WG, et al: Virus-simulating structures in the optic nerve head in Creutzfeldt–Jakob disease. Am J Ophthalmol 1979;87:827–833.
310. de Seze J, Hache JC, Vermersch P, et al: Creutzfeldt–Jakob disease. Neurophysiologic visual impairments. Neurology 1998;51:962–967.
311. Steinhoff BJ, Räcker S, Herrendorf G, et al: Accuracy and reliability of periodic sharp wave complexes in Creutzfeldt–Jakob disease. Arch Neurol 1996;53: 162–166.
312. Hsich G, Kenney K, Gibbs CJ, et al: The 14-3-3 brain protein in cerebrospinal fluid as a marker for transmissible spongiform encephalopathies. N Engl J Med 1996;335:924–930.
313. Zerr I, Bodemer M, Gefeller O, et al: Detection of 14-3-3 protein in the cerebrospinal fluid supports the diagnosis of Creutzfeldt–Jakob disease. Ann Neurol 1998;43:32–40.
314. Bahn MM, Kido DK, Lin W, et al: Brain magnetic resonance diffusion abnormalities in Creutzfeldt–Jakob disease. Arch Neurol 1997;54:1411–1415.

315. Demaerel P, Heiner L, Robberecht W, et al: Diffusion-weighted MRI in sporadic Creutzfeldt–Jakob disease. Neurology 1999;52:205–208.
316. Na DL, Suh CK, Choi SH, et al: Diffusion-weighted magnetic resonance imaging in probable Creutzfeldt–Jakob disease. Arch Neurol 1999;56:951–957.
317. Jibiki I, Fikushimja T, Kobayashi K, et al: Utility of 123-I-IMP SPECT brain scans for the early detection of site-specific abnormalities in Creutzfeldt–Jakob disease (Heidenhain type): a case study. Neuropsychobiology 1994;1994:29.
318. Brown P, Cathala F, Castaigne P, et al: Creutzfeldt–Jakob disease: clinical analysis of a consecutive series of 230 neuropathologically verified cases. Ann Neurol 1986;20:597–602.
319. Galetta SL: A stimulating view of human visual cortex (editorial). Neurology 2000;54:785–786.
320. Lee HW, Hong SB, Seo DW, et al: Mapping of functional organization in human visual cortex. Electrical cortical stimulation. Neurology 2000;54:849–854.
321. Andreasen N, Hesse C, Davidsson P, et al: Cerebrospinal fluid beta-amyloid (1-42) in Alzheimer disease. Differences between early- and late-onset Alzheimer disease and stability during the course of the disease. Arch Neurol 1999;56:673–680.
322. Mayeux R, Sano M: Treatment of Alzheimer's disease. N Engl J Med 1999;341:1670–1679.
323. Case Records of the MGH: Case 28-1999. N Engl J Med 1999;341:901–908.
324. Bahn MM, Parchi P: Abnormal diffusion-weighted magnetic resonance images in Creutzfeldt-Jakob disease. Arch Neurol 1999;56:577–583.

CHAPTER 10

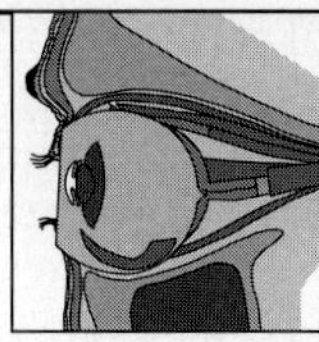

Transient Visual Loss

Blurring and loss of vision lasting for seconds or minutes are common visual complaints. This chapter suggests one approach to patients with these symptoms: to distinguish (1) the more innocent nonischemic ocular conditions from (2) those resulting from potentially catastrophic retinal or cerebral ischemia, and (3) other causes. The diagnosis and treatment of the neuro-ophthalmic causes of transient visual loss will be detailed, with particular emphasis on the presentation and management of carotid disease.

APPROACH: NONISCHEMIC, ISCHEMIC, AND OTHER CAUSES

The distinction between nonischemic, ischemic, and other causes of transient visual loss can often be made on historical grounds.[1]

Nonischemic Causes

Patients with nonischemic causes of transient visual loss may be recognized by their longstanding and vague but innocuous visual complaints. The term *transient visual blurring* is more accurate as these patients generally have only mild visual changes. Most often they are concerned by a reduced quality to their vision with a superimposed, momentary, worsening or change that causes their vision to vary during the course of the day. They often have difficulty determining which eye is having the problem. Patients will typically report problems with reading small print or seeing words on the television or computer screen. They rarely describe a visual field defect. They are generally concerned but are not alarmed by their altered vision. Other neurologic complaints or new headaches are absent.

Ischemic Causes

Episodic sudden visual acuity or field loss with normal vision between events would be more consistent with an ischemic cause. Patients tend to be more definitive in their description of the visual loss with regard to the onset of symptoms, the number of episodes, and their duration. When field deficits occur, they may respect the vertical or horizontal meridian, and when bilateral may be homonymous, consistent with a vascular cause. Bruno et al[2] found that patients with altitudinal or lateralized transient monocular visual loss were likely to have identifiable ischemic causes. Pain, headache, scalp tenderness, jaw claudication, accompanying neurologic signs or symptoms and the presence of cerebrovascular risk factors suggest an ischemic cause of the transient visual loss. Migraine, suggested by symptoms of headache, nausea, or vomiting, should also be considered. Previous migraines, a history of affected family members, or accompanying positive phenomena such as scintillations, prisms, or colored lights also support the diagnosis of migrainous visual loss. When numerous recurrent unexplained episodes of visual loss occur, particularly in young people, a vascular cause should also be considered.

Other Causes

A history of seizures, loss of consciousness, or abnormal motor activity would suggest ictal or postictal visual loss. The patient with a history of optic neuritis might complain of transient visual loss with a rise in body temperature (Uhthoff's phenomenon). Vision loss with eye movements is consistent with gaze evoked amaurosis and suggests an underlying orbital mass. Patients with papilledema may have transient visual obscurations that occasionally will be gaze evoked.

EXAMINATION OF THE PATIENT WITH TRANSIENT VISUAL LOSS

In addition to documenting afferent visual function, particular attention should be paid to the slit-lamp examination to search for any tear surface or corneal abnormalities and to the funduscopic examination for evidence of retinal emboli or disc swelling. Focal signs on the neurologic examination should also be excluded. On the general examination, palpation of the temporal arteries and auscultation of the carotid arteries and heart should be performed.

NONISCHEMIC TRANSIENT VISION LOSS

Many patients that describe variable blurring of their vision have an ocular (nonischemic) cause (Table 10–1). While the symptoms may be quite disruptive and difficult to treat, there are almost no critical diagnoses to make except transient elevation of intraocular pressure or corneal edema.

TABLE 10–1. Nonischemic Causes of Transient Visual Loss

Tear film abnormalities
Dry eye
Blepharitis
Corneal epithelial disease
Dry eye
Epithelial irregularity
Corneal endothelial dysfunction
Transient elevation of intraocular pressure
Intermittent angle closure
Uveitis
Fluctuating blood sugar
Anterior chamber abnormalities
Uveitis
Hyphema
Vitreous floaters
Afterimages
Optic disc anomalies (transient visual obscurations)
Optic nerve head drusen (transient visual obscurations)

(Adapted from Volpe NJ, Liu GT, Galetta SL: Transient visual loss. Curr Concepts Ophthalmol 1998;6:55–59, with permission.)

Ocular Surface Abnormalities

Tear film or corneal abnormalities are probably the most common nonischemic causes of transient visual loss. Patients with tear film abnormalities typically describe a pattern in which visual blurring occurs many times per week, often at the end of the day and often under one environmental circumstance. For instance, they may complain of blurring of the vision in the afternoon at work, in the evening when they sit down to read, or after a walk on a windy day. Visual blurring in the setting of tear film irregularities may persist for a few hours. Repeat blinking or lubrication of the eyes in this setting will often improve the vision. The penlight examination of the eye will almost always be unrevealing. Even with slit-lamp biomicroscopy, obvious abnormalities may not be present although there may be abnormal tear film break up, blepharitis, or corneal and conjunctival fluorescein staining. Patients with blepharitis may have the greatest problem in the morning with increased accumulation of abnormal meibomian gland secretions overnight. Bathing the eyes usually leads to prompt improvement. If dryness or tear film abnormality leads to epithelial breakdown, there may be associated foreign body sensation, pain, or redness. Those with dry eyes will frequently have a positive Schirmer's test (see Chapter 2).

Other Ocular Causes

Subacute transient attacks of narrow-angle glaucoma may cause episodes of transient visual blurring accompanied by halos.[3] During asymptomatic periods intraocular pressure may be normal, but slit-lamp examination and gonioscopy will reveal shallow occludable anterior chambers. Recurrent spontaneous anterior chamber hemorrhages may also cause episodic visual blurring.[4, 5] Such recurrent hemorrhages can occur in patients with juvenile xanthogranuloma, those with a malpositioned intraocular lens with iris contact, and patients with iris neovacularization.

In addition, patients with corneal endothelial dysfunction can develop blurred vision. These episodes often last for hours and occur most commonly in the morning. The diagnosis can be made by examining patients during symptomatic periods. Osmotic changes in the lens can occur with widely fluctuating blood glucose levels, such as in patients with diabetes or those taking corticosteroids. This blurring is associated with a change in refractive error, for instance, an increase in myopia with elevation in blood glucose level, but there is no reliable change in the appearance of the lens on slit-lamp examination. Pinholes usually improve the visual acuities in these cases. Alteration in the vitreous, particularly acute posterior vitreous detachments and increased opacities in the vitreous associated with uveitis, can also cause transient visual blurring. Posterior opacities can move or float over the macula and alter visual acuity. Most patients describe typical floaters, but some report a more fixed opacity that blurs vision.

ISCHEMIC TRANSIENT VISUAL LOSS

The mechanism in these instances is temporary interruption of the blood supply of the retina, optic nerve, or retrochiasmal visual pathways (Table 10–2). In patients with transient monocular blindness, carotid disease, cardiac emboli, and giant cell arteritis should be considered and distinguished from migraine or vasospasm. Bilateral visual loss may be due to involvement of both eyes, but hemianopic visual loss due to middle cerebral artery or vertebrobasilar ischemia should also be excluded. Since many of these patients are at risk for permanent visual loss or stroke, they must be identified and treated expeditiously.

Vascular Anatomy. The aortic arch gives rise to the great vessels supplying the head and neck. The first branch of the aorta is the innominate artery, which divides to form the right subclavian and right common carotid arteries. The next branch off of the aorta is the left common carotid artery. Each carotid artery enters the neck, eventually traveling through the temporal bone to enter the cavernous sinus (Fig. 10–1). The sympathetic pathway finds its way to the eye by following the carotid and its branches (see Chapter 13). Upon exiting the cavernous sinus, the carotid gives off its first major branch, the ophthalmic artery. In 10% of patients, the ophthalmic artery originates from the cavernous carotid. The ophthalmic artery provides the blood supply to the optic nerve, retina, and other structures of the eye. The muscular branches supply the extraocular muscles. The central retinal artery enters the substance of the optic nerve to supply the most anterior portion of the optic nerve head and retina. Most of the optic nerve head derives its supply from two or more long posterior ciliary arteries. The optic nerve head represents a potential watershed area between these posterior ciliary arteries (see Chapter 5 for more details).

The blood supplies of the optic radiations and occipital cortex are reviewed in detail in Chapter 8.

TABLE 10–2. Ischemic Causes of Transient Vision Loss

Carotid embolic disease
Cardiac embolic disease
Valvular disease
Mural thrombus (atrial fibrillation)
Atrial myxoma
Migraine
Temporal arteritis
Vertebrobasilar insufficiency
Hematologic abnormalities
Hypercoaguable state
Polycythemia

(Adapted from Volpe NJ, Liu GT, Galetta SL: Transient visual loss. Curr Concepts Ophthalmol 1998;6:55–59, with permission.)

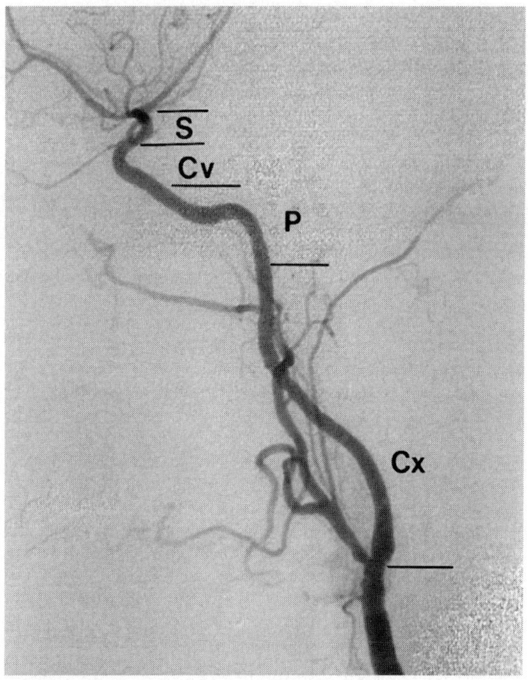

FIGURE 10–1. Angiogram of a normal carotid artery. S = supraclinoid, Cv = cavernous, P = petrous, and Cx = cervical portions. (From Bennett J, Volpe NJ, Liu GT, Galetta SL: Neurovascular neuro-ophthalmology. In Albert D, Jakobiec FA (eds): Principles of Ophthalmology, pp 4238–4274. Philadelphia, WB Saunders, 2000, with permission.)

Carotid Disease

Extracranial internal carotid artery disease is the most common cause of the ischemic form of transient visual loss, as approximately 60% of patients with transient monocular blindness will have angiographically proven carotid stenosis or occlusion.[6, 7] In this setting, transient visual loss is more often labeled as transient monocular blindness, amaurosis fugax ("fleeting blindness"), or a retinal transient ischemic attack. The origin of the internal carotid artery at the bifurcation may be narrowed by atherosclerotic plaque formation (Fig. 10–2) and related mural thrombi, plaque ulceration, and intraplaque hemorrhage.[8, 9] Nonatherosclerotic causes of carotid disease include carotid dissection (see Chapter 13), fibromuscular dysplasia, Takayasu's arteritis, carotid trauma, and radiation arteritis.[10]

Carotid-related amaurosis fugax most frequently results from emboli from the diseased proximal internal carotid artery segment to the retinal artery circulation.[11] Another mechanism for monocular visual loss due to occlusive carotid disease is low flow,[12] particularly when collateral circulation to the eye from the circle of Willis and external carotid artery circulation are also compromised. In these cases symptoms may be induced when carotid blood

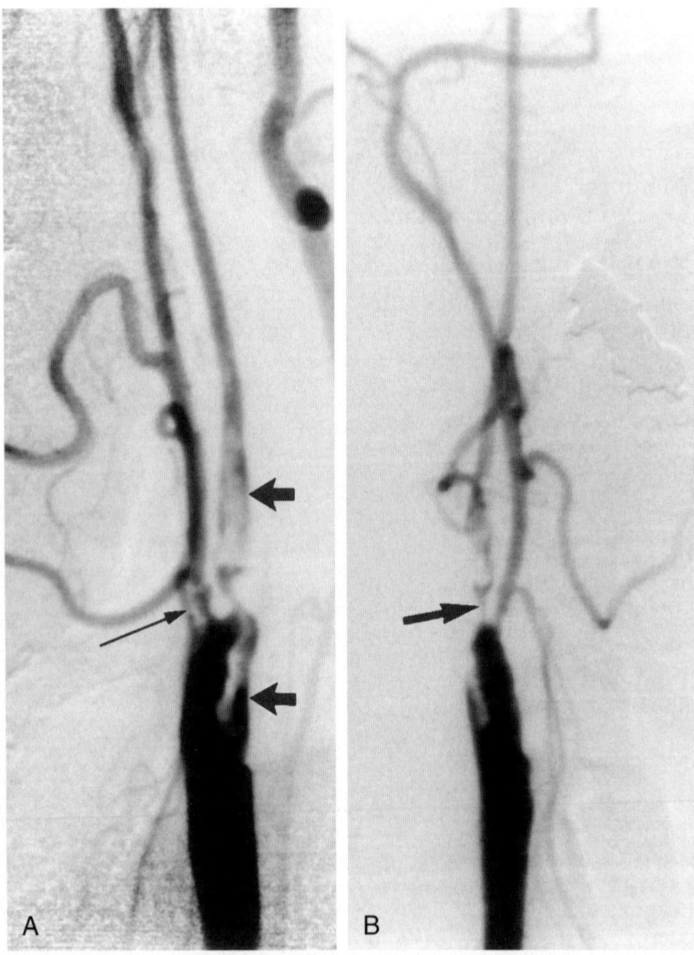

FIGURE 10–2. Right common carotid artery angiogram in a patient with amaurosis fugax and carotid artery stenosis. **A.** Magnified view of the right common carotid artery injection demonstrating filling defects within the common carotid (*lower arrow*), internal carotid (*upper arrow*), and external carotid arteries (*thin arrow*). These filling defects represent extensive clots within the carotid circulation. **B.** Oblique view showing the high-grade stenosis of the internal carotid artery (*arrow*) with the filling defect from the clot above. The small caliber of the cervical portion of the right internal carotid artery extending superiorly should be noted. (From Balcer LJ, Galetta SL, Yousem DM, et al: Pupil-involving third nerve palsy and carotid stenosis: rapid recovery following endarterectomy. Ann Neurol 1997;41:273–276, with permission.)

TABLE 10–3. Typical Features of Embolic Transient Monocular Blindness

Abrupt onset
Painless
Typically lasts 1 to 5 minutes
Darkening or fogging (not blurring) of visual field
Altitudinal pattern (shade closing) of vision loss
Vision returns gradually over minutes

(Adapted from Volpe NJ, Liu GT, Galetta SL: Transient visual loss. Curr Concepts Ophthalmol 1998;6:55–59, with permission.)

flow is decreased because of changes in posture or eating,[13] or when distal blood flow is insufficient, as in chronic ocular ischemia or bright-light amaurosis (see below).

The risk of stroke per annum with amaurosis fugax had been previously estimated to be 2%, with a 1% risk of permanent visual loss.[14] This compares with the 5% to 8% yearly risk of stroke associated with cerebral transient ischemic attacks (TIAs).[15] It is unclear why transient monocular visual loss has less of a stroke risk than those with hemispheric TIAs.[16] Possible explanations include: (1) local ophthalmic disease rather than carotid disease, and (2) mechanisms of transient visual loss other than arteriosclerotic disease such as vasospasm.

Symptoms. The characteristics of this type of vision loss are summarized in Table 10–3. Its onset is usually sudden and is often described as a shade or curtain that obscures vision in one eye. Visual loss may be altitudinal, peripheral, central, or even vertical.[15] A nasal visual field defect may suggest an embolic mechanism because of the tendency of these particles to lodge in the temporal retinal circulation.[17] Most episodes last 5 minutes or less. Rarely, scintillating scotomas or tiny bright lights may be experienced.[5] Pain is uncommon and its presence should raise the possibility of temporal arteritis (see below).

Rarely, patients may complain of transient monocular blindness after exposure to sunlight or even after viewing a white wall.[18] This phenomenon of bright-light-induced amaurosis fugax in patients with carotid occlusive disease is well documented.[19] Presumably, impaired blood flow to the outer retinal segment compromises the regeneration of retinal pigments required for visual perception. In one study,[20] the visual evoked response was attenuated when the patients were exposed to a light source for 30 seconds or more.

In patients with carotid stenosis, ipsilateral eye symptoms may be accompanied by those of ipsilateral cerebral ischemia. These include contralateral hemiparesis, sensory loss, or even hemianopsia. Ischemia of the dominant hemisphere may cause language deficits.

Other History. A screening history for other evidence of arteriosclerotic vascular disease, hypertension, smoking, diabetes, and cardiac arrhythmias should be obtained. In addition, symptoms suggestive of temporal (giant cell) arteritis (see below) should be excluded.

Neuro-ophthalmic Signs. Retinal emboli are the most common associated finding, and there are two main types seen in carotid disease: (1) cholesterol (Hollenhorst plaques), which have a refractile, metallic gold appearance and are typically a sign of carotid disease[21]; and (2) platelet–fibrin emboli, which are creamy white/grey longitudinal intravascular opacifications that fill the entire lumen.[17, 21] Platelet–fibrin emboli are likely a result of either carotid thrombosis or thrombosis associated with recent myocardial infarction. Retinal emboli and their clinical characteristics and implications are discussed in more detail in Chapter 4.

Severe carotid disease may produce hypoperfusion of the globe and *chronic ocular ischemia*. This is associated with a variety of signs involving the posterior and anterior segments of the eye (Fig. 10–3; see Color Plate 44). Anterior ischemia may lead to episcleral and conjunctival injection. Corneal edema may obscure vision, while cells and flare in the anterior chamber may be mistaken for an inflammatory process. If new vessels form on the iris, neovascular glaucoma may ensue. In the retina, a venous stasis retinopathy characterized by microaneurysms and mid-

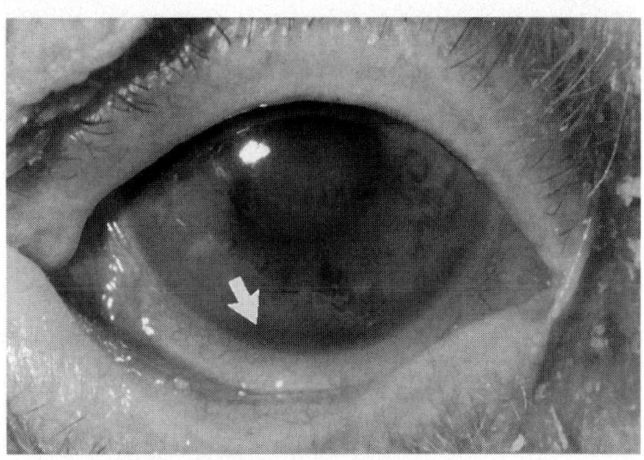

FIGURE 10–3. Ocular ischemic syndrome due to carotid stenosis, characterized by a cloudy cornea, cataract, iris rubeosis, and hyphema (*arrow*) (see Color Plate 44).

peripheral dot and blot hemorrhages may be evident (Fig. 10–4). The retinal abnormalities are similar to those seen in diabetic retinopathy, except they are preferentially located in the mid-periphery instead of the posterior pole and they tend to be unilateral, corresponding to the side of the more obstructed carotid.[22] Optic nerve head swelling is typically not seen until the very late stages of posterior segment ischemia. When vision is severely affected, the visual prognosis is poor.[23]

Rarely, signs of *orbital ischemia* may follow severe carotid disease, with proptosis, chemosis, conjunctival injection, ophthalmoparesis, and retinal ischemia heralding its onset.[24, 25] Orbital ischemia and infarction are uncommon because of the rich anastomoses between the ophthalmic and external carotid arteries.

Other neuro-ophthalmic findings associated with carotid disease include retinal artery occlusions (see Chapter 4) and Horner syndrome (see Chapter 13). Ocular motor palsies have been reported following carotid occlusion and dissection.[24, 26, 27] Presumably, ischemia of the extraocular muscles or nerves is responsible for the ophthalmoparesis, which may be transient, usually resolving within days to weeks. These motility disturbances do not occur in isolation as patients typically have severe unilateral severe visual loss and hemispheric signs of variable degree. Although anterior ischemic optic neuropathy (AION) has also been described in association with carotid disease,[28] the causative relationship is uncertain because AION is more likely the result of small vessel posterior ciliary artery occlusion rather than artery-to-artery emboli or low-flow state.

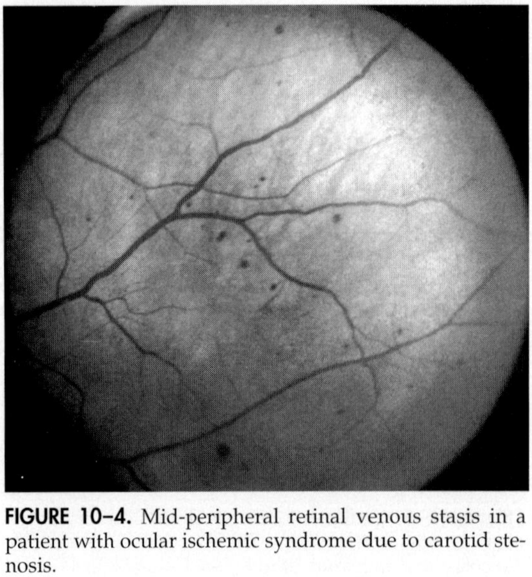

FIGURE 10–4. Mid-peripheral retinal venous stasis in a patient with ocular ischemic syndrome due to carotid stenosis.

General Examination. The presence or absence of a carotid bruit is generally not helpful. The incidence of carotid bruits increases with age. They may be predictive of future cardiac and cerebrovascular events,[29, 30] especially when further evaluation reveals an underlying carotid stenosis.[31] However, the accuracy of this physical finding is low, and therefore the presence of a bruit cannot be used to diagnose carotid stenosis. Furthermore, in one study[32] over one third of patients with high-grade carotid stenosis did not have a bruit. Thus the absence of a bruit cannot be used to exclude operable carotid artery disease.[33, 34]

Diagnostic Tests. The laboratory evaluation of the patient with suspected ischemic monocular visual loss[35] begins with noninvasive assessment of the carotid using either ultrasound or magnetic resonance imaging-angiography. Carotid ultrasound and Doppler are effective screening tools for identification and estimation of the degree of internal carotid artery stenosis.[36] When atherosclerotic plaques are present, B-mode ultrasound can often provide morphologic details.[37] Doppler waveforms allow analysis of blood flow velocity.[38] Because of technical limitations, one major drawback is the technique's relative inability to differentiate between 99% stenosis and total occlusion.[39]

Magnetic resonance imaging-angiography (MRA) is another effective noninvasive test available to detect carotid disease.[40, 41] Results are generally reported within a range: mild (0 to 30% occluded), moderate (30% to 70% occluded), and severe (70% to 99% occluded). Sometimes the occlusion is complete, and the source is presumed to be a stump embolus. MRA in particular is best at identifying ulcerative areas with stenotic plaques. Unlike carotid ultrasound, MRA also provides a view of the intracranial circulation. Its major limitation is that it tends to overestimate stenoses.[41] However, a normal MRA is very helpful because it makes any clinically important carotid disease very unlikely.

Conventional angiography still remains the most accurate method for the evaluation and quantitation of carotid stenoses (Fig. 10–2).[42] The specificity and sensitivity of angiography exceed those of any noninvasive test. Disadvantages of angiography include potential allergy to intravenous contrast and risk of stroke and renal failure. In one study,[43] the angiographic stroke rate was 1.2%. Many surgeons prefer formal angiography prior to endarterectomy, although that may change as ultrasound and MRI techniques continue to improve. Some may operate on stenotic arteries when the ultrasound and MRA examinations are in agreement, thus eliminating the complications associated with conventional angiography.

Other useful studies in the evaluation of retinal ischemia include a complete blood count and cholesterol, triglyceride, and serum glucose levels. A careful historical review and erythrocyte sedimentation rate should always be obtained in an elderly patient with amaurosis as transient visual loss may be the initial manifestation of giant cell arteritis (see below). A cardiac source embolus should be excluded (see below). In select patients, neuroimaging of the brain and transcranial doppler studies may be obtained. Color doppler imaging is a new noninvasive technique that provides anatomic and velocity information about the orbital arteries.[44] It may ultimately prove helpful in the differential diagnosis of amaurosis, but more experience is needed with this technique.

In many elderly patients the workup outlined above will be unrevealing. In this setting atheroma may be arising from the more proximal vessels such as the aorta, or acephalgic migraine should be considered. In younger patients vasospasm and hypercoagulable states, due to abnormal antiphospholipid antibodies, protein C, protein S, and antithrombin III levels, need to be excluded.

Treatment (Medical). If not contraindicated, aspirin therapy should be begun in all patients with amaurosis fugax. Aspirin, an antiplatelet agent, has been shown to reduce the risk of stroke in men and woman in this setting.[45] If episodes continue to occur, then larger doses of aspirin (doses may vary between 40 and 1300 mg), clopidogrel (75 mg po qd), ticlopidine (250 mg po bid), and warfarin can be considered as alternatives in patients without surgical carotid disease (see below). If crescendo TIAs are present or suspected, then heparinization and an inpatient workup and treatment should be considered.[46] Medical treatment is generally agreed upon in patients with mild to moderate stenosis or high-grade stenosis in which medical problems prohibit endarterectomy.

Treatment (Surgical). Together the North American Symptomatic Carotid Endarterectomy Trial (NASCET),[47, 48] the European Carotid Surgery Trial,[49] and the Veterans Administration Cooperative Symptomatic Carotid Stenosis Trial[50] established a benefit for carotid surgery, during which occlusive lesions are removed, for stenoses greater than 70% in individuals suffering a retinal or hemisphere TIA. The procedure should also be considered in selected symptomatic patients with 50% to 70% stenosis, for instance, those without underlying medical complications.[48] Patients with both symptomatic extracranial and mild to moderate intracranial internal carotid artery stenoses may still benefit from endarterectomy.[51] Technical details of the procedure are detailed elsewhere.[52, 53]

The perioperative complication rate for major stroke and death was 2.1% in the NASCET study, emphasizing the importance of the skills of the angiographer, anesthetist, and vascular or neurosurgeon in patients requiring carotid endarterectomy. The low complication rate in the NASCET study likely reflects the exclusion patients greater than 80 years of age, with significant intracranial disease, cardiac emboli, and life threatening disease.[54] In addition to stroke[55] and TIA,[56] other recognized complications of carotid endarectomy include seizures,[57] intracerebral hemorrhage[58] and cerebral edema[59] from hyperperfusion,[60] hypertension,[61] and lower cranial nerve palsies.[62]

In contrast, the surgical management of asymptomatic carotid stenosis remains controversial.[63–66] Previous studies[67, 68] had produced conflicting results, but in a more definitive study[43] endarterectomy was shown to benefit patients with asymptomatic carotid stenosis of greater than 60%. A meta-analysis of the results suggested endarterectomy in patients with asymptomatic stenosis reduced the incidence of ipsilateral stroke, but the absolute benefit was small.[69] Individuals with asymptomatic retinal emboli or carotid bruits detected on a routine examination, or vascular disease elsewhere (cardiac or peripheral vascular disease), should probably undergo carotid doppler examination. Endarterectomy may be considered in those with stenosis, taking into account the age and general health of the patient as well as the operative statistics of the surgeon. Massive screening programs of asymptomatic patients are clearly not cost effective.

Percutaneous transluminal angioplasty and stenting of the internal carotid artery are currently being considered as possible alternatives to carotid endarterectomy.[70–74] Neither requires general anesthesia or a surgical incision, therefore, these procedures may be ideal for patients with coexisting coronary disease, who may be poor surgical candidates.[75] On the other hand, angioplasty is associated with the theoretical possibilities of dislodging a thrombus, which can embolize to the cerebral circulation, or causing a carotid dissection.[76] Restenosis may also occur. At this time these procedures are controversial and are still being studied.[77–80]

In eyes with chronic ischemia, the intraocular pressure should be lowered if high. Endarterectomy is performed in surgical candidates with high-grade stenosis. Extracranial–intracranial arterial bypass or external carotid endarterectomy have been occasionally performed with anecdotal success. Panretinal photocoagulation to prevent iris neovascularization remains controversial,[23] but most authors favor it. Occasionally the signs of ocular ischemia will spontaneously regress without specific therapy.

Cardiac Emboli

Less commonly, cardiac emboli, due to atrial fibrillation, valvular disease, atrial myxomas,[81] and mitral valve prolapse,[82] for instance, can reach the retinal circulation. Retinal *calcific emboli* are usually seen in patients with cardiac valvular disease. These emboli are grey-white and ovoid in appearance and usually lodge near the optic nerve head. They usually result in retinal infarction. Less commonly they arise from a carotid source.

A careful cardiac examination should be directed at detection of an irregular pulse suggestive of atrial fibrillation or a murmur consistent with significant cardiac valvular disease. Cardiac evaluation, including electrocardiography, 24-hour cardiac monitoring, and transthoracic echocardiography, is also suggested. Recently, transesophageal echocardiography has proven useful to identify a cardiac source of emboli in certain patients with unexplained ocular ischemia.[83] It has particular advantage over conventional echocardiography in viewing the left atrial appendage, the aorta, and the interatrial septum and in detecting a patient foramen ovale.

Migraine

Transient visual loss in migraine is exceedingly common and takes many different forms. The three most frequently encountered are scintillating scotomas, hemianopias, and monocular visual loss. While the retinal form of migraine is likely vasospastic, the cause of the visual loss in other types of migraine is less certain. Purely negative phenomena, while they can occur in the aura of migraine, are usually accompanied by positive phenomena (Table 10–4). The reader is referred to Chapter 19 for a detailed discussion of the pathophysiology, diagnosis, and treatment of migraine.

In migraine with aura (classic migraine), a typical migraine headache with hemicranial throbbing, nausea, and photophobia follows the visual disturbance. Many older patients, many with a history of migraine as a younger adult, will develop migrainous visual auras without headache (acephalgic migraine). Often these events are difficult to distinguish from the ischemic embolic events described above. When positive visual phenomena and gradual build up of aura symptoms over 15 to 30 minutes occurs, migraine is more readily differentiated from an occipital lobe TIA.

Scotomas. The best example of combined negative and positive visual phenomena in migraine is an enlarging scintillating scotoma (Fig. 12–2). An area of blurry, wavy, or absent vision surrounded by teichopsia is characteristic. Scintillating scotomas and positive visual phenomena associated with migraine are described in detail in Chapter 12.

Hemianopias. Other migraine patients may develop a true hemianopia in the aura phase without positive visual phenomena. Fortunately, transient isolated hemianopias, particularly in young patients, are more commonly the result of migraine and less frequently the result of a hemispheric embolic TIA. In the migraine setting they often build up over several minutes then resolve over 15 to 30 minutes. Many patients with migrainous transient hemianopia will recognize the visual distur-

TABLE 10–4. Typical Features of Migraine-Related Transient Vision Loss

Gradual onset and duration of up to 1 hour
Positive visual phenomena
Photopsias
Scintillating scotoma
Often followed by headache but may be acephalgic
Associated photophobia and nausea
Previous history of migraine

(Adapted from Volpe NJ, Liu GT, Galetta SL: Transient visual loss. Curr Concepts Ophthalmol 1998;6:55–59, with permission.)

bance in one only eye, typically the one with the temporal visual field defect, making their condition sometimes difficult to discern from ischemic transient monocular blindness.

Retinal Migraine. The last important migraine variant of transient visual loss, retinal migraine, is the least common but the most difficult to distinguish from amaurosis fugax. The typical symptom is complete loss of vision in one eye for over 30 seconds or 1 minute. Patients generally do not describe a shade coming down over their vision as occurs with emboli. Episodes result from widespread retinal vasospasm and last for several minutes. Ophthalmoscopy may reveal the constricted retinal vessels, although usually it is very difficult to make such an observation. One such example is given in Chapter 19, where retinal migraine is also discussed. Since the symptoms of retinal migraine may be difficult to distinguish from embolic amaurosis fugax, it remains a diagnosis of exclusion. One feature of vasospastic amaurosis is its tendency to recur several times a day without residual vision loss. Such a rate would be very atypical for embolic transient monocular blindness.

Treatment. Migraine therapies are discussed in detail in Chapter 19.

Nonmigrainous Retinal Vasospasm

Vasospastic vision loss may also occur outside of the context of migraine. These patients will have no associated pain or headache, and they may complain of several episodes of monocular visual loss per day. Rarely during an event, temporary narrowing of the retinal vessels may be witnessed.[84] The diagnosis is one of exclusion with negative cardiac and carotid evaluations. However, retinal vasospasm may occur with increased frequency in patients with connective tissue disorders such as systemic lupus erythematosus. If a vasospastic cause of the vision loss is suspected, symptoms may be improved with calcium channel blockers.[85, 86] We prefer using verapamil 120 to 360 mg per day, but amlodipine or propranolol are alternative medications that may be effective in this situation. If necessary, aspirin may also be added to the regimen.

Retinal vasospasm and transient monocular visual loss have also been reported in association with cocaine abuse.[87]

Amaurosis Fugax in Adolescents and Young Adults

In patients under age 45, the ischemic ocular causes of transient blurring are relatively uncommon. Most of these patients have vasospastic migraine, and almost none of them will go on to develop significant visual or neurologic deficits.[88] That being said, important diagnoses to exclude in young patients with transient monocular blindness include atrial septal defect, cardiac valvular disease, carotid dissection, hypercoagulable states, and connective tissue disorders such as fibromuscular dysplasia.[89]

Giant Cell Arteritis

In patients over the age of 55 with transient monocular or binocular vision loss, the diagnosis of giant cell (temporal) arteritis must be considered. Many patients with temporal arteritis who develop infarction of the optic nerve and blindness report multiple episodes of blurring or darkening of their vision prior to the permanent event.[90, 91] In fact, repeated episodes of amaurosis makes embolic causes less likely and temporal arteritis more likely. Transient visual loss may be positional in the setting of tenuous blood flow[92] or as a result of viewing bright light (bright light amaurosis, see above).[93] A careful historical review with attention to headaches, scalp tenderness, jaw claudication, fever, weight loss, and polymyalgia symptoms must be performed. In patients with giant cell arteritis and amaurosis fugax, the fundus is usually normal but on occasion a cotton-wool spot (nerve fiber infarct) may be seen.[94] Fluorescein angiography may demonstrate abnormal choroidal perfusion in some cases (see Fig. 5–40).

Further details regarding the pathology, diagnosis, and management of giant cell arteritis are discussed in Chapter 5.

Cortical Transient Ischemic Attacks

Signs of TIAs last for minutes to hours; usually any neurologic deficit of a vascular nature that lasts for more than a day is a stroke. One study found that patients with TIAs that lasted longer than 1 hour were more likely to be associated with proximal arterial stenosis or cardiogenic emboli and have evidence of recent infarcts. TIAs characterized by isolated homonymous hemianopias are uncommon. Most are accompanied by evidence of ischemia to neighboring structures in the same vascular distribution.

In addition to cardiogenic emboli and hypercoagulable states, other causes are discussed below by location.

Anterior Circulation. Other responsible causes in this distribution include extracranial or intracranial (cavernous) internal carotid artery stenosis and middle cerebral artery atheromatous disease. Ischemia in this distribution typically also leads to motor, sensory, or language disturbances.

Posterior Circulation. Vertebrobasilar insufficiency, due to vertebral or basilar artery stenosis, for example, can be associated with transient visual loss that is fleeting and bilateral. In this setting there is reduced perfusion to the occipital lobes resulting in momentary altered vision. These TIAs are often associated with other symptoms of posterior circulation blood flow insufficiency such as ataxia, vertigo, slurred speech, and double vision. However, in some instances the visual loss may be isolated.

Following exclusion of carotid or vertebrobasilar disease or cardiac source emboli, as well as a hypercoagulable state, patients with cortical TIAs usually receive anticoagulation using aspirin or another antiplatelet agent.

OTHER CAUSES OF TRANSIENT VISUAL LOSS

Table 10–5 summarizes other causes of transient vision loss that may be confused with vascular amaurosis fugax. This last section will discuss these and other causes of transient visual loss.

Transient Visual Obscurations

Papilledema may be associated with episodes of grey, black, or white vision lasting for seconds. The hallmark of this type of transient visual loss is its fleeting nature and its association with changes in position, such as sitting up. These transient visual obscurations also occur in patients with pseudopapilledema due to optic nerve head drusen or colobomas, for instance.[95] The mechanism is likely transient ischemia or axonal compression at the elevated, crowded optic nerve head. Transient visual obscurations are also discussed in Chapter 6.

Uhthoff's Phenomenon

Patients with optic neuropathy, resolved or otherwise, may complain of transient visual loss in the affected eye when body temperature is elevated. Symptoms resolve when the body temperature normalizes, and there are no permanent visual sequelae. This phenomenon is most common following optic neuritis, and is discussed in more detail in Chapter 5.

Gaze Evoked Amaurosis

Eye movements may cause temporary visual loss in the setting of intraorbital optic nerve compression. Responsible lesions include optic nerve sheath meningiomas, optic gliomas, papilledema,[96] and intraconal masses such as cavernous hemangiomas.[97] Either horizontal or vertical eye movements may induce visual loss,[98] depending on the location of the culprit lesion. Vision typically decreases seconds after eccentric gaze and returns to normal seconds after returning to straight-ahead gaze.[99] One report[100] described reading-induced visual dim-

TABLE 10–5. Other Causes of Transient Visual Loss

Type of Vision Loss	Symptom	Most Common Setting	Alternative Settings
Transient visual obscuration (TVO)	Fleeting greying vision associated with postural change	Papilledema	Other elevated optic disc anomalies
Uhthoff's symptom	Loss of vision associated with increased body temperature	Optic neuritis (active or recovered)	Other optic neuropathies
Gaze-evoked amaurosis	Loss of vision associated with eye movement in one direction	Optic nerve sheath meningioma	Orbital masses

(Adapted from Volpe NJ, Liu GT, Galetta SL: Transient visual loss. Curr Concepts Ophthalmol 1998;6:55–59, with permission.)

ming. Either transient axonal or vascular compression have been suggested as possible mechanisms.[99]

Epileptic Visual Loss

Although ictal and postictal visual losses are unusual, the phenomena are well recognized. The visual deficits are almost always binocular, and patients may complain of homonymous hemianopias or complete blindness. In the absence of other seizure activity or a history of epilepsy, clinically these patients can be difficult to differentiate from those with migrainous visual loss.

Ictal Visual Loss. Ictal amaurosis is highly characteristic of benign occipital lobe epilepsy, a childhood seizure condition.[101, 102] The average age of onset is 6 years of age, and other clinical features include postictal headache, nausea, and vomiting; psychomotor or hemiclonic seizures; occipital spike- and slow-wave activity with eyes closed; good response to anticonvulsant medication; and spontaneous remission by age 19.[103] Neuroimaging is typically normal.

Other related groups of patients with ictal visual loss have been described.[101] For example, Gilliam and Wyllie[104] reported seven children or young adults with this phenomenon, but in contrast to those with benign occipital lobe epilepsy, most of their patients had magnetic resonance imaging evidence of a stroke, trauma, or neoplasm. No interictal visual field defects were readily identified. Interictal electroencephalography demonstrated posterior spike- and slow-wave complexes limited to the occipital, parieto-occipital, or temporo-occipital regions. Barry et al[105] described five patients, some middle aged and elderly, with hemianopias or complete cortical blindness lasting for minutes, hours, or days. They used the term *status epilepticus amauroticus* to describe the patients with the longer-lasting symptoms. Most had other clinical evidence of seizures such as mental status change or forced eye deviation. Ictal occipital or temporo-occipital discharges were recorded. Finally, occipital lobe seizures and transient cortical visual loss may be a manifestation of nonketotic hyperglycemia.[106]

Postictal Visual Loss. Similar to a Todd's paralysis, visual loss may occur for hours or days following a seizure. In hemianopic cases, the visual deficit is usually contralateral to the cortical seizure focus. Postictal visual loss is much less common than the ictal variety.

REFERENCES

1. Volpe NJ, Liu GT, Galetta SL: Transient visual loss. Curr Concepts Ophthalmol 1998;6:55–59.
2. Bruno A, Corbett JJ, Biller J, et al: Transient monocular visual loss patterns and associated vascular abnormalities. Stroke 1990;21:34–39.
3. Ravits J, Seybold M: Transient monocular visual loss from narrow-angle glaucoma. Arch Neurol 1984; 41:991–993.
4. Kosmorsky GS, Rosenfeld SL, Burde RM: Transient monocular obscuration—? amaurosis fugax: a case report. Br J Ophthalmol 1985;69:688–690.
5. Burde RM: Amaurosis fugax. An overview. J Clin Neuro-ophthalmol 1989;9:185–189.
6. Adams HP, Putnam SF, Corbett JJ, et al: Amaurosis fugax: the results of arteriography in 59 patients. Stroke 1983;14:742–744.
7. Kollaritis CR, Lubow M, Hissong SL: Retinal stroke: Incidence of carotid disease. JAMA 1972;222:1273–1276.
8. Hayward JK, Davies AH, Lamont PM: Carotid plaque morphology: a review. Eur J Vasc Endovasc Surg 1995;9:368–374.
9. Garcia JH, Khang-Loon H: Carotid atherosclerosis. Definition, pathogenesis, and clinical significance. Neuroimag Clin North Am 1996;6:801–810.
10. Russo CP, Smoker WRK: Nonatheromatous carotid artery disease. Neuroimag Clin North Am 1996;6: 811–830.
11. Fisher CM: Observation of the fundus oculi in transient monocular blindness. Neurology 1959;9:333–336.
12. Lepore FE: Visual obscurations: evanescent and elementary. Semin Neurol 1986;6:167–175.
13. Levin LA, Mootha VV: Postprandial transient visual loss. A symptom of critical carotid stenosis. Ophthalmology 1997;104:397–401.
14. Poole CJM, Russell RWR: Mortality and stroke after amaurosis fugax. J Neurol Neurosurg Psychiatry 1985;48:902–905.
15. Wray SH: Visual aspects of extracranial internal carotid artery disease. In: Bernstein EF (ed): Amaurosis Fugax, pp 72–80. New York, Springer-Verlag, 1988.
16. Streifler JY, Eliasziw M, Benavente OR, et al: The risk of stroke in patients with first-ever retinal vs. hemispheric transient ischemic attacks and high-grade carotid stenosis. Arch Neurol 1995;52:246–249.
17. Arruga J, Saunders MD: Ophthalmologic findings in 70 patients with evidence of retinal embolism. Ophthalmology 1982;89:1336–1347.
18. Sempere AP, Duarte J, Coria F, et al: Loss of vision induced by the color white: a sign of carotid occlusive disease (letter). Stroke 1992;23:1179.
19. Furlan AJ, Whisnant JP, Kearns TP: Unilateral visual loss in bright light: an unusual symptom of carotid artery occlusive disease. Arch Neurol 1979;36:675–676.
20. Donnan GA, Sharbrough FW, Whisnant JP: Carotid occlusive disease: effect of bright light on visual evoked reponse. Arch Neurol 1982;1982:687–689.
21. Howard RS, Russell RW: Prognosis of patients with retinal embolism. J Neurol Neurosurg Psychiatry 1987;50:1142–1147.

22. McCrary JA: Venous stasis retinopathy of stenotic or occlusive carotid origin. J Clin Neuro-ophthalmol 1989;9:195–199.
23. Mizener JB, Podhajsky P, Hayreh SS: Ocular ischemic syndrome. Ophthalmology 1997;104:859–864.
24. Galetta SL, Leahey A, Nichols CW, et al: Orbital ischemia, ophthalmoparesis, and carotid dissection. J Clin Neuro-ophthalmol 1991;11:284–287.
25. Borruat F-X, Bogousslavsky J, Uffer S, et al: Orbital infarction syndrome. Ophthalmology 1993;100:562–568.
26. Wilson WB, Leavengood JM, Ringel SP, et al: Transient ocular motor paresis associated with acute internal carotid artery occlusion. Ann Neurol 1989;25: 286–290.
27. Balcer LJ, Galetta SL, Yousem DM, et al: Pupil-involving third nerve palsy and carotid stenosis: rapid recovery following endarterectomy. Ann Neurol 1997;41:273–276.
28. Waybright EA, Selhorst JB, Combs J: Anterior ischemic optic neuropathy with internal carotid artery occlusion. Am J Ophthalmol 1982;93:42–47.
29. Roederer GO, Langlois YE, Jager KA, et al: The natural history of carotid arterial disease in asymptomatic patients with cervical bruits. Stroke 1984;15:605–613.
30. Chambers BR, Norris JW: Outcome in patients with asymptomatic neck bruits. N Engl J Med 1986; 315:860–865.
31. Mackey AE, Abrahamowicz M, Langlois Y, et al: Outcome of asymptomatic patients with carotid disease. Neurology 1997;48:896–903.
32. Sauve JS, Thorpe KE, Sackett DL, et al: Can bruits distinguish high-grade from moderate symptomatic carotid stenosis? The North American Symptomatic Carotid Endarterectomy Trial. Ann Intern Med 1994;120:633–637.
33. David TE, Humphries AW, Young JR, et al: A correlation of neck bruits and arteriosclerotic carotid arteries. Arch Surg 1973;107:729–734.
34. Sauvé J-S, Laupacis A, Østbye T, et al: Does this patient have a clinically important carotid bruit? JAMA 1993;270:2843–2845.
35. The Amaurosis Fugax Study Group: Current management of amaurosis fugax. Stroke 1990;21:201–208.
36. Carroll BA: Carotid ultrasound. Neuroimag Clin North Am 1996;6:875–897.
37. Sidhu PS, Allan PL: The extended role of carotid artery ultrasound. Clin Radiol 1997;52:643–653.
38. Prestigiacomo CJ, Connolly ES, Jr., Quest DO: Use of carotid ultrasound as a preoperative assessment of extracranial carotid artery blood flow and vascular anatomy. Neurosurg Clin North Am 1996;7:577–587.
39. Sidhu PS, Allan PL: Ultrasound assessment of internal carotid artery stenosis. Clin Radiol 1997;52: 654–658.
40. Lamparello PJ, Riles TS: MR angiography in carotid stenosis. A clinical perspective. Magn Reson Clin North Am 1995;3:455–465.
41. Rosovsky MA, Litt AW, Krinsky G: Magnetic resonance carotid angiography of the neck. Clinical implications. Neuroimag Clin North Am 1996;6:863–874.
42. Dean BL, Borden N: Imaging of carotid artery disease. Conventional angiography. Neuroimag Clin North Am 1996;6:843–851.
43. Executive Committee for the Asymptomatic Carotid Atherosclerosis Study: Endarterectomy for asymptomatic carotid artery stenosis. JAMA 1995;273:1421–1428.
44. Hu H-H, Sheng W-Y, Yen M-Y, et al: Color doppler imaging of orbital arteries for detection of carotid occlusive disease. Stroke 1993;24:1196–1203.
45. Bousser MG, Eschwege E, Haguenau M, et al: "AICCA" controlled trial of aspirin and dipyramidole in secondary prevention of atheromatous cerebral ischemia. Stroke 1983;14:5–12.
46. Adams HP, Jr., Davis PH: Management of transient ischemic attacks. Compr Ther 1995;21:355–361.
47. North American Symptomatic Carotid Endarterectomy Trial Collaborators: Beneficial effect of endarterectomy in symptomatic patients with high-grade carotid stenosis. N Engl J Med 1991;325:445–453.
48. Barnett HJM, Taylor DW, Eliasziw M, et al: Benefit of carotid endartectomy in patients with symptomatic moderate or severe stenosis. N Engl J Med 1998; 339:1415–1425.
49. European Carotid Surgery Trialists' Collaborative Group: MRC European Carotid surgery trial: interim results for symptomatic patients with severe (70–99%) or with mild (0–29%) carotid stenosis. Lancet 1991;337:1235–1243.
50. Mayberg MR, Wilson SE, Yatsu F, et al: Carotid endartectomy and prevention of cerebral ischemia in symptomatic carotid stenosis. JAMA 1991;266:3289–3294.
51. Kappelle LJ, Eliasziw M, Fox AJ, et al: Importance of intracranial atherosclerotic disease in patients with symptomatic stenosis of the internal carotid artery. The North American Symptomatic Carotid Endarterectomy Trail. Stroke 1999;30:282–286.
52. Pritz MB: Carotid endarterectomy. Semin Neurol 1998;18:493–500.
53. Riggs PN, DeWeese JA: Carotid endarterectomy. Surg Clin North Am 1998;78:881–900.
54. North American Symptomatic Carotid Endarterectomy Trial (NASCET) Steering Committee: North American Symptomatic Carotid Endarterectomy Trial. Methods, patient characteristics, and progress. Stroke 1991;22:711–720.
55. Ruckley CV: Stroke after carotid endarterectomy. Br J Surg 1999;86:3–4.
56. Rothwell PM, Slattery J, Warlow CP: A systematic review of the risks of stroke and death due to endarterectomy for symptomatic carotid stenosis. Stroke 1996;27:260–265.
57. Kieburtz K, Ricotta JJ, Moxley RT: Seizures following carotid endarterectomy. Arch Neurol 1990;47:568–570.
58. Mansoor GA, White WB, Grunnet M, et al: Intracerebral hemorrhage after carotid endarterectomy associated with ipsilateral fibrinoid necrosis: a consequence of the hyperperfusion syndrome? J Vasc Surg 1996; 23:147–151.
59. Breen JC, Caplan LR, DeWitt LD, et al: Brain edema after carotid surgery. Neurology 1996;46:175–181.
60. Sundt TM, Sharbrough FW, Piepgras DG, et al: Correlation of cerebral blood flow and electroencephalographic changes during carotid endarterectomy. With results of surgery and hemodynamics of cerebral ischemia. Mayo Clin Proc 1981;56:533–543.
61. Biller J, Feinberg WM, Castaldo JE, et al: Guidelines for carotid endarterectomy: a statement for healthcare professionals from a Special Writing Group of the Stroke Council, American Heart Association. Circulation 1998;97:501–509.
62. Ballotta E, Da Giau G, Renon L, et al: Cranial and cervical nerve injuries after carotid endarterectomy: a prospective study. Surgery 1999;125:85–91.

63. Frey JL: Asymptomatic carotid stenosis: surgery's the answer, but that's not the question (editorial). Ann Neurol 1996;39:405–406.
64. Barnett HJM, Eliasziw M, Meldrum HE, et al: Do the facts and figures warrant a 10-fold increase in the performance of carotid endartectomy on asymptomatic patients? Neurology 1996;46:603–608.
65. Perry JR, Szalai JP, Norris JW, et al: Consensus against both endarterectomy and routine screening for asymptomatic carotid artery stenosis. Arch Neurol 1997;54:25–28.
66. Warlow C: Carotid endarterectomy for asymptomatic carotid stenosis. Better data, but the case is still not convincing [editorial]. BMJ 1998;317:1468.
67. The Casanova Study Group: Carotid surgery versus medical therapy in asymptomatic carotid stenosis. Stroke 1991;22:1229–1235.
68. Hobson RW, Weiss DG, Fields WS, et al: Efficacy of carotid endarterectomy for asymptomatic carotid stenosis. N Engl J Med 1993;328:221–227.
69. Benavente O, Moher D, Pham B: Carotid endarterectomy for asymptomatic carotid stenosis: a meta-analysis. BMJ 1998;317:1477–1480.
70. Urwin RW, Higashida RT, Halbach VV, et al: Endovascular therapy for the carotid artery. Neuroimag Clin North Am 1996;6:957–973.
71. Kachel R: Results of balloon angioplasty in the carotid arteries. J Endovasc Surg 1996;3:22–30.
72. Gomez CR: The role of carotid angioplasty and stenting. Semin Neurol 1998;18:501–511.
73. Abrahamsen J, Roeder OC, Justesen P, et al: Percutaneous transluminal angioplasty in selected patients with severe carotid artery stenoses: the results of a consecutive series of 24 patients. Eur J Vasc Endovasc Surg 1998;16:438–442.
74. Henry M, Amor M, Masson I, et al: Angioplasty and stenting of the extracranial carotid arteries. J Endovasc Surg 1998; 5:293–304.
75. Bladin CF, Davis SM, Burton K, et al: The use of percutaneous transluminal angioplasty (PTA) for the treatment of extracranial atherosclerotic vascular disease. The Australian Association of Neurologists (AAN). Aust NZ J Med 1998;28:654–656.
76. Crawley F, Brown MM, Clifton AG: Angioplasty and stenting in the carotid and vertebral arteries. Postgrad Med J 1998;74:7–10.
77. Ferguson RD, Ferguson JG: Carotid angioplasty. In search of a worthy alternative to endarterectomy. Arch Neurol 1996;53:696–698.
78. Ferguson GG: Angioplasty for carotid disease. No. Arch Neurol 1996;53:698–700.
79. McGuinness CL, Burnand KG: Percutaneous transluminal angioplasty of the internal carotid artery. Br J Surg 1996:83:1171–1173.
80. Bergeron P: Carotid angioplasty and stenting: is endovascular treatment for cerebrovascular disease justified? (editorial). J Endovasc Surg 1996;3:129–131.
81. Furlong BR, Verdile VP: Myxomatous embolization resulting in unilateral amaurosis. Am J Emerg Med 1995;13:46–49.
82. Lesser RL, Heineman M-H, Borkowski H, et al: Mitral valve prolapse and amaurosis fugax. J Clin Neuro-ophthalmol 1981;1:153–160.
83. Wisotsky BJ, Engel HM: Transesophageal echocardiography in the diagnosis of branch retinal artery obstruction. Am J Ophthalmol 1993;115:653–656.
84. Burger SK, Saul RF, Selhorst JB, et al: Transient monocular blindness caused by vasospasm. N Engl J Med 1991;12:870–873.
85. Winterkorn JMS, Teman AJ: Recurrent attacks of amaurosis fugax treated with calcium channel blocker. Ann Neurol 1991;30:423–425.
86. Winterkorn JMS, Kupersmith MJ, Wirtschafter JD, et al: Treatment of vasospastic amaurosis fugax with calcium channel blockers. N Engl J Med 1993;329: 396–398.
87. Libman RB, Masters SR, de Paola A, et al: Transient monocular blindness associated with cocaine abuse. Neurology 1993;43:228–229.
88. Tippin J, Corbett JJ, Kerber RE, et al: Amaurosis fugax and ocular infarction in adolescents and young adults. Ann Neurol 1989;26:69–77.
89. Slavin ML, Wall M, Weinstein J: Amaurosis fugax in the young. Surv Ophthalmol 1997;41:481–487.
90. Liu GT, Glaser JS, Schatz NJ, et al: Visual morbidity in giant cell arteritis: clinical characteristics and prognosis for vision. Ophthalmology 1994;101:1779–1785.
91. Finelli P: Alternating amaurosis fugax and temporal arteritis. Am J Ophthalmol 1997;123:850–851.
92. Diego M, Margo CE: Postural visual loss in giant cell arteritis. J Neuro-ophthalmol 1998;18:124–126.
93. Galetta SL, Balcer LJ, Liu GT: Giant cell arteritis with unusual flow related neuro-ophthalmologic manifestations. Neurology 1997;49:1463–1465.
94. Melberg MS, Grand MG, Dieckert JP, et al: Cotton wool spots and the early diagnosis of giant cell arteritis. Ophthalmology 1995;102:1611–1614.
95. Sadun AA, Currie JN, Lessell S: Transient visual obscurations with elevated optic discs. Ann Neurol 1984;16:489–494.
96. O'Duffy D, James B, Elston J: Idiopathic intracranial hypertension presenting with gaze-evoked amaurosis. Acta Ophthalmol Scand 1998;76:119–120.
97. McDonald WI: The symptomatology of tumours of the anterior visual pathway. Can J Neurol Sci 1982; 8:381–390.
98. Manor RS, Ben Sira I: Amaurosis at downward gaze. Surv Ophthalmol 1987;31:411–416.
99. Orcutt JC, Tucker WM, Mills RP, et al: Gaze-evoked amaurosis. Ophthalmology 1987;94:213–218.
100. Manor RS, Yassur Y, Hoyt WF: Reading-evoked visual dimming. Am J Ophthalmol 1996;121:212–214.
101. Jaffe SJ, Roach ES: Transient cortical blindness with occipital lobe epilepsy. J Clin Neuro-ophthalmol 1988;8:221–224.
102. Andermann F, Zifkin B: The benign occipital epilepsies of childhood: an overview of the idiopathic syndromes and of the relationship to migraine. Epilepsia 1998;39:S9–23.
103. Gastaut H: A new type of epilepsy: benign partial epilepsy of childhood with occipital spike-waves. Clin Electroencephalogr 1982;13:13–22.
104. Gilliam F, Wyllie E: Ictal amaurosis: MRI, EEG, and clinical features. Neurology 1995;45:1619–1621.
105. Barry E, Sussman NM, Bosley TM, et al: Ictal blindness and status epilepticus amauroticus. Epilepsia 1985;26:577–584.
106. Harden CL, Rosenbaum DH, Daras M: Hyperglycemia presenting with occipital seizures. Epilepsia 1991;32:215–220.

CHAPTER 11

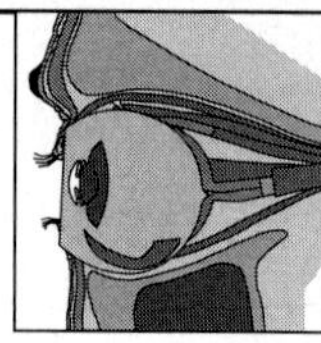

Functional Visual Loss

Functional (nonorganic) visual loss is frequently encountered in ophthalmic and neurologic practice, occurring in 0.5%[1] to 5% of patients presenting with vision loss according to some estimates.[2–4] Patients with functional visual loss may be misdiagnosed because of the paucity of objective findings on examination, particularly ophthalmoscopy. Identifying such patients is extremely important in order to avoid unnecessary laboratory testing and secondary gain.

Although the characterization of the psychological profile of patients with functional vision loss is helpful, a familiarity with diagnostic strategies is more important for the ophthalmologist or neurologist. In this chapter, terminology will be clarified, then patient types and their potential interactions with the examiner will be described. The methods used to diagnose functional vision loss will be reviewed in detail, followed by a brief description of other neuro-ophthalmologic manifestations of nonorganic disease.

TERMINOLOGY

Historically, numerous terms have been used to describe functional visual loss, including *hysteria, hysterical visual loss, malingering, nonphysiologic visual loss, factitious visual loss, nonorganic visual loss, psychogenic visual loss, Münchausen syndrome,* and *conversion disorder of vision*. Ambiguity results for two different reasons. First, there has been no universal agreement about a term to describe nonorganic visual loss. The term *functional visual loss* denotes the symptomatic and measured loss of vision that is unassociated with an identifiable lesion of the visual pathways. Furthermore, patients with functional visual loss have no explanation for their complaints on the basis of contemporary knowledge of the visual pathways. Thus the term *functional visual loss* is equivalent to *factitious, nonorganic,* and *nonphysiologic* visual loss.

The second level of confusion exists when the terminology attempts to identify the underlying cause of the nonorganicity. For instance, *malingering* implies that there is a willful alteration of subjective symptoms and responses on examination. Usually this is an attempt to secure secondary gain such as time away from work or monetary gain from an insurance settlement. Such patients with volitional alteration of the examination can be labeled as malingerers if the examiner chooses to begin a long and arduous confrontation between him- or herself, the patient, lawyers, and insurance companies. The examiner may simply report the vision loss as functional and incompatible with a specific organic lesion. This approach is particularly wise when the initial factors driving the feigned loss are unclear.

Other diagnoses, such as hysteria, conversion disorder, Münchausen syndrome, hypochondriasis, or somatization disorder, may be considered in patients who are not clearly seeking secondary gain. The use of each of these terms is dependent on an understanding of the patient's potential psychiatric problems. For instance, Münchausen syndrome is a factitious disorder in which the patient intentionally produces physical signs and symptoms.[5] When Münchausen syndrome is associated with visual loss, patients can have associated eyelid swelling, conjunctival injection, or hemorrhages (Fig. 11–1). This may be the result of

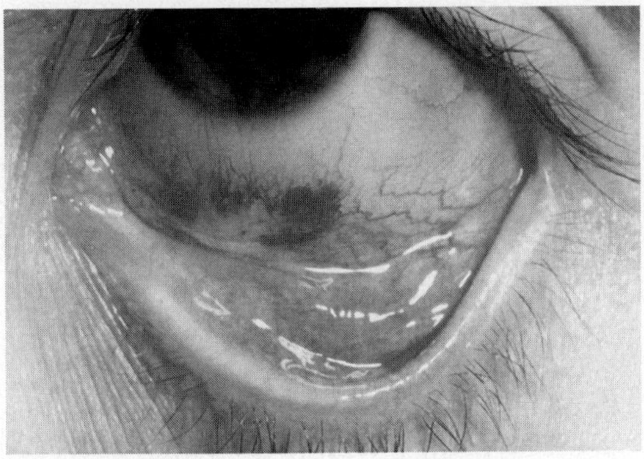

FIGURE 11–1. Conjunctival injection and abrasion secondary to digital trauma in a patient with Münchausen syndrome and associated functional visual loss.

self-inflicted trauma or self-instilled eye irritant. These patients generally have some psychogenic factor driving them to assume the role of a sick person.

The physical symptoms of a patient with a conversion disorder and vision loss may reflect an inner conflict. The label *conversion disorder* incorporates many of the patients who, in the past, were diagnosed as having hysteria or hysterical vision loss. *Hysteria* derives from the root "hyst," referring to the uterus. This terminology had its beginnings in ancient Greece where many conditions were thought to occur only in women, and the uterus was thought to have a will of its own. Until the 19th century this was a popular notion. Charcot was the first to ascribe "hysterical symptoms" to a mental disorder, and he felt it was likely that a specific brain lesion was present in these patients.[6] Babinski expanded on the notion that these symptoms were likely "caused by suggestion and cured by persuasion." Freud popularized the concept that like all else, "hysterical" vision loss had its basis in the inner unconscious battle between the ego, id, and superego. He then popularized the term *conversion disorder*, implying an emotional symptom lead to a physical finding.[6] These patients, although less deliberate than the malingerer, may realize both primary (reduction of stress from inner conflict) and secondary (more attention) gain.[7,8]

Finally, *hypochondriacs* are patients who excessively report signs and symptoms and believe they are seriously ill. They also attempt to convince the examiner that their symptoms and problems are serious. In somatization disorders, patients who are depressed or suffering from an anxiety disorder report numerous vague complaints. These may include symptoms of vision loss that ultimately prove to be nonorganic.

Since the terminology is inexact and overlapping, we prefer the umbrella term of *functional visual loss* and attempt to determine if there are secondary gain issues. It is important to understand the terminology used to identify each of the types of psychogenic illness associated with functional visual loss but prefer that ultimately others more expert in psychiatric illness apply the specific label. Although the techniques used to identify patients that are malingering versus those that are truly suffering from some psychogenic process are the same, the interventions or treatment required may differ immensely.

CLINICAL PRESENTATION

Setting

Some insight into and understanding of types of patients with functional visual loss, as well as the attitudes of both the examiner and the patient toward their interaction, are essential. This understanding will help to make a potentially difficult interaction tolerable and nonconfrontational.

The distortion of the patient–physician relationship in this setting may be very difficult for the physician to accept and manage. Instead of using knowledge and skill to diagnose and treat a real problem, the examiner instead often becomes frustrated and confrontational as he or she becomes increasingly suspicious regarding the nature of the patient's disorder. To paraphrase Thompson,[6] what usually is an allied relationship between doctor and patient against the common enemy of vision loss becomes an adversarial relationship in which the patient complains of vision loss, and the physician is out to prove otherwise. Many times the physician fails to make the correct diagnosis because of this distortion in the doctor–patient relationship. More concerning is the fact that as many as half of the patients with functional visual loss have this superimposed upon true or organic pathology. Any underlying problems may be unrecognized because the examiner is so put off by the patient's behavior.[9]

Patient Characteristics

Patients with functional visual loss can come from any socioeconomic group. There is no clear sex or race predilection. A large proportion of one series consisted of blue-collar workers.[9] Another series found a high prevalence of functional visual loss in Cambodians living in California, and the authors postulated a relationship to previous stress during incarceration in prison camps.[10]

Although it is to some extent linked to the above discussion of terminology, the types of patients encountered, along with the type of interaction they are likely to have with the examiner, have been characterized by Thompson under a slightly different scheme. He offered descriptive subgroups: the *deliberate malingerer, worried impostor, impressionable exaggerator,* and *suggestible innocent.*[6] Characteristics of each of these patients are summarized in Table 11–1. This schema is useful in distinguishing patients as it avoids the term *hysteria.* It can assist with the interaction with the patient and can guide the examiner when giving advice to the patient, the family, and the referring doctor.

Classically, "la belle indifference" has been described as an important feature in all patients with hysterical vision loss (and used to distinguish it from malingering). However, we agree with other series[11, 12] that suggest this finding is present only in a minority of patients and is most likely to occur in those characterized by the "suggestible innocent" profile. These patients with more subtle manifestations of functional visual loss might improve simply by reducing the amount of stress in their lives. Keltner et al[9] found that 51 of 59 adults were clearly seeking financial gain. They presumably fit best in the "deliberate malingerer" subgroup, but some patients may have been "worried impostors," afraid to might miss some deserved benefit. Many adults with functional visual loss are consciously aware of their alteration of their examination.

Types of Complaints

The diagnosis of functional visual loss will be made only if the examiner has a high degree of suspicion. Therefore, unless the patient comes with functional visual loss as the referring diagnosis or the patient is being seen for an insurance company or lawyer, the examiner must depend on the history then the examination. With increasing experience, recognition of typical settings for organic and inorganic disease often suggests to the clinician that functional visual loss should be highly considered. For instance, head trauma is an important cause of traumatic optic neuropathy (see Chapter 5) and also is a common setting for functional visual loss. However, the characteristic severe blow to the brow or cheek that causes traumatic optic neuropathy is usually not described by the patient with functional visual loss. Similarly, a blow to the back of the head or a whiplash-type injury is unlikely to produce a traumatic optic neuropathy. In this setting, the examiner knows to be on guard.

Patients with functional visual loss often offer rather alarming chief complaints that frequently identify the potential for secondary

TABLE 11–1. Types of Patients Encountered With Functional Visual Loss

	Patient's Feelings	Patient's Behavior	Characteristics of Interaction
Deliberate malingerer	Malicious intent	Deliberate nonorganic responses	Confrontational; contest between patient and doctor
Worried impostor	Concerned that something is being missed	Aware of symptom exaggeration; self doubt leads patient to believe symptoms	Tries to convince examiner of severity; often will accept diagnosis of "healthy eyes"
Impressionable exaggerator	Certain something is wrong with eyes	Does not want to hide serious problem; awareness of nonorganic symptoms is result of wanting to be sure nothing is missed	Wants to help by making diagnosis easy; yields poor effort, might improve with suggestion
Suggestible innocent	Convinced that something is wrong after minor injury	Indifferent about inconsistencies of exam or behavior ("la belle indifference")	Complacent; open to suggestions about improvement

From Thompson HS: Functional visual loss. Am J Ophthalmol 1985;100:209–213.

gain; for instance, "I am blind in my eye since the accident" or "I cannot see since I got that chemical in my eye." However, as the examiner investigates further, the complaints become very vague, and patients are often unable to characterize the vision loss as anything more than absent or "blurry." They will often answer, "I do not know" or "I cannot be sure" to questions directed at better characterizing the nature of the vision loss. They less commonly describe the symptoms characteristic of true optic neuropathy such a loss of brightness, darkening, pieces of vision missing, central blind spots, and altitudinal visual field loss. They are very unlikely to report metamorphopsia as patients with maculopathies might.

Impact

The major societal impact of functional visual loss is financial, in the form of undeserved benefits paid for fraudulent claims. Most of the patients in Keltner et al's series[9] were unemployed. Convincing the examiner of a visual defect could result in a lifetime disability check as opposed to either dependency on public assistance or ultimate need to secure employment. The exact monetary amount is difficult to estimate. Keltner et al[9] noted that as many as one third of claims from the Workers Compensation program may have been fraudulent. The problem is likely one that costs society millions of dollars per year. Ophthalmologists and optometrists can declare a patient legally blind, and because of the financial impact are obligated to be absolutely certain that functional visual loss is not present.

FUNCTIONAL VISUAL LOSS IN CHILDREN

The presentation of functional visual loss in children may be different from that in adults. First, the clinical suspicion for true or organic vision loss in children must be higher since the pediatric eye examination may be marked by poor cooperation or a lack of understanding of test procedures. Even when functional visual loss is "confidently" diagnosed the patients must be followed closely for development of organic findings over time. Second, malingering, confrontational behavior, and pending insurance claims are infrequent in children. Lastly, children are less sophisticated and highly suggestible.

Clinical Setting

Functional visual loss has been estimated to occur in approximately one child per 1000 per year, and the most commonly encountered demographic group is pubescent girls (ages 9 to 11).[1, 9, 13–16] There are often other accompanying symptoms such as headache.[14] As with adults, functional visual loss may accompany organic visual loss. Rada et al[17] reported that one fourth of children with functional visual loss have some true underlying organic disease.

Causes

Mantyjarvi[16] found that only a few children had an underlying psychological illness causing the functional visual loss. In some children functional visual loss resulted from a lack of parental attention or conflict with parents. Divorce or a move to a different school or city are common external stresses. Although not malingering, many children realize the secondary gain of increased parental attention as a result of their complaints of defective vision. In others, deterioration in school performance may trigger complaints of functional visual loss.[14] In this setting there is often a mismatch between visual difficulty encountered at school and that noted at home. For instance, when the child is observed unknowingly, there may be no visual difficulty watching television or at play. Similar behavior may be seen in children who want to have glasses because their friends have them.

A true conversion disorder may be present when the child is neither conscious of the loss of function or of the potential secondary gain. Thus the functional visual loss allows the child to avoid a situation in which conflict occurs. In Catalano's series,[14] 4 of 23 children had been physically or sexually abused. In unusual circumstances, a parent drives the complaint of functional visual loss, thereby indirectly assuming the sick role (*Münchausen's by proxy*).

APPROACH TO THE PATIENT WITH FUNCTIONAL VISUAL LOSS

Subjectivity

Every measure of visual function that requires the patient to respond or describe something is, by definition, subjective. In other words, patient cooperation and effort are required to obtain optimal results, especially with regard to testing of visual acuity, stereopsis, color vision, and visual fields.

Diagnosis

The diagnosis of functional visual loss is suggested when the examiner can demonstrate that a patient's behavior and responses to testing are inconsistent with an organic lesion. The diagnosis is confirmed when the examiner is able to prove, by some of the methods described below, that the patient has better vision than he or she claims. Although tempting, the diagnosis of functional visual loss should not be made unless normal acuity and visual fields can be established, and the pupillary and funduscopic examinations are also normal.

Alteration of the Patient–Physician Relationship

Often the examiner can immediately recognize that a patient's behavior is inappropriate. This type of behavior frequently suggests the vision loss is functional and often sets the tone of the patient–physician interaction. The patient maybe overly stoic or overly dramatic. Hostile, suspicious, flirtatious, and excessively cooperative behavior should make the examiner suspicious of functional visual loss. However, prejudices should not interfere with or alter the examiner's empathetic attitude. The caring and genuinely concerned examiner will be the most successful at applying the tests that ultimately prove functional visual loss. Disbelieving or confrontational behavior is likely to make the patient uncooperative with testing.[18, 19]

PATTERNS OF FUNCTIONAL VISUAL LOSS

In most patients with nonorganic loss of vision, acuity and visual fields are both affected.[1, 7, 18, 20, 21] Although it is somewhat artificial, the various techniques used to identify functional visual loss will be described according to the level of visual dysfunction and whether the visual loss is monocular or binocular. It is essential that the examiner becomes familiar and comfortable with a few of the techniques that are used to identify functional visual loss. The testing should be performed in a routine and skillful manner without making the patient suspicious that the agenda is to prove functional visual loss.

It is important for the reader to note that while these techniques aim to prove that the vision is better than the patient claims, some of them are able to establish the actual level of vision in the supposed bad eye or eyes.

Total Blindness

Observation. Throughout the course of the doctor–patient encounter the examiner must carefully observe the patient for behavior incompatible with the degree of alleged vision loss. Truly blind persons will always proceed cautiously around office furniture and equipment. They feel their way, and they will often bump into objects. Patient with functional visual loss, particularly deliberate malingerers, will move quickly and purposely bump objects but never fall or harm themselves. An examination chair can be put in their path as a test. In addition, most truly blind patients will look at the examiner in the direction of the examiner's voice. The deliberate malingerer might not look at or even avoid the examiner, assuming that without vision, auditory clues would be inadequate to locate the other individuals in the room. Many patients with functional visual loss will wear sunglasses for no apparent reason,[22] and we have seen patients who took on the physical appearance, behavior, and head movements of famous blind people commonly seen in the media.

Pupillary Reactions. In the presence of clear ocular media, patients who are bilaterally blind (no light perception) because of retinal, optic nerve, chiasmal, or optic tract disturbances will have pupils that are unreactive to light. Only cortical blindness is associated with normal pupillary reactivity. Therefore a patient who complains of total blindness, with intact pupillary responses, but no cortical lesion, is likely to be functional. A complaint of photophobia with orbicularis contraction when the bright indirect ophthalmoscope light is shined in the eye is incompatible with an ocular cause of blindness.

Optokinetic Nystagmus (OKN). An optokinetic stimulus such as a drum or tape (see Chapter 2) produces a horizontal jerk nystagmus in patients with intact vision and an ocular motor system. The patient must look at and be able to see the figures or stripes on the drum or tape. The response is involuntary and implies a level of acuity equal to that necessary to resolve the stripes or other targets. Patients can voluntarily block this response if they look away from or beyond the stimulus. Excessive convergence on the part of the patient may also dampen the response. The use of a +3.00-diopter lens in front of the eye may force attention to the near stimulus and elicit a response. In the majority of cases, an intact OKN response confirms visual acuity to be at least 20/400. Although it is potentially possible to estimate a level of acuity by reducing the size of the object or stripe or using neutral density filters,[23] we do not recommend this approach.[22]

Tests of Proprioception. Truly blind patients have no difficulty performing tests that appear to require vision but are actually proprioceptive tasks. For instance, a patient can be asked to simply look at his or her hand. A blind person can do this easily, but a patient with functional visual loss will often look away from his or her hand. The patient also can be asked to bring the tips of the first finger from each hand together from a distance.[7] This can be done without any vision and is easily performed by most blind patients. Patients with functional visual loss will often miss by inches. Finally, a blind person asked to sign his or her name will have no difficulty signing, while a functional patient will often produce a signature that is unlike his or her true signature and clearly is not along a horizontal line.

Mirror Test. When a large mirror is placed in front of the face of a sighted person and rocked back and forth, an involuntary nystagmoid movement that results from forced fixation on the image in the mirror is produced.[24] A patient with functional visual loss will be unable to avoid this movement provided he or she is looking at the image in the mirror. Acuity better than hand motion is present if this response occurs.

Surprise. Although generally too confrontational to recommend in most settings, actions that are designed to surprise and elicit a response from a patient can be quite effective. Various techniques have been described, and all generally involve some behavior atypical in a normal physician–patient interaction. The examiner can make faces or write shocking words and watch the patient for a response. A smile, gasp, or surprised look by the patient confirms that he or she can see and often ends with a "you got me, doc."

Evoked Potentials. Electrophysiologic testing has a definite role in the testing of patients with functional visual loss. In a patient with purported complete blindness, the flash evoked visual potential can be used to document intact visual pathways.[13, 25–27] In cooperative patients the pattern-reversal visual evoked potential can provide information about the level of acuity. However, in patients with suspected functional visual loss, an abnormal visual evoked potential is difficult to interpret.[27] The patient can voluntarily alter the amplitude and latency of the P100 peak by defocusing, not wearing corrective lenses, or looking away from the stimulus.[28–30] Unfortunately, the opposite is also true, as normal responses have been documented in patients with organic visual loss.[31]

Severe Unilateral Vision Loss

Techniques used on patients with severe bilateral vision loss can be applied to patients with severe unilateral vision loss by patching or covering the "good" eye. In fact, gross differences in behavioral observations and tests of proprioception when the examiner tests each eye separately are often the most compelling findings in this situation. The methods outlined below tend to emphasize the advantage the examiner has because of his or her understanding of binocularity and afferent visual pathway anatomy. It is most important to observe the patient carefully while performing these tests since a "smart" patient may close the "good" eye periodically to try to figure out what the examiner is trying to do.

Afferent Pupillary Defect. Most patients with severe unilateral vision loss, with no history of amblyopia and with clear media, have a relative afferent pupillary defect (RAPD). Regardless of the localization of unilateral vision loss (optic nerve or chiasm), if the level of acuity is 20/200 or worse, an RAPD is usually present. Certainly nearly all patients with counting fingers or worse vision in one eye, with normal vision in the other, will have a RAPD. The examiner should exercise caution because the RAPD in many ways is a subjective observation and may be absent in asymmetric but bilateral cases of optic neuropathy with very disparate levels of acuity. The absence of an RAPD should not be used to rule out an optic neuropathy, especially if there is a chance of pre- or coexisting optic neuropathy in the other eye.

Stereopsis. In cooperative but unsuspecting patients, measurement of stereopsis can be invaluable in testing for functional visual loss because the results may prove the patient has better vision than he or she claims.[24] Levy and Glick[32] have determined the minimum level of acuity in each eye required to achieve each of the levels of stereoacuity on the Titmus test (Fig. 11–2). Therefore, a patient with a claim of reduced acuity to the 20/400 level in one eye but who sees 8 or 9 circles in stereo on the Titmus test certainly has functional visual loss. Unfortunately, some patients quickly close an eye and realize the test requires binocular vision and subjectively further alter their responses. As with the visual acuity testing strategy described below, it is often effective to begin the stereoacuity testing with the most difficult circles (the ninth) and act somewhat surprised if the patient denies appreciation of elevation of the circle. The great advantages of the stereoacuity testing are its widespread availability and the fact that a specific level of acuity can be proven.

Duochrome Test. Several variations of the duochrome test have been described. Two pieces of equipment commonly available in eye lanes are required. The first is the red/green filter on the projector eye chart (Fig. 11–3). This filter is commonly used to refine refraction but in this setting is used to separate the right and left portions of the chart (left is green and right is red). The test is effective as described only if the red filter is incomplete. Next the red/green glasses used for the Worth 4 dot response are utilized. The test takes advantage of the fact that the eye looking through the red lens will see both sides of the chart. The eye looking through the green lens will see only the letters on the green side of the chart. The red lens is therefore put in front of the bad eye. If the patient reads the entire line (including those on the "red" half) better than their alleged level of visual acuity then the examiner knows that the "bad" eye is seeing as it is the only eye that can see the red half of the chart. A "poor man's" version of this test can be performed by simply writing letters in red or with a pink highlighter. These letters cannot be seen with the eye that has the red lens and therefore the green lens is placed over the bad eye. If the patient reads the letters, then they were seen with the "affected" eye. This technique, using a somewhat objectionable series or words, is a powerful combination.

Color Plates and the Red/Green Lenses. Another test that takes advantage of the readily available red/green lenses and can be used to prove at least 20/400 vision involves use of the Ishihara color plates.[33] These plates cannot

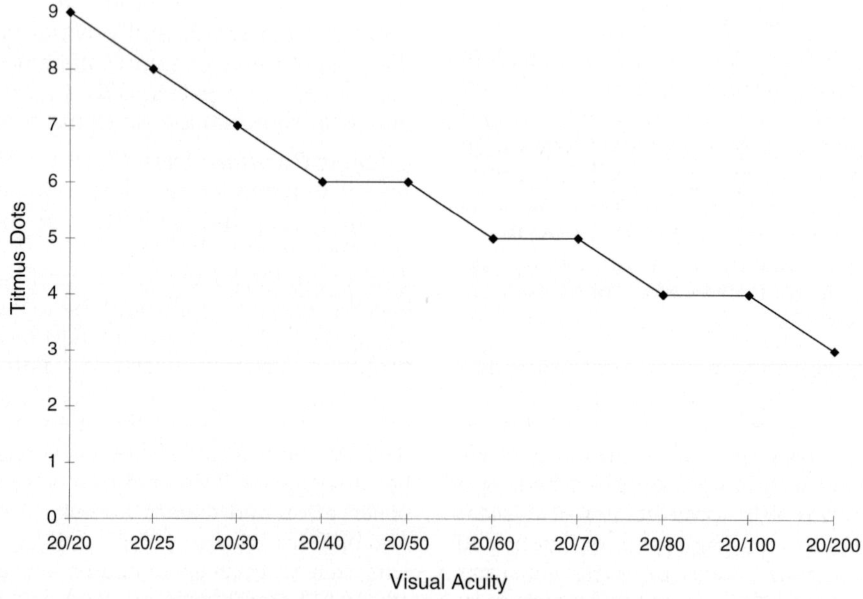

FIGURE 11–2. Correlation of level of stereoacuity with visual acuity. Individuals who can perceive the eighth of nine Titmus stereo dots must have at least 20/25 acuity in each eye. Similarly, the ability to perceive the first six of nine stereo dots correctly requires at least 20/50 in each eye. (Adapted from Levy NS, Glick EB: Stereoscopic perception and Snellen visual acuity, Am J Ophthalmol 1974;78:722–724, with permission from Elsevier Science.)

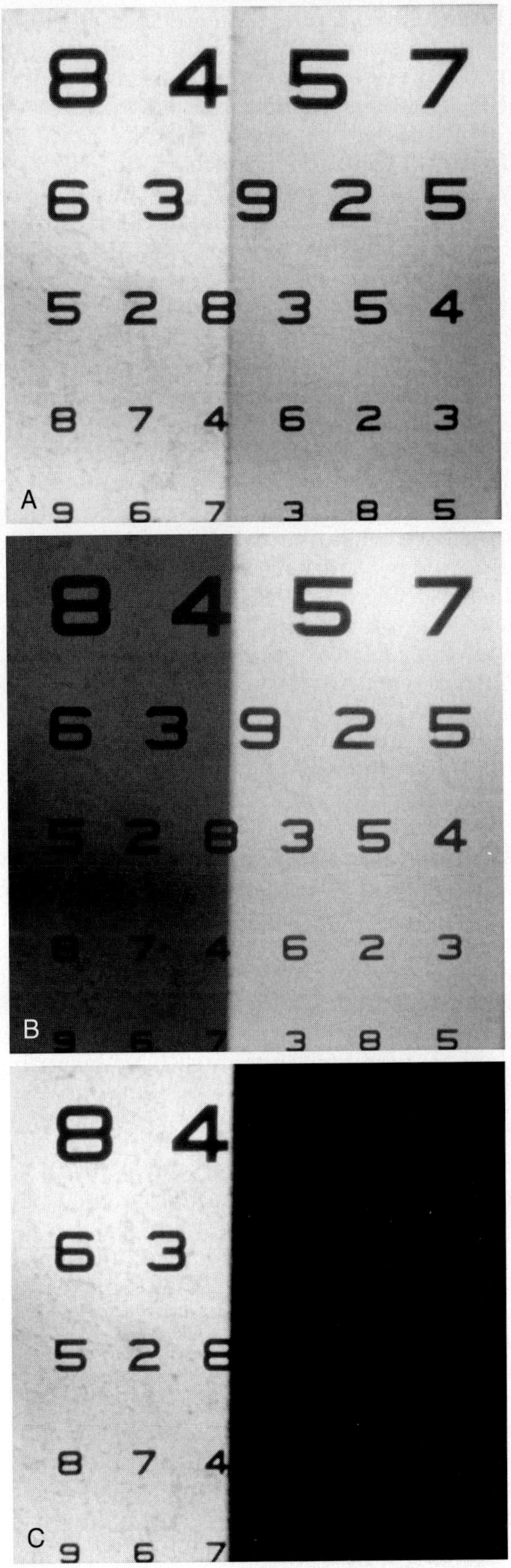

be seen through a green lens, therefore if the red lens is put on over the "bad" eye and the patient reads the plates then at least 20/400 vision is present in the eye that the patient claims has poor vision.

Polarized Eye Chart. Some commercially available projector charts come with a slide containing polarized letters. These charts along with the readily available polarized glasses used for stereoacuity testing can be used to dissociate the eyes and demonstrates that each eye is reading the letters.[34] The projected letters can be seen by the right eye, left eye, or both eyes and if the examiner moves quickly before the patient tries closing the good eye (not easily seen by the examiner because of the glasses) better acuity with the bad eye can usually be demonstrated.

Prism Shift Test. A normal prism shift test depends on the presence of binocular vision. To perform this test the examiner chooses a Snellen letter that is smaller than the acuity at which the patient alleges to see in the affected eye. For example, if the patient sees 20/200 with the affected eye, the test can be performed with a 20/50 letter or smaller. The patient then views the target binocularly, and a four-diopter base-in loose prism is placed in front of the alleged bad eye. If the patient truly sees the target with both eyes then a compensatory movement of both eyes toward the apex of the prism is followed by a convergence movement of the fellow eye back toward center as the patient refuses the image. If the alleged bad eye is truly defective, a prism over it will not result in any compensatory eye movements because the patient is fixing only with the other eye.

Prism Dissociation. Several variations of the prism dissociation test have been described.[35] This test uses a vertical prism to separate the images from the two eyes, and the goal is to have the patient unknowingly read the letters

FIGURE 11–3. The duochrome test is performed using the red/green glasses as the eye chart is projected through the red/green filter. The test is effective only if the red filter is incomplete. The left half of the screen is green, the right side is red. Through clear lenses (**A**) the red and green portions of the chart are seen. Through a red lens, (**B**) both sides of the chart are seen. Through a green lens, (**C**) only the letters on the left side are seen. The test for functional vision loss is done by placing the green lens over the good eye and demonstrating that the bad eye sees if the entire line is read.

that correspond to the line seen by the bad eye. To perform this test the examiner needs to fool the patient into believing that both images are being seen by the good eye. This can be accomplished by momentarily holding the vertical prism only partially over the visual axis over the good eye, while covering the bad eye, intermittently causing monocular diplopia. The prism is then completely moved over the good eye while the bad eye is uncovered. This results in true binocular diplopia with each eye seeing the same but separate lines of Snellen acuity. For example, if an eight-diopter base-up prism is held over the good eye, the patient is then asked to read the higher line. If the patient reads the upper line, the examiner has established the acuity of the bad eye at that level.

Magic Drop Test. "Suggestible innocent" patients may believe that a magic drop placed in their eye is going to temporarily improve their vision. It is important to emphasize that the improvement is only temporary since many patients are not going to be ready to "give up" their "poor" vision immediately. A topical anesthetic, with the bottle's label hidden, can be used. As it is instilled, it may be helpful for the examiner to say that if the vision improves with this drop, it will "help to understand better what part of the eye is having the problem." Putting the patient's distance refraction and a pinhole in a trial frame while the patient reads with the "magic drop" often helps the patient to see even better. This test is very effective in children because of their suggestibility, as moments later vision amazingly improves and then reverts to predrop level. This is another test that establishes a better level of vision that what the patient claims.

Moderate Monocular Vision Loss

Each of the methods outlined above for more severe unilateral vision loss is helpful in patients with complaints of more moderate visual acuity loss in the range of 20/40 to 20/100. However, in this situation the examiner often encounters a more sophisticated patient and finds the job of "proving" that the patient has better vision more difficult. Many times better acuity cannot be demonstrated, and the presence of nonphysiologic visual field loss must be relied upon to suggest nonorganicity.

Visual Acuity Testing. The relationship of the testing distance and the visual acuity that the patient is able to see can be used to confirm functional visual loss. A person who sees 20/100 should be able to read the 20/50 line from 10 feet from the chart (ie, 10/50 = 20/100). By varying testing distances, nonorganic responses can usually be demonstrated. Significant mismatches between distance and near acuities can also be considered evidence of functional visual loss. Finally, the method by which acuity is tested may be used to "prove" the patient has better vision. For instance, one of the most reliable ways to demonstrate better visual acuity is to start testing at the 20/10 line of the chart. Then the size of the letters is slowly increased while the examiner tries to outlast the patient. Prolonged periods of silence while the patient struggles can be followed by "are you sure you cannot see that" then by "OK, the letters will become twice the size now." If a chart is used that has three or four 20/20 lines, by the time the sixth line (20/25) is reached the patient often tires, acquiesces, and reads the line.

Another relatively simple test of visual acuity can be performed while testing near vision. A reading card with a paragraph of prose is used, and the patient is asked to read 20/20 size print with both eyes and near correction. The patient reads smoothly because the good eye is open. The patient is then asked to do the same thing with a pen held vertically between the eyes and the reading material. If the patient continues to read smoothly without having to move his or her head to look around the pen, then both eyes must have been able to see.

Fogging. The fogging technique involves blurring the good eye with lenses while the patient views the acuity chart binocularly. The acuity level achieved thereby represents the function of the supposed bad eye. One technique uses the phoropter, and the examiner makes numerous lens changes for several seconds involving the dials for both eyes. Eventually a small amount of sphere or cylinder over the bad eye and a +6.00-diopter lens over the good eye are achieved. This maneuver blurs the vision of the good eye. The patient is then asked quietly but quickly to read the Snellen line in question. This technique is outstanding with suggestible patients, but in our experience many patients are sophisticated enough to be aware of the blurring of the good eye and close it.

An alternative method of using paired cylinders is subtler and may be more effective.[6, 13] The blurring of the good eye is less obvious to the patient with this technique than with high-plus lenses. To perform this test a trial frame is used, and a plus and minus cylinder of 3.00 diopters are placed on the same axis over the good eye with one lens in the posterior, nonrotating slot where spheres are usually placed. The correct distance refraction is placed over the bad eye, and the patient is asked to start reading the chart. At that point the examiner claims to need to "adjust the trial frame." While repositioning the trial frame on the patient's nose, the examiner rotates the cylinder in the front of the trial frame on the good eye 20 degrees. This effectively blurs the good eye without being obvious to the patient. The patient then continues to read with the bad eye. One disadvantage of this test is that it cannot be performed with the phoropter, which usually aids in distracting the patient and confusing from which eye he or she is seeing.

Constricted Visual Fields. Although patients with functional acuity loss may not complain of defective peripheral vision, visual field testing commonly reveals constricted visual fields.[19] These are characterized on Goldmann perimetry or automated visual field analysis by preserved small central islands of vision[36] (Fig. 11–4). On the Goldmann visual field the size of the field often does not vary much with the size of the stimulus. With confrontation techniques, such patients see clearly only when objects are directly in front of their face.

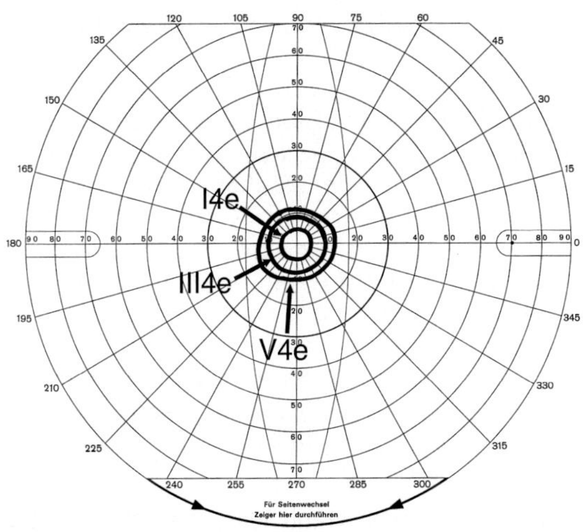

FIGURE 11–4. Goldmann visual field demonstrating generalized constriction. Note that each stimulus is associated with approximately the same size visual field.

Nonspecific generalized constriction of the visual fields is also characteristic of many organic conditions including end-stage glaucoma, bilateral occipital lobe damage, atrophic papilledema, and retinitis pigmentosa. Patients with functional visual loss can be distinguished from true cases of generalized constriction by the following maneuvers:

1. *Tubular visual fields.* The test is based on the principle that the normal visual field increases in size as the eye is moved farther away from the testing plane. It is generally performed with a tangent screen (Fig. 11–5) although simple confrontation methods can also be used. A monocular field is tested first at 1 meter, and the screen is marked with the patient's responses. The patient is then moved to 2 meters and the size of the stimulus is doubled. The field is retested, and many patients with functional visual loss will demonstrate tunneling without physiologic visual field expansion.
2. *Pantomime.* Patients who claim to have a small central visual field can often be fooled with the "Simon says trick." In this test the examiner claims to be doing a neurologic examination, and the patient's vigilance decreases because it appears as if vision is not being tested. The examiner holds both of his or her hands up beyond the central 30 degrees of the patient's visual field as they face each other. The examiner then begins with verbal commands such as "open and close your hands" or "hold up two fingers on each hand." At the same time the examiner is doing what he or she has asked the patient to perform. Suddenly the examiner makes a different type of hand or finger movement without a verbal command to the patient. If the patient mimics the movement accurately, intact visual fields beyond the central 30 degrees are confirmed.
3. *Nonphysiologic constriction.* Some patients may demonstrate nonphysiologic constriction of isopters with a field associated with larger stimuli actually smaller than the field with smaller stimuli (Fig. 11–6). It is occasionally helpful to begin perimetry with the smallest isopter so the examiner can demonstrate a normal-sized visual field before the patient begins voluntarily to constrict the field. For instance, a patient with a 10-degree I1e (the smallest, dimmest stimulus) field in the Goldmann perimeter is unlikely

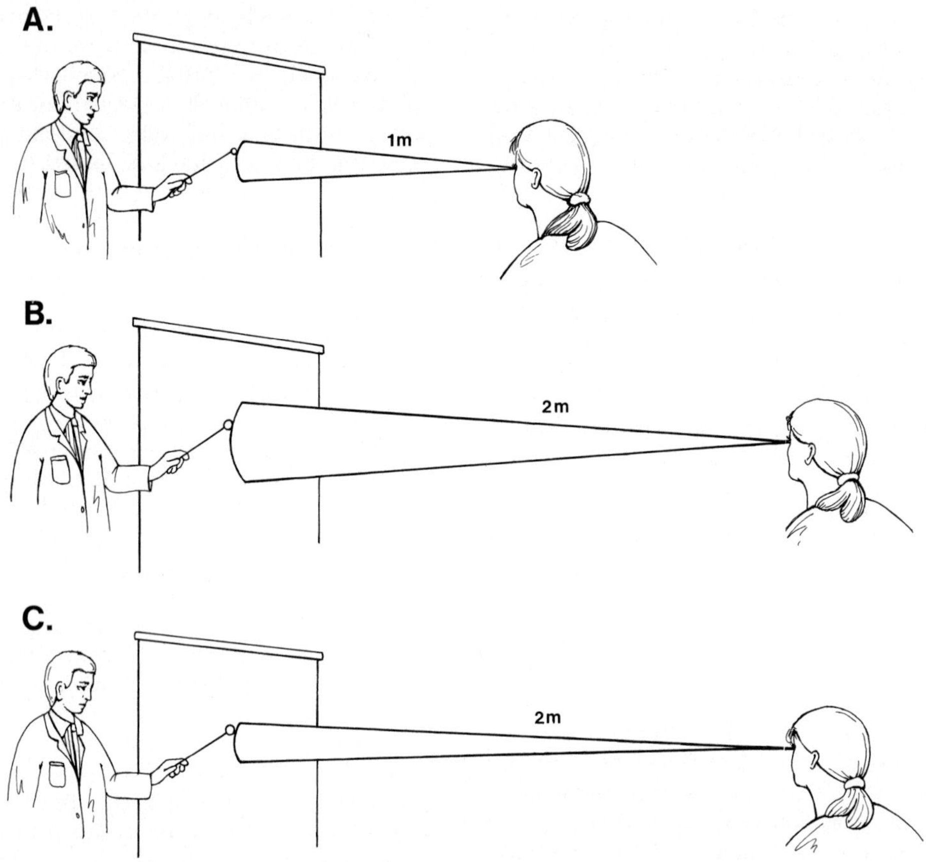

FIGURE 11–5. Testing for tubular visual fields with the tangent screen. **A.** The field is tested at one meter with a 9-mm white object and the results marked on the screen with chalk. **B.** When the patient with organic visual field loss is moved to 2 meters from the screen and the stimulus sized doubled (18-mm white) the field expands to twice the size. **C.** The patient with functional visual loss demonstrates tubular fields as the field does not expand as the testing distance is increased from 1 to 2 meters and the target size is doubled.

to be suffering from organic visual loss. The test can also be repeated with encouragement, such as telling the patient that he or she does not have to wait until the entire stimulus is seen with certainty before pushing the buzzer. A different result on retest is suggestive of functional visual loss.

4. *Spiraling*. A classic alteration of the visual field on Goldmann perimetry is called *spiraling* (Fig. 11–7). In this case the patient, often the "worried impostor" type, becomes more and more hesitant to respond to the same stimulus as it is sequentially presented along radial angles. The resultant field nonphysiologically spirals to the center.

Moderate Binocular Vision Loss

Patients with mild to moderate functional visual acuity loss of 20/40 to 20/60 in both eyes can be some of the most difficult patients to deal with. This slight level of acuity reduction is often sufficient to qualify for disability benefits, yet the patient is able to continue with daily activities, including driving and recreation. They claim binocular vision loss, and the patients are simply unwilling ever to report being able to see the smaller lines on the eye chart. Tests described above that depend on the tricking the patient with purported monocular visual loss into using the supposed bad eye cannot be used effectively. Except for the potential acuity meter technique, for the most part the examiner must depend largely on nonphysiologic responses during visual acuity and field testing as described above to make the diagnosis.

Potential Acuity Meter. The potential acuity meter can be used in this setting to demonstrate better vision.[37] This apparatus projects the Snellen acuity letters directly onto the ret-

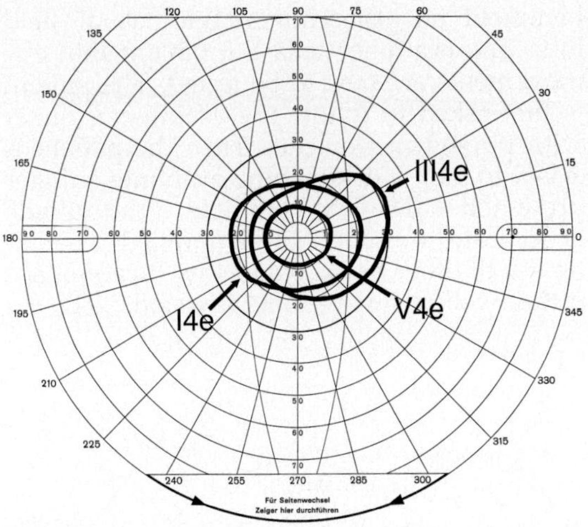

FIGURE 11–6. Goldmann visual field demonstrating "criss-crossing" of isopters, Note that there are parts of the visual field that are larger when testing with the smaller III4e stimulus compared to the larger V4e stimulus, and the I4e field is larger than the V4e field. This is nonphysiologic.

ina and is more commonly used to establish the potential visual acuity in patients with cataracts. The functional patient is informed that a problem has been found and that the diagnosis will be confirmed with this next test. It can be explained that the problem is likely in the retina, and it will be "bypassed with the potential acuity meter and the eye chart will be shined directly on the optic nerve." The patient will often read to a normal level in this circumstance.

Functional Visual Field Loss

Tunneling of the visual fields and spiraling are often associated with functional visual loss, and as described above suggest the nonorganic nature of vision loss in many patients. However, in some patients, visual field deficits are the sole or primary manifestation of functional visual loss.

Perimetry. Visual field defects can be presented or "created" on any type of perimeter. That is, functional visual fields can be found in patients tested with sophisticated automated threshold perimetry as well as standard kinetic perimetry.[38–46] Visual field defects such as hemianopias and quadrantanopias can be fabricated on the automated perimeter, and in such cases the reliability parameters such as false positives and negatives are not helpful in identifying a voluntary alteration of the field.[42] However, the presence of an intereye difference in the mean threshold light sensitivity of 8.7dB in patients with organic visual loss has been shown nearly always produce an RAPD.[47] Therefore if such a difference exists, and there is no RAPD, functional visual field loss is likely present.

Bitemporal Hemianopia. Functional visual loss can present as a bitemporal hemianopia.[44, 48] Patients, presumably unaware of the anatomic basis of the visual fields and the localization of bitemporal hemianopia to the chiasm, may complain of loss of side vision, loss of peripheral vision, or tunnel vision. The key to the diagnosis here is the discrepancy between visual field tests when performed monocularly versus binocularly.[39, 41, 48] Standard perimetry is performed on each eye and results in a bitemporal hemianopia. The test is then repeated with both eyes open. Patients never realize the extent of the nasal field of the contralateral eye. This area of intact vision disappears when the eyes are tested together because they assume the temporal visual field is only seen by the ipsilateral eye.

Monocular Temporal Hemianopia. Similar strategies can be applied in patients complaining of only monocular temporal visual field defects, the so-called missing half defect.[39, 41, 48, 49] Despite the full nasal field of the normal other eye, binocular visual field testing fails to show an intact temporal field on the side of the "af-

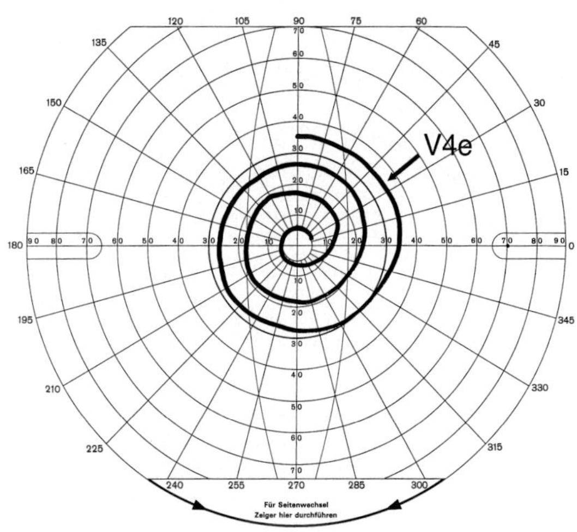

FIGURE 11–7. Goldmann visual field demonstrating nonphysiologic spiraling. As the test proceeds along adjacent radii, the patient responds later and later. The field "spirals" to the center.

fected" eye (Fig. 11–8).[50] A similar strategy may be employed using computerized perimetry as well.[51] Such nonphysiologic results confirm there is some nonorganicity to the complaints. However, they do not prove necessarily that the monocular field defect is not real.

Saccades. The presence of accurate saccadic movement by an eye into an allegedly blind hemifield suggests nonorganic visual field loss. The examiner tells the patient that eye movements are next to be tested. The patient is first asked to follow the examiner's finger with pursuit movements. Then the patient is asked to look quickly at the examiner's finger presented in the blind hemifield; if the saccade is accurate, an intact field is implied. The patient will often hesitate and say "I cannot see it that well in my peripheral vision." The ex-

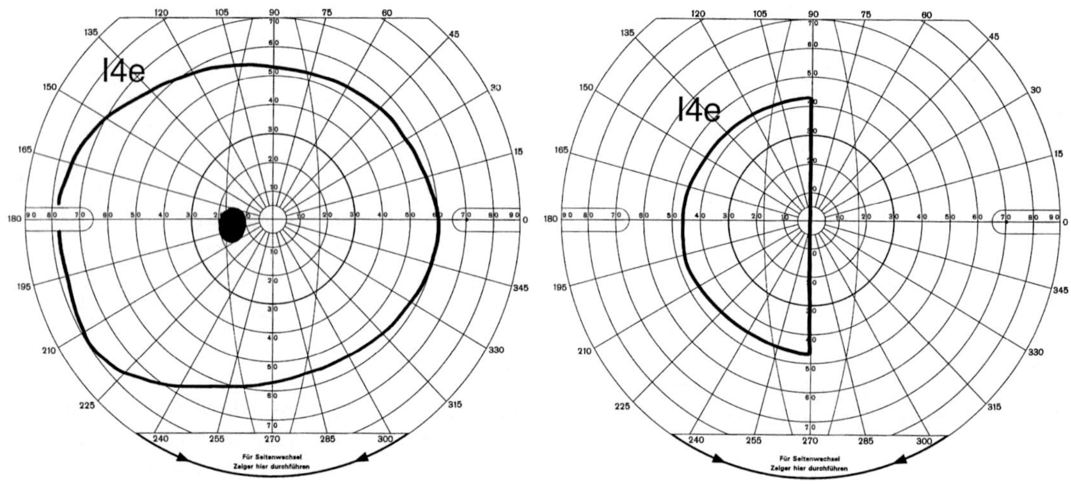

A Left eye Right eye

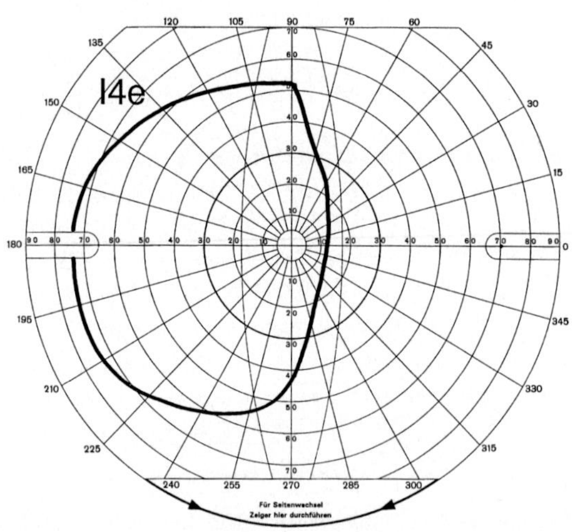

B Both eyes

FIGURE 11–8. Testing for nonorganic temporal visual field defect using binocular Goldmann visual fields. The patient complains of temporal field loss in the right eye, which is documented in **A.** Note the visual field of the left eye is normal. **B.** The patient is then tested binocularly and believes that the right side of the visual field is seen only by the right eye. Therefore, a persistent temporal defect is present despite the presence of intact right-sided (nasal) visual field in the left eye.

aminer responds by saying "I know, therefore I want you to look at it with your central vision" and precise saccadic eye movements sometimes follow.

Central Scotomas. Central scotomas are exceedingly rare manifestations of functional visual loss, but they have been reported. Patients with functional visual loss for the most part lack the sophistication required to know that a profound reduction of central acuity may occur despite intact peripheral fields. When a central scotoma is found an extensive search for a maculopathy or optic neuropathy must be undertaken. Finally, patients complaining only of paracentral visual field defects can be tested using the red Amsler's grid and the red/green glasses.[52] If the scotoma disappears when the red lens is over the affected eye, and the green lens is over the good eye, then the patient is functional. The grid can only be seen through the red lens, and the patient's assumption that he or she can see it because the good eye is being used is incorrect.

Findings and Diagnosis of Functional Visual Loss in Children

Children with functional visual loss most commonly present with moderate binocular deficits with visual acuities in the range of 20/40 to 20/100. The child often seems to exert tremendous effort as he or she attempts to read the eye chart. Guesses are often completely wrong.

Diagnosis. In contrast to adults, who often have to be "tricked" into seeing better, children are much more easily coaxed into exhibiting normal vision with relatively simple maneuvers such as plano glasses or verbal encouragement. Many of the tests outlined above are also effective in children with functional visual loss. The technique described above in which the examiner starts with the smallest letters and acts surprised as he or she moves slowly up the chart to letters of increasing size (frequently combined with a low-power lens) often demonstrates better vision. "Magic drops" such as topical anesthetics, with the appropriate convincing, will often be quite effective. Stereoacuity testing is another very effective way to demonstrate better vision since most young patients fail to realize the test requires binocular vision.

Overview of Efferent Nonorganic Neuro-ophthalmic Disorders

Efferent nonorganic neuro-ophthalmic disorders are much less common than afferent problems and can affect ocular motility or alignment, the eyelids, or the pupil. The most commonly encountered problems are voluntary nystagmus and convergence spasm. These topics will be mentioned briefly, as they are described in more detail in other chapters.

Factitious Pupillary Abnormalities. Nonorganic pupillary abnormalities can only result from the patient instilling something in the eye to make either the pupil larger or smaller. The distinction of pharmocologic dilation of the pupil from other causes of the fixed dilated pupil such as third nerve palsy and Adie's pupil is described in Chapter 13. The key features of the pharmacologically dilated pupil are the wide dilation to 7 to 8 mm and the absence of constriction when 1% pilocarpine is instilled. The majority of pharmacologically dilated pupils are due to a chemical (often never identified) getting into an eye inadvertently. This is in contradistinction to a patient who knowingly places something in the eye in an attempt to create concern. These patients often have knowledge of various available drops that can dilate pupils and also know that this examination finding will likely be interpreted as a neurologic emergency. For these reasons, many of these patients are health care workers.

Factitious Ptosis. Factitious ptosis is relatively easily distinguished from true ptosis by the position of the eyebrow. Patients with true ptosis will be struggling to hold their eye open and will use the frontalis muscle to try and elevate the lid, thereby elevating the brow. The patient with factitious ptosis creates it with orbicularis contraction, thereby lowering the brow toward the eye.[53] Ptosis is discussed in greater detail in Chapter 14.

Factitious Ophthalmoplegia: Convergence Spasm. Spasm of the near reflex, or convergence spasm, is characterized by esotropia (intermittent convergence), abduction limitation, accommodation (blurred distance vision), and miosis.[54] The condition is often associated with ocular discomfort and is always intermittent. Its differentiation from sixth nerve palsies and its differential diagnosis and management are reviewed in Chapter 15.

Factitious Nystagmus. Voluntary "nystagmus" occurs when a patient willingly initiates rapid back-to-back saccadic eye movements.[55] The movement, unlike true nystagmus, can be produced on command and can be sustained for only a few moments. The condition is recognized by its voluntary nature and by the frequently associated orbicularis contraction, eyelid flutter, and convergence. This eye movement disorder is also discussed in Chapter 17.

Management of the Patient With Nonorganic Symptoms

Differential Diagnosis. It is paramount in this setting to be absolutely certain about the diagnosis of functional visual loss and to exclude any true disease that requires treatment. When normal vision can be proven, and the examination is otherwise normal, the examiner may be more comfortable regarding the absence of organicity. However, in many instances a true underlying disorder cannot be excluded.

The most common diseases that need to be considered in the differential diagnosis of functional visual loss include amblyopia, optic neuropathies, retinal degenerations, and cortical visual loss. Thus, when the diagnosis is uncertain, magnetic resonance imaging with contrast should be performed. Electroretinography should then be considered in all patients to exclude retinal dysfunction. When unrevealing, neuroimaging with nuclear medicine techniques to assess brain function (single proton emission computed tomography (SPECT) or positron emission tomography (PET)) can be performed. Moster et al[56] reported two cases of cortical visual loss that were initially thought to be functional because of normal conventional neuroimaging. Ultimately the patients were determined to have cortical dysfunction based on occipital lobe hypoperfusion on SPECT. In addition, more occult forms of optic neuropathy, including hereditary conditions, inflammations associated with systemic illness, and nutritional causes, should be excluded. These can be screened for by examining family members, careful systemic evaluation by an internist, and appropriate blood tests.

Management of Functional Visual Loss in Adults. The successful management of patients with nonorganic neuro-ophthalmic symptoms begins with physician empathy and encouragement. For the most part, there is nothing to gain by confronting the patient. The best approach for the examiner is to acknowledge to the patient that a thorough examination of his or her eyes suggests that he or she is healthy. In particular, emphasis can be placed on statements that the patient is likely to agree with, such as the peripheral vision seems good, and the optic nerves appear healthy. The examiner can continue along these lines by saying that there is no evidence of serious neurologic illness such as a brain tumor, stroke, or multiple sclerosis. Finally, the examiner can state that he or she has seen similar patients who often improve with time as the "brain" once again realizes the visual potential of the eye.

Specific interventions have been reported to "improve" vision in patients with functional visual loss. These include the use of various drops, low-power spectacle prescription, contact lenses, and "retinal rest." Retinal rest[24] was a treatment used by physicians in the military after a diagnosis of a strained or tired retina was made. The patient's eyes were patched, the eyes covered, and the patient isolated from all auditory stimuli with minimal contact with others. Vision was checked everyday and usually improved spontaneously. Outside of a military structure, it seems unlikely that this strategy could be applied. However, for some highly suggestible patients this treatment option seems ideal. Hypnosis and psychoanalysis have also been reported to be successful treatments of functional visual loss.[57–59] In Kathol et al's series,[60] 22 of the 42 patients had a diagnosable psychiatric condition or personality disorder. In contrast, in our experience (given the high prevalence of deliberate malingerers) and that of others,[6, 8, 13] the vast majority of patients neither require nor benefit from psychiatric intervention.

Fortunately, many patients with functional visual loss do not continue to revisit the physician demanding an explanation or pleading for help. Kathol et al[13] found that most of the patients that were seen in follow-up were less bothered by their "vision loss" although they continued to demonstrate nonphysiologic responses on testing. Sletteberg et al[1] found that half of their patients had spontaneous resolution, but 22% of their patients were still "disabled" because of their vision loss.

Patients who indeed have organic visual deficits but have superimposed nonphysiologic vision loss are often the most problematic. In such patients it can be very difficult to determine the exact amount of organic vision loss, making diagnostic and therapeutic decisions very difficult. There are no easy guidelines to help manage such patients. This may be the one time when discussion with the patient about concerns about his or her nonphysiologic responses is worthwhile (particularly for the "worried impostor," see Table 11–1). Explaining to the patient that avoiding a risky treatment or intervention might result in improvement of the nonorganic component of the vision loss.

Management of Functional Visual Loss in Children. As with adults, the most productive interaction between the child with functional visual loss and the examiner occurs when the latter demonstrates empathetic, optimistic, and encouraging behavior. Once the diagnosis of functional visual loss without organicity in child has been made, we often speak to the parents without the child present. We explain that we cannot find anything wrong with the child's eyes or visual pathways. We tell them that we believe the child is not "making this up," but rather may have the visual problem as a result of some external trigger or stress. We emphasize to the parents that they should optimistically encourage their child, rather than accuse the child of dragging them to unnecessary doctor's visits and tests. Then we talk to the child in front of the parents, and explain to the child in an encouraging manner that we believe his or her vision will improve over the next few weeks. We schedule a follow-up visit in approximately 3 months, and suggest to the child the vision will likely improve by then.

In general, the prognosis for "visual recovery" in children with functional visual loss is excellent. In Mantyjarvi's series of children,[16] one third improved spontaneously. Catalano et al[14] found that one third of their patients were better within 1 day, and three quarters were better by 2 months.

REFERENCES

1. Sletteberg O, Bertelsen T, Hovding G: The prognosis of patients with hysterical visual impairment. Acta Ophthalmol 1989;67:159–163.
2. Rowland WD, Rowe AW: Marked concentric contraction of the visual fields: a study of 100 consecutive cases. Trans Am Acad Ophthalmol 1929;34:107–114.
3. Schaegel TF, Jr, Quilala FV: Hysterical amblyopia. Statistical analysis of forty-two cases found in a survey of eight hundred unselected eye patients at a state medical center. Arch Ophthalmol 1955;54:875–884.
4. Yasuna ER: Hysterical amblyopia. Its differentiation from malingering. Am J Ophthalmol 1946;29:570–578.
5. Asher R: Munchausen's syndrome. Lancet 1951;1: 339–341.
6. Thompson HS: Functional visual loss. Am J Ophthalmol 1985;100:209–213.
7. Weller M, Wiedemann P: Hysterical symptoms in ophthalmology. Doc Ophthalmol 1989;73:1–33.
8. Rada RT, Meyer GG, Kellner R: Visual conversion reaction in children and adults. J Nerv Ment Dis 1978; 166:580–587.
9. Keltner JL, May WN, Johnson CA, et al: The California syndrome: Functional visual complaints with potential economic impact. Ophthalmology 1985;92:427–435.
10. Drinnan MJ, Marmor MF: Functional vision loss in Cambodin refugees: a study of cultural factors in ophthalmology. Eur J Ophthalmol 1991;1:115–118.
11. Stephens JH, Kamp M: On some aspects of hysteria: A clinical study. J Nerv Ment Dis 1962;134:305–315.
12. Ziegler FJ, Imboden JM, Meyer E: Contemporary conversion reactions: A clinical study. Am J Psychiatry 1960;116:901–909.
13. Kathol RG, Cox TA, Corbett JJ, et al: Functional visual loss. Follow-up of 42 cases. Arch Ophthalmol 1983; 101:729–735.
14. Catalano RA, Simon JA, Krohel GB, et al: Functional visual loss in children. Ophthalmology 1986;93:385–390.
15. Clarke WN, Noel L-P, Bariciak M: Functional visual loss in children: A common problem with an easy solution. Can J Ophthalmol 1996;31:311–313.
16. Mantyjarvi MI: The amblyopic schoolgirl syndrome. J Pediatr Ophthalmol Strabismus 1981;18:30–33.
17. Rada RT, Krill AE, Meyer GG, et al: Visual conversion reaction in children. II. Follow up. Psychosomatics 1973;14:271–276.
18. Keltner JL: The California syndrome: A threat to all. Arch Ophthalmol 1988;106:1053–1054.
19. Newman NJ: Neuro-ophthalmology and psychiatry. Gen Hosp Psychiatry 1993;15:102–114.
20. Barris MC, Kaufman DI, Barbiero D: Visual impairment in hysteria. Doc Ophthalmol 1992;82:369–382.
21. Kathol RG, Cox TA, Corbett JJ, et al: Functional visual loss. I. A true psychiatric disorder? Psychol Med 1983;13:307–314.
22. Miller NR, Keane JR: Neuro-ophthalmologic manifestations of nonorganic disease. In: Miller NR, Newman NJ (eds): Walsh and Hoyt's Clinical Neuro-ophthalmology, 5th edition, pp 1765–1786. Baltimore, Williams & Wilkins, 1998.
23. Gruber H: Decrease of visual acuity in patients with clear media and normal fundi: Objective screening methods for differentiation and documentation. Doc Ophthalmol 1984;56:327–335.
24. Kramer KK, La Piana F, Appleton B: Ocular malingering and hysteria: Diagnosis and management. Surv Ophthalmol 1979;24:89–96.
25. Wildberger H: Contrast evoked potentials in the evaluation of the suspected malingering. Doc Ophthalmol 1981;27:425–430.
26. Steele M, Seiple WH, Carr RE, et al: The clinical utility of visual-evoked potential acuity testing. Am J Ophthalmol 1989;108:572–577.
27. Towle VL, Sutcliffe E, Sokol S: Diagnosing functional visual deficits with the P300 component of the visual evoked potential. Arch Ophthalmol 1985;103:47–50.

28. Uren SM, Stewart P, Crosby PA: Subject cooperation and the visual evoked response. Invest Ophthalmol Vis Sci 1979;18:648–652.
29. Morgan RK, Nugent B, Harrison JM, et al: Voluntary alteration of pattern visual evoked responses. Ophthalmology 1985;92:1356–1363.
30. Bumgartner J, Epstein CM: Voluntary alteration of visual evoked potentials. Ann Neurol 1982;12:475–480.
31. Hess CW, Meienberg O, Ludin HP: Visual evoked potentials in acute occipital blindness. J Neurol 1982; 227:193–200.
32. Levy NS, Glick EB: Stereoscopic perception and Snellen visual acuity. Am J Ophthalmol 1974;78:722–724.
33. Savir H, Segal M: A simple test for detection of monocular functional visual impairment. Am J Ophthalmol 1988;106:500.
34. Fahle M, Mohn G: Assessment of visual function in suspected ocular malingering. Br J Ophthalmol 1989; 73:651–654.
35. Slavin ML: The prism dissociation test in detecting unilateral functional visual loss. J Clin Neuro-ophthalmol 1990;10:127–130.
36. Linhart WO: Field findings in functional disease. Am J Ophthalmol 1956;42:75–84.
37. Levi L, Feldman RM: Use of the potential acuity meter in suspected functional visual loss. Am J Ophthalmol 1992;114:502–503.
38. Stewart JFG: Automated perimetry and malingerers: Can the Humphrey be outwitted? Ophthalmology 1995;102:27–32.
39. Keane JR: Hysterical hemianopia: The missing half field defect. Arch Ophthalmol 1979;97:865–866.
40. Ellenberger CJ: Tunnel vision. Neurology 1984;34:129.
41. Gittinger JW, Jr: Functional monocular temporal hemianopsia. Am J Ophthalmol 1986;101:226–231.
42. Smith TJ, Baker RS: Perimetric findings in functional disorders using automated techniques. Ophthalmology 1987;94:1562–1566.
43. Glovinsky Y, Quigley HA, Bissett RA, et al: Artificially produced quadrantanopsia in computed visual field testing. Am J Ophthalmol 1990;110:90–91.
44. Fish RH, Kline LB, Hanumanthu VK, et al: Hysterical bitemporal hemianopia "cured" with contact lenses. J Clin Neuro-ophthalmol 1990;10:76–78.
45. Macleod JD, Manners RM, Heaven CJ, et al: Visual field defects: How easily can they be fabricated using the automated perimeter? Neuro-ophthalmology 1994;14:185–188.
46. Thompson JC, Komorsky GS, Ellis BD: Field of dreamers and dreamed-up fields: Functional and fake perimetry. Ophthalmology 1996;103:117–125.
47. Johnson LN, Hill RA, Bartholomew MJ: Correlation of afferent pupillary defect with visual field loss on automated perimetry. Ophthalmology 1988;95:1649–1655.
48. Mills RP, Glaser JS: Hysterical bitemporal hemianopia. Arch Ophthalmol 1981;99:2053.
49. Gittinger JW, Jr: Functional hemianopsia: A historical perspective. Surv Ophthalmol 1988;32:427–432.
50. Keane JR: Patterns of hysterical hemianopia. Neurology 1998;51:1230–1231.
51. Martin TJ: Threshold perimetry of each eye with both eyes open in patients with monocular functional (nonorganic) and organic visual loss. Am J Ophthalmol 1998;125:857–864.
52. Slavin ML: The use of red Amsler grid and red-green lenses in detecting spurious paracentral visual field defects. Am J Ophthalmol 1987;103:338–339.
53. Keane JR: Neuro-ophthalmic signs and symptoms of hysteria. Neurology 1982;32:757–762.
54. Keane JR: Convergence spasm. Neurology 1983;33: 1637.
55. Shults WT, Stark L, Hoyt WF, et al: Normal saccadic structure of voluntary nystagmus. Arch Ophthalmol 1977;95:1399–1404.
56. Moster ML, Galetta SL, Schatz NJ: Physiologic functional imaging in "functional" visual loss. Surv Ophthalmol 1996;40:395–399.
57. Greenleaf E: The red house: hypnotherapy of hysterical blindness. Am J Clin Hypnosis 1971;13: 155–161.
58. Ames TH: Analysis of blindness as a symptom of hysteria. Arch Ophthalmol 1914;43:357–367.
59. Wilkins LG, Field PB: Helpless under attack: hypnotic abreaction in hysterical loss of vision. Am J Clin Hypnosis 1968;10:271–275.
60. Kathol RG, Cox TA, Corbett JJ, et al: Functional visual loss. II. Psychiatric aspects in 42 patients followed for 4 years. Psychol Med 1983;13:315–324.

CHAPTER 12

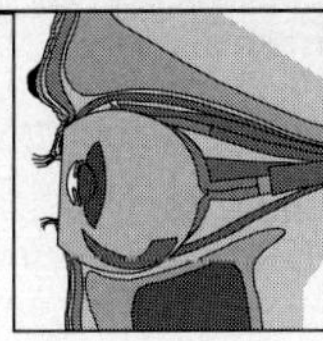

Visual Hallucinations and Illusions

Visual hallucinations and illusions comprise some of the most vivid and sometimes bizarre symptoms in neuro-ophthalmology. *Hallucinations* are defined as perceptions that occur in the absence of a corresponding external sensory stimulus.[1] Visual hallucinations can be classified as unformed/simple (eg, dots, flashes, zig-zags) or formed/complex (actual objects or people). In contrast, *illusions* are misinterpretations of a true sensory stimulus.[2] Visual hallucinations and illusions are generally positive phenomena, in contrast to visual loss, which is a negative phenomenon.

The causes of visual hallucinations and illusions can grouped into several major categories: migraine, release phenomena (in the setting of impaired vision), entopic phenomena, alcohol and drugs, seizures, central nervous system lesions, psychiatric disease, neurogenerative disease, and narcolepsy. These are summarized in Table 12–1, which also describes distinguishing features of each. This chapter will detail the various categories, but first theories on the pathogenesis of hallucinations and the history, examination, and diagnostic and therapeutic considerations in patients with hallucinations and illusions will be reviewed.

HALLUCINATIONS: THEORIES ON PATHOGENESIS

Hughlings Jackson proposed that the central nervous system is organized into three levels: the higher cortical level; the middle structures (eg, the basal ganglia), and the lowest level, of which the spinal cord is one part.[1] In this scheme, hallucinations were thought to occur when damage to the cortical level disinhibited activity of the middle level.

Subsequent authorities refined this notion that hallucinations can be release phenomena. West[3] theorized that in the normal waking state, the constant bombardment of external and internal stimuli inhibits the emergence of "previous perceptions." However, "impairment of information (sensory) input then permits the emergence or release of previously recorded percepts which can be woven into hallucinations." Cogan[4] presented patients with various ocular, optic nerve, chiasmal, tract, and occipital lesions who developed formed and complex visual sensations, and, like West, concluded that "a major factor in releasing the hallucinations is loss of the normally inhibiting visual control through blindness, hemianopia, or loss of cognitive functions." Similarly, in Fischer's "sensory/motor ratio" theory, an imbalance between internal and external sensory input is a necessary and sufficient condition for hallucinations.[5] ffytche and Howard[138] suggested that the quality of the release hallucinations are often reflective of dysfunction (and sometimes normal function) of striate and extrastriate cortex. For instance, color hallucinations may originate from area V4.

All hallucinations are not necessarily release phenomena, however. Clearly, some are due to abnormal biochemical states in the setting of alcohol, drugs, hallucinogens, or metabolic disturbances.[6] Dysfunction of the centrally acting neurotransmitters norepinephrine, dopa-

TABLE 12–1. Major causes of Visual Hallucinations and Illusions and Their Distinguishing Features and Clinical Setting

Cause	Distinguishing Feature(s) of Visual Hallucinations or Illusions	Clinical Setting
Migraine	Fortification spectra Scintillating scotomas Develops and migrates over minutes Persistent positive visual phenomena	Headache Personal or family history of migraine
Release phenomena Variable over time	Continuous	Visual loss
Entopic phenomena	Phosphenes	Vitreoretinal traction Observation of normal phenomena
Alcohol and drugs	Colors Small insects or animals "Flashbacks"	Accompanying auditory or tactile hallucinations History of substance abuse
Seizures	Stereotyped Brief	Other motor or sensory manifestations of seizures Abnormal EEG
Neurodegenerative		Clinical evidence of Parkinson's or Alzheimer's disease
Focal neurologic lesions		
Peduncular hallucinations		Other evidence of a midbrain lesion
Palinopsia		Other evidence of an occipital lobe lesion
Cerebral diplopia and polyopia		Other evidence of an occipital lobe lesion
Upside down vision		Other evidence of a vestibular lesion
Psychiatric		Auditory hallucinations Delusions History of psychiatric disease
Narcolepsy		Sleep attacks Daytime somnulence

mine, and serotonin has been implicated in the pathogenesis of visual hallucinations.[6] In Marrazzi's "neurophysiological dissociation" theory, it is proposed that hallucinogenic drugs have their effect by producing a functional dissociation between primary sensory cortex and cortical association areas.[5]

Other mechanisms include irritation of cortical neurons, as in epilepsy, and cognitive deficits, which can cause confusion between real stimuli and imagination.[2] Visual hallucinations related to migraine may result from cortical ischemia or neuronal depression, without frank visual loss. Entopic visual phenomena are images produced by the structures of the eye. Brain stem lesions causing visual hallucinations may affect ascending cholinergic and serotonergic pathways, resulting in associated sleep disturbances.[7] In the psychodynamic approach, hallucinations are thought to be similar to dreams, and Freud thought impairment of the ego allowed unconscious or preconscious material to enter consciousness and be misinterpreted as an external stimulus.[1,2]

HISTORY AND EXAMINATION IN PATIENTS WITH VISUAL HALLUCINATIONS OR ILLUSIONS

The history is paramount in these patients because the diagnosis is frequently made based on the clinical setting and the detailed description of the visual symptoms. All too often the examination is unrevealing. The patient should be asked to detail the hallucinations or illusions, with particular attention to their content, complexity, and static or dynamic features. It is always helpful to have him or her draw what is perceived. One can ask whether the visual symptoms are monocular or binocular, but usually the patient has never checked or cannot determine this. In addition, their frequency, duration, and repetitiveness should be established.

Accompanying neurologic symptoms also can be very helpful in the diagnosis. For instance, a visual hallucination followed by a headache suggests migraine, while one followed by limb twitching and then loss of consciousness is suspicious of a seizure. The patient should be asked whether he or she knows if the perception is a hallucination or not. Insight is characteristic of release visual hallucinations (see below), for instance, while a schizophrenic with psychotic hallucinations might not be able to differentiate the hallucination from reality. Investigation into predisposing underlying conditions, such as metabolic disturbances, visual loss, psychiatric illnesses, alcohol intake, and drug use (illicit, recreational, or otherwise), is also extremely important.

The neuro-ophthalmic examination of a patient with visual hallucinations or illusions is directed toward excluding afferent pathway disease or another responsible lesion of the nervous system. Particular attention should be paid to visual acuity, color vision, pupillary reactivity, and the funduscopic examination. Even mild visual loss in the setting of macular degeneration or optic atrophy can be associated with release hallucinations, and these may be missed without a careful examination. We also prefer to perform formal visual field testing in almost every patient with a visual hallucination or illusion to exclude a field deficit. The neurologic examination, for example, should exclude an altered sensorium due a mass lesion or toxic/metabolic disturbance; a hemiparesis or hemisensory loss suggestive of a hemispheric mass lesion; ataxia, third nerve palsy, or vertical gaze paresis consistent with a mesencephalic process (see peduncular hallucinations, below); nystagmus and imbalance associated with a brain stem or vestibular lesion; and evidence of Parkinson's or Alzheimer's disease.

DIAGNOSTIC AND TREATMENT CONSIDERATIONS (OVERVIEW)

Diagnosis

In one approach to the patient with visual hallucinations and illusions, the general categories (Table 12–1) should be considered first. Then, the patient's description of the visual phenomena is often very suggestive a particular cause. Finally, the history and examination give the clinical setting and frequently supply clues to establish the proper diagnosis. For example, in a patient with a normal examination, a crescent of pulsating zig-zag lines seen in visual periphery, followed by a headache with nausea and vomiting, is most likely the result of a migraine. Brief episodes of flashing lights followed by loss of consciousness are more consistent with epilepsy. An individual who complains of seeing people or objects that are not there may suffer sensory deprivation associated with bilateral visual loss. This patient most likely has release hallucinations.

Treatment Overview

In hallucinations due to migraine or epilepsy, the treatment is directed at the underlying disorder. In psychiatric and neurodegenerative disorders, treatment of the primary disorder is also important, but the addition of a neuroleptic is often required in these two conditions. In general, hallucinations associated with illicit or prescription drug use should be treated by removing the offending agent. In contrast, release visual hallucinations are very difficult to treat. Sometimes affected patients require low-dose neuroleptics, but often patient reassurance is the best management.

MIGRAINE

A variety of visual hallucinations are characteristic of migraine.[8] These include enlarging scintillating scotomas and fortification spectra, or stars, sparks, flashes, or simple geometric forms.[9] Visual illusions, experienced less commonly by migraineurs than hallucinations, include palinopsia (persistence of visual images), polyopia (multiple images), micropsia (shrunken images), macropsia (enlarged images), metamorphopsia (distortion of shape), and Alice-in-Wonderland syndrome (disortion of bodily image).[10, 11] These are summarized in Table 12–2.

The visual hallucinations and illusions associated with migraine are typically part of the aura. The International Headache Society defines a typical aura as one that develops over more than 4 minutes, lasts less than 1 hour, and precedes or rarely accompanies or follows the headache.[12] Usually the migraine headache occurs contralateral to the hemifield containing the visual aura.[13] A "prolonged aura" lasts more than 60 minutes but no longer than 7 days.[12] When auras are of longer duration, or when an infarction is demonstrated radiographically, a diagnosis of "migrainous infarction" is satisfied.[12] Migraine with aura was previously termed *classic migraine*.

TABLE 12–2. Hallucinations, Illusions, and Distortions Associated With Migraine

Hallucinations
Complex
Dots
Fortification spectra
Halos
Heat waves
Lights
Lines
Prisms
Scintillating scotomas
Shapes (geometric)
Sparkles
Squiggles
Illusions/Distortions
Alice in Wonderland syndrome
Macropsia
Metamorphopsia
Micropsia
Palinopsia
Polyopia

Although some published studies demonstrate that visual auras occur at relatively similar frequencies in adults and children with migraine, that is not the uniform experience. Between 33% and 53% of adults with migraine have visual symptoms.[14, 15] In two studies in children with migraine, visual auras were experienced by 31%[16] and 41%.[10] However, in a study by Kinast et al[17] only 15% had auras, but whether the symptoms were visual, sensory, or motor was not specified. It is also our impression and that of some experienced pediatric neurologists[18, 19] that a visual aura is relatively uncommon in children with migraine. Although it is possible that younger children are unable to appreciate or describe a visual aura, even the most articulate pediatric patients usually deny any visual phenomena. We have found migraine without aura to be much more common in children, and that few pediatric patients, including adolescents, have visual symptoms.

Traditional theories proposed that vasoconstriction-induced cortical ischemia caused migraine aura, and recent experiments measuring regional cerebral blood flow and volume have confirmed decreased regional cerebral blood flow during the aura phase.[20, 21] More recent theories, however, attribute the hypoperfusion to the decreased metabolic demand of cortical neurons resulting from uncharacterized neuronal and biochemical triggers (trigeminovascular theory).[13] The pathophysiology of migraine and aura is discussed in more detail in Chapter 19.

The remainder of this section will first detail the various visual hallucinations and illusions associated with migraine. For the most part, the hallucinations and illusions in migraine are positive visual phenomena. Negative visual phenomena associated with migraine, such as transient monocular blindness or hemifield loss, are detailed in Chapter 10. The treatment of migraine is discussed in Chapter 19.

Fortification Spectra and Scintillating Scotomas

A visual aura consisting of fortification spectra or a scintillating scotoma, followed by a headache, is almost pathognomonic of migraine.[13] The *fortification spectra* phenomenon, the most common visual aura, is characterized by an arc of jagged, serrated, or zig-zag lines (Fig. 12–1).[22] Patients often relate that the lines, also termed *teichopsia,* shimmer, scintillate, vibrate, flicker, or pulse at 3 to 30 Hz.[23] The term *fortification* refers to the similarity of the visual phenomena with early European military fortifications.[8] The term *spectra* is used because many patients will describe colored jagged edges. The shimmering aspect gives the appearance of light reflecting off of small prisms and produces the various colors of a rainbow.

In addition to the typical appearance, the "buildup" or "march" of the fortification spectra is also highly characteristic (Fig. 12–2). Patients usually notice the visual phenomenon

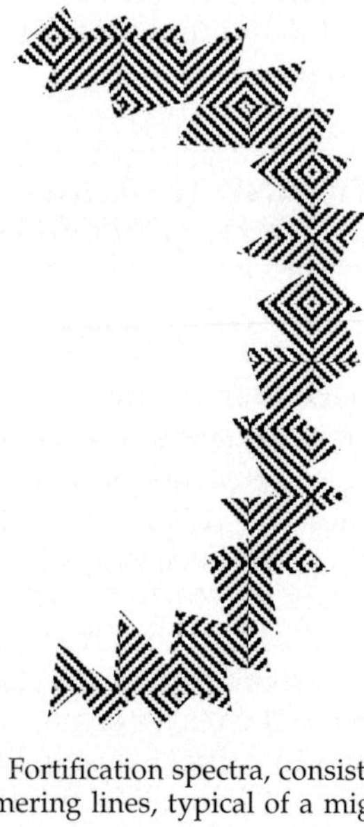

FIGURE 12–1. Fortification spectra, consisting of an arc of jagged, shimmering lines, typical of a migraine aura.

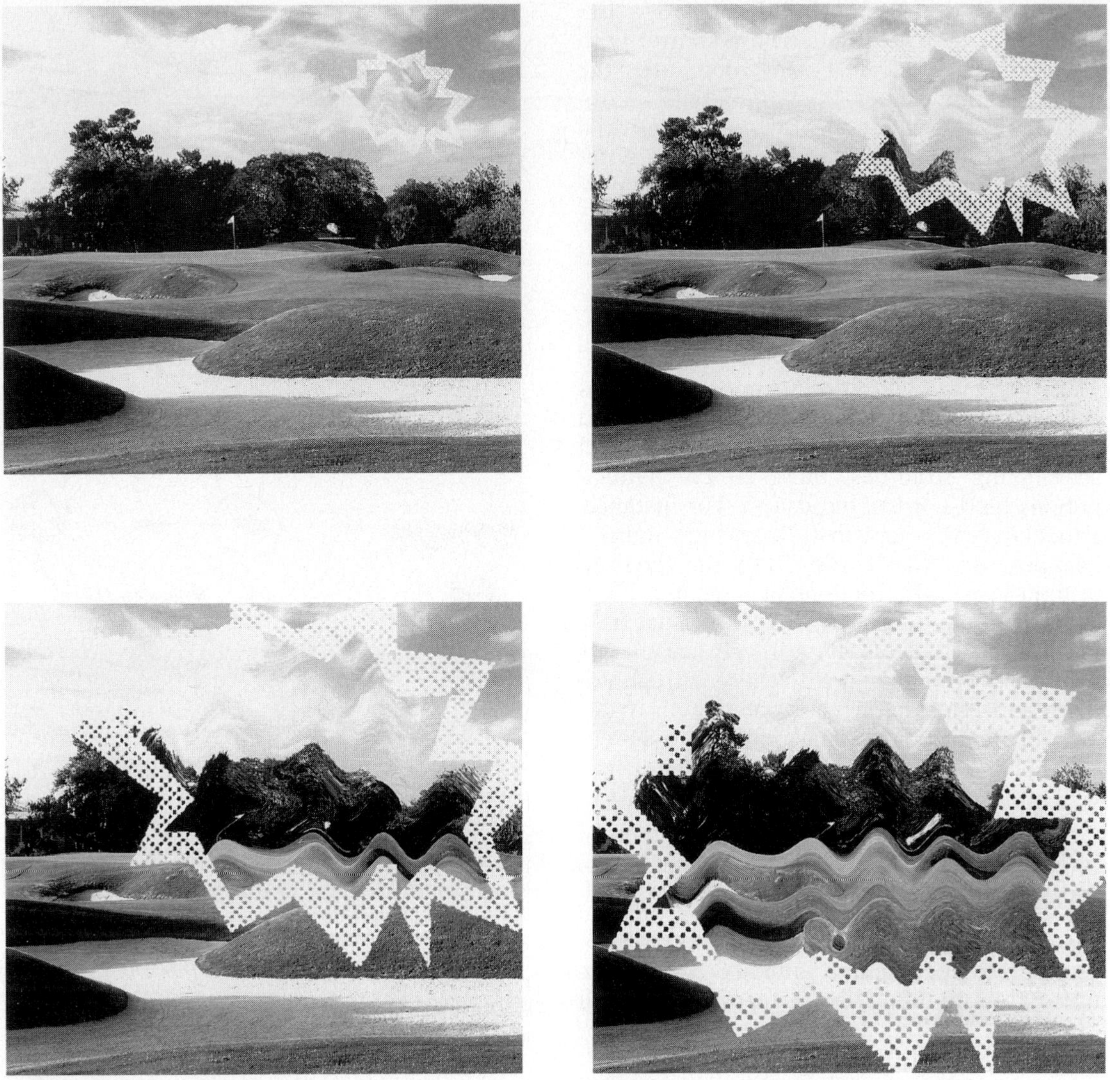

FIGURE 12–2. Characteristic buildup of a migrainous scintillating scotoma experienced by one of the authors. **Top left**. A small pulsating object was seen in the upper right quadrant of both eyes. **Top right**. The object gradually enlarged to consume the homonymous quadrant, and the border of it consisted of small, colored, shimmering prisms. Within the center, the vision was blurry (as if looking through water), but not absent. **Bottom left**. The area gradually enlarged, and crossed the midline. **Bottom right**. The visual disturbance consumed the entire visual field. Eventually it disintegrated at its borders and within the blurry center. Its resolution was followed by a holocephalic headache accompanied by nausea.

paracentrally, and the open part of the arc of the fortification spectra faces centrally. Often vision within the arc is scotomatous or defective, and patients will describe this area as grey, cloudy, or blurry. The combination of the positive fortification spectra on the outside and the negative area in the middle is termed a *scintillating scotoma*. These are often circular, but may also be kidney-bean shaped. Over minutes, the diameter of the arc enlarges, and drifts toward the periphery, and the scotoma, when present, also enlarges. Often the entire visual field is affected, as the fortification spectra or scintillating scotoma frequently crosses the vertical and horizontal meridians. The entire sequence may take 15 to 20 minutes, after which the fortification spectra or scintillating scotoma breaks up and disappears. The phenomenon is usually homonymous but also can be monocular. However, often it is difficult for even the best observers to describe whether the phenomenon is perceived in one or both eyes.

Although highly suggestive of migraine, fortification spectra and scintillating scotomas may also be triggered by seizure foci such as arteriovascular malformations (AVMs) or neoplasms. However, the "buildup" is less frequent and the hallucinations are shorter with irritative mass lesions. Furthermore, after the hallucination resolves, the patient with an underlying mass lesion will often have a residual visual field defect. Rarely, scintillations without "buildup" also can be associated with posterior cerebral artery ischemia.[8]

Simple Positive Visual Phenomena in Migraine

Many patients with migraine report seeing less complex phenomena, some of which are listed in Table 12–2. Unlike fortification spectra and scintillating scotomas, these simple hallucinations tend not to "build up." For instance, patients may describe "dancing lights," "shapes," or a "flash bulb."[8] In some, the flash of light lasts only fractions of a second; however, they may migrate across the visual field (Fig. 12–3). Patients with these complaints should not be confused with those with photopsias and phosphenes associated with disorders of the anterior visual pathway (see entopic phenomena, below).

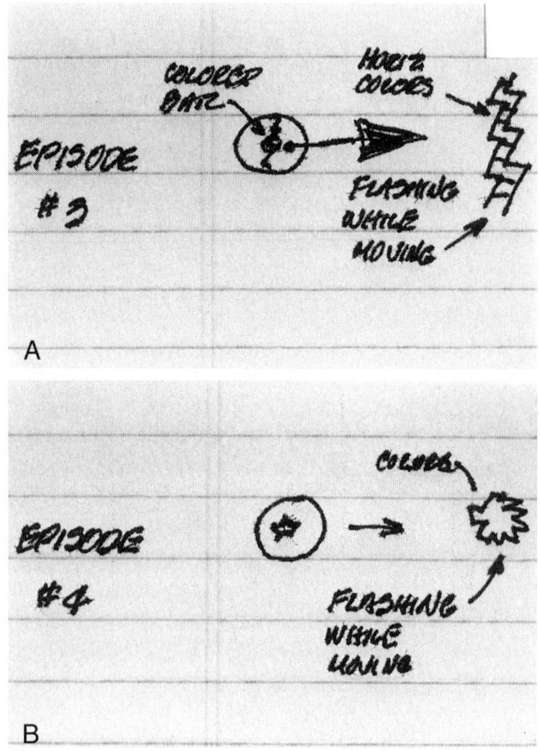

FIGURE 12–3. Migration of a characteristic simple visual phenomena drawn and described by a migraineur. He wrote that in one episode (**A**), "a colored bar appeared at the center of the eye and began flashing and flickering, then moved from the center of the eye to the left. This lasted about 10 minutes. After the bar reached the side of the eye, it took the shape of an arc and continued to flicker for about 10 minutes." In another episode (**B**), "when looking down on the floor, eight-pointed colorful starlike figures appeared (one at a time), flickering and bright. One of the starlike figures (depicted in drawing), appeared at the center of the eye and worked itself toward the left outside of the eye, blinking and flickering as it moved."

Complex Visual Hallucinations in Migraine

Visual hallucinations containing complex objects such as people and animals (*zoopsia*) are unusual in migraine visual aura, but are well described. Hachinski et al[10] described an 18-year-old girl with migraine who saw herself lying on a railroad track while a train passed over her. In her left visual field she experienced irregular multicolored scotomas. The visual hallucinations lasted 10 minutes and the accompanying migraine headache lasted 3 hours.

When complex visual hallucinations occur in migraine, they are usually unaccompanied by auditory and abnormal thought content[13]; however, Fuller et al[24] reported an exceptional 69-year-old man with migraine and complex visual and auditory hallucinations as well as paranoid delusions. He felt his wife and brother-in-law had been killed, and the "ward staff were systematically butchering other patients on the ward." He saw "red and squirmy piranha fish on the floor of his room and would try to stamp on them, after which they would disappear." This history would be more suggestive of a psychiatric disorder or drug use, and migraine would have to be a diagnosis of exclusion.

A unique patient with migraine auras characterized by complete *achromatopsia* (no perception of color), *prosopagnosia* (inability to recognize faces), and *visual agnosia* (inability to recognize objects) has also been described.[25] These higher cortical visual disorders are discussed in Chapter 9.

Visual Distortions and Illusions in Migraine

Metamorphopsia. Distortion of the shapes of objects may be experienced by patients with migraine (objects may appear too fat, too thin, too short, or too tall, for instance); however, metamorphopsia is a much more common complaint among patients with macular disease.

Micropsia/Macropsia. In a variation of metamorphopsia, patients with migraine may complain that objects appear too small (*micropsia*) or too large (*macropsia*). We have seen a patient who described one episode in which a telephone, which was located across the room, appeared as if it were right next to her because is looked much larger than normal. In *teleopsia,* objects seem too far away. People may appear too small in *lilliputianism*. These symptoms can also be caused by seizures.

Alice in Wonderland Syndrome. Lippman[26] described seven patients with classic migraine who experienced episodes of distorted body image. Each had fascinating hallucinations characterized by enlargement, diminution, or distortion of part of or the whole body, and each patient knew the sensations were not real. One 38-year-old woman reported attacks of feeling "about 1 foot high" accompanied by headache. Another elderly woman complained of migraine headaches preceded by the feeling of her left ear "ballooning out 6 inches or more." His Patient 7 reported headaches accompanied by "experiences," in which half his body changed size. He told Lippman he felt "as if someone had drawn a vertical line separating the two halves; the right half seems to be twice the size of the left half," and he wondered how he was going to get his hat on when one side of his head was so much bigger than the other. The patient also reported that "after a few minutes of feeling large, the right half seems to shrink until it is smaller than the left," and felt the process had been coming and going all day long.

Subsequently, other similar patients have been described,[27] and many reports emphasize the syndrome's occurrence in children with migraine.[10, 28] Hachinski et al[10] described a 6-year-old child who thought people around her were smaller than normal. Once, while playing in the snow, this same child felt that she was "unusually large" and that an ordinary snowball had become "huge and turned blue."

Lippman[26] recalled that Lewis Carroll (Charles Lutwidge Dodgson), also a migraineur, had described similar hallucinations in his book, *Alice in Wonderland*. It has been speculated that Dodgson had experienced distortions in body image during his migraine events, and incorporated the hallucinations into the fictional story about the young girl who, during her adventures in Wonderland, shrinks and grows numerous times. Rolak[11] has pointed out the similarity between original illustrations in Dodgson's book (Figs. 12–4 and 12–5) and some of the descriptions catalogued by Lippman.[26]

Metamorphopsia, micropsia/macropsia, and Alice in Wonderland syndrome are supposedly more common in children than in adults.[13] Although this has also been our experience, nevertheless, we have found these symptoms tend to be relatively uncommon in all age groups. The cause of these atypical hallucinations has been attributed to migrainous ischemia involving the nondominant posterior parietal lobule.[11] Ischemia of the anterior occipital and posterior temporal lobes has also been considered, but is thought to be less likely.[11] Almost all cases of Alice in Wonderland syndrome have been associated with migraine, but three affected children with encephalopathy due to infectious mononucleosis have been reported.[29]

Other Distortions and Illusions. Migraine may also produce the perception of multiple images, and should be included in the differential diagnosis of cerebral diplopia.[30] Kosmorsky,[31] in a report of his own acephalgic migraine, described the duplication of images within a scintillating scotoma. The double vision was present with either eye covered, and did not change with either monocular or binocular viewing. Migraineurs may also complain of *palinopsia* (see below), the persistence of visual images. However, palinopsia is more characteristically a symptom of parieto-occipital lobe damage.

Persistent Positive Visual Phenomena

Patients with migraine rarely may have symptoms consistent with persistent visual aura. Ten patients with migraine who developed persistent positive visual phenomena lasting months to years have been reported.[32] None had major psychiatric disease. The visual complaints were similar in their simplicity and involvement of the entire visual field and usually consisted of diffuse small particles such as TV static, snow, lines of ants, dots, and rain (Table 12–3 and Fig. 12–6). Some patients reported greater awareness of the visual phenomena when looking at the sky or at a light-colored wall. Complex phenomena such as

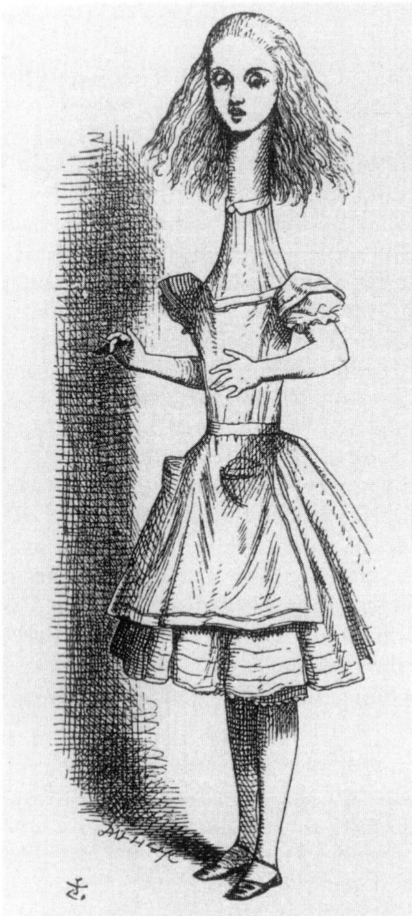

FIGURE 12–4. This original illustration from Lewis Carroll's "Alice in Wonderland" matches the descriptions of two of Lippmann's[26] patients who experienced distortions in body image, in particular, excessive height. Patient 3, a 23-old woman, described the following: "I experienced the sensation that my head had grown to tremendous proportions and was so light that it floated up to the ceiling, although I was sure it was still attached to my neck. I used to try to hold it down with my hands. This sensation would pass with the migraine but would leave me with a feeling that I was very tall. When walking down the street I would think I would be able to look down on the tops of others' heads, and it was very frightening and annoying not to see as I was feeling. The sensation was so real that when I would see myself in a window or full-length mirror, it was quite a shock to realize that I was still my normal height of under five feet." Patient 6 said "I get tired out from pulling my head down from the ceiling. My head feels like a balloon; my neck stretches and my head goes to the ceiling. I've been pulling it down all night long." (Illustration borrowed with permission from Dover Publications, Mineola, NY.)

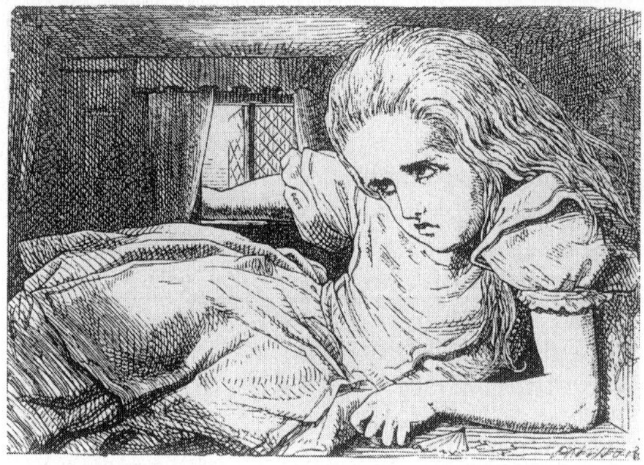

FIGURE 12–5. This original illustration from Lewis Carroll's "Alice in Wonderland" matches the descriptions of one of Lippmann's[26] patients who experienced distortions in body image, in particular, excessive height. (Illustration borrowed with permission from Dover Publications, Mineola, NY.)

palinopsia, micropsia, and formed hallucinations were exceptional. Some characterized these unformed visual hallucinations as bothersome, uncomfortable, or emotionally disabling, but not interfering with visual function. Other patients were unconcerned by them. Neurologic and ophthalmologic examinations were normal in all patients, and electroencephalograms were normal in eight of eight patients tested. Magnetic resonance imaging (MRI) was normal without evidence of infarc-

TABLE 12–3. Persistent Positive Visual Phenomena in Migraine

Simple, Unformed
A million dots
Black cracks and lines
Blobs of white and gray
Blue squares
Bubbles
Carpet background
Circles
Clouds
Comets
Dots
Black and white
Colored
Grainy vision
Heat waves
Lights
Flashing
Flickering
Lines of ants
Photopsias
Rainlike pattern
Snow
Squiggles
TV static
Complex
Micropsia
Palinopsia
People's heads

(From Liu GT et al: Neurology 1995;45:664–668, with permission.)

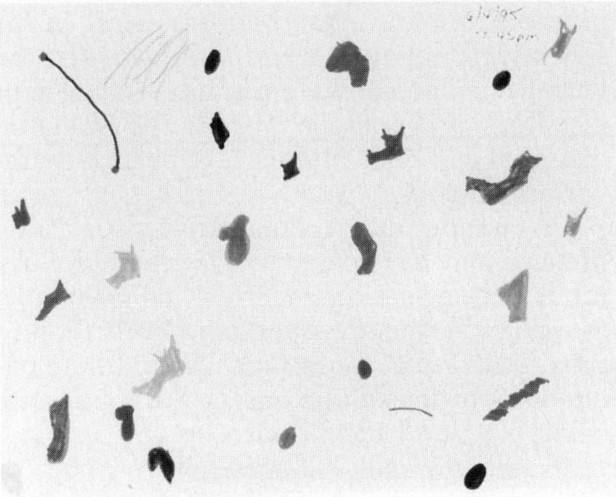

FIGURE 12–6. A young girl's depiction of persistent positive visual phenomena associated with her migraine.

tion in all patients except one who had nonspecific biparietal white matter lesions and another with a small venous angioma. In this series, medications such as tricyclic agents, calcium channel and beta blockers, and analgesics were unhelpful.

Three patients with migraine and hemifield persistent visual symptoms have been described. Haas[33] reported two individuals with "prolonged migraine aura status"; the first was a 70-year-old man with a long-standing history of migraine headaches who developed a constant "pinwheel of bright whirling color, mainly yellow and red" in the left homonymous hemifield accompanied by left hand paresthesias and clumsiness. The episode lasted 5 weeks, and resolved with aspirin and cyproheptadine. The second patient was an 18-year-old boy with a history of migraine with aura who experienced 7 months of "concentric gray circles like ripples in a pond" and "clustered sets of concentric circles in the right visual field," unaccompanied by headache. Both patients had normal neurologic and ophthalmologic examinations, but only the first had computed tomography of the brain and encephalography (EEG), both of which were normal. Luda et al[34] reported a 65-year-old woman with "sustained visual aura" who had a 50-year history of migraine with aura who then developed 12 months of "scintillating geometric figures (in the shape of either rings or chains)" in the right visual hemifield. Carbamazepine, diazepam, flunarizine, nimodipine, and citicoline were unhelpful. Examination, EEG, and brain MRI were normal.

Persistent positive visual phenomena may result from spontaneous cortical discharges. Alternatively, selective dysfunction of inhibitory and modulating neurons in extrastriate areas, due to subclinical ischemia, for example, may have allowed spontaneous discharges from the lateral geniculate or visual cortex, resulting in release visual hallucinations (see below), as suggested by West[3] and Cogan.[4]

While most migraine medications, anticonvulsants, and antidepressants are ineffective in the treatment of these persistent visual hallucinations, Rothrock[35] reported the successful management of two affected patients with divalproex sodium.

Acephalgic Migraine

In patients with *acephalgic migraine,* the aura is unaccompanied by headache. In Alvarez's study,[17] 12% of men and 0.7% of women had "scotomas without a headache." The diagnosis of acephalgic migraine is suggested by a previous history of migraine, the occurrence of a positive or negative visual phenomenon typical of migraine, and the absence of cerebrovascular causes for the event. Both visual hallucinations and illusions as well as transient monocular and binocular visual loss can occur.[36]

When acephalgic migraine is experienced by older adults, distinguishing the event from a transient ischemic attack may be very difficult.[37] Fisher[38] described a group of patients over 40 years of age who experienced visual symptoms initially thought to be transient ischemic attacks. However, 50% had headache, the visual symptoms were more consistent with migraine, and angiography was unrevealing. He emphasized that in adults with positive and negative visual phenomena seemingly consistent with a vascular event, migraine can be considered but must be a diagnosis of exclusion. The gradual buildup of the visual disturbance typically favors the diagnosis of migraine.

Acephalgic migraine in children is very unusual, occurring in only 14 of 710 (2%) migraineurs in one series.[39] In the subanalysis of this report, 5 of 14 had only visual auras, while the remaining 9 had mixed acephalgic migraine and migraine with aura. Thus, in this childhood series, acephalgic migraine without any history of headache was distinctly uncommon (5 of 710 (1%)).

The workup and treatment of acephalgic migraine are discussed in Chapter 19.

VISUAL LOSS (RELEASE HALLUCINATIONS AND THE CHARLES BONNET SYNDROME)

Cogan popularized the notion that visual hallucinations may be associated with loss of vision.[4] In his report entitled "Visual Hallucinations as Release Phenomena," he presented patients with blindness of varying degree and cause, including monocular blindness due to optic neuropathy, chiasmal visual loss affecting both eyes, and homonymous heminanopia due to retrochiasmal lesions. Each had formed or unformed visual hallucinations, typically within the defective area of vision. For instance, one woman with a right homonymous hemianopia complained of "zig-zag lines, colored triangles, and formed images suggesting that people and traffic were moving in on her from the right side." In general, the complexity of the hallucinations had no localizing value. When present, the hallucinations in his patients were usually continuous, variable, and more intense when the eyelids were closed (Table 12–4). He contrasted these from the episodic stereotyped visual hallucinations associated with seizure activity. Cogan suggested that interference of the normal visual input, from any lesion in the afferent visual pathway, might allow a "release of brain activity."

Lepore[40] studied 104 patients with retinal or neural afferent pathway disease, and found 57% reported spontaneous visual phenomena. Elementary disturbances such as photopsias and geometric forms, as well as complex ones such as people, animals, or vehicles were described. Like Cogan,[4] Lepore found their complexity did not correlate with lesion site. Furthermore, hallucinations occurred even in individuals with only minor amounts of visual loss. For example, spontaneous visual phenomena were described by three of Lepore's patients with pseudotumor cerebri, 20/20 vision, and only minimal enlargement of the physiologic blind spot. Many patients in his series were relieved when informed that the visual phenomena were common sequelae of visual loss and not reflective of any psychiatric disturbance. Other authors have provided similar accounts.[138]

TABLE 12–4. Characteristics of Release Visual Hallucinations

Formed or unformed
Within the defective area of vision
Complexity nonlocalizing
Usually continuous
Nonstereotyped
More intense when eyes closed

As described by Cogan.[4]

The notion that spontaneous visual phenomena may be released by a lack of inhibitory input may also explain visual hallucinations associated with severe sensory deprivation in prisoners of war, for instance. In addition, patients with dense, bilateral cataracts, despite being alert and lucid, may experience vivid, pleasurable visual hallucinations.[41] Many of the cataract-associated hallucinations seem to occur when the patient is not receiving external stimuli, such as in a quiet room or just before the patient goes to sleep. In further support of the sensory deprivation concept, the hallucinations often resolve following cataract extraction.

Release visual hallucinations rarely can occur in children as well. A 3 1/2-year-old boy with an optic pathway glioma became completely blind following tumor debulking surgery, and 1 week later reported he saw his brother, Santa Claus, and animals for 3 days.[42]

Patients may find these visual images pleasant or disturbing, and be embarassed to volunteer them to their physician. In some cases, however, the release hallucinations are the presenting symptom of new visual loss.[43, 44] We examined a 51-year-old woman who complained of seeing "a picture within a picture—like the new kind of television sets" in her lower left visual field (Fig. 12–7) as a presentation of a new incomplete left inferior quadrantanopia due to a right parieto-occipital infarction.[45] She described a rectangular scene with a red background filled with several people milling about, and it differed completely from what she saw in her larger intact field. Multiple broad horizontal lines swept upward over the scene, and the patient said this effect mimicked a television set with malfunctioning "vertical hold."

Various aspects of release hallucinations associated with homonymous hemianopias have been investigated. Kölmel[46] described patients who experienced simple hallucinations consisting of colored geometric phosphenes organized either vertically or horizontally in the hemianopic field, and their lesions were confined primarily to the occipital lobe. In contrast, a second group he reported[47] with complex hallucinations saw either static or moving

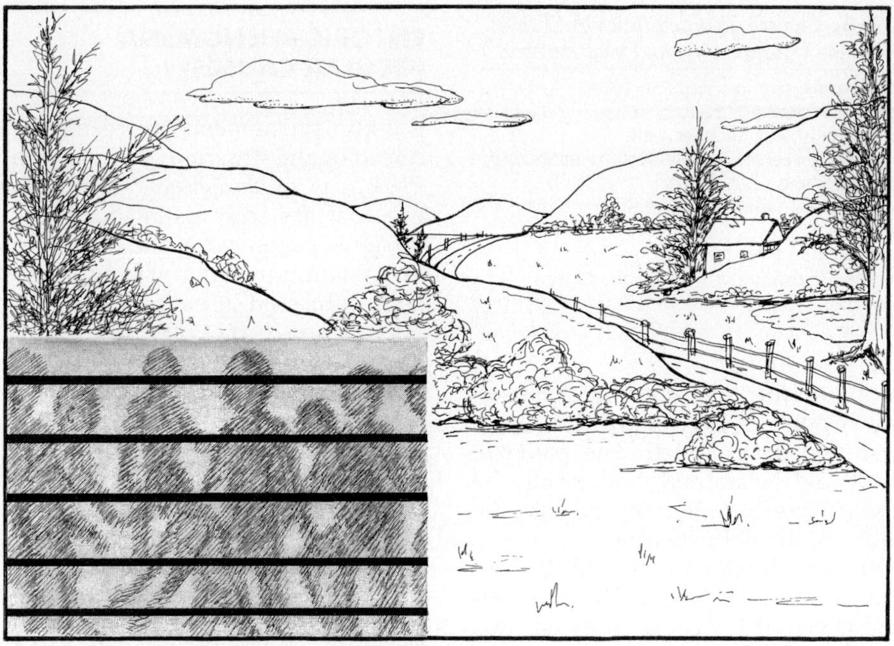

FIGURE 12–7. Artist's rendition of a patient's "picture within a picture" release hallucination due to a right parieto-occipital infarction. She complained of seeing "people milling about" and malfunctioning "vertical hold" in the lower left quandrant of vision. (From Benegas NM et al: Neurology 1996;47:1347–1348, with permission.)

objects, animals, and humans in the blind hemifield. The lesions in these cases also involved the occipital lobe, but frequently also extended partially into the posterior parietal or temporal lobes. Vaphiades et al[48] found that persons with hemianopias due to large lesions involving the middle cerebral artery territory alone tended not to have visual hallucinations. They suggested that complete destruction of visual association areas, which may contain "stored representation of visual features," or their connections, precluded the development of hemianopic release hallucinations. Anderson and Rizzo[49] hypothesized that hallucinations in the hemianopic field resulted from "pathological activation of neural ensembles in the regions bordering an occipital lesion." Kölmel[47] made the additional observation that saccadic eye movements in any direction caused temporary resolution of the visual hallucinations, perhaps because of suppression of visual information during the saccade. Vaphiades et al[48] found that only saccades away from the hemianopia had this affect, and suggested that this shift of the visual hallucinations into the intact visual field was enough to suppress them temporarily.

The use of the term *Charles Bonnet syndrome,* which has been applied to some patients with visual hallucinations associated with visual loss,[50] probably should be avoided. Charles Bonnet was a Swiss naturalist and philosopher who, in 1769, described his 89-year-old grandfather's affliction with cataracts, blindness, and visions of men, women, birds, and buildings.[51] Since then, the label Charles Bonnet syndrome has been used as a "wastebasket" term to describe patients with visual hallucinations without psychiatric disease or drug use (so-called isolated visual hallucinations).[52, 53] In fact, most patients with Charles Bonnet syndrome are elderly and have visual deficits of varying degree due to age-related macular degeneration, diabetic retinopathy, glaucoma, and corneal disease, for example.[54, 55] However, visual loss is not a criterion for the diagnosis (Table 12–5). Therefore, to describe visual hallucinations due to visual loss, we favor the use of the term *release visual hallucinations* rather than the Charles Bonnet syndrome.

Evaluation

In a patient with visual hallucinations with known visual loss, release phenomena should be suspected but is a diagnosis of exclusion. Stereotyped images and accompanying motor

TABLE 12–5. Clinical Characteristics of Charles Bonnet Syndrome ("Isolated Visual Hallucinations")

Visual hallucinations
Both simple and complex
Can arise suddenly and unexpectedly
More common, but necessarily, in elderly patients and those with visual loss
Insight into the unreal nature of the hallucinations
Intact sensorium
Absence of delusions
No hallucinations in any other sensory modality

activity or autonomic symptoms suggest seizures. Any history of psychiatric disease or drug use should be excluded. The patient's mentation should be normal, and ideally he or she should have complete insight into the unreal nature of the hallucinations.

An electroencephalogram should be obtained to rule out seizure activity. Neuroimaging is unnecessary if the cause of visual loss is ocular. However, if the cause of the visual loss is extraocular, we would recommend neuroimaging to ensure there was no change in the original lesion, such as a hemorrhage, new stroke, or tumor growth. Neuroimaging would also be indicated if the electroencephalogram were abnormal. Finally, because release hallucinations can be the presenting symptoms of new visual loss,[43] careful assessment of afferent visual function, such as acuity, color vision, and visual fields, should be performed, and the appropriate workup should be undertaken if a new visual deficit is detected.

Treatment

The best treatment of release visual hallucinations is physician recognition, reassurance, and patient education.[51] Patients with depressive symptoms may benefit from appropriate pharmacologic therapy. Psychotherapy, neuroleptics, and anticonvulsants are generally unhelpful in this disorder, but in one reported patient,[50] haloperidol successfully diminished the hallucinations.

Ironically, in some patients with hallucinations associated with progressive visual loss, the hallucinations resolve as their vision worsens. Some patients experience reduction of symptoms with increased lighting, which perhaps increases visual stimuli. Similarly, rapid eye movements, which may help release hallucinations by filling in scotomas in visual scenes, can be helpful.

ENTOPIC PHENOMENA (OCULAR CAUSES)

Entopic phenomena are visual images produced by the structures of the eye Table 12–6.[56] *Photopsias*, or *phosphenes*, are entopic phenomena that are truly hallucinogenic, in that an image is perceived in the absence of any true visual stimulus. They are unformed flashes of light witnessed in patients with a blow to the eye, traction on the retina, retinal inflammation or degeneration, and optic neuropathy (particularly optic neuritis and papilledema).[41] *Moore's lightning streak* is a brief vertical lightning flash usually appearing in the temporal field. It is a special type of phosphene attributed to vitreoretinal traction related to advancing vitreous changes and shrinkage.[56] The streak is often seen as the individual walks into a dark room. *Flick phosphenes* are flashes of light occurring during during eye movements. The phenomenon is best observed by dark-adapted eyes and while the eyelids are closed.[57] One possible mechanism is deformation of the posterior face of the vitreous and mechanical stimulation of the retina.[56] This explanation may also account for *pressure phosphenes*, which can occur when mechanical pressure is applied to the eye. *Accommodative phosphenes of Czermak* may be seen during prolonged accommodation, perhaps due to ciliary muscle traction on the peripheral retina.[56]

Many entopic phenomena are not true hallucinations. Some are actually opacified posterior vitreous floaters or hemorrhages seen by the patient. *Scheerer's phenomenon* is the normal perception of moving stars or small lights, particular when an individual looks at a bright field snow or the blue sky,[57] and is thought to be the result of leukocytes traveling in the retinal capillaries.[58] *Purkinje figures* are images of the vessels of the eye, best seen when a bright light is pressed and moved against a closed eyelid, casting shadows of the retinal circulation on the photoreceptors.

TABLE 12–6. Entopic Phenomena

Phosphenes, photopsias
Moore's lightning streak
Flick
Pressure
Accommodative, of Czermak
Media opacities
Scheerer's phenomena
Purkinje figures

Entopic phenomena can be difficult to distinguish from the photopsias seen in outer retinal disease (see Chapter 4) and migraine.

ALCOHOL AND DRUGS

Alcohol, illicit drug use (cocaine, lysergic acid diethylamide, (LSD), phencyclidine (PCP)), and medications (digoxin, levodopa) may also cause visual hallucinations and illusions. The discussion below is not intended to be exhaustive, but instead the goal is to highlight substances that are commonly responsible for these visual disturbances.

Alcohol Withdrawal

Following prolonged or heavy ethanol consumption, periods of abstinence may be characterized by alcohol withdrawal. Symptoms include generalized tremor, hallucinosis, delirium tremens, and withdrawal seizures.[59] Tremor and hallucinations tend to be the earliest withdrawal symptoms, typically occurring within hours of withdrawal and becoming most pronounced at 24 to 36 hours.[60] Hallucinations may be auditory or visual and usually occur with a clear sensorium,[59] in contrast to the confusion associated with delirium tremens, which is a later withdrawal symptom. Resumption of alcohol intake, and administration of benzodiazepines, beta-adrenergic receptor antagonists, or alpha-2-adrenergic receptor agonists, are effective means of suppressing the tremor and hallucinations.[60]

Hallucinogens

Cocaine, LSD, psilocybin, psilocin, and PCP are drugs classified as a "hallucinogens," "illusionogens," or "psychedelics" because, in addition to mood alteration, their ingestion often produces hallucinations and distortion of sensory stimuli.[61] The effects occur at nontoxic doses and without alteration in consciousness. Synesthetic hallucinations are also associated with psychedelic use, and these are characterized by colorful visual phenomena induced by a loud noise, or an auditory hallucination in response to a bright light.[1]

Some visual phenomena associated with hallucinogen use can persist. So-called hallucinogen persisting perception disorder is associated with visual phenomena occurring well after discontinuation of the drug. For instance, "flashbacks" are visual images that recur after the hallucinogen has worn off, and many are repetitions of previous hallucinations experienced during drug use. Levi and Miller[62] reported similar individuals with persistent visual hallucinations and illusions months to years after marijuana, LSD, or cocaine use. Visual complaints included shimmering of images, visual perseveration of stationary objects, streaking of moving objects, and strobe-light-like images. We have also seen such patients, and neuro-ophthalmic examinations, neuroimaging, EEG, and single photon emission tomography were all unrevealing. It is not uncommon for this syndrome to be provoked by a prescribed medication with central nervous system side effects.

Cocaine. The classic hallucination associated with chronic cocaine use is the sensation of animals, bugs, or insects moving under the skin ("cocaine bugs," or parasitosis).[63] However, other purely visual hallucinations and illusions can occur with cocaine (Table 12–7), and these were experienced by 15% of cocaine users in Siegel's study.[64] "Snow lights" refers to the sensation of sunlight reflecting off of snow crystals. This phenomenon, and others such as vibrating or pulsating geometric shapes, and polyopia and dysmorphia, have an uncanny resemblance to migraine visual aura (see above). Cocaine use is also associated with olfactory, tactile, and gustatory hallucinations. One possible mechanism for the hallucinations and illusions in cocaine use implicates cocaine's excitatory affect on cortical structures.[64] Caution should applied when individuals using cocaine complain of photophobia, halos around lights, and difficulty focusing. These symptoms are more likely the result of pupillary mydriasis caused by a cocaine-related increase in sympathetic tone.

TABLE 12–7. Cocaine Visual Hallucinations and Illusions

"Cocaine bugs" in or under the skin
"Snow lights"
Mistaken sensation of objects moving in the periphery
Geometric patterns (circles, zig-zags, lines) that can pulsate or vibrate
Complex hallucinations
Objects
Scenes
Polyopia
Dysmorphopsia
Pulsation or movement of real objects

LSD. Common visual hallucinations associated with LSD use include moving patterns of bright color[65] and pulsating geometric shapes. Individuals may experience complex hallucinations consisting of people and scenes against a background of geometric forms. About one fifth of LSD users report having seen Satan's face floating freely or over someone else's body, while about one tenth report having seen rapid aging of their friend's or a stranger's face.[66] Flashbacks occurred in 64% of LSD users in one study,[66] and halos of light around objects, light following moving objects, geometric designs within familiar objects, and distortion in the sizes and shapes of faces and images were reported. In addition, Kawasaki and Purvin[67] described three patients with persistent palinopsia up to 3 years following LSD ingestion. LSD can inhibit serotonin in the central nervous system, and it also has an effect on postsynaptic dopamine receptors, but the exact mechanism for producing hallucinations is unclear.[61]

Psilocybin and Psilocin. These are the active ingredients in hallucinogenic mushrooms. Hallucinations are usually visual, but can also be tactile or auditory.[68] Faces of friends or strangers can be reported to change shape or color or age dramatically.[69] Kaleidoscopic images or flashes of colors may be seen, but fully formed visual hallucinations consisting of people and Martians have also been described.[70]

PCP. A toxic psychosis, characterized by auditory or visual hallucinations, delusions, abnormal behavior, and sometimes disorientation, may occur with PCP use.[71] The visual hallucinations often consist of brightly colored objects. Although PCP-induced psychosis resembles acute schizophrenia, PCP use can often be recognized by the accompanying hypertension and nystagmus.[72]

Others. Mescaline,[73] amphetamines, cannabinoids, opiate agonists, and synthetic opiods may also be associated with visual hallucinations.[61] Cannabinoid, the active ingredient in marijuana and hashish, typically causes hallucinations only when there is excessive intoxication.

Digoxin

Toxic and sometimes even normal levels of the cardiac glycoside digoxin are characteristically associated with xanthopsia, the illusion of objects exhibiting abnormal colors. Yellow and green are typical colors in digoxin toxicity. Patients may also complain about blurry or snowy vision, and their visual symptoms are typically worse in brighter lighting conditions. These visual symptoms are summarized in Table 12–8. On examination, patients with digoxin toxicity may actually have decreased acuity, central scotomas, generalized visual field depression, color vision defects, and pupillary mydriasis.[74] Electroretinography (ERG) often reveal evidence of cone dysfunction, suggesting the retina is the site of toxicity, perhaps at the level of Na^+K^+-ATPase pumps in retinal cells.[75] Symptoms and ERG abnormalities usually improve following lowering of the digoxin dose.

Several elderly patients have been described with visual symptoms consistent with digoxin toxicity, but the serum concentrations of digoxin were below or within the usual therapeutic range.[76, 77] We have been a similar patient who within weeks of starting digoxin developed constant flickering lights. The abnormalities were absent with eyes closed and worse when fluorescent room lights were on. Digoxin level was normal, but ERG demonstrated delay in cone timing. The symptoms abated completely when the digoxin was stopped and another antiarrhythmic begun.

Levodopa

Levodopa is the mainstay of treatment for Parkinson's disease, however, its use may be complicated by visual hallucinations in 5% to 30%.[78] In some instances individuals taking levodopa can develop a pure psychosis.[79] Their underlying Parkinson's disease, elderly age, and use of other potentially psychotropic medications likely predispose them to hallucinations. Patients often report seeing people in the room who are not really there, and animals

TABLE 12–8. Ophthalmic Symptoms of Digoxin Toxicity

Blurred vision, trouble reading
Dim, hazy, misty, snowy vision
Xanthopsia and other dyschromatopsias
Flashing, scintillating lights (photopsias)
Moving spots and shapes
Diplopia
Pain with eye movements

(From Piltz JR et al: J Clin Neuro-ophthalmol 1993:277, with permission.)

can be described.[80] The mechanism is likely related to its effect on central dopamine receptors.

Levodopa-induced hallucinations can produce a vexing management dilemma, often necessating a compromise. Although hallucinatory symptoms usually improve following lowering of the levodopa dose, doing so typically aggravates motor symptoms such as rigidity and bradykinesia. Occasionally longer-acting preparations of levodopa/carbidopa combinations may be used to lower the total amount of levodopa given. Bromocriptine, pergolide, topinerole, and pramipexole can be added to ameliorate motor symptoms, but because these medications are also dopaminergic, they too are associated with hallucinations (see Table 12–9). When hallucinations are unacceptable, clozapine and risperidone, antipsychotic medications with little or no extrapyramidal side effects, can be used.[81, 139] Sometimes the patient chooses to accept a lower dose of levodopa to resolve the hallucinations and accept a minor amount of motor worsening.

Other Prescription Medications

A list of prescription medications that can cause visual hallucinations is given in Table 12–9.

SEIZURES

Visual hallucinations due to irritative cortical foci tend to be brief, intermittent, and stereotypically repetitive, and are often accompanied by other motor and sensory phenomena.[41] Secondary generalization, loss of consciousness, and ictal discharges on EEG also support a diagnosis of epilepsy. It is a useful generalization that occipital lobe seizures tend to be associated with simple visual hallucinations, while complex visual hallucinations are more likely the result of temporal lobe foci. Negative visual phenomena in epilepsy, in particular ictal and postictal visual loss, are discussed in Chapter 10.

Visual hallucinations are much more common in occipital lobe epilepsy than in seizures produced by temporal and parietal lobe foci. In general, they have no lateralizing value. Frontal lobe discharges, unless they generalize, are rarely associated with visual hallucinatons. The following discussion will be subdivided by cerebral localization, with particular emphasis on hallucinations associated with occipital lobe epilepsy.

Occipital Lobe Epilepsy

Simple visual hallucinations were the most common presentation (60%) in patients with

TABLE 12–9. Prescription Medications That Can Cause Visual Hallucinations

Acyclovir	Indomethacin
Amantadine	Isosorbide
Atropine eye drops	Levodopa
Baclofen	Lorazepam
Benztropine	Metaproterenol
Bromocriptine	Methyldopa
Carbamazepine	Methylphenidate
Chlordiazepoxide	Methylprednisolone
Chlorpheniramine	Minocycline
Cimetidine	Pemoline
Clomiphene citrate[135]	Pergolide
Clonazepam	Phenylephrine
Clonidine	Proamipexole
Cyclosporine[136]	Procainamide
Cyclopentolate eye drops	Propranolol
Dantrolene	Ranitidine
Dextromethorphan	Ropinirole
Digoxin	Sildenafil
Diphenhydramine	Sulfasalazine
Disopyramide	Timolol eye drops
Ephedrine	Triazolam
Imipramine and other antidepressants	Trihexphenidyl

(Adapted from Leikin et al: Med Toxicol Adverse Drug Exp 1989;4:342, with permission.)

occipital lobe epilepsy in Williamson et al's study.[82] These individuals reported flashing colored lights, white phosphenes, and steady white or colored lights. In the series of patients with occipital lobe epilepsy by Salanova et al,[83] simple visual hallucinations such as flashes, colored lights, stars, wheels, or triangles were frequently reported, and they were usually contralateral to the epileptogenic side. Complex hallucinations, thought to represent seizure spread to the temporal lobe, were reported by less than 10% in this study, and these consisted of familiar faces, pictures, and people. Similar findings were described in another series by Aykut-Bingol et al.[84]

In these studies,[82–84] the visual phenomena were often accompanied by other manifestations of seizures, such as rapid bilateral blinking or eye flutter or eye deviation with or without head deviation. When automatisms or motor manifestations appeared, seizure spread to the temporal lobe or motor cortex, respectively, was thought to have occurred. Hemianopic visual field defects were detected in approximately 60%, but patients were often unaware of their visual field deficits. The majority of patients in these series had an identifiable lesion in the occipital lobe, usually a neoplasm, but scarring related to old trauma, cysts, old strokes, and cortical dysplasia were also found. Children with occipital seizures often have cerebral palsy, cerebral dysgenesis, or a genetic disorder, and many have cortical visual loss.[140]

Since occipital lobe seizures may present solely with visual hallucinations, without other neurologic manifestations, the disorder may be very difficult to distinguish clinically from those in acephalgic migraine or release phenomena.[85] Panayiotopoulos[86] compared the visual hallucinations of 50 migraine patients with those of 20 patients with occipital epilepsy. He concluded the following: (1) the hallucinations produced by seizures tended to be more multicolored with circular or spherical patterns; (2) in contrast, the hallucinations in the migraineurs were more often black and white, with occasional color on the borders, and linear or zig-zag; and (3) no seizure patients experienced scintillating scotomas or fortification spectra. The author believed these observations could be helpful in distinguishing hallucinations between the two groups. However, we would use these as only general guidelines, as we have seen several exceptions to these observations. In cases such as these formal visual field testing may also be useful, as a hemianopic visual field defect would be suggestive of a structural lesion and a possible ictal focus.

Two exceptional individuals with continuous visual hallucinations due to occipital lobe status epilepticus have been reported. Walker et al[85] reported a 31-year-old man with an 18-year history of prolonged periods of flashing lights (like "sunlight shimmering on the sea") in his left visual field, associated with a headache, lasting up to 2 days. Elencephalograms obtained during this portion of the events demonstrated 4- to 5-Hz activity over the right occipital region. Near the end of each episode, the shimmering lights would enlarge and increase in frequency until the entire left visual field became white. Then he would experience complex hallucinations consisting of familiar faces. The episodes concluded with complete loss of vision, then loss of consciousness, then occasionally a grand mal seizure, indicating spread of the epileptic activity. MRI demonstrated slight atrophy of the right hemisphere and abnormal parietal gyral pattern. He was treated successfully with antiepileptic agents. Thomas et al[87] reported a pregnant woman who experienced intermittent episodes of nystagmus, bright spots in the left visual field, complex hallucinations consisting of people in the left visual field, and "strange structures that continuously changed shape." The neurologic exam revealed prosopagnosia and left visual and spatial agnosia. Neuroimaging was normal, but EEG revealed low-amplitude spikes arising from the right occipital region, with spread into the left occipital and right temporal lobes. Over 2 days she developed complex partial status epilepticus, characterized by repetitive visual phenomena occurring every 15 minutes, and a left homonymous hemianopia between episodes. After a cesarean section, the seizures stopped and the exam normalized. The cause of the seizures was uncertain.

Benign childhood epilepsy with occipital paroxysms is one of the benign, location-related seizure disorders in the pediatric age group.[88] This subtype made up 4.2% of all epilepsies with onset before age 13 in one study.[89] Nocturnal seizures with tonic deviation of the eyes and vomiting were the typical presenting features in younger children, while visual hallucinations and diurnal fits were more common in older children. The characteristic EEG finding is repetitive spike and slow-wave occipital discharges that diminish with open eyelids.[89] Overall, the prognosis for spontaneous remission is good. The visual hallucinations are typically unformed, but Gastaut and Zifkin[90] described three unusual children who experienced ictal visualization of numbers.

Temporal Lobe Epilepsy

Visual hallucinations in temporal lobe epilepsy are uncommon but not rare (Fig. 12–8). In two large reviews[91, 92] of patients with temporal lobe epilepsy, visual hallucinations occurred in 18% and 16%, respectively. Compared with patients with occipital lobe epilepsy, those with temporal lobe discharges are less likely to present solely with visual hallucinations, and complex visual phenomena are more common.[93] Auras consisting of bad smells or tastes, visceral sensations, or déjà vu episodes are frequent accompaniments. Temporal lobe seizures are also characterized by focal motor activity (eg, eye deviation, head turning, limb movements) in 80%, automatisms (eg, lip pursing, chewing, swallowing, finger movements, gesturing, verbalizations) in 95%, and autonomic changes (eg, pupillary dilation, salivation, blushing, pallor, urinary incontinence) in 83%.[92]

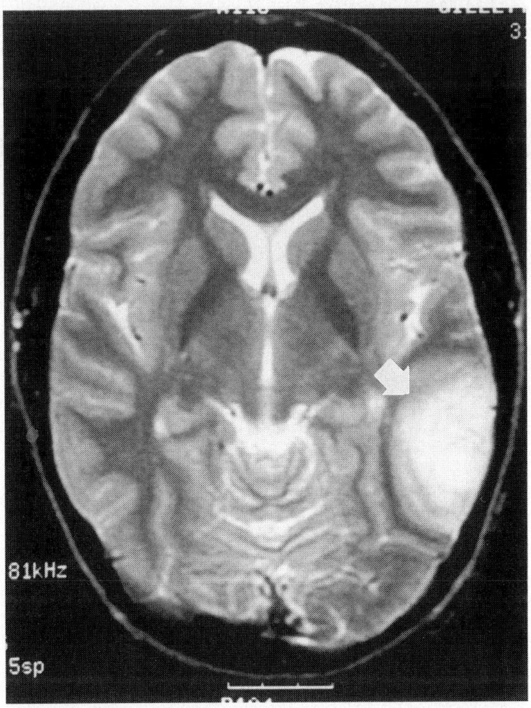

FIGURE 12–8. T_2-weighted MR Image of a woman with epileptic, simple positive visual phenomena in her right visual field as presentation of a left temporal lobe glioma (*arrow*).

Distortions of bodily image, such as missing body parts and autoscopic phenomena (see below), have also been reported in association with temporal lobe seizures.[94] Left ictal *hemimacropsia,* the illusory enlargement the left half of the visual field, was described in one patient with right temporal lobe seizures.[95]

Parietal Lobe Epilepsy

Visual hallucinations due to parietal lobe seizure foci are very uncommon,[96] but illusions of change or distortion in body shape, similar to Alice in Wonderland syndrome of migraine, can be associated with parietal lobe discharges. Elongation, shortening, swelling, or shrinking of a body part or the whole body may be experienced. The phenomenon is thought to arise from epileptic involvement of the nondominant inferior parietal lobule and superior part of the postcentral gyrus.[97]

Rousseaux et al[98] described a teenager with left parietal epileptiform discharges who complained of visual hallucinations containing written words. He had a fluent aphasia due to head trauma 6 months earlier, and neuroimaging had demonstrated a porencephalic cavity area resulting from a hemorrhage in the left temporoparietal area.

Other Unusual Ictal Visual Hallucinations

Seizures rarely may also cause *macropsia, micropsia,* and *palinopsia,*[99] visual illusions described elsewhere in this chapter.

Autoscopic Phenomena. Devinsky et al[100] described 10 patients and reviewed 33 previously reported patients with seizures and *autoscopic phenomena,* in which the individual sees a copy of his or her body, or in which the individual leaves his or her body to view it from another vantage point. The latter is also known as an "out-of-body experience," and the person's body is typically viewed from above. In the first type, the body double is usually wearing the same clothing, has the same facial expression, and has the same gesticulations as the patient. Autoscopic phenomena are not associated with any particular seizure type, as patients with tonic–clonic, simple partial, and complex partial seizures were reported in this review. They are also associated with cocaine or alcohol addiction; schizophrenia, migraine; focal lesions of the parietal, temporal, and occipital lobes; near-death experiences; and release phenomena.

Visual Allesthesia. This phenomenon, in which visual information from one homonymous field is transferred to the other, may have several causes, but in one well-documented case by Jacobs,[101] epileptogenic activity was implicated. The patient had a right parieto-occipital AVM and an incomplete left homonymous hemianopia, and intermittently saw images in the defective left field transposed from the good right field. Sometimes the images were palinopic, persisting in the left field up to 15 minutes after the real objects were no longer visible. A right parieto-occipital focus was demonstrated, and anticonvulsants led to resolution of the visual allesthesia. Jacobs attributed the visual phenomena to interhemispheric transfer of visual information from the good to irritated parieto-occipital lobe. We have seen a patient with a left occipital lobe meningioma who experienced visual allesthesia while reading. The right page of her book would often shift to the left.

NEURODEGENERATIVE DISEASE

Parkinson's Disease

As many as one quarter to one third of patients with Parkinson's disease may complain of visual hallucinations.[102] Typically they describe complex images of familiar or strange people, and the hallucinations are usually nonthreatening and felt to be real. Although the use of levodopa is the most common cause of visual hallucinations in patients with Parkinson's disease, other contributory factors include anticholinergic medications, advancing age, sleep disturbances, psychoses, and dementia.[102] Hallucinations in this group of patients can be severely disabling, and are often predictive of the need for nursing home placement.[103]

Alzheimer's Disease

Visual hallucinations occur in 3% to 33% of patients with Alzheimer's disease, and they are the most common type (up to 85%) of hallucination associated with the disorder.[104] The visual hallucinations in Alzheimer's disease tend to be complex, as in one report[105] patients were reported to see "people in the backyard," "ducks sitting in the backyard," "animals at home and babies in bed." Alzheimer patients with visual hallucinations tend to perform more poorly on mini-mental status examinations than those without hallucinations. This association with poorer cognitive performance may explain why the patients with Alzheimer's disease and visual hallucinations also frequently display delusional and paranoid ideation, auditory hallucinations, and verbal outbursts.[104] One theory[106] relating Alzheimer's disease with hallucinations implicates the propensity for neurofibrillary tangles and neuritic plaques to affect the hippocampus, amygdala, and adjacent mesial temporal cortex, areas also implicated in the generation of visual hallucinations in temporal lobe epilepsy (see above).

Low doses of neuroleptics, such as haloperidol, fluphenazine, and resperidone, can be used to treat hallucinations in patients with Alzheimer's disease.[107] Anticholinergic and extrapyramidal side effects should be monitored.

SPECIAL VISUAL HALLUCINATIONS AND ILLUSIONS RELATED TO CENTRAL NERVOUS SYSTEM LESIONS

Peduncular Hallucinations

Peduncular hallucinations, consisting of vivid and lifelike visual images of concrete objects, are rare sequelae of ventral midbrain injury. Affected patients often report seeing animals, and the hallucinations are frequently accompanied by signs of third nerve dysfunction, ataxia, and sleep and cognitive disturbances. Table 12–10 summarizes the clinical characteristics of peduncular hallucinations. The usual cause is infarction in the distribution of the

TABLE 12–10. Clinical Characteristics of Peduncular Hallucinations

Generally visual, but can involve other sensory modalities
Involve the entire visual field
Frequently contain animals or people
Great variability (not stereotyped)
Last from seconds to hours
May occur over a period lasting days to weeks
Variable patient insight
Sleep and cognitive disturbances
Third nerve palsy and ataxia common

paramedian penetrating arteries arising from the proximal posterior cerebral arteries. However, an 8-year-old with peduncular hallucinations due to a craniopharyngioma cyst causing extrinsic compression of the midbrain also has been reported.[108] The term *peduncular* refers to the French "pédonculaire," meaning the midbrain,[109] rather than the cerebral peduncles, per se.

The original description is attributed to Lhermitte,[110] who reported a patient with visual hallucinations containing cats, chickens, and people, left ophthalmoplegia, and dysmetria suggestive of a destructive lesion of the midbrain and pons. However, there was no pathologic verification. Later van Bogaert described the clinical[111] and pathologic[112] findings in a similar patient, who developed bilateral ptosis, a complete right third nerve palsy, a sluggish left pupil, left dysmetria, gait ataxia, and mildly increased reflexes and Babinski sign on the left. She complained of seeing a dog's head on her pillow, a horse's picture on the wall, a green serpent, and lines crossing the wall. The objects did not move, and they appeared and disappeared spontaneously. Occasionally she said white walls appeared pink and yellow, and sometimes her hands looked black. She was not frightened by the perceptions, but was convinced they were real. On pathologic examination, the patient was found to have a paramedian midbrain infarction involving the left red nucleus, left third nerve root, and left cerebral peduncle. Only the left side of the brain was studied. Attributing the abnormal visual perceptions to the midbrain damage, van Bogaert coined the term *peduncular hallucinations* (translation of van Bogaert's papers[111, 112] courtesy of Dr. François-Xavier Borruat). Others[108, 109, 113–115] have subsequently reported similar patients.

The mechanism, other than the association with a ventral midbrain lesion, is unclear. van Bogaert's[111, 112] and Geller and Bellur's[113] patients had relatively large lesions involving the red nuclei, third nerve fascicles, and cerebral peduncles. In contrast, in the clinicopathologic study by McKee et al[114] the patient had only bilateral destruction of the medial substantia nigra pars reticulata, suggesting that involvement of this structure is crucial for the development of peduncular hallucinations. The substantia nigra pars reticulata, owing to connections with the pedunculopontine nucleus, may have a role in regulating REM sleep, and via connections with the striatum and limbic structures, may also participate in cognitive functions. McKee et al[114] hypothesized disruption of these connections may be responsible for the sleep and cognitive disturbances sometimes seen in association with peduncular hallucinations. Other authors have considered peduncular hallucinations as release phenomena,[4, 108] but afferent vision is usually unaffected.

The best treatment for peduncular hallucinations is uncertain, but in one report,[115] agitation was treated with "a moderate dose of neuroleptic agent."

Palinopsia

Palinopsia (or *palinopia*) is an illusory visual phenomenon that Bender et al[116] defined as "the persistence or recurrence of visual images after the exciting stimulus object has been removed." Alternatively, having looked at an object then turned away from it, they may report the image of the object follows their visual tracking (*visual perseveration*), like a "movie" or "strobe light." The persistent image may be incorporated appropriately into the scene being perceived, as in Meadows and Munro's[117] patient, who saw a Santa Claus beard superimposed upon peoples' faces at a party. *Illusory visual spread* is an associated phenomenon in which objects or patterns enlarge to involve adjacent structures. Palinopic images should be distinguished from common afterimages produced by retinal overstimulation by a bright light, for example.

The most common cause of palinopsia is parieto-occipital damage with incomplete homonymous hemianopic field loss. The abnormal visual phenomenon typically, but not always, appears within the field defect. Some authors have observed that palinopsia occurs early in the course of a progressive field defect, or as a severe visual field defect resolved.[116] The right hemisphere is most commonly affected, and the damage may be caused by vascular insults, trauma, and neoplasms.[118] Palinopsia rarely occurs during migraine aura, and it may also be associated with drugs such as mescaline or LSD (see above).[118] Palinopsia has also been reported in otherwise normal individuals and in patients with eye and optic nerve disease but without drug use or cerebral lesions.[141]

The mechanism of palinopsia is uncertain. Epileptic discharges have been implicated but seem unlikely in most cases because affected patients typically lack seizure activity on EEG and do not respond to anticonvulsants. It is possible they represent a type of hallucinatory release phenomenon in the defective visual field, although not all patients with palinopsia have identifiable field defects. The predilection for responsible parieto-occipital lesions to be right sided may be artifactual because similar left-sided lesions may render patients too aphasic to communicate the abnormal visual phenomenon.

Cerebral Diplopia and Polyopia

Occipital lesions may rarely cause multiplicity of visual images, in either monocular or binocular viewing conditions. The visual disturbance is unrelated to ocular misalignment and does not resolve with use of a pinhole occluder. Specifically, the term *cerebral diplopia* refers to the duplication of images on a cortical basis, while *cerebral polyopia* describes the perception of multiple images.[119] Homonymous field defects are frequently associated findings when the cause is an occipital disturbance,[142] but cerebral diplopia and polyopia may also be described by migraineurs. The exact mechanism is uncertain. Although this phenomenon and palinopsia are similar and likely share common mechanisms,[120] technically cerebral diplopia and polyopia refer to the multiplicity of a viewed image, while palinopsia describes the persistence of an image that is no longer being viewed.

Tilted and Upside-Down Vision Associated With Vestibular Disease

Because otolith receptors play an important role in the perception of verticality, an illusion that the environment is tilted or upside-down may follow damage to the peripheral or central vestibular system or its cortical connections. Visual images may be rotated or flipped 180 degrees.[121] Affected patients with posterior fossa lesions also usually have telltale ocular motor evidence of otolith dysfunction, such as skew deviation, ocular tilt, or ocular torsion (see Chapter 15). Their subjective visual vertical may be misaligned when compared with true vertical defined by the earth's gravitational force.

Lesions causing the illusion that the room is tilted or upside-down are usually in the brain stem and are vascular in nature. Reported causes include transient vertebrobasilar ischemia,[122–125] compression of the lateral medulla by a dolichoectatic vertebral artery,[126] midbrain cavernoma,[127] basilar migraine,[121] and infarctions involving the lateral medulla (Wallenberg syndrome),[128] the territory of the medial branch of the posterior inferior cerebellar artery,[129] and the pons.[122, 127]

Cortical processes may also be responsible for tilted or upside down-vision. Migraine and epilepsy should always be considered when evidence of a posterior fossa lesion is lacking, although responsible supratentorial lesions have also been reported. Brandt et al[130] found that 23 of 52 patients with middle cerebral artery infarctions developed subjective visual vertical tilts. The authors attributed the altered perception of verticality to damage to the posterior insula, likely the homologue to parieto-insular vestibular cortex in monkeys. Solms et al[131] described a patient with bifrontal abscesses who experienced transient episodes of upside-down vision, and they cite other similar cases in the literature. The mechanism in that case is unclear. A case of 90% rotation of the visual environment after placement of a ventriculoperitoneal shunt in the right parieto-occipital lobe has also been reported.[143]

PSYCHIATRIC DISEASE

Hallucinations and delusions (false beliefs) are the hallmarks of psychosis. Of all psychiatric disorders with psychotic features, schizophrenia is the one most commonly associated with visual hallucinations. Psychosis in schizophrenia is suggested when complex visual hallucinations are accompanied by auditory hallucinations, particularly voices.[57] The visual hallucinations are characteristically formed, and are present with eyes opened or closed.[1] Affected individuals typically have a clear consciousness, but they display lack of insight into the unreal nature of their hallucinations.

Hallucinations are less common in affective disorders, however, psychosis occurs in a small minority of patients. In a study of 1,715 hospitalized individuals with affective disorders,[132] visual hallucinations were reported by 3.0% of those with primary unipolar depression, 1.5% of those with secondary unipolar depression, 3.0% with bipolar depression, and 5.8% of those with bipolar mania.

Antipsychotic medication is the mainstay of treatment for hallucinations in psychiatric diseases.

HYPNAGOGIC HALLUCINATIONS IN NARCOLEPSY

Narcolepsy is characterized by the clinical tetrad of (1) *sleep attacks,* which are episodes of unwanted sleep; (2) *cataplexy,* an abrupt and reversible decrease or loss of muscle tone; (3) *sleep paralysis,* which occurs during sleep–wake transitions, and (4) *hypnagogic hallucinations,* which can be auditory or visual. Patients usually find hypnagogic hallucinations unpleasant or dreadful, and a common sensation is a threatening person at the door. Hypnagogic hallucinations occur at sleep onset, either at night or during daytime sleep episodes, and are frequently accompanied by sleep paralysis.[133]

Patients with narcolepsy also typically exhibit excessive daytime somnulence. The age range of affected patients is 5 to 55 years, but the largest number of individuals are in their second decade. The diagnosis is usually a straightforward one, but cases should be confirmed with polysomnography to document REM sleep at the onset of daytime or nightime sleep episodes. Central nervous system stimulants, such as methylphenidate, are the mainstay of treatment.[133]

Hypnogogic hallucinations are not necessarily pathologic. Normal individuals may experience both formed and unformed visual images upon wakening (*hypnopompic*) or upon going to sleep (*hypnagogic*).

METABOLIC

In unexplained cases, and in hospitalized patients, electrolyte imbalance, hypoxemia, and fevers should be considered as causes of visual hallucinations. Endocrine abnormalities and toxic levels of various chemicals, such as carbon dioxide, mercury, and bromide, can also produce hallucinations.[1]

VISUAL HALLUCINATIONS IN NORMAL INDIVIDUALS

Aside from the aforementioned hypnogogic and hypnopompic phenomena associated with sleep/wake states, other visual hallucinations can occur in normal people. In a *grief reaction,* individuals may perceive the image of the spouse or close friend who recently died.[134] Life-threatening stress and fatigue may be other causes.[1]

REFERENCES

1. Asaad G, Shapiro B: Hallucinations: theoretical and clinical overview. Am J Psychiatry 1986;143:1088–1097.
2. Carter JL: Visual, somatosensory, olfactory, and gustatory hallucinations. Psychiatr Clin North Am 1992;15:347–358.
3. West LJ: A general theory of hallucinations and dreams. In: West LJ (ed): Hallucinations, pp 275–291, New York, Grune & Stratton, 1962.
4. Cogan DG: Visual hallucinations as release phenomena. Graefes Arch Klin Exp Ophthalmol 1973;188: 139–150.
5. Slade P: Hallucinations [editorial]. Psychol Med 1976;6:7–13.
6. Weller M, Wiedemann P: Visual hallucinations. An outline of etiological and pathogenetic concepts. Int Ophthalmol 1989;13:193–199.
7. Manford M, Andermann F: Complex visual hallucinations. Clinical and neurobiological insights. Brain 1998;121:1819–1840.
8. Hupp SL, Kline LB, Corbett JJ: Visual disturbances of migraine. Surv Ophthalmol 1989;33:221–236.
9. Sacks O: Migraine aura and classical migraine. In: Migraine: Understanding a Common Disorder, 2nd edition, pp 55–110. Berkeley, University of California Press, 1985.
10. Hachinski VC, Porchawka J, Steele JC: Visual symptoms in the migraine syndrome. Neurology 1973; 23:570–579.
11. Rolak LA: Literary neurologic syndromes. Alice in Wonderland. Arch Neurol 1991;48:649–651.
12. Headache classification committee of the International Headache Society: Classification and diagnostic criteria for headache disorders, cranial neuralgias and facial pain. Cephalgia 1988;8(Suppl 7):1–96.
13. Kaufman DM, Solomon S: Migraine visual auras. A medical update for the psychiatrist. Gen Hosp Psychiatry 1992;14:162–170.
14. Alvarez WC: The migrainous scotoma as studied in 618 persons. Am J Ophthalmol 1960;49:489–504.
15. Lance JW, Anthony M: Some clinical aspects of migraine: a prospective survey of 500 patients. Arch Neurol 1966;15:356–361.
16. Congdon PJ, Forsythe WI: Migraine in childhood: a study of 300 children. Dev Med Child Neurol 1979;21:209–216.
17. Kinast M, Lueders H, Rothner AD, et al: Benign focal epileptiform discharges in childhood migraine. Neurology 1982;32:1309–1311.
18. Dodge PR, Griffith JF: Some transient ocular manifestations of neurologic disease in children. In: Smith JL (ed): Neuro-Ophthalmology, pp 316–325. St. Louis, CV Mosby, 1976.
19. Barlow CF: The expression of childhood migraine. In: Headache and Migraine in Childhood, pp 46–75. Philadelphia, JB Lippincott, 1984.
20. Olesen J, Friberg L, Olsen TS, et al: Timing and topography of cerebral blood flow, aura, and headache during migraine attacks. Ann Neurol 1990;28: 791–798.
21. Cutrer FM, Sorensen AG, Weisskoff RM, et al: Perfusion-weighted imaging defects during spontaneous migrainous aura. Ann Neurol 1998;43:25–31.

22. Plant GT: The fortification spectra of migraine. Br Med J 1986;293:1613–1617.
23. Fazekas F, Koch M, Schmidt R, et al: The prevalence of cerebral damage varies with migraine type: a MRI study. Headache 1992;32:287–291.
24. Fuller GN, Marshall A, Flint J, et al: Migraine madness: recurrent psychosis after migraine. J Neurol Neurosurg Psychiatry 1993;56:416–418.
25. Lawden MC, Cleland PG: Achromatopsia in the aura of migraine. J Neurol Neurosurg Psychiatr 1993;56: 708–709.
26. Lippman CW: Certain hallucinations peculiar to migraine. J Nerv Ment Dis 1952;116:346–351.
27. Todd J: The syndrome of Alice in Wonderland. Can Med Assoc J 1955;73:701–704.
28. Golden GS: The Alice in Wonderland syndrome in juvenile migraine. Pediatrics 1979;63:517–519.
29. Copperman SM: 'Alice in Wonderland' syndrome as a presenting symptom of infectious mononucleosis in children. Clin Pediatr 1977;16:143–146.
30. Sinoff SE, Rosenberg M: Permanent cerebral diplopia in a migraineur. Neurology 1990;40:1138–1139.
31. Kosmorsky G: Unusual visual phenomenon during acephalgic migraine [letter]. Arch Ophthalmol 1987;105:613.
32. Liu GT, Schatz NJ, Galetta SL, et al: Persistent positive visual phenomena in migraine. Neurology 1995;45: 664–668.
33. Haas DC: Prolonged migraine aura status. Ann Neurol 1982;11:197–199.
34. Luda E, Bo E, Sicuro L, et al: Sustained visual aura: a totally new variation of migraine. Headache 1991;31:582–583.
35. Rothrock JF: Successful treatment of persistent migraine aura with divalproex sodium. Neurology 1997;48:261–262.
36. O'Connor PS, Tredici TJ: Acephalgic migraine: fifteen years experience. Ophthalmology 1981;88:999–1003.
37. Wijman CAC, Wolf PA, Kase CS, et al: Migrainous visual accompaniments are not rare in late life. The Framingham study. Stroke 1998;29:1539–1543.
38. Fisher CM: Late-life migraine accompaniments as a cause of unexplained transient ischemic attacks. Can J Neurol Sci 1980;7:9–17.
39. Shevell MI: Acephalgic migraines of childhood. Pediatr Neurol 1996;14:211–215.
40. Lepore FE: Spontaneous visual phenomena with visual loss: 104 patients with lesions of the retinal and neural afferent pathways. Neurology 1990;40: 444–447.
41. Gittinger JW, Miller NR, Keltner JL, et al: Sugarplum fairies. Visual hallucinations. Surv Ophthalmol 1982;27:42–48.
42. White CP, Jan JE: Visual hallucinations after acute visual loss in a young child. Dev Med Child Neurol 1992;34:259–261.
43. Brust JCM, Behrens MM: "Release hallucinations" as the major symptoms of posterior cerebral artery occlusion: a report of 2 cases. Ann Neurol 1977;2: 432–436.
44. Hoksbergen I, Pickut BA, Mariën P, et al: SPECT findings in an unusual case of visual hallucinosis. J Neurol 1996;243:594–598.
45. Benegas NM, Liu GT, Volpe NJ, et al: "Picture within a picture" visual hallucinations. Neurology 1996;47: 1347–1348.
46. Kölmel HW: Coloured patterns in hemianopic fields. Brain 1984;107:155–167.
47. Kölmel HW: Complex visual hallucinations in the hemianopic field. J Neurol Neurosurg Psychiatry 1985;48:29–38.
48. Vaphiades MS, Celesia GG, Brigell MG: Positive spontaneous visual phenomena limited to the hemianopic field in lesions of central visual pathways. Neurology 1996;47:408–417.
49. Anderson SW, Rizzo M: Hallucinations following occipital lobe damage: the pathological activation of visual representations. J Clin Exp Neuropsychol 1994;16:651–663.
50. Siatkowski RM, Zimmer B, Rosenberg PR: The Charles Bonnet syndrome. Visual perceptive dysfunction in sensory deprivation. J Clin Neuro-ophthalmol 1990;10:215–218.
51. Fernandez A, Lichtshein G, Vieweg WV: The Charles Bonnet syndrome: a review. J Nerv Ment Dis 1997; 185:195–200.
52. Gold K, Rabins PV: Isolated visual hallucinations and the Charles Bonnet syndrome: a review of the literature and presentation of six cases. Compr Psychiatry 1989;30:90–98.
53. Teunisse RJ, Zitman FG, Raes DCM: Clinical evaluation of 14 patients with the Charles Bonnet syndrome (isolated visual hallucinations). Compr Psychiatry 1994;35:70–75.
54. Teunisse RJ, Cruysberg JRM, Verbeek AL, et al: The Charles Bonnet syndrome: a large prospective study in The Netherlands. A study of the prevalence of the Charles Bonnet syndrome and associated factors in 500 patients attending the University Department of Ophthalmology at Nijmegen. Br J Psychiatr 1995; 166:254–257.
55. Teunisse RJ, Cruysberg JR, Hoefnagels WH, et al: Visual hallucinations in psychologically normal people: Charles Bonnet's syndrome. Lancet 1996;347: 794–797.
56. Adamczyk DT: Visual phenomena, disturbances, and hallucinations. Optom Clin 1996;5:33–52.
57. Lessell S: Higher disorders of visual function: positive phenomena. In: Glaser JS, Smith JL (eds): Neuro-Ophthalmology, pp 27–44. St. Louis, CV Mosby, 1975.
58. Sinclair SH, Azar-Cavanagh M, Soper KA, et al: Investigation of the source of the blue field entoptic phenomenon. Invest Ophthalmol Vis Sci 1989;30: 668–673.
59. Thomas PK: Alcohol and disease: central nervous system. Acta Med Scand 1985;703 (Suppl):251–264.
60. Charness ME, Simon RP, Greenberg DA: Ethanol and the nervous system. N Engl J Med 1989;321:442–454.
61. Leikin JB, Krantz AJ, Zell-Kanter M, et al: Clinical features and management of intoxication due to hallucinogenic drugs. Med Toxicol Adverse Drug Exp 1989;4:324–350.
62. Levi L, Miller NR: Visual illusions associated with previous drug abuse. J Clin Neuro-ophthalmol 1990; 10:103–110.
63. Mitchell J, Vierkant AD: Delusions and hallucinations of cocaine abusers and paranoid schizophrenics: a comparative study. J Psychol 1991;125:301–310.
64. Siegel RK: Cocaine hallucinations. Am J Psychiatry 1978;135:309–314.
65. Kulig K: LSD. Emerg Med Clin North Am 1990;8: 551–558.
66. Schwartz RH, Comerci GD, Meeks JE: Clinical and laboratory observations. LSD: patterns of use by chemically dependent adolescents. J Pediatr 1987; 111:936–938.

67. Kawasaki A, Purvin V. Persistent palinopsia following ingestion of lysergic acid diethylamide (LSD). Arch Opthalmol 1996;114:47–50.
68. Francis J, Murray VSG: Review of enquiries made to the NPIS concerning psilocybe mushroom ingestion. 1978–1981. Hum Toxicol 1983;2:349–352.
69. Schwartz RH, Smith DE: Hallucinogenic mushrooms. Clin Pediatr 1988;27:70–73.
70. Peden NR, Macaulay KEC, Bissett AF, et al: Clinical toxicology of magic mushroom ingestion. Postgrad Med J 1981;57:543–545.
71. McCarron MM, Schulze BW, Thompson GA, et al: Acute phencyclidine intoxication: clinical patterns complications and treatment. Ann Emerg Med 1981; 10:290–297.
72. McCarron MM, Schulze BW, Thompson GA, et al: Acute phencyclidine intoxication: incidence of clinical finding in 1000 cases. Ann Emerg Med 1981;10: 237–242.
73. Schwartz RH: Mescaline: a survey. Am Fam Phys 1988;37:122–124.
74. Piltz JR, Wertenbaker C, Lance SE, et al: Digoxin toxicity. J Clin Neuro-ophthalmol 1993;13:275–280.
75. Weleber RG, Shults WT: Digoxin retinal toxicity. Clinical and electrophysiologic evaluation of a cone dysfunction syndrome. Arch Ophthalmol 1981;99: 1568–1572.
76. Butler VP, Odel JG, Rath E, et al: Digitalis-induced visual disturbances with therapeutic serum digitalis concentrations. Ann Intern Med 1995;123:676–680.
77. Wolin MJ: Digoxin visual toxicity with therapeutic blood levels of digoxin. Am J Ophthalmol 1998; 125:406–407.
78. Banerjee AK, Falkai PG, Savidge M: Visual hallucinations in the elderly associated with the use of levodopa. Postgrad Med J 1989;65:358–361.
79. Friedman JH: The management of the levodopa psychoses. Clin Neuropharmacol 1991;14:283–295.
80. Cummings JL: Behavioral complications of drug treatment of Parkinson's disease. J Am Geriatr Soc 1991;39:708–716.
81. Alexander GE: Parkinson's disease. In: Johnson RT, Griffin JW (eds): Current Therapy in Neurologic Disease, 5th edition, pp 268–274. St. Louis, CV Mosby, 1997.
82. Williamson PD, Thadani VM, Darcey TM, et al: Occipital lobe epilepsy: clinical characteristics, seizure spread patterns, and results of surgery. Ann Neurol 1992;31:3–13.
83. Salanova V, Andermann F, Olivier A, et al: Occipital lobe epilepsy: electroclinical manifestations, electrocorticography, cortical stimulation and outcome in 42 patients treated between 1930 and 1991. Brain 1992;115:1655–1680.
84. Aykut-Bingol C, Bronen RA, Kim JH, et al: Surgical outcome in occipital lobe epilepsy: implications for pathophysiology. Ann Neurol 1998;44:60–69.
85. Walker MC, Smith SJM, Sisodiya SM, et al: Case of simple partial status epilepticus in occipital lobe misdiagnosed as migraine: clinical, electrophysiological, and magnetic resonance imagining characteristics. Epilepsia 1995;36:1233–1236.
86. Panayiotopoulos CP: Elementary visual hallucinations in migraine and epilepsy. J Neurol Neurosurg Psychiatr 1994;57:1371–1374.
87. Thomas P, Barrè P, Chatel M: Complex partial status epilepticus of extratemporal origin: report of a case. Neurology 1991;41:1147–1149.
88. Deonna T, Ziegler A-L, Despland PA: Paroxysmal visual disturbances of epileptic origin and occipital epilepsy in children. Neuropediatrics 1984;15: 131–135.
89. Panayiotopoulos CP: Benign childhood epilepsy with occipital paroxysms. A 15-year prospective clinical and electroencephalographic study. Ann Neurol 1989;26:51–56.
90. Gastaut H, Zifkin BG: Ictal visual hallucinations of numerals. Neurology 1984;34:950–953.
91. Currie S, Heathfield KWG, Henson RA, et al: Clinical course and prognosis of temporal lobe epilepsy. Brain 1971;94:173–190.
92. King DW, Ajmone Marsan C: Clinical features and ictal patterns in epileptic patients with EEG temporal lobe foci. Ann Neurol 1977;2:138–147.
93. Sowa MV, Pituck S: Prolonged spontaneous complex visual hallucinations and illusions as ictal phenomena. Epilepsia 1989;30:524–526.
94. Ionasescu V: Paroxysmal disorders of the body image in temporal lobe epilepsy. Acta Psychiatr Scand 1960;35:171–181.
95. Mendez MF: Ictal hemimacropsia. Neurology 1992; 42:1119–1120.
96. Williamson PD, Boon PA, Thadani VM, et al: Parietal lobe epilepsy: diagnostic considerations and results of surgery. Ann Neurol 1992;31:193–201.
97. Sveinbjornsdottir S, Duncan JS: Parietal and occipital lobe epilepsy: a review. Epilepsia 1993;34:493–521.
98. Rousseaux M, Debrock D, Cabaret M, et al: Visual hallucinations with written words in a case of left parietotemporal lesion. J Neurol Neurosurg Psychiatry 1994;57:1268–1271.
99. Müller T, Büttner T, Kuhn W, et al: Palinopsia as sensory epileptic phenomenon. Acta Neurol Scand 1995;91:433–436.
100. Devinsky O, Feldmann E, Burrowes K, et al: Autoscopic phenomena with seizures. Arch Neurol 1989; 46:1080–1088.
101. Jacobs L: Visual allesthesia. Neurology 1980;30:1059–1063.
102. Sanchez-Ramos JR, Ortoll R, Paulson GW: Visual hallucinations associated with Parkinson disease. Arch Neurol 1996;53:1265–1268.
103. Goetz CG, Stebbins GT: Mortality and hallucinations in nursing home patients with advanced Parkinson's disease. Neurology 1995;45:669–671.
104. Lerner AJ, Koss E, Patterson MB, et al: Concomitants of visual hallucinations in Alzheimer's disease. Neurology 1994;44:523–527.
105. Lopez OL, Becker JT, Brenner RP, et al: Alzheimer's disease with delusions and hallucinations: neuropsychological and electroencephalographic correlates. Neurology 1991;41:906–912.
106. Gilley DW, Whalen ME, Wilson RS, et al: Hallucinations and associated factors in Alzheimer's disease. J Neuropsychiatry Clin Neurosci 1991;3:371–376.
107. Kawas C, Morrison A: Alzheimer's disease and other dementias. In: Johnson RT, Griffin JW (eds): Current Therapy in Neurologic Disease, 5th edition, pp 303–306. St. Louis, CV Mosby, 1997.
108. Dunn DW, Weisberg LA, Nadell J: Peduncular hallucinations caused by brainstem compression. Neurology 1983;33:1360–1361.
109. Caplan LR: "Top of the basilar" syndrome. Neurology 1980;30:72–79.
110. Lhermitte J: Syndrome de la calotte du pédoncule cérébral. Les troubles psycho-sensoriels dans les lé-

sions due mésocéphale. Rev Neurol (Paris) 1922;38: 1359–1365.
111. van Bogaert L: Syndrome inférieur du noyau rouge, troubles psycho-sensoriels d'origine mésocéphalique. Rev Neurol (Paris) 1924;40:417–423.
112. van Bogaert L: L'hallucinose pédonculaire. Rev Neurol (Paris) 1927;47:608–617.
113. Geller TJ, Bellur SN: Peduncular hallucinosis: magnetic resonance imaging confirmation of mesencephalic infarction during life. Ann Neurol 1987;21: 602–604.
114. McKee AC, Levine DN, Kowall NW, et al: Peduncular hallucinosis associated with isolated infarction of the substantia nigra pars reticulata. Ann Neurol 1990; 27:500–504.
115. Kölmel HW: Peduncular hallucinations. J Neurol 1991;238:457–459.
116. Bender MB, Feldman M, Sobin AJ: Palinopsia. Brain 1968;91:321–328.
117. Meadows JC, Monro SSF: Palinopsia. J Neurol Neurosurg Psychiatry 1977;40:5–8.
118. Michel EM, Troost BT: Palinopsia: cerebral localization with computed tomography. Neurology 1980;30: 887–889.
119. Lopez JR, Adornato BT, Hoyt WF: 'Entomopia': A remarkable case of cerebral polyopia. Neurology 1993;43:2145–2146.
120. Gottlieb D: The unidirectionality of cerebral polyopia. J Clin Neuro-ophthalmol 1992;12:257–262.
121. River Y, Ben Hur T, Steiner I: Reversal of vision metamorphopsia. Clinical and anatomical characteristics. Arch Neurol 1998;55:1362–1368.
122. Ropper AH: Illusion of tilting of the visual environment: report of five cases. J Clin Neuro-ophthalmol 1983;3:147–151.
123. Steiner I, Shahin R, Melamed E: Acute upside down reversal of vision in transient vertebrobasilar ischemia. Neurology 1987;37:1685–1686.
124. Mehler MF: Complete visual inversion in vertebrobasilar ischaemic disease. J Neurol Neurosurg Psychiatry 1988;51:1236–1237.
125. Stracciari A, Guarino M, Ciucci G, et al: Acute upside down reversal of vision in vertebrobasilar ischaemia [letter]. J Neurol Neurosurg Psychiatry 1993;56:423.
126. Slavin ML, LoPinto RJ: Isolated environmental tilt associated with lateral medullary compression by dolichoectasia of the vertebral artery. Is there a cause and effect relationship? J Clin Neuro-ophthalmol 1987;7:29–33.
127. Tiliket C, Ventre-Dominey J, Vighetto A, et al: Room tilt illusion. A central otolith dysfunction. Arch Neurol 1996;53:1259–1264.
128. Hörnsten G: Wallenberg's syndrome. Part I, General symptomatology with special references to visual disturbances and imbalance. Acta Neurol Scand 1974;50:434–446.
129. Charles N, Froment C, Rode G, et al: Vertigo and upside down vision due to an infarct in the territory of the medial branch of the posterior inferior cerebellar artery caused by dissection of a vertebral artery. J Neurol Neurosurg Psychiatr 1992;55:188–189.
130. Brandt T, Dieterich M, Danek A: Vestibular cortex lesions affect the perception of verticality. Ann Neurol 1994;35:403–412.
131. Solms M, Kaplan-Solms K, Saling M, et al: Inverted vision after frontal lobe disease. Cortex 1988;24: 499–509.
132. Black DW, Nasrallah A: Hallucinations and delusions in 1715 patients with unipolar and bipolar affective disorders. Psychopathology 1989;22:28–34.
133. Billiard M: Narcolepsy. Clinical features and aetiology. Ann Clin Res 1985;17:220–226.
134. Schneck JM: S. Weir Mitchell's visual hallucinations as a grief reaction [letter]. Am J Psychiatry 1989; 146:409.
135. Purvin VA: Visual disturbance secondary to clomiphene citrate. Arch Ophthalmol 1995;113:482–484.
136. Steg RE, Garcia EG: Complex visual hallucinations and cyclosporine neurotoxicity. Neurology 1991;41: 1156.
137. Kölmel HW: Visual illusions and hallucinations. Baillieres Clin Neurol 1993;2:243–264.
138. ffytche DH, Howard RJ: The perceptual consequences of visual loss: "positive" pathologies of vision. Brain 1999;122:1247–1260.
139. The Parkinson Study Group: Low-dose clozapine for the treatment of drug-induced psychosis in Parkinson's disease. N Engl J Med 1999;340:757–763.
140. Libenson MH, Caravale B, Prasad AN: Clinical correlations of occipital epileptiform discharges in children. Neurology 1999;53:265–269.
141. Pomeranz HD, Lessell S: Palinopsia and polyopia in the absence of drugs or cerebral disease. Neurology 2000;54:855–859.
142. Jones MR, Waggoner R, Hoyt WF: Cerebral polyopia with extrastriate quadrantopia: report of a case with magnetic resonance documentation of V2/V3 cortical infarction. J Neuro-ophthalmol 1999;19:1–6.
143. Girkin CA, Perry JD, Miller NR: Visual environmental rotation: a novel disorder of visiospatial integration. J Neuro-ophthalmol 1999;19:13–16.

PART III

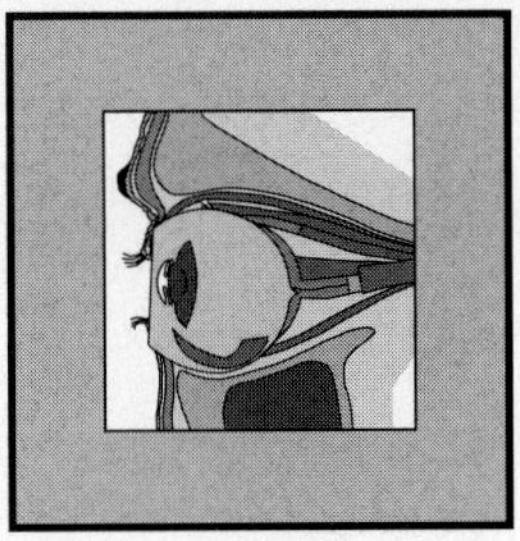

EFFERENT NEURO-OPHTHALMIC DISORDERS

CHAPTER 13

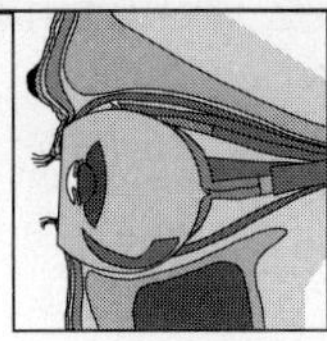

Pupillary Disorders

Pupillary disorders usually fall into one of three major categories: (1) abnormally shaped pupils, (2) abnormal pupillary reaction to light, or (3) unequally sized pupils (anisocoria). Occasionally pupillary abnormalities are isolated findings, but in many cases they are manifestations of more serious intracranial pathology.

The pupillary examination is discussed in detail in Chapter 2. Pupillary neuroanatomy and physiology will be reviewed here, then the various pupillary disorders, grouped roughly into one of the three categories listed above, will be discussed.

NEUROANATOMY AND PHYSIOLOGY

The major functions of the pupil are to vary the quantity of light reaching the retina, to minimize the spherical aberrations of the peripheral cornea and lens, and to increase the depth of field (the depth within which objects will appear sharp).[1] In most individuals the two pupils are equal in size, and each is situated slightly nasal and inferior to the center of the cornea (Fig. 13–1).[2]

The iris contains the two muscles that control the size of the pupil. Contraction of the dilator muscle leads to pupillary enlargement (mydriasis), while sphinctor muscle contraction causes pupillary constriction (miosis). The sphincter muscle wraps 360 degrees around the pupillary margin, and the dilator muscle similarly encircles the pupil but is more peripherally located.

Normally, light directed in either eye leads to bilateral pupillary constriction, and this pupillary light reflex is mediated by a parasympathetic pathway (see Fig. 13–2 for details). Light entering the eye causes retinal photoreceptors to hyperpolarize, in turn causing activation of retinal interneurons and ultimately the retinal ganglion cells, the axons of which travel through the optic nerve, chiasm, and optic tract to reach the pretectal nuclei (afferent arc). Interneurons then connect the pretectal nuclei to the Edinger–Westphal nuclei. Although these connections are bilateral, the input into the Edinger–Westphal nuclei is predominantly from the contralateral pretectal nucleus. Since the afferent pupillary fibers leave the optic tract before the lateral geniculate nucleus, isolated lesions of the geniculate, optic radiations, and visual cortex do not affect pupillary size or reactivity. Efferent parasympathetic fibers, arising from the Edinger–Westphal nucleus, exit the midbrain within the third nerve (efferent arc). Within the subarachnoid portion of the third nerve, pupillary fibers tend to run on the external surface, making them more vulnerable to compression or infiltration and less susceptible to vascular insult. Within the anterior cavernous sinus, the third nerve divides into two portions. The pupillary fibers follow the inferior division into the orbit, where they then synapse at the ciliary ganglion, which lies in the posterior part of the orbit between the optic nerve and lateral rectus muscle (Fig. 13–3). The ciliary ganglion issues postganglionic cholinergic short ciliary nerves, which travel to the globe, then between the sclera and choroid, to innervate the ciliary body and iris sphincter muscle. Fibers to the ciliary body outnumber those to the iris sphincter muscle by 30:1.

The near response consists of pupillary constriction, accommodation (change in the shape

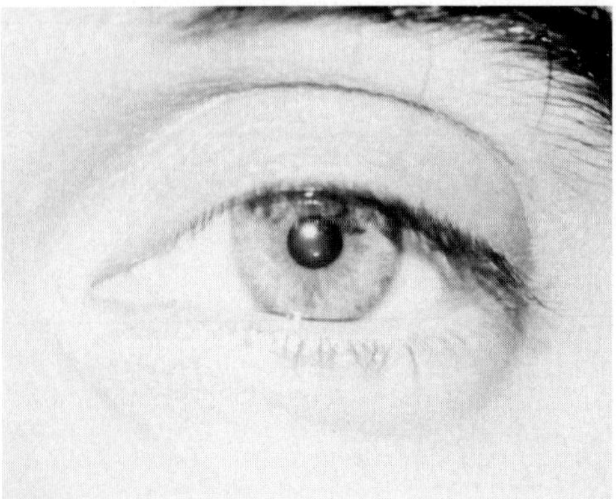

FIGURE 13–1. A normal left eye. Note the pupil is slightly nasal to the center of the cornea.

of the lens), and convergence of the eyes (see Chapter 2). Although the pathways are unclear, likely the supranuclear control for the near response arises from diffuse cortical locations. Stimulation of the peristriate cortex (areas 19 and 22) in primates can evoke a near reponse,[3] but more recent evidence suggests the lateral suprasylvian area is also related to the control of lens accommodation.[4] The signals converge in the rostral superior colliculus, near which a group of midbrain near-reponse neurons coordinates the pretectum for accommodation and miosis, the mesencephalic reticular formation for accommodation and vergence, and the raphe interpositus for visual fixation.[4,5] The final signal for pupillary miosis at near is still mediated by the Edinger–Westphal nuclei.

Pupillary dilation is the function of the oculosympathetic system (the ocular part of the sympathetic nervous system), which consists of three neurons beginning in the posterolateral hypothalmus and ending at the iris and eyelids (see Fig. 13–4 for details). The first-order neuron projects from the hypothalamus through ill-defined brain stem pathways to synapse on the intermediolateral cell column in the spinal cord at C8–T2 (ciliospinal center of Budge). The second-order neuron (preganglionic) leaves the spinal cord and travels over the apex of the lung before ascending with the internal carotid artery to synapse at the superior cervical ganglion. In the region of the lung apex, the sympathetic pathway lies in close proximity to the lower brachial plexus. The third-order neuron (postganglionic) travels along the internal carotid into the cavernous sinus, after which the sympathetic pathways follow the sixth nerve and then the nasociliary nerve (a branch of the first division of the trigeminal nerve) into the orbit.[6] This neuron releases the neurotransmitter norepinephrine at the iris dilator muscle.

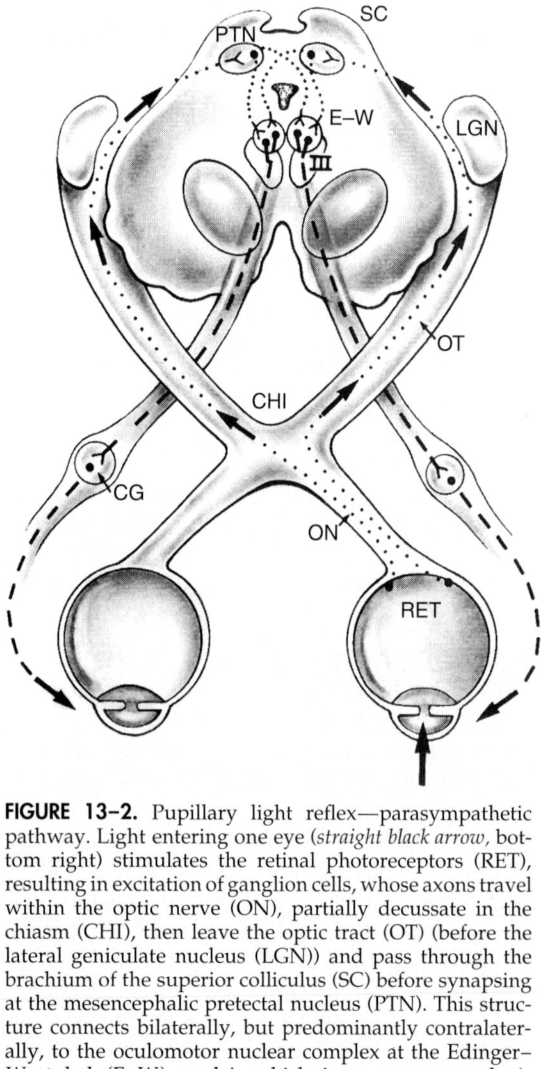

FIGURE 13–2. Pupillary light reflex—parasympathetic pathway. Light entering one eye (*straight black arrow,* bottom right) stimulates the retinal photoreceptors (RET), resulting in excitation of ganglion cells, whose axons travel within the optic nerve (ON), partially decussate in the chiasm (CHI), then leave the optic tract (OT) (before the lateral geniculate nucleus (LGN)) and pass through the brachium of the superior colliculus (SC) before synapsing at the mesencephalic pretectal nucleus (PTN). This structure connects bilaterally, but predominantly contralaterally, to the oculomotor nuclear complex at the Edinger–Westphal (E–W) nuclei, which issue parasympathetic fibers that travel within the third nerve (inferior division) and terminate at the ciliary ganglion (CG) in the orbit. Postsynaptic cells innervate the pupillary sphincter, resulting in miosis. Note light in one eye causes bilaterally pupillary constriction. (From Liu GT: Disorders of the eyes and eyelids: Disorders of the pupil. In Samuels MA, Feske S (eds): The Office Practice of Neurology, p 61. New York, Churchill Livingstone, 1996, with permission. Adapted from Slamovits TL, Glaser JS. The pupils and accommodation. In: Glaser JS (ed): Neuro-opthalmology, 2nd edition, p 460. Philadelphia, JB Lippincott, 1990, with permission.)

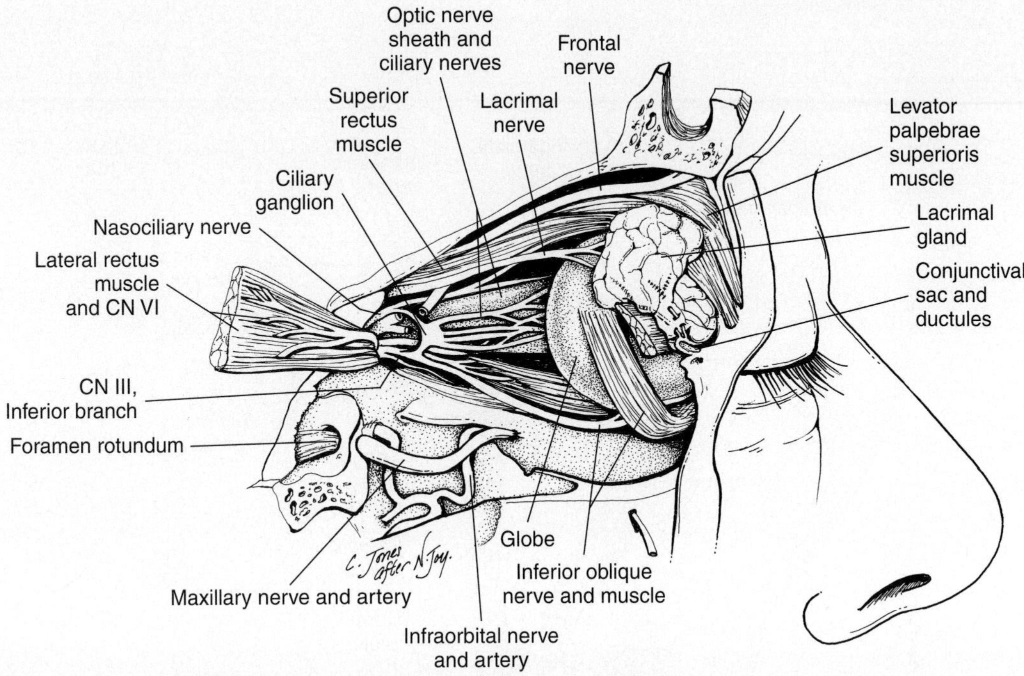

FIGURE 13–3. Ciliary ganglion depicted in a lateral view of a dissection of the orbit. Note the ciliary ganglion lies between the optic nerve and the lateral rectus muscle, receives fibers from the inferior branch of the third nerve, and issues short ciliary nerves to the orbit, orbital muscles, and lacrimal gland. (Redrawn with permission from Moore KL. Clinically Oriented Anatomy, 3rd edition, p 708. Baltimore, Williams & Wilkins, 1992, with permission.)

PHARMACOLOGIC TESTING OF THE PUPILS

As will be discussed, pharmacologic testing helps confirm the clinical diagnosis of many pupillary abnormalities. Some general guidelines need to be followed in this regard. Since corneal reflex evaluation and applanation tonometry may alter corneal permeability to the drug, they should not be performed on the same day as pharmacologic testing. In general, the drops should be instilled in the inferior cul-de-sac, with care taken to use the same size drop in each eye. Drop administration should be repeated 1 to 5 minutes later. The pupil sizes then can be measured 30 to 45 minutes after instillation of the last set of drops. Baseline and test pupillary sizes are best measured in the same lighting conditions.

ABNORMALLY SHAPED PUPILS

Irregularly shaped pupils may be congenital or acquired (Table 13–1). Congenital conditions include:

1. *Aniridia,* in which the iris is hypoplastic, creating a large pupillary opening. Associated ocular findings often include cataracts, glaucoma, and impaired vision due to macular or optic nerve hypoplasia.[7] Patients with aniridia, genitourinary anomalies, mental retardation, and a defect in chromosome 11 are predisposed to Wilms' tumor.[8]
2. *Ectopia lentis et pupillae,* a rare heritable condition limited to the eyes in which lens dislocations may be associated with oval, ellipsoid, or slitlike displaced pupils.[8, 9]
3. An *iris coloboma* is a notch inferiorly or inferonasally in the iris (Fig. 13–5). This anomaly may be accompanied by chorioretinal or optic nerve colobomas, which like the iris abnormality are defects in closure of the embryonic fissure. Colobomas may occur in isolation in healthy individuals or in patients with chromosomal duplication or deletions. They may also be seen in complex congenital disorders such as CHARGE association (C = coloboma, H = heart disease, A = atresia or stenosis of the choanae, R = retarded growth and development or central nervous system anomalies, G = genital hypoplasia, and E = ear anomalies or deafness).[10]

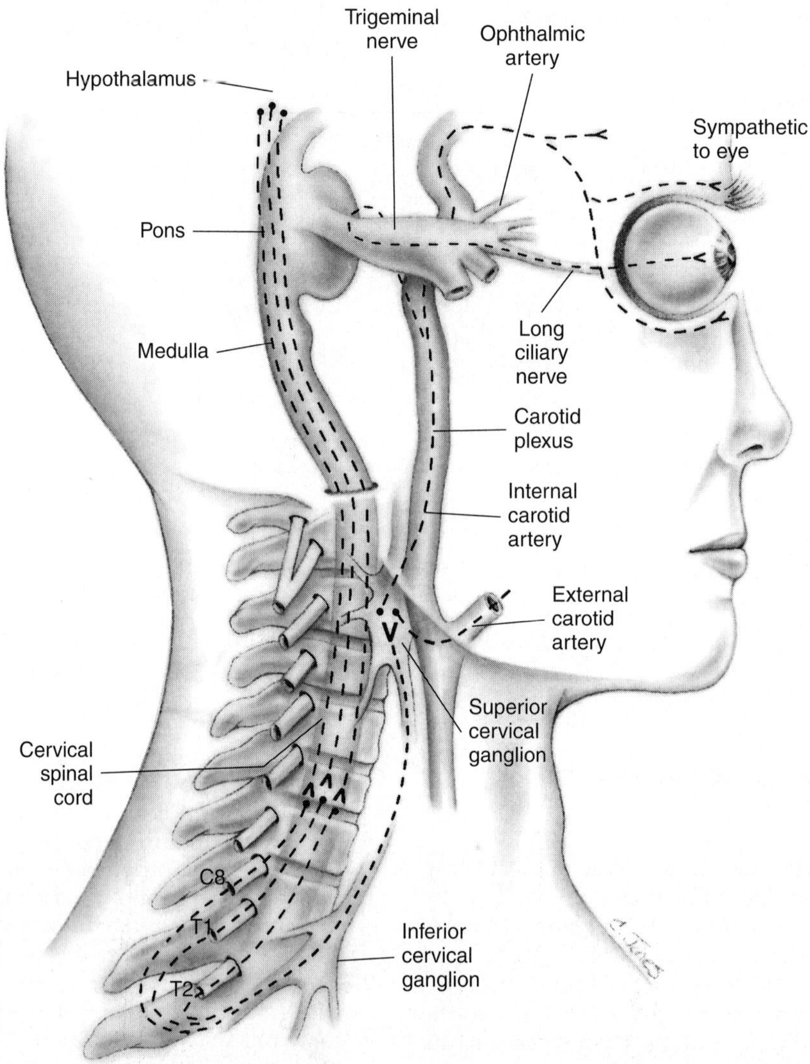

FIGURE 13–4. Sympathetic innervation of the pupil and eyelids. First-order hypothalamic (central) neurons descend through the brain stem (midbrain, pons, medulla) and cervical spinal cord. These fibers then synapse with preganglionic neurons, whose cell bodies lie in the intermediolateral grey column and whose axons exit the cord ipsilaterally at C8, T1, and T2 via the ventral roots. These second-order fibers then travel rostrally via the sympathetic chain, traverse the superior mediastinum, pass through the stellate ganglion, and terminate in the superior cervical ganglion, which lies at posterior to the angle of the mandible. The postganglionic axons ascend within the carotid plexus, which surrounds the internal carotid artery, to reach the cavernous sinus. The sympathetic branches ultimately reach the iris by first joining the sixth nerve, followed by connections to the branches of the first division of the trigeminal nerve, and then the long ciliary nerve. Sudomotor fibers (eg, for sweating) to the lower face follow the external carotid and then the facial arteries. Sympathetic fibers to Müller's muscles (upper eyelid elevators and lower eyelid depressors) also travel within the carotid plexus into the cavernous sinus, then may join branches of the third nerve before reaching the upper and lower eyelids (Redrawn from Liu GT: Disorders of the eyes and eyelids: Disorders of the pupil. In Samuels MA, Feske S (eds): The Office Practice of Neurology, p 62. New York, Churchill Livingstone, 1996, with permission.)

TABLE 13–1. Causes of Abnormally Shaped Pupils

Congenital Causes
Aniridia
Ectopia lentis et pupillae
Iris coloboma
Anterior chamber cleavage anomalies
Ectopic pupils
Persistent pupillary membranes
Acquired Causes
Iritis
Trauma (accidental or surgical)
Neurologic (eg, tonic pupils, midbrain damage, tadpole-shaped pupils)

4. *Anterior chamber cleavage anomalies*, such as Peters (central corneal defects) or Rieger syndrome (peripheral corneal defects), also may be associated with misshapen pupils accompanied by abnormal adhesions between the cornea and iris.[7, 11, 12]
5. *Ectopic pupils* (misplaced—also called *corectopia*) may be inherited as an isolated ocular finding.[13] Patients with these anomalies may require further genetic evaluation. An idiopathic tractional corectopia, in which a fibrous structure tethers the pupillary margin to the peripheral cornea and causes a misplaced pupil, has also been described.[14]
6. *Persistent pupillary membranes* may cause spokelike opacities across the pupil. These derive from persistence of the tunica vasculosa lentis, which supplies blood to the developing crystalline lens and normally disappears by the 34th week of gestation.[15]

Acquired causes of abnormally shaped pupils include:

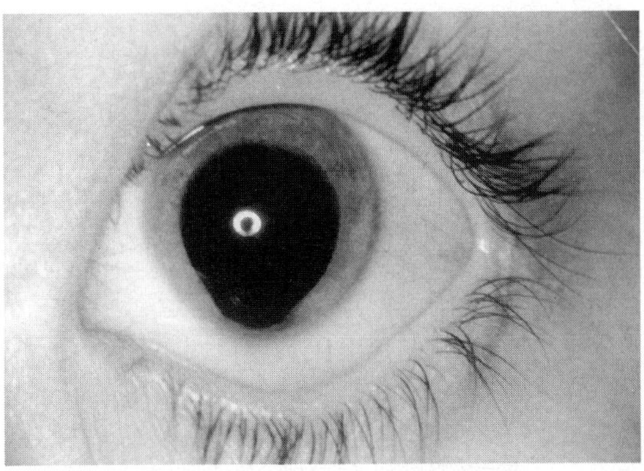

FIGURE 13–5. Iris coloboma, characterized by the inferior iris defect. (Photo courtesy of Dr. David Kozart. From Liu GT: Pupillary abnormalities in childhood. Contemp Pediatr 1995;12 (Nov):83-98, with permission.)

1. *Iritis.* Inflammation of the iris (iritis), seen in juvenile rheumatoid arthritis, for instance, may lead to adhesions between the iris and lens (posterior synechiae) and cause pupillary distortion (Fig. 13–6).
2. *Trauma* may result in an iris tear or rupture of the iris sphincter. The ocular trauma may be accidental, or the iris may be damaged during cataract surgery.
3. *Neurologic causes* such as tonic pupils, neurosyphilis, severe damage to the midbrain, which can rarely cause pupillary ectopia (Fig. 13–7), tadpole-shaped pupils, and other conditions (eg, herniation) associated with coma. These entities are all described in more detail below.

DEFECTIVE PUPILLARY LIGHT REACTION ASSOCIATED WITH VISION LOSS

In these cases the direct pupillary reaction to light is abnormal because of a disturbance within the afferent arc of the pupillary light reflex. In most such instances, there is associated visual loss.

Relative Afferent Pupillary Defect (RAPD)

The swinging flashlight test and the detection and grading of RAPDs are discussed in Chapter 2. Abnormal visual acuity and color vision, a central scotoma, and on RAPD collectively are highly suggestive of an optic neuropathy, although a large macular lesion could produce similar findings. In bilateral optic nerve disease, an RAPD may not be present unless the visual loss is highly asymmetric. An individual with severe unilateral visual loss, no RAPD, and a normal ocular examination may have nonorganic visual loss. An RAPD is not associated with visual loss due to corneal, lens, and vitreous opacities and refractive errors, but an amblyopic eye may have an RAPD.[16] Nevertheless, an amblyopic eye with an RAPD often requires further investigation to exclude an acquired optic neuropathy. When anisocoria is present, care should be taken to avoid overcalling an RAPD.[207]

Asymmetric chiasmal syndromes may be associated with an RAPD, especially if an eye has subnormal visual acuity. Isolated optic tract lesions may have a contralateral RAPD, despite normal visual acuities, because the defec-

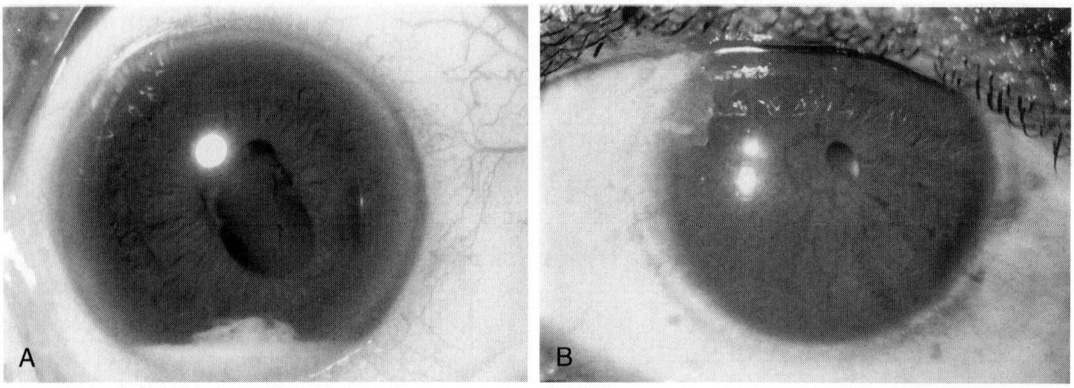

FIGURE 13–6. Misshapen pupils due to abnormal attachments between the iris and lens (iris synechiae) resulting from inflammation or the iris (iritis). **A.** Note the pus layered out at the bottom of the anterior chamber (hypopyon). (Photo courtesy of Dr. Stephen Orlin. From Liu GT: Pupillary abnormalities in childhood. Contemp Pediatr 1995;12 (Nov):83-98, with permission.) **B.** Small misshapen pupil due to syphilitic iritis.

tive temporal field in the contralateral eye is 61% to 71% larger than the nasal field of the ipsilateral eye, the nasal retina has a greater photoreceptor density, and the ratio of crossed to uncrossed fibers in the chiasm is 53:47.[17] Less commonly, when an optic tract lesion is associated with an incongrous homonymous hemianopia with greater involvement of the nasal field, the RAPD will be in the ipsilateral eye. *Behr's pupil* (a large contralateral pupil) and *Wernicke's hemianopic pupil*, one which reacts more briskly to light projected from within the intact hemifield than to light within the abnormal field, have been associated with optic tract syndromes. However, in clinical practice they are rarely identified, and the reliability of both signs has been questioned.[18]

Exceptional cases of RAPDs without visual loss can be associated with lesions in the midbrain pretectum,[19–22] which contains afferent pupillary fibers and the pretectal nuclei, but no visual fibers (Fig. 13–8). The RAPD is usually contralateral to the lesion. Most of these patients have other signs of dorsal midbrain involvement, such as upgaze paresis, ataxia, or fourth nerve dysfunction.

Amaurotic (Deafferented) Pupil

In the absence of any optic nerve or retinal function, or both, the eye is completely blind (ie, has no light perception (NLP)). The pupil is unreactive to even the brightest direct light stimuli because it is deafferented. If the fellow eye is normal and light is directed at it, the pupillary reaction in the affected eye (consensual) should be intact. An amaurotic pupil con-

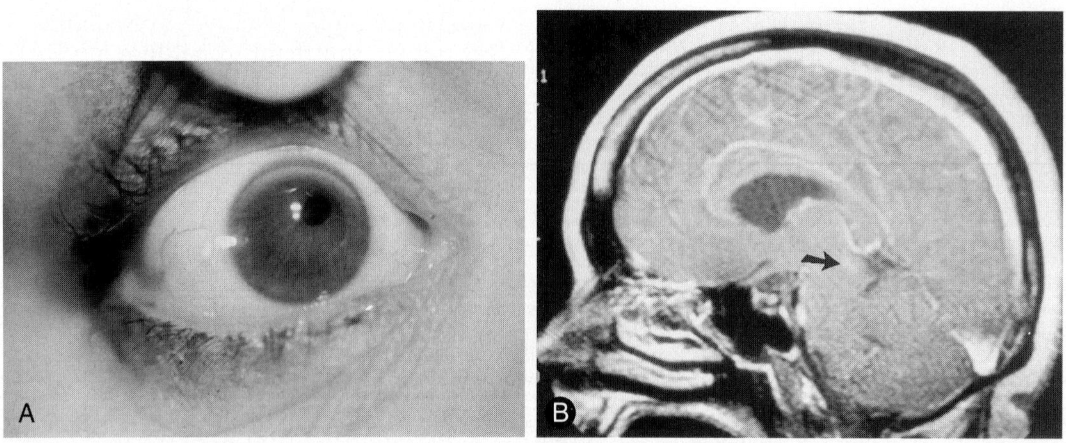

FIGURE 13–7. Pupil corectopia due to cysticercosis. **A.** The pupil of the right eye is displaced supranasally. **B.** T_1-weighted gadolinium-enhanced sagittal MRI scan from the same patient shows enhancement (*arrow*) in the sylvian aqueduct.

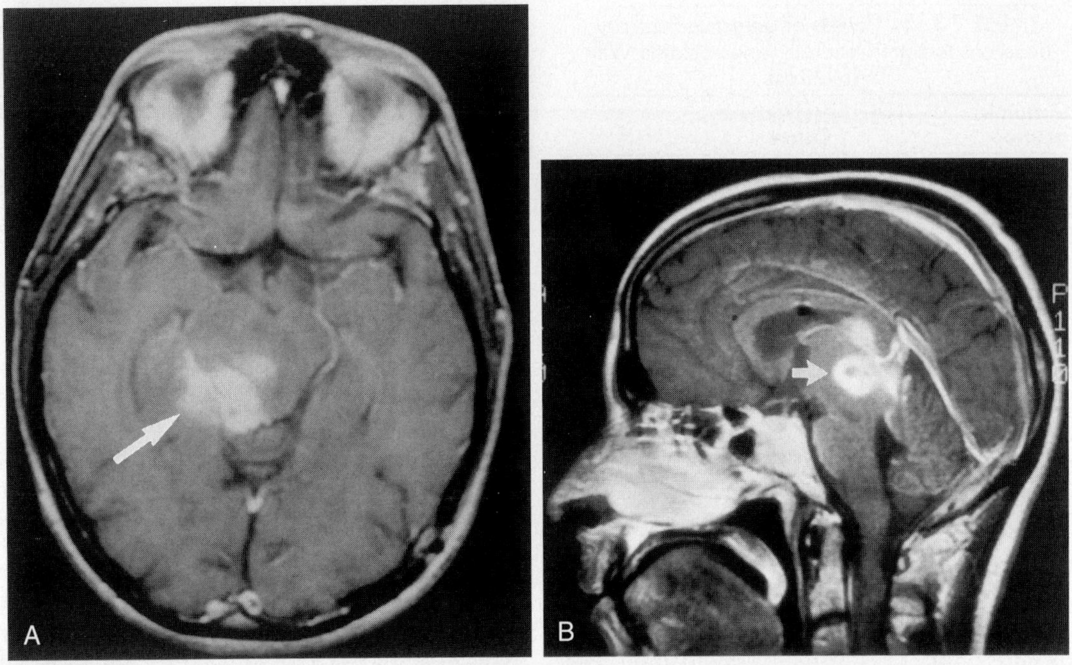

FIGURE 13–8. Thalamic and midbrain glioma responsible for a relative afferent pupillary defect with normal vision. T_1-weighted gadolinium-enhanced axial MRI scan, and (**A**) sagittal T1-weighted gadolinium enhanced MRI scan (**B**) showing tumor (*arrows*) and edema involving the dorsal midbrain, thalamus, and anterior medullary velum. (From King JT, Galetta SL, Flamm ES: Relative afferent pupillary defect with normal vision in a glial brainstem tumor. Neurology 1991;41:945-946, with permission.)

firms blindness if the patient claims not to see anything out of that eye. However if the pupil reacts to direct light in an eye with purported blindness, the visual loss is either nonorganic or has a cortical basis, or the patient is a poor observer. Bilateral deafferentiation will result in an increase in the resting size of both pupils, as less total light is able to reach the midbrain pretectum.

Deafferented pupils can also react during attempted gaze at near targets, and thus exhibit light–near dissociation (Table 13–2). Even individuals who are bilaterally blind can attempt to look at their thumb placed a few inches in front of their face and stimulate the near reflex, as the task can be accomplished using proprioceptive clues.

DEFECTIVE PUPILLARY LIGHT REACTION UNASSOCIATED WITH VISION LOSS

Defective pupillary light reactivity in most of these cases owes to dysfunction within the efferent arc of the pupillary light reflex, a so-called motor pupil. Lesions in the midbrain pretectum may also cause similar dysfunction. The major causes of this pupillary abnormality are highlighted in Table 13–3. A dilated pupil accompanied by eye movement or eyelid abnormalities suggests a lesion proximal to the ciliary ganglion (preganglionic), while an isolated dilated pupil would be more likely associated with a postganglionic process.

TABLE 13–2. Important Causes of Pupillary Light–Near Dissociation

Cause	Distinguishing Feature(s)
Deafferention	Associated visual loss
Tonic pupil	Tonic redilation; denervation hypersensitivity (see Table 13–4)
Tectal lesions (Parinaud syndrome)	Associated upgaze paresis
Argyll Robertson pupils	Small; no pupillary response to direct or consensual light stimulation
Aberrant regeneration of the third nerve	Miosis during adduction; other signs of third nerve paresis
Diabetes	Irregularly shaped pupil; history of retinal photocoagulation; other evidence of autonomic neuropathy

TABLE 13–3. Causes of Defective Pupillary Reactions to Light Generally Unassociated With Visual Loss

Anatomic Location	Cause
Dorsal midbrain	Tectal pupil (Parinaud syndrome)
	Argyll Robertson pupil
Third nerve	Third nerve palsy
Ciliary ganglion	Tonic pupil (Adie syndrome)
Synapse	Pharmacologic dilation
	Botulism
Iris sphincter	Trauma
	Angle-closure glaucoma
	Iritis

Anatomically, responsible lesions can be located in the dorsal midbrain or anywhere along the efferent parasympathetic pathway of the pupillary light reflex (see Fig. 13–2).

Pretectal Pupils

Lesions affecting the dorsal midbrain, causing the pretectal, or Parinaud, syndrome (see Chapter 16), may interfere with pupillary reactivity by disrupting ganglion cell axons entering the pretectal region. The pretectal nuclei may also be involved. Bilaterally the pupils may be midposition to large and exhibit light–near dissociation due to intact supranuclear influences upon midbrain accommodative centers (Fig. 13–9). Usually both pupils are involved, although size and light reactivity may be asymmetric. Occasionally the near response may also be defective, as accommodative and convergence insufficiency can be observed. The diagnosis is suggested when other features of Parinaud syndrome, such as upgaze paresis, convergence retraction nystagmus, and eyelid retraction, are evident. Common causes include pineal region tumors and hydrocephalus, so abnormal pupils suggestive of a tectal lesion would mandate neuroimaging.

Argyll Robertson Pupils

Argyll Robertson pupils[23] also exhibit light–near dissociation with a brisk near response, but typically are miotic, are slightly irregular, and dilate poorly in the dark (Fig. 13–10). The pupil does not react to light regardless of which eye is stimulated. Technically, to have an Argyll Robertson pupil, the involved eye must have some vision, to ensure the light–near dissociation is not due to a deafferented pupil. This pupillary abnormality is highly suggestive of syphilis and should therefore prompt serologic and fluorescent treponemal antibody absorption (FTA-ABS) testing. However, it is nonspecific and may also be caused by diabetes. The lesion responsible for Argyll Robertson pupils is uncertain but may result from a disturbance in the midbrain light-reflex pathway between the pretectal and Edinger–Westphal nuclei.

Third Nerve Palsy

Because the third nerve carries parasympathetic fibers originating from the Edinger–Westphal nuclei, injury to the third nerve often results in an ipsilateral poorly reactive or unreactive pupil.

Signs and Symptoms. In a *pupil-involving third nerve palsy,* the pupil is large and does not

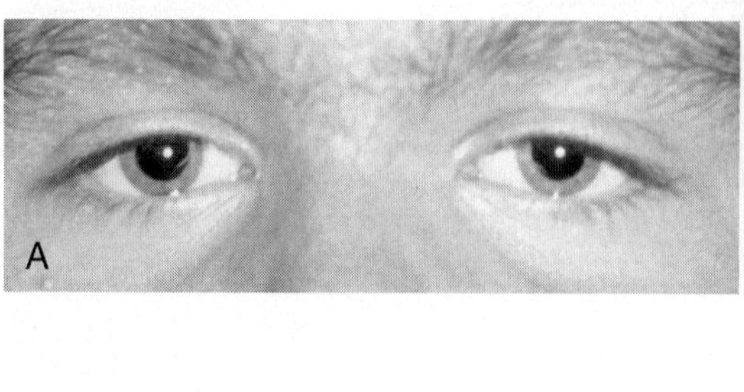

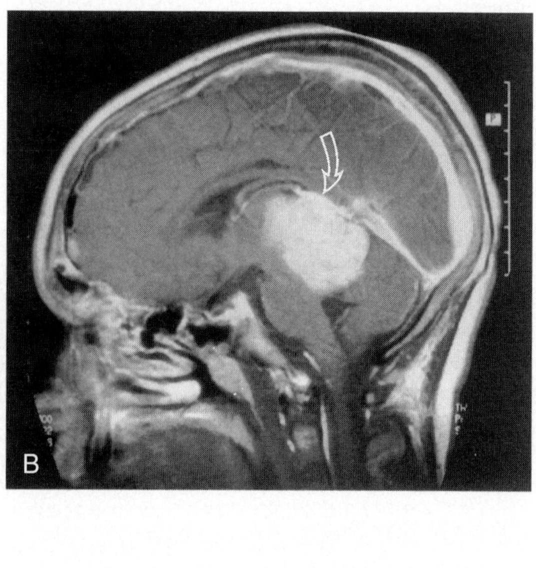

FIGURE 13–9. Tectal pupils associated with Parinaud syndrome due to a pineal region germinoma. **A.** This 10-year-old boy presented with headache, gait unsteadiness, precocious puberty, acne, and blurry vision. On examination he was also found to have upgaze paresis, accommodative insufficiency, and pupils that were large, poorly reactive to light, but reactive to near stimuli (light–near dissociation). **B.** Sagittal gadolinium-enhanced MRI scan demonstrating a large enhancing pineal region mass (*arrow*) compressing the dorsal midbrain.

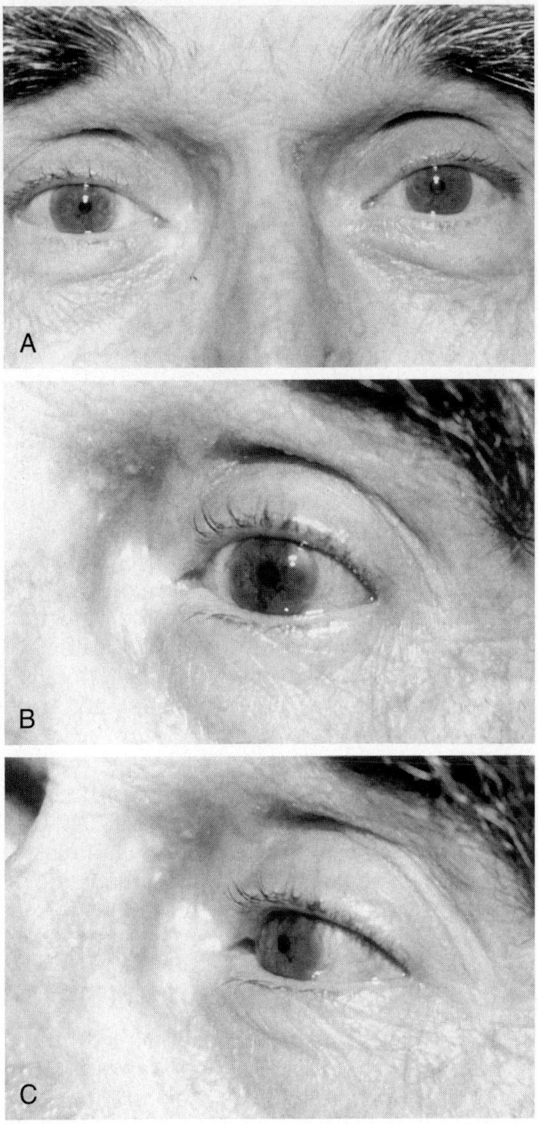

FIGURE 13–10. Argyll Robertson pupils in tabes dorsalis (absent deep tendon reflexes, loss of vibratory sense and proprioception in the lower extremities, and Charcot joints). The pupils are small (**A**), poorly reactive to light (**B**), but constrict to near stimuli (**C**). (The patient was seen courtesy of Dr. J. Lawton Smith.) (From Liu GT: Disorders of the eyes and eyelids: Disorders of the pupil. In Samuels MA, Feske S (eds): The Office Practice of Neurology, p 66. New York, Churchill Livingstone, 1996, with permission.)

constrict to light or near stimuli, either directly or consensually (internal ophthalmoplegia) (Fig. 13–11). Usually either ptosis or a deficit in adduction, depression, or elevation of the eye, or a combination of these findings, will assist in the diagnosis of a third nerve palsy, but in very rare instances a dilated pupil is the only manifestation. In inferior division third nerve palsies, the pupil and inferior rectus muscles are involved. In a *pupil-sparing third nerve palsy*, the eye movements or lid are affected, but the pupil retains normal size and reactivity.

Because a dilated pupil exposes spherical aberrations of the lens and cornea, some patients with pupil-involving third nerve palsies complain of blurry vision in that eye. Because this is a refractive problem, a pinhole occluder may resolve the cloudy vision. This simple maneuver helps exclude other causes of visual loss associated with a third nerve palsy, such as Terson syndrome or an or optic neuropathy.

Abnormal miosis during attempted ocular adduction or depression may be a sign of *aberrant regeneration* (or *synkinesis* or *misdirection*) following a third nerve palsy (Fig. 13–12).[24] The phenomenon results when fibers that had previously supplied the medial rectus or inferior rectus regenerate and accidentally reach the ciliary ganglion, then connect with postganglionic neurons, which innervate the pupil. In these situations the pupil does not react to direct or consensual light stimulation but contracts during ocular adduction or depression. Segmental contraction of the iris sphincter during eye movements (Czarnecki's sign[25]) may also be observed in these instances. Furthermore, because postganglionic accommodative fibers far outnumber those dedicated to the pupillary light reflex (see tonic pupil, below), pupillary miosis during accommodation is more likely to recover than constriction to direct light (light–near dissociation). These pupillary signs are sometimes accompanied by other manifestations of aberrant regeneration of the third nerve, such as elevation of the ptotic eyelid during adduction or depression of the eye.

Etiology. Pupil involvement is commonly seen in nuclear, fascicular, and especially subarachnoid third nerve palsies. As alluded to earlier, the external location of the pupillary fibers of

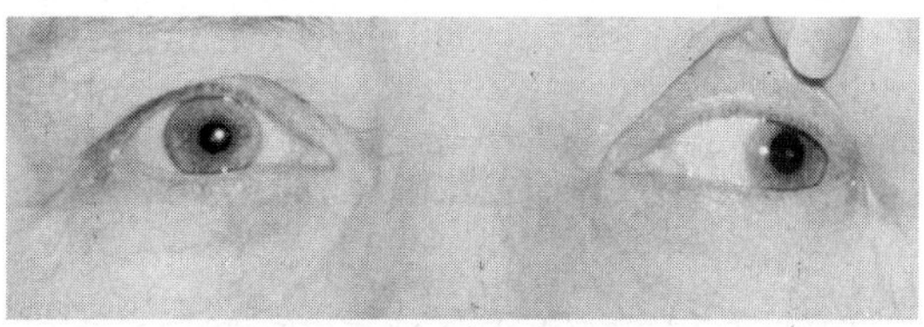

FIGURE 13–11. Pupil-involving left third nerve palsy following basilar artery aneurysm clipping. The ptotic left eyelid is being held up, revealing the exotropic left eye and dilated left pupil.

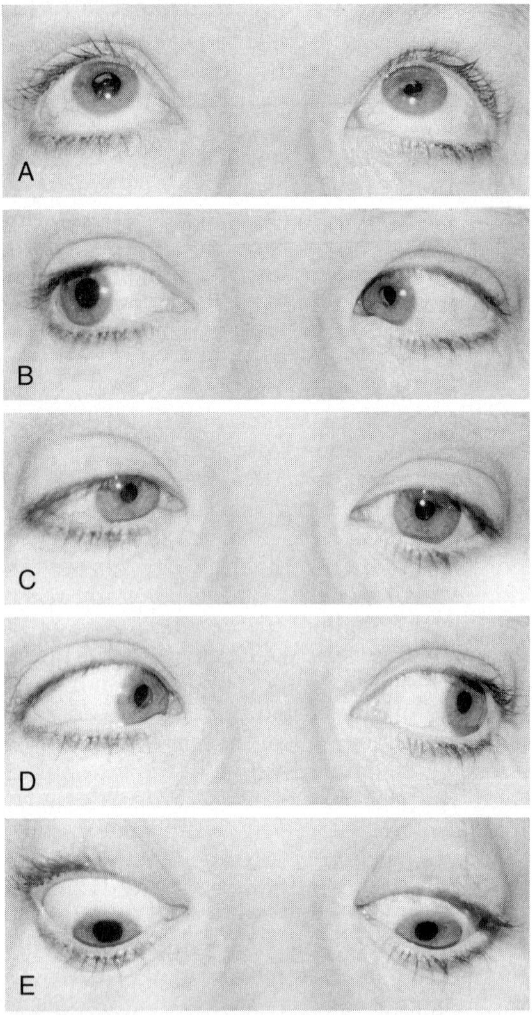

FIGURE 13–12. Pupillary constriction in adduction due to aberrant regeneration of the right third nerve. Pituitary apoplexy had caused ptosis and complete ophthalmoplegia of the right eye (see Fig. 7–21), which recovered. The right pupil remained slightly enlarged, but was reactive to light. Note in upgaze (**A**), rightward gaze (**B**), and downgaze (**E**), the right pupil is larger than the left. However, the right pupil constricts during adduction of the right eye (**D**), and constricts more than the left when viewing a near target (**C**).

the third nerve renders them particularly vulnerable to compression and infiltration in subarachnoid processes such as meningitis, aneurysmal compression (posterior communicating or internal carotid), and uncal herniation (Hutchinson's pupil). *Pupil-sparing third nerve palsies* in middle-age to elderly patients are usually related to diabetes or hypertension, but occasionally can be seen even in fascicular or subarachnoid third nerve palsies from other causes. However, an aneurysm that presents initially with external ophthalmoparesis or ptosis alone typically will involve the pupil within several days.[26]

Aberrant regeneration typically occurs in traumatic or compressive third nerve palsies, sometimes with congenital or tumor-related third nerve palsies, but *never* in diabetic or hypertensive third nerve palsies.

Pharmacologic Testing. A chronically dilated pupil due to a third nerve palsy may be difficult to distinguish from a tonic pupil (see below). Although the latter redilates slowly after constriction, both may exhibit light–near dissociation, segmental paresis of the iris sphincter, and denervation hypersensitivity.[27,28] The last characteristic, demonstrated by pupillary constriction following instillation of dilute (0.125%) pilocarpine eye drops, does not seem to depend on whether the lesion is anatomically before or after the ciliary ganglion (ie, pre- or postganglionic), or whether there is aberrant regeneration. Jacobson[29–31] has offered the following explanations for denervation hypersensitivity in preganglionic third nerve lesions: (1) transsynaptic degeneration of postganglionic axons; (2) the greater sensitivity of larger pupils than smaller ones to dilute pilocarpine; and (3) upregulation of acetylcholine receptors because of decreased cholinergic stimulation following third nerve injury. Denervation hypersensitivity in acute pupil-involving third nerve palsies, due to unclear mechanisms, is less common but has been observed.[32]

Management. If the patient has isolated pupillary dilation along with other signs of a third nerve palsy, an aneurysm of the posterior communicating artery should be considered until proven otherwise. In this situation it is often useful to obtain an emergent computed tomography (CT) or magnetic resonance imaging (MRI) scan before proceeding with angiography since other compressive lesions may be found, eliminating the need for an invasive procedure. However, if the scan cannot be obtained immediately, we would proceed directly to angiography. If the scan is negative, even if it includes MRI-angiography (MRA), conventional angiography is still necessary to exclude an aneurysm. Keane and Ahmadi have documented two patients with third nerve palsy and posterior communicating artery aneurysms measuring 5 to 6 mm missed by MRA.[33] A recent study evaluating the accuracy of three-dimensional MRA in the detection of intracranial aneurysms found a mean sensitivity of 63% among five observers using conventional angiography as the gold standard.[34] Furthermore, higher diagnostic sensitivity was found for anterior communicating and middle cerebral aneurysms compared to internal carotid artery aneurysms.

The reader is referred to a more detailed discussion regarding the differential diagnosis and management of third nerve palsies, in addition to issues regarding pupil-involving versus pupil-sparing third nerve palsies as well as aberrant regeneration in Chapter 15.

Tonic Pupils

Clinical Symptoms and Signs. (See Table 13–4.) Patients with a tonic pupil often discover that they have a unilateral, partially dilated pupil while looking in the mirror, or a friend notices the pupillary inequality. Affected individuals are usually otherwise healthy and more commonly female. They may be symptomatic with photophobia or difficulty reading with that eye. In general, the disorder is painless although occasionally patients will complain of a cramping sensation in the affected eye resulting from ciliary body spasm.

Characteristically the pupil is large, exhibits light–near dissociation (Fig. 13–13), and redilates slowly after constriction (hence the term "tonic"). In some patients, especially in early cases, the near response may also be defective, or the individual may have difficulty refixing from near to far visual targets ("tonic" accommodation). Corneal sensation may be depressed. On a slit-lamp examination, the pupil may be irregular, with sectoral paralysis (immobility of parts of the pupil during light stimulation),[35] vermiform movements, and loss of pupillary ruff (the normal border of the pupil)[36] (Fig. 13–14). After 1 or 2 months, a tonic pupil may become miotic and smaller than the fellow pupil. In most patients the disorder is unilateral, but in about 10% of cases, the other pupil may become involved months or years later.[37]

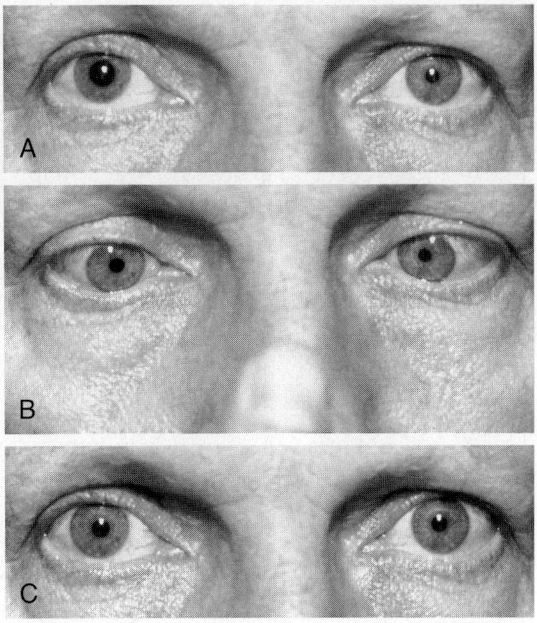

FIGURE 13–13. Idiopathic right tonic pupil. The right pupil is mid-position and larger than the left (**A**), poorly reactive to light, but reactive to near stimulus (the examiner's thumb) (**B**). The patient complained of blurry vision in the right eye while attempting to read, consistent with accommodation paresis. After instillation of 0.125% pilocarpine eye drops at 0 and 5 minutes into both conjunctivae 30 minutes later, the right pupil was found to have constricted while the left was unchanged ((**C**) compared with (**A**)), indicating denervation hypersensitivity on the right. (From Liu GT: Disorders of the eyes and eyelids: Disorders of the pupil. In Samuels MA, Feske S (eds): The Office Practice of Neurology, p 65. New York, Churchill Livingstone, 1996, with permission.)

TABLE 13–4. Clinical Features of Tonic Pupils

Presentation
Anisocoria noticed by the patient or others
Painless
Difficulty reading
Difficulty refocusing from near to far stimuli
Photophobia
More common in women
Examination
Initially large in size, but in chronic cases can become more miotic
Light–near dissociation (sometimes miosis at near response is also lost acutely)
Tonic redilation
Anisocoria worse in the dark (when unilateral)
Sectoral paralysis
Vermiform movements of the iris
Loss of pupillary ruff
Accommodative insufficiency
Depressed corneal sensation
Bilateral in 10% of cases
Pharmacologic testing
Denervation sensitivity, demonstrated by pupillary constriction following instillation of dilute (0.125%) pilocarpine

Pathophysiology. The pupillary abnormality results from damage to the ciliary ganglion or the postganglionic short ciliary nerves (see Fig. 13–3), which innervate the pupillary sphincter and ciliary muscles (the latter is important for accommodation). Partial preservation of the

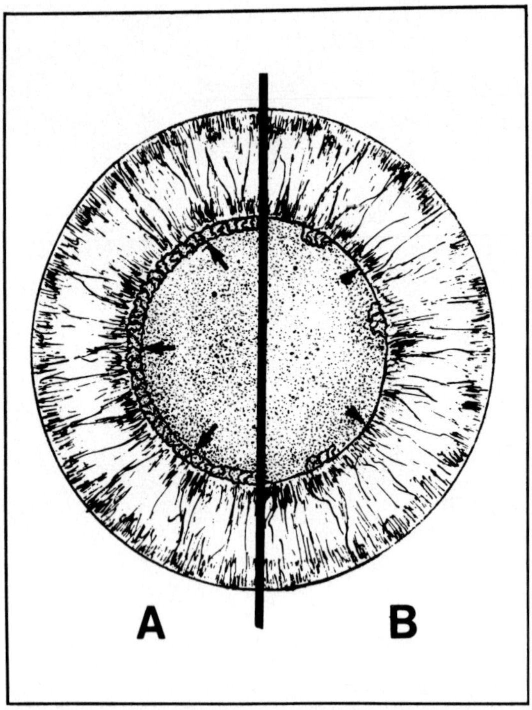

FIGURE 13–14. Normal (**A**) and abnormal, atrophic (**B**) pupillary ruff (*arrows*). The latter may be seen in patients with tonic pupils. (From Gilmore PC, Carlow TJ. Diabetic oculomotor paresis with pupil fixed to light. Neurology 1980;30:1229-1230, with permission.)

pupil's parasympathetic innervation results in areas of segmental contraction adjacent to sector paralysis. When normal portions of the pupil contract, they pull and twist paralyzed segments toward them. Accommodation paresis accounts for the difficulty with near vision, and the photophobia results from the poor pupillary constriction to light. The light–near dissociation can be explained by the 30 : 1 ratio of accommodative fibers arising from the ciliary ganglion relative to those responsible for pupillary constriction.[37] Hence damage to the ciliary ganglion or short ciliary nerves would have a greater chance of disabling pupillary constriction to light than disrupting miosis associated with accommodation. Furthermore, as neuronal cell bodies in the ciliary ganglion sprout new axons following injury, postganglionic accommodative fibers may mistakenly reinnervate the iris sphincter. This misdirection results in excess pupillary constriction during accommodation.

Etiology. The causes of tonic pupils fall into three major groups:

1. *Adie syndrome,* which is a symptom complex consisting of tonic pupil(s) and absent deep tendon reflexes. The cause has yet to be elucidated, but the disorder may be explained by concurrent involvement of the ciliary and dorsal root ganglia or root entry zone. This is the most common cause of a tonic pupil. Ross syndrome is a rare, related condition characterized by the triad of tonic pupil, hyporeflexia, and segmental anhidrosis. It is probably related to injury to sympathetic and parasympathetic ganglion cells or their postganglionic projections.[38–40]
2. *Local ocular processes* that affect the ciliary ganglion or short ciliary nerves, such as eye or orbital trauma, or viral illnesses (eg, varicella), or ischemia (eg, giant cell arteritis or other vasculitides[41] or strabismus surgery). Orbital tumors have also been reported in association with tonic pupils (Fig. 13–15).[42] Retinal photocoagulation (laser) in patients with diabetic retinopathy may damage the ciliary nerves underlying the retina.[43] The resultant pupil is typically irregularly shaped and poorly reactive to light (Fig. 13–16). Other factors contributing to a poorly reactive pupil in diabetics can include laser damage to the iris sphincter muscle as well as autonomic neuropathy.
3. *Widespread autonomic dysfunction,* uncommonly, tonic pupils may occur in association with neurosyphilis, advanced diabetes mellitus, dysautonomias (eg, Shy–Drager and Riley–Day syndromes), amyloidosis, sarcoidosis, Guillain–Barré syndrome, Miller Fisher variant (see below), or Charcot–Marie–Tooth and Dejerine–Sottas neuropathies.[37] In one large series of Lambert–Eaton myasthenic syndrome, 6 of 50 patients (12%) had sluggish pupillary reactions to light, and 2 of these displayed tonic pupil physiology.[44]

Pharmacologic Testing. Because of iris sphincter denervation cholinergic hypersensitivity, chronically tonic pupils will constrict following administration of dilute (0.125%) pilocarpine (see Fig. 13–13).[45] Pilocarpine is a cholinergic substance that can act directly on the iris dilator muscle at higher concentrations. However, normal pupils typically have little or no reponse to dilute pilocarpine. The test should be considered positive when the pupil in question constricts more than the fellow pupil (assuming the fellow pupil is normal). The solution can be premixed or made readily by combining 0.1 cc of 1% pilocarpine with 0.7 cc

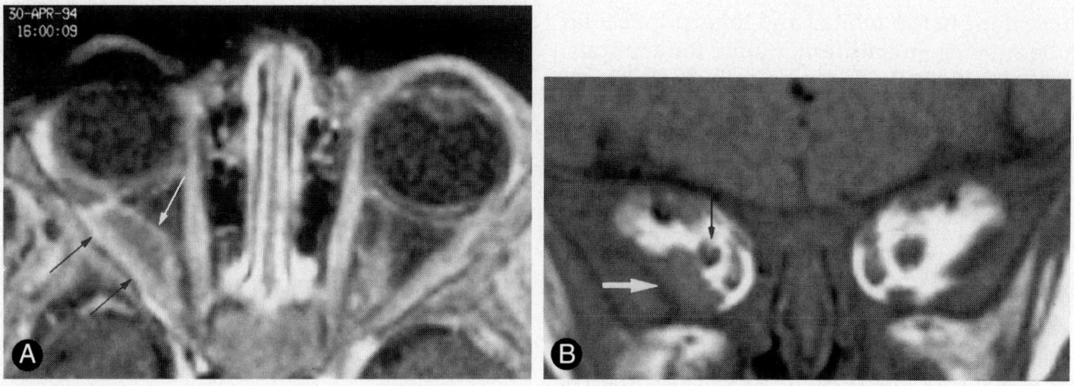

FIGURE 13–15. Posterolateral orbital mass that caused a tonic pupil in an infant. The lesion, which presumably compressed the ciliary ganglion or short ciliary nerves, was demonstrated to be a glial–neural hamartoma at biopsy. **A.** Axial contrast-enhanced MRI scan (TR = 600, TE with fat saturation) reveals enhancement on the periphery (*white arrow*) of the mass. There is normal contrast enhancement of the rectus muscles, and thus the right lateral rectus (*black arrows*) can be distinguished from the mass that lies along it. **B.** Coronal MRI scan (TR = 700, TE = 15) reveals the mass (*white arrow*) in the inferolateral aspect of the right orbit and obscuring the inferior and lateral rectus muscles, which are visible in the normal left orbit. The mass abuts the optic nerve sheath complex (*black arrow*), which is slightly displaced superiorly. (From Brooks-Kayal AR, Liu GT, Menacker SJ, et al: Tonic pupil and orbital glial-neural hamartoma in infancy. Am J Ophthalmol 1995;119:809-811, with permission from Elsevier Science.)

of sterile saline in a 1-cc tuberculin syringe. With the needle removed, the syringe can be used as a dropper, with care taken to administer the same size drops into each eye.

Some caution is also necessary in interpreting the dilute pilocarpine test since some patients with preganglionic parasympathetic dysfunction (see above) will also respond to dilute pilocarpine.[31]

Management. Since tonic pupils may be a manifestation of neurosyphilis, FTA-ABS or microhemagglutination assay—*Treponema Pallidum* (MHA-TP) testing should be obtained in those patients without a defined cause for their dilated pupil.[46] No further laboratory workup is indicated, as tonic pupils usually have a benign cause. The presence or absence of deep tendon reflexes should be noted.

Symptomatic treatment is sometimes helpful. Refractive correction may be prescribed for reading in those with accommodative insufficiency, for instance. Rarely, some patients find the anisocoria bothersome cosmetically, and these individuals might find pupil-forming contact lenses or dilute pilocarpine helpful. Dilute pilocarpine may also aid accommodation, and in addition may relieve photophobia. However, some patients find the induced pupillary miosis intolerably painful.

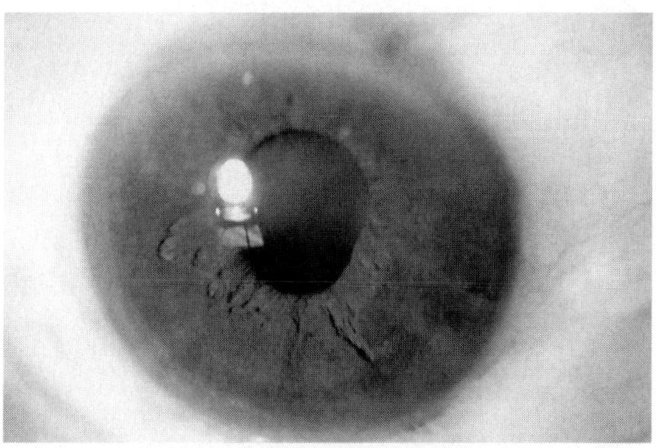

FIGURE 13–16. Irregularly shaped pupil in a diabetic patient who had undergone panretinal photocoagulation and whose diabetes was complicated by peripheral and autonomic neuropathy.

Pharmacologically Dilated Pupils

Pupils dilated surreptitiously or as part of an ophthalmic evaluation with anticholinergic agents such as atropine, tropicamide, or cyclopentolate are generally large (>7 to 8 mm) and unreactive to light or near stimulation.[47] Pharmacologically dilated pupils can also occur accidentally in an individual who has contact with atropine-like drugs, a scopolamine patch, or plants such as jimson weed or blue nightshade, who then touches his eye. Other patients may consciously place mydriatic solutions in their eye as part of a functional illness (Münchausen syndrome, for example). Pupils that are overly generous and unreactive but appear normal on slit-lamp examination should suggest pharmacologic dilation, because third nerve-related and tonic pupils tend to be smaller. In addition, unlike tonic pupils, pharmacologically dilated pupils do not react to near targets.

Pharmacologic Testing. One percent pilocarpine drops will fail to constrict pharmacologically dilated pupils (examined after 30 minutes) because the postsynaptic receptors have been blocked.[48] However, 1% pilocarpine would be effective in normal pupils, as well as third nerve-related mydriasis, tonic pupils, and other pre- and postganglionic parasympathetic disorders because in these cases the receptors at the iris constrictor muscle are either normal or hypersensitive. This test should be applied with caution, as dilated pupils due to traumatic iridoplegia and acute narrow-angle glaucoma would also fail to constrict with 1% pilocarpine (see below).[47] The 1% pilocarpine test should also be interpreted carefully if it is performed near the termination of pharmacologic blockade, since the affected pupil may constrict.

Neuromuscular Junction Blockade

Patients with botulism, who have defective release of acetylcholine, can develop bilaterally dilated pupils and accommodative paresis with varying degrees of ptosis and ophthalmoparesis. The eye findings are often accompanied by bulbar or generalized weakness.[49, 50] In general, the pupils are unaffected in myasthenia gravis, which affects nicotinic and not muscarinic cholinergic synapses. Both botulism and myasthenia gravis are discussed in more detail in Chapter 14.

Ocular Causes of Unreactive Pupils

The clinical history or slit-lamp examination may suggest the following conditions. Depending on disease severity, the pupillary constriction with 1% pilocarpine may be defective.

1. *Ocular trauma.* Following trauma to the eye, the pupil may be fixed and unreactive (traumatic iridoplegia). Responsible mechanisms include tears or stunning of the iris sphincter muscle, tearing of short ciliary nerves, or compression of the ciliary nerves or ganglion by blunt trauma or a retrobulbar hemorrhage.
2. *Angle-closure glaucoma.* This disorder, an ophthalmic emergency, should be considered when the pupil is mid-dilated and fixed, and the patient acutely complains of visual loss, nausea, vomiting, eye pain, and a rainbow-colored halo seen around lights. Ocular pressures can be very high (>60 mm Hg), and visual acuity may be markedly impaired. Slit-lamp examination will identify the characteristic shallow anterior chamber, cornea edema, and ciliary or conjunctival injection. Pupillary nonreactivity is the result of sphincter muscle ischemia. If left untreated, the pupil may remain fixed, and the iris can become atrophic.
3. *Iritis.* When affected by iritis, the pupil can be small, irregular, and poorly reactive (see Fig. 13–6B). Cells and flare in the anterior chamber, iris synechiae, and keratic precipitates seen on slit-lamp examination help establish the diagnosis. Photophobia is the major complaint, and there is less pain and the onset is more gradual than in angle-closure glaucoma. Because of the synechiae, the pupil dilates poorly and irregularly, even with mydriatics.

ANISOCORIA

The most common cause of asymmetric pupils (anisocoria) is nonpathologic *simple* (*essential, physiologic*) *anisocoria* (Fig. 13–17). The latter occurs in 15% to 30% of the normal population,[51, 52] and is characterized by normal pupillary constriction and dilation as well as

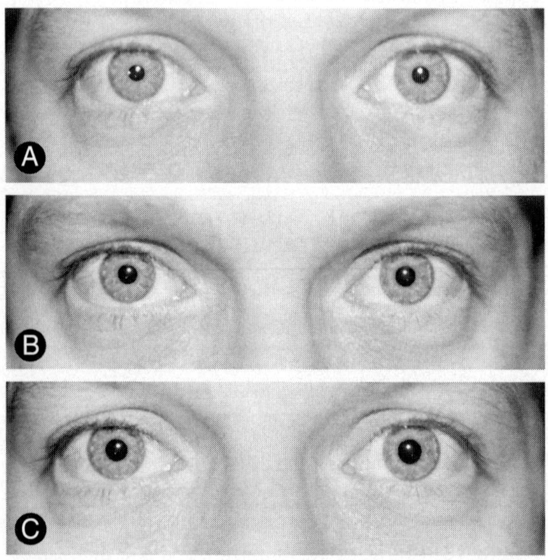

FIGURE 13–17. Physiologic anisocoria. The amount of pupillary inequality is roughly the same in (**A**) bright light, (**B**) in ambient light, and (**C**) in the dark.

little change in the net amount of anisocoria under light and dark conditions.[1] The pupillary inequality in these cases is rarely more than 1 mm.[53] Often the simple anisocoria will be evident on old photographs or a driver's license, which can be viewed critically with a slit-lamp or 20-diopter lens. No further testing is necessary in these instances. It is rare for the pupil asymmetry to change sides in physiologic anisocoria (see idiopathic alternating anisocoria, below).

If the anisocoria is not physiologic, the next issue to resolve is which pupil is the abnormal one, assuming the problem is unilateral. The process combines examination of the pupillary light reactions and measurements of the anisocoria in light and dark.[53] If the pupillary inequality is greater in the light, and if one pupil is sluggish to light stimulation, then this pupil is the abnormal one. Likely the lesion lies in the efferent arc of the pupillary light reflex, or there may be pharmacologic blockade or iris damage. These pupillary abnormalities are discussed above in the sections on pupils with defective reactions to light, and the differential diagnosis includes those entities listed in Table 13–3.

A greater difference in darkness, with normal pupillary reactivity to light, implies either oculosympathetic paresis on the side with the smaller pupil or, less commonly, simple anisocoria, which may be less evident in light due to mechanical limitations of the iris.[54]

Figure 13–18 outlines an algorithm for evaluating anisocoria when only one pupil is abnormal.

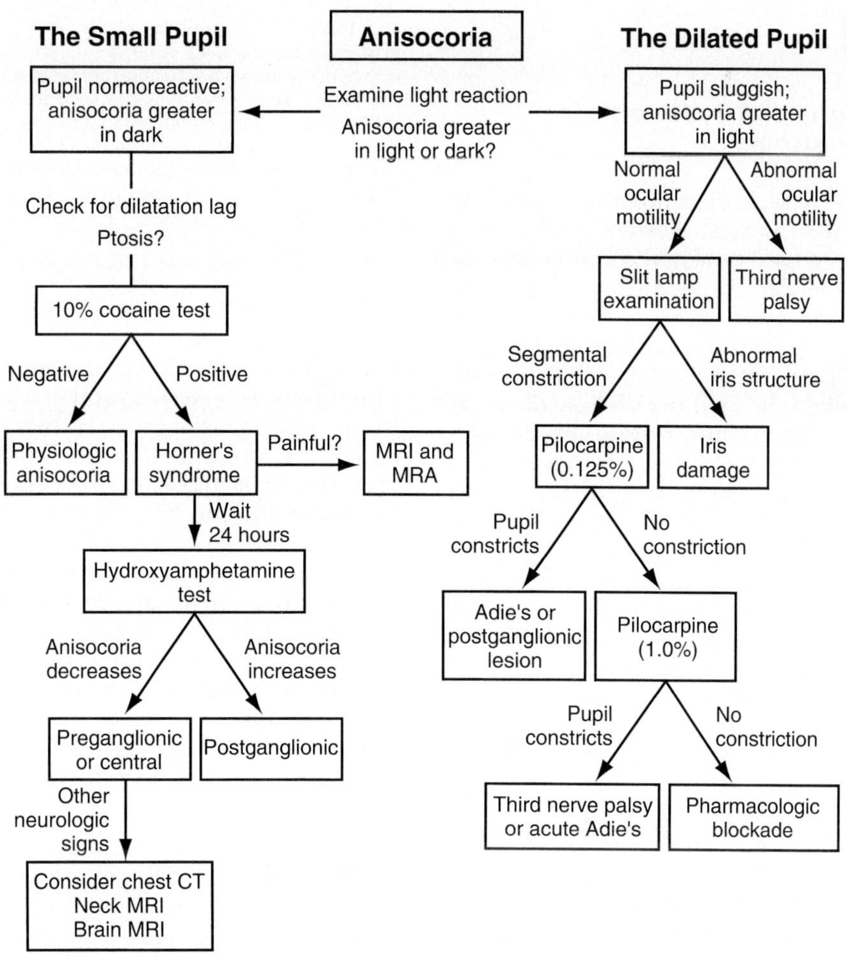

FIGURE 13–18. A diagnostic approach to anisocoria. The chart guides the workup of an abnormal pupil and assumes the other pupil is normal. (From Galetta SL, Liu GT, Volpe NJ: Neuro-ophthalmology. In: Evans R (ed): Diagnostic Testing in Neurology, Neurol Clinics, Vol. 14, p 212, with permission. Adapted from Thompson HS, Pilley SF: Unequal pupils: a flow chart for sorting out the anisocorias. Surv Ophthalmol 1976;21:45, with permission.)

DISORDERS OF PUPILLARY DILATION—OCULOSYMPATHETIC DISRUPTION (HORNER SYNDROME)

Horner syndrome, characterized primarily by unilateral miosis, facial anhidrosis, and mild upper and lower eyelid ptosis (Fig. 13–19),[55, 56] is the most important neuro-ophthalmic cause of a small pupil that dilates poorly when the lights are turned off. Table 13–5 lists the differential diagnosis of other entities which should be considered, and most of them have been discussed previously in other sections of this chapter.

Horner syndrome is caused by interruption of any of the three oculosympathetic neurons (see Fig. 13–4). The causes and management will be discussed according to which neuron has been affected, and the management of Horner syndrome in childhood also will be reviewed.

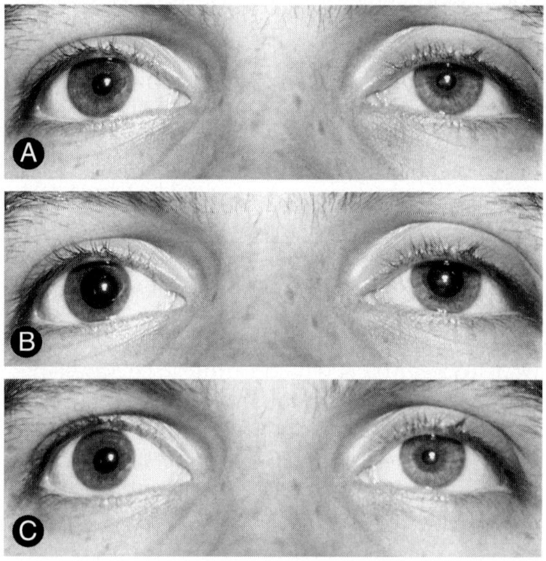

FIGURE 13–19. Left Horner syndrome due to cervical spinal cord trauma. **A.** In room light, the left pupil is miotic, and there is left upper lid ptosis. **B.** The anisocoria is greater in the dark. **C.** After instillation of 10% cocaine into both conjunctivae at 0 and 1 minutes, 45 minutes later, the normal right pupil was found to have dilated while the left pupil remained the same, confirming oculosympathetic paresis on the left. (From Liu GT: Disorders of the eyes and eyelids: Disorders of the pupil. In Samuels MA, Feske S (eds): The Office Practice of Neurology, p 67. New York, Churchill Livingstone, 1996, with permission.)

Clinical Signs and Symptoms in Horner Syndrome

Because of the lack of sympathetic input to the iris dilator muscle, Horner syndrome is strongly suggested when the anisocoria increases in the dark or if dilation lag of the miotic pupil is observed (Table 13–6). Dilation lag may be demonstrated at the bedside by turning the lights off and observing the pupils with a dim light directed from below the nose. The normal pupil dilates briskly, but it takes time for the sympathetically denervated pupil to reach its final resting state in the dark.[57] Typically, measurements of pupil size are made at 5 and 15 seconds to document this dilation disparity in darkness, and there is usually more anisocoria at the earlier measurement. The pupil in Horner syndrome reacts normally to light and near stimuli.

The upper lid ptosis is always mild and rarely ever covers the visual axis. The lower lid may be slightly elevated (lower eyelid, or upside-down, ptosis). The upper and lower eyelid ptosis may give the false impression that the eye is set back in the orbit (pseudoenophthalmos).

Horner syndrome by itself does not cause visual symptoms. However, disruption in sympathetic input to the eye may produce several other ocular signs. There may be conjunctival congestion or transient ocular hypotony. Because iris melanocytes require oculosympathetic input, congenital Horner syndromes can be associated with an ipsilateral lighter colored iris (*iris heterochromia*).[58] In rare instances, heterochromia may also result from acquired instances of Horner syndrome.[59] Also, neurotrophic corneal endothelial failure has been reported in association with Horner syndrome.[208]

Theoretically, lesions of the third-order neuron distal to the carotid bifurcation result in loss of sweating on the medial aspect of the forehead and side of the nose, while more proximal lesions, including those of the first- and second-order neurons, decrease sweating in the whole half of the face.[60] Hemibody sweating would also be anticipated from first-order neuron dysfunction. However, the ex-

TABLE 13–5. Differential Diagnosis of a Small Pupil That Dilates Poorly

Oculosympathetic paresis (Horner syndrome)
Iritis
Pharmacologic miosis
Tonic pupil (chronic)
Argyll Robertson pupil

TABLE 13–6. Clinical Features of Oculosympathetic Paresis (Horner Syndrome)

Presentation
Anisocoria noticed by the patient or others
Unassociated with visual loss

Examination[64]
Pupillary miosis
Anisocoria worse in the dark
Pupillary dilation lag
Minimal ptosis of the upper lid
"Inverse" or "upside-down" ptosis of the lower lid
Pseudoenophthalmos
Anhidrosis
Conjunctival congestion
Ocular hypotony, transient
Iris heterochromia (in congenital cases, typically)

Pharmacologic testing
Greater than 1 mm of relative anisocoria following instillation of 10% cocaine eye drops into both eyes
In postganglionic lesions, increase in the relative anisocoria by at least 1 mm following instillation of 1% hydroxyamphetamine drops into both eyes

pected patterns are present inconsistently, and the air conditioning in most hospitals and offices often masks any anhidrosis, making it a less important practical sign of Horner syndrome compared with the ptosis and miosis. If desired, the exact pattern of sweating may be outlined with alizarin powder, which turns dark purple when it comes in contact with perspiration.[40]

Etiology and Localization of Horner Syndrome

Table 13–7 outlines the differential diagnosis of Horner syndrome according to localization and frequency. The various causes have been analyzed in large series, and the most common localization varies, most likely due to selection bias. In a study of inpatients with acquired oculosympathetic palsy,[61] 63% had involvement of the first-order neuron, reflecting a large proportion of patients with strokes. The second-order neuron (preganglionic) was the most common lesion site in two other studies,[62,63] while the third-order neuron (postganglionic) was most frequent in another, reflecting the authors' interest in vascular headaches.[64] The ganglion referred to is the superior cervical ganglion, thus "preganglionic" refers to the second-order neuron, "postganglionic" to the third-order neuron.

The presence of other clinical signs or symptoms may help localize the Horner syndrome. Sweat patterns have been mentioned already. Brain stem or spinal cord signs suggest involvement of the first-order neuron. Arm pain, or a history of neck or shoulder trauma, surgery, or catheterization point to injury of the second-order neuron. Horner syndrome accompanied by ipsilateral facial pain or headache is characteristic of disorders that affect the third-order neuron.

The ciliospinal reflex may also help with localization in Horner syndrome. The reflex consists of bilateral pupillary dilation in response to a noxious stimulus, such as a pinch, on the face, neck, or upper trunk. Reeves and Posner[65] showed that when there is a lesion of the first-order oculosympathetic neuron, the reflex is still intact. In contrast, in patients with injury to the second- or third-order neurons, which contain the efferent arm of the reflex, the pupil usually fails to dilate ipsilaterally.

Injury of the First-Order Neuron (Central Horner Syndrome)

Central Horner syndrome can be caused by lesions involving the descending oculosympathetic pathway in the hypothalamus, brain stem, or spinal cord.

TABLE 13–7. Causes of Oculosympathetic Paresis (Horner Syndrome), According to Affected Neuron and Frequency

	Common	Uncommon
First-order (central) neuron	Lateral medullary stroke Spinal cord lesion	Hypothalmic, midbrain, or pontine injury
Second-order (preganglionic) neuron	Pancoast tumor Brachial plexus injury Iatrogenic trauma	Cervical disc disease
Third-order (postganglionic) neuron	Carotid dissection Carotid thrombosis Cluster headache Cavernous sinus lesion	Intraoral trauma

Hypothalamic Lesions. Injury to the neuronal cell bodies in the hypothalamus is relatively infrequent. The most common causes of dysfunction in this area are tumors or hemorrhages involving the thalamus or hypothalamus (Fig. 13–20). Less commonly, a Horner syndrome is the result of hypothalamic infarction.[66, 67] Isolated infarction of the hypothalamus is an unusual event because of a rich blood supply to the hypothalamus, consisting of branches from the anterior cerebral artery and thalamoperforating arteries arising from the proximal portions of the posterior cerebral arteries near the basilar bifurcation, as well as short hypothalamic arteries that derive from the posterior segment of the posterior communicating artery. However, in some individuals with persistence of the fetal circulation, the hypothalamus is supplied directly by branches of the internal carotid artery.[66, 67] In such cases, large, deep cerebral infarcts may involve the hypothalamus when this artery is occluded, and these patients may have prominent sensory or motor signs or a hemianopia contralateral to the Horner syndrome.

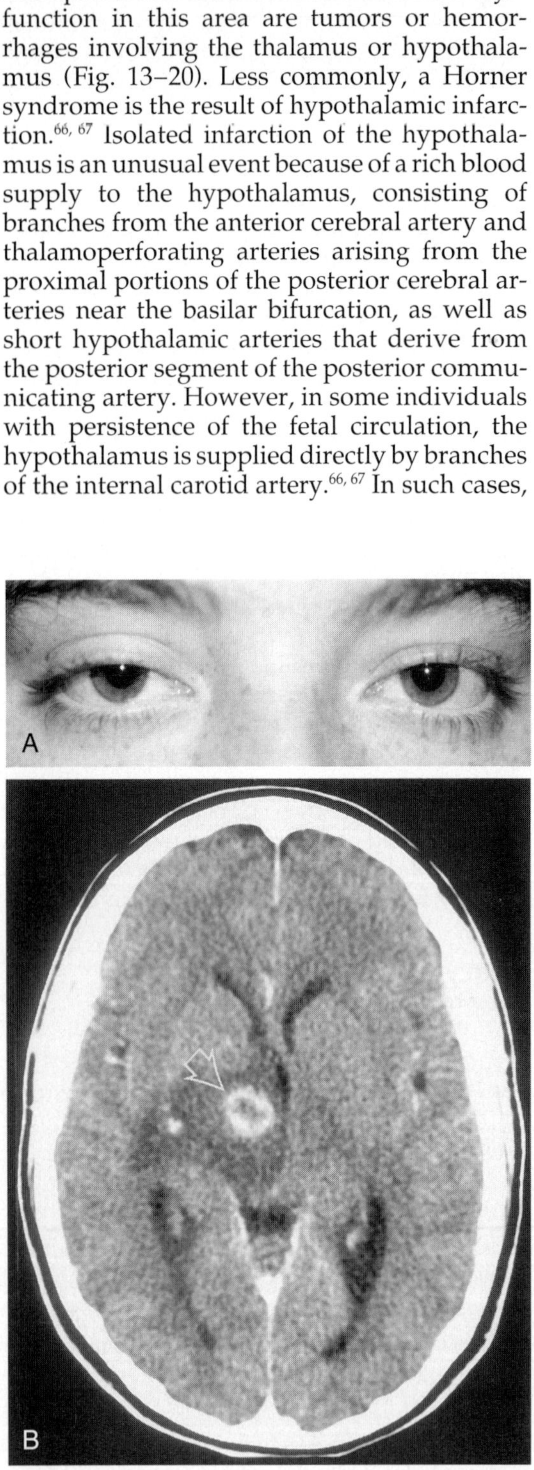

FIGURE 13–20. A. Right Horner syndrome due to T-cell lymphoma involving the right thalamus and hypothalamus. **B.** Ring-enhancement (*arrow*) and edema are seen on the axial CT scan.

Mesencephalic and Pontine Lesions. A lesion in the dorsal midbrain at the pontomesencephalic junction may cause a Horner syndrome and a contralateral fourth nerve palsy by interrupting the descending sympathetic tract and adjacent fourth nerve nucleus or fascicle (Fig. 13–21).[68] In a large series of isolated pontine infarcts,[69] for unclear reasons Horner syndrome was not a feature in any of the cases. However, large pontine hemorrhages may affect the descending sympathetic fibers, causing uni- or bilateral pinpoint pupils.

Wallenberg Syndrome. The most common central cause of a Horner syndrome is a lateral medullary stroke (Wallenberg syndrome), caused by infarction in lateral medullary or posterior inferior cerebellar artery (PICA) distributions. Horner syndrome, ipsilateral to the lesion, occurs in at least three quarters of cases.[70, 71] Ocular motor abnormalities are very frequent and are reviewed in detail in other chapters. These include skew deviation (Chapter 15), lateropulsion and defective smooth pursuit (Chapter 16), and torsional or horizontal nystagmus (Chapter 17). Other characteristic findings are (1) ipsilateral appendicular and gait ataxia, due to involvement of the inferior cerebellar peduncle, (2) ipsilateral corneal and facial anesthesia, owing to damage to the trigeminal spinal nucleus and tract, (3) contralateral body anesthesia, resulting from involvement of the ascending spinothalamic tract, (4) vertigo, caused by damage to the vestibular nuclei, and (5) nausea and vomiting, dysphagia, and ipsilateral palate, pharyngeal, and vocal cord paralysis due to involvement of the nucleus ambiguus.[72] Not infrequently the infarct extends rostrally into the lower pons, producing abducens and facial weakness, due to involvement of the sixth and seventh cranial nerves, respectively. Motor and tongue weakness and corticospinal tract signs are uncommon and would reflect medial medullary involvement.

Typically in patients with Wallenberg syndrome, MRI reveals a wedge-shaped defect in the lateral medulla (Fig. 13–22), and in a minority of cases (approximately 20%) there is also a cerebellar infarction in the distal PICA territory.[70] Most cases result from occlusion of the intracranial vertebral artery or one of its

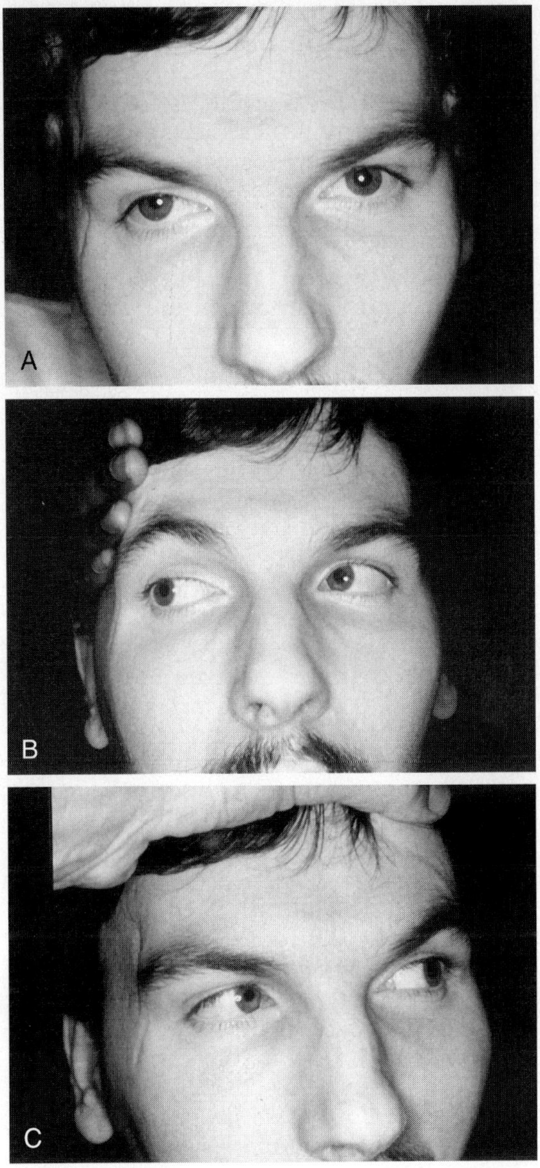

FIGURE 13–21. Right Horner syndrome and left fourth nerve palsy due to a midbrain lesion. **A.** Right head tilt and right eye ptosis and miosis. The left hypertropia is worse in rightward gaze (**B**) compared with leftward gaze (**C**). (Photos courtesy of Lawrence Gray, O.D.)

branches due to local atheromatous disease.[73] However, emboli from the heart, proximal vertebral artery, or aortic arch should also be considered.

Spinal Cord Injury. Any injury to the spinal cord that affects the descending sympathetic pathway or the ciliospinal center of Budge at C8 through T2 can cause a Horner syndrome ipsilateral to the lesion (Fig. 13–23). The most common causes are syringomyelia and trauma

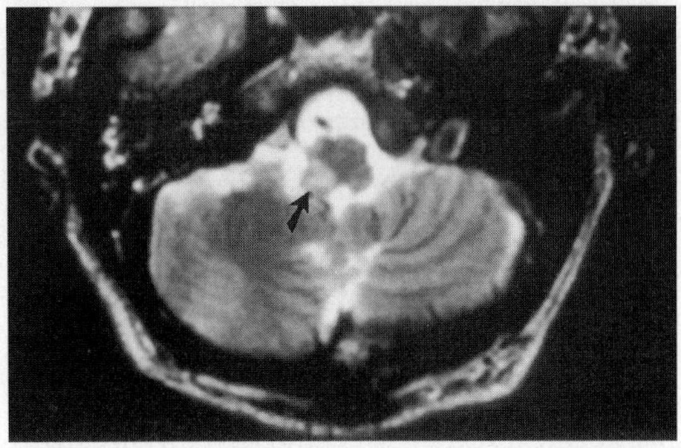

FIGURE 13–22. Wallenberg stroke. Axial T_2-weighted MRI scan demonstrating a lateral medullary infarction (*arrow*) on the right. The patient had an ipsilateral Horner syndrome, skew deviation, lateropulsion to the right, left-beating nystagmus in left gaze, right face hypesthesia, and diminished pain and temperature sensation on the left side of the body. (From Galetta SL, et al: Cyclodeviation in skew deviation. Am J Ophthalmol 1994;118:509-514, with permission from Elsevier Science.)

to the cord, but other recognized causes include myelitis, tumors, multiple sclerosis, and infarction.[74] Quadra- or paraparesis, a sensory level, bladder and bowel difficulty, hyperreflexia, and extensory plantar responses will aid in localization. In Brown–Séquard hemicord syndrome, Horner syndrome may be present ipsilateral to the weakness and loss of light touch sensation, and contralateral to the pain and temperature sense loss.[75] In cases with cer-

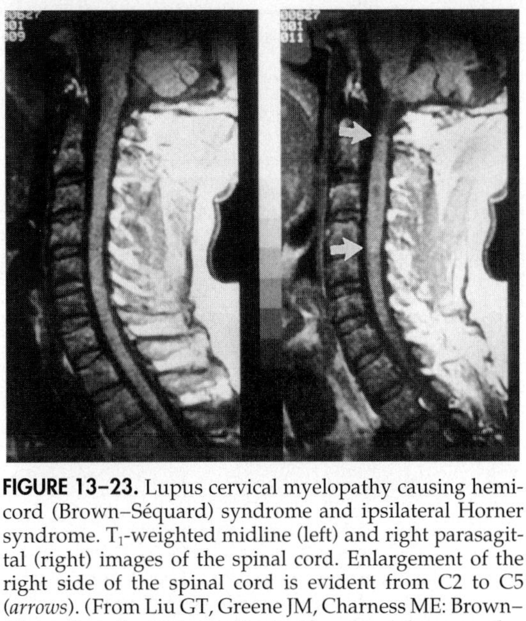

FIGURE 13–23. Lupus cervical myelopathy causing hemicord (Brown–Séquard) syndrome and ipsilateral Horner syndrome. T_1-weighted midline (left) and right parasagittal (right) images of the spinal cord. Enlargement of the right side of the spinal cord is evident from C2 to C5 (*arrows*). (From Liu GT, Greene JM, Charness ME: Brown–Séquard syndrome in a patient with systemic lupus erythematosus. Neurology 1990;40:1474-1475, with permission.)

vical injury associated with a cyst, very rarely the Horner syndrome may alternate when the patient turns from side to side[74] (see also oculosympathetic spasm, below).

Injury of the Second-Order Neuron (Preganglionic Horner Syndrome)

Thoracic (lung and mediastinal) and neck tumors, brachial plexus or radicular injury, and iatrogenic trauma are the most common causes of impairment of this neuron. Maloney et al[63] emphasized the association of Horner syndrome and ipsilateral arm pain as a presentation of a tumor in the superior pulmonary sulcus (Pancoast syndrome[76]) (Fig. 13–24). Owing to irritation of the sympathetic chain, some patients with Pancoast syndrome may exhibit ipsilateral facial flushing and hyperhydrosis of the face before developing Horner syndrome.[77]

Iatrogenic causes of second-order Horner syndrome include radical neck dissection, lung or mediastinal surgery, coronary artery bypass surgery,[78] chest tube placement,[79] internal jugular catherization,[80] Swan–Ganz catheterization,[81] hydromediastinum due to migration of a central venous catheter,[82] and lumbar epidural anesthesia.[83]

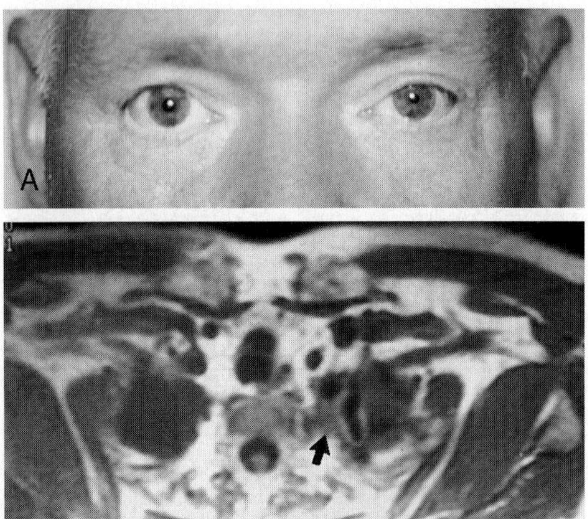

FIGURE 13–24. A. Left Horner syndrome due to apical lung (Pancoast) tumor. **B.** The lesion (*arrow*) in the upper thorax is demonstrated on the axial CT scan. (From Balcer LJ, Galetta SL. Pancoast syndrome. N Engl J Med 1997;337:1359, with permission from the Massachusetts Medical Society.)

Injury of the Third-Order Neuron (Postganglionic Horner Syndrome)

Many of the processes that affect the third-order neuron produce Horner syndrome and ipsilateral facial pain or headache, and this combination has been loosely termed *Raeder's paratrigeminal syndrome or neuralgia.*[84] Carotid artery dissection or thrombosis, vascular headache syndromes, and cavernous sinus lesions are the major disorders to consider in this subgroup.

Carotid Dissection. This disorder should always be considered in the setting of Horner syndrome associated with ipsilateral headache or pain, carotidynia, and dysgeusia, as well as signs and symptoms consistent with ipsilateral ocular or cerebral ischemia.[85, 86] Dissection of the carotid artery results when intraluminal blood enters the arterial wall and separates its component layers.[87] Accumulation of blood in the resulting dissecting aneurysm may compromise the true arterial lumen (Fig. 13–25).[88, 89] Ischemic symptoms result either from carotid stenosis or from embolism of thrombotic fragments; the latter is probably more common.[90] About 5% to 10% of cases are bilateral,[89] and dissection is the cause of at least 5% of cerebral ischemic episodes in young adults.[91] Cases in children are uncommon but have been reported.[92] Arterial dissections may be spontaneous or secondary to minor trauma, or arise in the setting of fibromuscular dysplasia, cystic medial necrosis, syphilis, pharyngeal infection, extension of aortic dissection, atheromatous disease, or cerebral aneurysm.[89, 93] Other predisposing conditions include collagen disorders such as Marfan syndrome or Ehlers–Danlos syndrome. Some result from obvious blunt and penetrating trauma to the head and neck, and motor vehicle accidents are the most common cause in such cases.[94]

Abrupt facial, ear, or neck pain usually signifies the onset of dissection of the extracranial carotid artery and may precede symptomatic ischemia to the eye or brain by hours to days. Patients may also complain of subjective bruits or pulsatile tinnitus.

The neuro-ophthalmic manifestations of carotid dissection are listed in Table 13–8.[87, 95–102, 209] Of these, Horner syndrome is most common, occurring in approximately 50% of patients.[89, 93] In some instances Horner syndrome with ipsilateral headache is the only manifestation.[85, 103] Cranial nerve palsies are not

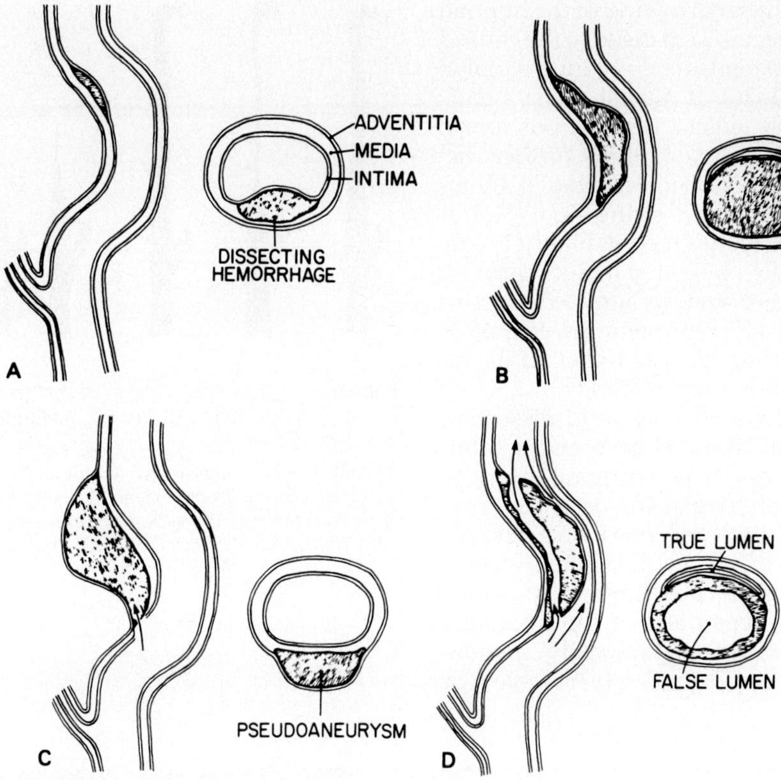

FIGURE 13–25. **A.** Lateral (left) and cross sectional (right) schematic views of the internal carotid artery demonstrate the initial phase of a dissecting aneurysm. The three basic arterial layers (intima, media, and adventitia) are delineated. The dissection is intramedial and subintimal. **B.** Comparable views demonstrate progression of the intramedial hemorrhage. The arterial lumen is reduced in size. **C.** Comparable views illustrate an intramedial hemorrhage that dissects into the subadventitial, rather than the subintimal (as in (A) and (B)), plane. A large pseudoaneurysm results. **D.** The dissecting hemorrhage eruptures through the intima, establishing communication with the true lumen. Recanalization may occur, thus enlarging the true and/or false lumen. (From Friedman WA, Day AL, Quisling RG, et al.: Cervical carotid dissecting aneurysms. Neurosurgery 1980;7:207-214, with permission.)

TABLE 13–8. Neuro-ophthalmic Complications of Carotid Dissection, According to Frequency

Common	Uncommon
Horner syndrome	Anterior ischemic optic neuropathy
Amaurosis fugax	Posterior ischemic optic neuropathy
	Central retinal artery occlusion
	Ophthalmic artery occlusion
	Transient ophthalmoparesis
	Third, fourth, or sixth nerve palsy
	Ocular ischemic syndrome
	Homonymous field defects
	Monocular or binocular scintillations

Adapted from Galetta SL, Leahey A, Nichols CW, et al: J Clin Neuro-ophthalmol 1991;11:284–287, with permission.

uncommon, and in one large series[101] occurred in 12% of patients. Lower cranial nerve (IX through XII) involvement can be explained by the geographic proximity of these structures to the carotid artery in the neck (see Fig 13–28). For example, tongue weakness and dysgeusia may result from ischemia, stretching, or compression of the hypoglossal nerve (XII) and chorda tympani, respectively.[104] On the other hand, ocular motor (III, IV, and VI)[100, 105] and trigeminal (V)[106] nerve palsies are likely ischemic due to emboli into nutrient vessels.[101] Some authors have attributed cases of ischemic optic neuropathy[107] and other cranial neuropathies[108] associated with carotid dissection to a low-flow state. This mechanism, however, seems less likely in the absence of concomitant cerebral hemispheric signs.

Conventional or MRA is essential for establishing the diagnosis and defining the extent of dissection. Lumen narrowing of the internal carotid usually begins 2 cm distal to the carotid bifurcation and extends rostrally for a variable distance (Fig. 13–26). It almost always ends before the artery enters the petrous bone, where mechanical support limits further dissection.[89] The most common finding is a long narrow irregular lumen ("string sign"[109]), but other patterns are highlighted in Figure 13–27. Axial MR T_1- and T_2-weighted images through the neck may demonstrate a characteristic crescentic hyperintensity, representing a mural hematoma, constricting the true lumen of the internal carotid artery (Fig. 13–26).[110]

Management options for carotid dissection include anticoagulation with heparin, antiplatelet agents, superficial temporal artery to middle cerebral artery anastomosis, direct exploration of the dissected internal carotid artery, and observation.[93, 210] Mokri et al[93] found excellent or complete clinical recovery in 85% of their patients, regardless of the treatment modality chosen. Angiographically demonstrated stenosis also completely resolved or

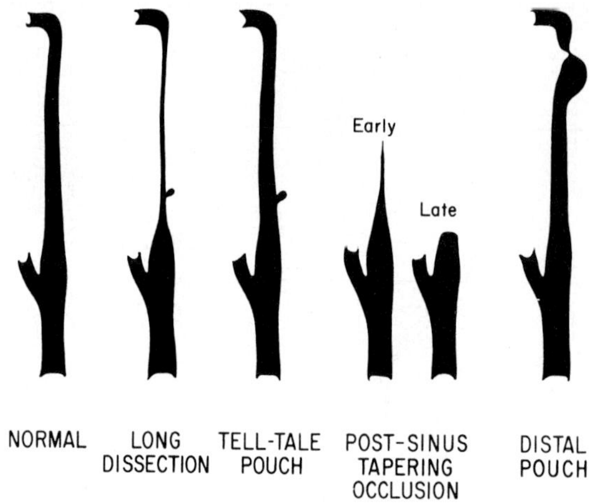

FIGURE 13–27. Diagrams of angiographic profiles in carotid dissection. (From Fisher CM, Ojemann RG, Robinson GH: Spontaneous dissection of cervico-cerebral arteries. Can J Neurol Sci 1978;5:9-19, with permission.)

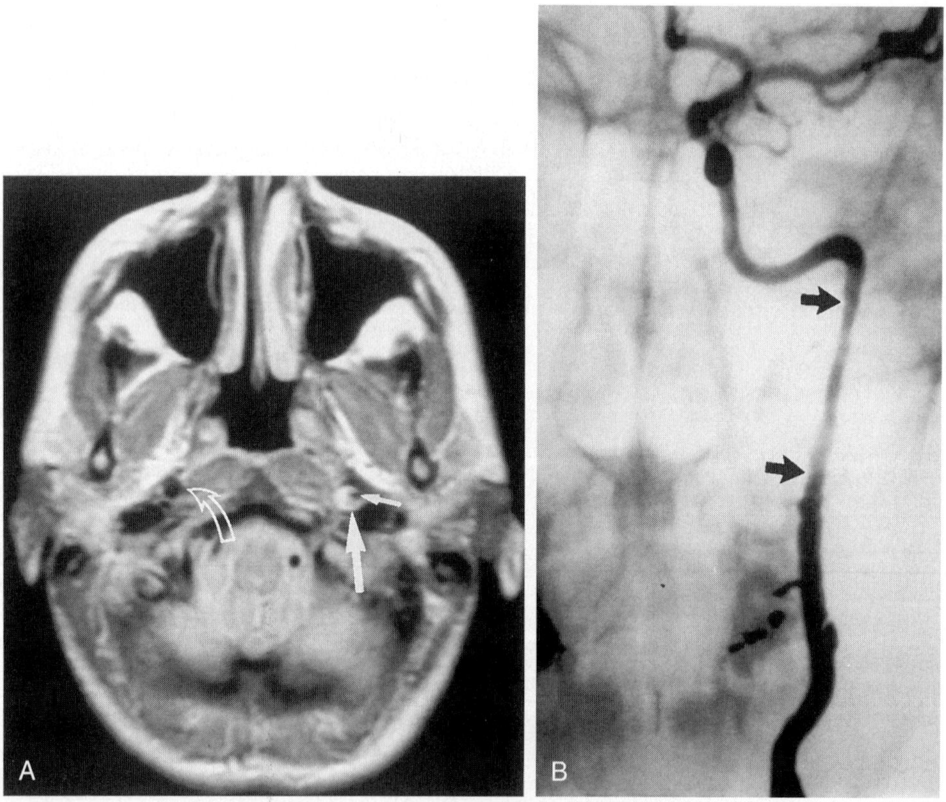

FIGURE 13–26. Painful Horner syndrome due to carotid dissection. **A.** Axial MRI (TR 2700, TE 17) through the neck demonstrating crescent-shaped hyperintensity (*large straight arrow*), consistent with dissecting hemorrhage, and narrowing of the lumen of the left internal carotid artery (*small arrow*) compared with the artery on the other side (*curved arrow*). **B.** Digital subtraction angiogram of the left carotid showing long narrowing (*arrows*) of the artery ("string-sign").

markedly improved in 85%. Recurrence, which usually affects another artery, is uncommon. After the first month, the risk of recurrent dissection is only 1% per year.[111] In patients with acute carotid dissection, treatment with intravenous heparin for 5 to 7 days followed by 3 to 6 months of warfarin is one approach.[89] In individuals in whom long-term anticoagulation is contraindicated, heparin therapy can be followed by an antiplatelet agent such as aspirin. In otherwise asymptomatic patients whose dissection is several weeks old, aspirin alone can be given.

Carotid Thrombosis. Carotid thrombosis, by interrupting the blood supply to the superior cervical ganglion or carotid plexus, can cause oculosympathetic paresis ipsilaterally, with or without pain.[112–115] The superior cervical ganglion derives its blood supply from small branches of the carotid artery and from the ascending pharyngeal and superior thyroid arteries, both of which arise from the external carotid artery. The sympathetic carotid plexus is supplied by small direct branches from the internal carotid artery. Hemispheric signs, such as weakness, sensory loss, and hemianopia, may be present contralaterally, and in such situations it may difficult to tell whether the Horner syndrome is third order or due to deep cerebral infarction involving the hypothalamus (as described above). Further details regarding thrombotic carotid disease are discussed in the chapter on transient visual loss (Chapter 10).

Intraoral Trauma. Iatrogenic or accidental intraoral trauma may cause a Horner syndrome by damaging the internal carotid artery or superior cervical ganglion, which are adjacent to the peritonsillar area (Fig. 13–28).[116] In an adult, the superior cervical ganglion, which is often 2 to 3 cm longitudinally,[13] lies approximately 30 to 40 degrees lateral and only 1.5 cm behind the palatine tonsil.[117] At this level the internal carotid artery, surrounded by the sympathetic plexus, is situated immediately lateral to the superior cervical ganglion (Fig. 13–28). Other neighboring structures include the internal jugular vein, external carotid artery, and the glossopharyngeal (IX), vagus (X), and hypoglossal (XII) nerves. Alternatively, trauma to the internal carotid artery with intimal disruption could subsequently lead to thrombus formation[118] or dissection, then sympathetic plexus ischemia. Accidental injury usually results from penetration by pencils,[119] sticks,[120] or other sharp objects.[121] Iatrogenic causes include tonsillectomy[122] or other intraoral surgery, and peritonsillar anesthesia.[123] Horner syndrome following trauma to the peritonsillar region may be an ominous sign, alerting the clinician to the possibility of internal carotid injury, thrombus formation, or dissection.

Cluster Headaches. These are characterized by "clusters" of ipsilateral headache or eye pain accompanied by ipsilateral Horner syndrome, rhinorrhea, conjunctival injection, and tearing. Although the oculosympathetic paresis is presumptively postganglionic, pharmacologic testing is often inconsistent.[124–126] More details regarding the clinical features, pathophysiology, and treatment of this disorder are discussed in Chapter 19.

Small-Vessel Ischemia. Not uncommonly, individuals with atherosclerosis associated with hypertension or diabetes, for instance, may develop a painless Horner syndrome. The mechanism is likely small-vessel ischemia involving the carotid plexus or vasa vasorium.

Cavernous Sinus, Superior Orbital Fissure, and Orbital Apex. A Horner syndrome and any combination of ipsilateral third, fourth, V_1, V_2, or sixth nerve involvement suggests a cavernous sinus process. Alternating anisocoria in light and dark is unique to this localization.[127] If, for example, a right-sided cavernous sinus mass causes a right Horner syndrome and a right third nerve palsy, in the light, because of the third nerve palsy, the right pupil may be *larger* than the left. In the dark, however, because of the oculosympathetic paresis, the right pupil may become *smaller* than the left.

Except for sparing of V_2, lesions of the superior orbital fissure are clinically difficult to distinguish from those of the cavernous sinus, and the causes are similar. The orbital apex syndrome consists of third, fourth, and sixth nerve paresis, V_1 distribution sensory loss, Horner syndrome, and visual loss due to optic nerve involvement. The differential diagnosis and management of lesions of the cavernous sinus, superior orbital fissure, and orbital apex are discussed in more detail in Chapters 15 and 18.

Autonomic Neuropathies. Unilateral and bilateral Horner syndrome due to sympathetic ganglion dysfunction may be a manifestation of autonomic neuropathy. Responsible underlying systemic disorders would include diabetes and amyloidosis, for instance. Oculosympa-

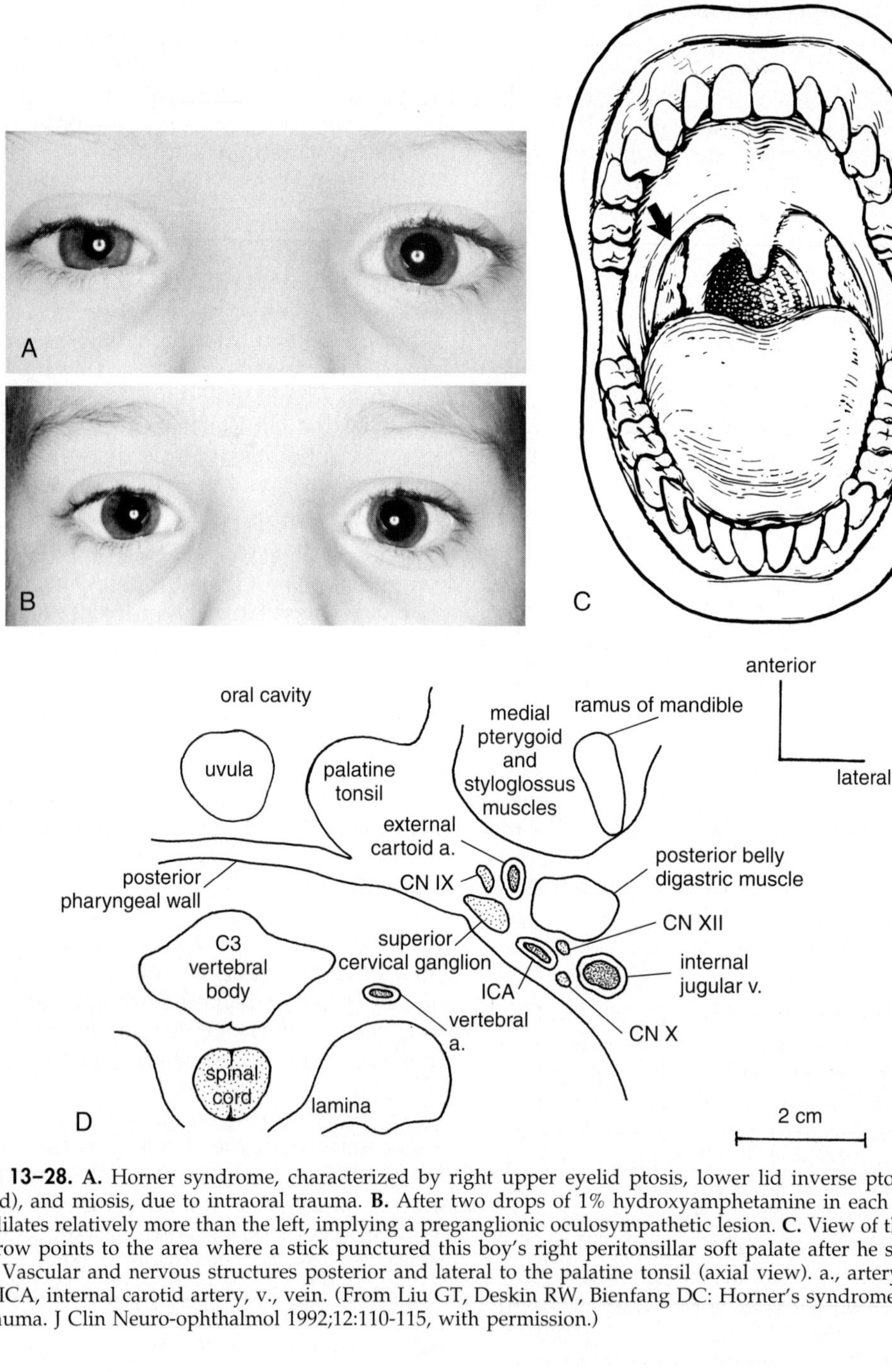

FIGURE 13–28. **A.** Horner syndrome, characterized by right upper eyelid ptosis, lower lid inverse ptosis (lower lid elevated), and miosis, due to intraoral trauma. **B.** After two drops of 1% hydroxyamphetamine in each eye, the right pupil dilates relatively more than the left, implying a preganglionic oculosympathetic lesion. **C.** View of the oral cavity. The arrow points to the area where a stick punctured this boy's right peritonsillar soft palate after he slipped on the ice. **D.** Vascular and nervous structures posterior and lateral to the palatine tonsil (axial view). a., artery, CN, cranial nerve, ICA, internal carotid artery, v., vein. (From Liu GT, Deskin RW, Bienfang DC: Horner's syndrome due to intraoral trauma. J Clin Neuro-ophthalmol 1992;12:110-115, with permission.)

thetic autonomic neuropathy may be a feature of Ross syndrome (see above), hereditary sensory and autonomic neuropathy (HSAN) type II, Anderson–Fabry disease, familial dysautonomia, multiple-system atrophy, pure autonomic failure, and dopamine-beta-hydroxylase deficiency.[128]

Congenital and Acquired Causes of Horner Syndrome in Childhood

The most important identifiable causes in young children with Horner syndrome are occult neuroblastoma and birth trauma. Iris heterochromia, although an excellent sign of congenital oculosympathetic paresis,[58] is not always present. In many cases of Horner syndrome in infants, however, no cause can be found despite extensive history taking and investigation.[129] Weinstein et al[130] speculated that these idiopathic cases might result from a congenital malformation or vascular insult of the superior cervical ganglion or some other structure in the oculosympathetic pathway. Like others,[131–133] we have found idiopathic cases to be the most common group in childhood (Table 13–9). One congenital case was reported in association with agenesis of the internal carotid artery.[211]

Neuroblastoma. Horner syndrome was found in 3.5% of neuroblastomas in one large series.[134] Neuroblastomas, believed to be of neural crest origin, are among the most common childhood solid tumors. When arising in the upper thorax or cervical sympathetic chain (Fig. 13–29), this tumor can present with Horner syndrome as well as with lower cranial nerve involvement, stridor due to tracheal displacement, or dysphagia owing to esophageal compression.[135, 136] In some instances, they may grow large enough to present as a visible neck mass.[137] There have been rare cases with Horner syndrome associated with neuroblastomas arising from the adrenal glands and in the lower thoracic sympathetic chain.[138] How distant tumors affect the oculosympathetic pathway is uncertain, but a more generalized disorder of sympathetic neuronal maturation has been proposed.[138, 139] A more differentiated, benign form of the tumor, termed *ganglioneuroma*[139] or *ganglioneuroblastoma*,[140] may also be associated with Horner syndrome when it occurs in the neck and upper thorax.

The adrenal glands are the most common location, being the site of tumor in about one half of cases.[141] Approximately one quarter of neuroblastomas present in the cervical region or mediastinum, and these tumors may have a better prognosis.[142] Thus Musarella et al[134] found patients with neuroblastoma associated with Horner syndrome to have an excellent survival rate of 78.6% at 3 years, due to the predominance of localized disease and favorable location among these patients. In the absence of metastases, treatment generally consists of surgical resection, then observation. The treatment and prognosis of neuroblastoma is discussed in more detail in the discussion of opsoclonus/myoclonus in Chapter 17.

Birth Trauma. A forceful pull of a child's arm during vaginal delivery (Fig. 13–30) may result in injury to the lower trunk of the brachial plexus (Klumpke's palsy). In such instances Horner syndrome may result from dislocation of the C8 and T1 dorsal and ventral nerve roots. In addition, muscles and skin supplied by the C8 and T1 nerve roots are affected, leading to weakness of wrist flexion and intrinsic muscles of the hand as well as anesthesia in the ulnar aspect of the forearm and hand. Traction on the carotid plexus during difficult forceps delivery is another birth-related injury that may cause Horner syndrome.[130]

Acquired Horner Syndrome in Childhood. The differential diagnosis of acquired causes of Horner syndrome in children is different than that in adults (Table 13–9).[143] Brain stem infarction, spontaneous carotid dissection, pulmonary tumors, and cluster headache are much less frequent in this age group.

Pharmacologic Testing in Horner Syndrome

Cocaine. The diagnosis of a Horner syndrome associated with a lateral medullary stroke, brachial plexus injury, or spinal cord trauma, for instance, is often straightforward because of the accompanying signs and symptoms. However, the distinction between ipsilateral ptosis and miosis due to oculosympathetic paresis and other causes, such as physiologic anisocoria combined with levator dehiscence–disinsertion on the side of the miotic pupil (so-called pseudo-Horner syndrome[144]), may require pharmacologic testing. Cocaine, which blocks reuptake of norepinephrine at the sympathetic nerve terminal in the iris dilator muscle, allows a relative increase of neurotransmitter available for the postsynaptic receptors. Iris dilator tone depends on the intactness of each neuron in the oculosympathetic pathway. Normally, cocaine will dilate the pupil and widen the palpebral fissure, and the pupillary dilation is more pronounced in individuals with light irises than in those with dark ones. However, interruption of any one of the three neurons results in decreased norepinephrine release by the third-order neuron, so cocaine will have little or no effect in such cases. Cocaine testing helps confirm the presence of a Horner syndrome, but does not aid in localization.

A 10% solution should be used since cocaine is a relatively weak pupillary dilator, and drop administration should be repeated 1 minute later. Pupil sizes should be assessed at baseline

TABLE 13–9. Horner Syndrome in Childhood: Differential Diagnosis According to Location, Cause, and Frequency as Seen in Various Series.

Localization	Cause	Series: Cleveland (1976)[143]	Iowa (1980)[130]	Toronto (1988)[131]	Phila. C.H.O.P. (1993–1996)	U.S.C.F. (1998)[133]	Toronto/Hopkins (1998)[132]
Idiopathic			4 (36%)	4 (40%)	6 (43%)	16 (70%)	31 (42%)
First-order (central) neuron	Neoplasm involving:						
	hypothalmus				2 (43%)		
	brain stem,						
	or spinal cord	1 (14%)					
	Spinal cord trauma						
	Syringomyelia						
	Arachnoid cyst			1 (10%)			
	Cerebral palsy			1 (10%)			
	Klippel–Feil				1 (7%)		
Second-order (preganglionic) neuron	Neuroblastoma	1 (14%)		2 (20%)	1 (7%)	2 (9%)	3 (5%)
	Chest surgery		2 (18%)	2 (20%)			
	Birth-related injury of nerve roots or brachial plexus	1 (14%)	1 (9%)				
	Metastatic disease	1 (14%)					
	Intrathoracic aneurysm	1 (14%)					
	Mediastinitis				1 (7%)		
	Cervical lymphadenopathy				1 (7%)		2 (3%)
	Neurofibroma				1 (7%)		
	Neck surgery				1 (7%)		
	Ganglioneuroma					1 (4%)	
Third-order (postganglionic) neuron	Birth-related injury		4 (36%)			4 (17%)	
	Otitis media						
	Intraoral trauma						
	Nasopharyngeal tumor	1 (14%)					1 (1%)
	Carotid artery occlusion	1 (14%)					
	Total	7	11	10	14	23	73

In the Cleveland series,[143] the presenting age was 10 years or younger. The Iowa[130] and University of California, San Francisco (UCSF), series[133] included only those patients with onset of Horner syndrome in the first year of life, while in the Toronto (1988) series,[131] all patients were 8 years of age or less. The Philadelphia series consists of all cases in patients less than 18 years of age seen by one of us (GTL) at the Children's Hospital of Philadelphia (CHOP) from July 1993 through November 1996. The Toronto/Hopkins series, which was also made up of patients less than 18 years of age, provided insufficient information to localize all cases. Thus, the list for that series is incomplete. All cases in the Iowa and Toronto (1988) series were confirmed with cocaine testing. In the Philadelphia series all idiopathic cases were confirmed pharmacologically and had unremarkable imaging and negative urine catecholamine screening.

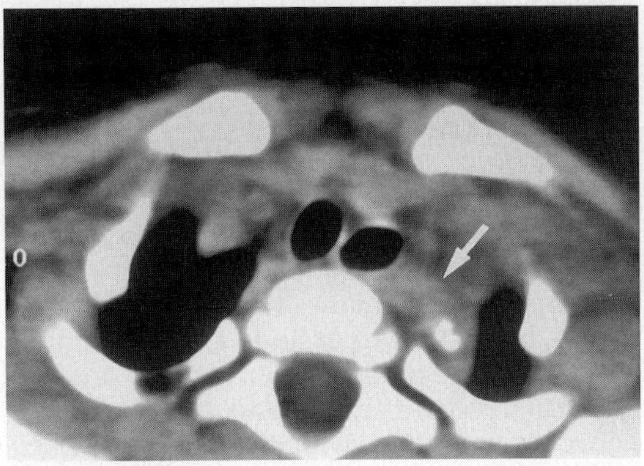

FIGURE 13–29. Neuroblastoma of the cervical region presenting with Horner syndrome. The axial CT scan through the lung apex reveals a left paraspinous calcified soft tissue mass (*arrow*).

and 40 to 60 minutes after the cocaine eye drops have been instilled. Sometimes neither pupil has responded, and this requires a readministration of drops and further observation for another 30 minutes. In a positive test, cocaine fails to dilate a sympathetically impaired pupil or does so very poorly, while the unaffected pupil dilates normally (see Fig. 13–19). Kardon and colleagues[145] and Van der Wiel and Van Gijn[146] suggest the most accurate way to interpret the cocaine test is to measure the postcocaine anisocoria. If the pupillary inequality following cocaine is greater than 1.0 mm, the test should be considered positive, and the greater the size difference, the more likely the positive result is correct. In simple anisocoria, both pupils will dilate with cocaine, but the pupillary inequality following cocaine should be small.

Hydroxyamphetamine. Because most postganglionic Horner syndromes tend to be benign, while preganglionic Horner syndromes may reflect an underlying neoplasm, the distinction between pre- and postganglionic lesions may have important management implications. If the cocaine test indicates oculosympathetic paresis, 24 to 48 hours later 1% hydroxyamphetamine drops can be applied topically to both eyes to aid in localization. Drop administration is repeated after 1 minute, and the pupillary sizes 45 minutes later are compared with baseline measurements. Hydroxyamphetamine enhances the release of presynaptic norepinephrine, and this property depends only on the intactness of the third-order neuron.[147] In normal individuals, hydroxyamphetamine produces a symmetric 2-mm mean increase in the size of pupils,[148] and the drug dilates lighter irises faster and more effectively than dark ones.[149] Hydroxyamphetamine also normally widens the palpebral fissure.

As a rule, in first or second-order Horner syndrome, both pupils will also dilate with hydroxyamphetamine, and sometimes the involved pupil actually dilates more than the normal one (see Fig. 13–28A,B).[150] In contrast, in third-order sympathetic interruption, the involved pupil theoretically should not dilate. However, in order to establish a Horner syndrome as third order, in practice it is probably more helpful to determine whether the relative anisocoria *increases* following administration of hydroxyamphetamine. Cremer et al[150] studied the amount of hydroxyamphetamine-induced mydriasis necessary to establish the presence of a postganglionic sympathetic defect. A 1-mm increase in the amount of anisocoria provides an 85.5% probability that the lesion is postganglionic. A 2-mm increase is associated with a 99% probability of a postganglionic defect. Cremer et al[150] and Van der Wiel and van Gijn[151] suggest using any increase in anisocoria of 1 mm or greater as indicative of a postganglionic lesion.

Unfortunately, the hydroxyamphetamine test is imperfect, as evidenced by the mixed results seen in various studies. Maloney and colleagues[63] found that the diagnostic specificity of the hydroxyamphetamine test for postganglionic Horner syndrome was only 84%. In

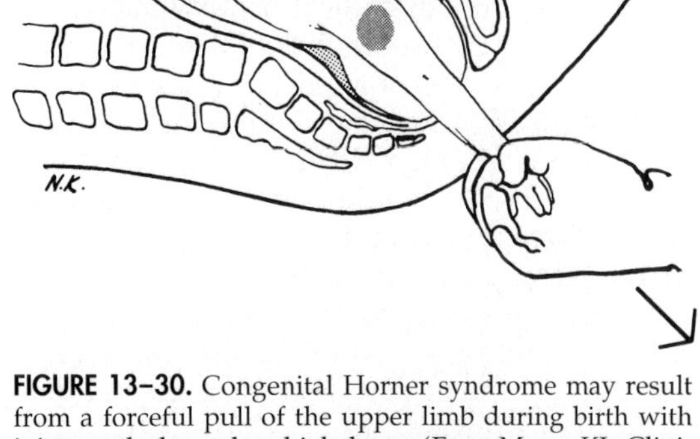

FIGURE 13–30. Congenital Horner syndrome may result from a forceful pull of the upper limb during birth with injury to the lower brachial plexus. (From Moore KL: Clinically Oriented Anatomy, 3rd edition, p 524. Baltimore, Williams & Wilkins, 1992, with permission.)

other words, 16% of patients who failed to dilate in fact had a preganglionic lesion. However, bilateral pupillary dilation accurately diagnosed a preganglionic lesion in 97% of cases. In the aforementioned study, Cremer et al[150] found an increase in the anisocoria in 93% of postganglionic cases. The anisocoria decreased or did not change in 90% of preganglionic patients. In another study Van der Wiel and van Gijn[151] found abnormally weak unilateral dilation was accurate in detecting postganglionic Horner syndrome but 60% of third-order lesions were missed by normal hydroxyamphetamine tests.

Caution also should be applied when hydroxyamphetamine is used in children with Horner syndrome. The normal development of the third-order oculosympathetic neuron and its synaptic connections depends on the integrity of the first and second neuron. In congenital preganglionic lesions, therefore, it is possible that hydroxyamphetamine will completely or partially fail to dilate the involved pupil because of transsynaptic degeneration of postganglionic fibers.[130]

Management of Horner Syndrome

The diagnosis of Horner syndrome is usually a clinical one based upon examination findings, with cocaine used only to confirm equivocal cases. Hydroxyamphetamine is becoming more difficult to acquire because of decreasing commercial availability. This, coupled with the high false-negative rate of the hydroxyamphetamine test, will encourage clinicians in most instances to localize the Horner syndrome and make management decisions largely based upon clinical grounds.

In adults with Horner syndrome, there are two situations that mandate radiologic investigation regardless of clinical or pharmacologic localization (because neither is perfect). First, in any middle-aged or elderly patient, especially one with a history of smoking, with an isolated, unexplained Horner syndrome, chest roentgenography should be performed to rule out an apical lung tumor. Second, Horner syndrome accompanied by ipsilateral headache or eye pain, with or without ipsilateral cerebral or ocular ischemic symptoms, requires MRI and MRA of the neck to exclude a carotid dissection or thrombosis.[110, 152–154] Axial T1-weighted MR images through the neck are especially important in this setting.

Other situations can be governed by suspected localization:

1. *First-order neuron.* If the process is thought to be first order because of the presence of cerebral, posterior fossa, or spinal cord signs, then the neurologic findings should guide the investigation. For instance, accompanying hemianesthesia or ataxia mandate brain MRI to exclude a brain stem lesion. On the other hand, a sensory level or paraparesis accompanying a Horner syndrome should be evaluated with spine MRI.
2. *Second-order neuron.* If a presumed preganglionic Horner syndrome is isolated or associated with brachial plexopathy, screening chest roentgenography or chest CT or MRI with attention to the lung apex and neck is indicated.
3. *Third-order neuron.* If the lesion can be localized to the postganglionic neuron, we recommend MRI and MRA of the neck only if the Horner syndrome is painfull since many postganglionic Horner syndromes have a benign cause (eg, vasculopathathy). Because of the proximity between sympathetic and vascular structures in the lateral and parapharyngeal space, Horner syndrome in the setting of intraoral trauma should also prompt evaluation of the neck and internal carotid artery. The presence of a third, fourth, or sixth nerve palsy or trigeminal neuropathy ipsilateral to the Horner syndrome should suggest MRI with special attention to the cavernous sinus, or if suspected, MRA to exclude carotid dissection.

Most individuals with Horner syndrome do not find the ptosis bothersome, as it is usually very mild and rarely affects vision. Cosmetic surgery may be considered in patients who find their appearance undesirable. The pupil abnormality should not cause subjective symptoms.

Congenital Horner Syndrome. Cocaine testing should be used to confirm the Horner syndrome in unexplained cases in young children. Then, in those without birth trauma, diagnostic testing should be performed to exclude neuroblastoma.[134] CT or MRI of the neck, chest, and abdomen and urinary catecholamine metabolite screening (vanillylmandelic acid (VMA) and homovanillic acid (HVA)) is a recommended protocol. Excess production of catecholamines or their metabolites occurs in 90% of neuroblastomas.[155] Hydroxyamphetamine is not helpful because of transsynaptic degeneration.

PUPILS IN OTHER NEUROLOGIC CONDITIONS

Coma

Pupillary signs may be extremely important in the evaluation of comatose patients, especially with regard to diagnosis and localization Fig. 13–31. As a rule, metabolic coma is more likely to be associated with normoreactive pupils than coma due to a structural lesion, although there are exceptions (see systemic medications, below).[156]

As stated above, hypothalamic lesions may cause small but reactive pupils due to oculosympathetic paresis, while thalamic and mesencephalic lesions may result in third nerve palsies, midposition or large pupils or, less likely, pupillary corectopia. Destructive lesions of the pons may disrupt the descending oculosympathetic pathways and result in bilateral pinpoint pupils. Diffuse anoxic brain damage can cause midbrain dysfunction and dilated pupils. Initially in brain death the pupils can be midposition or dilated and unreactive to light.[157,158] With more time after death, however, all pupils become midposition, reflecting the equal parasympathetic and sympathetic dysfunction.

Ipsilateral pupillary dilation may be the first sign of transtentorial uncal herniation before other signs of third nerve paresis develop. In this setting, mechanisms for third nerve dysfunction include direct compression by the herniating uncus beneath the tentorial edge, compression by the posterior cerebral artery or hippocampal gyrus, compression of the oculomotor complex in the midbrain, or displacement and kinking of the nerve over the clivus.[159] Further clinical progression may be monitored by examining the opposite pupil, which initially may be midposition with a depressed light reaction, then slightly miotic, and finally dilated.[160] Transiently the pupils may acquire an oval shape.[161] Uncommonly in transtentorial herniation, the opposite pupil is paradoxically the first to dilate.[162]

In metabolic encephalopathies, the pupils may be small but remain reactive to light until midbrain dysfunction ensues. In hepatic encephalopathy, for example, oculocephalic eye movements and pupillary reactivity are normal despite severe alteration in consciousness. However, in stage IV hepatic encephalopathy,

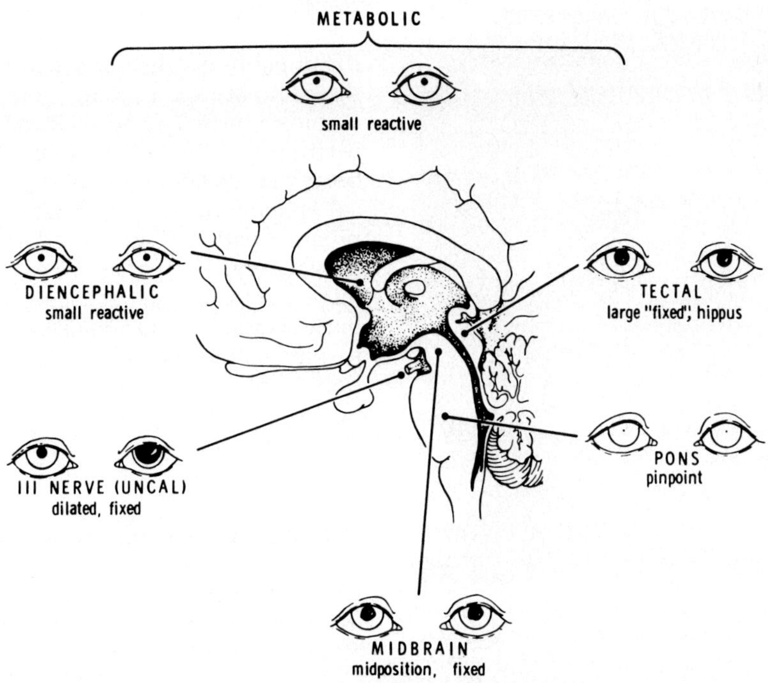

FIGURE 13–31. Pupils in comatose patients. (From Plum F, Posner JB: Pupils: In: The Diagnosis of Stupor and Coma, 3rd edition, p 46. New York, Oxford University Press, 1980, with permission.)

cerebral edema and downward herniation can cause coma, fixed and dilated pupils, and ophthalmoplegia.[163, 164]

Systemic Medications

Opiate intoxication causes pinpoint pupils resembling those seen with large pontine lesions.[156] Theoretically in these instances the pupils should be reactive to light, but they can be so miotic that any constriction is difficult to appreciate, even with a magnifying glass.

Poisoning with any substance, such as atropine or a tricyclic antidepressant, with anticholinergic properties may cause dilated and fixed pupils. These pupils will not react to 1% pilocarpine. Glutethimide and barbiturate intoxication can also fix the pupils.[156]

Migraine

A dilated pupil and ipsilateral headache may be alarming for both the patient and physician, and certainly in these instances a third nerve palsy should be excluded. However, transient isolated mydriasis or so-called benign episodic mydriasis, with normal vision and pupillary reactivity to light, may occasionally accompany migraine headaches (Fig. 13–32).[165] Eyelid or motility disturbances, which might otherwise suggest ophthalmoplegic migraine, are absent. The dilated pupil is due either to parasympathetic insufficiency of the iris sphincter or sympathetic hyperactivity of the iris dilator.[166] In unusual cases, the mydriasis can have the clinical and pharmacologic characteristics of a tonic pupil,[167] or be tadpole shaped (see below).[168]

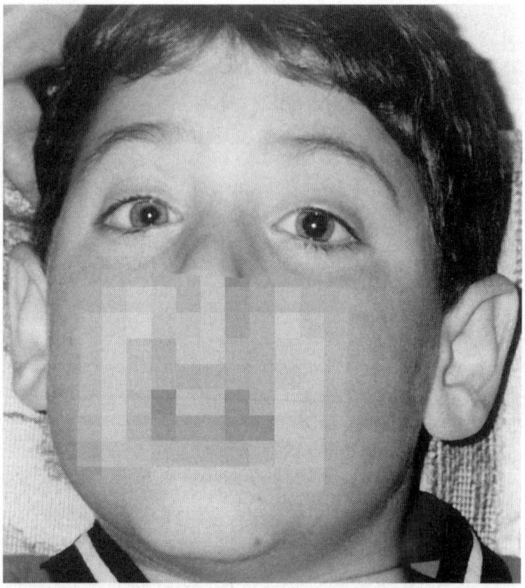

FIGURE 13–32. Benign episodic mydriasis in migraine. This boy developed transient episodes of left unilateral pupillary dilation accompanied by ipsilateral headache. Ocular motility, pupillary reactivity, and eyelids were normal. The photo was taken by his mother during one such episode.

Drummond[169] studied the pupils of a population of migraineurs during headache-free periods. Pupil asymmetry was greater in the migraine sufferers than in controls, but there was no correlation with the side of miotic pupil and of the headache. In addition, some pupils exhibited dilation lag and did not dilate after instillation of 4% cocaine eye drops. Drummond hypothesized that vasodilation or swelling of the arterial wall in the carotid canal could lead to minor oculosympathetic deficits in patients with frequent or severe migraine attacks. Other studies[170] have found similar oculosympathetic defects. The differential diagnosis of oculosympathetic paresis and ipsilateral headache is discussed in more detail above.

The neuro-ophthalmic complications of migraine are discussed in more detail in Chapters 11 and 19.

Seizures

Presumably because of diffuse stimulation of the sympathetic system, generalized tonic–clonic seizures may be associated with bilateral mydriasis. Ictal unilateral mydriasis may be observed ipsilateral or contralateral to a cortical epileptic focus.[171, 172] Rarely, unilateral pupillary dilation (without other signs of third nerve palsy) may persist for a few hours postictally.[173] Ictal miosis has also been described, both bilaterally and unilaterally, contralateral to the seizure focus.[174, 175] Proposed explanations implicate stimulation or inhibition of cortical centers with parasympathetic or sympathetic connections to the eye.[174, 175]

Other Neuromuscular Diseases

Pupillary abnormalities in disorders of the neuromuscular junction have been described above in the section on unreactive pupils.

Guillain–Barré Syndrome and the Miller Fisher Variant. Pupillary dysfunction is purportedly uncommon in Guillain–Barré syndrome, but this may reflect insufficient attention to the pupils in patients with this syndrome without ophthalmoplegia.[176] In contrast, pupillary abnormalities are more frequent and better characterized in the Miller Fisher variant (ophthalmoplegia, ataxia, and areflexia). Two of Fisher's first three patients had pupils that were poorly reactive to light.[177] Subsequently, there have been several other papers dealing with internal ophthalmoplegia in this condition. Okajima et al[178] reported a patient with the Miller Fisher variant and unequal and unreactive pupils. Pharmacologic testing revealed a preganglionic sympathetic defect in addition to an unlocalizable parasympathetic defect. Keane[179] described two patients with Miller Fisher variant and bilaterally dilated pupils with light–near dissociation and cholinergic hypersensitivity. Radziwill[180] reported another such patient, but in addition circulating antibodies to GQ1b gangliosides, which they surmised may also be in the ciliary ganglia, were also demonstrated. These disorders are detailed in Chapter 14.

Pupils in Alzheimer's Disease and Progressive Supranuclear Palsy

Scinto et al,[181] based upon the hypothesis that patients with Alzheimer's disease may be hypersensitive to acetylcholine receptor antagonists, tested the response to dilute (0.01%) tropicamide in patients with and without the disorder. They found that patients with Alzheimer's disease were markedly hypersensitive in their pupillary dilation response, compared with controls. The authors suggested that dilute tropicamide might be used antemortem to confirm the diagnosis of Alzheimer's disease.[182] Since then, however, there have been a number of studies refuting this.[183–188] For instance, Loupe et al[183] were unable to use the pupillary response to dilute tropicamide to distinguish between individuals in four groups: young and elderly control subjects, and patients with Alzheimer's disease using tacrine (an oral acetylcholinesterase inhibitor) and those not on the drug. Scinto's study has been criticized over methodologic issues such as lack of controlling for corneal permeability and blink rate, for instance.[189, 190]

Litvan and FitzGibbon[191] also studied the pupillary response to dilute tropicamide in patients with progressive supranuclear palsy (PSP), another degenerative disorder characterized by cholinergic deficits. They found that the pupils of normal individuals and those with PSP both dilated the same amount. They concluded that pupillary dilation to tropicamide was nonspecific and that caution should be applied before using this test to detect Alzheimer's disease.

OTHER PUPILLARY PHENOMENA

Westphal–Piltz Reflex

Pupillary constriction in darkness is a normal occurrence when individuals close their eyes to go to sleep (Westphal–Piltz reflex). This phenomenon is thought to be secondary to decreased inhibition of the oculomotor complex.

Paradoxic Pupillary Constriction in the Dark

Pupillary miosis followed by slow redilation when the lights are turned off may suggest a retinal dystrophy such as in congenital stationary night blindness or congenital achromatopsia.[192, 193] The mechanism is uncertain, but a transient delay or "noise" in the rod bleaching signal, allowing the small but normal cone bleaching signal to constrict the pupils when the lights are turned off, has been proposed.[194] A child with paradoxic pupillary constriction, poor vision, nystagmus, or a family history of retinal disorders should undergo electroretinography.

Tournay's Pupillary Phenomenon

Anisocoria induced by lateral gaze, which occurs in no more than 10% of the normal population, is referred to as *Tournay's pupillary phenomenon*.[195, 196] The pupil of the abducting eye is larger, and either that pupil has dilated or the pupil of the adducting eye has constricted. The mechanism is unclear, but an anomalous connection between the medial rectus subnucleus and the Edinger–Westphal nucleus may be responsible.[197]

Abduction Miosis

In this rare phenomenon, the pupil constricts during ocular abduction. The finding may be congenital, perhaps due to an anastomosis between the sixth nerve and ciliary ganglion, or acquired following concurrent injury to the third and sixth nerves with aberrant regeneration of abducens fibers into the parasympathetic pupilllary pathway.[198, 199] Miosis is also an important feature of abduction limitation associated with convergence spasm.

Oculosympathetic Spasm

Irritation of the oculosympathetic pathway may result in unilateral pupillary mydriasis, occasionally accompanied by ipsilateral facial flushing, lid retraction, and hyperhydrosis. Oculosympathetic spasm is typically a delayed phenomenon associated with chronic cervical cord lesions such as syringomyelia or infarction, and the cause is unknown.[200] Cysts in this area may cause alternating anisocoria characterized by the presence of a Horner syndrome when the patient lies on the side of the lesion. The anisocoria reverses, presumably because of oculosympathetic spasm, when the patient lies on the other side.[74]

Cyclic Oculomotor Spasms

This disorder, which is also discussed in Chapter 15, is characterized by a complete or partial third nerve palsy that alternates with lid elevation, miosis, and a downward and inward movement of the eye.[201] Most cases are seen in infancy, and a cause is found only infrequently.[202]

Idiopathic Alternating Anisocoria

In this rare condition, one pupil dilates, then several hours later the pupil returns to normal size, but the other pupil dilates.[203] The cycle can occur several times in one day. The eyelids and ocular motility remain normal, and there are no other neurologic abnormalities. The mechanism is unclear.

Tadpole-Shaped Pupils

Thompson et al[168] described an unusual group of patients who exhibited episodic mydriasis with segmental pupillary distortion. This phenomenon occurred over minutes and was frequently accompanied by an ache or other abnormal sensations in the affected eye. Clinical settings included ipsilateral Horner syndrome, tonic pupils, and migraine. The authors coined the descriptive term *tadpole-shaped pupils* and attributed them to abnormal segmental spasm of the iris dilator muscle.

Spasm of the Near Reflex

In this condition, miosis is associated with convergence, accommodation, and pseudo-(induced) myopia.[204] It is usually indicative of a functional disorder.[205] The esotropia tends to be variable, and the myopia usually resolves after cycloplegia. The miosis upon attempted abduction is highly characteristic and may resolve upon occlusion of the fellow eye by disrupting the binocular input necessary for convergence.[206] Spasm of the near reflex is discussed in more detail in Chapter 15.

REFERENCES

1. Slamovits TL, Glaser JS: The pupils and accommodation. In: Glaser JS (ed): Neuro-ophthalmology, 2nd edition, pp 459–486. Philadelphia, JB Lippincott, 1990.
2. Liu GT: Disorders of the eyes and eyelids: Disorders of the pupil. In: Samuels MA, Feske S (eds): The Office Practice of Neurology, pp 60–68. New York, Churchill Livingstone, 1996.
3. Jampel RS: Representation of the near-response in the cerebral cortex of the Macaque. Am J Ophthalmol 1959;48:573–582.
4. Ohtsuka K, Sato A: Descending projections from the cortical accommodation area in the cat. Invest Ophthalmol Vis Sci 1996;37:1429–1436.
5. Mays LE, Gamlin PD: Neuronal circuitry controlling the near response. Curr Opin Neurobiol 1995;5:763–768.
6. Parkinson D: Further observations on the sympathetic pathways to the pupil. Anat Rec 1988;220:108–109.
7. Nelson LB: Pediatric Ophthalmology, pp 77–93. Philadelphia, WB Saunders, 1984.
8. Martyn LJ, DiGeorge A: Selected eye defects of special importance in pediatrics. Pediatr Clin North Am 1987;34:1517–1542.
9. Byles DB, Nischal KK, Cheng H: Ectopia lentis et pupillae. A hypothesis revisited. Ophthalmology 1998;105:1331–1336.
10. Hayashi N, Valdes-Dapena M, Green WR: CHARGE association: histopathological report of two cases and a review. J Pediatr Ophthalmol Strabismus 1998;35:100–106.
11. Jorgenson RJ, Levin LS, Cross HE, et al: The Rieger syndrome. Am J Med Genet 1978;2:307–318.
12. Fitch N, Kaback M: The Axenfeld syndrome and the Rieger syndrome. J Med Genet 1978;15:30–34.
13. Miller NR: Walsh and Hoyt's Clinical Neuro-ophthalmology, 4th edition, pp 385–556. Baltimore, William & Wilkins, 1985.

14. Atkinson CS, Brodsky MC, Hiles DA, et al: Idiopathic tractional corectopia. J Pediatr Ophthalmol Strabismus 1994;31:387–390.
15. Burton BJ, Adams GG: Persistent pupillary membranes (letter). Br J Ophthalmol 1998;82:711–712.
16. Portnoy JZ, Thompson HS, Lennarson L, et al: Pupillary defects in amblyopia. Am J Ophthalmol 1983;96: 609–614.
17. Bell RA, Thompson HS: Relative afferent pupillary defect in optic tract hemianopsias. Am J Ophthalmol 1978;85:538–540.
18. Savino PJ, Paris M, Schatz NJ, et al: Optic tract syndrome. A review of 21 patients. Arch Ophthalmol 1978;96:656–663.
19. Forman S, Behrens MM, Odel JG, et al: Relative afferent pupillary defect with normal visual function. Arch Ophthalmol 1990;108:1074–1075.
20. King JT, Galetta SL, Flamm ES: Relative afferent pupillary defect with normal vision in a glial brainstem tumor. Neurology 1991;41:945–946.
21. Eliott D, Cunningham ET, Miller NR: Fourth nerve paresis and ipsilateral relative afferent pupillary defect without visual sensory disturbance. A sign of contralateral dorsal midbrain disease. J Clin Neuro-ophthalmol 1991;11:169–172.
22. Girkin CA, Perry JD, Miller NR: A relative afferent pupillary defect without any visual sensory deficit. Arch Ophthalmol 1998;116:1544–1545.
23. Ravin JG: Argyll Robertson. 'Twas better to be his pupil than to have his pupil. Ophthalmology 1998; 105:867–870.
24. Sebag J, Sadun AA: Aberrant regeneration of the third nerve following orbital trauma. Synkinesis of the iris sphincter. Arch Neurol 1983;40:762–764.
25. Czarnecki JSC, Thompson HS: The iris sphincter in aberrant regeneration of the third nerve. Arch Ophthalmol 1978;96:1606–1610.
26. Kissel JT, Burde RM, Klingele TG, et al: Pupil-sparing oculomotor palsies with internal carotid–posterior communicating artery aneurysms. Ann Neurol 1983;13:149–154.
27. Coppeto JR, Monteiro MLR, Young D: Tonic pupils following oculomotor nerve palsies. Ann Ophthalmol 1985;17:585–588.
28. Cox TA, Goldberg RA, Rootman J: Tonic pupil and Czarnecki's sign following third nerve palsy. J Clin Neuro-ophthalmol 1991;11:55–56.
29. Jacobson DM: Pupillary responses to dilute pilocarpine in preganglionic 3rd nerve disorders. Neurology 1990;40:804–808.
30. Jacobson DM, Olson KA: Influence of pupil size, anisocoria, and ambient light on pilocarpine miosis. Implications for supersensitivity testing. Ophthalmology 1993;100:275–280.
31. Jacobson DM: A prospective evaluation of cholinergic supersensitivity of the iris sphincter in patients with oculomotor nerve palsies. Am J Ophthalmol 1994;118:377–383.
32. Slamovits TL, Miller NR,Burde RM: Intracranial oculomotor nerve paresis with anisocoria and pupillary parasympathetic hypersensitivity. Am J Ophthalmol 1987;104:401–406.
33. Keane JR, Ahmadi J: Third nerve palsies and angiography. Arch Neurol 1991;48:470.
34. Korogi Y, Takahashi M, Mabuchi M, et al: Intracranial aneurysms: diagnostic accuracy of three dimensional time of flight MR angiography. Radiology 1994;193: 181–186.
35. Thompson HS: Segmental palsy of the iris sphincter in Adie's syndrome. Arch Ophthalmol 1978;96:1615–1620.
36. Gilmore PC, Carlow TJ: Diabetic oculomotor paresis with pupil fixed to light. Neurology 1980;30:1229–1230.
37. Loewenfeld IE: Lesions in the ciliary ganglion and short ciliary nerves: the tonic pupil ("Adie's" syndrome). In: The Pupil. Anatomy, Physiology, and Clinical Applications. Vol 1, pp 1080–1130. Detroit, Wayne State University Press, 1993.
38. Drummond PD, Edis RH: Loss of facial sweating and flushing in Holmes–Adie syndrome. Neurology 1990;40:847–849.
39. Drummond PD, Lance JW: Site of autonomic deficit in harlequin syndrome: local autonomic failure affecting the arm and face. Ann Neurol 1993;34: 814–819.
40. Wolfe GI, Galetta SL, Teener JW, et al: Site of autonomic dysfunction in a patient with Ross' syndrome and postganglionic Horner's syndrome. Neurology 1995;45:2094–2096.
41. Bennett JL, Pelak VA, Mourelatos Z, et al: Acute sensorimotor polyneuropathy with tonic pupils and an abduction deficit: an unusual presentation of polyarteritis nodosa. Surv Ophthalmol 1999;43:341–344.
42. Brooks-Kayal AR, Liu GT, Menacker SJ, et al: Tonic pupil and orbital glial-neural hamartoma in infancy. Am J Ophthalmol 1995;119:809–811.
43. Rogell GD: Internal ophthalmoplegia after argon laser panretinal photocoagulation. Arch Ophthalmol 1979;97:904–905.
44. O'Neill JH, Murray NMF, Newsom-Davis J: The Lambert-Eaton myasthenic syndrome. A review of 50 cases. Brain 1988;111:577–596.
45. Bourgon P, Pilley SFJ, Thompson HS: Cholinergic supersensitivity of the iris sphincter in Adie's tonic pupil. Am J Ophthalmol 1978;85:373–377.
46. Fletcher WA, Sharpe JA: Tonic pupils in neurosyphilis. Neurology 1986;36:188–192.
47. McCrary JA, Webb NR: Anisocoria from scopolamine patches. JAMA 1982;248:353–354.
48. Thompson HS, Newsome DA, Loewenfield IE: The fixed dilated pupil: Sudden iridoplegia or mydriatic drops? A simple diagnostic test. Arch Ophthalmol 1971;86:21–27.
49. Miller NR, Moses H: Ocular involvement in wound botulism. Arch Ophthalmol 1977;95:1788–1789.
50. Terranova W, Palumbo JN, Breman JG: Ocular findings in botulism type B. JAMA 1979;241:475–477.
51. Lam BL, Thompson HS, Corbett JJ: The prevalence of simple anisocoria. Am J Ophthalmol 1987;104:69–73.
52. Roarty JD, Keltner JL: Normal pupil size and anisocoria in newborn infants. Arch Ophthalmol 1990;108: 94–95.
53. Thompson HS, Pilley SFJ: Unequal pupils. A flow chart for sorting out the anisocorias. Surv Ophthalmol 1976;21:45–48.
54. Lam BL, Thompson HS, Walls RC: Effect of light on the prevalence of simple anisocoria. Ophthalmology 1996;103:790–793.
55. Wilkins RH, Brody IA: Horner's syndrome. Arch Neurol 1968;19:540–542.
56. Thompson HS: Johann Friedrich Horner (1831–1886). Am J Ophthalmol 1986;102:792–795.
57. Pilley SF, Thompson HS: Pupillary "dilatation lag" in Horner's syndrome. Br J Ophthalmol 1975;59: 731–735.

58. Jaffe N, Cassady JR, Filler RM, et al: Heterochromia and Horner syndrome associated with cervical and mediastinal neuroblastoma. J Pediatr 1975;87:75–77.
59. Diesenhouse MC, Palay DA, Newman NJ, et al: Acquired heterochromia with Horner syndrome in two adults. Ophthalmology 1992;99:1815–1817.
60. Morris JGL, Lee J, Lim CL: Facial sweating in Horner's syndrome. Brain 1984;107:751–758.
61. Keane JR: Oculosympathetic paresis. Analysis of 100 hospitalized patients. Arch Neurol 1979;36:13–16.
62. Giles CL, Henderson JW: Horner's syndrome: an analysis of 216 cases. Am J Ophthalmol 1958;46: 289–296.
63. Maloney WF, Younge BR, Moyer NJ: Evaluation of the causes and accuracy of pharmacologic localization in Horner's syndrome. Am J Ophthalmol 1980; 90:394–402.
64. Grimson BS, Thompson HS: Drug testing in Horner's syndrome. In: Glaser JS, Smith JL (eds): Neuro-ophthalmology. Symposium of the University of Miami and the Bascom Palmer Eye Institute. Vol. VIII, pp 265–270. St. Louis, CV Mosby, 1975.
65. Reeves AG, Posner JB: The ciliospinal response in man. Neurology 1969;19:1145–1152.
66. Stone WM, de Toledo J, Romanul FCA: Horner's syndrome due to hypothalamic infarction. Clinical, radiologic, and pathologic correlations. Arch Neurol 1986;43:199–200.
67. Austin CP, Lessell S: Horner's syndrome from hypothalamic infarction. Arch Neurol 1991;48:332–334.
68. Guy J, Day AL, Mickle JP, et al: Contralateral trochlear nerve paresis and ipsilateral Horner's syndrome. Am J Ophthalmol 1989;107:73–76.
69. Bassetti C, Bogousslavsky J, Barth A, et al: Isolated infarcts of the pons. Neurology 1996;46:165–175.
70. Sacco RL, Freddo L, Bello JA, et al: Wallenberg's lateral medullary syndrome. Arch Neurol 1993;50: 609–614.
71. Kim JS, Lee JH, Suh DC, et al: Spectrum of lateral medullary syndrome. Correlation between clinical findings and magnetic resonance imaging in 33 subjects. Stroke 1994;25:1405–1410.
72. Brazis PW: Ocular motor abnormalities in Wallenberg's lateral medullary syndrome. Mayo Clin Proc 1992;67:365–368.
73. Norrving B, Cronqvist S: Lateral medullary infarction: prognosis in an unselected series. Neurology 1991;41:244–248.
74. Loewenfeld IE: Impairment of sympathetic pathways. In: The Pupil. Anatomy, Physiology, and Clinical Applications. Vol 1, pp 1131–1187. Detroit, Wayne State University Press, 1993.
75. Liu GT, Greene JM, Charness ME: Brown–Séquard syndrome in a patient with systemic lupus erythematosus. Neurology 1990;40:1474–1475.
76. Balcer LJ, Galetta SL: Pancoast syndrome. N Engl J Med 1997;337:1359.
77. Arcasoy SM, Jett JR: Superior pulmonary sulcus tumors and Pancoast's syndrome. N Engl J Med 1997;337:1370–1376.
78. Barbut D, Gold JP, Heinemann MH, et al: Horner's syndrome after coronary artery bypass surgery. Neurology 1996;46:181–184.
79. Bertino RE, Wesbey GE, Johnson RJ: Horner syndrome occurring as a complication of chest tube placement. Radiology 1987;164:745.
80. Garcia EG, Wijdicks EFM, Younge BR: Neurologic complications associated with internal jugular vein cannulation in critically ill patients: a prospective study. Neurology 1994;44:951–952.
81. Teich SA, Halprin SL, Tay S: Horner's syndrome secondary to Swan–Ganz catheterization. Am J Med 1985;78:168–170.
82. Milam MG, Sahn SA: Horner's syndrome secondary to hydromediastinum. A complication of extravascular migration of a central venous catheter. Chest 1988;94:1093–1094.
83. Biousse V, Guevara RA, Newman NJ: Transient Horner's syndrome after lumbar epidural anesthesia. Neurology 1998;51:1473–1475.
84. Grimson BS, Thompson HS: Raeder's syndrome. A clinical review. Surv Ophthalmol 1980;24:199–210.
85. Kline LB, Vitek JJ, Raymon BC: Painful Horner's syndrome due to spontaneous carotid artery dissection. Ophthalmology 1987;94:226–230.
86. Kline LB: The neuro-ophthalmologic manifestations of spontaneous dissection of the internal carotid artery. Semin Ophthalmol 1992;7:30–37.
87. Galetta SL, Leahey A, Nichols CW, et al: Orbital ischemia, ophthalmoparesis, and carotid dissection. J Clin Neuro-ophthalmol 1991;11:284–287.
88. Friedman WA, Day AL, Quisling RG, et al: Cervical carotid dissecting aneurysms. Neurosurgery 1980; 7:207–214.
89. Hart RG, Easton JD: Dissections of cervical and cerebral arteries. Neurol Clin 1983;1:155–182.
90. Lucas C, Moulin T, Deplanque D, et al: Stroke patterns of internal carotid artery dissection in 40 patients. Stroke 1998;29:2646–2648.
91. Hart RG, Easton JD: Dissections [editorial]. Stroke 1985;16:925–927.
92. Schievink WI, Mokri B, Piepgras DG: Spontaneous dissections of cervicocephalic arteries in childhood and adolescence. Neurology 1994;44:1607–1612.
93. Mokri B, Sundt TM, Houser OW, et al: Spontaneous dissection of the cervical internal carotid artery. Ann Neurol 1986;19:126–138.
94. Mokri B, Piepgras DG, Houser OW: Traumatic dissections of the extracranial internal carotid artery. J Neurosurg 1988;68:189–197.
95. Maitland CG, Black JL, Smith WA: Abducens nerve palsy due to spontaneous dissection of the internal carotid artery. Arch Neurol 1983;40:448–449.
96. Duker JS, Belmont JB: Ocular ischemic syndrome secondary to carotid artery dissection. Am J Ophthalmol 1988;106:750–752.
97. Newman NJ, Kline LB, Leifer D, et al: Ocular stroke and carotid artery dissection. Neurology 1989;39: 1462–1464.
98. Rivkin MJ, Hedges TR, Logigian EL: Carotid dissection presenting as posterior ischemic optic neuropathy. Neurology 1990;40:1469.
99. Ramadan NM, Tietjen GE, Levine SR, et al: Scintillating scotomata associated with internal carotid artery dissection: report of three cases. Neurology 1991;41: 1084–1087.
100. Schievink WI, Mokri B, Garrity JA, et al: Ocular motor nerve palsies in spontaneous dissections of the cervical internal carotid artery. Neurology 1993;43:1938–1941.
101. Mokri B, Silbert PL, Schievink WI, et al: Cranial nerve palsy in spontaneous dissection of the extracranial internal carotid artery. Neurology 1996;46:356–359.
102. Biousse V, Touboul P-J, D'Anglejan-Chatillon J, et al: Ophthalmologic manifestations of internal carotid artery dissection. Am J Ophthalmol 1998;126: 565–577.

103. Leira EC, Bendixen BH, Kardon RH, et al: Brief, transient Horner's syndrome can be the hallmark of a carotid artery dissection. Neurology 1998;50:289–290.
104. Lieschke GJ, Davis S, Tress BM, et al: Spontaneous internal carotid artery dissection presenting as hypoglossal nerve palsy. Stroke 1988;19:1151–1155.
105. Vargas ME, Desrouleaux JR, Kupersmith MJ: Ophthalmoplegia as a presenting manifestation of internal carotid artery dissection. J Clin Neuro-ophthalmol 1992;12:268–271.
106. Francis KR, Williams DP, Troost BT: Facial numbness and dysesthesia. New features of carotid artery dissection. Arch Neurol 1987;44:345–346.
107. Biousse V, Schaison M, Touboul P-J, et al: Ischemic optic neuropathy associated with internal carotid artery dissection. Arch Neurol 1998;55:715–719.
108. Koennecke H-C, Seyfert S: Mydriatic pupil as the presenting sign of common carotid artery dissection. Stroke 1998;29:2653–2655.
109. Fisher CM, Ojemann RG, Robinson GH: Spontaneous dissection of cervico-cerebral arteries. Can J Neurol Sci 1978;5:9–19.
110. Goldberg HI, Grossman RI, Gomori JM, et al: Cervical internal carotid artery dissecting hemorrhage: diagnosis using MR. Radiology 1986;158:157–161.
111. Schievink WI, Mokri B: Recurrent spontaneous cervical-artery dissection. N Engl J Med 1994;330: 393–397.
112. O'Doherty DS, Green JB: Diagnostic value of Horner's syndrome in thrombosis of the carotid artery. Neurology 1958;8:842–845.
113. Sears ML, Kier L, Chavis RM: Horner's syndrome caused by occlusion of the vascular supply to sympathetic ganglia. Am J Ophthalmol 1974;77:717–724.
114. Monteiro MLR, Coppeto JR: Horner's syndrome associated with carotid artery atherosclerosis. Am J Ophthalmol 1988;105:93–94.
115. Bollen AE, Krikke AP, de Jager AEJ: Painful Horner syndrome due to arteritis of the internal carotid artery. Neurology 1998;51:1471–1472.
116. Liu GT, Deskin RW, Bienfang DC: Horner's syndrome due to intra-oral trauma. J Clin Neuro-ophthalmol 1992;12:110–115.
117. Schnitzlein HN, Murtagh FR: Imaging Anatomy of the Head and Spine. A Photographic Atlas of MRI, CT, Gross, and Microscopic Anatomy in Axial, Coronal, and Sagittal Planes, p 77. Baltimore, Urban & Schwarzenberg, 1985.
118. Pitner SE: Carotid thrombosis due to intraoral trauma. An unusual complication of a common childhood accident. N Engl J Med 1966;274:764–767.
119. Woodhurst WB, Robertson WD, Thompson GB: Carotid injury due to intraoral trauma; case report and review of the literature. Neurosurgery 1980;6: 559–563.
120. Pruett RC: Horner's syndrome following intra-oral trauma. Arch Ophthalmol 1967;78:420–421.
121. Bazak I, Miller A, Uri N: Oculosympathetic paresis caused by foreign body perforation of pharyngeal wall. Postgrad Med J 1987;63:681–683.
122. Shissas CG, Golnik KC: Horner's syndrome after tonsillectomy. Am J Ophthalmol 1994;117:812–813.
123. Campbell RL, Mercuri LG, Van Sickels J: Cervical sympathetic block following intraoral local anesthesia. Oral Surg Oral Med Oral Pathol 1979;47:223–226.
124. Salvesen R, Bogucki A, Wysocka-Bakowska MM, et al: Cluster headache pathogenesis: a pupillometric study. Cephalalgia 1987;7:273–284.
125. Salvesen R, Sand T, Zhao J-M, et al: Cluster headache: pupillometric patterns as a function of the degree of anisocoria. Cephalalgia 1989;9:131–138.
126. Khurana RK: Bilateral Horner's syndrome in cluster type headaches. Headache 1993;33:449–451.
127. Trobe JD, Glaser JS, Post JD: Meningiomas and aneurysms of the cavernous sinus. Arch Ophthalmol 1978;96:457–467.
128. Smith SA, Smith SE: Bilateral Horner's syndrome: detection and occurrence. J Neurol Neurosurg Psychiatry 1999;66:48–51.
129. Leung A: Congenital Horner's syndrome. Ala J Med Sci 1986;23:204–205.
130. Weinstein JM, Zweifel TJ, Thompson HS: Congenital Horner's syndrome. Arch Ophthalmol 1980;98:1074–1078.
131. Woodruff G, Buncic JR, Morin JD: Horner's syndrome in children. J Pediatr Ophthalmol Strab 1988;25:40–44.
132. Jeffery AR, Ellis FJ, Repka MX, et al: Pediatric Horner syndrome. J Am Assoc Pediatr Ophthalmol Strabismus 1998;2:159–167.
133. George NDL, Gonzalez G, Hoyt CS: Does Horner's syndrome in infancy require investigation? Br J Ophthalmol 1998;82:51–54.
134. Musarella M, Chan HSL, DeBoer G, et al: Ocular involvement in neuroblastoma: prognostic implications. Ophthalmology 1984;91:936–940.
135. Ogita S, Tokiwa K, Takahashi T, et al: Congenital cervical neuroblastoma associated with Horner syndrome. J Pediatr Surg 1988;23:991–992.
136. Abramson SJ, Berdon WE, Ruzal-Shapiro C, et al: Cervical neuroblastoma in eleven infants—a tumor with favorable prognosis. Clinical and radiologic (US, CT, MRI) findings. Pediatr Radiol 1993;23:253–257.
137. Casselman JW, Smet MH, Van Damme B, et al: Primary cervical neuroblastoma: CT and MR findings. J Comput Assist Tomogr 1988;12:684–686.
138. Gibbs J, Appleton RE, Martin J, et al: Congenital Horner syndrome associated with non-cervical neuroblastoma. Dev Med Child Neurol 1992;34:642–644.
139. McRae D, Shaw A: Ganglioneuroma, heterochromia iridis, and Horner's syndrome. J Pediatr Surg 1979;14:612–614.
140. Al-Jassim AHH: Cervical ganglioneuroblastoma. J Laryngol Otol 1987;101:296–301.
141. Coldman AJ, Fryer CJH, Elmwood JM, et al: Neuroblastoma: influence of age at diagnosis, stage, tumor site, and sex on prognosis. Cancer 1980;46:1896–1901.
142. Carlsen NLT, Schroeder H, Bro PV, et al: Neuroblastomas treated at the four major child oncologic clinics in Denmark 1943–1980: an evaluation of 180 cases. Med Pediatr Oncol 1985;13:180–186.
143. Sauer C, Levinsohn MW: Horner's syndrome in childhood. Neurology 1976;26:216–220.
144. Thompson BM, Corbett JJ, Kline LB, et al: Pseudo-Horner's syndrome. Arch Neurol 1982;39:108–111.
145. Kardon RH, Denison CE, Brown CK, et al: Critical evaluation of the cocaine test in the diagnosis of Horner's syndrome. Arch Ophthalmol 1990;108: 384–387.
146. Van der Wiel HL, Van Gijn J: The diagnosis of Horner's syndrome. Use and limitations of the cocaine test. J Neurol Sci 1986;73:311–316.
147. Thompson HS, Mensher JH: Adrenergic mydriasis in Horner's syndrome. Am J Ophthalmol 1971;72: 472–480.
148. Cremer SA, Thompson HS, Digre KB, et al: Hydroxyamphetamine mydriasis in normal subjects. Am J Ophthalmol 1990;110:66–70.

149. Heitman K, Bodé DD: The paredrine test in normal eyes. J Clin Neuro-ophthalmol 1986;6:228–231.
150. Cremer SA, Thompson HS, Digre KB, et al: Hydroxyamphetamine mydriasis in Horner's syndrome. Am J Ophthalmol 1990;110:71–76.
151. Van der Wiel HL, Van Gijn J: Localization of Horner's syndrome. Use and limitations of the hydroxyamphetamine test. J Neurol Sci 1986;59:229–235.
152. Stern MJ, Patel M, Davis J, et al: Painful Horner syndrome associated with occlusion of the extracranial internal carotid artery: MR imaging. J Comput Assist Tomogr 1989;13:918–920.
153. Digre KB, Smoker WR, Johnston P, et al: Selective MR imaging approach for evaluation of patients with Horner's syndrome. Am J Neuroradiol 1992;13: 223–227.
154. Brown J, Danielson R, Donahue SP, et al: Horner's syndrome in subadventitial carotid artery dissection and the role of magnetic resonance angiography. Am J Ophthalmol 1995;119:811–813.
155. Halperin EC, Constine LS, Tarbell NJ, et al: Neuroblastoma. In: Pediatric Radiation Oncology, 2nd edition, pp 171–214. New York, Raven Press, 1994.
156. Plum F, Posner JB: Pupils. In: The Diagnosis of Stupor and Coma, 3rd edition, pp 41–47. Philadelphia, FA Davis, 1980.
157. Wijdicks EFM: Determining brain death in adults. Neurology 1995;45:1003–1011.
158. Quality standards subcommittee of the American Academy of Neurology: Practice parameters for determining brain death in adults (summary statement). Neurology 1995;45:1012–1014.
159. Ropper AH, Cole D, Louis DN: Clinicopathologic correlation in a case of pupillary dilation from cerebral hemorrhage. Arch Neurol 1991;48:1166–1169.
160. Ropper AH: The opposite pupil in herniation. Neurology 1990;40:1707–1709.
161. Fisher CM: Oval pupils. Arch Neurol 1980;37: 502–503.
162. Chen R, Sahjpaul R, Del Maestro RF, et al: Initial enlargement of the opposite pupil as a false localising sign in intraparenchymal frontal haemorrhage. J Neurol Neurosurg Psychiatry 1994;57:1126–1128.
163. Rothstein JD, Herlong HF: Neurologic manifestations of hepatic disease. Neurol Clin 1989;7:563–578.
164. Liu GT, Urion DK, Volpe JJ: Cerebral edema in acute fulminant hepatic failure: clinicopathologic correlation. Pediatr Neurol 1993;9:224–226.
165. Woods D, O'Connor PS, Fleming R: Episodic unilateral mydriasis and migraine. Am J Ophthalmol 1984;98:229–234.
166. Jacobson DM: Benign episodic unilateral mydriasis. Ophthalmology 1995;102:1623–1627.
167. Purvin VA: Adie's tonic pupil secondary to migraine. J Neuro-ophthalmol 1995;15:43–44.
168. Thompson HS, Zackon DH, Czarnecki JSC: Tadpole shaped pupils caused by segmental spasm of the iris dilator muscle. Am J Ophthalmol 1983;96:467–477.
169. Drummond PD: Cervical sympathetic deficit in unilateral migraine headache. Headache 1991;31: 669–672.
170. De Marinis M, Assenza S, Carletto F: Oculosympathetic alterations in migraine patients. Cephalalgia 1998;18:77–84.
171. Pant SS, Benton JN, Dodge PR: Unilateral pupillary dilatation during and immediately following seizures. Neurology 1966;16:837–840.
172. Zee DS, Griffen J, Price DL: Unilateral pupillary dilatation during adversive seizures. Arch Neurol 1974; 30:403–405.
173. Gadoth N, Margalith D, Bechar M: Unilateral pupillary dilatation during focal seizures. J Neurol 1981; 225:227–230.
174. Afifi AK, Corbett JJ, Thompson HS, et al: Seizure-induced miosis and ptosis: association with temporal lobe magnetic resonance imaging abnormalities. J Child Neurol 1990;5:142–146.
175. Rosenberg ML, Jabbari B: Miosis and internal ophthalmoplegia as a manifestation of partial seizures. Neurology 1991;41:737–739.
176. Ropper AH, Wijdicks EFM, Truax BT: Pupillary abnormalities. Clinical features of the typical syndrome. In: Guillain–Barré Syndrome, p 92. Philadelphia, FA Davis, 1991.
177. Fisher M: An unusual variant of acute idiopathic polyneuritis (syndrome of ophthalmoplegia, ataxia and areflexia). N Engl J Med 1956;255:57–65.
178. Okajima T, Imamura S, Kawasaki S, et al: Fisher's syndrome: a pharmacological study of the pupils. Ann Neurol 1977;2:63–65.
179. Keane JR: Tonic pupils with acute ophthalmoplegic polyneuritis. Ann Neurol 1977;2:393–396.
180. Radziwill AJ, Steck AJ, Borruat F-X, et al: Isolated internal ophthalmoplegia associated with IgG anti-GQ1b antibody. Neurology 1998;50:307.
181. Scinto LFM, Daffner KR, Dressler D, et al: A potential noninvasive neurobiological test for Alzheimer's disease. Science 1994;266:1051–1054.
182. Scinto LF, Rentz DM, Potter H, et al: Pupil assay and Alzheimer's disease: a critical analysis (letter). Neurology 1999;52:673–674.
183. Loupe DN, Newman NJ, Green RC, et al: Pupillary response to tropicamide in patients with Alzheimer disease. Ophthalmology 1996;103:495–503.
184. Reitner A, Baumgartner I, Thule C, et al: The mydriatic effect of tropicamide and its diagnostic use in Alzheimer's disease. Vision Res 1997;37:165–168.
185. Growdon JH, Graefe K, Tennis M, et al: Pupil dilation to tropicamide is not specific for Alzheimer disease. Arch Neurol 1997;54:841–844.
186. Graff-Radford NR, Lin S-C, Brazis PW, et al: Tropicamide eyedrops cannot be used for reliable diagnosis of Alzheimer's disease. Mayo Clin Proc 1997;72: 495–504.
187. Ferrario E, Molaschi M, Villa L, et al: Is videopupillography useful in the diagnosis of Alzheimer's disease? Neurology 1998;50:642–644.
188. Kaneyuki H, Mitsuno S, Nishida T, et al: Enhanced miotic response to topical dilute pilocarpine in patients with Alzheimer's disease. Neurology 1998;50: 802–804.
189. Newman NJ: The eyes don't have it in Alzheimer's disease (editorial). Mayo Clin Proc 1997;72:581–582.
190. Kardon RH: Drop the Alzheimer's drop test (editorial). Neurology 1998;50:588–591.
191. Litvan I, FitzGibbon EJ: Can tropicamide eye drop response differentiate patients with progressive supranuclear palsy and Alzheimer's disease from healthy subjects? Neurology 1996;47:1324–1326.
192. Price MJ, Thompson HS, Judisch GF, et al: Pupillary constriction to darkness. Br J Ophthalmol 1985;69: 205–211.
193. Myers GA, Barricks ME, Stark L: Paradoxic pupillary constriction in a patient with congenital stationary night blindness. Invest Ophthalmol Vis Sci 1985;26: 736–740.
194. Barricks ME, Flynn JT, Kushner BJ: Pardoxical pupillary responses in congenital stationary night blindness. Arch Ophthalmol 1977;95:1800–1804.

195. Sharpe JA, Glaser JS: Tournay's phenomenon—a reappraisal of anisocoria in lateral gaze. Am J Ophthalmol 1974;77:250–255.
196. Loewenfeld IE, Friedlaender RP, McKinnon PFM: Pupillary inequality associated with lateral gaze (Tournay's phenomenon). Am J Ophthalmol 1974; 78:449–469.
197. Cox TA, Law FCH: The clinical significance of Tournay's pupillary phenomenon. J Clin Neuro-ophthalmol 1991;11:186–189.
198. Pfeiffer N, Simonsz HJ, Kommerell G: Misdirected regeneration of abducens nerve neurons into the parasympathetic pupillary pathway. Graefes Arch Clin Exp Ophthalmol 1992;230:150–153.
199. Wilhelm H, Wilhelm B, Mildenberger I: Primary aberrant regeneration of abducens nerve fibers into the pupillary pathway. Neuro-ophthalmology 1994;14: 85–89.
200. Kline LB, McCluer SM, Bonikowski FP: Oculosympathetic spasm with cervical spinal cord injury. Arch Neurol 1984;41:61–64.
201. Loewenfeld IE, Thompson HS: Oculomotor paresis with cyclic spasms. A critical review of the literature and a new case. Surv Ophthalmol 1975;20:81–124.
202. Bateman DE, Saunders M: Cyclic oculomotor palsy: description of a case and hypothesis of the mechanism. J Neurol Neurosurg Psychiatry 1983;46: 451–453.
203. Brodsky MC, Sharp GB, Fritz KJ, et al: Idiopathic alternating anisocoria. Am J Ophthalmol 1992;114: 509–510.
204. Goldstein JH, Schneekloth BB: Spasm of the near reflex: a spectrum of anomalies. Surv Ophthalmol 1996;40:269–278.
205. Griffin JF, Wray SH, Anderson DP: Misdiagnosis of spasm of the near reflex. Neurology 1976;26:1018–1020.
206. Newman NJ, Lessell S: Pupillary dilatation with monocular occlusion as a sign of nonorganic oculomotor dysfunction. Am J Ophthalmol 1989;108:461–462.
207. Lam BL, Thompson HS: An anisocoria produces a small relative afferent pupillary defect in the eye with the smaller pupil. J Neuro-ophthalmol 1999;19: 153–159.
208. Zamir E, Chowers I, Banin E, et al: Neurotrophic corneal endothelial failure complicating acute Horner syndrome. Ophthalmology 1999;106:1692–1696.
209. Lee SK, Kwon SU, Ahn H, et al: Acute isolated monocular blindness and painless carotid artery dissection. Neurology 1999;53:1155–1156.
210. Guillon B, Brunereau L, Biousse V, et al: Long-term follow-up of aneurysms developed during extracranial internal carotid artery dissection. Neurology 1999;53:117–122.
211. Ryan FH, Kline LB, Gomez C: Congenital Horner's syndrome resulting from agenesis of the internal carotid artery. Ophthalmology 2000;107:185–188.

CHAPTER 14

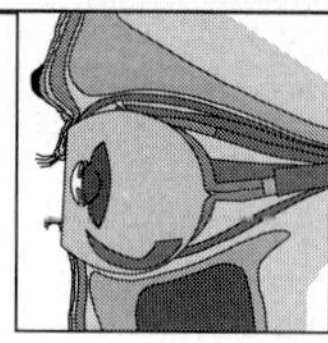

Eyelid and Facial Nerve Disorders

The eyelids protect the eye and help maintain the corneal tear film. *Ptosis* (drooping), *retraction* (abnormal elevation), *facial weakness* (causing insufficient eyelid closure), *abnormal blinking* (absent or excessive), and other *abnormal eyelid and facial movements* are the most important eyelid and facial nerve disorders in neuro-ophthalmology. This chapter will review the relevant neuroanatomy, examination of the eyelids and facial nerve, and differential diagnosis of these and other eyelid abnormalities. At the end of the chapter, diseases that are commonly associated with ptosis or facial weakness will be discussed.

NEUROANATOMY

Upper Eyelid

Upper Eyelid Muscles and Their Innervations. The *levator palpebrae superioris muscle,* with minor contributions from *Müller's* and the *frontalis muscles,* maintains the normal position of the upper eyelid. The aponeurosis of the levator muscle attaches to the anterior surface and the superior edge of the superior tarsal plate (Fig. 14–1). Both levator muscles are controlled by the central caudal nucleus (CCN) of the oculomotor nuclear complex (third cranial nerve) (see Chapter 15), while the frontalis is innervated by the facial nerve (see below). Within the CCN, which is a single midline subnucleus, neurons to both levators are intermixed. Müller's muscle is innervated by oculosympathetic neurons (see Chapter 13), while the frontalis receives fibers from the facial nerve. Eyelid position depends mainly on the resting tone of the levator muscles, which varies according to the patient's state of arousal, with individuals having wider palpebral fissures when alert compared to when they are drowsy. Experimental lesions of the frontal lobes, angular gyrus, and temporal lobes may produce ptosis, and experimental stimulation of areas within frontal, temporal, and occipital lobes may produce eyelid opening, but the exact nature of the cortical control of the eyelids is unclear.[1] There is some evidence to suggest that the right hemisphere may be dominant for this function (see cerebral ptosis, below).

Coordination With Vertical Eye Movements. With only some minor differences in speed and conjugacy, the eyelids move with the eyes during both slow and rapid vertical eye movements.[2] The major nonpathologic exception to this occurs while the eye blinks, at which time the levator is temporarily inhibited, and the orbicularis oculi contracts. Recent evidence suggests that vertical eye movements and lid position are coordinated in the midbrain by the nucleus of the posterior commissure (nPC), whose neurons pass through the supra oculomotor area (supra III, or M-group) to inhibit the CCN (Fig. 14–2).[3,4] This supraoculomotor area lies inferior to the nPC. Thus in upgaze, the levator muscles contract and the eyelids open, while during downgaze, nPC neurons fire, allowing eyelid relaxation. Each nPC lies dorsolaterally to the third nerve nuclei, and interconnecting neurons between the nPC on each side travel through the posterior commissure in the dorsal midbrain. More details re-

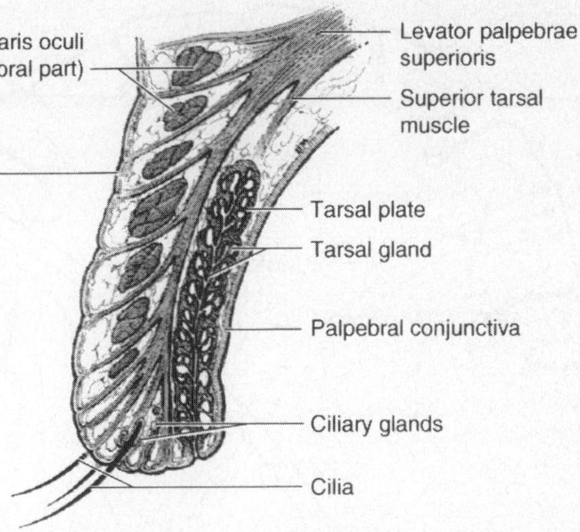

FIGURE 14–1. Sagittal drawing of the upper eyelid. The levator palpebrae superioris muscle attaches to the anterior surface and superior edge of the superior tarsal plate. (From Moore KL: Clinically Oriented Anatomy, 4th edition, p 900. Baltimore, Lippincott Williams & Wilkins, 1999, with permission.)

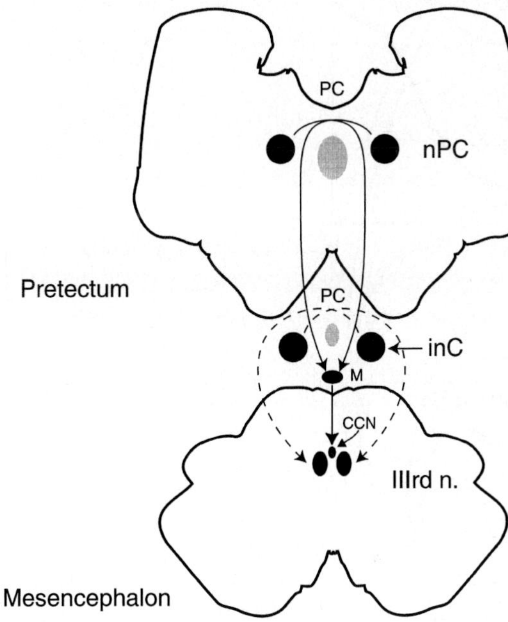

FIGURE 14–2. Theoretical scheme of lid–eye coordination. The inhibitory pathways from the nucleus of the posterior commissure (nPC) cross within the posterior commissure (PC), then connect to an intermediary region called the M-group (M) (supraoculomotor area, or supra III). The M-group exerts control over the central caudal nucleus (CCN) in the oculomotor nuclear complex (IIIrd n.). Note fibers from the interstitial nucleus of Cajal (inC) mediating vertical gaze (also see Fig. 16–17) also pass through the posterior commissure before innervating the third and fourth nerve nuclei. Thus lesions of the posterior commissure may cause both vertical gaze paresis and eyelid retraction.

garding the anatomy of the third nerve are discussed in Chapter 15.

Facial Nerve

Supranuclear Pathways. The supranuclear neurons destined to innervate the facial nerve nucleus lie in the precentral gyrus of the frontal lobe.[5] Discharges from this region initiate voluntary movements to command such as smiling or puckering of the lips. Somatotopically, these supranuclear neurons are located most laterally in the frontal cortex just below the representation for the hand. Leaving the precentral gyrus, the axons of the facial motor area coalesce and become part of the corticobulbar tracts that descend through the middle of the internal capsule on their way to the medial part of the cerebral peduncle. Immediately below this midbrain level, most of the supranuclear fibers cross over to the opposite side of the pons to innervate the facial nerve nucleus. However, some fibers synapse on the ipsilateral facial nerve nucleus, providing the upper face with innervation from both cerebral hemispheres. This unusual anatomic feature explains why supranuclear lesions involving the descending motor pathways results in weakness of the contralateral lower face only (Fig. 14–3).

Pons. The motor nucleus of the facial nerve resides in the lateral midpons.[6] Motor axons leaving the facial nucleus course dorsomedi-

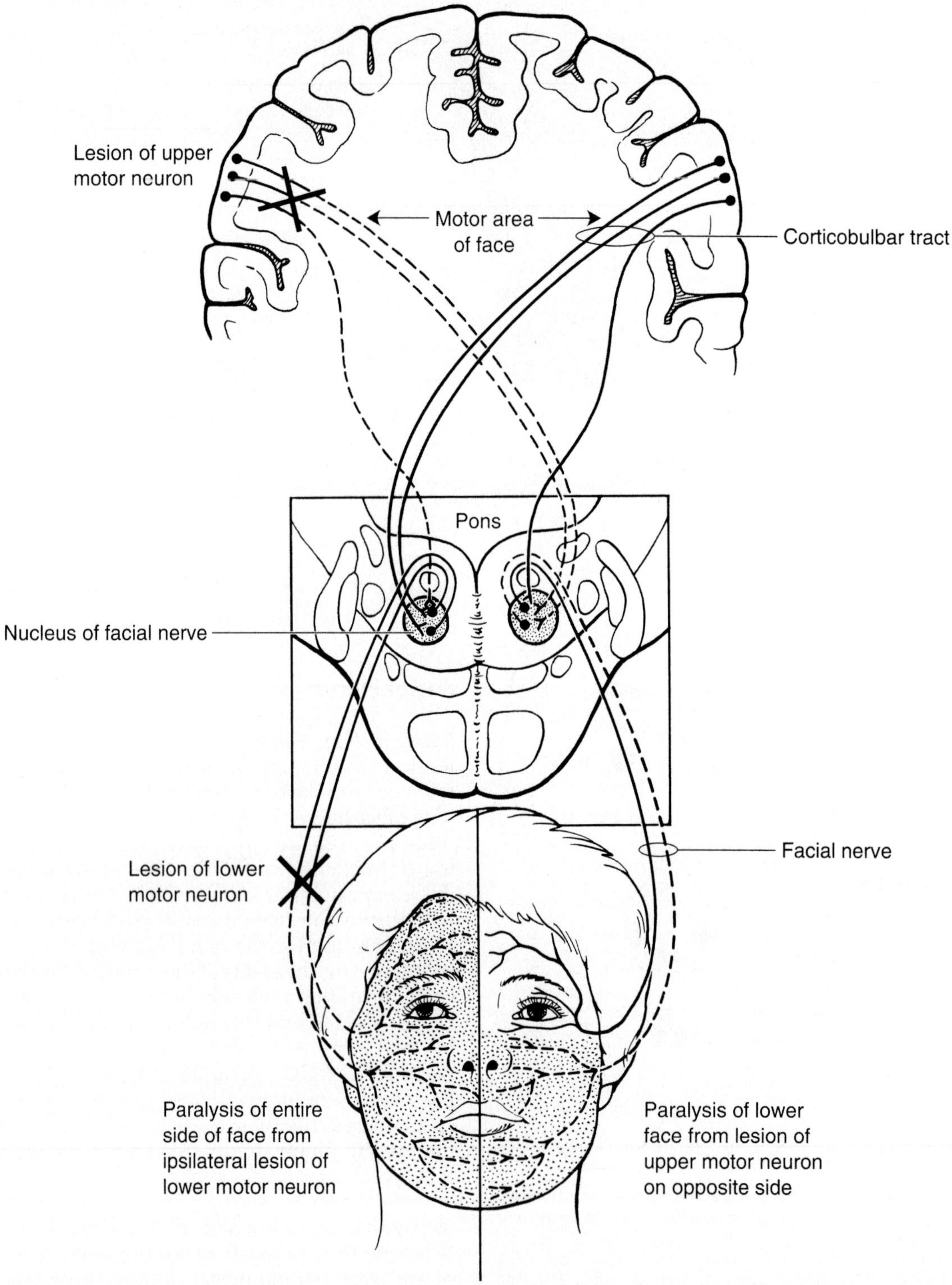

FIGURE 14–3. Facial motor axons descend from the precentral gyrus as part of corticobulbar tracts to the cerebral peduncle. Below midbrain level, most supranuclear fibers decussate to innervate the contralateral facial nerve nucleus. Some fibers destined to innervate the upper face synapse in the ipsilateral facial nucleus. Thus, the upper face is innervated by both hemispheres, which explains why supranuclear lesions result in weakness of the lower face only. Modified from Gilman S, Newman SH: Manter and Gatz's Essentials of Clinical Neuroanatomy and Neurophysiology, 7th edition. Philadelphia, FA Davis, 1987, with permission.)

ally toward the fourth ventricle to loop around the sixth nerve nucleus, thus forming the facial colliculus. After bending around the sixth nerve nucleus, the motor fibers extend laterally to exit the pons (Fig. 14–4). The parasympathetic component of the facial nerve originates from the superior salvatory nucleus, which lies just superior to the facial motor nucleus. This nucleus supplies the sublingual, submandibular, and lacrimal glands and forms one part of the nervus intermedius (Fig.14–5). The other component of the nervus intermedius is sensory, containing those fibers subserving taste to the anterior two thirds of the tongue and somatic sensation to the external auditory meatus and postauricular region. Taste fibers synapse in the nucleus solitarius, while those of somatic sensation terminate in the spinal tract of the fifth nerve. Afferents to the facial nucleus are also derived from the trigeminal nucleus as part of the corneal reflex and the acoustic pathways as part of the stapedius reflex, in which the eyes blink reflexively to a loud noise (see below).

Cerebellopontine Angle. At the ventrolateral angle of the pons, the facial motor root and the vestibuloacoustic nerve exit the brain stem together. Between these two nerves lies the nervus intermedius carrying sensory and parasympathetic information. In the cerebellopontine angle, the anterior inferior cerebellar artery (AICA) courses between the seventh and eighth nerves in its course to supply the lateral pons and anterior cerebellum.[7] The close proximity of the fifth, seventh, and eighth nerves in the cerebellopontine angle helps predict their involvement in tumors in this region. As the facial nerve motor branch enters the internal auditory meatus, it is joined to the nervus intermedus and lies superior and anterior to the vestibuloacoustic nerve. After exiting the internal auditory meatus, the facial nerve separates from the acoustic nerve to enter its own canal, the fallopian or facial canal[8] (Fig. 14–6). Here the facial nerve incorporates the geniculate ganglion and the first branch of the facial nerve, known as the greater superficial petrosal nerve.[9] This nerve travels forward

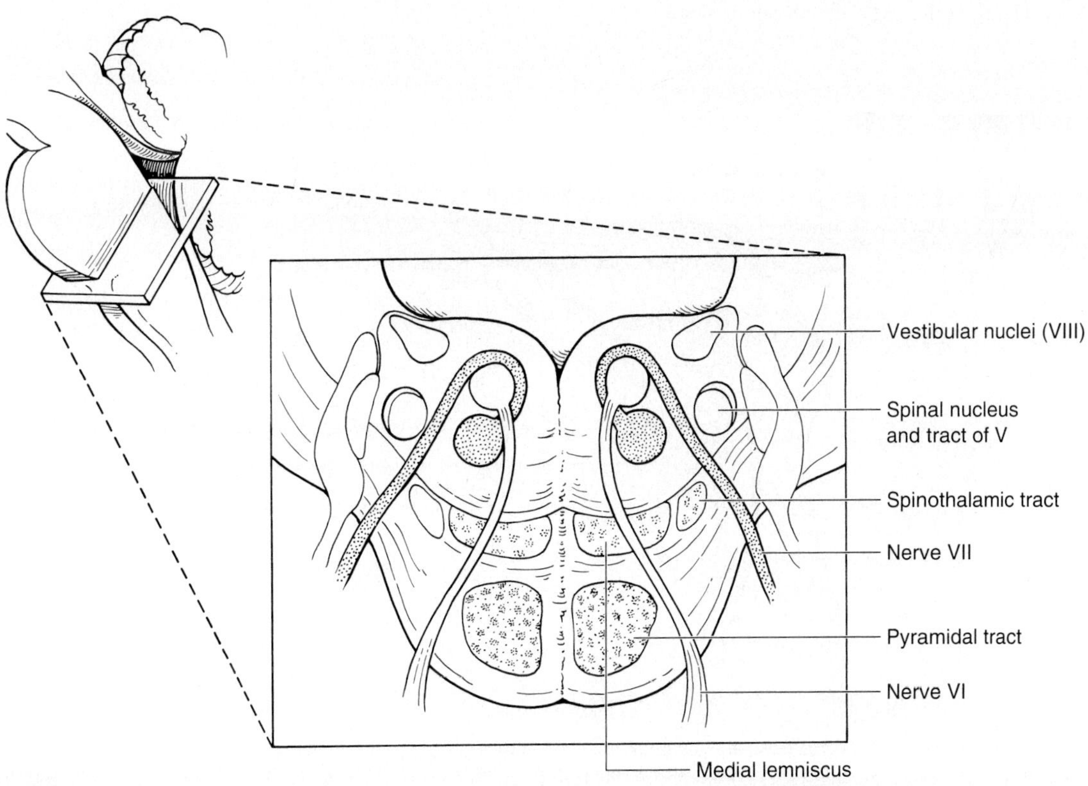

FIGURE 14–4. Cross section of the lower pons. There is close proximity of the sixth, seventh, and eighth cranial nerve nuclei. Their location in relation to the pyramidal or corticospinal tracts should also be noted. (From Handler LF, Galetta SL, Wulc AE et al: Facial paralysis: diagnosis and management. In: Bosniak S. (ed): Principles and Practice of Ophthalmic Plastic and Reconstructive Surgery, p 467. Philadelphia, WB Saunders, 1996, with permission.)

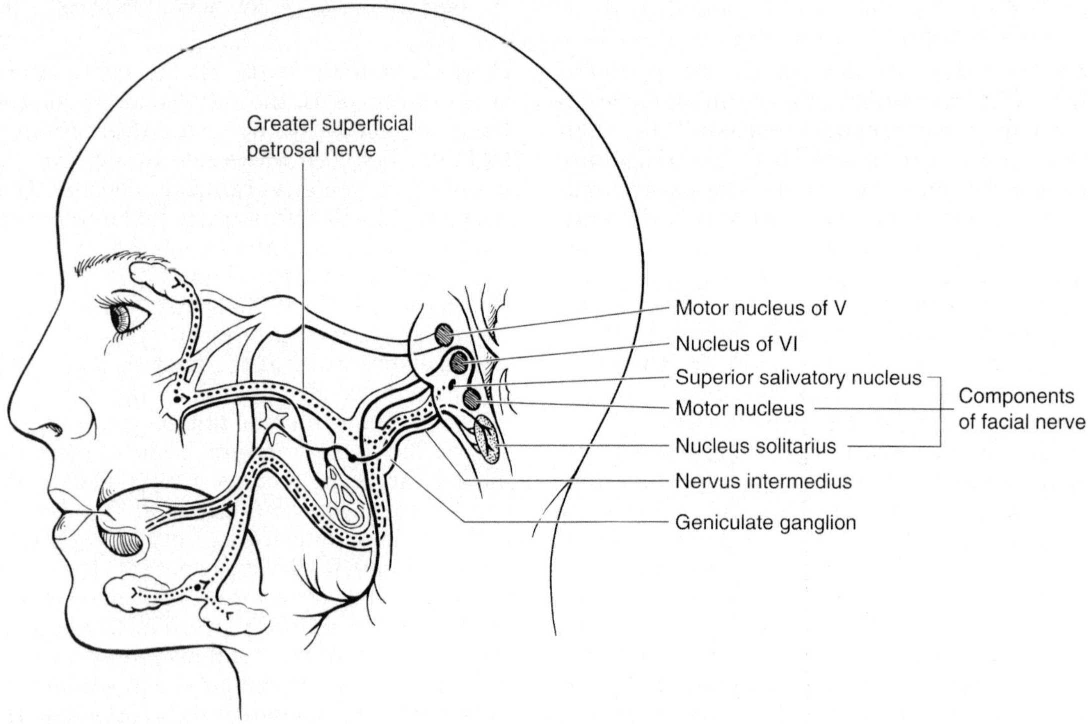

FIGURE 14–5. Facial nerve separated into motor fibers and nervus intermedius. The nervus intermedius contains both parasympathetic and sensory fibers. (From Handler LF, Galetta SL, Wulc AE et al: Facial paralysis: diagnosis and management. In Bosniak S. (ed): Principles and Practice of Ophthalmic Plastic and Reconstructive Surgery, p 467. Philadelphia, WB Saunders, 1996. Modified from Dejong RN: The Neurologic Examination, 4th edition, p 181. New York, Harper & Row, 1979, with permission.)

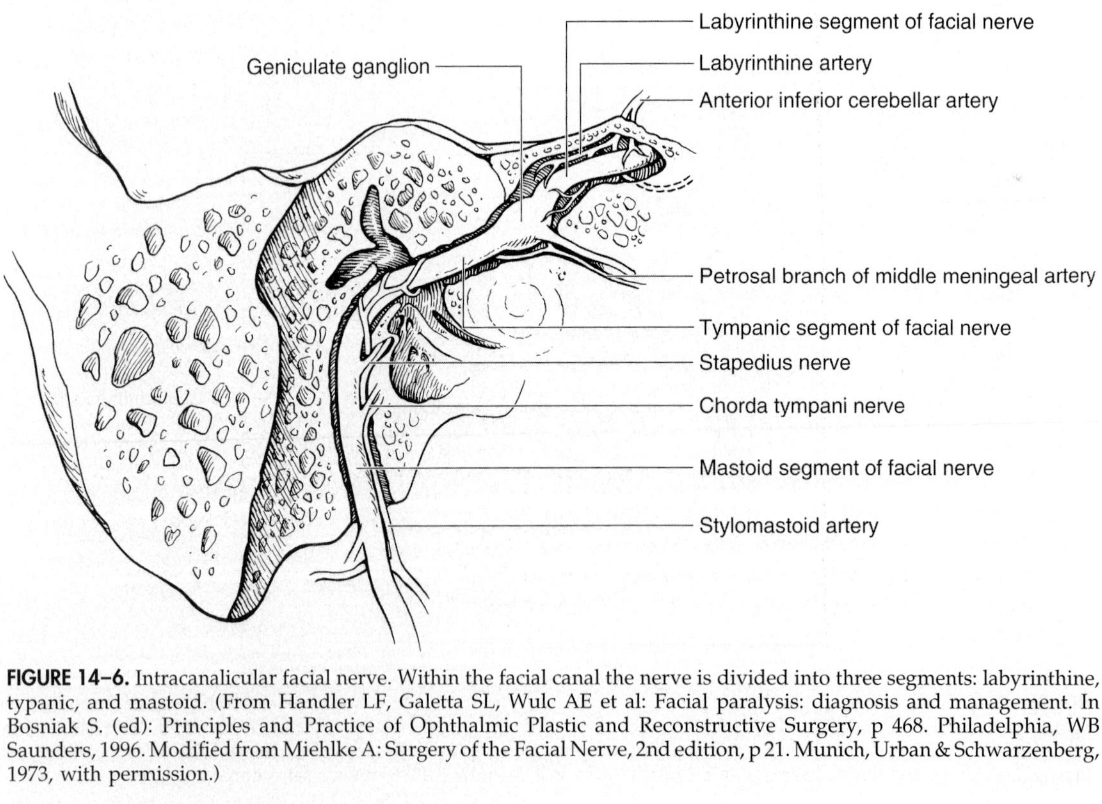

FIGURE 14–6. Intracanalicular facial nerve. Within the facial canal the nerve is divided into three segments: labyrinthine, typanic, and mastoid. (From Handler LF, Galetta SL, Wulc AE et al: Facial paralysis: diagnosis and management. In Bosniak S. (ed): Principles and Practice of Ophthalmic Plastic and Reconstructive Surgery, p 468. Philadelphia, WB Saunders, 1996. Modified from Miehlke A: Surgery of the Facial Nerve, 2nd edition, p 21. Munich, Urban & Schwarzenberg, 1973, with permission.)

along the floor of the middle cranial fossa to synapse in the sphenopalatine ganglion. Postganglionic parasympathetic fibers continue forward to innervate the lacrimal gland and nasopalatine glands.[10]

At the level of the lateral semicircular canal, the nerve to stapedius takes its origin at the proximal portion of this segment, while the chorda tympani nerve branches off more distally.[8] The chorda tympani nerve is a mixed nerve, carrying taste fibers from the anterior two thirds of the tongue, parasympathetic fibers to the submaxillary and sublingual glands, and pain and temperature sensation from the external auditory meatus.[10]

Extracranial Course. The motor branches of the facial nerve exit the skull base via the stylomastoid foramen. Nerve twigs are immediately provided to the posterior auricular, posterior belly of the digastric, and stylohyoid muscles. The facial nerve then bends again to proceed forward to penetrate the posterior aspect of the parotid gland. Within the substance of the parotid gland, the facial nerve divides into upper and lower divisions. These divisions may be further subdivided from top to bottom into temporal, zygomatic, buccal, mandibular, and cervical branches (Fig. 14–7).[11] The vast interconnections amongst these branches provide the substrate for aberrant regeneration to ensue after facial palsy (see below).[9]

Vascular Supply. From the brain stem to the internal auditory meatus, the facial nerve derives its blood supply from the AICA. The labyrinthine artery, a branch of the AICA, sup-

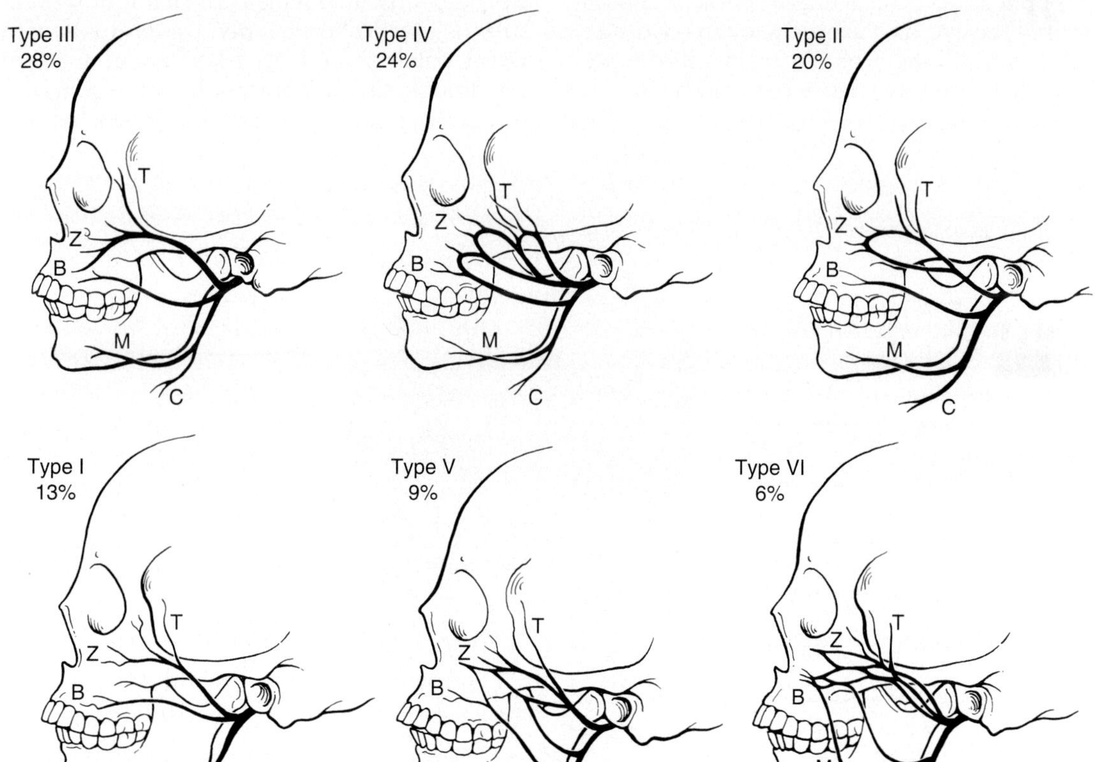

FIGURE 14–7. Branches of the facial nerve. Initially, the facial nerve divides into upper and lower segments within the parotid gland. The facial nerve then divides to form the temporal (T), zygomatic (Z), buccal (B), mandibular (M), and cervical (C) branches. The facial nerve divides into six common patterns. The frequency of each pattern is listed. (From Handler LF, Galetta SL, Wulc AE et al: Facial paralysis: diagnosis and management. In Bosniak S. (ed): Principles and Practice of Ophthalmic Plastic and Reconstructive Surgery, p. 468. Philadelphia, WB Saunders, 1996, with permission. Data from Davis RA, Anson BJ, et al: Surgical anatomy of the facial nerve and parotid gland based on a study of 350 cervical facial halves. Surg Gynecol Obstet 1956;102:385.)

plies the nerve in the internal auditory meatus. Moving distally, the petrosal branch of the middle meningeal artery enters the facial canal at the level of the geniculate ganglion and supplies blood to the tympanic portion of the nerve (Fig. 14–6). Anastomotic connections are made to the tympanic region by the stylomastoid artery, which extends up the vertically oriented mastoid segment. The weakest link in the arterial supply to the facial nerve is just proximal to the geniculate ganglion, and this region represents the most likely site for ischemic injury to the nerve.[12]

Muscles Innervated by the Facial Nerve. All the muscles of facial expression are supplied by the facial nerve (Fig. 14–8).[13] The major muscles are the *frontalis,* which lifts the eyebrow, the *orbicularis oculi,* which closes the eyelids, the *orbicularis oris,* which closes the mouth and purses the lips, and the *zygomaticus major,* which lifts the angle of the mouth upward. The orbicularis oculi acts as a sphincter muscle around the eye, as it is organized in concentric circles around the orbital margin and the eyelids. There are three major parts of the orbicularis oculi: (1) the thick orbital part, for the most vigorous eyelid closure; (2) the thin palpebral part, for closing the eyelids lightly, and (3) the lacrimal part, which pulls the eyelids and lacrimal puncta medially.[13]

HISTORY AND EXAMINATION

When a patient complains of ptosis, historical details such as duration, acuteness of symptoms, and presence of eye pain or diplopia are important considerations in making the diagnosis. Qualities such as fatiguability and associated dysarthria, and swallowing or breathing difficulty may suggest underlying myasthenia gravis. Patients with eyelid retraction should be asked about symptoms such as temperature intolerance, tachycardia, and proptosis, which might indicate underlying thyroid-associated ophthalmopathy. Headache or difficulty with upgaze, consistent with a dorsal midbrain syndrome, should be excluded. Individuals with facial palsy should be asked about medical conditions, such as diabetes, hypertension, sar-

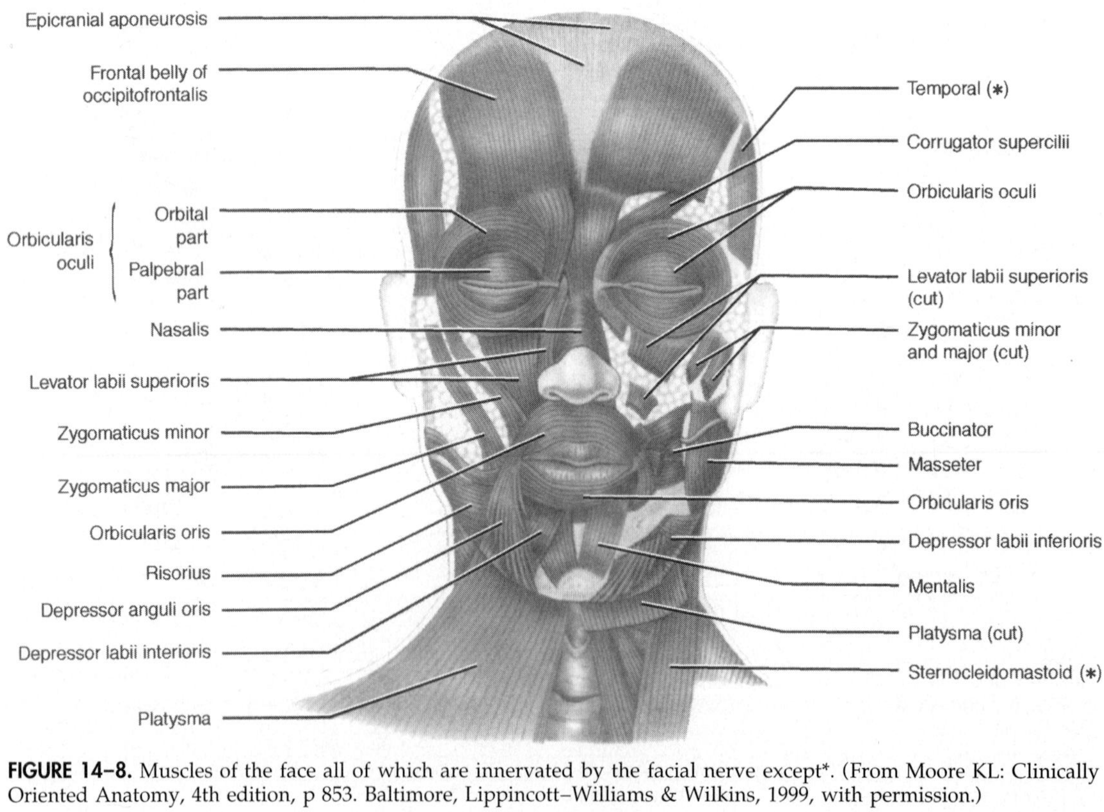

FIGURE 14–8. Muscles of the face all of which are innervated by the facial nerve except*. (From Moore KL: Clinically Oriented Anatomy, 4th edition, p 853. Baltimore, Lippincott–Williams & Wilkins, 1999, with permission.)

coidosis, Lyme disease, and pregnancy, which may predispose them to acquired seventh nerve injury. In those with abnormal blinking or facial movements, historical evidence of basal ganglia diseases, old Bell's palsy, or multiple sclerosis, for example, should be investigated. A history consistent with allergies, photophobia, dry eye, or corneal damage may suggest an ocular cause of excessive eyelid closure.

The techniques of the eyelid and facial nerve examination are detailed in Chapter 2. However, some important guidelines will be discussed here. The eyelids and facial nerve should first be observed at rest. Eyelid position in relationship to the limbus and corneal light reflex should be noted, and the palpebral fissures measured. The postion of the nasolabial fold and the nostrils should be evaluated because the nasolabial fold may disappear or be displaced in facial palsy, and the nostril may be ptotic or decreased circumferentially.

Eyelid fatigue, curtaining, and lid twitch should be tested for if the eyelid is ptotic. Although these signs are suggestive of myasthenia gravis, they are not specific for the disease.[14] Hering's law of equal innervation, referring to the yoking of agonist muscles, applies to both levator muscles. Thus ptosis on one side may be accompanied by lid retraction on the other due to the excess tonus required to keep the ptotic lid open (Fig. 14–9A). This is the case especially if the ptotic eye is the dominant and fixating one. In addition, if the ptotic eyelid is manually elevated, the retracted eyelid of the fellow eye droops (curtaining) (Fig. 14–9B). Similarly, if ptosis is bilateral, if either eyelid is manually elevated, the ptosis on the other side worsens (enhanced ptosis) (Fig. 14–10). Hering's law applies to ptosis caused by neuromuscular junction deficits as well as to ptosis resulting from oculomotor and other more proximal lesions.[15,16] Conversely, there may be pseudoptosis associated with contralateral pathologic eyelid retraction (Fig. 14–11).

The pupils and eye movements should also be observed. Levator and orbicularis oculi function should be assessed. Facial nerve function can be tested by having the patient lift the eyebrows, close the eyelids, and smile. In facial palsies, the ear should be examined for the presence of vesicles. When there are involuntary facial movements, the presence of subtle facial weakness or movements of other head and neck structures should be excluded. As suggested above, corneal abrasion or ulceration, iritis with photophobia, blepharitis, dry eye, and eyelid follicles should be ruled out in patients with excessive blinking. The tarsal conjunctiva should be examined for follicles in all patients with ptosis and ocular irritation.

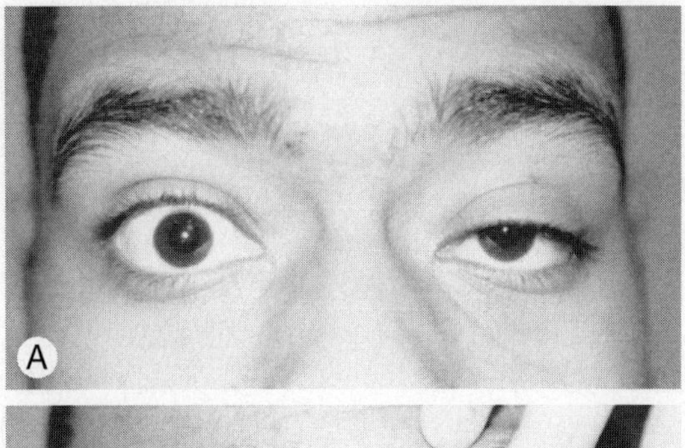

FIGURE 14–9. **A.** Pseudoretraction of the right upper eyelid associated with ptosis of the left upper eyelid in ocular myasthenia gravis. This is a consequence of Hering's law. Note how the eyebrows are elevated, indicating frontalis contraction as the patient attempts to keep the eyelids open. **B.** When the ptotic eyelid is elevated manually, the pseudoretracted lid falls. Note the eyebrows have relaxed. **C.** After intravenous administration of edrophonium, the left ptosis and right pseudoretraction resolve.

Physiologic Blink Reflexes. In the *corneal blink reflex,* bilateral eyelid closure is elicited by touching one cornea with cotton, for instance. The ophthalmic division of the trigeminal nerve (V_1) is the afferent limb of this reflex, with first-order neurons synapsing primarily in the chief sensory nucleus within the pontine tegmentum. Second-order neurons project

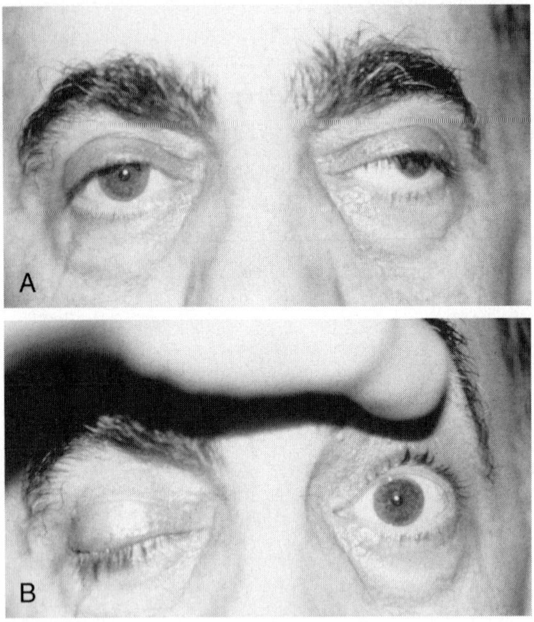

FIGURE 14–10. Enhanced ptosis in myasthenia gravis. **A.** Bilateral ptosis and exotropia. **B.** When a ptotic eyelid is manually elevated, the contralaterally retracted eyelid droops as a consequence of Hering's law.

from the chief sensory nucleus to both facial nerve nuclei. Tactile stimulation of the eyelids or eyelashes or tapping the forehead (*glabellar reflex*), which also elicit bilateral eyelid closure, are likely mediated by the same pathway.[17] These reflexes normally habituate with repetitive stimulation.[18] In the *corneomandibular reflex,* corneal stimulation elicits a bilateral eyelid blink and a brisk anterolateral jaw movement (palebromandibular synkinesia).[19]

The *reflex blink to visual threat,* useful for evaluating visual fields in young children or uncooperative adults, can be elicited by a threatening gesture such as a menacing hand. Care should be taken not to push air onto the cornea, thereby provoking a corneal blink reflex. The reflex blink to visual threat requires an intact afferent visual pathway and occipital lobe as well as parietal and frontal lobe areas which mediate visual attention.[20] The reflex is likely a learned one,[21] as infants younger than 2 to 4 months of age may not exhibit it.[22]

Other normal blink reflexes include *blinking to sudden bright light or dazzle,* which is entirely brain stem mediated.[23–25] In the *stapedius reflex,* the eyes blink reflexively to a loud noise.

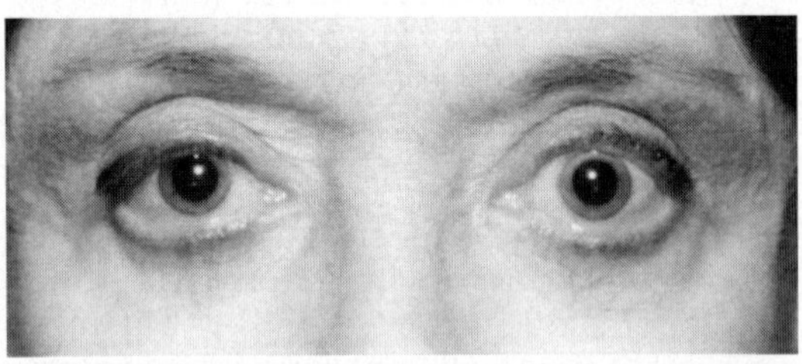

FIGURE 14–11. Pseudoptosis of the right upper eyelid associated with pathologic upper eyelid retraction of the left upper eyelid in thyroid associated ophthalmopathy. This is a consequence of Hering's law.

PTOSIS

Approach

The cause of ptosis should be determined by considering age (congenital versus acquired in adulthood), abruptness of onset, the appearance of the eyelid, the severity of the ptosis, pupillary size, and accompanying neurologic signs.[26] Acquired, painless ptosis of sudden onset strongly suggests a neurologic cause such as Horner syndrome or third nerve palsy, especially in unilateral cases with pupillary involvement. Gradually progressive bilateral ptosis would be more consistent with a myopathic or neuromuscular junction disorder. Nonneurologic causes of ptosis, such as levator dehiscence, are more common than the causes listed above, and these disorders should be suspected in isolated cases. In addition, ptosis may be suspected incorrectly when in fact the upper eyelid of the other eye is pathologically retracted. When the ptosis is severe, a third nerve palsy or myasthenia gravis is the more likely cause as the lid droop of a Horner syndrome, for instance, is quite mild.

Measurement of levator palpebrae superioris function is also frequently helpful in narrowing the differential diagnosis (see Fig. 2–21). Ptosis produced by levator dehiscence and Horner syndrome is usually associated with normal levator function. In contrast, levator function is reduced in ptosis associated with myasthenia gravis, congenital ptosis, third nerve palsies, and myopathic conditions.

A detailed differential diagnosis of ptosis is outlined in Table 14–1,[27] but this section will concentrate on the most common causes.

Congenital

Isolated and With Elevator Palsy. Isolated, nonprogressive ptosis in the neonate or child is usually due to congenital maldevelopment

TABLE 14–1. Differential Diagnosis of Ptosis

Congenital	Acquired
Isolated	**Myogenic**
With double-elevator palsy	Chronic progressive external ophthalmoplegia (CPEO)
Anomalous synkineses (including Marcus Gunn jaw-winking)	Kearns–Sayre syndrome (CPEO "plus")
Lid or orbital tumors (hemangioma, dermoid)	Myotonic dystrophy
Birth trauma (third nerve palsy, Horner syndrome)	Oculopharyngeal dystrophy
Neurofibromatosis (neurofibroma)	Topical steroid eyedrops
Neonatal myasthenia (transient)	**Disorder of neuromuscular transmission**
Congenital fibrosis syndrome	Myasthenia gravis
	Lambert–Eaton syndrome
	Botulism
	Neurogenic
	Horner syndrome
	Oculomotor nerve palsy
	"Cortical" ptosis
	Obtundation, drowsiness, coma
	Apraxia of eyelid opening
	Mechanical
	Inflammatory (edema, allergy, chalazion, hordeolum, blepharitis, conjunctivitis)
	Cicatricial
	Tumor (lid, orbit)
	Blepharochalasis
	Levator Dehiscence–Disinsertion Syndrome
	Aging
	Inflammation (ocular, lids, orbit)
	Surgery (ocular, orbital, postcataract)
	Trauma
	Contact lens use
	Pseudoptosis
	Dermatochalasis
	Duane's retraction syndrome
	Microphthalmos/phthisis bulbi
	Enophthalmos
	Pathologic lid retraction of the opposite eye
	Chronic (old) Bell's palsy
	Voluntary blepharospasm
	Hypotropia
	Hysteria

Adapted from Thompson BM, Corbett JJ, Kline LB, et al: Pseudo-Horner's syndrome. Arch Neurol 1982;39:108–111, with permission.

of the levator palpebrae or its tendon. This also causes incomplete lowering of the eyelid in downgaze, resulting in lid lag (Fig. 14–12). The upper eyelid crease is typically shallow or absent. Commonly the involved eye has superior rectus or complete elevator palsy, and if both eyes are ptotic, neither eye may have normal upgaze. This frequent association between the eyelid and motility deficit has been attributed to a common embryologic origin of and insult to the levator palpebrae and superior rectus muscles.[28] Some studies have demonstrated myopathic or dysgenetic features in the levator muscle.[29]

Marcus Gunn Jaw-Winking. Patients with Marcus Gunn jaw-winking have a ptotic eyelid that retracts during contraction of the external pterygoid muscle (eg, nursing, chewing, mouth opening, or moving the jaw forward or side to side), presumably from anomolous innervation of the levator by the trigeminal nucleus (trigemino-oculomotor synkinesis). Cases are usually unilateral, but rarely patients are bilaterally affected. We have seen bilateral involvement where one eyelid was retracted and the other ptotic, and this pattern alternated when the child sucked a pacifier (Fig. 14–13). Associated ophthalmologic abnormalities include amblyopia, superior rectus weakness, double elevator palsy, and anisometropia.[30, 31] Eyelid surgery can be considered when the jaw-winking or ptosis creates a functional or cosmetic problem.[32]

Other Congenital Causes. Neurofibromas and lid tumors such as hemangiomas should also be suspected in children with ptosis. Usually

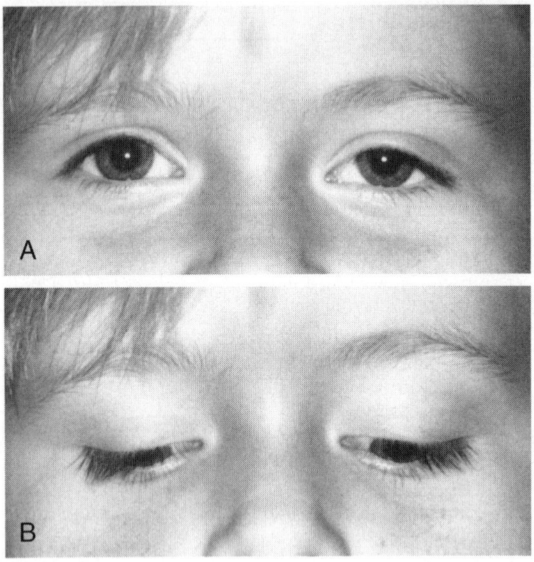

FIGURE 14–12. Congenital left ptosis characterized by a droopy eyelid (**A**), which incompletely lowers in downgaze (**B**).

there is a palpable upper eyelid mass in these cases. Congenital oculomotor palsies (see Chapter 15), Horner syndrome (see Chapter 13), and congenital fibrosis syndromes (see Chapter 15) should also be considered in this age group.

Acquired

Myopathic. Patients with myopathic ptosis often give a long history of droopy lids. Occasionally the ptosis will be the only manifestation of a myopathic condition. However, many patients have other neurologic signs. These patients often have levator function between 5 and 11 mm. Important myogenic causes of ptosis include the mitochondrial disorders chronic progressive external ophthalmoplegia and Kearns–Sayre syndrome, myotonic dystrophy, and oculopharyngeal dystrophy. These entities are discussed in detail at the end of this chapter.

Neuromuscular Junction. Fatiguable or variable unilateral or bilateral ptosis suggests a

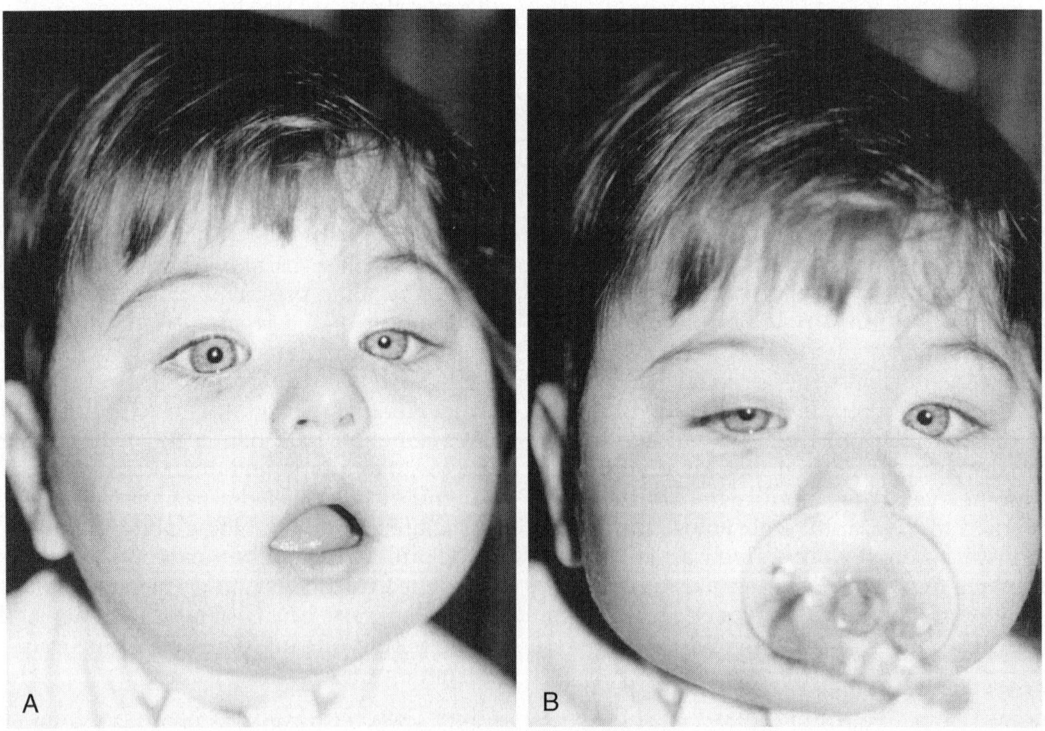

FIGURE 14–13. Bilateral Marcus Gunn jaw-winking phenomenon. **A.** This baby had left ptosis with the mouth open. **B.** When she sucked on a pacifier, the left ptosis alternated with right ptosis.

disorder of neuromuscular transmission, such as myasthenia gravis, Lambert-Eaton myasthenic syndrome, and botulism. These are also discussed in detail at the end of this chapter.

Neuropathic

Third Nerve Palsy. Prominent unilateral ptosis with adduction, elevation, and depression deficits, with or without pupillary mydriasis, suggests an infranuclear third nerve palsy (see Chapter 15). There has been a single case report of a posterior communicating aneurysm manifesting as unilateral ptosis in isolation.[33] A unilateral nuclear oculomotor lesion causes bilateral ptosis (*nuclear ptosis*), worse ipsilaterally, ipsilateral third nerve dysfunction, and contralateral superior rectus weakness (see Chapter 15).[34]

In the setting of a resolved third nerve palsy, a ptotic eyelid that elevates (retracts) when the eye infraducts or adducts implies aberrant regeneration of the eyelid. This levator synkinesis phenomenon is discussed in more detail in Chapter 15.

Horner Syndrome. Mild unilateral ptosis accompanied by miosis and pupillary dilation lag in the dark implies Horner syndrome (see Chapter 13). The ptosis never completely covers the eye in Horner syndrome. The lower eyelid may be elevated in so-called lower eyelid ptosis. The small palpebral fissure due to the combination of the upper and lower eyelid ptosis gives the eye a pseudoenophthalmic appearance.

Cerebral (or Cortical) Ptosis. A unilateral cerebral hemispheric lesion may uncommonly cause unilateral or bilateral ptosis without third nerve or sympathetic involvement or apraxia (see below).[1, 35] The side of the unilateral ptosis or the lower lid in bilateral cases can be either ipsilateral or contralateral to the lesion. The ptosis is usually transient, lasting only for a few days. In a series of 13 patients with bilateral cerebral ptosis, all patients had an acute right frontotemporoparietal lobe lesion and conjugate gaze deviation to the right.[36] Three other patients with right-sided lesions were reported who had bilateral ptosis and upgaze palsy.[37] These observations suggest some supranuclear cortical control of the levator muscles, perhaps with right hemispheric dominance.

Apraxia of Eyelid Opening. Nonparalytic, deficient voluntary eyelid elevation (*apraxia of eyelid opening*) can mimic levator paralysis until the patient opens the eyes without ptosis after a sudden command or stimulation.[38] Patients contract their frontalis muscles while attempting to open their eyes. No ocular myopathy or sympathetic dysfunction is present.[39] This disorder should be distinguished from blepharospasm, which often accompanies it.[40] In blepharospasm (see facial nerve section) there is obvious contraction of the orbicularis oculi, which does not visibly occur in apraxia of eyelid opening. However, in some patients with apraxia of eyelid opening, there may be electromyographically demonstrable (but not visible) orbicularis oculi contractions of the pretarsal portion during attempted eyelid opening.[41, 42]

Apraxia of eyelid opening occurs insidiously in association with extrapyramidal disorders such as progressive supranuclear palsy (PSP),[43, 44] Parkinson's disease (PD), Shy–Drager syndrome,[39] Huntington's disease,[38] and Wilson's disease. Rarely this disorder can be seen acutely with right hemispheric lesions[45, 46] and bifrontal lobe disease,[47] and chronically with amyotrophic lateral sclerosis.[48] The exact lesions responsible for apraxia of eyelid opening are uncertain.[40]

In patients with pyramidal and extrapyramidal diseases, some authors have questioned the use of the term "apraxia," which should be used only in the context of intact motor systems. Therefore a more appropriate term such as "involuntary levator palpebrae inhibition of supranuclear origin" has been suggested.[39] Others have termed it an eyelid "dystonia."[49]

Botulinum injections of the pretarsal portion of the orbicularis oculi are sometimes recommended,[50, 51] based on the motor persistence of this muscle alluded to above.[41, 42] Levodopa has been used in some isolated cases.[52]

Levator Dehiscence–Disinsertion Syndrome (Aponeurotic Ptosis). This is the most common cause of acquired ptosis in adults. In many elderly patients the aponeurosis of the levator muscle may spontaneously dehisce or disinsert from the tarsal plate of the upper eyelid. The eyelids are usually affected bilaterally. The upper eyelid crease is often high or indistinct, and levator function is still relatively preserved (Fig. 14–14). In younger and middle-aged patients, the most common cause of levator dehiscence is contact lens wear.[53] Eyelid manipulation during lens removal is thought to cause or exacerbate the disinsertion. Other important causes of levator dehisence include

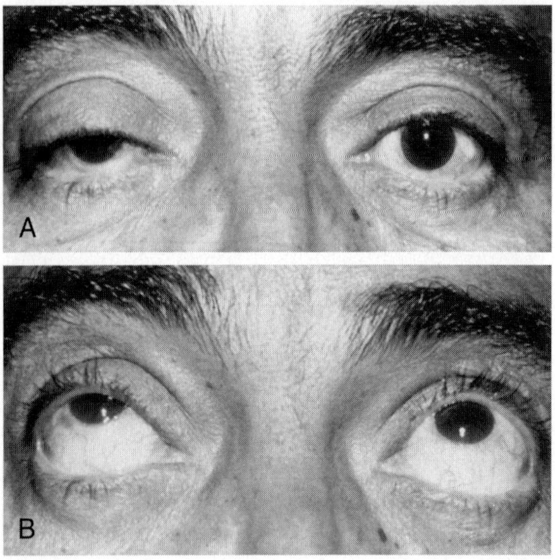

FIGURE 14–14. Levator dehiscence–disinsertion syndrome (aponeurotic ptosis). **A.** Ptosis of the right upper eyelid with a high upper eyelid crease. **B.** Relative preservation of right levator function.

trauma, ocular surgery (such as cataract or orbital surgery), allergies, and eyelid edema.

Pseudoptosis. Disorders in this group are characterized by an eyelid that falsely appears to be drooping and therefore mimics ptosis. The various causes are listed in Table 14–1, but the most important ones include contralateral lid retraction and ipsilateral eyelid relaxation secondary to Hering's law (see Fig. 14–11), enophthalmos, hypotropia, and dermatochalasis, the hanging of skin over the eyelid due to loss of skin elasticity and orbital fat herniation.

Treatment

Other than treating the primary cause, ptosis can be managed with taping the eyelids open or with eyelid "crutches" attached to eyeglasses. Most patients find the latter uncomfortable. Surgical management of ptosis is more effective in chronic cases, and popular procedures include shortening of the levator muscle or aponeurosis, or Müller's muscle resection.

EYELID RETRACTION

In primary gaze, the upper eyelid normally reaches just below the limbus. Eyelid retraction is diagnosed if there is sclera showing between the lower edge of the upper eyelid and the limbus. Table 14–2 lists a differential diagnosis of eyelid retraction.[54, 55] The three most important neuro-ophthalmic causes of eyelid retraction are thyroid-associated ophthalmopathy, dorsal midbrain lesions, and contralateral ptosis. This section will discuss the first two. Eyelid retraction due to contralateral ptosis is a consequence of Hering's law and has already been discussed above. Based on this relatively small differential diagnosis, we recommend for any patient with acquired eyelid retraction without contralateral ptosis or known thyroid disease to undergo thyroid function testing (TFT). If the thyroid workup is unrevealing, or if there is a history of headache, blurred vision, or ataxia, and there are other signs of dorsal midbrain disease, then neuroimaging of the brain is warranted.

Thyroid-Associated Ophthalmopathy

Upper eyelid retraction may be the only ocular abnormality in these patients. The retraction can either be uni- or bilateral (Fig. 14–15). The eyelid tends to more retracted temporally than medially. The exact mechanism of the eyelid retraction is unclear, but (1) fibrous contraction, thickening, shortening, or hyperactivity

TABLE 14–2. Differential Diagnosis of Eyelid Retraction

Neurogenic
Dorsal midbrain syndrome
Collier's eyelid retraction
Eyelid lag in downgaze
Contralateral ptosis
Marcus Gunn jaw-winking
Aberrant regeneration of the third nerve
Ocular neuromyotonia
Third nerve palsy with cyclic spasms
Facial nerve paresis
Eyelid nystagmus
Extrapyramidal disease
Ipsilateral superior rectus weakness and enhanced innervation to the superior rectus/levator complex
Hypo- and hyperkalemic periodic paralysis
Myogenic
Thyroid-associated ophthalmopathy (Graves)
Congenital
Mechanistic
Proptosis
Axial myopia
Ocular or orbital surgery
Eyelid scarring

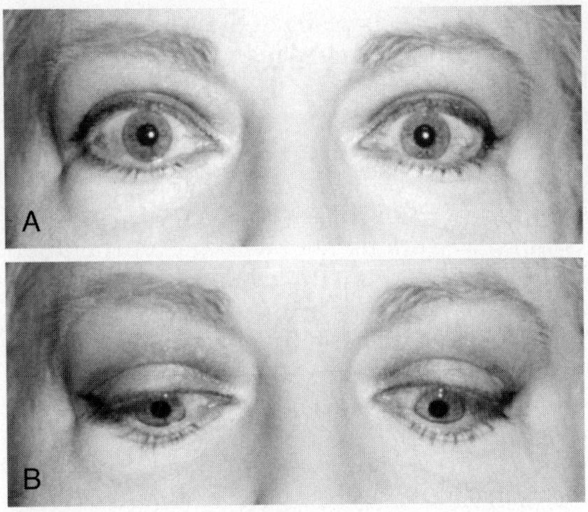

FIGURE 14–15. Eyelid retraction (**A**) and lid lag(**B**)— the lids fail to relax in downgaze—related to thyroid-associated ophthalmopathy. Note the characteristic upper and lower eyelid swelling and conjunctival injection.

of the levator palpebrae muscle; (2) sympathetic overdrive and overaction of Müller's muscle; (3) proptosis; and (4) secondary upper eyelid retraction due to a restricted inferior rectus and limited upgaze have all been proposed as contributory factors.[56,57] Retraction is often accompanied by lid lag (von Graefe sign), in which the upper eyelid fails or is slow to follow the eye in downgaze (Fig. 14–15). In thyroid-associated ophthalmopathy, the cause of lid lag is likely related to the causes of the lid retraction. The lower lid is also frequently retracted.

Exposure keratopathy and dry eye can complicate thyroid-related lid retraction and lag, especially in individuals with infrequent blinking. Artificial tears are usually sufficient, but some thyroid patients with lid retraction require surgical levator recession or division, aponeurosis division, or excision of Müller's muscle.[56]

Further details regarding the features, diagnosis, and management of thyroid-associated ophthalmopathy are discussed in Chapter 18.

Pretectal Eyelid Retraction (Collier's Sign)

Eyelid retraction may be prominent sign in the pretectal (or Parinaud's or dorsal midbrain) syndrome. The patients have a characteristic stare (Fig. 14–16), often accompanied by upgaze paresis. The lid retraction is typically symmetric, except in the plus–minus lid syndrome (see below). Also, it usually is exacerbated on attempted upgaze, and normally the lids relax on downgaze. However, in some exceptional instances there is lid lag in downgaze (see below).

The other elements of the pretectal syndrome, which include supranuclear vertical gaze paresis (Chapter 16), pupillary light–near dissociation (Chapter 13), and convergence retraction nystagmus (Chapter 17) are discussed elsewhere.

Because the lid retraction typically occurs in patients with upgaze paresis, some authors have attributed the finding to combined excess superior rectus innervation and levator activity.[58] However, Schmidtke and Büttner-Ennever[3] postulated that neurogenic lid retraction can result either from a unilateral lesion of the nPC or from interruption of the posterior commissure, both of which would result in decreased inhibition of levator neurons in the CCN (see Fig. 14–2).

Eyelid Lag in Downgaze. As alluded to earlier in this chapter, eyelid position is normally coordinated with vertical eye movements so that in upgaze the eyelids elevate, and in downgaze the eyelids typically relax and fall. In dorsal midbrain lesions, this relationship can be disrupted, causing the eyelids to remain elevated while the eyes infraduct.[59] Dramatic examples include the setting-sun sign (tonic downward eye deviation with lid retraction) in infants with hydrocephalus, thalamic hemorrhage (see Chapter 16), and rare comatose patients with phasic vertical eye movements and persistent eyelid elevation.[60] Lid lag in some instances may be difficult to detect because patients with pretectal dysfunction may have

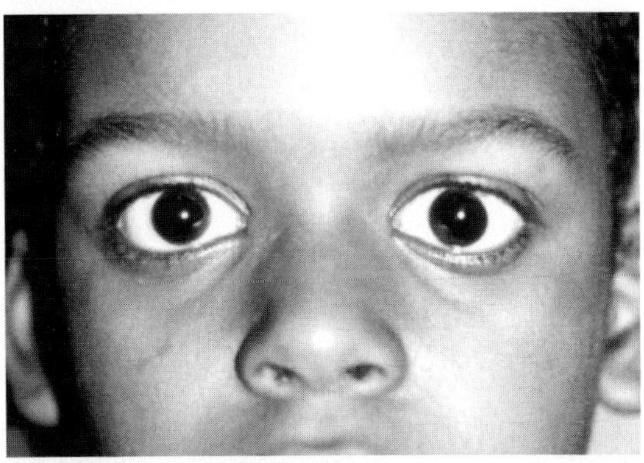

FIGURE 14–16. Eyelid retraction due to dorsal midbrain astrocytoma (Collier's sign).

downgaze paralysis early in their course that precludes the ability to detect lid lag.

Although lid lag and lid retraction in such instances may share the same mechanism, patients have been observed who do not have lid retraction in primary gaze but have lid lag in downgaze (Fig. 14–17).[61] This suggests there may be separate central mechanisms for these eyelid abnormalities. One possible lesion for lid lag without retraction involves the inhibitory connections from the supranuclear downgaze centers to the central caudal nucleus (see Fig. 14–2).

Plus–Minus Eyelid Syndrome. A unilateral lesion involving nPC and the oculomotor fascicle would produce an ipsilateral third nerve palsy with ptosis and contralateral lid retraction (*plus–minus lid syndrome*) (Fig. 14–18).[62] The ipsilateral lid retraction is masked by the infranuclear third nerve palsy. This eyelid pattern of ptosis and contralateral lid retraction can be mimicked in an individual with ptosis who fixates with the ptotic eye, thereby increasing the innervation to both levators (Hering's law). In this case manual elevation of the ptotic eyelid would eliminate the contralateral lid retraction. It may also be seen in a patient with ptosis and contralateral superior rectus weakness who is fixating with the nonptotic eye and increasing the innervation to the levator/superior rectus complex. This possibility can be investigated by covering the fixating nonptotic eye.

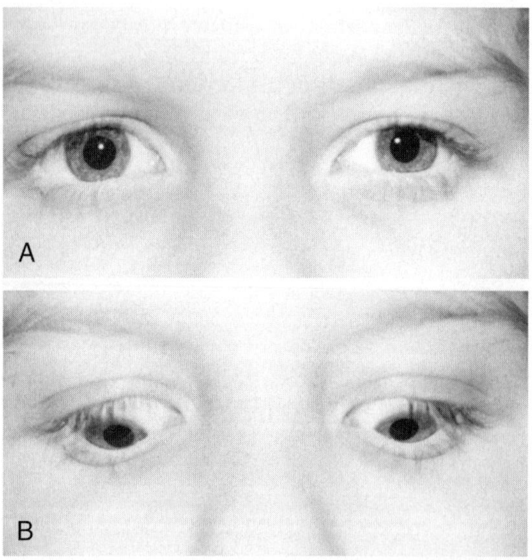

FIGURE 14–17. Child with pineal region germinoma and supranuclear upgaze paresis with normal lid position in primary gaze (**A**) but lid lag in downgaze (**B**).

Miscellaneous Causes

Eyelid retraction in association with Marcus Gunn jaw-winking and aberrant regeneration of the third nerve with levator synkinesis has already been mentioned in the section on ptosis. Other neuro-ophthalmic causes include extrapyramidal diseases, neuromyotonia, and oculomotor paresis with cyclic spasm[63] (see Chapter 15). Mechanistic causes such as proptosis, axial myopia, eyelid scarring, and ocular or orbital surgery (such as overcorrection of ptosis) should be considered. A congenital, idiopathic variety has also been described.[64]

FACIAL WEAKNESS

Although idiopathic Bell's palsy is a common cause of facial weakness, it is important to explore the differential diagnosis of facial palsies. This was emphasized in a study by May,[65] in which only 53% of patients who were referred to one practice with a diagnosis of Bell's palsy had the disorder. Approximately 10% had a treatable, progressive, or life-threatening lesion. Bell's palsy is a diagnosis of exclusion, and other supranuclear, nuclear, infranuclear, and neuromuscular causes of facial weakness must be considered.

Approach

When weakness of the face is present, determining whether the palsy is central or peripheral is the first important diagnostic consideration. Asking the patient to look up causes contraction of the frontalis muscle. If frontalis function is intact, a central palsy is likely, while impaired frontalis contraction suggests a peripheral cause (see Fig. 14–3). The clinical setting and accompanying signs then aid in refining the localization and determining the exact cause.

A detailed differential diagnosis based on this approach is given in Table 14–3. For example, nuclear facial nerve palsies are usually associated with other pontine disturbances. Also, peripheral facial nerve palsies are frequently accompanied by defective taste and tearing as well as hyperacusis. Furthermore, synkinesis and the misdirection phenomenon

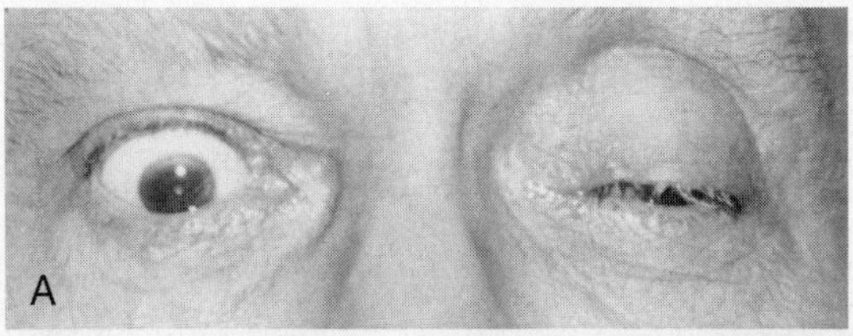

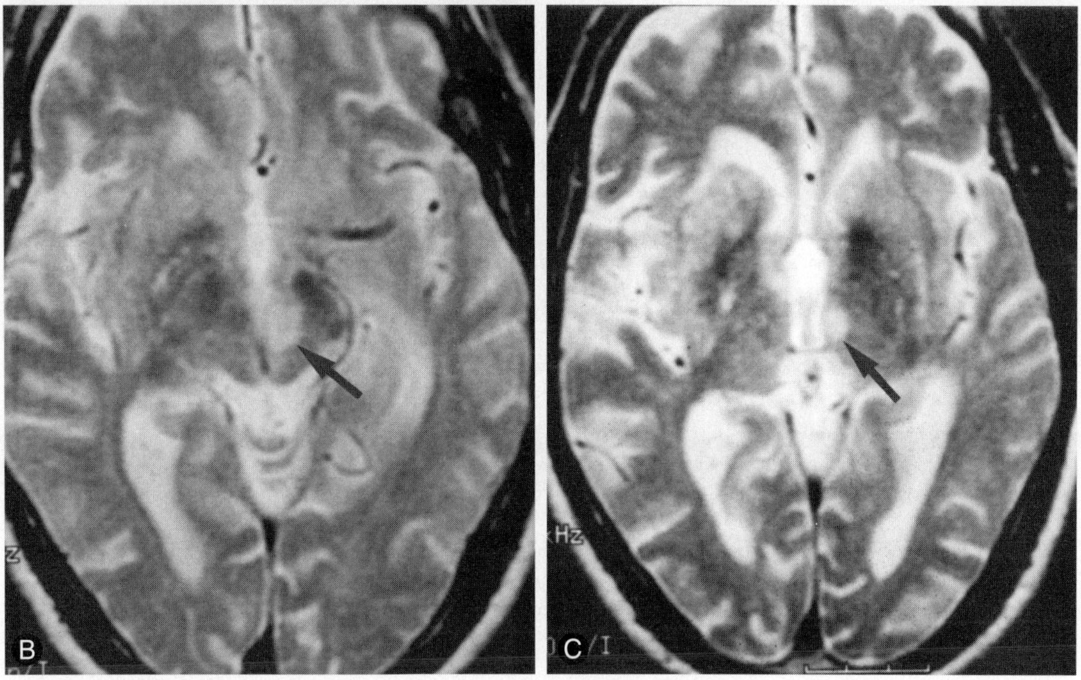

FIGURE 14–18. Plus–minus lid syndrome. **A.** Complete left ptosis from third nerve palsy and contralateral eyelid retraction. The right eye is moderately hypotropic in primary gaze. **B,C.** T_2-weighted axial MRI scans showing high signal abnormality involving the region of left third nerve fascicle (arrow) (**B**) and more rostrally, the region of the nucleus of posterior commissure (arrow) (**C**).

(see next section) are late sequela of peripheral rather than central facial palsies. In addition, idiopathic Bell's palsy rarely may affect both sides of the face, but acquired bilateral facial weakness should alert the examiner to the possibility of Lyme disease, sarcoidosis, carcinomatous meningitis, Guillain–Barré syndrome, and myasthenia gravis.[66] Congenital causes of bilateral facial weakness include Möbius syndrome and myotonic dystrophy.

The remainder of this section highlights some of the important causes of facial weakness, grouped by localization.

Central

Supranuclear. Supranuclear cortex and internal capsule lesions that produce lower facial weakness are usually associated with weakness of the ipsilateral arm. Since the facial nucleus also receives input from the basal ganglia region there may be a dissociation of voluntary and spontaneous facial movements. Thus, patients with lower facial weakness resulting from corticobulbar tract dysfunction typically show better facial movement when told a joke rather than simply asking them to smile.[67] On the other hand, thalamic, basal ganglia, dorsal midbrain, and supplementary motor area lesions may lead to normal voluntary smiling, but defective contralateral facial nerve function during reflex smiling.[68, 69]

A supranuclear paralysis of voluntary eyelid closure has been described. Lessell[70] reported a patient with presumed amyotrophic lateral sclerosis, with evidence of bilateral pyramidal tract involvement, who could not close his eyelids voluntarily but blinked to visual threat. Ross Russell[71] described three individuals with Creutzfeldt–Jakob disease with pyramidal tract degeneration documented on postmortem examination who similarly could not blink on command but blinked to threat. In both reports, the patients also continued to blink spontaneously and in response to corneal stim-

(*Text continued on page 482.*)

TABLE 14–3. Topical Diagnosis of Lesions of the Facial Nerve

Level	Signs	Probable Diagnosis
Supranuclear		
Cortex and internal capsule	Tone and upper face intact, loss of volitional movement with intact spontaneous expression, slurred speech (tongue weakness), hemiparesis on side of facial involvement. Paresis of upper extremity begins with involvement of thumb, finger, and hand movement.	Lesion of motor cortex or internal capsule on side opposite facial involvement
Extrapyramidal	Increased salivary flow, impaired, spontaneous facial movement, intact volitional facial movement, masked face of parkinsonism or dystonia, progressive hemifacial spasm.	Tumor or vascular lesion of basal ganglia; parkinsonism; Meige's syndrome (cervical facial dystonia)
Midbrain	Ipsilateral hemiparesis involving face, arm, and leg, and contralateral oculomotor palsy.	Weber syndrome (lesion of cerebral peduncle and third nerve)
	Bilateral facial paresis with other cranial nerve deficits, emotional lability, hyperactive gag reflex, marked hyperflexia.	Pseudobulbar palsy associated with multiple infarcts
Nuclear		
Pontine nucleus	Involvement of cranial nerves VII and VI on side of lesion with gaze palsy on side of facial paresis; associated ataxia, cerebellovestibular signs, and contralateral hemiparesis.	Involvement of pons at level of seventh and sixth nerve nuclei by pontine glioma; multiple sclerosis; infection; or infarction
	Cranial nerve VII and VI palsy noted from time of birth with or without other congenital anomalies. Facial motor involvement usually incomplete with sparing of corner of mouth or lower lip common. Involvement of the lower lip with complete or partial sparing of upper face. Anomalies of the pinna, canal, or mandible associated with facial palsy indicate developmental defect of facial nerve.	Developmental facial palsy (noted at birth); oculofacial syndrome; Möbius syndrome; thalidomide toxicity; nondevelopmental facial or abducens nerve anomalies most often result from infranuclear lesions
Infranuclear (Intracranial)		
Cerebellopontine angle	Impairment of hearing, especially discrimination out of proportion to pure tone scores; possible ataxia, abnormalities of tearing or taste, stapes reflex decay, decreased corneal sensation; facial motor deficit (late sign).	Acoustic schwannoma
	Abnormalities in trigeminal, acoustic–vestibular, and facial nerve function, starting with facial pain or numbness. Lesion noted on CT (enhancement with contrast) may show evidence of calcification.	Meningioma
	Abnormalities of facial and acoustic–vestibular nerve function; may start with facial twitching; erosion or lytic area evident on plain radiographs of temporal bone.	Cholesteatoma or facial schwannoma arising in temporal bone
	Abnormalities of cranial nerves VII, VIII, IX, X, XI, and XII; pulsatile tinnitus and purple-red pulsating mass bulging through the tympanic membrane.	Glomus jugulare tumor

TABLE 14–3. Topical Diagnosis of Lesions of the Facial Nerve *Continued*

Level	Signs	Probable Diagnosis
	Abnormalities of abducens nerve in addition to above.	Glomus jugulare tumor extending to petrous apex to involve middle fossa
Subarachnoid	Multiple cranial nerve involvement in rapid succession.	Carcinomatous meningitis, leukemia, Guillian–Barré syndrome, mononucleosis, diphtheria, tuberculosis, sarcoidosis, malignant external otitis, Lyme disease
Skull base	Conductive or sensorineural hearing loss, acute or recurrent facial palsy; positive family history, abnormalities of bone density on skull radiograph.	Osteopetrosis
Infranuclear (Transtemporal bone)		
Internal auditory canal and labyrinthine segment of facial nerve	Ecchymosis around pinna and mastoid prominence (Battle's sign); hematotympanum with sensorineural hearing loss (tuning fork lateralizes to normal side), vertigo, nystagmus (fast component away from involved side); sudden complete facial paralysis following head trauma; usually associated with basilar skull fracture, loss of consciousness, and CSF leak. Transection of facial nerve is more likely with this injury than with longitudinal fracture.	Temporal bone fracture (transverse, longitudinal, or combination)
Geniculate ganglion	Dry eye, decreased taste and salivation. Erosion of geniculate ganglion area or middle fossa is demonstrated by CT of temporal bone.	Schwannoma, meningioma, cholesteatoma, hemangioma, arteriovenous malformation
	Ear pain, vesicles on pinna, dry eye, decreased taste and salivary flow; sensorineural hearing loss, nystagmus, vertigo, red chorda tympani nerve. Facial palsy may be complete, incomplete, or progress to complete over 14 days.	Herpes zoster cephalicus (Ramsay Hunt syndrome)
	Same as above without vesicles, no other cause evident. Facial palsy may be complete, incomplete, or progress to complete over 10 days.	Idiopathic (Bell's) palsy (viral–inflammatory immune disorder)
	Same as above but no recovery in 6 months.	Tumor
	Ecchymosis around pinna and mastoid (Battle's sign), hematotympanum; conductive hearing loss (tuning fork lateralizes to involved ear); no vestibular involvement unless stapes subluxed into vestibule (causes fluctuating sensorineural hearing loss and vertigo with nystagmus).	Longitudinal fracture of temporal bone; may be proximal or at geniculate ganglion (dry eye), or distal to geniculate ganglion (tearing symmetric) (tear test valid only in acute injury)
Tympanomastoid	Decreased taste and salivation, loss of stapes reflex and symmetrical tearing; sudden-onset facial palsy, which may be complete or incomplete or may progress to complete.	
	Pain, vesicles, red chorda tympani.	Herpes zoster cephalicus
	Pain without vesicles, red chorda tympani.	Bell's palsy

Table continued on following page

TABLE 14–3. Topical Diagnosis of Lesions of the Facial Nerve *Continued*

Level	Signs	Probable Diagnosis
	Red, bulging tympanic membrane, conductive hearing loss; usually history of upper respiratory illness. Lower face may be involved more than upper.	Acute suppurative otitis media
	Foul drainage through perforated tympanic membrane; history of recurrent ear infection, drainage, and hearing loss.	Chronic suppurative otitis media, most likely associated with cholesteatoma
	Pulsatile tinnitus, purple-red pulsatile mass noted through tympanic membrane.	Glomus tympanicum or jugulare
	Recurrent facial paralysis, positive family history, facial edema, fissured tongue; may present with simultaneous bilateral facial paralysis.	Melkersson–Rosenthal syndrome
Infranuclear (Extracranial)		
	Incomplete facial nerve paresis; hearing, balance, tearing, stapes reflex, taste, salivary flow spared.	Penetrating wound of face; sequelae of parotid surgery; malignancy of parotid, tonsil, or oronasopharynx; rarely, with benign lesion of parotid gland compressing facial nerve
	Uveitis, salivary gland enlargement, fever.	Sarcoidosis (Heerfordt syndrome), Lyme disease, lymphoma
Various Sites		
	Bilateral facial paralysis from birth.	Möbius syndrome
	Bilateral facial paralysis, acquired.	Guillain–Barré syndrome, sarcoidosis, mononucleosis, leukemia, idiopathic (Bell's) palsy
	Facial paralysis, especially simultaneous bilateral facial paralysis with ascending areflexic quadriparesis; sensory changes usually mild with spinal fluid typically showing albuminocytologic dissociation (elevated protein without cells).	Guillain–Barré syndrome
	Deficits of cranial nerves VI and VII or VII, VI, and III, possible in association with marked increase in jaw jerk or gag reflex.	Carcinoma of nasopharynx; metastatic carcinoma from breast, ovary, or prostate; meningitis; leukemia; diabetes mellitus
Pseudobulbar palsy	Inappropriate or exaggerated laughing or crying; may be associated with marked increase in jaw jerk or gag reflex.	Demyelinating, degenerative, or vascular lesion involving bilateral corticobulbar pathways

CSF = cerebrospinal fluid; CT= computed tomography.
Adapted from May M, Galetta SL: The facial nerve. In Tasman W, Jaeger EA (eds): Duane's Clinical Ophthalmology, pp 5–7. Philadelphia, JB Lippincott, 1988, with permission.

ulation and loud noise. Lessell[70] and Ross Russell[71] argued that the deficiency in voluntary eyelid closure resulted from bilateral damage to cortical motor neurons and not from a facial dyspraxia (ie, difficulty with motor planning or initiation).

Nuclear

Möbius Syndrome. Congenital facial diplegia is the hallmark of this syndrome (Fig. 14–19). Abducens palsy is the most commonly associated feature, occurring in 82% of cases in the series reported by Henderson.[72] In addition, total external ophthalmoplegia was present in 25% of the cases in this series, oculomotor palsy in 21%, and bilateral ptosis in 10%. The abducens weakness is almost always bilateral, but of varying degree. When the lateral rectus palsy is severe, there is usually complete conjugate gaze paresis.

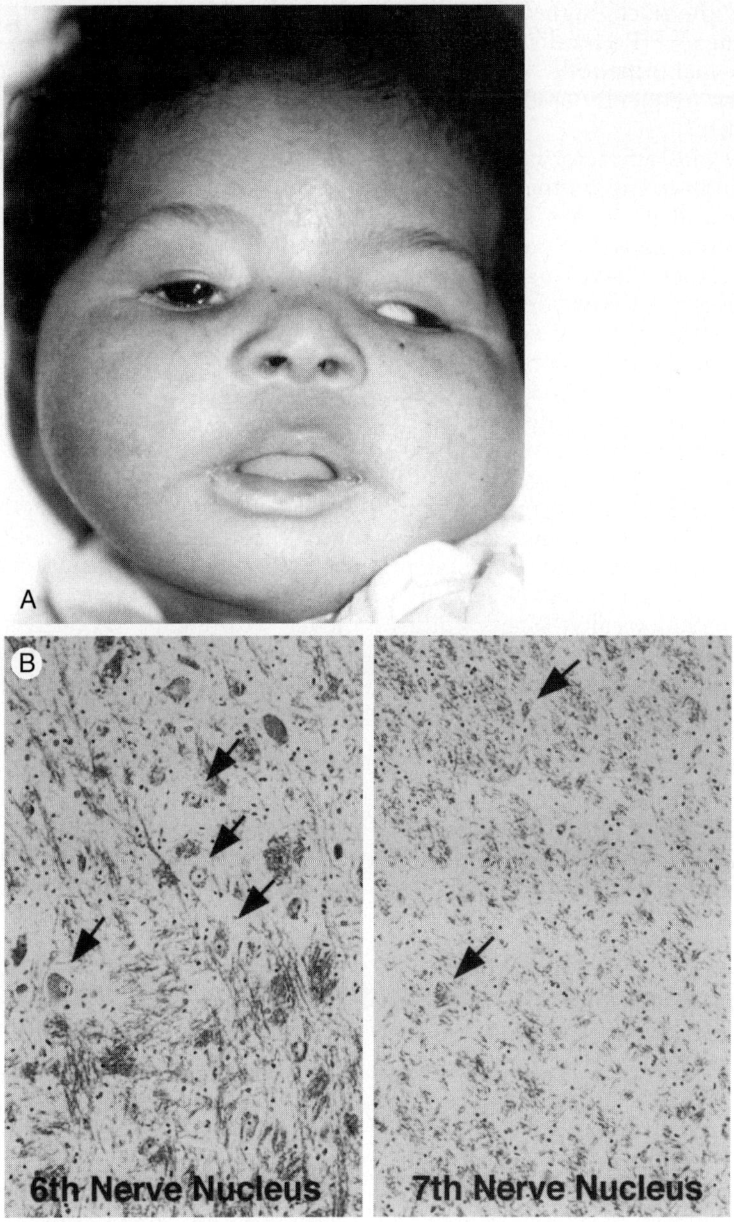

FIGURE 14–19. Child with Möbius syndrome characterized by bifacial weakness. **A.** In contrast to most patients with Möbius syndrome, this patient had bilateral oculomotor palsies but sparing of the abducens nerves. **B.** Photomicrographs of the sixth and seventh nerve nuclei. (Left) The sixth nerve nucleus shows a normal population of large neurons. (Right) The seventh nerve nucleus shows a subtotal depletion of neurons without secondary reactive changes. The arrow points to a remaining large neuron. Several smaller neurons are also seen in the background. The pathologic findings were the same on both sides of the brainstem. (A and B, Kluver stain, × 200.) (From Tran DB et al: Möbius syndrome with oculomotor nerve paralysis but without abducens paralysis. J Neuro-ophthalmol 1998;18:281–283, with permission.)

Parents may not notice the facial weakness if it is subtle, and often the child is brought to medical attention solely because of an esotropia. When the disorder involves only ocular motility and the upper face, the major issues—strabismus surgery, amblyopia, corneal surface protection, and cosmesis—can be handled primarily by ophthalmologists and plastic surgeons. However, lower facial weakness may complicate an infant's ability to suck a bottle or nipple. Less commonly lower cranial nerves, such as the ninth, tenth, and twelfth nerves, are involved, causing dysphagia, arrhythmias, and aspiration.[73] In such cases the disorder can be associated with much higher morbidity and mortality rates.[74, 75] Pectoralis muscle defects and limb malformations (eg, Poland anomaly) are also frequently associated with Möbius syndrome.[76]

No one theory can satisfactorily explain all cases of Möbius syndrome, as the disorder is usually sporadic and likely has many possible causes.[77, 78] In one subset of patients, electrophysiologic studies[79] have suggested and pathologic studies[75, 80] have demonstrated aplasia or hypoplasia of cranial nerve nuclei. In a second group, abnormal peripheral portions of the cranial nerves can be found. In the third subset, more widespread destruction of the brain stem, perhaps due to a prenatal vascular insult, has been suggested radiologically and neuropathologically.[81, 82] Neuroimaging in this group can demonstrate brain stem hypoplasia and calcification, and brain stem atrophy and mineralized necrotic foci have been found histopathologically.[83] These studies support the notion that Möbius syndrome in some cases could be the result of in-utero brain stem vascular insufficiency. In one hypothesis, during the development of the posterior circulation, a potential transient watershed area within the brain stem exists, while the blood flow in the basilar artery changes from a rostrocaudal to a caudal to rostral pattern. Brain stem ischemia may result if the blood flow during this transition is disrupted.[83] Uncommonly the disorder is inherited, and one family harbored a defective gene in chromosome 3q.[84] Also, attempted abortion with misoprostol, a synthetic prostaglandin analogue, is associated with an increased risk of Möbius syndrome in infants.[85]

Fascicular. In the pons, the seventh nerve fascicle may be disrupted dorsally in the facial colliculus syndrome (see Chapter 16), which is characterized by a facial palsy and ipsilateral conjugate gaze paresis. Facial weakness in combination with ipsilateral deafness, facial numbness, and Horner syndrome signifies a lesion in the lateral pons. More ventral pontine injury, where the seventh nerve fascicle travels near the corticospinal tracts, may lead to ipsilateral facial paresis and contralateral hemiparesis (Millard–Gubler syndrome).[86]

Peripheral

Cerebellopontine Angle

Acoustic Neuroma. These usually present with a seventh cranial nerve palsy late in their course as the facial nerve is displaced and compressed by the expanding cerebellopontine tumor. Common symptoms of acoustic neuroma include tinnitus, hearing loss, and cerebellar and vestibular signs. On MRI, the mass is hypointense on T_1-weighted images and hyperintense on T_2-weighted images, and diffusely enhances. Treatment consists of neurosurgical excision.

Subarachnoid

Lyme Disease. Lyme disease, caused by the tick-borne spirochete *Borrelia burgdorferi,* may cause unilateral or bilateral facial palsy at some point in its course in approximately 10% of patients.[87] Approximately 60% of patients will recall the diagnostic skin lesion of erythema chronicum migrans, an erythematous raised area that spreads centripetally, leaving a central clear zone and lasting several weeks if left untreated. Flulike symptoms, including chills, fever, arthralgias, headaches, and myalgias, may occur concomitant with the lesion. The diagnosis may be made by finding a positive serum enzyme-linked immunosorbent assay titer and may be confirmed by the results of a Western blot. A spinal tap can direct treatment in one suggested approach to patients with facial palsy and a positive Lyme titer: those with normal cerebrospinal fluid (CSF) can be treated with oral doxycycline, while those with pleocytosis have meningitis and should be given a course of intravenous ceftriaxone for 1 month. The facial palsy has an excellent prognosis regardless of the antibiotic regimen chosen.

Sarcoidosis. Unilateral and bilateral facial nerve palsies may be a presenting symptom of neurosarcoidosis.[88] MRI may demonstrate meningeal enhancement, and CSF examination may reveal elevated protein or lymphocytosis, or both. A serum angiotensin converting enzyme (ACE) level and chest roentgenography may be helpful in establishing sarcoidosis as the etiology of the facial palsy. The diagnosis and treatment of neurosarcoid is discussed in more detail in Chapters 5 and 7. Sarcoidosis may also cause a peripheral facial nerve palsy by involving the parotid gland (Heerfordt's syndrome).

Metastatic Lesions. A history of cancer and the presence of a rapidly progressive facial palsy are highly suggestive of a metastatic lesion. The nerve or the meninges may be infiltrated. MRI may show enhancement of the dura or of the facial nerve, disruption of the blood–brain barrier, or both. Serial lumbar punctures may be necessary for the cytologic diagnosis of meningeal carcinomatosis.

Transtemporal Bone

Trauma. The facial nerve is vulnerable in its bony course within the temporal bone at its exit point from the stylomastoid foramen and along its course to innervate the muscles of facial expression. The nerve itself can be either lacerated or traumatized bluntly. Fractures parallel to the long aspect of the petrous portion of the temporal bone (Fig. 14–20) are often accompanied by fractures of the ossicles or the labyrinth.

The facial nerve may be injured by mandibular fractures or during surgery of the mandible. The facial nerve branches are particularly vulnerable to undermining in the vicinity of the zygoma and lateral orbit during a face lift.

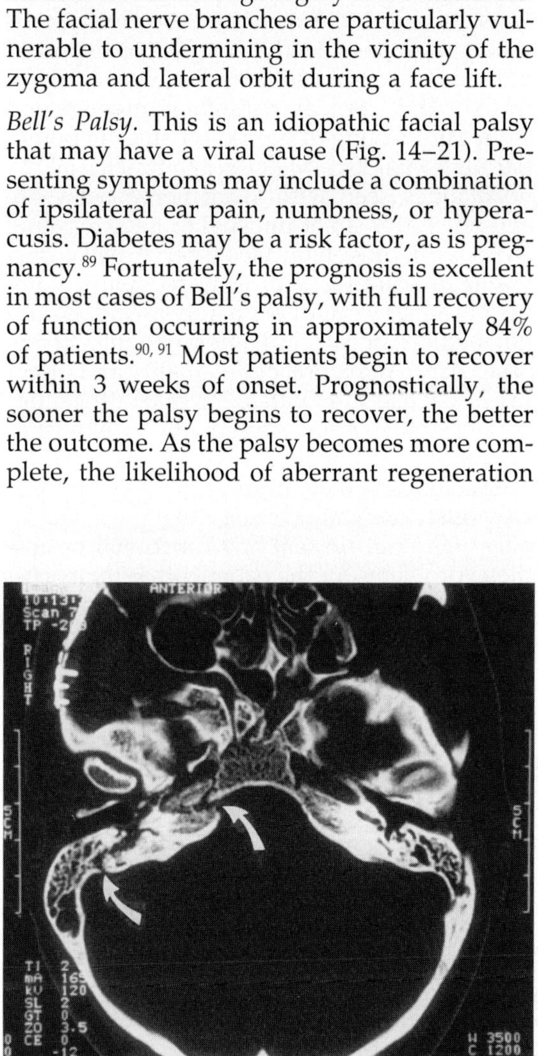

FIGURE 14–20. CT-demonstrated temporal bone traumatic fracture causing facial nerve palsy in patient depicted in Fig. 2–24.

Bell's Palsy. This is an idiopathic facial palsy that may have a viral cause (Fig. 14–21). Presenting symptoms may include a combination of ipsilateral ear pain, numbness, or hyperacusis. Diabetes may be a risk factor, as is pregnancy.[89] Fortunately, the prognosis is excellent in most cases of Bell's palsy, with full recovery of function occurring in approximately 84% of patients.[90, 91] Most patients begin to recover within 3 weeks of onset. Prognostically, the sooner the palsy begins to recover, the better the outcome. As the palsy becomes more complete, the likelihood of aberrant regeneration increases.[65] The prognosis for recovery in Bell's palsy is worse in patients with hyperacusis, decreased tearing, age greater than 60 years, diabetes, hypertension, and psychiatric disease.[92] Bell's palsy may recur in 10% to 20% of affected people.

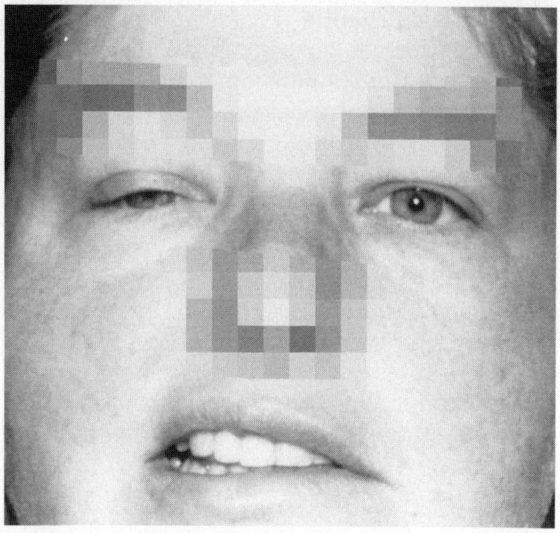

FIGURE 14–21. Left peripheral facial weakness in Bell's palsy.

The treatment of idiopathic Bell's palsy remains controversial. Although corticosteroids are frequently used, most studies have failed to demonstrate any effect on the natural course of the disorder.[90, 93] Because of the purported viral etiology of Bell's palsy, in some patients acyclovir has been used. One study[94] compared acyclovir 800 mg tid for 10 days versus prednisone 1mg/kg of body weight for 10 days and tapered to 0 over the next 6 days. Recovery was better in the prednisone group. Another study[95] found acyclovir combined with prednisone was better than prednisone alone. Facial nerve surgical decompression is ineffective and no longer routinely used.[93] We tend to use the combination of acyclovir with prednisone when the patient is seen early in his or her course. If there is any concern regarding the possibility of Lyme disease, we would use acyclovir alone pending further studies (see below).

Ramsay Hunt Syndrome. Ramsay Hunt syndrome, or cephalic herpes zoster, is characteristically preceded by a prodrome of severe pain in the affected ear and is followed by a vesicular rash involving the pinna and external auditory canal.[96] The facial palsy may be accompanied by hearing loss, vestibular impariment, or encephalitis in severe cases. The prognosis for herpes zoster cephalicus is poorer than that for Bell's palsy in terms of complete recovery of facial function, with only 60% of patients having complete return of function.[97]

Otitis Media. Acute otitis media with or without mastoiditis may occur and, when chronic, may affect the facial nerve as it courses through the temporal bone. In elderly diabetic patients, malignant external otitis is usually caused by a necrotizing *Pseudomonas* infection that progresses fulminantly. Both intravenous antibiotics and surgery, with wide debridement of necrotic bone and granulation tissue, are necessary. The facial nerve is vulnerable within the fallopian canal and can be affected by adjacent suppuration, abscess formation, or cholesteatoma. The association of a sixth cranial nerve palsy with facial palsy in petrous apex infection (Gradenigo syndrome[98]) is well described and usually reponds to antibiotic treatment.

Neuromuscular Junction, Myopathic, and Neuropathic Causes of Facial Weakness

Patients with myasthenia gravis and botulism may present with bilateral facial weakness. Almost all patients with ptosis or ophthalmoparesis due to myasthenia gravis also have orbicularis oculi weakness. Myotonic dystrophy is also characterized by bilateral weakness of the facial muscles. Facial weakness is also commonly seen in Guillian–Barré syndrome and Miller Fisher syndrome. These disorders are discussed in more detail at the end of this chapter.

Evaluation

One suggested approach is given in Table 14–4. A central facial palsy always requires neuroimaging in the workup. The evaluation of peripheral palsies, on the other hand, is usually directed toward excluding inflammatory and infectious causes. The history and examination are critical in determining the extent of the evaluation performed in patient with an isolated facial palsy.

Treatment

Aside from diagnosis and treatment of the underlying cause of the facial palsy, from an ocular standpoint, the major concern with facial paralysis is poor eyelid closure and exposure keratitis. The cornea may become compromised, and corneal pathology may extend from mild drying to ulceration and the potential for visual loss. Many of the functional abnormalities seen with facial nerve palsy are age related. It is not unusual to have a young child with congenital facial nerve palsy or a young individual with acquired palsy completely adapt to his or her paralysis and require no medical or surgical intervention. On the other hand, reduction of the quality and quantity of the tear film with aging makes the older patient much more susceptible to exposure keratitis. Additionally, there are various degrees of facial palsy, from partial to complete. Obviously one should realize that partial facial palsy may not present any functional or aesthetic problems for the patient other than occasional drying, whereas a complete loss of facial function would make the individual more susceptible to exposure and its related complica-

TABLE 14–4. Diagnostic Considerations in Facial Nerve Palsy

Clinical Problem	Test
Central facial palsy	Brain MRI
Peripheral facial palsy	
Bilateral palsy	Brain MRI, lumbar puncture, EMG (exclude Guillain–Barré syndrome, myotonia), edrophonium test (exclude myasthenia)
Progressive palsy, dizziness, or associated hearing loss	MRI of cerebellopontine angle
Acute unilateral palsy	Blood glucose level, syphilis serology, and CBC; Lyme titer (endemic area or exposure history); angiotensin-converting enzyme (exclude sarcoid)
Chronic palsy	Chest radiograph (exclude sarcoid, tumor), brain MRI

CBC = complete blood count; EMG = electromyography; MRI = magnetic resonance imaging.
From Handler LF, Galetta SL, Wulc AE et al: Facial paralysis: diagnosis and management. In: Bosniak S, (ed): Principles and Practice of Ophthalmic Plastic and Reconstructive Surgery, pp 465–483. Philadelphia, WB Saunders, 1996, with permission.

tions. Keratitis is more severe in patients who have neurotrophic keratitis (caused by trigeminal dysfunction), and such patients should be observed even more closely. In this section we review the medical and surgical management of facial nerve palsy.

Medical. The treatment of all patients with facial nerve palsy includes some type of topical lubricant. There are many artificial tear products available in the over-the-counter market. These drops should be the primary treatment in all cases. Some patients will need topical lubrication throughout the course of their disease regardless of any additional medical or surgical treatment. Artificial tears given four times a day is an appropriate starting point. Some patients will want to try several different tear film products as their comfort levels of each type of drop vary widely. Also, the dosage schedule will need to be tailored to the individual's needs. The unpreserved lubricating drops can be used as frequently as every 1/2 hour to 1 hour based on the patient's need for lubrication. Initial bedtime coverage would include a petroleum-based ointment and again there are numerous brands of lubricating ointments on the market that could fill this need. Individuals that have severe keratitis may need day- and night-time applications of the ointment. Once the keratitis has begun to heal the patient may be switched to drops daily and ointment at night. The advantage to this regimen is that the ointment is quite disruptive to visual acuity, whereas the less viscous drops are not. Certain environmental aberrations such as windy weather and dry air may prompt the patient to switch ointments for short periods of time in order to maintain corneal comfort.

The next level of management involves additional coverage to the eye at bedtime. As mentioned above, these individuals should be using a protective ointment. Sometimes patients need to have a "moisture bubble" taped over the eye at night after applying the ointment. Options include standard swimming goggles or a small oval of cellophane wrap. Taping the eyelid closed is not always successful. The tape comes off, and if the patient is not skilled at taping the lids, they might tape the lids in an open position. This unfortunate situation might precipitate further irritation of the cornea. Moisture chambers, which are fitted to standard glass frames and molded to the face to create a tight seal, may eventually be required for daytime protection as well.

Surgical. When medical therapies are ineffective or not tolerated or when corneal damage makes more definitive measures imperative, surgical intervention may be indicated. Initial surgical therapy is usually with a temporary tarsorrhaphy, in which the eyelids are temporarily sewn together either partially or completely.[99] We have a low threshold for performing temporary tarsorrhaphies in patients with newly acquired seventh nerve palsies with severe keratitis, especially those with defective trigeminal nerve function as well. If the seventh nerve defect persists then consideration can be given to permanent lateral tarsorrhaphy, medial tarsorraphy, lateral canthoplasty, or ectropion repair. These may produce scarring and reduced peripheral vision. Another group of procedures have been developed using various prosthetic devices to improve eyelid function and closure. These include silicone bands, eyelid springs, and eyelid gold weight implants.[100] Silicone bands have been abandoned because of difficulty in assessing the balance between eyelid closing and opening forces. Eyelid springs work well but are often complicated by infection, extrusion, local granuloma formation, and need for readjustment.

Implantation of a gold eyelid weight is a commonly performed procedure for eyelid animation, and it is our preferred procedure.[101] During this procedure a small gold weight (usually around 1 g) is sutured to the orbital septum or upper eyelid tarsus to aid passively in gravity-assisted eyelid closure. Preoperatively, test weights can be taped to the upper eyelid to determine the effects of various-sized gold weights. The key is to have adequate weight to close the eye but not enough to cause severe ptosis. Implantation is accomplished through a small upper eyelid incision and the implant is sutured directly to the tarsus[102] or orbital septum through preplaced holes in the implant. Gold is the ideal material because it is heavy, and the color matches the color of fat, rendering it difficult to see through the skin. As well, gold weight implants are compatible with magnetic resonance imaging (MRI) since they are nonmagnetic. This is particularly important in patients with seventh nerve palsy secondary to an intracranial tumor that will require serial neuroimaging studies. Success rates for this procedure are reported to be as high as 90%,[100, 102–104] with failures generally falling into two groups: unacceptable ptosis or inadequate closure. More rare complications include infections, eyelid contour changes, and ectropion.[105] Gold weights rarely spontaneously extrude.[101] They can, however, be surgically removed relatively easily.

ABNORMAL BLINKING

A blink is a temporary closure of both eyelids and normally does not interfere with the continuity of vision. The mean ± SD spontaneous blink rate is 16 ± 9 blinks per minute. Physiologic blinking helps keep the cornea moist and protects the eye from excess light and foreign objects. This section will be subdivided into two parts: absent or decreased blinking and excessive blinking.

Absent or Decreased Blinking

Spontaneous Blinking. Decreased spontaneous blink rates may be characteristic of thyroid-associated ophthalmopathy, parkinsonism (eg, Parkinson's disease or progressive supranuclear palsy).[44, 106] In patients with parkinsonism, however, reflex blink rates may be increased (see below).

Corneal and Supraorbital Blink Reflexes. If the left ophthalmic division is defective, neither eye will blink to left corneal or forehead stimulation; if the right cornea or forehead is stimulated in this setting, both eyes will blink. This scenario must be contrasted to the case of a left facial nerve palsy in which only the right eye will blink fully whether either cornea or the forehead is stimulated.

In a well-studied phenomenon,[107, 108] patients with acute unilateral hemispheric lesions may have a diminished blink reflex when the contralateral cornea or forehead is stimulated. The responsible lesions tend to be large strokes. The defective blink reflex is usually temporary, lasting only 1 or 2 weeks following the ictus. These observations suggest the contralateral hemisphere exerts a supranuclear influence upon the blink reflex, and a cortical lesion may inhibit it.

Blink to Visual Threat. Patients with hemianopias from occipital and parietal lesions may not blink when approached with a menacing gesture in the defective field. A cardinal feature of cortical blindness is a completely absent blink to visual threat. Those with left-sided visual attention from a right parietal or frontal lesion or with diffusely decreased visual attention from Balint's syndrome (see Chapter 9) may have decreased blink to threat in their inattentive fields.[20]

Excessive Blinking

Increased blink rates are associated with schizophrenia and Tourette syndrome (see below). In addition, reflex blinking can be increased in parkinsonism. In this setting, when tapped on the forehead, the patient persistently blinks with each tap (the glabellar or Myerson's sign).

Blepharospasm and Hemifacial Spasm

Blepharospasm. Essential blepharospasm is an idiopathic dystonic disorder characterized by involuntary intermittent bilateral eyelid closure. It ranges from increased blink frequency to severe, sustained spasms of the orbicularis oculi. Initially only one eye may be affected, but within weeks to months both orbicularis oculi are involved. Wind, sunlight, or stress may exacerbate the spasms, but more chronic cases are characterized by spontaneous eyelid closure. Some more severely affected patients complain of functional blindness. Women are affected more than men, and blepharospasm usually begins in the fourth to sixth decades of life.[109] The cause is unclear, but enhanced blink reflex excitability, perhaps due to a loss of supranuclear inhibition, has been proposed.[110] Usually the patient has no underlying cause for the disorder, but blepharospasm may occur in parkinsonism,[44] months or years following an episode of Bell's palsy,[111] and in association with a lower pontine lesion.[112] Blepharospasm accompanied by dystonic movements of the lower face or neck (oromandibular dystonia) is termed *Meige syndrome.*

Hemifacial Spasm. In hemifacial spasm, the whole face on one side contracts, with eyelid closure and elevation of the corner of the mouth. The movement disorder is thought to be due to either (1) hyperexcitability of the facial motor nucleus, either idiopathically or because of an ischemic or mass lesion in the pons; or (2) compression of the facial nerve near its exit from the brain stem, causing myelin sheath injury and ephaptic transmission between individual nerve fibers.[113] A tortuous AICA or dolichoectatic artery of the posterior circulation is believed to be responsible for the majority of cases of hemifacial spasm. MRI and

MRI-angiography are helpful in demonstrating vascular compression of the pons or facial nerve.[114, 323]

Treatment. The treatment of choice in patients with debilitating blepharospasm or hemifacial spasm is localized subcutaneous injections of botulinum-A toxin around the eyelids to weaken the orbicularis oculi, other muscles involved in eyelid closure, and facial movements.[50, 112, 115, 116] Botulinum-A is produced by *Clostridium botulinum* and causes temporary paralysis of injected muscles by interfering with acetylcholine release from nerve terminals. Injection of botulinum into the eyebrow and upper and lower eyelids in blepharospasm patients, and into these same structures and into the lower facial musculature in hemifacial spasm patients, has a high degree of initial success, with relief of eyelid spasm and patient acceptance.

We usually begin with injections of 2.5 units of botulinum per injection site (Fig. 14–22) and agree that avoidance of the middle portion of the upper eyelid reduces the risk of ptosis. The exact sites of the injections can be varied from patient to patient depending on the areas in which the patient has the most spasms. A recent study has evaluated these standard injection sites and compared them to injection sites further from the eyelid margin and in the brow.[117] This study found that for blepharospasm patients, standard injections had the longest duration but were associated with increased transient ocular side effects, including irritation and epiphora. In the hemifacial spasm patients, brow treatment was as effective as standard treatment.

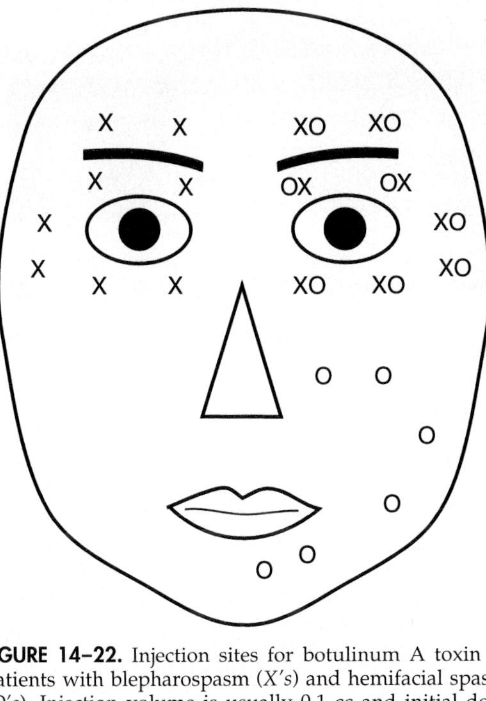

FIGURE 14–22. Injection sites for botulinum A toxin in patients with blepharospasm (*X's*) and hemifacial spasm (*O's*). Injection volume is usually 0.1 cc and initial dose is 2.5μm of botulinum A toxin.

Clinical experience has traditionally been that initial treatments are the most successful and with time, the effect of each injection may be less or tend to last for a shorter period. Reduced efficacy may be the result of antitoxin development, binding of the nonactive large protein chain, or a resprouting of motor endplates.[118, 119] In this setting a larger amount of botulinum can be given with each injection (5 units). Other studies, however, have failed to demonstrate a reduced effectivity or shorter duration of treatment with time.[120, 121] Greater than 90% of patients report a marked decrease in the squeezing action of the eyelids and twitching in the lower part of the face.[115, 122–127] The effect generally lasts between 1 and 4 months and tends to persist longer in hemifacial spasm compared to blepharospasm. Because of its transient effect, the procedure must be repeated indefinitely.

Complications of botulinum injections include lagophthalmos and exposure keratitis, which generally lasts several days and can be treated with lubricants and taping if necessary. Patients may develop tearing from keratitis or poor tear pump function. Sagging of the eyelid skin and brow may occur. More concerning complications result from deep penetration and include ptosis and double vision.[117] Ptosis develops in about 8% of patients[128] and double vision occurs in 2% of patients. The inferior oblique muscle is the most commonly affected muscle.[129] Systemic complications do not occur although systemic antibody production has been reported in patients receiving botulinum injections for hemifacial spasm or blepharospasm.[130]

If botulinum toxin fails, medications such as benzodiazepines, anticholinergic agents, dopamine agonists, anticonvulsants, and presynaptic dopamine-depleting agents may help some patients,[131] but their use is usually limited by side effects. In patients with refractory hemifacial spasm, a Teflon sponge can be placed between the AICA and facial nerve. Other more drastic measures include myectomy, during which the orbicularis oculi and other muscles used in eyelid closure are excised (either surgically[127] or chemically[132]), or neurectomy, a procedure in which branches of the facial nerve are cut.[125]

The importance of support groups for these patients has recently been emphasized in a report by Anderson and associates,[127] who found support group intervention was the most effective therapy in blepharospasm. Ultimately most patients (70%) continue to receive botulinum injections, while a few (7%) spontaneously improve, and others benefit from pharmacotherapy, surgery, or psychotherapy.[126]

Other Causes of Excessive Blinking

Physiologic Facial Synkineses. Following injury of the peripheral facial nerve, abnormal reinnervation patterns may be observed as motor function recovers. Eyelid closure upon smiling or vice versa (Fig. 14–23) is caused by incorrect reinnervation by orbicularis oculi and zygomaticus motor neurons.[133] Tearing in anticipation of eating food (crocodile tears) occurs when nerve fibers destined to supply the salivary glands are misdirected to the lacrimal gland. Other proposed mechanisms, such as ephaptic transmission and central reorganization of synaptic inputs to facial motor neurons, are unlikely (see discussion of oculomotor synkinesis, Chapter 15).

Eyelid Tics. These are brief, stereotyped, repetitive, and involuntary eyelid blinks, winks, or blepharospasm.[131] Affected patients may have a preceding urge before their tics, and they may be able to suppress them. Often idiopathic and considered benign motor tics, they can also be associated with encephalitis, drugs, toxins, stroke, head truama, and static encephalopathies. Usually they do not require treatment. However, in some instances eyelid tics are a first manifestation of Tourette syndrome. This is a childhood disorder, affecting boys more than girls, in which eyelid and facial tics can be associated with tics in the limbs or body.[134] Characteristic behavioral manifestations of Tourette syndrome include obsessive–compulsive disorder, grunting, throat clearing, barking, copralalia, and echolalia.[135]

Myokymia and Neuromyotonia. Small unilateral contractions of the facial muscles characterize *facial myokymia,* which, when associated with ipsilateral facial contracture and weakness (spastic–paretic facial contracture), indicate a pontine lesion rostral to the seventh nerve nu-

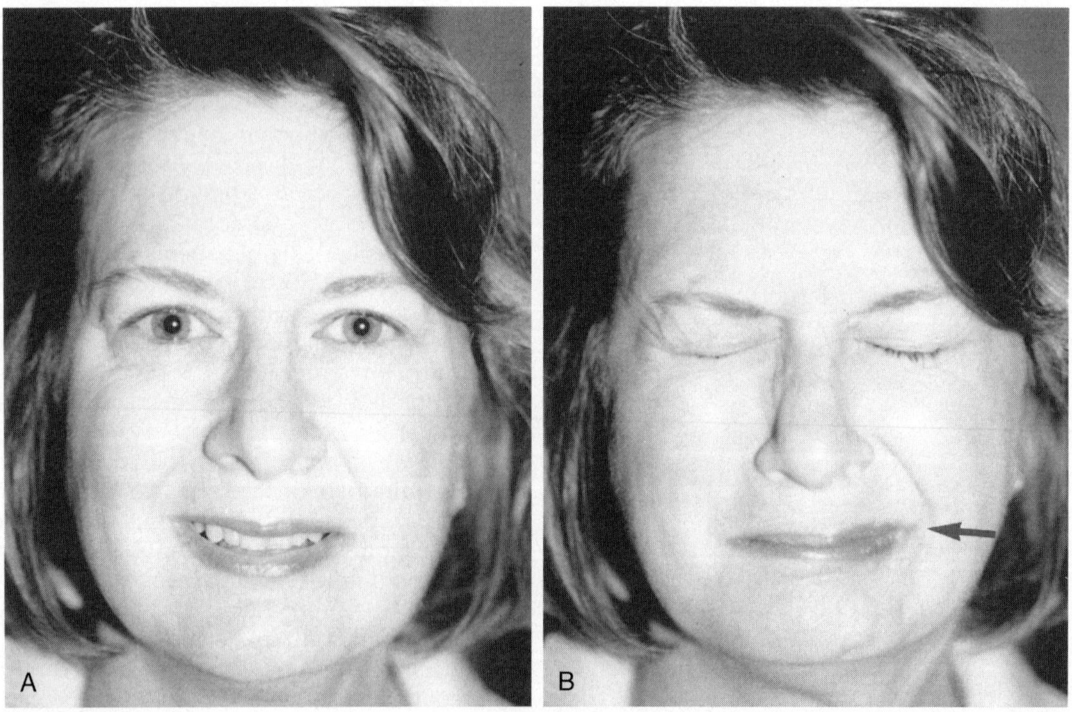

FIGURE 14–23. Facial synkinesis (aberrant regeneration). **A.** Patient with old left facial palsy following removal of left acoustic neuroma. **B.** Upon attempted eyelid closure, the orbicularis oris on the left (*arrow*) also contracts.

cleus. Multiple sclerosis and brain stem tumors are the typical causes.[136, 137] Other causes of facial myokymia include stroke, syringobulbia, hydrocephalus, acoustic neuroma, Guillain–Barré syndrome, hypoxic injury, and meningitis. *Eyelid myokymia,* which refers to small, annoying twitches of the upper or lower eyelids, is very common. This condition is benign and usually due to stress, fatigue, nicotine, or caffeine. Most patients require only reassurance, as eyelid myokymia usually abates spontaneously. Occasionally it persists, and in this situation it may be treated with benzodiazepines or botulinum. *Facial neuromyotonia,* which is similar to myokymia but is defined as a delay in muscle relaxation after a voluntary contraction, has been reported as a complication of radiation and responds to carbemazepine.[138]

Abnormal Facial Movements in Other Movement Disorders. Blepharospasm and other involuntary movements of the face may be seen in Parkinson's disease, progressive supranuclear palsy, Huntington's disease, and Wilson's disease.

Drug-Induced Facial Dyskinesias. Use of antiemetics such as metoclopramide or neuroleptics such as haloperidol, as well as antihistamines may lead to tardive dyskinesia, which may involve the face and eyes.[139] In such cases, patients develop stereotyped, writhing unilateral or bilateral eyelid closure. The diagnosis is usually evident after eliciting the medication history. Treatment consists of withdrawing the offending agent, sometimes combined with the use of botulinum injections in refractory cases.

Focal Motor Seizures. Unilateral facial movements or eyelid closure that is repetitive, brief, and followed by weakness (Todd's paralysis) would suggest a focal motor seizure involving the face. Spread to the hands or limbs, or generalization to involve the other side of the face or body with loss of consciousness would make this diagnosis obvious. Evaluation would consist of electroencephalography (EEG) and neuroimaging to detect a structural seizure focus, followed by treatment with anticonvulsants.

Palpebromandibular Synkinesia. Spontaneous eyelid blinking associated with anterolateral jaw movements may be seen in bilateral cortical disease or upper brain stem lesions sparing the pons.[19]

OTHER ABNORMAL EYELID AND FACIAL MOVEMENTS

Oculomasticatory Myorhythmia

This movement disorder is characterized by slow (1 Hz) pendular convergent–divergent nystagmus associated with rhythmic movements of the muscles of mastication, face, and extremities. It is considered virtually pathognomonic of Whipple's disease, which is caused by the bacillus *Tropheryma whippelii* (see Chapter 16).

Eyelid Nystagmus

A slow downward drift of the eyelids followed by a quick corrective upward flick may be observed in myasthenia gravis and brain stem lesions, particularly mesencephalic ones.[140] Naturally, eyelid nystagmus may also be observed with vertical nystagmus of the eyes, particularly upbeat. Eyelid nystagmus may be observed in medullary lesions with lateral gaze shifts. Other terms for this phenomenon include *lid hopping* and *upper-lid jerks.* The mechanism is unclear, but typically eyelid nystagmus is evoked by convergence[141] or horizontal gaze.[3]

DISEASES COMMONLY ASSOCIATED WITH PTOSIS AND/OR FACIAL WEAKNESS

Diseases to be discussed here include three neuromuscular junction disorders: myasthenia gravis, Lambert–Eaton myasthenic syndrome, and botulism; several myopathic disorders: chronic external ophthalmoplegia and Kearns–Sayre syndrome, myotonic dystrophy, and oculopharyngeal dystrophy; and polyneuropathies such as Guillain–Barré syndrome, Miller Fisher syndrome, and chronic inflammatory demyelinating polyneuropathy. These are all neuromuscular conditions whose neuro-ophthalmic presentation can be predominantly ptosis and/or facial weakness.

Myasthenia Gravis

This neurotransmission disorder is characterized by fatiguable muscular weakness. The eyelids and extraocular muscles are involved in over 90% of patients. Fifty percent present with ptosis or ocular motility abnormalities only,[142] and of this group, approximately half will remain "ocular myasthenics," while the other half will develop generalized symptoms, usually within 2 years.[143] There is an approximately 22% spontaneous remission rate.[144]

Myasthenia has a prevalence of 50 to 125 cases per million population, with a sex- and age-related bimodal distribution consisting of women in their twenties to thirties and men in their sixties and seventies.[145] One study[146] suggested younger patients had a better prognosis than those who presented when older than 50. Rarely, another member of the family also has a history of myasthenia.

Pathophysiology. A reduction in the number of available acetylcholine receptors of skeletal muscles (Fig. 14–24) results in a defect in neuromuscular transmission and weakness. A humorally mediated autoimmune attack directed against acetylcholine receptors causes their blockade, accelerated degradation, and complement-mediated damage.[145, 147, 148] Both production of high-affinity IgG antibodies and sensitization of antiacetylcholine receptor antibody $CD4^+$ T helper cells are observed.[149]

Usually the cause of this autoimmune disorder is unknown. However, in some cases it is drug-induced in association with the use of D-penicillamine, for instance. Antiacetylcholine receptor antibodies may be produced, and when the D-penicillamine is removed, often symptoms and receptor antibody levels normalize.[150] Several drugs, such as aminoglycosides, beta blockers, and quinidine, may exacerbate myasthenia gravis by their direct effects on the neuromuscular junction and neuromuscular blockade.[151–153]

Thymus hyperplasia and thymoma, the latter in approximately 15% of adult patients, are related findings. Myasthenia gravis also occurs frequently in association with other autoimmune disturbances such as hyperthyroidism (3% to 8% of patients with myasthenia[145]) and systemic lupus erythematosus.

Preferential Involvement of Extraocular Muscles. Kaminski et al[154] have reviewed the possible reasons why the eye muscles are frequently involved and sometimes solely affected in myasthenia gravis. These include (1) only mild extraocular muscle weakness is enough to cause ocular misalignment and symptomatic diplopia, (2) the high firing frequencies of extraocular muscles may predispose them to myasthenic fatigue, (3) extraocular muscle fibers may be more susceptible to neuromuscular blockade, and (4) extraocular muscles may contain antigens specific to them that make them more susceptible to immune attack. Although the fetal gamma subunit of the acetylcholine receptor in extraocular muscles was proposed as one such antigen,[155] in one study[156] the frequency of this subunit was found to be as common in eye as in other muscles. Alternatively, it is possible that there is another, yet unidentified autoantibody in myasthenia gravis that preferentially affects the extraocular muscles.[157]

Symptoms and Signs

Symptoms. Variable and fatiguable ptosis, diplopia, chewing difficulties, dysarthria, dysphagia, dyspnea, and systemic weakness are the

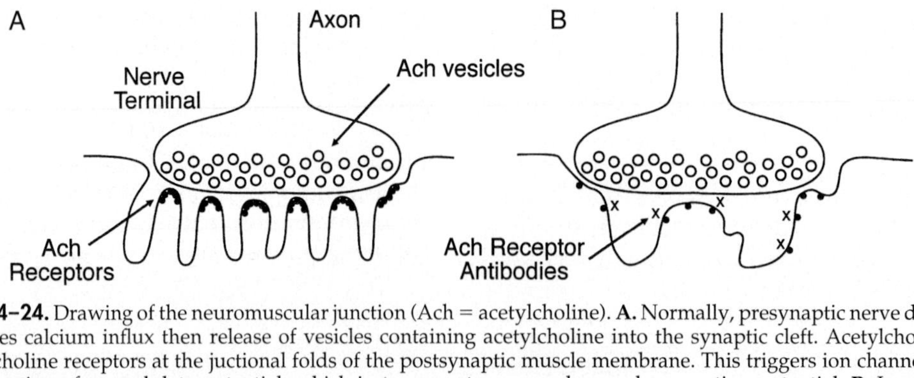

FIGURE 14–24. Drawing of the neuromuscular junction (Ach = acetylcholine). **A.** Normally, presynaptic nerve depolarization causes calcium influx then release of vesicles containing acetylcholine into the synaptic cleft. Acetylcholine binds to acetylcholine receptors at the juctional folds of the postsynaptic muscle membrane. This triggers ion channel opening and generation of an endplate potential, which in turn creates a muscle membrane action potential. **B.** In myasthenia gravis, a humorally mediated autoimmune attack by antibodies (*X's*) directed against acetylcholine receptors causes their blockade, accelerated degradation, and complement-mediated damage. This results in a defect in neuromuscular transmission and muscle weakness.

hallmarks of myasthenia gravis. Most patients' symptoms exhibit diurnal variation, as their weakness is better in the morning or after sleep than at the end of the day, when they are weakest.

Neuro-ophthalmic Signs. Eyelid abnormalities are frequently the most prominent ocular sign, and these include ptosis, fatiguability, Cogan's lid twitch, curtaining, and orbicularis oculi weakness (Table 14–5). None of these are pathognomonic of myasthenia,[158, 159] but when they are all present, this diagnosis should be strongly considered. Pupil-sparing ophthalmoplegia of any pattern may also be seen.

1. *Ptosis.* Myasthenic eyelid drooping, due to weakness of the levator palpebrae muscles, can be symmetric or asymmetric. The patient may adopt a chin-up position to look underneath the ptotic eyelids and raise the eyebrows and furrow the brow to keep the eyelids open (Fig. 14–25). When asymmetric, the eyelid that is affected more may alternate over time (so-called alternating ptosis). The pattern of ptosis and contralateral pseudoretraction reflects Hering's law and the patient's increased effort to control both levator muscles.
   Levator function in myasthenia is related to the amount of ptosis; those with prominent ptosis will have the most impaired levator function. Normal levator function in the setting of marked ptosis argues against the diagnosis of myasthenia.[160] Documentation of a change in levator function is one objective method to assess an improvement of ptosis.
2. *Fatigability.* If the patient is asked to maintain upgaze, the eyelids may tire and droop because of levator fatigue. Although characteristic of myasthenia, fatigable ptosis may sometimes also be seen in other causes of ptosis.[324]
3. *Cogan's lid twitch.* If a patient with myasthenic ptosis looks downward for 3 to 5 seconds, then looks up quickly into primary gaze, the eyelid appears to overshoot upward, then quickly falls.[159, 161] One purported mechanism for the overshoot is a buildup of acetylcholine in the neuromuscular junctions of levator muscle fibers while the eyelid is resting in downgaze. Following upward refixation, the levator quickly fatigues, and the eyelid droops.
4. *Curtaining and enhanced ptosis.* In asymmetric ptosis, when the more ptotic eyelid is manually elevated, the fellow eyelid often droops (*curtaining*) (see Fig. 14–9). This sign is nonspecific, and can be seen in many other situations with asymmetric ptosis such as a third nerve palsy. When the ptosis is symmetric, elevation of one eyelid will worsen the other eyelid (enhanced ptosis) (see Fig. 14–10). As discussed earlier, these eyelid signs are consequences of Hering's law, as manual elevation of a ptotic eyelid reduces the patient's required effort to elevate the eyelids, and the other eyelid falls.
5. *Orbicularis oculi weakness.* In almost all patients with myasthenic ptosis or ophthalmoplegia, the orbicularis oculi are also weak, causing weakness of eyelid closure. In the related *lid peak sign,* if a patient with myasthenic weakness of the orbicularis

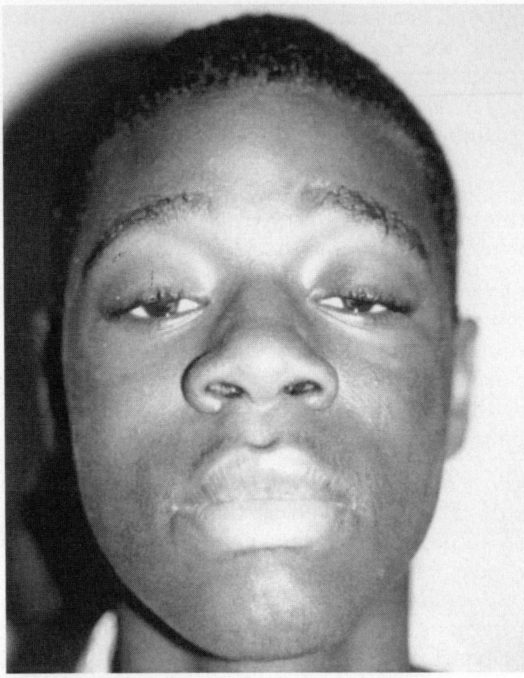

FIGURE 14–25. Severe bilateral ptosis in myasthenia gravis with chin-up position. In an attempt to lift the eyelids, the frontalis muscle is contracted and the brow is elevated.

TABLE 14–5. Common Eyelid Signs in Ocular Myasthenia Gravis

Ptosis—asymmetric or symmetric
Cogan's lid twitch
Curtaining (enhanced ptosis)
Fatigue
Weakness of eyelid closure

oculi is asked to maintain vigorous closure of the eyelids, the orbicularis may tire, allowing the palpebral fissures to open.

6. *Lid hopping.* During attempted lateral gaze, the eyelids may appear to hop or jump.[162]

The pupils are normal, and this should distinguish myasthenic ptosis from that of Horner syndrome or a third nerve palsy.

Ophthalmoparesis. Myasthenic ocular motility abnormalities, which are very common, are reviewed in Chapter 15. These can mimic any pupil-sparing third nerve palsy, or fourth or sixth nerve palsy, or supranuclear or nuclear gaze paresis.

Other Signs. The lower facial muscles may be sufficiently involved so the patient is unable to smile, whistle, pucker, or hold air in the cheeks.[163] Chewing difficulties may occur secondary to masseter weakness. When the oropharyngeal muscles are affected, speech may be nasal, and tongue protrusion may be weak. Neck flexor muscles are typically affected more than neck extensors in myasthenia. Any limb muscle may be weak. Deep tendon reflexes are decreased only in patients with severe weakness. Since myasthenia involves only the neuromuscular system, mental status and sensation are normal. *Myasthenic crisis* refers to life-threatening impairment of respiration.[145]

Although more useful for clinical studies than in everyday practice, the Osserman grading scheme can be used to classify severity of myasthenia: grade I = ocular involvement only; IIa = mild generalized; IIb = moderate generalized; III = acute fulminant; or IV = severe-late.

Diagnostic Testing

Edrophonium Test. Edrophonium, an acetylcholinesterase inhibitor with rapid onset and short duration of effect, may be administered to slow the breakdown and increase the availability of acetylcholine in the neuromuscular junction. In patients with myasthenia gravis, many of the eyelid, ocular motor, or systemic signs may objectively improve, thereby verifying the diagnosis (see Fig. 14–9).[164] The edrophonium test is positive in 80% to 90% of patients with myasthenia gravis.[165,166] The test should be performed only in those with obvious ptosis or ophthalmoparesis, in whom improvement can easily be observed.[167]

Edrophonium may be drawn up in a 1-cc tuberculin syringe and administered intravenously in 2-mg increments separated by 30 to 60 seconds up to a total of 10 mg. The advantage of the incremental method of edrophonium adminstration is that the full 10-mg dose may not be required to produce a positive response. Furthermore, overmedicating the patient and occasionally missing the point of ocular recovery can be avoided. The test can be terminated at any point or after the patient has received the full 10-mg dose if no response has occurred. If an intravenous line is used instead of a tuberculin syringe, flushing the line with normal saline is necessary to ensure that the edrophonium has been delivered to the bloodstream.

Optimally, an edrophonium test requires a team effort, with one individual administering the drug, another documenting the clinical findings, and a third monitoring the blood pressure and pulse. Occasionally patients develop salivation and mild gastrointestinal discomfort. Atropine 0.4 mg should be ready in a separate syringe and administered intravenously if symptomatic bradycardia occurs. Cardiac monitoring or avoiding the test is suggested in patients with a history of heart disease or arrhythmia.

In patients with myasthenic ptosis, the response to edrophonium is often dramatic and occurs within seconds or minutes of injection. Paradoxical worsening of ptosis should not be considered a positive test. The edrophonium test in patients with ocular dysmotility is discussed in more detail in Chapter 15. Eyelid twitching, tearing, and abdominal cramping are signs that the edrophonium has taken effect.[168] The edrophonium lasts for just a few minutes. Placebo injections are not necessary in patients with ptosis, which is almost never functional.

The edrophonium test unfortunately has many false negative and false positive results. For unclear reasons, some individuals with myasthenia, confirmed by other test parameters (see below), may have an equivocal or no response to edrophonium. In contrast, clinical improvement with edrophonium may be observed in other disorders of neuromuscular transmission such as Lambert–Eaton myasthenic syndrome (see below), botulism, and organophosphate toxicity. In addition, patients whose ptosis and eye movements unequivocally improved with edrophonium, who later were found to have skull base tumors, have been described.[158] Therefore, a positive edrophonium test should not be the sole basis for making a diagnosis of myasthenia gravis.

Intramuscular neostigmine may be used instead of edrophonium in children who may be too uncooperative for an IV infusion or too agitated to monitor over a short period of time or in adults whose signs are subtle and require a longer period of observation. [168,169] For adults, 1.5 mg of neostigmine and 0.6 mg of atropine sulfate are drawn up into a syringe and injected intramuscularly. The dose for children of neostigmine is .04 mg/kg, not to exceed a total of 1.5 mg.[170] The effect of intramuscular neostigmine usually begins by 15 minutes and is maximal by 30 minutes.[170]

Ice Pack or Sleep Test. If the patient has a cardiac history, one could try the noninvasive ice pack or sleep tests.[171, 172] In the ice pack test, a bag of ice is placed over the affected lid for 1 minute and then response of the lid is assessed. Eight out of 10 patients with myasthenia gravis displayed unequivocal improvement of levator strength in one study.[171] One of the myasthenic patients with a negative edrophonium test had a positive ice pack test, demonstrating its added benefit as a diagnostic test.[171] Another study found 80% of patients with myasthenic ptosis had a positive ice pack test, while all 20 patients with nonmyasthenic ptosis had a negative test.[173] The precise mechanism by which cooling improves myasthentic weakness is unclear. Enhanced transmitter release, reduced acetycholinesterase activity, and increased receptor sensitization with lower temperature are possible mechanisms.[171] However, similar improvement of ptosis may occur with warm packs as well, suggesting it is the resting, rather than the temperature, that is important. In the sleep test, the patient is allowed to sleep for approximately 30 minutes to see if rest improves the ptosis.[172]

Antibody Testing. Antiacetycholine receptor antibodies are detected in 50% to 75% of ocular myasthenic patients and in 80% to 90% with generalized disease.[174–176] These antibodies are entirely specific for myasthenia gravis,[174] but their levels do not correlate with the presence or severity of the disease. Antibody tests that measure the accelerated degradation or blockage of acetylcholine receptors may occasionally be positive in seronegative individuals.[145] Also, antibodies against components of striated muscle may be detected in myasthenia gravis. They have a low sensitivity but high specificity for myasthenia gravis,[148] and they also suggest the presence of thymoma.

Electromyography. A decrement of the compound muscle action potential during electromyographic repetitive nerve stimulation (2 to 5 Hz) of limb or facial muscles is diagnostic in many cases of myasthenia gravis.[177] However, this technique is relatively insensitive in ocular myasthenia, as it is positive in only approximately one third of such patients. Additional single-fiber electromyography (EMG) may be helpful in ocular myasthenia if the repetitive stimulation, edrophonium test, and antibody studies are nondiagnostic or cannot be performed. Normally, two muscle fibers innervated by the same motor axon will exhibit a variation, called *jitter*, in the time interval between their two action potentials during successive impulses. Jitter, detected by single-fiber EMG, can be increased in myasthenia gravis and other disorders of neuromuscular transmission.[178] Normally, a limb muscle is studied first, and if negative, one of the facial muscles, for instance, the orbicularis oris, oculi, or frontalis, is next evaluated. Patients who have only ocular symptoms but have abnormal EMG when a limb muscle is tested are still considered to have only ocular myasthenia. By testing the orbicularis oculi muscles, one study found abnormal findings in 13 out of 14 (93%) myasthenic patients.[166] However, caution should be used when using single-fiber EMG to distinguish between ocular myasthenia gravis and chronic progressive external ophthalmoparesis (CPEO). One study[179] found that patients with CPEO may have abnormal jitter, while none of the patients with CPEO had abnormal single-fiber EMG in a more recent paper.[166] Although extraocular muscles can be evaluated using single-fiber EMG,[180] they are not normally studied by this technique in most neurophysiology laboratories. In patients with mild myasthenia, the combination of single-fiber EMG, antiacetylcholine receptor antibody studies, and the edrophonium test should provide the laboratory confirmation of myasthenia gravis in at least 95% of patients.[165]

Imaging. If there is any concern that the eyelid and ocular motility abnormalities are suggestive of more central rather than neuromuscular origin, then MRI of the brain is manditory. Computerized tomography (CT) or MRI of the chest should be performed to exclude a thymoma in all cases.

Treatment. Patients with myasthenia gravis are treated with acetylcholinesterase inhibitors, plasmapheresis, intravenous gamma globulin, immunodulators, or thymectomy, either alone or in combination (Table 14–6).[181] Treatment decisions are based on the presence of bulbar or generalized symptoms, age, and disease severity.

Medical Treatment. As a first-line agent in patients with ocular or mild generalized myasthenia, pyridostigmine, an acetylcholinesterase inhibitor, can be given orally at a starting dose of 30 mg every 4 hours while awake. The medication can be increased by 30 mg per dose, up to 120 to 150 mg every 4 hours, and a timespan preparation can be given at nighttime to aid breathing, bulbar function, and weakness overnight and upon awakening. The response to pyridostigmine is variable, and it seems most effective at alleviating many of the bulbar and systemic symptoms, somewhat effective at improving ptosis, but relatively ineffective for diplopia. Tachyphylaxis and overmedication, inducing cholinergic crisis, rarely occur.[182] The most common side effects are diarrhea and cramping, which resolve with lowering the dosage or can be alleviated with loperamide, glycopyrrolate, or diphenoxylate with atropine. The latter two drugs decrease respiratory secretions.

Because corticosteroids are the most effective immunosuppressive agents for myasthenia gravis,[183] they are frequently used in patients with ocular myasthenia who fail pyridostigmine. Their use must be weighed against the possible short- and long-term steroid-related side effects. One suggested regimen starts patients at low alternate day doses (eg, prednisone 10 mg qod), with slow weekly increases to achieve 60 mg qod.[148] H_2 blockers for ulcer prophylaxis are often added, and a tuberculin skin test is recommended before starting corticosteroids to exclude prior exposure to tuberculosis. The prednisone dose can be tapered once therapeutic efficacy is reached, typically after a few months. Starting with lower doses decreases the potential for steroid-induced worsening of symptoms in moderate to severe generalized myasthenia, but this complication rarely occurs in patients with predominantly ocular findings.[184] Therefore, in patients with purely ocular myasthenia, another alternative is to start patients at higher initial doses at 40 to 80 mg qd. Symptoms usually begin to improve more rapidly within the first 2 to 4 weeks. When the maximal effect, which may not be evident for 3 to 6 months, is reached, the dose can be tapered slowly. Every other dose is reduced by 5 mg per week, until a complete alternate day dosing is achieved. Then the remaining dose is reduced by 5 mg per week as well. Most patients on corticosteroids chronically require a small amount of alternate-day dosing. A critical dose where worsening may occur is usually around 20 mg every other day. Failed attempts at dose reduction can be followed by slower dose reduction rates, an increased ending dose, the addition of another immunosuppressive, or thymectomy (see below).[185]

TABLE 14–6. Therapeutic Options in Ocular Myasthenia Gravis

Symptomatic relief—pharmacologic
Pyridostigmine
Symptomatic relief—conservative
Eyelid crutches
Patching
Disease suppression
Corticosteroids
Azathioprine
Cyclosporine
Potential cure
Thymectomy

Some authorities have argued that lid crutches for ptosis and patching for diplopia are better conservative measures than corticosteroids in patients with ocular myasthenia. However, we have found that many patients find these alternatives unacceptable, especially those who require stereoscopic vision for their occupation, and prefer using corticosteroids with careful monitoring for side effects. Surgical correction of ptosis in general is not recommended because of the variability of the eyelid drooping.

In patients with severe refractory symptoms, other immunosuppressants such as azathioprine or cyclosporine may be used as supplementary agents or for steroid-sparing effects. Azathioprine is given in 2- to 3-mg/kg/day doses, with a time to onset of effect of 3 to 12 months and time to maximal effect of 1 to 2 years.[145,186] Bone marrow and liver function should be monitored for possible side effects. Cyclosporine can be given at 2.5 mg/kg bid, with a time to onset of effect of 2 to 12 weeks and a time to maximal effect of 3 to 6 months. For this drug, blood pressure, renal function, and drug levels should be monitored.[187] Some authors[188] have advocated their judicious use with corticosteroids in patients with difficult-to-manage ocular myasthenia. However, because of their toxic side effect profile, our practice has been to eschew these medications unless generalized symptoms are present. Similarly, because of the cost, requirement of an inpatient stay, and need for repeated treatments, we have not used plasmapheresis or intravenous gamma globulin[189, 190] in patients with solely ocular myasthenia. These modalities are more appropriate for patients whose systemic symptoms of dyspnea, dysphagia, and generalized weakness are debilitating enough to require hospitalization.

Surgical. Besides spontaneous remission, thymectomy represents the only potential cure for myasthenia gravis.[191] Possible mechanisms for improvement include eliminating a source of continued antigenic stimulation[192]; removing a possible reservoir of B cells, which secrete acetylcholine receptor antibodies; and correcting a disturbance of immune regulation.[145] The procedure traditionally is performed via a trans-sternal approach.[193, 194] The transcervical approach, which requires only a incision at the base of the neck, has become popular because of less associated discomfort and quicker recovery.[195] Pathologically the thymus typically exhibits lymphoid hyperplasia.

Patients without thymoma less than 60 years of age who have generalized symptoms are ideal candidates for thymectomy. Those with bulbar or respiratory weakness may require preoperative plasmapheresis to reduce the postoperative recovery period. Sixty percent of patients will experience complete remission without symptoms or need for medication over several years.[178, 196] Another 30 percent are able to reduce their dose of pyridostigmine or immunosuppressive agent. Surgery earlier in the disease course and less severe disease appear to be associated with better outcomes.[197] As the morbidity associated with thymectomy, especially via the transcervical route, decreases with improvement in surgical techniques, we have lowered our threshold for recommending this procedure in patients with solely ocular myasthenia who are refractive to medical therapy.[198, 199] In addition, it has recently been suggested that patients older than 60 may safely undergo and benefit from the procedure.[200]

Thymoma associated with myasthenia is another indication for thymectomy, which is usually performed trans-sternally to ensure complete removal of the tumor. Postoperatively the myasthenia in these patients tends to be more unstable, severe, and difficult to manage, and such patients often require a combination of different medical therapies. However, one recent study[201] suggested the long-term outcome in myasthenic patients with thymoma was no different than in those without thymoma.

Myasthenia Gravis in Children. *Juvenile* (or *infantile) myasthenia gravis* has the same pathophysiology as the adult type, with idiopathic production of acetylcholine receptor antibodies.[202] Fourteen to 30% of children experience spontaneous remission,[203] and in one study[204] this always occurred within 40 months of disease onset in prepubertal patients. In one small exceptional series,[205] all of four children with solely ocular myasthenia had a spontaneous remission. As in adults, about half of children presenting with ocular myasthenia will eventually generalize.[206] Forty percent of children with ocular myasthenia have detectable acetylcholine receptor antibodies, whereas 70% of children with generalized symptoms are seropositive.[206] Younger prepubertal children have a higher incidence of seronegativity.[207] When an edrophonium test is performed, a total of 0.2 mg/kg can be infused intravenously in divided doses, not exceeding 10 mg.

Pyridostigmine is first-line therapy in ocular or generalized juvenile myasthenia, but as in adults, the results are often unsatisfactory. Long-term corticosteroids, because of their effects on bone growth, and chronic immunosuppression with azathioprine or cyclosporine, are problematic in young patients. The effect of intravenous gamma globulin is usually only transient. Transsternal thymectomy has been performed in children with generalized myasthenia gravis with a remission rate of approximately 67%,[208–211] but controversy exists because some authors have opined that the thymus may be important for proper development of the immune system,[212] especially within the first year of life. However, Herrmann et al[213] cite numerous studies in which no subsequent immunodeficiency was found in children undergoing thymectomy for myasthenia gravis, as part of early cardiac surgery, and for suspected thymoma. To date, we have not recommended thymectomy for any child with solely ocular myasthenia gravis.

In transient *neonatal myasthenia gravis,* about 12% of infants of mothers with myasthenia may exhibit poor sucking, a weak cry, and hypotonia due to passive transfer of acetylcholine receptor antibodies. As the antibody titer declines over the first days or weeks of life, the child spontaneously improves. *Congenital myasthenic syndromes* share a different mechanism from antibody-mediated myasthenia gravis although children present similarly with weakness evident shortly after birth. These syndromes have been traced to genetic abnormalities of the presynaptic, synaptic, or postsynaptic portions of the neuromuscular junction.[214] Neither circulating autoantibodies nor abnormal thymus glands are found. Engel[215–219] and, others[220] have characterized several congenital myasthenic syndromes, and examples include (1) a defect in acetylcholine resynthesis and packaging (presynaptic), (2) a congenital endplate acetylcholinesterase deficiency (synaptic), (3) a slow-channel syndrome (postsynaptic), (4) a congenital endplate acetylcholine receptor deficiency (postsynaptic), and (5) high conductance and fast closure of the acetylcholine receptor channel (postsynaptic). Except for the slow-channel syndrome, which is autosomal dominant, the congenital myasthenic syndromes have autosomal recessive inheritance.[221]

Lambert–Eaton Myasthenic Syndrome

Lambert–Eaton myasthenic syndrome (LEMS), which is much rarer than myasthenia gravis, is a presynaptic neurotransmission disorder. The syndrome has two major forms: paraneoplastic and primary autoimmune, but their presentations and pathophysiology are similar. Most patients are elderly, but individuals in all age groups can be affected. LEMS is commonly mistaken for myasthenia gravis because patients with both disorders may present with weakness and ptosis. However, LEMS is distinguished clinically by the presence of autonomic symptoms and lack of obvious ophthalmoplegia.

About half of all newly diagnosed patients with LEMS have the paraneoplastic form with an underlying malignancy. Most of these patients harbor a small cell carcinoma of the lung, but LEMS is also associated with large cell neuroendocrine carcinomas and adenocarcinomas of the lung, lymphoproliferative disorders, renal cell carcinoma, and parotid tumors. As in many paraneoplastic disorders, the presentation of LEMS may precede or followthe cancer diagnosis. Rare individuals with LEMS and paraneoplastic cerebellar degeneration[222–224] and others with LEMS and antibody-positive myasthenia gravis[225] have been reported. LEMS can also be seen in association with other autoimmune diseases such as systemic lupus erythematosis, pernicious anemia, diabetes mellitus, and thyroid disease.[226] LEMS due to diltiazem, a calcium channel blocker, has also been described.[227]

Pathophysiology. In both the paraneoplastic or primary autoimmune types, LEMS is caused by antibodies directed against voltage-gated calcium channels on the presynaptic portion of the neuromuscular junction.[228, 229] Various subtypes of these antibodies, designated P/Q, L, N, T, and MysB, have been described.[230] Acetylcholine release, which is dependent upon the influx of calcium into the nerve terminal, is therefore impaired. Exercise or high rates of stimulation increase the intracellular calcium concentration, thereby enhancing acetylcholine release.

Symptoms. Most patients present with progressive fatiguable proximal weakness, usually starting in their legs. Autonomic symptoms are also common and include dry mouth, impotence, blurred vision, dry eyes, and constipation. Neuro-ophthalmic symptoms are typically not prominent but may consist of droopy eyelids and transient diplopia. Respiratory difficulty and bulbar symptoms such as dysphagia and dysarthria are also uncommon.

Signs. The neurologic examination in LEMS is characterized by proximal muscle weakness and absent or depressed reflexes most apparent in the weakest limbs.[231] The increase in muscle strength after exercise is actually difficult to demonstrate clinically. An improvement in deep tendon reflexes after sustained contraction is more easily found. Sensation is typically normal.

Neuro-ophthalmic Signs. Patients with LEMS may have mild bilateral ptosis, usually without noticeable ophthalmoparesis. In contrast to patients with myasthenia gravis, some patients may have improvement in their ptosis, mimicking lid retraction, with sustained upgaze.[232, 233] In O'Neill et al's series,[226] about one half had ptosis, and despite the complaint of diplopia in half of patients, no eye movement abnormalities were found. Two studies of patients with LEMS, with normal eye movements on neuro-ophthalmic exam, had improvement in saccadic velocity after exercise documented with oculography.[234, 235] Autonomic dysfunction may be reflected in dry eye and sluggish pupillary reactivity.

Diagnosis. Although the characteristic combination of clinical signs and symptoms may suggest LEMS, the diagnosis must be confirmed by EMG. A decreased resting compound muscle action potential (CMAP) that increases with maximal voluntary contraction is the classic EMG finding. Repetitive stimulation at 3 Hz, which is typically performed to demonstrate decrement of the CMAP amplitude in myasthenia gravis, may also show a decremental response in LEMS. However, repetitive stimulation at 50 Hz may produce an incremental response. Single-fiber EMG may demonstrate jitter (see above) and neuromuscular blockade. Immunoassay for the antibodies directed against voltage-gated calcium channels may also be performed and is sensitive but not specific for LEMS.[229] Edrophonium testing, which is also nonspecific, may lead to some improvement in weakness. CT and MRI of the chest and abdomen, followed by bronchoscopy in smokers, is recommended to exclude cancer.[236]

Treatment. Management of patients with LEMS typically has three forms: identification and treatment of the underlying malignancy, enhancement of neurotransmission, and immunomodulation.[231,236,237] Treatment of the cancer, via chemotherapy, surgery, or radiation, and is the most important step.[238] Although not widely available, 3,4-diaminopyridine, which prolongs the activation of voltage-gated calcium channels at the nerve terminal, thereby enhancing the release of acetylcholine, has been reported as an effective treatment in LEMS.[239, 325] Guanidine, which has a similar mechanism of action, and acetylcholinesterase inhibitors also may be used to enhance neurotransmission. Immunomodulation may be achieved with plasmapheresis, intravenous immunoglobulin,[240, 241] or immunosuppression with prednisone or azathioprine.[242] Neurologic improvement can be observed in many cases, with survival over months to years after treatment.

Botulism

Botulism is caused by a clostridial toxin from *C. botulinum* that blocks the release of acetylcholine from the presynaptic nerve terminal. Breast-fed infants less than 1 year of age living in endemic areas are most commonly affected. Ingestion of honey or home-canned or -bottled products that have not been sterilized,[243] or wounds[244] can result in clostridial infection.

The time from onset of symptoms to medical presentation is usually days to a week. Infants usually present with generalized hypotonia and poor suck for several days. In all ages, pharyngeal weakness, respiratory difficulty, and decreased limb strength may occur.

Neuro-ophthalmic complications such as bifacial weakness, ophthalmoplegia, and ptosis are very common.[244–246] Poorly reactive pupils are also frequently seen, and this finding and constipation often help differentiate patients with botulism in the emergency setting from myasthenia gravis or Guillian–Barré syndrome, the two major other disorders in the differential diagnosis of acute paralysis. High-frequency repetitive stimulation studies demonstrating post-tetanic potentiation and stool tests for botulinum toxin and culture can help confirm the diagnosis.

Chronic Progressive External Ophthalmoplegia, Kearns–Sayre Syndrome, and Related Mitochondrial Disorders

Chronic Progressive External Ophthalmoplegia and Kearns–Sayre Syndrome. In chronic progressive external ophthalmoplegia (CPEO), the ptosis is usually symmetric and accompanied by bilateral ophthalmoparesis and orbicularis oculi weakness. Patients with Kearns–Sayre syndrome (KSS) have the combination of (1) CPEO, (2) onset before age 20, (3) pigmentary retinopathy, and (4) at least one of the following: heart block, ataxia, or CSF protein above 100 mg/dL. CPEO and KSS are both mitochondrial myopathies.

Pathophysiology. These disorders are caused by mitochondrial DNA deletions.[247, 248] Most cases are sporadic, and these are associated with single, large deletions that vary in size from 1.3 to 9.1 kb. The most common deletion is 4.9 kb from positions 8470 to 13460. Approximately half of patients with CPEO and 90% of those with KSS have demonstrable mitochondrial deletions.[249]

Less common, familial varieties of CPEO have also been described that are inherited either autosomal dominantly or recessively. In autosomal dominant patients, multiple mitochondrial DNA deletions are identified either on 3p or 10q.[250–252] Overlap mitochondrial syndromes with ptosis, ophthalmoplegia, and pigmentary retinopathy consistent with KSS combined with other features suggestive of other mitochondrial disorders such as the syndrome of mitochondrial myopathy, encephalopathy, lactic acidosis, and strokelike episodes (MELAS, see Chapter 8), and the syndrome of myoclonus, epilepsy, and ragged-red fibers (MERRF), have been associated with a point mutation at mitochondrial DNA position 3243 (MELAS mutation).[253]

Symptoms. Except in KSS, symptoms can start at almost any age. Slowly progressive ptosis can be a patient's prominent complaint. Because the ophthalmoplegia is typically symmetric and chronically progressive, usually there is no diplopia. Family members or friends may be the first to notice the difficulty with eye movements. Visual loss due to retinal complications in KSS is uncommon but mild when it occurs. Historical evidence of longstanding muscle weakness, such as difficulty with running, jumping, or climbing, may be present.

Signs. In CPEO, symmetric ptosis with levator dysfunction and diffuse ophthalmoparesis are the most common features (Fig. 14–26). The pupils are spared. Patients often have asymptomatic orbicularis, neck, and limb weakness.[249] The pigmentary retinopathy in KSS (Fig. 14–27; see Color Plates 45 and 46), which has been described as salt-and-pepper in appearance, is discussed in more detail in Chapter 4. Patients with KSS may have sensorineural hearing loss, dementia, or ataxia.

Systemic Complications in Kearns–Sayre Syndrome. The major cardiac complication in KSS is heart block, but short stature and hypoparathyroidism have also been observed.[254, 255]

Diagnosis. A definitive diagnosis of CPEO or KSS can be made on muscle biopsy, in which histologic and ultrastructural abnormalities of skeletal muscle mitochondria can be demonstrated[256] and from which genetic testing can be performed. Usually a deltoid or quadriceps muscle is biopsied. Ragged-red fibers, which are red-staining granules in the subsarcolemmal zones and within the muscle fibers,[255] can be seen on modified Gomori trichrome staining (Fig. 14–28; see Color Plate 47). Electron microscopy may reveal excessive proliferation of normal-looking mitochondria, giant mitochondria with disoriented cristae, intramitochondrial paracrystalline inclusions ("parking lots"), and electron-dense osmiophilic inclusions.[257]

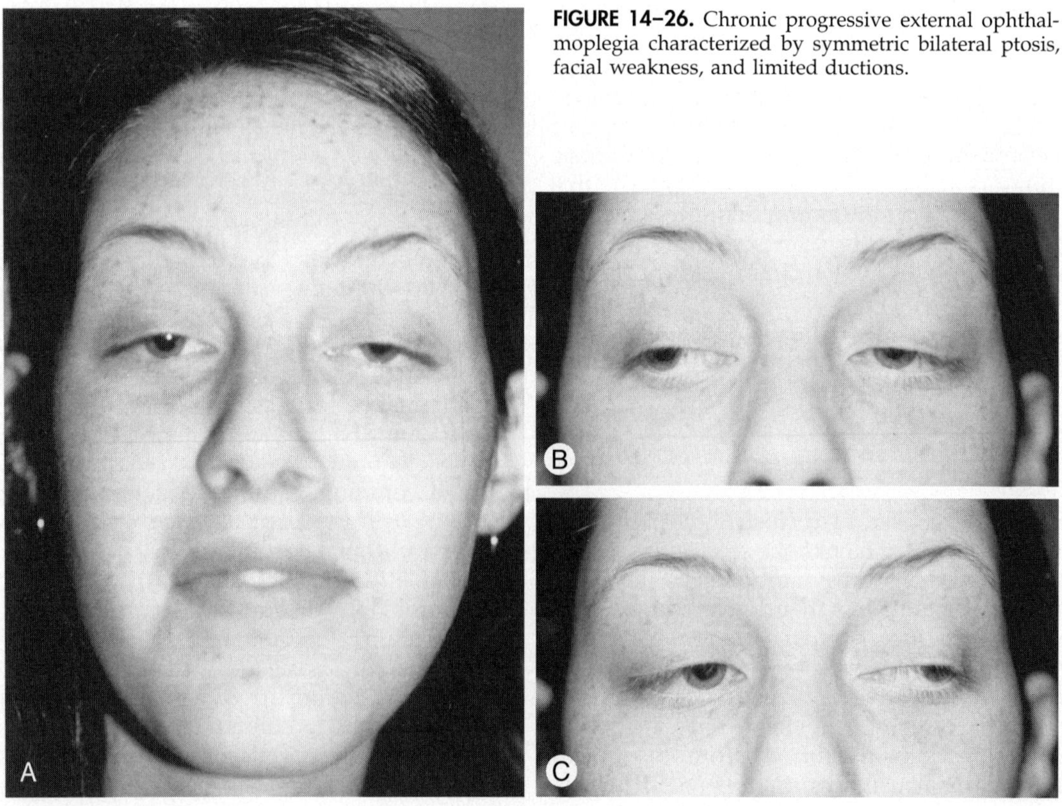

FIGURE 14–26. Chronic progressive external ophthalmoplegia characterized by symmetric bilateral ptosis, facial weakness, and limited ductions.

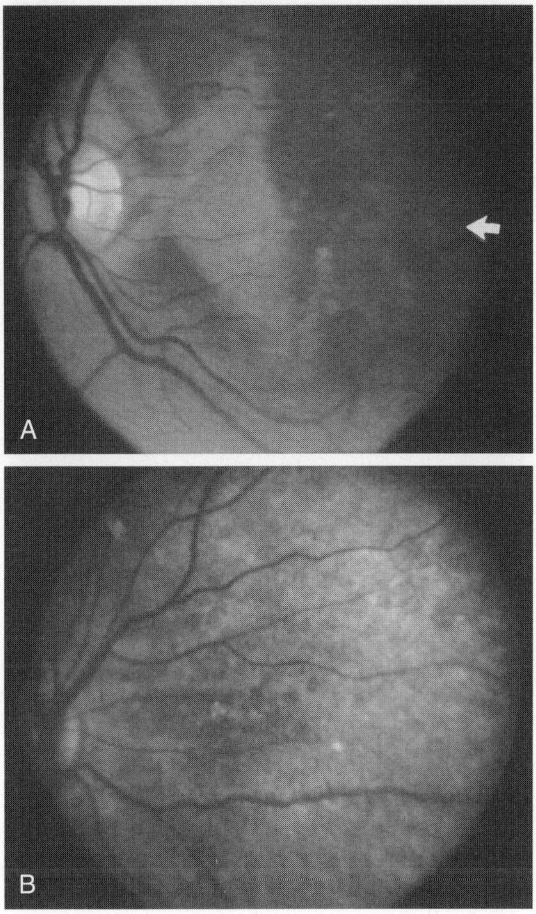

FIGURE 14–27. Fundus photographs in Kearns–Sayre syndrome. A. Posterior pole photograph demonstrating a healthy-appearing optic nerve but extensive pigmentary degeneration with atrophy and pigment clumping (*arrow*). (See Color Plate 45.) B. Photograph of nasal periphery demonstrating diffuse pigmentary mottling with atrophy and hyperpigmentation ("salt and pepper" configuration). (See Color Plate 46.)

Other ancillary testing may provide supportive evidence before the muscle biopsy is performed and test results are available. Conventional EMG usually demonstrates myopathic patterns. However, as alluded to earlier in the section on myasthenia gravis, single-fiber EMG in CPEO may also show increased jitter.[179] This highlights the difficulty in using single-fiber EMG to differentiate CPEO from myasthenia gravis.

In KSS, nonspecific MRI findings such as atrophy and white matter and basal ganglia hyperintensities on T_2-weighted images may be seen.[258, 259] Magnetic resonance proton spectroscopy may reveal elevated brain lactate levels, which has been attributed to the impairment in oxidative metabolism.[260, 261] CT may demonstrate basal ganglia hypointensities[255] or calcification.

Other abnormalities on diagnostic evaluation include elevation of serum lactate and abnormally increased CSF protein in KSS. At postmortem, spongy degeneration of the brain may be seen histopathologically.

Treatment. Treatment measures are symptomatic and biochemical. Ptosis surgery is often helpful. However, overwidening of the palpebral fissures should be avoided in individuals who are unable to elevate their eye under the upper eyelid to protect the cornea. Strabismus surgery can be performed in the rare individual with strabismus and diplopia.[262] Vitamins and coenzyme Q can be given but often are of little benefit.

Mitochondrial Neurogastrointestinal Encephalopathy Syndrome. A familial *m*itochondrial *n*eurogastrointestinal *e*ncephalomyopathy (MNGIE) syndrome, caused by multiple mitochondrial DNA deletions, is now well-recognized.[263–269] Other acronyms, such as POLIP (for polyneuropathy, ophthalmoplegia, leukoencephalopathy, and intestinal pseudo-obstruction), had also been used previously.[270] Affected patients are usually young to middle-aged adults. Characteristic clinical features are symmetric ptosis, ophthalmoparesis, intestinal pseudo-obstruction, and a mixed demyelinating and axonal neuropathy. Short stature, deafness, cachexia, white matter abnormalities on MRI, optic atrophy, and retinal pigmentary degeneration have also been observed.[268, 269]

Myotonic Dystrophy

Myotonic dystrophy is a hereditary bilateral myopathy that is associated with weakness

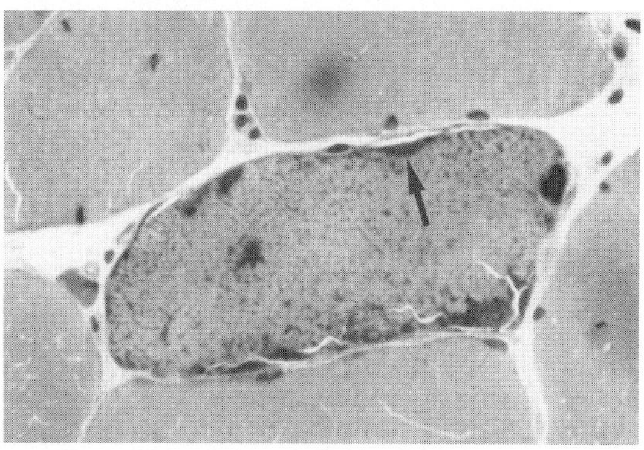

FIGURE 14–28. Muscle biopsy (modified Gomori trichrome) demonstrating ragged red fibers (*arrow*) in Kearns–Sayre syndrome. (See Color Plate 47.)

and atrophy of the muscles of the face and extremities. This disorder, however, is distinguished from other neuromuscular disorders by muscle myotonia, a continued contraction despite attempted relaxation, and multiorgan involvement.

Pathophysiology. Myotonic dystrophy is inherited in an autosomally dominant fashion, typically from the mother. It is caused by an unstable cytosine–thymine–guanine trinucleotide (CTG triplet) repeat on chromosome 19q13.3. Anticipation among successive generations is observed, as the offspring typically are more severely affected than the parent. This phenomenon is explained by an increase in the number of triplet repeats among more affected offspring. The abnormal gene codes for a cyclic AMP-dependent protein kinase enzyme. A defect in phosphorylation of skeletal muscle ion channels may affect the excitability of the muscle membranes and result in myotonia.[271]

Symptoms. Patients often complain of progressive distal and proximal weakness. Neuro-ophthalmic symptoms include ptosis, lack of facial expression, and rarely, diplopia. They may have a history of heart disease and cognitive deficits. Patients may present in the neonatal period with weakness and difficulty sucking and swallowing.

Signs. Bilateral ptosis is associated with bifacial weakness and "hatchet facies" due to temporalis muscle wasting. The upper lip may be "tented."[272] Ocular motor abnormalities have been described, including external ophthalmoplegia. Subclinical saccadic slowing has been demonstrated oculographically, but it is controversial whether this phenomenon is a peripheral or central one.[273–277] A characteristic "Christmas tree" cataract, consisting of multicolored iridescent flecks, is found in almost all patients and can cause visual acuity loss. Less commonly, central macular lesions, pigmentary retinal degeneration, and hypotony may occur.[278]

Patients with myotonic dystrophy are diffusely weak. Action myotonia is elicited by having the patient grasp an object then have difficulty relaxing. Percussion myotonia can be observed following mechanical depression of the tongue or thenar eminence, for example. Many have cognitive delay, decreased IQ, or other mental status abnormalities. Typical systemic findings in males include temporal balding and testicular atrophy. Patients also may have cardiac abnormalities such as arrhythmias, conduction defects, and congestive heart failure.

Diagnosis. The diagnosis is suspected clinically in a patient with weakness, myotonia, the typical facies, and similarly affected family members. Electrical myotonia can be elicited during EMG. Characteristic is a "dive bomber" sound, reflecting continuous discharges and difficulty with muscle relaxation.

The disorder should be distinguished from other myotonic neuromuscular disorders such as hyperkalemic period paralysis, paramyotonia congenita, and myotonia congenita.[271] Except for lid retraction and lag in hyperkalemic periodic paralysis, neuro-ophthalmic signs and symptoms in these conditions are less prominent than in myotonic dystrophy.

Other Muscular Dystrophies

Oculopharyngeal Muscular Dystrophy. Patients with this disorder usually present in middle age with progressive bilateral ptosis and dysphagia. Several subtypes have been described:

1. An autosomal oculopharyngeal muscular dystrophy recognized among French Canadian and Bukhara Jewish families. Ophthalmoplegia is a feature only late in the disease, and facial weakness and proximal limb weakness may also develop. The pathologic hallmark is a filamentous intranuclear inclusion in affected muscles. The genetic defect has been mapped to chromosome 14q11.2–13, and a guanine–cytosine–guanine (GCG) triplet repeat has been demonstrated.[279]
2. Another type, in which ophthalmoplegia is more prominent, and affected patients display clinical, electrophysiologic, and pathologic evidence of myopathy and neuropathy.[280]

Guillian–Barré Syndrome and Related Polyneuropathies

Guillian–Barré Syndrome. Today Guillain–Barré syndrome (GBS) is the most common cause of acute flaccid paralysis in the United States. Facial paresis occurs in approximately 50 percent.[281]

Pathophysiology. Most cases of GBS are caused by acute inflammatory demyelination of peripheral nerves (AIDP), the pathogenesis of which is likely to be autoimmune. Areas of demyelination are typically segmental and characterized by focal, perivascular infiltrates of lymphocytes and macrophages.[282, 283] However, less common forms such as acute motor axonal neuropathy (AMAN), acute motor and sensory axonal neuropathy (AMSAN), and the Miller Fisher variant (discussed separately below) are well recognized.[284–286] CNS involvement is uncommon.[287]

Up to three quarters of patients with GBS have a preceding infection, which is usually gastrointestinal or respiratory.[286] Approximately one quarter of patients have serologic or stool-culture evidence of recent *Campylobacter jejuni* infection, and a majority of these have diarrhea in the weeks before the onset of GBS. Patients with *C. jejuni* infection and GBS also have a greater likelihood of testing positive for GM_1 antibodies directed against gangliosides in peripheral nerve,[288] having AMAN or secondary axonal degeneration in association with AIDP,[289] as well as exhibiting slower recovery and greater residual neurologic disability.[290] Other common antecent infections include human immunodeficiency virus (HIV), cytomegalovirus, Epstein–Barr virus, and *Mycoplasma pneumoniae*.[291] Associated diseases include Hodgkin's lymphoma[292] and systemic lupus erythematosus. A history of recent surgery is also a risk factor for GBS, although infrequent.

Symptoms. Patients usually present with motor weakness, often ascending, which progresses over days to weeks. Paresthesias in affected limbs occur frequently, but are usually a less prominent complaint. Pain in the thighs or back may occur.

Signs. GBS is highlighted by areflexia and symmetric motor weakness affecting the limbs and trunk. Bulbar and respiratory muscles are often involved. Sensory loss is mild.[293] Uni- or bilateral facial weakness occurs in about one half of patients. The third, fourth, and sixth nerves may be affected, leading to ophthalmoplegia in about 15%.[281] Ptosis, when it occurs, is usually a result of third nerve palsy. However, in one series[294] 8% of patients with GBS had ptosis without ophthalmoparesis or pupillary abnormalities. Without third nerve palsy, the pupils are usually spared (see discussion in Chapter 13). When the spinal fluid protein level is very high, papilledema may observed (see discussion in Chapter 6). Rare cases of optic neuritis have been reported.[295]

Respiratory failure may require mechanical ventilatory support in about one third of cases.[281] Medical complications include pneumonia, urinary tract infections, sepsis, cardiac arrhythmias, blood pressure fluctuations, cardiac arrest from autonomic instability,[296] and deep vein thromboses and pulmonary emboli from immobility.

Diagnosis. Spinal fluid examination is helpful and classically demonstrates an elevated protein without pleocytosis (albuminocytologic dissociation). The typical EMG findings of AIDP are conduction block or slowing of motor nerve conduction velocity.[297] However, both the CSF examination and EMG may be normal within the first few days of the illness, and therefore in such cases they should be repeated approximately one week later if GBS is still strongly suspected. Detection of specific ganglioside autoantibodies, such as GM_1, GT_{1a}, GQ_{1b} (see below), and GD_{1b}, is often helpful.[298] Anti-GQ_{1b} can be detected in patients with GBS and ophthalmoparesis and usually not in those with normal eye movements.[299] The differential diagnosis for acute flaccid paralysis includes myasthenia gravis, poliomyelitis, botulism, tick bite paralysis, porphyria, hexacarbon abuse, diphtheria, and lead toxicity.[300]

Treatment. Large studies have demonstrated that patients with acute respiratory deficiency or inability to walk improve more rapidly with early plasmapheresis.[301] Alternatively, intravenous immunoglobulin therapy (IVIG), which is safer and easier to use, may also be administered. Some studies suggest that IVIG is as effective plasmapheresis.[302, 303] A number of other advances have improved the morbidity and mortality of patients with GBS. These include hospitalization of patients in intensive care settings, ventilatory management and pulmonary toilet, nutrition, pain control, deep vein thrombosis prophylaxis, blood pressure and cardiac monitoring, avoidance of decubiti with positioning, and improved bowel and bladder care.

Most patients recover over weeks to months[304] although some require hospitalization for up to a year. Many patients have persistent minor weakness, areflexia, or paresthesias that do not interfere with ordinary activities.[281]

Miller Fisher Syndrome. This variant of GBS, first characterized by Miller Fisher in 1956,[305] is highlighted by ataxia, ophthalmoplegia, and areflexia. In contrast to the usual AIDP form of GBS, eye movement abnormalities are prominent in the Miller Fisher syndrome, and diplopia is often the first complaint.[294] The ophthalmoplegia typically consists of various combinations of third, fourth, and sixth nerve involvement, and some patients develop complete loss of eye movements. Pupillary dysfunction can also occur (see discussion in Chapter 13). Facial nerve palsy is frequently observed, but usually systemic weakness is less salient than in AIDP. However, similar areflexia, electrophysiologic abnormalities, cytoalbuminal dissociation in the CSF, association with antecedent infections, and clinical course justify Miller Fisher as a subgroup of GBS.

Over 90% of patients with Miller Fisher syndrome have GQ_{1b} IgG autoantibodies in their serum, and titers decrease during clinical improvement.[299, 306] In some cases this autoantibody is produced following *C. jejuni* infection,[307] and there is evidence for GQ_{1b}-like lipopolysaccharides on *C. jejuni* that could be the immunogens for their synthesis.[308, 309]

There is considerable debate whether the lesions in Miller Fisher are entirely peripheral or if the CNS is also affected. Extra-axial enhancement of the ocular motor nerves on MRI suggests that in some cases the external ophthalmoplegia is caused by a peripheral process.[310, 311] GQ_{1b} gangliosides are found in the paranodal regions of the extramedullary portions of the ocular motor nerves,[299] suggesting a basis for attack at this site. However, other MRI studies[312] have showed white matter lesions in the brain stem, implying that the process may be both central and peripheral in some cases. Furthermore, one report demonstrated GQ_{1b} and GT_{1b} antibodies from sera of patients with Miller Fisher syndrome binds to cells in the molecular layer of human cerebellum.[313] This may be the mechanism for the ataxia seen in these patients. Cases with brain stem lesions but without peripheral nerve involvement (ie, normal reflexes and EMG) probably do not fall under the rubric of GBS. Instead these patients might be more appropriately diagnosed with Bickerstaff's brain stem encephalitis (see Chapter 15).[314]

Patients with Miller Fisher syndrome are treated the same as those with AIDP. The prognosis for full recovery after weeks to months is good.[315]

Chronic Inflammatory Demyelinating Polyneuropathy. Patients with chronic inflammatory demyelinating polyneuropathy (CIDP) develop slowly progressive symmetric distal and proximal weakness, sensory loss, and areflexia in patterns similar to those with GBS. Facial weakness may be present in about 15%,[316, 317] and rarely the ocular motor nerves are affected.[318] Progression occurs over several months, and approximately half have a monophasic course while the other half experience relapses and remissions.[317] Rarely there is clinical evidence of CNS demyelination and optic atrophy.[319] Papilledema may occur when the protein level is severely elevated in the CSF (see discussion in Chapter 6).

In about one third of patients there may be a history of an antecedent viral illness or vaccination.[316] Concurrent illnesses such as Hodgkin's disease, benign monoclonal gammopathy, inflammatory bowel disease, chronic hepatitis, diabetes, and HIV, for instance, may also occur. Either demyelinating or axonal features or both on EMG or sural nerve biopsy can confirm the diagnosis. As in GBS, the spinal fluid protein is elevated without pleocytosis. Treatment options include corticosteroids, azathioprine, cyclosporine, plasma-pheresis, and intravenous immunoglobulin.[320–322]

REFERENCES

1. Caplan LR: Ptosis. J Neurol Neurosurg Psychiatry 1974;37:1–7.
2. Wouters RJ, van den Bosch WA, Stijnen T, et al: Conjugacy of eyelid movements in vertical eye saccades. Invest Ophthalmol Vis Sci 1995;36:2686–2694.
3. Schmidtke K, Büttner-Ennever JA: Nervous control of eyelid function. A review of clinical, experimental and pathological data. Brain 1992;227–247.
4. Büttner-Ennever JA, Jenkins C, Armin-Parsa H, et al: A neuroanatomical analysis of lid–eye coordination in ptosis and downgaze paralysis. Clin Neuropathol 1996;15:313–318.
5. Crosby EC, DeJonge BR: Experimental and clinical studies of the central connections and the central relations of the facial nerve. Ann Otol 1963;72: 735–755.
6. Carpenter M: Core Text of Neuro-anatomy, p 151. Baltimore, William & Wilkins, 1985.
7. Martin RG, Grant JL, Peace D: Microsurgical relationship of the anterior inferior cerebellar artery and the facial–vestibulocochlear nerve complex. Neurosurgery 1980;6:483.
8. Malone B, Maisel RH: Anatomy of the facial nerve. Am J Otol 1988;9:494–504.
9. May M, Galetta SL: The facial nerve and related disorders of the face. In: Glaser JS (ed): Neuro-Ophthalmology, 3rd edition, pp 293–326. Philadelphia, Lippincott, Williams & Wilkins, 1999.
10. Miehike A: Surgery of the Facial Nerve, pp 7-21, Philadelphia, W.B. Saunders, 1973.
11. Davis RA, Anson BJ, Puddinger JM, et al: Surgical anatomy of the facial nerve and parotid gland based

upon a study of 350 cervical facial halves. Surg Gynecol Obstet 1956;102:385–412.

12. Blunt MJ: The possible role of vascular changes in the etiology of Bell's palsy. J Laryngol 1956;70:701–713.
13. Moore KL: Clinically Oriented Anatomy, 3rd edition. Baltimore, Williams & Wilkins, 1992.
14. Ragge NK, Hoyt WF: Midbrain myasthenia: fatigable ptosis, 'lid twich' sign, and ophthalmoparesis from a dorsal midbrain glioma. Neurology 1992;42:917–919.
15. Averbuch-Heller L, Poonyathalang A, von Maydell RD, et al: Hering's law for eyelids: still valid. Neurology 1995;45:1781–1783.
16. Eggenberger E, Kayabasi N: Hering's law for eyelids (letter). Neurology 1996;47:1352.
17. Fine EJ, Sentz L, Soria E: The history of the blink reflex. Neurology 1992;42:450–454.
18. Zametkin AJ, Stevens JR, Pittman R: Ontogeny of spontaneous blinking and of habituation of the blink reflex. Ann Neurol 1979;5:453–457.
19. Pullicino PM, Jacobs L, McCall WD, et al: Spontaneous palpebromandibular synkinesia: a localizing clinical sign. Ann Neurol 1994;35:222–228.
20. Liu GT, Ronthal M: Reflex blink to visual threat. J Clin Neuro-ophthalmol 1992;12:47–56.
21. Bracha V, Zhao L, Wunderlich DA, et al: Patients with cerebellar lesions cannot acquire but are able to retained conditioned eyeblink reflexes. Brain 1997; 120:1401–1403.
22. Mac Keith RC: The eye and vision in the newborn infant. In: Gardiner P, Mac Keith RC, Smith V (eds): Aspects of Developmental and Paediatric Ophthalmology. Clinics in Developmental Medicine, pp 9–14. London, Spastics International, 1969.
23. Hill K, Cogan DG, Dodge PR: Ocular signs associated with hydranencephaly. Am J Ophthalmol 1961; 51:267–275.
24. Keane JR: Blinking to sudden illumination. A brain stem reflex present in neocortical death. Arch Neurol 1979;36:52–53.
25. Tavy DLJ, van Woerkom CAM, Bots GTAM, et al: Persistence of the blink reflex to sudden illumination in a comatose patient. Arch Neurol 1984;41:323–324.
26. Oosterhuis HJ: Acquired blepharoptosis. Clin Neurol Neurosurg 1996;98:1–7.
27. Thompson BM, Corbett JJ, Kline LB, et al: Pseudo-Horner's syndrome. Arch Neurol 1982;39:108–111.
28. Sevel D: Ptosis and underaction of the superior rectus muscle. Ophthalmology 1984;91:1080–1085.
29. Clark BJ, Kemp EG, Behan WMH, et al: Abnormal extracellular material in the levator palpebrae superioris complex in congenital ptosis. Arch Ophthalmol 1995;113:1414–1419.
30. Doucet TW, Crawford JS: The quantification, natural course, and surgical results in 57 eyes with Marcus Gunn (jaw-winking) syndrome. Am J Ophthalmol 1981;92:702–707.
31. Pratt SG, Beyer CK, Johnson CC: The Marcus Gunn phenomenon. A review of 71 cases. Ophthalmology 1984;90:27–30.
32. Khwarg SI, Tarbet KJ, Dortzbach DK, et al: Management of moderate-to-sever Marcus Gunn jaw-winking ptosis. Ophthalmology 1999;106:1191–1196.
33. Good EF: Ptosis as the sole manifestation of compression of the oculomotor nerve by an aneurysm of the posterior communicating artery. J Clin Neuro-ophthalmol 1990;10:59–61.
34. Barton JJ, Kardon RH, Slagel D, et al: Bilateral central ptosis in acquired immunodeficiency syndrome. Can J Neurol Sci 1995;22:52–55.
35. Krohel GB, Griffen JF: Cortical blepharoptosis. Am J Ophthalmol 1978;85:632–634.
36. Lepore F: Bilateral cerebral ptosis. Neurology 1987; 37:1043–1046.
37. Averbuch-Heller L, Stahl JS, Remler BF, et al: Bilateral ptosis and upgaze palsy with right hemispheric lesions. Ann Neurol 1996;40:465–468.
38. Goldstein JE, Cogan DG: Apraxia of lid opening. Arch Ophthalmol 1965;73:155–159.
39. Lepore FE, Duvoisin RC: "Apraxia" of eyelid opening: an involuntary levator inhibition. Neurology 1985;35:423–427.
40. Boghen D: Apraxia of lid opening: a review. Neurology 1997;48:1491–1494.
41. Aramideh M, Ongerboer de Visser BW, Koelman JHTM, et al: Motor persistence of orbicularis oculi muscle in eyelid-opening disorders. Neurology 1995;45:897–902.
42. Micheli F, Scorticati C, Diaz S: Lid-opening apraxia (letter). Neurology 1995;45:1788–1789.
43. Dehaene I: Apraxia of eyelid opening in progressive supranuclear palsy (letter). Ann Neurol 1984;15: 115–116.
44. Golbe LI, Davis PA, Lepore FE: Eyelid movement abnormalities in progressive supranuclear palsy. Mov Disord 1989;4:297–302.
45. Johnston JC, Rosenbaum DM, Picone CM, et al: Apraxia of eyelid opening secondary to right hemispheric infarction. Ann Neurol 1989;25:622–624.
46. Verghese J, Milling C, Rosenbaum DM: Ptosis, blepharospasm, and apraxia of eyelid opening secondary to putaminal hemorrhage. Neurology 1999;53:652.
47. Adair JC, Williamson DJG, Heilman KM: Eyelid opening apraxia in focal cortical degeneration (letter). J Neurol Neurosurg Psychiatry 1995;58:508–509.
48. Abe K, Fujimura H, Tatsumi C, et al: Eyelid "apraxia" in patients with motor neuron disease. J Neurol Neurosurg Psychiatry 1995;59:629–632.
49. Krack P, Marion MH: "Apraxia of lid opening," a focal eyelid dystonia: clinical study of 32 patients. Mov Disord 1994;9:610–615.
50. Aramideh M, Ongerboer de Visser BW, Brans JWM, et al: Pretarsal application of botulinum toxin for treatment of blepharospasm. J Neurol Neurosurg Psychiatry 1995;59:309–311.
51. Jankovic J: Pretarsal injection of botulinum toxin for blepharospasm and apraxia of eyelid opening. J Neurol Neurosurg Psychiatry 1996;60:704.
52. Dewey RB, Maraganore DM: Isolated eyelid-opening apraxia: report of a new levodopa-responsive syndrome. Neurology 1994;44:1752–1754.
53. Kersten RC, de Conciliis C, Kulwin DR: Acquired ptosis in the young and middle-aged adult population. Ophthalmology 1995;102:924–928.
54. Stout AU, Borchert M: Etiology of eyelid retraction in children: a retrospective study. J Pediatr Ophthalmol Strab 1993;30:96–99.
55. Bartley GB: The differential diagnosis and classification of eyelid retraction. Ophthalmology 1996;103: 168–176.
56. Olver JM, Fells P: 'Henderson's' relief of eyelid retraction revisited. Eye 1995;9:467–471.
57. Guimarães FC, Cruz AAV: Palpebral fissure height and downgaze in patients with Graves upper eyelid retraction and congenital blepharoptosis. Ophthalmology 1995;102:1218–1222.
58. Keane JR: The pretectal syndrome: 206 patients. Neurology 1990;40:684–690.

59. Galetta SL, Gray LG, Raps EC, et al: Pretectal eyelid retraction and lag. Ann Neurol 1993;33:554–557.
60. Keane JR: Spastic eyelids: failure of levator inhibition in unconscious states. Arch Neurol 1975;32:695–698.
61. Galetta SL, Raps EC, Liu GT, et al: Eyelid lag without eyelid retraction in pretectal disease. J Neuro-ophthalmol 1996;16:96–98.
62. Gaymard B, Lafitte C, Gelot A, et al: Plus-minus lid syndrome. J Neurol Neurosurg Psychiatry 1992;55: 846–848.
63. Lam BL, Nerad JA, Thompson HS: Paroxysmal eyelid retractions. Am J Ophthalmol 1992;114:105–107.
64. Collin JR, Allen L, Castronuovo S: Congenital eyelid retraction. Br J Ophthalmol 1990;74:542–544.
65. May M: The Facial Nerve. New York, Thieme–Stratton, 1986.
66. Keane JR: Bilateral seventh nerve palsy: analysis of 43 cases and review of the literature. Neurology 1994;44:1198–1202.
67. Urban PP, Wicht S, Marx J, et al: Isolated voluntary facial paresis due to pontine ischemia. Neurology 1998;50:1859–1862.
68. Hopf HC, Müller-Forell W, Hopf NJ: Localization of emotional and volitional facial paresis. Neurology 1992;42:1918–1923.
69. Ross RT, Mathiesen R: Volitional and emotional supranuclear facial weakness. N Engl J Med 1998; 338:1515.
70. Lessell S: Supranuclear paralysis of voluntary lid closure. Arch Ophthalmol 1972;88:241.
71. Ross Russell RW: Supranuclear palsy of eyelid closure. Brain 1980;103:71.
72. Henderson JL: The congenital facial diplegia syndrome: clinical features, pathology, and etiology. Brain 1939;62:381–403.
73. Carr MM, Ross DA, Zuker RM: Cranial nerve defects in congenital facial palsy. J Otolaryngol 1997;26: 80–87.
74. Igarashi M, Rose DF, Storgion SA: Moebius syndrome and central respiratory dysfunction. Pediatr Neurol 1997;16:237–240.
75. Tran DB, Wilson MC, Fox CA, et al: Möbius syndrome with oculomotor nerve paralysis but without abducens paralysis. J Neuro-ophthalmol 1998;18: 281–283.
76. Abramson DL, Cohen MM, Mulliken JB: Möbius syndrome: classification and grading system. Plastic Reconstr Surg 1998;102:961–967.
77. Sudarshan A, Goldie WD: The spectrum of congenital facial diplegia (Moebius syndrome). Pediatr Neurol 1985;1:180–184.
78. Kumar D: Moebius syndrome. J Med Genet 1990; 27:122–126.
79. Jaradeh S, D'Cruz O, Howard JF, Jr, et al: Mobius syndrome: electrophysiologic studies in seven cases. Muscle Nerve 1996;19:1148–1153.
80. Lammens M, Moerman P, Fryns JP, et al: Neuropathological findings in Moebius syndrome. Clin Genet 1998;54:136–141.
81. Saint-Martin C, Clapuyt P, Duprez T, et al: Möbius sequence and severe pons hypoplasia: a case report. Pediat Radiol 1998;28:932.
82. Ghabrial R, Versace P, Kourt G, et al: Möbius' syndrome: features and etiology. J Pediatr Ophthalmol Strabismus 1998;35:304–311.
83. D'Cruz OF, Swisher CN, Jaradeh S, et al: Möbius syndrome: evidence for a vascular etiology. J Child Neurol 1993;8:260–265.
84. Kremer H, Kuyt LP, van den Helm B, et al: Localization of a gene for Möbius syndrome to chromosome 3q by linkage analysis in a Dutch family. Hum Mol Genet 1996;5:1367–1371.
85. Pastuszak AL, Schüler L, Speck-Martins CE, et al: Use of misoprostol during pregnancy and Möbius syndrome in infants. N Engl J Med 1998;338:1881–1885.
86. Silverman IE, Liu GT, Volpe NJ, et al: The crossed paralyses: the original brainstem syndromes of Millard–Gubler, Foville, Weber, and Raymond–Cestan. Arch Neurol 1995;52:635–638.
87. Clark JR, Carlson RD, Sasak CT: Facial paralysis in Lyme disease. Laryngoscope 1985;95:1341–1345.
88. Zajicek JP, Scolding NJ, Foster O, et al: Central nervous system sarcoidosis-diagnosis and management. Q J Med 1999;92:103–117.
89. Paolino E, Granieri E, Tola MR: Predisposing factor in Bell's palsy: a case control study. J Neurol 1985;232:363–365.
90. Wolf SM, Wagner JH, Davidson S, et al: Treatment of Bell palsy with prednisone: a prospective, randomized study. Neurology 1978;28:158–161.
91. Peitersen E: The natural history of Bell's palsy. Am J Otol 1982;4:107–111.
92. Adour KK, Wingerd J: Idiopathic facial paralysis (Bell's palsy): factors affecting severity and outcome in 446 patients. Neurology 1974;24:1112–1116.
93. May M, Klein SR, Taylor FH: Idiopathic (Bell's) facial palsy: natural history defies steroid or surgical treatment. Laryngoscope 1985;95:406–409.
94. De Diego JI, Prim MP, De Sarriá MJ, et al: Idiopathic facial paralysis: a randomized, prospective, and controlled study using single-dose prednisone versus acyclovir three times daily. Laryngoscope 1998;108: 573–575.
95. Adour KK, Ruboyianes JM, von Doersten PG, et al: Bell's palsy treatment with acyclovir and prednisone compared with prednisone alone: a double-blind, randomized, controlled trial. Ann Otol Rhinol Laryngol 1996;105:371–378.
96. Hunt JR: On herpetic inflammations of the geniculate ganglion. A new syndrome and its complications. J Nerve Ment Dis 1907;34:73–96.
97. Portenoy RK, Duma C, Foley KM: Acute herpetic and postherpetic neuralgia. Clinical review and current management. Ann Neurol 1986;20:651–664.
98. Gradenigo G: A special syndrome of endocranial otitic complications. Ann Otol Rhinol Laryngol 1904;13:637.
99. Seiff SR, Chang J: Management of ophthalmic complications of facial nerve palsy. Otolaryngol Clin North Am 1992;25:669–690.
100. May M: Gold weight and wire spring implants as alternatives to tarsorrhaphy. Arch Otolaryngol Head Neck Surg 1987;113:656–660.
101. Catalano PJ, Bergstein MJ, Biller HF: Comprehensive management of the eye in facial paralysis. Arch Otolaryngol Head Neck Surg 1995;121:81–86.
102. Seiff SR, Sullivan JH, Freeman LN, et al: Pretarsal fixation of gold weights in facial nerve palsy. Ophthal Plast Reconstr Surg 1989;5:104–109.
103. Kartush JM, Linstrom CJ, McCann PM, et al: Early gold weight eyelid implantation for facial paralysis. Otolaryngol Head Neck Surg 1990;103:1016–1023.
104. Townsend DJ: Eyelid reanimation for the treatment of paralytic lagophthalmos: historical perspectives and current applications of the gold weight implant. Ophthal Plast Reconstr Surg 1992;8:196–201.

105. Dinces EA, Mauriello JA, Jr., Kwartler JA, et al: Complications of gold weight eyelid implants for treatment of fifth and seventh nerve paralysis. Laryngoscope 1997;107:1617–1622.
106. Karson CN, LeWitt PA, Calne DB, et al: Blink rates in parkinsonism. Ann Neurol 1982;12:580–583.
107. Kimura J: Effect of hemispheral lesions on the contralateral blink reflex. A clinical study. Neurology 1974;24:168–174.
108. Berardelli A, Accornero N, Cruccu G, et al: The orbicularis oculi response after hemispheral damage. J Neurol Neurosurg Psychiatry 1983;46:837–843.
109. Castelbuono A, Miller NR: Spontaneous remission in patients with essential blepharospasm and Meige syndrome. Am J Ophthalmol 1998;126:432–435.
110. Hasan S, Baker RS, Sun WS, et al: The role of blink adaptation in the pathophysiology of benign essential blepharospasm. Arch Ophthalmol 1997;115:631–636.
111. Baker RS, Sun WS, Hasan SA, et al: Maladaptive neural compensatory mechanisms in Bell's palsy-induced blepharospasm. Neurology 1997;49:223–229.
112. Aramideh M, Ongerboer de Visser BW, Holstege G, et al: Blepharospasm in association with a lower pontine lesion. Neurology 1996;46:476–478.
113. Ishikawa M, Ohira T, Namiki J, et al: Electrophysiological investigation of hemifancial spasm after microvascular decompression: F waves of the facial muscles, blink reflexes, and abnormal muscle response. J Neurosurg 1997;86:654–661.
114. Adler CH, Zimmerman RA, Savino PJ, et al: Hemifacial spasm: evaluation by magnetic resonance imaging and magnetic resonance tomographic angiography. Ann Neurol 1992;32:502–506.
115. Osako M, Keltner JL: Botulinum A toxin (Oculinum) in ophthalmology. Surv Ophthalmol 1991;36:28–46.
116. Price J, O'Day J: Efficacy and side effects of botulinum toxin treatment for blepharospasm and hemifacial spasm. Aust NZ J Ophthalmol 1994;22:255–260.
117. Price J, Farish S, Taylor H, et al: Blepharospasm and hemifacial spasm. Randomized trial to determine the most appropriate location for botulinum toxin injections. Ophthalmology 1997;104:865–868.
118. Holds JB, Alderson K, Fogg SG, et al: Motor nerve sprouting in human orbicularis muscle after botulinum A injection. Invest Ophthalmol Vis Sci 1990; 31:964–967.
119. Alderson K, Holds JB, Anderson RL: Botulinum-induced alteration of nerve-muscle interactions in the human orbicularis oculi following treatment for blepharospasm. Neurology 1991;41:1800–1805.
120. Jankovic J, Schwartz KS: Longitudinal experience with botulinum toxin injections for treatment of blepharospasm and cervical dystonia. Neurology 1993;43:834–836.
121. Ainsworth JR, Kraft SP: Long-term changes in duration of relief with botulinum toxin treatment of essential blepharospasm and hemifacial spasm. Ophthalmology 1995;102:2036–2040.
122. Elston JS: Long-term results of treatment of idiopathic blepharospasm with botulinum toxin injections. Br J Ophthalmol 1987;71:664–668.
123. Engstrom PF, Arnoult JB, Mazow ML, et al: Effectiveness of botulinum toxin therapy for essential blepharospasm. Ophthalmology 1987;94:971–975.
124. Dutton JJ, Buckley EG: Long-term results and complications of botulinum A toxin in the treatment of blepharospasm. Ophthalmology 1988;95:1529–1534.
125. Kennedy RH, Bartley GB, Flanagan JC, et al: Treatment of blepharospasm with botulinum toxin. Mayo Clin Proc 1989;64:1085–1090.
126. Mauriello JA, Jr., Dhillon S, Leone T, et al: Treatment selections of 239 patients with blepharospasm and Meige syndrome over 11 years. Br J Ophthalmol 1996;80:1073–1076.
127. Anderson RL, Patel BC, Holds JB: Blepharospasm: past, present, and future. Ophthal Plast Reconstr Surg 1998;14:305–317.
128. Kalra HK, Magoon EH: Side effects of the use of botulinum toxin for treatment of benign essential blepharospasm and hemifacial spasm. Ophthalmic Surg 1990;21:335–338.
129. Wutthiphan S, Kowal L, O'Day J, et al: Diplopia following subcutaneous injections of botulinum A toxin for facial spasms. J Pediatr Ophthalmol Strabismus 1997;34:229–234.
130. Siatkowski RM, Tyutyunikov A, Biglan AW, et al: Serum antibody production to botulinum A toxin. Ophthalmology 1993;100:1861–1866.
131. Evidente VGH, Adler CH: Hemifacial spasm and other craniofacial movement disorders. Mayo Clin Proc 1998;73:67–71.
132. Wirtschafter JD, McLoon LK: Long-term efficacy of local doxorubicin chemomyectomy in patients with blepharospasm and hemifacial spasm. Ophthalmology 1998;105:342–346.
133. Baker RS, Stava MW, Nelson KR, et al: Aberrant reinnervation of facial musculature in a subhuman primate: a correlative analysis of eyelid kinematics, muscle synkinesis, and motoneuron localization. Neurology 1994;44:2165–2173.
134. Jankovic J: The neurology of tics. In: Marsden CD, Fahn S (eds): Movement Disorders 2, pps 383–405. London, Butterworths, 1987.
135. Jankovic J, Stone L: Dystonic tics in patients with Tourette's syndrome. Mov Disord 1991;6:248–252.
136. Andermann F, Cosgrove JBR, Lloyd-Smith DL, et al: Facial myokymia in multiple sclerosis. Brain 1961; 84:31–44.
137. Jacobs L, Kaba S, Pullicino P: The lesion causing continuous facial myokymia in multiple sclerosis. Arch Neurol 1994;51:1115–1119.
138. Màrit-Fabregas J, Montero J, López-Villegas D, et al: Post-irradiation neuromyotonia in bilateral facial and trigeminal nerve distribution. Neurology 1997;48: 1107–1109.
139. Mauriello JA, Carbonaro P, Dhillon S, et al: Drug-associated facial dyskinesias—a study of 238 patients. J Clin Neuro-ophthalmol 1998;18:153–157.
140. Brodsky MC, Boop FA: Lid nystagmus as a sign of intrinsic midbrain disease. J Neuro-ophthalmol 1995;5:236–240.
141. Sanders MD, Hoyt WF, Daroff RB: Lid nystagmus evoked by ocular convergence: an ocular electromyographic study. J Neurol Neurosurg Psychiatry 1968; 31:368–371.
142. Grob D, Arsura EL, Brunner G, et al: The course of myasthenia gravis and therapies affecting outcome. Ann NY Acad Sci 1987;505:472–499.
143. Bever C, Aquino AV, Penn AS, et al: Prognosis of ocular myasthenia gravis. Ann Neurol 1983;14: 516–519.
144. Oosterhuis HJGH: The natural course of myasthenia gravis: a long term follow up study. J Neurol Neurosurg Psychiatry 1989;52:1121–1127.
145. Drachman DB: Myasthenia gravis. N Engl J Med 1994;330:1797–1810.

146. Donaldson DH, Ansher M, Horan S, et al: The relationship of age to outcome in myasthenia gravis. Neurology 1990;40:786–790.
147. Drachman DB, Adams RN, Josifek LF, et al: Functional activities of autoantibodies to acetylcholine receptors and the clinical severity of myasthenia gravis. N Engl J Med 1982;307:769–795.
148. Seybold ME: Myasthenia gravis: diagnostic and therapeutic perspectives in the 1990's. The Neurologist 1995;1:345–360.
149. Wang Z-Y, Okita DK, Howard J, et al: Th1 epitope repertoire on the α subunit of human muscle acetylcholine receptor in myasthenia gravis. Neurology 1997;48:1643–1653.
150. Liu GT, Bienfang DC: Penicillamine-induced ocular myasthenia gravis in rheumatoid arthritis. J Clin Neuro-ophthalmol 1990;10:201–205.
151. Argov Z, Mastaglia FL: Disorders of neuromuscular transmission caused by drugs. N Engl J Med 1979; 301:409–413.
152. Barrons RW: Drug-induced neuromuscular blockade and myasthenia gravis. Pharmacotherapy 1997;17: 1220–1232.
153. Wittbrodt ET: Drugs and myasthenia gravis. An update. Arch Intern Med 1997;157:399–408.
154. Kaminski HJ, Maas E, Spiegel P, et al: Why are eye muscles frequently involved in myasthenia gravis? Neurology 1990;40:1663–1669.
155. Kaminski HJ, Ruff RL: Ocular muscle involvement by myasthenia gravis (editorial). Ann Neurol 1997; 41:419–420.
156. MacLennan C, Beeson D, Buijs A-M, et al: Acetylcholine receptor expression in human extraocular muscles and their susceptibility to myasthenia gravis. Ann Neurol 1997;41:423–431.
157. Newsom-Davis J: Myasthenia gravis and the Miller-Fisher variant of Guillain-Barré syndrome. Curr Opin Neurol 1997;10:18–21.
158. Moorthy G, Behrens MM, Drachman DB, et al: Ocular pseudomyasthenia or ocular myasthenia "plus": a warning to clinicians. Neurology 1989;39:1150–1154.
159. Schmidt D: Signs in ocular myasthenia and pseudomyasthenia. Differential diagnostic criteria. A clinical review. Neuro-ophthalmology 1995;15:21–58.
160. Nunery WR, Cepela M: Levator function in the evaluation and management of blepharoptosis. Ophthalmol Clin North Am 1991;4:1–16.
161. Cogan DG: Myasthenia gravis; a review of the disease and a description of lid twitch as a characteristic sign. Arch Ophthalmol 1965;74:217–221.
162. Weinberg DA, Lesser RL, Vollmer TL: Ocular myasthenia: a protean disorder. Surv Ophthalmol 1994; 39:169–210.
163. Massey JM: Acquired myasthenia gravis. Neurol Clin 1997;15:577–595.
164. Seybold ME: The office tensilon test for ocular myasthenia. Arch Neurol 1986;43:842–843.
165. Kelly JJ, Daube J, Lennon VA: The laboratory diagnosis of mild myasthenia gravis. Ann Neurol 1982; 12:238–242.
166. Milone M, Monarco ML, Evoli A, et al: Ocular myasthenia: diagnostic value of single fiber EMG in the orbicularis oculi muscle. J Neurol Neurosurg Psychiatry 1993;56:720–721.
167. Daroff RB: The office Tensilon test for myasthenia gravis. Arch Neurol 1986;43:843–844.
168. Glaser JS, Bachynski B: Infranuclear disorders of eye movement. In: Glaser JS (ed): Neuro-Ophthalmology, pp 396–397. Philadelphia, JB Lippincott, 1990.
169. Miller NR, Morris JE, Maguire M: Combined use of neostigmine and ocular motility measurements in the diagnosis of myasthenia. Arch Ophthalmol 1982; 100:761–763.
170. Hyder DJ, Liu GT: Myasthenia gravis. In: Schwartz MW (ed): CHOP's 5 Minute Pediatric Consult, pp 508–509. Baltimore, Williams & Wilkins, 1997.
171. Sethi K, Rivner MH, Swift TR: Ice pack test for myasthenia gravis. Neurology 1987;37:1383–1385.
172. Odel JG, Winterkorn JMS, Behrens MM: The sleep test for myasthenia gravis: a safe alternative to tensilon. J Clin Neuro-ophthalmol 1991;11:228–292.
173. Golnik KC, Pena R, Lee AG, et al: An ice test for the diagnosis of myasthenia gravis. Ophthalmology 1999;106:1282–1286.
174. Lindstrom JM, Seybold ME, Lennon VA, et al: Antibody to acetylcholine receptor in myasthenia gravis. Prevalence, clinical correlates, and diagnostic value. Neurology 1976;26:1054–1059.
175. Soliven BC, Lange DT, Penn AS: Seronegative myasthenia gravis. Neurology 1988;38:514.
176. Vincent A, Newsom DJ: Anti-acetylcholine receptor antibodies. J Neurol Neurosurg Psychiatry 1980; 43:590–600.
177. Lange DJ: Electrophysiologic testing of neuromuscular transmission. Neurology 1997;48(Suppl 5): S18–S22.
178. Herrmann C, Lindstrom JM, Keesey JC, et al: Myasthenia gravis—current concepts. West J Med 1985; 142:797–809.
179. Krendel DA, Sanders DB, Massey JM: Single fiber electromyography in chronic progressive external ophthalmoplegia. Muscle Nerve 1987;10:299–302.
180. Uyama J, Mimura O, Ikeda N, et al: Single fiber electromyography of extraocular muscles in myasthenia gravis. Neuro-ophthalmology 1993;13:253–261.
181. Sanders DB, Scoppetta C: The treatment of patients with myasthenia gravis. Neurol Clin 1994;12: 343–368.
182. Rowland LP: Controversies about the treatment of myasthenia gravis. J Neurol Neurosurg Psychiatry 1980;43:644–659.
183. Lewis RA, Selwa JF, Lisak RP: Myasthenia gravis: immunological mechanisms and immunotherapy. Ann Neurol 1995;37:S51–62.
184. Kupersmith MJ, Moster M, Bhuiyan S, et al: Beneficial effects of corticosteroids on ocular myasthenia gravis. Arch Neurol 1996;53:802–804.
185. Miano MA, Bosley TM, Heiman-Patterson TD, et al: Factors influencing outcome of prednisone dose reduction in myasthenia gravis. Neurology 1991; 41:919–921.
186. Palace J, Newsom-Davis J, Lecky B, et al: A randomized double-blind trial of prednisolone alone or with azathioprine in myasthenia gravis. Neurology 1998;50:1778–1783.
187. Tindall RSA, Rollins JA, Phillips JT, et al: Preliminary results of a double-blind, randomized, placebo-controlled trial of cyclosporine in myasthenia gravis. N Engl J Med 1987;316:719–724.
188. Sommer N, Sigg B, Melms A, et al: Ocular myasthenia gravis: response to long term immunosuppressive treatment. J Neurol Neurosurg Psychiatry 1997; 62:156–162.
189. Gajdos P, Chevret S, Clair B, et al: Clinical trial of plasma exchange and high-dose intravenous immunoglobulin in myasthenia gravis. Ann Neurol 1997;41:789–796.

190. Howard JF: Intravenous immunoglobulin for the treatment of acquired myasthenia gravis. Neurology 1998;51 (Suppl 5):S30-S36.
191. Buckingham JM, Howard FM, Bernatz PE, et al: The value of thymectomy in myasthenia gravis: a computer-assisted matched study. Ann Surg 1976; 184:453–458.
192. Levinson AI, Wheatley LM: The thymus and the pathogenesis of myasthenia gravis. Clin Immunol Immunopathol 1996;78:1–5.
193. Mulder DG: Extended transsternal thymectomy. Chest Surg Clin North Am 1996;6:95–105.
194. Jaretzki A: Thymectomy for myasthenia gravis: analysis of the controversies regarding technique and results. Neurology 1997;48 (Suppl 5):S52-S63.
195. Ferguson MK: Transcervical thymectomy. Chest Surg Clin North Am 1996;6:105–115.
196. Mulder DG, Herrmann C, Keesey JC, et al: Thymectomy for myasthenia gravis. Am J Surg 1983;146: 61–66.
197. Nieto IP: Prognostic factors for myasthenia gravis treated by thymectomy. Ann Thorac Surg 1999; 67:1568–1571.
198. Schumm F, Wiethölter H, Fateh-Moghadam A, et al: Thymectomy in myasthenia with pure ocular symptoms. J Neurol Neurosurg Psychiatry 1985;48: 332–337.
199. Lanska DJ: Indications for thymectomy in myasthenia gravis. Neurology 1990;40:1828–1829.
200. Tsuchida M: Efficacy and safety of extended thymectomy for elderly patients with myasthenia gravis. Ann Thorac Surg 1999;67:1563–1567.
201. Bril V, Kojic J, Dhanani A: The long-term clnical outcome of myasthenia gravis in patients with thymoma. Neurology 1998;51:1198–1200.
202. Fenichel GM: Myasthenia gravis. Pediatr Ann 1989; 18:432–438.
203. Anlar B, Ozdirim E, Renda Y, et al: Myasthenia gravis in childhood. Acta Paediatr 1996;85:838–842.
204. Andrews PI, Massey JM, Howard JF, et al: Race, sex, and puberty influence onset, severity, and outcome in juvenile myasthenia gravis. Neurology 1994; 44:1208–1214.
205. Schmidt D: Prognosis of ocular myasthenia in childhood. Neuro-ophthalmology 1983;3:117–124.
206. Afifi AK, Bell WE: Tests for juvenile myasthenia gravis: comparative diagnostic yield and prediction of outcome. J Child Neurol 1993;8:403–411.
207. Andrews PI, Massey JM, Sanders DB: Acetylcholine receptor antibodies in juvenile myasthenia gravis. Neurology 1993;43:977–982.
208. Seybold ME, Howard FM, Duane DD, et al: Thymectomy in juvenile myasthenia gravis. Arch Neurol 1971;25:385–392.
209. Ryniewicz B, Badurska B: Follow-up study of myasthenic children after thymectomy. J Neurol 1977; 217:133–138.
210. Rodriguez M, Gomez MR, Howard FM, et al: Myasthenia gravis in children: long-term follow-up. Ann Neurol 1983;13:504–510.
211. Adams C, Theodorescu D, Murphy EG, et al: Thymectomy in juvenile myasthenia gravis. J Child Neurol 1990;5:215–218.
212. Sarnat HB, McGarry JD, Lewis JE: Effective treatment of infantile myasthenia gravis by combine prednisone and thymectomy. Neurology 1977;27:550–553.
213. Herrmann DN, Carney PR, Wald JJ: Juvenile myasthenia gravis: treatment with immune globulin and thymectomy. Pediatr Neurol 1998;18:63–66.
214. Vincent A, Newland C, Croxen R, et al: Genes at the junction—candidates for congenital myasthenic syndromes. Trends Neurosci 1997;20:15–22.
215. Engel AG: Congenital myasthenic syndromes. J Child Neurol 1988;3:233–246.
216. Engel AG, Uchitel OD, Walls TJ, et al: Newly recognized congenital myasthenic syndrome associated with high conductance and fast closure of the acetylcholine receptor channel. Ann Neurol 1993;34:38–47.
217. Engel AG, Ohno K, Milone M, et al: Congenital myasthenic syndromes caused by mutations in acetylcholine receptor genes. Neurology 1997;48 (Suppl 5): S28-S35.
218. Engel AG, Ohno K, Wang H-L, et al: Molecular basis of congenital myasthenic syndromes: mutations in the acetylcholine receptor. Neuroscientist 1998;4: 185–194.
219. Engel AG, Ohno K, Sine SM: Congenital myasthenic syndromes. Recent advances. Arch Neurol 1999; 56:163–167.
220. Sieb JP, Dörfler P, Tzartos S, et al: Congenital myasthenic syndromes in two kinships with end-plate acetylcholine receptor and utrophin deficiency. Neurology 1998;50:54–61.
221. Beeson D, Palace J, Vincent A: Congenital myasthenic syndromes. Curr Opin Neurol 1997;10:402–407.
222. Satoyoshi E, Kowa H, Fukunaga N: Subacute cerebellar degeneration and Eaton-Lambert syndrome with bronchogenic carcinoma. A case report. Neurology 1973;23:764–768.
223. Blumenfeld AM, Recht LD, Chad DA, et al: Coexistence of Lambert–Eaton myasthenic syndrome and subacute cerebellar degeneration: differential effects of treatment. Neurology 1991;41:1682–1685.
224. Mason WP, Graus F, Lang B, et al: Small-cell lung cancer, paraneoplasic cerebellar degeneration and the Lambert–Eaton myasthenic syndrome. Brain 1997;120:1279–1300.
225. Fettel MR, Shin HS, Penn AS, et al: Combined Eaton–Lambert syndrome and myasthenia gravis (abstract). Neurology 1978;398.
226. O'Neill JH, Murray NMF, Newsom-Davis J: The Lambert–Eaton myasthenic syndrome. A review of 50 cases. Brain 1988;111:577–596.
227. Ueno S, Hara Y: Lambert–Eaton myasthenic syndrome without anti-calcium channel antibody: adverse effect of calcium antagonist diltiazem. J Neurol Neurosurg Psychiatry 1992;55:409–410.
228. Lennon VA, Kryzer TJ, Griesmann GE, et al: Calcium-channel antibodies in the Lambert-Eaton syndrome and other paraneoplastic syndromes. N Engl J Med 1995;332:1467–1474.
229. Motomura M, Johnston I, Lang B, et al: An improved diagnostic assay for Lambert-Eaton myasthenic syndrome. J Neurol Neurosurg Psychiatry 1995;58: 85–87.
230. Dalmau JO, Posner JB: Paraneoplastic syndromes. Arch Neurol 1999;56:405–408.
231. McEvoy KM: Diagnosis and treatment of Lambert–Eaton myasthenic syndrome. Neurol Clin North Am 1994;12:387–399.
232. Breen LA, Gutmann L, Brick JF, et al: Paradoxical lid elevation with sustained upgaze: a sign of Lambert–Eaton syndrome. Muscle Nerve 1991;14:863–866.
233. Brazis PW: Enhanced ptosis in Lambert–Eaton myasthenic syndrome. J Neuro-ophthalmol 1997;17: 202–203.
234. Cruciger MP, Brown B, Denys EH, et al: Clinical and subclinical oculomotor findings in the Lambert–

Eaton syndrome. J Clin Neuro-ophthalmol 1983; 33:1157–1163.

235. Dell'Osso LF, Ayyar DR, Daroff RB, et al: Edrophonium test in Lambert–Eaton syndrome: quantitative oculography. Neurology 1983;33:1157–1163.
236. Sanders DB: Lambert–Eaton myasthenic syndrome: clinical diagnosis, immune-mediated mechanisms, and update on therapies. Ann Neurol 1995; 37(S1):S63-S73.
237. Case records of the Massachusetts General Hospital: Case 32-1994. N Engl J Med 1994;331:528–535.
238. Chalk CH, Murray NMF, Newsom-Davis J, et al: Response of the Lambert–Eaton myasthenic syndrome to treatment of associated small-cell lung carcinoma. Neurology 1990;40:1552–1556.
239. McEvoy KM, Windebank AJ, Daube JR, et al: 3,4-Diaminopyridine in the treatment of Lambert–Eaton-myasthenic syndrome. N Engl J Med 1989;321:1567–1571.
240. Bird SJ: Clinical and electrophysiologic improvement in Lambert–Eaton syndrome with intravenous immunoglobulin therapy. Neurology 1992;42:1422–1423.
241. Rich MM, Teener JW, Bird SJ: Treatment of Lambert–Eaton syndrome with intravenous immunoglobulin. Muscle Nerve 1997;20:614–615.
242. Grisold W, Drlicek M, Liszka-Setinek U, et al: Antitumour therapy in paraneoplastic neurological disease. Clin Neurol Neurosurg 1995;97:106–111.
243. Case records of the Massachusetts General Hospital: Case 22-1997. N Engl J Med 1997;337:184–190.
244. Miller NR, Moses H: Ocular involvement in wound botulism. Arch Ophthalmol 1977;95:1788–1789.
245. Terranova W, Palumbo JN, Breman JG: Ocular findings in botulism type B. JAMA 1979;241:475–477.
246. Hedges TR, Jones A, Stark L, et al: Botulin ophthalmoplegia. Clinical and oculographic observations. Arch Ophthalmol 1983;101:211–213.
247. Zeviani M, Moraes CT, DiMauro S, et al: Deletions of mitochondrial DNA in Kearns–Sayre syndrome. Neurology 1988;38:1339–1346.
248. Moraes CT, DiMauro S, Zeviani M, et al: Mitochondrial DNA deletions in progressive external ophthalmoplegia and Kearns–Sayre syndrome. N Engl J Med 1989;30:1293–1299.
249. Newman NJ: Mitochondrial disease and the eye. Ophthalmol Clin North Am 1992;5:405–424.
250. Moslemi A-R, Melberg A, Holme E, et al: Clonal expansion of mitochondrial DNA with multiple deletions in autosomal dominant progressive external ophthalmoplegia. Ann Neurol 1996;40:707–713.
251. Suomalainen A, Majander A, Wallin M, et al: Autosomal dominant progressive external ophthalmoplegia with multiple deletions of mtDNA. Clinical, biochemical, and molecular genetic features of the 10q-linked disease. Neurology 1997;48:1244–1253.
252. Moslemi A-R, Melberg A, Holme E, et al: Autosomal dominant progressive external ophthalmoplegia. Distribution of multiple mitochondrial DNA deletions. Neurology 1999;53:79–84.
253. Chang TS, Johns DR, Walker D, et al: Ocular clinicopathologic study of the mitochondrial encephalomyopathy overlap syndromes. Arch Ophthalmol 1993; 111:1254–1262.
254. Pellock JM, Behrens M, Lewis L, et al: Kearns–Sayre syndrome and hypoparathyroidism. Ann Neurol 1978;3:455–458.
255. Case records of the Massachusetts General Hospital: Case 34-1987. N Engl J Med 1987;317:493–501.
256. Mitsumoto H, Aprille JR, Wray SH, et al: Chronic progressive external ophthalmoplegia (CPEO): clinical, morphologic, and biochemical studies. Neurology 1983;33:452–461.
257. DiMauro S, Bonilla E, Lombes A, et al: Mitochondrial encephalomyopathies. Neurol Clin 1990;8:483–506.
258. Leutner C, Layer G, Zierz S, et al: Cerebral MR in ophthalmoplegia plus. AJNR Am J Neuroradiol 1994;15:681–687.
259. Kamata Y, Mashima Y, Yokoyama M, et al: Patient with Kearns–Sayre syndrome exhibiting abnormal magnetic resonance imaging of the brain. J Neuro-ophthalmol 1998;18:284–288.
260. Matthews PM, Andermann F, Silver K, et al: Proton MR spectroscopic differences in regional brain metabolic abnormalities in mitochondrial encephalomyopathies. Neurology 1993;43:2484–2490.
261. Kuwabara T, Watanabe H, Tanaka K, et al: Mitochondrial encephalomyopathy: elevated visual cortex lactate unresponsive to photic stimulation—a localized ^{1}H-MRS study. Neurology 1994;44:557–559.
262. Sorkin JA, Shoffner JM, Grossniklaus HE, et al: Strabismus and mitochondrial defects in chronic progressive external ophthalmoplegia. Am J Ophthalmol 1997;123:235–242.
263. Faber J, Fich A, Steinberg A, et al: Familial intestinal pseudoobstruction dominated by a progressive neurologic disease at a young age. Gastroenterology 1987;92:786–790.
264. Cervera R, Bruix J, Bayes A, et al: Chronic intestinal pseudoobstruction and ophthalmoplegia in a patient with mitochondrial myopathy. Gut 1988;29:544–547.
265. Case records of the Massachusetts General Hospital: Case 12-1990. N Engl J Med 1990;322:829–841.
266. Threlkeld AB, Miller NR, Golnik KC, et al: Ophthalmic involvement in myo-neuro-gastrointestinal encephalopathy syndrome. Am J Ophthalmol 1992; 114:322–328.
267. Johns DR, Threlkeld AB, Miller NR, et al: Multiple mitochondrial DNA deletions in myo-neuro-gastrointestinal encephalopathy syndrome (letter). Am J Ophthalmol 1993;115:108–109.
268. Hirano M, Silvestri G, Blacke DM, et al: Mitochondrial neurogastrointestinal encephalomyopathy (MNGIE): clinical, biochemical, and genetic features of an autosomal recessive mitochondrial disorder. Neurology 1994;44:721–727.
269. Papadimitriou A, Comi GP, Hadjigeorgiou GM, et al: Partial depletion and multiple deletions of muscle mtDNA in familial MNGIE syndrome. Neurology 1998;51:1086–1092.
270. Simon LT, Horoupian DS, Dorman LJ, et al: Polyneuropathy, ophthalmoplegia, leukoencephalopathy, and intestinal pseudo-obstruction: POLIP syndrome. Ann Neurol 1990;28:349–360.
271. Ptacek LJ, Johnson KJ, Griggs RC: Genetics and physiology of the myotonic muscle disorders. N Engl J Med 1993;328:482–489.
272. Dyken PR, Harper PS: Congenital dystrophia myotonica. Neurology 1973;23:465–473.
273. Verhagen WIM, ter Bruggen JP, Huygen PL: Oculomotor, auditory, and vestibular responses in myotonic dystrophy. Arch Neurol 1992;49:954–960.
274. Anastasopoulos D, Kimmig H, Mergner T, et al: Abnormalities of ocular motility in myotonic dystrophy. Brain 1996;119:1923–1932.
275. Verhagen WI, Huygen PL: Abnormalities of ocular motility in myotonic dystrophy [letter]. Brain 1997;120:1907–1909.

276. Versino M, Romani A, Bergamaschi R, et al: Eye movement abnormalities in myotonic dystrophy. Electroenceph Clin Neurophysiol 1998;109:184–190.
277. Osanai R, Kinoshita M, Hirose K: Saccadic slowing in myotonic dystrophy and CTG repeat expansion. J Neurol 1998;245:674–680.
278. Winchester CL, Ferrier RK, Sermoni A, et al: Characterization of the expression of DMPK and SIX5 in the human eye and implications for pathogenesis in myotonic dystrophy. Hum Mol Genet 1999;8: 481–492.
279. Blumen SC, Brais B, Korczyn AD, et al: Homozygotes for oculopharyngeal muscular dystrophy have a severe form of the disease. Ann Neurol 1999; 46:115–118.
280. Hardiman O, Halperin JJ, Farrell MA, et al: Neuropathic findings in oculopharyngeal muscular dystrophy. A report of seven cases and a review of the literature. Arch Neurol 1993;50:481–488.
281. Ropper AH: The Guillain–Barré syndrome. N Engl J Med 1992;326:1130–1136.
282. Asbury AK, Arnason BG, Adams RD: The inflammatory lesion in idiopathic polyneuritis. Medicine 1969;48:173–215.
283. Prineas JW: Pathology of the Guillain–Barré syndrome. Ann Neurol 1981;9(suppl):6–19.
284. Feasby TE, Gilbert JJ, Brown WF, et al: An acute axonal form of Guillain-Barré polyneuropathy. Brain 1986;109:1115–1126.
285. Griffin JW, Li CY, Ho TW, et al: Guillain–Barré syndrome in northern China: the spectrum of neuropathological changes in clinically defined cases. Brain 1995;118:577–595.
286. Asbury AK: Guillain–Barré syndrome. In: Stern MB, Brown MJ, Galetta SL, Asbury AK (eds): Penn Neurology 2000: Management of Common Neurological Problems, pp 99–114, Irvington, NY, Alpha Medica Press, 2000.
287. Maier I, Schmidbauer M, Pfausler B, et al: Central nervous system pathology in patients with the Guillain–Barré syndrome. Brain 1997;120:451–464.
288. Sheikh KA, Nachamkin I, Ho TW, et al: *Campylobacter jejuni* lipopolysaccharides in Guillain–Barré syndrome. Molecular mimicry and host susceptibility. Neurology 1998;51:371–378.
289. Hadden RDM, Cornblath DR, Hughes RAC, et al: Electrophysiological classification of Guillain–Barré syndrome: clinical associations and outcome. Ann Neurol 1998;44:780–788.
290. Rees JH, Soudain SE, Gregson NA, et al: *Campylobacter jejuni* infection in Guillain–Barré syndrome. N Engl J Med 1995;333:1374–1379.
291. Jacobs BC, Rothbarth PH, van der Meché FGA, et al: The spectrum of antecedent infections in Guillain–Barré syndrome. A case-control study. Neurology 1998;51:1110–1115.
292. Case records of the Massachusetts General Hospital: Case 39-1990. N Engl J Med 1990;323:895–908.
293. Asbury AK: Diagnostic considerations in Guillain–Barré syndrome. Ann Neurol 1981;9(suppl):1–5.
294. Ropper AH, Wijdicks EFM, Truax BT: Clinical features of Guillain–Barré syndrome. In: Guillain–Barré Syndrome, pp 56-152, Philadelphia, FA Davis, 1991.
295. Nadkarni N, Lisak RP: Guillain–Barré syndrome (GBS) with bilateral optic neuritis and central white matter disease. Neurology 1993;43:842–843.
296. Ropper AH, Wijdicks EFM: Blood pressure fluctuations in the dysautonomia of Guillain–Barré syndrome. Arch Neurol 1990;47:706–708.
297. Ropper AH, Wijdicks EFM, Shahani BT: Electrodiagnostic abnormalities in 113 consecutive patients with Guillain–Barré syndrome. Arch Neurol 1990; 47:881–887.
298. Case records of the Massachusetts General Hospital: Case 39-1999. N Engl J Med 1999;341:1996–2003.
299. Chiba A, Kusunoki S, Obata H, et al: Serum anti-GQ_{1b} antibody is associated with ophthalmoplegia in Miller Fisher syndrome and Guillain–Barré syndrome. Clinical and immunohistochemical studies. Neurology 1993;43:1911–1917.
300. Asbury AK, Cornblath DR: Assessment of current diagnostic criteria for Guillain–Barré syndrome. Ann Neurol 1990;27(suppl):S21-S24.
301. The Guillain–Barré Syndrome Study Group: Plasmapheresis and acute Guillain–Barré syndrome. Neurology 1985;35:1096–1104.
302. van der Meché FGA, Schmitz PIM, The Dutch Guillain–Barré Study Group: A randomized trial comparing intravenous immune globulin and plasma exchange in Guillain–Barré syndrome. N Engl J Med 1992;326:1123–1129.
303. Plasma exchange/Sandoglobulin Guillain–Barré syndrome trial group: Randomised trial of plasma exchange, intravenous immunoglobulin, and combined treatments in Guillain–Barré syndrome. Lancet 1997;349:225–230.
304. The Italian Guillain–Barré study group: The prognosis and main prognostic indicators of Guillain–Barré syndrome. A multicentre prospective study of 297 patients. Brain 1996;119:2053–2061.
305. Fisher M: An unusual variant of acute idiopathic polyneuritis (syndrome of ophthalmoplegia, ataxia and areflexia). N Engl J Med 1956;255:57–65.
306. Yuki N, Sato S, Tsuji S, et al: Frequent presence of anti-GQ_{1b} antibody in Fisher's syndrome. Neurology 1993;43:414–417.
307. Ohtsuka K, Nakamura Y, Hashimoto M, et al: Fisher syndrome associated with IgG antiGQ_{1b} antibody following infection by a specific serotype of *Campylobacter jejuni.* Ophthalmology 1998;105:1281–1285.
308. Yuki N, Taki T, Takahashi M, et al: Molecular mimicry between GQ_{1b} ganglioside and lipopolysaccharides of *Campylobacter jejuni* isolated from patients with Fisher's syndrome. Ann Neurol 1994;36: 791–793.
309. Jacobs BC, Endtz HPH, van der Meche FGA, et al: Serum anti-G_{Q1b} IgG antibodies recognize surface epitopes on *Campylobacter jejuni* isolated from patients with Miller Fisher syndrome. Ann Neurol 1995;37:260–264.
310. Nagaoka U, Kato T, Kurita K, et al: Cranial nerve enhancement on three-dimensional MRI in Miller Fisher syndrome. Neurology 1996;47:1601–1602.
311. Tanaka H, Yuki N, Hirata K: Trochlear nerve enhancement on three-dimensional magnetic resonance imaging in Fisher syndrome. Am J Ophthalmol 1998;126:322–324.
312. Fargus A, Roig M, Vazquez E, et al: Brainstem involvement in a child with ophthalmoplegia, ataxia, areflexia syndrome. Pediatr Neurol 1998;18:73–75.
313. Kornberg AJ, Pestronk A, Blume GM, et al: Selective staining of the cerebellar molecular layer by serum IgG in Miller-Fisher and related syndromes. Neurology 1996;47:1317–1320.
314. Al-din AN, Anderson M, Bickerstaff ER, et al: Brainstem encephalitis and the syndrome of Miller Fisher. A clinical study. Brain 1982;105:481–495.

315. Berlit P, Rakicky J: The Miller Fisher syndrome. Review of the literature. J Clin Neuro-ophthalmol 1992;12:57–63.
316. McCombe PA, Pollard JD, McLeod JG: Chronic inflammatory demyelinating polyradiculoneuropathy. Brain 1987;110:1617–1630.
317. Barohn RJ, Kissel JT, Warmolts JR, et al: Chronic inflammatory demyelinating polyradiculopathy. Clinical characteristics, course, and recommendations for diagnostic criteria. Arch Neurol 1989;46: 878–884.
318. Arroyo JG, Horton JC: Acute, painful, pupil-sparing third nerve palsy in chronic inflammatory demyelinating polyneuropathy. Neurology 1995;45:846–847.
319. Lee AG, Galetta SL, Lepore FE, et al: Optic atrophy and chronic acquired polyneuropathy. J Neuro-ophthalmol 1999;19:67–69.
320. Faed JM, Day B, Pollock M, et al: High-dose intravenous human immunoglobulin in chronic inflammatory demyelinating polyneuropathy. Neurology 1989;39:422–425.
321. van Doorn PA, Vermeulen M, Mulder PGH, et al: Intravenous immunoglobulin treatment in patients with chronic inflammatory demyelinating polyneuropathy. Clinical and laboratory characteristics associated with improvement. Arch Neurol 1991; 48:217–220.
322. Gorson KC, Allam G, Ropper AH: Chronic inflammatory demyelinating polneuropathy: clinical features and response to treatment in 67 consecutive patients with and without a monoclonal gammopathy. Neurology 1997;48:321–328.
323. Kao Y-F, Lan M-Y, Chou M-S, et al: Intracranial fatigable ptosis. J Neuro-ophthalmol 1999;19:257–259.
324. Ho SL, Cheng PW, Wong WC, et al: A case-controlled MRI/MRA study of neurovascular contact in hemifacial spasm. Neurology 1999;53:2132–2139.
325. Sanders DB, Massey JM, Sanders LL, et al: A randomized trial of 3,4-diaminopyridine in Lambert-Eaton myasthenic syndrome. Neurology 2000;43: 603–607.

CHAPTER 15

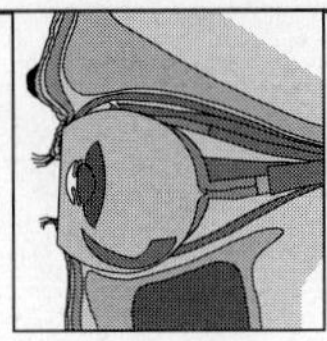

Eye Movement Disorders: Third, Fourth, and Sixth Nerve Palsies and Other Causes of Diplopia and Ocular Misalignment

This chapter will cover the diagnosis and management of the causes of double vision and ocular misalignment. Although the bulk of the discussion will concentrate on third, fourth, and sixth nerve palsies, other supranuclear, nuclear, neuromuscular junction, myopathic, and restrictive disorders will be detailed or alluded to. The relevant anatomy of the ocular motor system will be discussed first, followed by signs and symptoms in patients with diplopia, and then the diagnosis and management. The differential diagnosis of the major entities that cause diplopia or ocular misalignment will then be reviewed.

Note: The following terms will be interchanged throughout this chapter: oculomotor = third = IIIrd nerve; trochlear = fourth = IVth nerve; abducens = sixth = VIth nerve. Also, the term *ocular motor nerves* refers to the IIIrd, IVth, and VIth nerves together.

ANATOMY

Overview

The three ocular motor cranial nerves (third, fourth, and sixth) innervate the six extraocular muscles of each eye (Fig. 15–1), the major eyelid elevator, and the pupillary constrictor. The *oculomotor (third) nerve* activates the medial rectus (adduction), inferior rectus (depression), superior rectus, and inferior oblique (elevation) muscles as well as the pupillary sphincter muscle (constriction) and levator palpebrae of the upper lid. The *trochlear (fourth) nerve* supplies the superior oblique muscle, which intorts the eye and depresses it in adduction. The *abducens (sixth) nerve* innervates the lateral rectus muscle, which abducts the eye (Fig. 15–2).

From the Central Nervous System to the Orbit

Supranuclear Control of the Third, Fourth, and Sixth Nerves. In a logical, hierarchical control of eye movements, the supranuclear centers in cortex and brain stem direct the actions of the ocular motor nerves. For horizontal saccades, each frontal eye field (FEF) activates the contralateral paramedian pontine reticular formation (PPRF). Neurons of the PPRF in turn, excite the adjacent sixth nerve nucleus, which, via the ascending medial longitudinal fasciculus (MLF), innervates the contralateral medial rectus subnucleus in the mesencephalon (see Fig. 16–2). Supranuclear centers for pursuit lie in the ipsilateral occipitoparietal region (see Fig. 16–3). Upgaze and downgaze saccades,

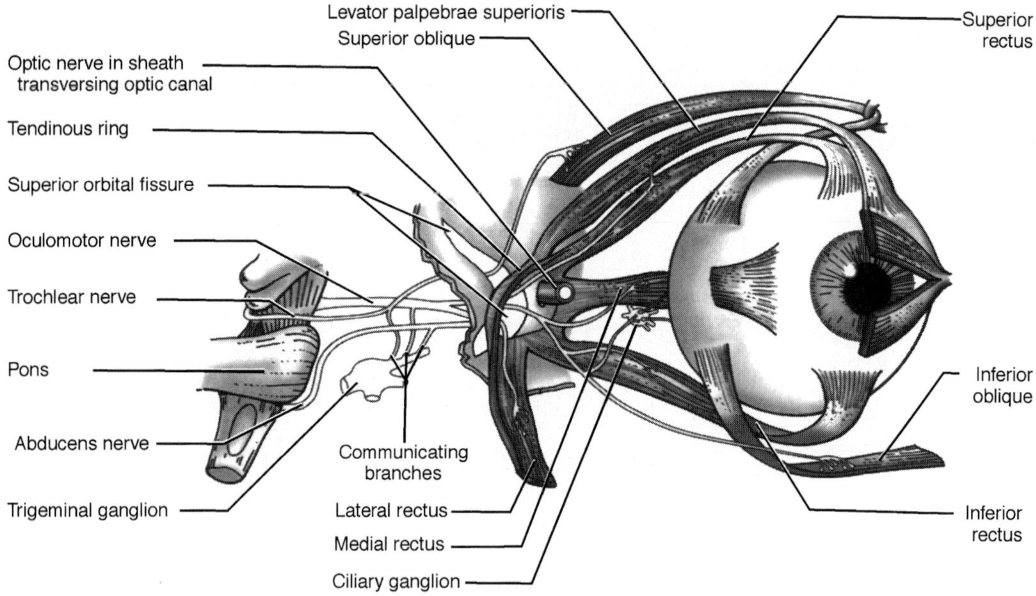

FIGURE 15–1. Innervation of the muscles of the globe. The oculomotor (III), trochlear (IV), and abducens (VI) nerves enter the orbit through the superior orbital fissure. The trochlear nerve supplies the superior oblique, the abducens nerve supplies the lateral rectus, and the oculomotor nerve supplies the remaining five muscles. (From Moore KL: Clinically Oriented Anatomy, 4th edition, p 911. Baltimore, Lippincott Williams & Wilkins, 1999, with permission.)

also under voluntary control by the FEFs, are initiated by neurons in the mesencephalic rostral interstitial nucleus of the medial longitudinal fasciculus (riMLF) and regulated by cells in the interstitial nucleus of Cajal (INC), areas that exert supranuclear control over the third and fourth nerve nuclei (see Figs. 16–16 and 16–17). The vestibular nuclei have direct connections with the third and fourth nerve nuclei, via the MLF. These and other supranuclear gaze centers are reviewed in detail in Chapter 16.

Nuclear and Fascicular Structures. The oculomotor (third) nuclear complex lies in the midbrain, anterior to the cerebral aqueduct (Fig. 15–3).[1] Each muscle innervated by the third nerve is subserved by individual subnuclei.[2, 3]

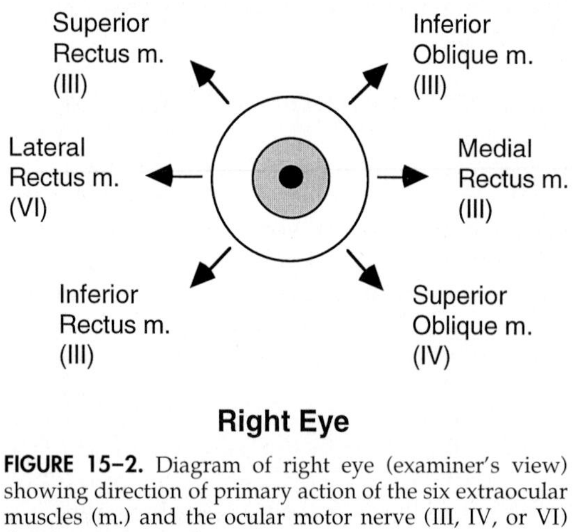

FIGURE 15–2. Diagram of right eye (examiner's view) showing direction of primary action of the six extraocular muscles (m.) and the ocular motor nerve (III, IV, or VI) that innervates each.

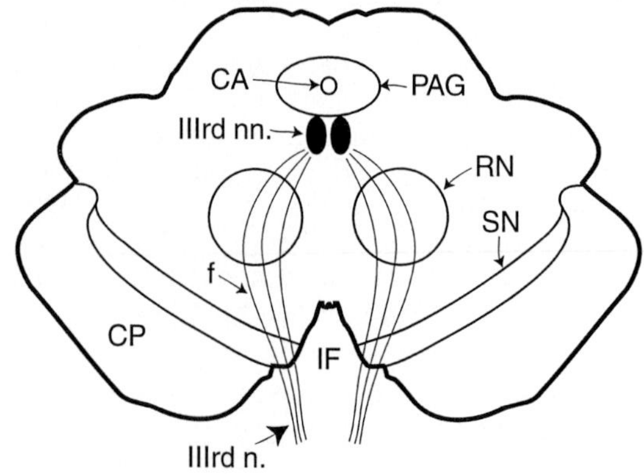

FIGURE 15–3. Diagram of axial section of the midbrain through the superior colliculus. CA = cerebral aqueduct, CP = cerebral peduncle, SN = substantia nigra, f = oculomotor nerve fascicle, IIIrd nn. = oculomotor nerve nucleus, IIIrd n. = oculomotor nerve, IF = interpeduncular fossa, PAG = periaqueductal grey, SC = superior colliculus, and RN = red nucleus.

Unique features, however, include the central caudal subnucleus, which subserves both levator muscles; the superior rectus subnuclei, which each innervate the contralateral superior rectus muscle (Fig. 15–4); and the Edinger–Westphal nuclei, which supply the preganglionic cholinergic neurons of the pupil. Fibers from the superior rectus subnuclei are thought to pass through the contralateral superior rectus subnucleus before joining the contralateral third nerve fascicle.[4] Pupillary and eyelid function and related abnormalities are discussed in Chapters 13 and 14, respectively. The paired oculomotor fascicles travel ventrally through the midbrain, each passing through the red nuclei and then the medial portion of the cerebral peduncles before exiting into the interpeducular fossa (Fig. 15–3). The neurons of each third nerve-innervated muscle are topographically organized within the fascicle (Fig. 15–5).

The trochlear nucleus lies ventral to the aqueduct in the pontomesencephalic junction (Fig. 15–6), caudal to the oculomotor complex. Fourth nerve axons decussate near the roof of the aqueduct and exit the brain stem dorsally just beneath the inferior colliculi, in an area called the anterior medullary vellum. Thus each trochlear nucleus innervates the contralateral superior oblique muscle.

The abducens nucleus lies immediately ventral to the genu of the facial nerve (facial colliculus in dorsal pons) (Fig. 15–7). This nucleus contains cell bodies for the motor neurons that will innervate the ipsilateral sixth nerve and interneurons that will climb within the MLF to innervate the contralateral medial rectus subnucleus (see Fig. 16–2). The fascicles travel ventrally, passing through the cortical spinal tracts, before exiting anterolaterally at the pontomedullary junction.

It should be emphasized that except for the superior rectus subnucleus and the trochlear nuclei, the ocular motor nuclei innervate ipsilateral eye muscles.

Extra-axial Structures. The three ocular motor nerves traverse the subarachnoid space at the

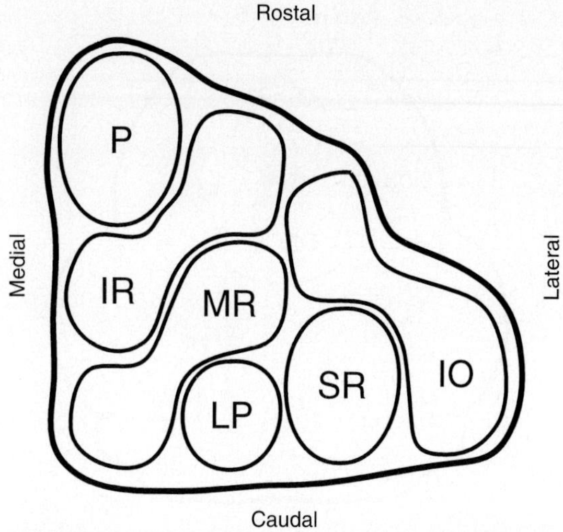

FIGURE 15–5. Cross-sectional diagram of topographic organization of the third nerve fascicle. Labeled fiber distributions: P = pupillary, IR = inferior rectus, MR = medial rectus, LP = levator palpebrae, SR = superior rectus, IO = inferior oblique. (Adapted from Ksiazek SM, et al: Ann Neurol 1989;26:714–718, and Castro O, et al: Arch Neurol 1990;47:235–237, with permission.)

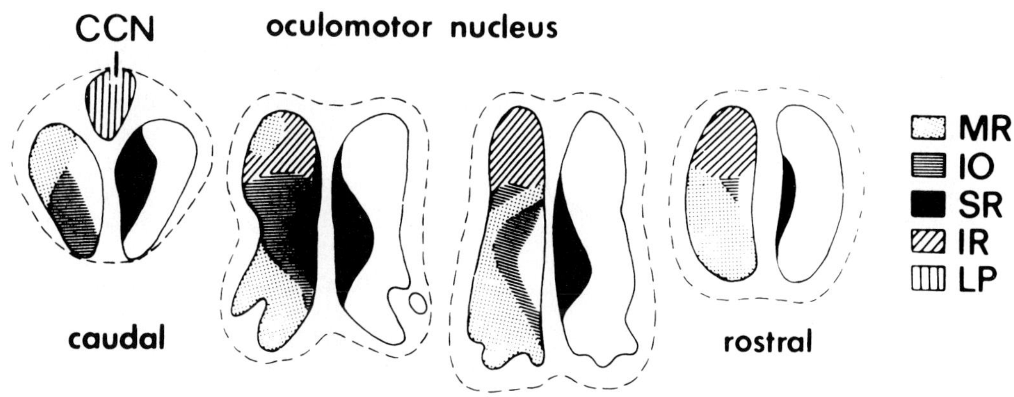

FIGURE 15–4. Axial sections of the oculomotor (IIIrd) nerve complex. Note each muscle innervated by the third nerve is subserved by individual subnuclei. The central caudal nucleus (CCN) innervates the levator palpebrae (LP). MR = medial rectus, IO = inferior oblique, SR = superior rectus, IR = inferior rectus. Note the Edinger–Westphal nucleus, which lies dorsally in the oculomotor complex, is not shown. (From Schmisdle K, Büttner-Ennever JA: Nervous control of eyelid function. A review of clinical, experimental and pathological data. Brain 1992;227–247, with permission.)

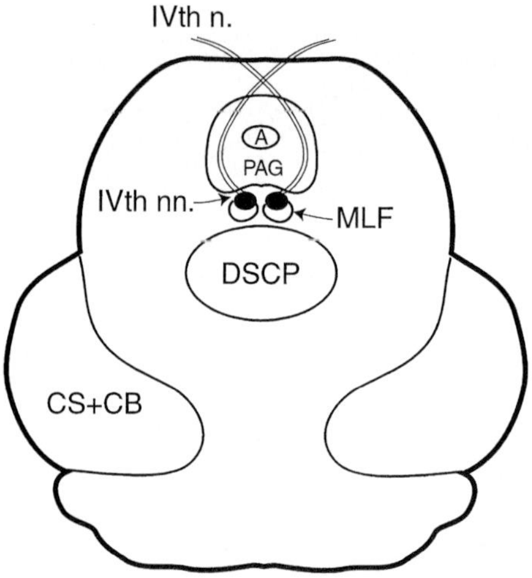

FIGURE 15–6. Axial section through the fourth nerve nuclei at the level of the pontomesencephalic junction. A = aqueduct, PAG = periaqueductal grey matter, IVth n. = fourth nerve, IVth nn. = fourth nerve nucleus, MLF = medial longitudinal fasciculus, CS + CB = corticospinal and corticobulbar tracts, and DSCP = decussation of the superior cerebellar peduncle (brachium conjunctivum).

skull base before reaching the cavernous sinus (Fig. 15–8). The third nerve enters the cavernous sinus by piercing the dura in its most superior portion just lateral to the posterior clinoid process. The fourth nerve travels for about 3.5 cm from behind the brain stem, running under the free edge of the tentorium before piercing the dura to lie immediately inferior

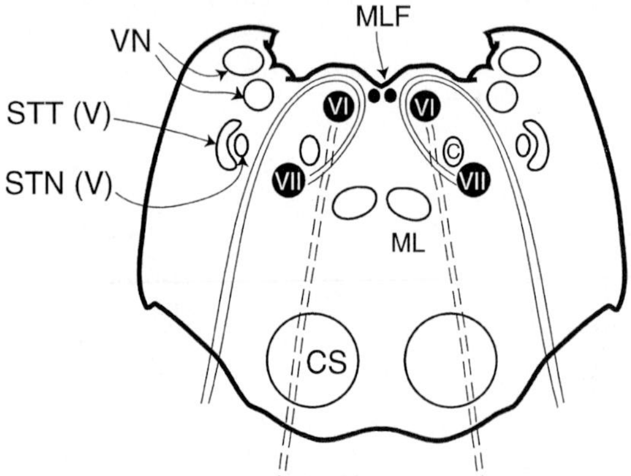

FIGURE 15–7. Axial section through the pons at the level of the sixth nerve nuclei. VI = sixth nerve, VII = seventh nerve, C = central tegmental tract, CS = corticospinal tract, VN = vestibular nuclei, ML = medial lemniscus, MLF = medial longitudinal fasciculus, STT (V) = spinal trigeminal tract of the fifth nerve, STN (V) = spinal trigeminal nucleus of the fifth nerve.

to the third nerve.[5] The sixth nerve ascends the clivus then travels underneath the petroclinoidal (Grüber's) ligament through Dorello's canal to enter the cavernous sinus. The transition from petrous to intracavernous segments of the internal carotid artery occurs as the vessel passes the petrolingual ligament, which is the posteroinferior attachment of the lateral wall of the cavernous sinus.[6]

The cavernous sinuses are triangular interconnecting structures that flank the lateral sides of the sella turcica. The walls of each sinus are created by dura mater extending from the superior orbital fissure to the posterior wall of the sella known as the dorsum sella. Inferiorly, the cavernous sinus region and pituitary fossa are in close proximity to the sphenoid and maxillary sinuses, while the optic chiasm lies superomedially (see Fig. 7–5). Each cavernous sinus contains a plexus of veins that drains the inferior and superior ophthalmic veins of the orbit and funnels posteriorly to the inferior and superior petrosal sinuses.[7] Communications are established to the opposite cavernous sinus by channels that cross the midline. Inferiorly, connections are made to the pterygoid plexus that subsequently drain into the internal jugular vein, while lateral anastomoses are made to the middle cerebral vein.[8–11]

The S-shaped intracavernous carotid artery gives rise to multiple important branches, including (1) the meningohypophysial trunk, which supplies blood to the tentorium and inferior pituitary gland; (2) the inferior lateral trunk; which nourishes the ocular motor nerves[12, 13]; and (3) the superior hypophysial artery, which provides blood to the rostral portion of the pituitary gland.[14]

The third and fourth nerves and the first and second divisions of the trigeminal nerve (V_1 and V_2) lie along the lateral wall of the cavernous sinus, while the internal carotid artery, the sixth nerve, and third-order oculosympathetic fibers from the superior cervical ganglion lie more medially (Fig. 15–9).[15] In the anterior portion of the cavernous sinus, the third nerve anatomically separates into superior and inferior divisions. The superior division innervates the superior rectus and levator muscles, while the inferior division supplies the inferior rectus, inferior oblique, medial rectus, and pupillary sphincter muscles. Within the anterior cavernous sinus, the fourth nerve crosses above the third nerve just before both nerves enter the superior orbital fissure.[11] Within the

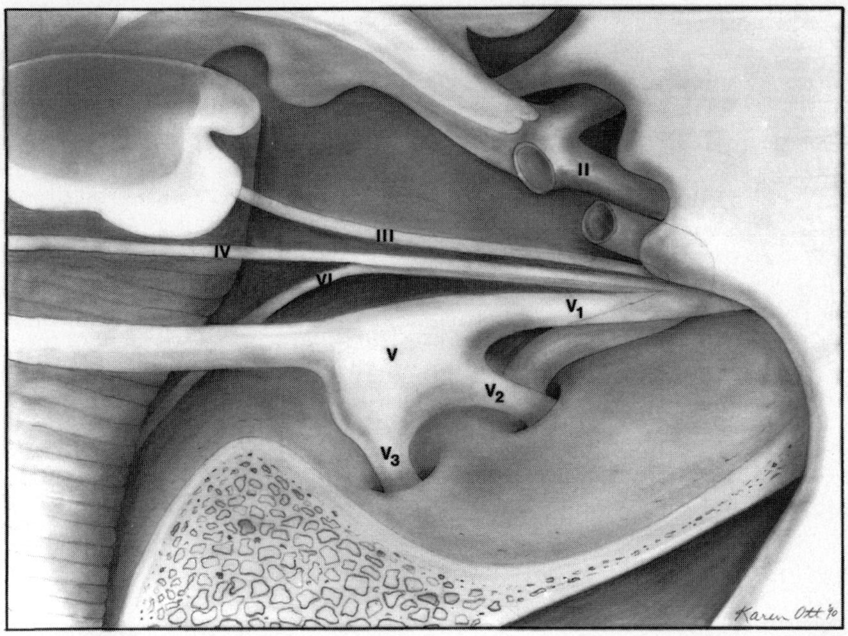

FIGURE 15–8. Lateral view of the right cavernous sinus with the temporal lobe and lateral wall dissected. The optic chiasm and third ventricle lie superomedially to this region and the divisions of the trigeminal nerve are entering their respective foramina. The third, fourth, and sixth nerves exit the brain stem (left), traverse the subarachoid space, then enter the cavernous sinus along with V_1 and V_2. (From Galetta SL, Cavernous sinus syndromes, in: Margo CE, Hamed LM, Mames RN (eds): Diagnostic Problems in Clinical Ophthalmology, p 610, Philadelphia: WB Saunders, 1994, with permission.)

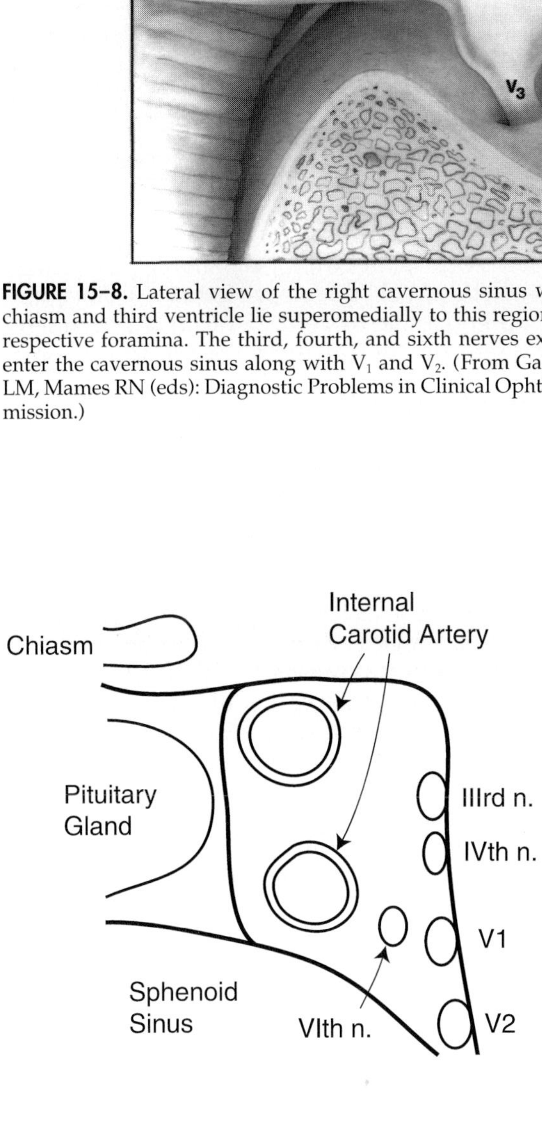

FIGURE 15–9. Diagram of the coronal view of the cavernous sinus. The third, fourth, and V1, and V2 cranial nerves line up vertically in the lateral wall of the cavernous sinus, whereas the sixth nerve lies freely next to the carotid artery.

cavernous sinus network, the sixth nerve lies freely just lateral to the cavernous carotid artery and enters the superior orbital fissure as it courses anteriorly. The postganglionic sympathetic fibers travel up the carotid artery and briefly join the sixth nerve within the cavernous sinus. This anatomic relationship accounts for the occasional case of abducens palsy and Horner syndrome associated with lesions of the cavernous sinus.[16]

The anatomy of the trigeminal nerve is critical in localizing lesions within the parasellar region.[17] Since the mandibular branch (V_3) of the trigeminal nerve travels through the foramen ovale, involvement of this branch indicates a process posterior to cavernous sinus. More anteriorly, the maxillary division leaves the skull base at the level of the cavernous sinus via the foramen rotundum. The ophthalmic branch of the trigeminal, along with the third, fourth, and sixth nerves and the oculosympathetic fibers, leaves the anterior cavernous sinus and enters the orbit through the superior orbital fissure (Figs. 15–1 and 15–10).

Orbit. Once in the orbit (Fig. 15–1), the ocular motor nerves reach their respective extraocu-

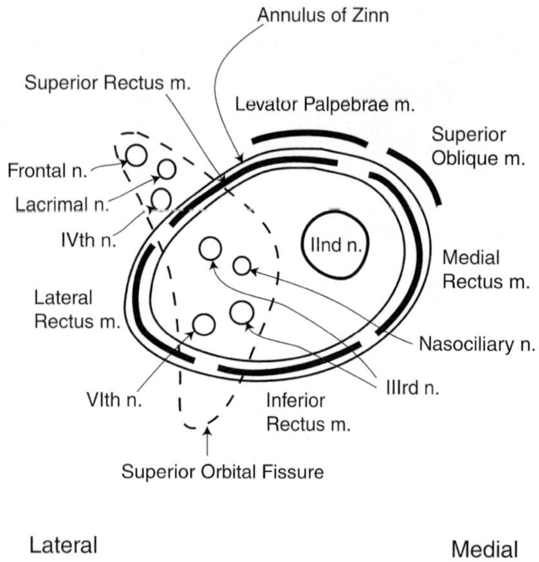

FIGURE 15–10. Diagram of the contents of the superior orbital fissure and annulus of Zinn in a coronal view of the back of the orbit.

lar muscles. The third and sixth nerves, along with the optic nerve, lie within the annulus of Zinn and muscle cone (Fig. 15–10). Like the frontal and lacrimal nerves (branches of V_1), the trochlear nerve passes above the annulus of Zinn. However, the orbital apex syndrome is usually considered to consist of optic nerve, third, fourth, sixth, and V_1 dysfunction. In contrast to the more direct orientation and attachments of the lateral, inferior, and superior rectus and inferior oblique muscles, the superior oblique muscle tendon courses through a pulley attached to the superonasal orbital wall then attaches to the globe on its posterior and temporal aspect (Fig. 15–1). This arrangement accounts for the down and in movement and intorsion of the eye produced by superior oblique contraction. Pupilloconstrictor fibers from the third nerve synapse in the ciliary ganglion, which lies within the lateral muscle cone (see Fig. 13–3) and issues postsynaptic fibers that innervate the pupil. Other details regarding orbital anatomy, including that of the extraocular muscles, are discussed in Chapter 18. Readers interested in detailed reviews of the anatomy and physiology of the extraocular muscles are referred to the reviews and articles by Porter, Baker, and their colleagues.[18–20]

Blood Supply of the Extra-axial Ocular Motor Nerves. The nutrient circulation to the third nerve[21, 22] arises from (1) small thalamomesencephalic perforators arising from the basilar and posterior cerebral arteries and the posterior circle of Willis, in the proximal subarachnoid space,[23] (2) as alluded to earlier, microscopic branches of the inferior lateral trunk of the intracavernous carotid within the cavernous sinus,[24] and (3) recurrent branches of the ophthalmic artery intraorbitally. A watershed region of the third nerve may exist between the proximal and intracavernous portions.[25] The cavernous and orbital blood supply of the fourth and sixth nerves is likely similar. The subarachnoid segment of the fourth nerve derives its blood supply from branches of the superior cerebellar artery.[26] The subarachnoid segment of the sixth nerve is likely supplied by branches from the posterior cerebral and superior cerebellar arteries.

SYMPTOMS

Patients with diplopia should be asked whether their double vision is (1) binocular, (2) horizontal or vertical, or (3) worse in left-, right-, up-, or downgaze, or distance or near.

1. *Binocularity* can be assessed by inquiring, "Does the double vision go away when you cover either eye?" Neurologic misalignment causes binocular diplopia, whereas ocular causes such as refractive error, for instance, lead to monocular diplopia.
2. *Horizontal or Vertical.* Horizontal double vision suggests dysfunction of the medial or lateral rectus muscles. Vertical diplopia implies an abnormality of vertically acting muscles such as the inferior rectus, superior rectus, inferior oblique, or superior oblique. Because the vertically acting muscles also tort the eye, their dysfunction can also cause diplopia with tilted images.
3. *Directionality.* In a patient with diplopia caused by extraocular muscle paralysis, the double vision will worsen when the patient attempts to look in the direction of action of the paretic muscle. For example, attempted leftward gaze worsens the horizontal diplopia due to weakness of the right medial rectus muscle. Thus, in some instances, history alone is often sufficient to localize the problem.

Some patients with ocular misalignment complain of blurry vision instead of frank diplopia, especially if the two images are close together or the person has intermittent fusion.

Asking if the blurry vision resolves with one eye covered is helpful in this regard.

Individuals with ocular misalignment who have no diplopia usually have either (1) defective vision in one or both eyes due to refractive error, cataract, optic neuropathy, or maculopathy, for instance, (2) long-standing childhood strabismus with strabismic amblyopia (defined as loss of two Snellen lines of visual acuity in the bad eye compared with the good eye) or suppression (the ability to ignore one of the images), (3) ptosis of one eyelid or (4) a large angle of strabismus, making the second image less confusing and easy to ignore.

The examiner should investigate other historical details such as duration of onset; whether the patient has had the motility deficit since childhood; presence of pain; fatigability; other neurologic symptoms such as dysphagia or weakness; underlying illnesses such as hypertension, diabetes, cerebrovascular disease, cardiac atherosclerotic disease, or multiple sclerosis; and habits such as smoking or alcohol use.

SIGNS

The ocular motility examination is detailed in Chapter 2. It should consist of testing for the following:

1. Obvious misalignment, ptosis, or pupillary abnormalities, first by inspection.
2. Ductions, which are discoordinated movements of each eye.
3. Vergences, which are coordinated movements of both eyes in opposite directions.
4. Saccades and pursuit.
5. Oculocephalic maneuver.
6. Ocular misalignment, assessed qualitatively or quantitatively using the cover/uncover, alternate cover, Maddox rod, Krimsky, or Hirschberg technique. Often the motility disturbance will be obvious after inspection and testing of vergences. However, more subtle problems will require quantification of the misalignment using prism-alternative cover or Maddox rod techniques. Although there are many exceptions, acquired incomitant deviations (in which the ocular misalignment is different in different directions) are usually a neurologic problem, while comitant deviations (same in every direction) are typically longstanding, often dating to childhood.
7. Other clues, such as head, face, and chin position (e.g., head tilt) or orbital signs such as proptosis or eyelid swelling.
8. Forced ductions when restrictive abnormalities are suspected.

Monocular diplopia that resolves with a pinhole test is likely due to refractive error, media opacity, or retinal abnormality, but psychogenic disturbances should also be considered.

APPROACH

Using the clues from the history and examination, the examiner's goals are to determine:

1. Whether the diplopia or misalignment is a neurologic, ocular, or childhood strabismus problem. If it is neurologic, then a lesion affecting the structures outlined in the anatomic pathways above, from supranuclear ones to muscle, may be implicated.
2. Which extraocular muscles are involved.
3. The cause. We suggest considering the most common causes of acquired misalignment by whether they typically cause horizontal[27] or vertical diplopia[28, 29] (Table 15–1).

Often the ophthalmoparesis and abnormal motility pattern are characteristic, and other historical features or accompanying neurologic findings aid in localization and diagnosis. A complete, isolated infranuclear third nerve palsy causes ipsilateral elevation, adduction, and depression weakness accompanied by abduction, hypodeviation, pupillary mydriasis, and ptosis. Patients with superior oblique paresis complain of vertical diplopia, often with a torsional component, and they have an ipsilateral hypertropia worse on contraversive

TABLE 15–1. Horizontal versus Vertical Diplopia: Major Causes

Horizontal Diplopia
Sixth nerve palsy
Third nerve palsy
Convergence insufficiency
Internuclear ophthalmoplegia
Myasthenia gravis
Vertical Diplopia
Fourth nerve palsy
Thyroid-associated ophthalmopathy
Myasthenia gravis
Skew deviation
Third nerve palsy

(contralateral conjugate) horizontal gaze and ipsilateral head tilt. Patients with lateral rectus palsy complain of binocular horizontal double vision worse on ipsiversive gaze and at distance. In many cases the limitation of abduction is evident, but in more subtle instances, alternate cover or Maddox rod testing would confirm an esotropia largest on ipsiversive gaze. Restrictive diplopia, due to orbital processes such as thyroid-associated ophthalmopathy, is associated with positive forced duction testing. Proptosis and periorbital swelling are also usually present in such cases.

Another important consideration when determining the cause of diplopia is the age of the patient. In adults, diabetes, hypertension, trauma, and aneurysms are common causes of oculomotor palsies (Table 15–2).[30–32] In contrast, in most pediatric series, the most common causes of acquired third, fourth, and sixth nerve palsies are trauma and neoplasms. Vascular and aneurysmal causes of oculomotor palsies are uncommon in children.[33]

TREATMENT OVERVIEW

The ophthalmoparesis in some of the disorders described, such as ischemic and traumatic oculomotor palsies, will often resolve spontaneously. Other cases, such as those due to myasthenia gravis or bacterial meningitis, will improve as the underlying cause is treated. In the meantime, patients with diplopia can wear an eye patch over one eye to resolve the double vision, or one lens of a pair of eyeglasses can be taped over. Some authors have advocated botulinum toxin injections into the antagonist muscle of a paretic one, even in supranuclear ocular motility disorders.[34] For instance, in a left lateral rectus palsy, the left medial rectus muscle is injected with botulinum to decrease adduction tone. Prisms may be used to facilitate image alignment, and are best for patients with relatively comitant deviations. Temporary Fresnel paste-on prisms can be used initially followed by ground-in prisms in chronic cases. Individuals with ophthalmoparesis who do not improve spontaneously, and whose exams remain stable for at least 6 months, may be candidates for corrective eye muscle surgery.

Children with oculomotor palsies, especially those under age 8, have the potential for developing strabismic amblyopia. Third nerve palsies have the complicating feature of ptosis with the potential for deprivational amblyopia. These children, when able, should be referred to a pediatric ophthalmologist for patching or lid elevation. Children patched for symptomatic diplopia should have the patch alternated daily between eyes to prevent occlusion amblyopia.

MONOCULAR DOUBLE VISION

Ophthalmic Causes of Monocular Double Vision

Most patients with monocular double vision either have an optical problem, a macular abnormality, or a nonorganic symptom. Generally, the description of double vision that persists with one eye closed is different in each of these circumstances. Patients with optical causes of monocular double vision generally describe blurring and a "ghost image" or extra line to things they are viewing. They do not see a discrete, second image but a lighter, partial second image that is attached to the main image and separates from it in one direction. The symptom almost always improves or disappears when the same object is viewed through a pinhole. Common causes of this type of dou-

TABLE 15–2. Causes of Acquired Third, Fourth, and Sixth Nerve Palsies in Adults

Cause	IIIrd (%)	IVth (%)	VIth (%)	Multiple (any combination of IIIrd, IVth, or VIth) (%)
Undetermined	24*	32*	26*	12
Vascular	20†	18	13	4
Head trauma	15	29†	15	17
Aneurysm	16	1	3	9
Neoplasm	12	5	22†	35*,†
Other	13	15	22	23

"Vascular" refers to associated diabetes mellitus, hypertension, or atherosclerosis.
* = Most common group.
† = Most common group with an identifiable cause.
Data from Richards DW, Jones FR, Younge BR: Am J Ophthalmol 1992;113:489–496.

ble vision include cataract, irregular astigmatism (particularly keratoconus), corneal scars, and tear film irregularities. If refraction with a rigid contact lens improves the double vision then the cause is likely to be an irregular corneal surface. Treatment of this type of double vision is cause specific (ie, refraction, rigid contact lens use, cataract extraction, or laser keratectomy).

Patients with macular causes of monocular double vision generally describe a break, bend, or distortion of the viewed edge leading to a double or distorted image. This type of monocular double vision generally does not improve when the object is viewed through a pinhole and, in fact, vision is often worse through a pinhole in this setting. Common macular causes of monocular double vision include epiretinal membranes and retinal or choroidal folds. In addition, it should be noted that binocular diplopia can result from macular disease as well. In this case, macular disease leads to significant image distortion or difference in image size compared to the other eye (*aniseikonia*). This image size or shape discrepancy prevents fusion of images despite normal alignment.[35, 36]

Finally, patients with nonorganic or functional vision loss often complain of monocular double vision. In our experience this is an ill-defined symptom that cannot be further characterized by the patient and may affect one or both eyes. Double vision may be reported only after the examiner asks specifically about double vision when trying to characterize a complaint of "blurred vision." In this setting patients may also complain of triple or quadruple vision. The symptom does not improve with pinhole or any other maneuver on the part of the examiner. Nonorganic vision loss is discussed further in Chapter 11.

Neurologic Causes of Monocular Double Vision

Rarely, acquired occipital lobe lesions or drugs may cause multiple images, akin to palinopsia. These types of visual hallucinations are discussed in Chapter 12.

SUPRANUCLEAR CAUSES OF DIPLOPIA

This section will review diplopia caused by supranuclear lesions: internuclear ophthalmoplegia, convergence spasm, convergence and divergence insufficiency, and pseudoabducens palsy, which cause horizontal diplopia, and skew deviation and monocular elevator palsy, which lead to vertical diplopia.

Internuclear Ophthalmoplegia

Disruption of the MLF in the pons or midbrain results in an *internuclear ophthalmoplegia* (*INO*) typified by an ipsilateral adduction deficit and contralateral abducting nystagmus (Figs. 15–11 and 15–12). The side of the adduction deficit determines the side of the INO.

Symptoms. Patients with INO may complain of horizontal diplopia, particularly when the adduction weakness is profound. Those patients with subtle paresis may have no symptoms or complain of blurred vision with eccentric gaze only. Since a skew deviation (see below) is frequently associated with lesions of the MLF, vertical diplopia may be another complaint.[37] Oscillopsia may result from either the abduction nystagmus or an impaired vertical vestibular ocular reflex.[37]

Signs. The hallmark finding of INO is impaired adduction of the eye (Fig. 15–11). There is a wide range of medial rectus dysfunction in INO. Subtle cases may be evident only upon fast eye movements from midline to eccentric gaze ("medial rectus float"). An optokinetic flag pulled along the horizontal plane may reveal slow adducting saccades in the affected eye during the fast phase of the nystagmus.[38] The demonstration of intact convergence in INO establishes the supranuclear localization of the medial rectus weakness and usually signifies a lesion of the MLF within the pons. In contrast, patients with MLF lesions close to the third nerve nucleus may have impaired convergence. However, some patients with INO have poor convergence because of the vertical misalignment produced by the associated skew deviation.[37] Therefore, the absence of convergence may not be a totally reliable sign to localize the lesion in a discrete part of the MLF pathway.

The eye that is contralateral to the MLF lesion typically exhibits an abducting nystagmus in end gaze. Evidence suggests that this abducting nystagmus is a phenomenon adapted in an attempt to increase the innervation to the weak adducting eye.[37, 39]

Since the otolith pathways project through the MLF, a skew deviation is commonly ob-

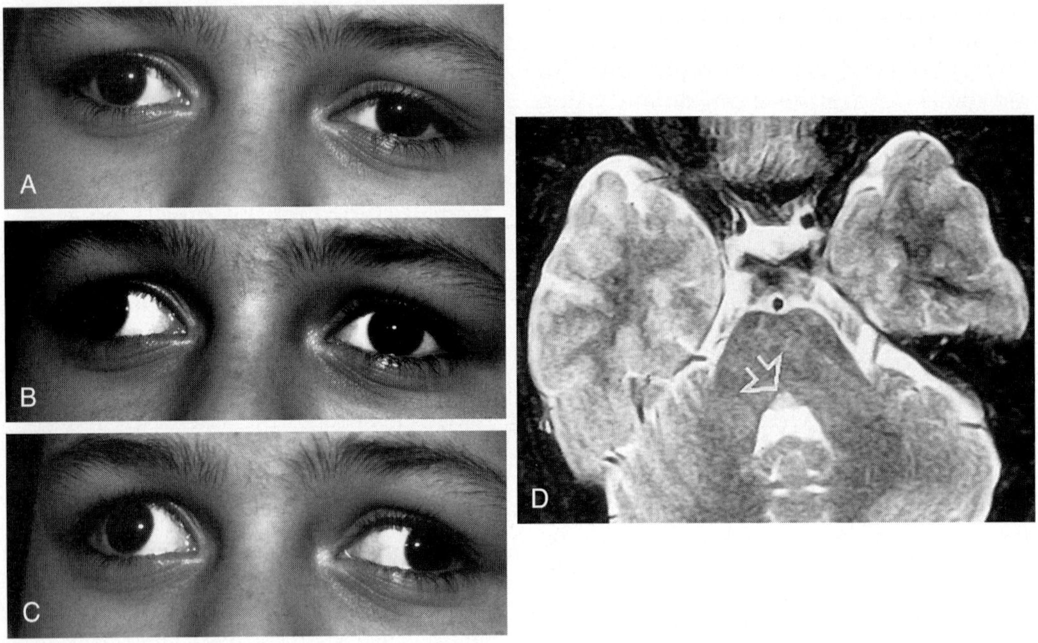

FIGURE 15–11. Bilateral INO in multiple sclerosis. **A.** Mild exotropia in primary gaze. Adduction deficits in attempted right gaze **(B)** and left gaze **(C)** with nystagmus of the abducting eye. **D.** T_2-weighted axial MRI scan demonstrating high-signal lesion (*arrow*) affecting the MLF bilaterally.

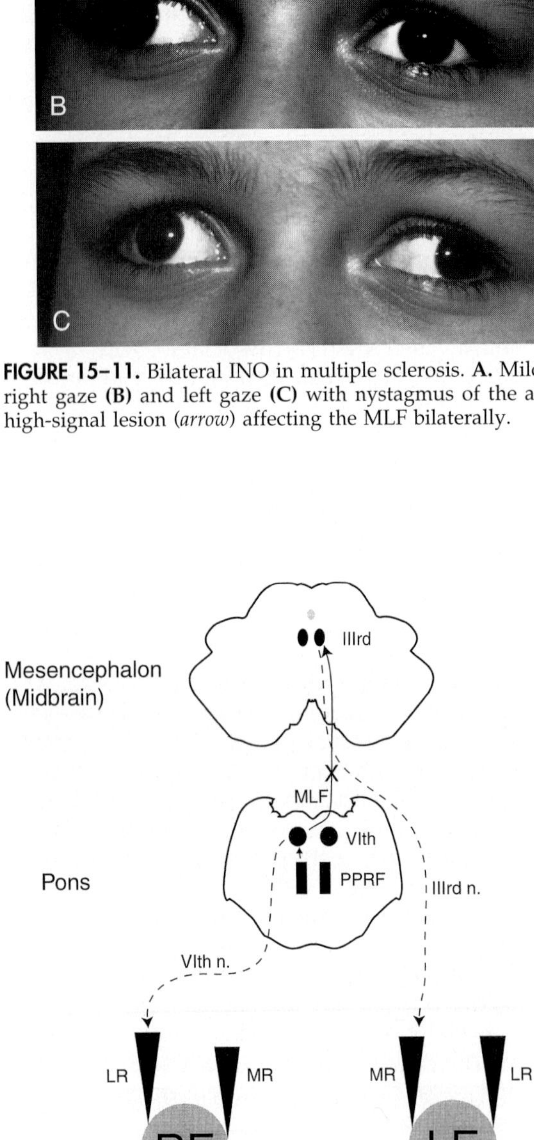

FIGURE 15–12. Diagram of the pathways and lesion for INO. Interneurons from the sixth nerve nucleus cross in the pons and ascend within the MLF to innervate the contralateral medial rectus subnucleus. A lesion within the MLF (x) will cause an ipsilateral adduction deficit.

served with an INO (see below). Typically, the hypertropic eye is on the same side as the adduction weakness. A dissociated form of vertical torsional nystagmus may also be observed because of disrupted connections from the posterior semicircular canal. This results in a downbeating nystagmus in the eye ipsilateral to the MLF lesion and torsional nystagmus in the contralateral eye.[40, 41] Bilateral lesions of the MLF usually produce additional eye findings, including impaired vertical pursuit and vertical gaze holding defects.[42] Severe bilateral INOs may also result in a large angle exotropia in primary gaze in so-called WEBINO (*w*all-*e*yed *b*ilateral INO).

Pathophysiology. Axons for the MLF arise from interneurons intermingled within the abducens nucleus (Fig. 15–12). These axons immediately cross the midline and ascend in the MLF. Lesions of the MLF produce impaired adduction of the ipsilateral eye. Since other important pathways travel in the MLF, a variety of other neuro-ophthalmologic signs may be found. The utricular pathway arising from the vestibular nucleus ascends in the MLF. Interruption of these vestibular connections results in ipsilateral hypertropia. Vestibular information also travels to and from the interstitial nucleus of Cajal.[37, 39, 42] Interruption of these connections in the MLF, particularly when bilateral, will impair (1) vertical pursuit, (2) the vertical vestibular ocular reflex, and (3) vertical gaze holding mechanisms.

Diagnosis. The diagnosis of INO is usually straightforward, especially when there is impaired medial rectus dysfunction in lateral gaze with normal convergence. One should carefully search for other orbital signs since isolated medial rectus lesions may occur from local conditions such as extraocular muscle entrapment. Exotropia resulting from strabismus can be distinguished by the presence of full extraocular movements in lateral gaze and normal saccades on gaze or optokinetic testing. Caution should be applied in this regard, however, because some patients with longstanding large angle exotropia may develop adduction weakness, perhaps on a restrictive basis, which may mimic an INO. Myasthenia gravis can rarely mimic an INO (see myasthenia gravis section later in this chapter). In such patients there are often eyelid signs to suggest this diagnosis.

Differential Diagnosis. A unilateral INO in an older patient usually results from a brain stem infarction, while bilateral INO in a young patient typically signifies a demyelinating process such as multiple sclerosis.[43, 44] However, a variety of lesions may be associated with INOs, including vascular malformations; tumors; head trauma[45, 46]; infections[47]; vasculitides such as systemic lupus erythematosus,[48–50] Behçet's disease,[51] and giant cell arteritis[52]; nutritional disorders such as Wernicke's disease; metabolic disorders such as hepatic encephalopathy; structural abnormalities (Arnold–Chiari malformation)[53]; drug intoxications such as toluene abuse[54]; and degenerative conditions, particularly progressive supranuclear palsy. We have seen transient INO in other metabolic disorders causing coma.

Variations. The combination of an INO with an ipsiversive conjugate palsy is a *pontine "one-and-a-half" syndrome* due to simultaneous ipsilateral involvement of the PPRF (or sixth nerve nucleus) and the MLF (see Chapter 16, and Figs. 16–8 and 16–9). Damage to the MLF in addition to the corticospinal tracts results in the *Raymond–Cestan syndrome,* characterized by an INO and contralateral hemiparesis.[55] Rarely, patients with impaired abduction will have adducting nystagmus. This has been sometimes referred to as a posterior INO of Lutz.[56] This combination of eye signs most likely results from an abducens palsy with the adducting nystagmus representing an adaptive response. A lesion of the MLF seems unlikely with this combination of eye signs.[37]

Convergence Spasm

This condition, characterized by convergence, accommodation, bilateral pupillary miosis, and pseudomyopia, may mimic bilateral sixth nerve palsies. The distinction is important because convergence spasm (or spasm of the near reflex) is almost always indicative of a functional disorder.[57, 58] Patients usually complain of double or blurry vision, and they often have obvious personality disorders or other hysterical symptoms. The hallmarks are pupillary constriction on attempted abduction and a variable esotropia (reflecting variable patient effort). Other features include normal abducting saccades, intact abduction during the oculocephalic maneuver or testing of monocular ductions, and resolution of the myopia following cycloplegia.[59] The miosis may resolve upon occlusion of the fellow eye by disrupting the binocular input necessary for convergence.[60]

Rarely, spasm of the near reflex may be seen in disease states such as metabolic encephalopathy,[61] Arnold–Chiari malformation, pituitary tumors, and trauma.[62] Treatment of the condition consists of cycloplegic eye drops (eg, atropine) to inhibit accommodation, or weak minus lenses.[59] Other possible treatments, however, include opacification of the medial third of the lenses.[63] However, patient reassurance that no organic disease exits is often the best approach.[57] Convergence spasm should be distinguished from convergence retraction nystagmus or pseudoabducens palsy from pretectal lesions.

Convergence Insufficiency

Patients with convergence insufficiency describe horizontal diplopia at near, typically after a period of reading. In a practical definition, patients with this condition are unable to maintain the esodeviation required for near tasks. Once an object is brought to within 10 cm of the bridge of their nose, affected patients are unable to converge. Medial rectus function is normal when ocular ductions are tested, but patients typically have an exodeviation worse at near. A common sequela of head trauma,[64] the condition may also be seen in association with dorsal midbrain lesions (Parinaud syndrome, see Chapter 16) may be a decompensation of long-standing exophoria or may be idiopathic. The exact anatomic lesion that causes convergence insufficiency is unknown.

Convergence exercises such as "pencil push-ups," in which the patient is asked to focus on the pencil eraser as it is repeatedly brought close to the eyes, and use of base-out prisms, which force convergence, can be tried. However, these measures may be inadequate for many individuals, who may require either base-in prisms for near tasks or strabismus surgery.

Divergence Insufficiency

This ocular motility deficit is characterized by acquired horizontal diplopia at distance but not near, a comitant esophoria or esotropia at distance, motor fusion at near, and full ocular ductions without evidence of a sixth nerve palsy. The abnormality has been attributed to a disturbance of a poorly defined supranuclear "divergence center" in the brain stem. It may also simply result from a decompensation of an esophoria.

Divergence insufficiency is typically benign, and affected patients are usually neurologically normal otherwise. However, since small bilateral sixth nerve palsies may mimic divergence insufficiency,[65] elevated intracranial pressure, masses, and pontine lesions[66, 67] must be excluded with neuroimaging. Small vessel ischemic disease is a relatively common finding on magnetic resonance imaging studies of older patients with this condition. Patients can be treated extremely effectively with base-out prisms or strabismus surgery.[68]

Pseudoabducens Palsy

This entity is reviewed in detail in Chapter 16 because it often accompanies the dorsal midbrain syndrome or thalamic lesions. Although the lateral rectus appears to be weak, oculocephalic maneuvers demonstrate full horizontal ductions. The esotropia is usually variable, and may represent excess convergence tone.

Skew Deviation

Skew deviation refers to a vertical misalignment of the eyes that commonly occurs from acute brain stem dysfunction.[69–72] Occasionally, skew deviation may also result from peripheral vestibular or cerebellar lesions.[73–77]

Symptoms and Signs. Patients may complain of binocular vertical diplopia, sometimes with a torsional component. The presence of other neurologic symptoms and signs often helps to distinguish skew deviation from other causes of vertical misalignment such as third and fourth nerve palsies.[78] For example, a vertical deviation of the eyes with signs of pontomedullary dysfunction, such as ataxia, usually suggests a skew deviation is present.

Ocular Tilt Reaction. The combination of skew deviation with ocular torsion and a head tilt is known as the *ocular tilt reaction* (*OTR*) (Fig. 15–13).[71] This triad of signs is typically observed with lesions of the lateral pontomedullary junction (Fig. 15–14) or the paramedian thalamic–mesencephalic region, and results from dysfunction of the utricular pathways that begin in the labyrinths and terminate in the rostral brain stem.[70–72] Although the exact neuroanatomic pathways that mediate the OTR or its prime component, skew deviation, remain uncertain, the localizing value of skew deviation has evolved from clinical and experimental observation (Table 15–3).

Pathophysiology. It appears that both the utricular and the semicircular canal pathways that regulate vertical gaze synapse in the vestibular nuclei and cross the midline to ascend in the MLF (Fig. 15–15).[70–72] There, the utricular

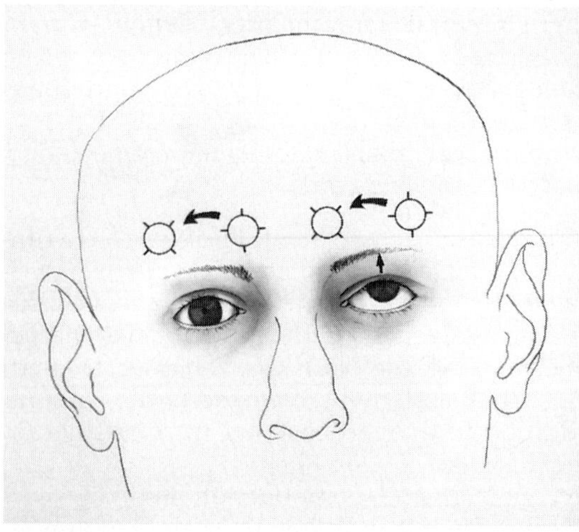

FIGURE 15–13. Diagram demonstrating the three components of the OTR: (1) right head tilt, (2) ocular counter roll, and (3) skew deviation. Note that the eyes roll toward the hypotropic eye.

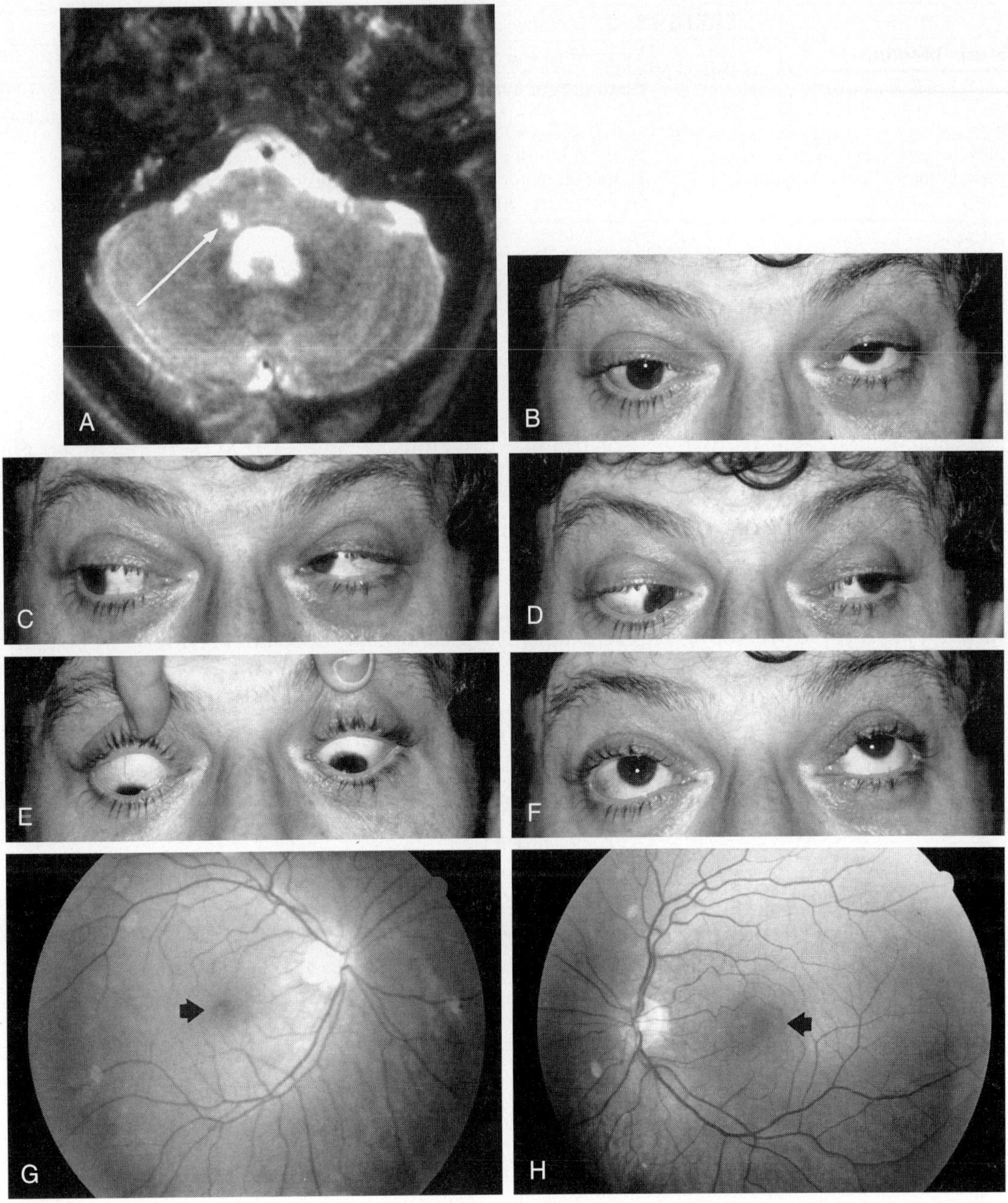

FIGURE 15–14. Pontomedullary lesion causing ocular tilt reaction. **A.** Axial T_2-weighted MRI scan showing right lateral pontomedullary infarction (*arrow*). **B.** Left hypertropia in primary gaze, which was worse in right gaze **(C–F)**. Excyclotorsion of the hypotropic right eye **(G)** (note downward displacement of macula (*arrow*) relative to the optic disc) and incyclotorsion of the hypertropic left eye **(H)** (note upward displacement of the macula (*arrow*), which normally lies below the horizontal meridian) were also present. (Courtesy of Stefania Bianchi-Marzoli, MD.)

pathway connects to the nuclei that activate the four vertically acting muscles, namely, the superior rectus, superior oblique, inferior rectus, and inferior oblique. Remember that the superior rectus subnucleus and trochlear nucleus control the contralateral superior rectus and superior oblique muscles, respectively. Thus, a right utricular nerve lesion would result in a left hypertropia as a result of impaired action of the left inferior rectus muscle and the right superior rectus muscle. If the lesion occurs in the MLF, the hypertropia will be ipsi-

TABLE 15–3. Localizing Value of Skew Deviation

Lesion Location	Type of Skew	Associated Signs
Lateral pontomedullary	Contralateral hypertropia	Ipsilateral excyclotorsion; ipsilateral facial numbness; ipsilateral Horner syndrome; lateropulsion
Midline cervicomedullary junction	Bilateral inferior rectus	Downbeat nystagmus
Medial longitudinal fasciculus	Ipsilateral hypertropia	Internuclear ophthalmoplegia
Rostral midbrain	Ipsilateral hypertropia	Vertical gaze palsy; conjugate cyclotorsion

lateral unless lateral pontomedullary structures are also affected; in this case the hypertropia may be contralateral to the INO.[72]

Skew deviation may also ensue following selective damage to the posterior or the anterior semicircular canal pathway.[72] For example, injury to the right posterior semicircular canal projections would lead to a left hypertropia and relative right eye excyclotorsion from impaired innervation to the left inferior rectus and right superior oblique muscles, receptively. Although both eyes are torted toward the hypotropic eye, the lower eye is usually more excyclorotated than the higher eye is incyclorotated, hence the term *relative excyclorotation*.[78] Bilateral damage to the crossing posterior semicircular pathway projection in the dorsal medulla could lead to an alternating hypertropia (ie, right hypertropia in right gaze from impaired action of the right inferior rectus muscle, and a left hypertropia in left gaze from disturbed function of the left inferior rectus muscle).[79, 80] Patients who have skew deviation from interruption of the semicircular canal pathway often have associated vertical nystagmus. For instance, interruption of the posterior semicircular canal pathway leads to a skew deviation in association with downbeat nystagmus in one eye and a torsional nystagmus in the fellow eye. Although brain stem strokes

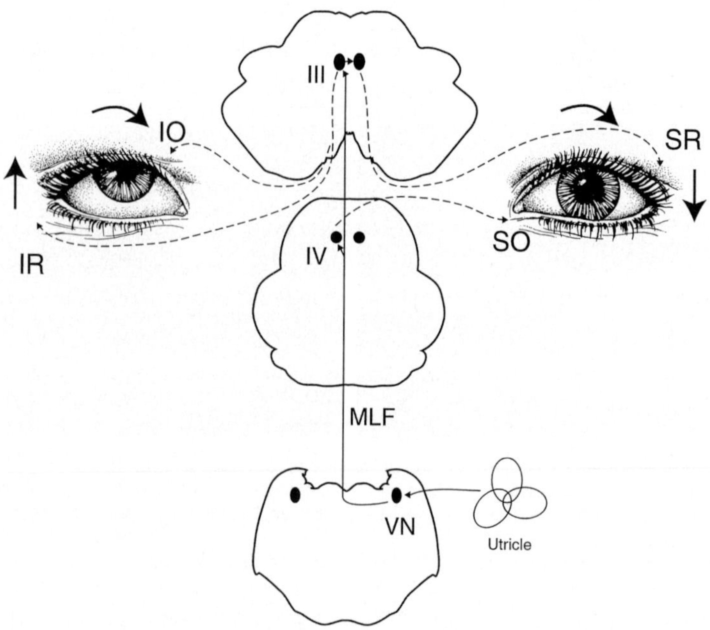

FIGURE 15–15. Diagram demonstrating the presumed projections of the utricular pathway for lateral head tilting. Note the utricular projections synapse in the vestibular nucleus (VN), which issues fibers that cross and ascend in the MLF to the subnuclei of the four vertically acting extraocular muscles. These subnuclei include the fourth nerve nucleus and the third nerve subnuclei controlling the superior rectus (SR), inferior rectus (IR), and the superior oblique muscles (IO). Note that the fourth nerve nucleus and the superior rectus subnucleus innervate their respective muscles of the contralateral eye. For example, a lesion within the utricular connection to the (*left*) VN or the (*right*) MLF will produce a right hypertropia, a counter-roll of the eyes to the left (as shown), and a left head tilt. The SO is labeled in the lower part of the eye for the sake of simplicity.

and tumors are the most common causes of skew deviation, this motility disturbance may be rarely observed as a false localizing sign of increased intracranial pressure, such as that caused by pseudotumor cerebri.[81, 82]

Diagnosis. The hypertropia of a skew deviation may be comitant (deviation is the same in all positions of gaze) or noncomitant (deviation varies with gaze position). When a skew deviation is noncomitant, it may be difficult to distinguish from an oculomotor palsy or extraocular muscle weakness. A fourth nerve palsy is the motility disorder that may be the most difficult to distinguish from a skew deviation since both conditions may be associated with a positive head-tilt[78] or three-step test (see fourth nerve palsies, below).[83] However, patients with skew deviation typically have binocular torsion as opposed to the excyclotorsion of one just eye seen in a fourth nerve palsy.[72, 84] Binocular torsion may be demonstrated by double Maddox rod testing (Fig. 15–16), fundus photography (see Fig. 15–14), indirect ophthalmoscopy, or measurement of the subjective visual vertical.[72, 85] Furthermore, the supranuclear nature of the hyperdeviation

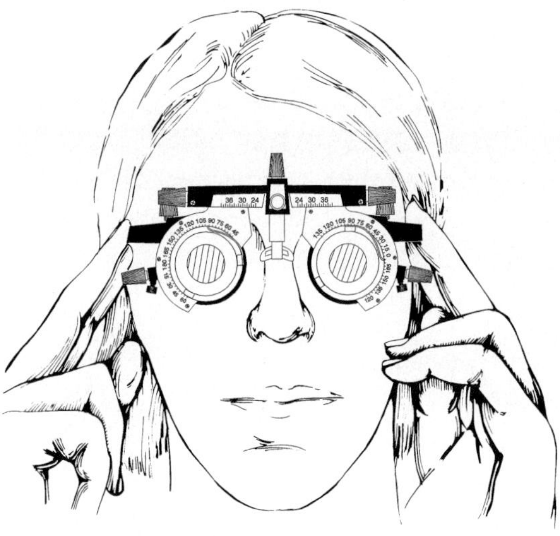

FIGURE 15–16. Drawing of double Maddox rod testing in a patient with a skew deviation (right hypertropia). Red Maddox rod lenses are placed over each eye in a trial frame, each at the 90° mark. As the patient is viewing a hand-held light at distance, two separate horizontal red lines will be seen, one from each eye. The patient is asked to align the two red lines so that they are parallel to each other and the floor by rotating the dials of the trial frame. In the example shown, the patient displayed asymmetric cyclotorsion of both eyes toward the left shoulder. In this case there was incyclotorsion of approximately 10° OD and excyclotorsion of approximately 15° OS.

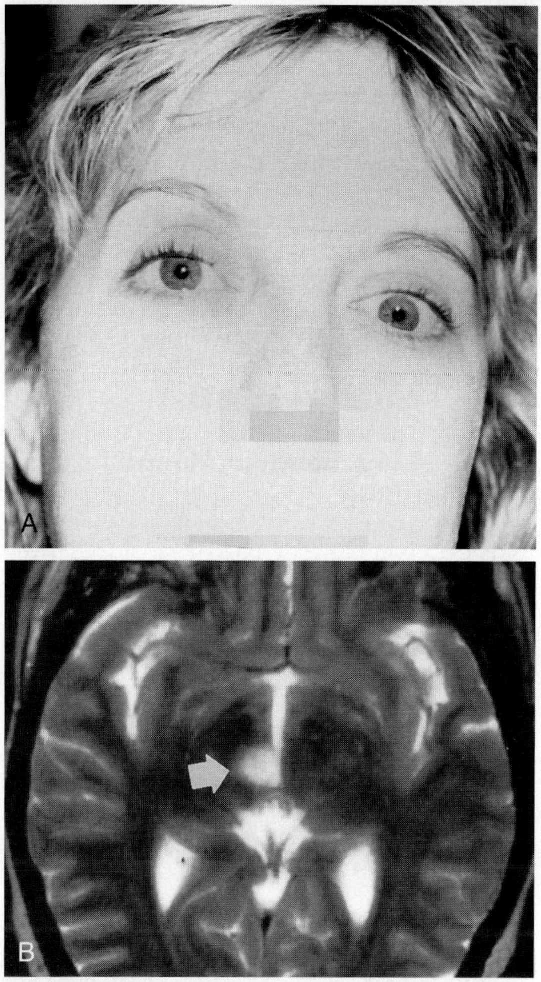

FIGURE 15–17. A. External photograph demonstrating a patient with an OTR (large right hypertropia and left head tilt due to a **(B)** right midbrain-thalamic infarction (*arrow*). The patient also had counter-rolling of the eyes toward the left shoulder on funduscopy.)

associated with skew deviation may be evident during oculocephalic testing or forced eyelid closure (Bell's phenomenon).[78]

Midbrain lesions involving the INC may also produce skew deviation with the hypertropic eye ipsilateral to the lesions. A full OTR may also ensue with midbrain lesions, producing a conjugate counter roll of the eyes toward the contralateral shoulder (Fig. 15–17).[86–88] The head tilt will be contralateral to the lesion as well. Alternating skew with lateral gaze may also be associated with midbrain lesions.[80]

Variations. Occasionally, irritative lesions of the midbrain will produce a paroxysmal skew deviation.[89–92] These patients have a contralateral hypertropia, ipsilateral head tilt, and a conjugate counter roll of the eyes toward the ipsilateral shoulder. This triad replicates the eye findings observed with the electrical stimulation of the INC in animals.[89] One patient has been documented with skew deviation from ictal activity of the vestibular cortex.[93]

Alternating skew deviation in the primary position is an unusual eye movement disorder that may be observed with midbrain lesions. The hypertropia may switch sides over several minutes in an aperiodic or periodic manner.[94,95] Periodic alternating deviation may also coexist with periodic alternating nystagmus.

Acquired Supranuclear Monocular Elevator Palsy

This "double elevator palsy" is caused by a pretectal, supranuclear lesion.[96–100] Function of both the superior rectus and inferior oblique muscles of one eye is affected by a unilateral lesion in the rostral mesencephalon. Such a lesion would disrupt the efferent fibers from the riMLF to the inferior oblique subnucleus, and the contralateral superior rectus subnucleus, which innervates the superior rectus muscle contralateral to it (see Fig. 16–17). Thus, a unilateral lesion produces a monocular elevation paresis. As the name of the condition implies, Bell's phenomenon and the oculocephalic responses are intact in the affected eye. If reflex eye movements are not preserved with a monocular elevator palsy, one should consider a fascicular third nerve palsy or a lesion along the distal path of the third nerve, including the orbit.

THIRD NERVE PALSIES

As indicated earlier, a complete, isolated infranuclear third nerve palsy causes ipsilateral elevation, adduction, and depression weakness accompanied by abduction, hypodeviation, pupillary mydriasis, and ptosis (Fig. 15–18). In adults, the most common identifiable cause of acquired third nerve palsy is vascular insufficiency due to diabetes, hypertension, or atherosclerosis.[30] The most feared cause of a third nerve palsy in adulthood is a posterior communicating artery aneurysm, which may compress the third nerve within the subarachnoid space. Other causes of isolated third nerve pal-

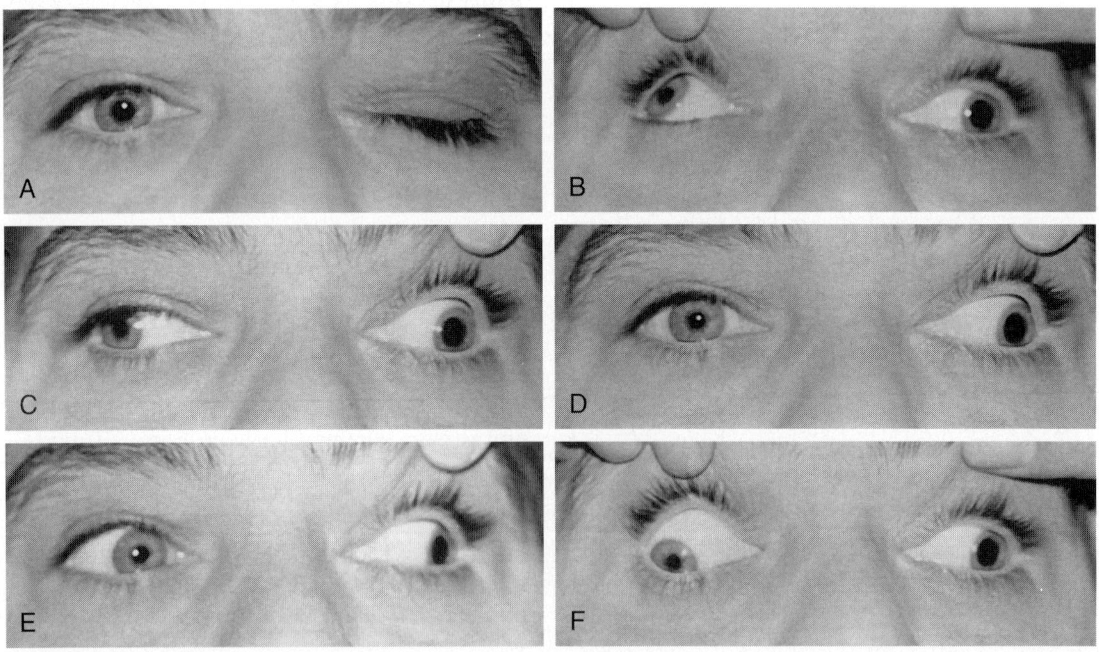

FIGURE 15–18. Complete pupil-involving left third nerve palsy. The left eye has complete ptosis **(A)**, defective upgaze **(B)**, absent adduction **(C)**, a down and out position in primary gaze with a large unreactive pupil **(D)**, intact abduction **(E)**, and deficient downgaze **(F)**. (From Liu GT: Disorders of the eyes and eyelids: Disorders of eye movements. In Samuels MA, Feske S (eds): The Office Practice of Neurology, p 53. New York, Churchill Livingstone, 1996, with permission.)

sies include trauma, meningitis, stroke, and mass lesion at the base of the skull. In children the most common cause of acquired third nerve palsy is trauma. This section will discuss other clinical features of third nerve palsies, then detail their various causes and workup in adults and children.

Other Clinical Features of Third Nerve Palsies

Complete versus Incomplete (or Partial). These terms refer to the extent of involvement of the eyelid and third nerve innervated extraocular muscles. These are nonlocalizing. Palsies of individual muscles can occur as a result of lesions at any level of the nerve.[101, 102]

Pupil Involvement versus Sparing. If the pupil is mydriatic and less reactive to light compared to the pupil of the fellow eye, it is said to be "involved." A normally reactive pupil that is the same size as the pupil of the fellow eye is "spared." These features are nonlocalizing.

Inferior versus Superior Division. As alluded to earlier, the third nerve divides into two divisions in the anterior cavernous sinus, so divisional ocular paresis classically localizes to this region or to the posterior orbit. However, examples of fascicular[103, 104] and subarachnoid[105] lesions causing involvement of third nerve inferior or superior division innervated muscles have been described.

Aberrant Regeneration. Patients with traumatic or chronic compressive third nerve palsies may develop *aberrant regeneration, misdirection,* or *synkinesis.* Common abnormal patterns include lid elevation during adduction or depression of the eye (pseudo-Graefe phenomenon) (Fig. 15–19) or depression and miosis of a pupil unreactive to light during adduction (see Fig. 13–12).[106, 107] Pupillary findings are discussed in more detail in Chapter 13. Less common patterns include defective vertical eye movements with retraction of the globe upon attempted vertical deviations, adduction of the eye during attempted vertical movement,[108] and transient synkinesis.[109, 110] Aberrant regeneration is not observed after microvascular ischemic nerve palsies, and in the absence of trauma, its presence should heighten suspicion for a compressive lesion.

Primary (spontaneous) and secondary (acquired) aberrant regeneration are usually considered separately because of their etiologic

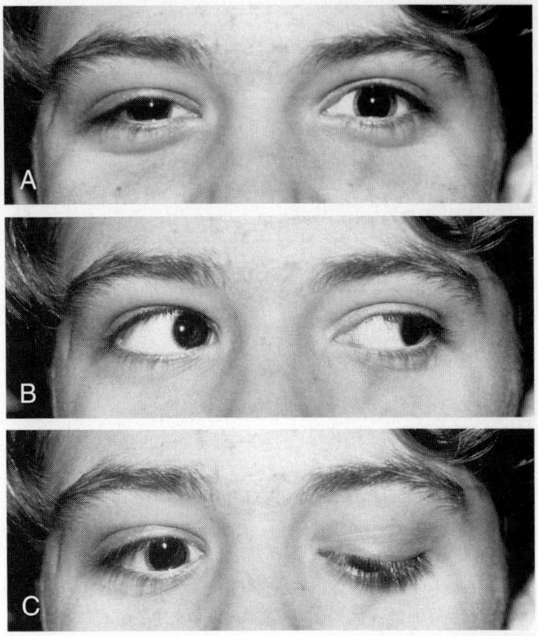

FIGURE 15–19. Aberrant regeneration of eyelid innervation in partially recovered traumatic right third nerve palsy. In primary gaze the right eyelid is ptotic **(A)**, but the right eyelid elevates in adduction **(B)** and in attempted downgaze **(C)**. The pupils had been dilated pharmacologically.

implications. The synkinesis is the first manifestation of third nerve dysfunction in primary aberrant regeneration. This type, manifesting as a ptotic eyelid that elevates in adduction or depression of the eye, is usually associated with expanding lesions in or around the cavernous sinus such as intracavernous meningiomas,[111–114] aneurysms,[114, 115] pituitary tumors,[108] and other extracavernous masses.[116, 117] On the other hand, secondary aberrant regeneration occurs in the recovery phase several weeks after an acute third nerve palsy due to trauma,[118] ophthalmoplegic migraine,[114, 119] pituitary apoplexy[110] (see Fig. 13–12), or inflammation,[109, 120] for instance.

In one purported mechanism, damaged, regenerating axons follow alternate pathways within the nerve sheath to innervate targets distinct from their original destination. Lid elevation in adduction would then be explained by misdirected third nerve fibers for the medial rectus muscle incorrectly innervating the levator muscle. Similarly, miosis during adduction could be attributed to medial rectus fibers mistakenly innervating the pupillary sphincter. However, cases of spontaneous and transient synkinesis might argue against hardwired misdirection. Alternative explanations include

(1) ephaptic transmission, a cross-talk between adjacent injured and intact nerve fibers, and (2) central synaptic reorganization within the oculomotor subnuclei.[114, 121]

Cyclic Oculomotor Spasms. In this eye movement disorder, a complete or third nerve palsy alternates with brief spasms of the third nerve innervated structures.[122] Often heralded by eyelid twitches,[123] the spastic phase is characterized by pupillary miosis, lid elevation, and adduction and depression of the eye. The condition is usually unilateral, persists during sleep, and persists for the lifetime of the patient.[123] Most cases are seen in congenital third nerve palsies, but rarely third nerve compression may be implicated.[124] Alternating phases of aberrant regeneration of the third nerve with an intermittent conduction block has been a proposed mechanism.[124]

Causes of third nerve palsies and their accompanying clinical features are discussed by location in the following sections.

Intra-axial Lesions

Nuclear Third Nerve Palsy. The classical unilateral lesion of the third nerve nucleus results in bilateral ptosis, worse ipsilaterally; ipsilateral mydriasis; ipsilateral palsy of the medial rectus, inferior rectus, and inferior oblique muscles; and bilateral superior rectus palsies. However, bilateral ptosis with various combinations of oculomotor paresis has been described from nuclear third nerve lesions.[125–133] Other cases of nuclear third nerve palsies have been described without levator involvement[134, 135] and with isolated inferior rectus palsy.[136, 137] Such patients without bilateral ptosis would be difficult to discern clinically from fascicular involvement only.

Fascicular Third Nerve Palsy. Lesions of the midbrain tegmentum can affect the oculomotor nerve fascicles as they travel ventrally, and are often associated with "crossed" neurologic signs.[138] Involvement of the fascicle as it passes through the crossing dentatorubrothalamic fibers produces an ipsilateral oculomotor palsy and contralateral ataxia (*Claude syndrome*) (Fig. 15–20). A lesion of the cerebral peduncle results in ipsilateral oculomotor palsy and contralateral hemiparesis (*Weber syndrome*), and a larger process also involving the red nucleus can cause the same findings plus contralateral involuntary limb movements or tremor (*Benedikt syndrome*). Third nerve palsy accompanied

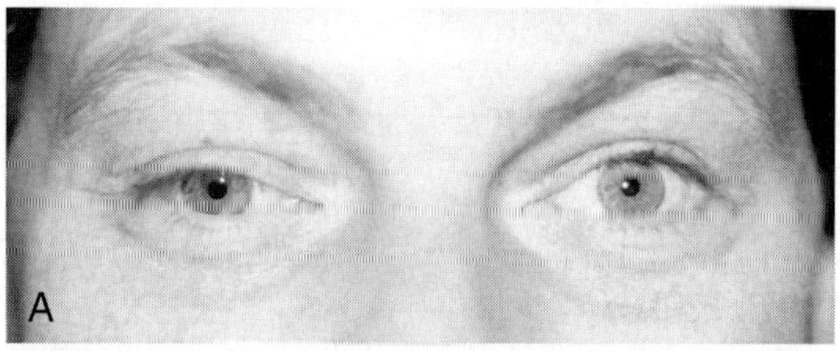

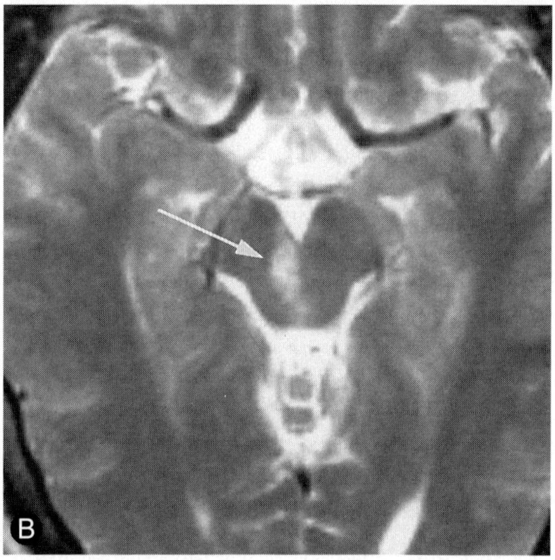

FIGURE 15–20. Fascicular right third nerve palsy **(A)** and contralateral ataxia (Claude syndrome) due to paramedian midbrain infarction (*arrow*) seen on T_2-weighted axial MRI **(B)**.

by vertical gaze paresis, lid retraction, skew deviation, and convergence retraction saccades would be suggestive of a dorsal midbrain process, as in the top of the basilar syndrome (see Chapter 16).[139] In this setting, emboli to the posterior cerebral arteries may also result in a homonymous hemianopsia and visual hallucinations. Secondary diencephalic lesions may cause additional memory disturbances, behavioral changes, and altered consciousness.

Fascicular oculomotor palsies may also be isolated,[140] and either pupil involvement or sparing may occur.[141–143] In incomplete oculomotor palsies, the pattern of ophthalmoplegia often reflects the topographical arrangement of the fibers to each extraocular muscle within the fascicle (see Fig. 15–5).[144–146] Divisional pareses may occur,[104, 147] and uncommonly, individual muscles may be affected.[148]

The usual cause of a nuclear or fascicular oculomotor palsy is infarction in the territory of a mesencephalic paramedian penetrating vessel arising from the proximal posterior cerebral artery,[149, 150] but other causes include metastatic tumors,[151] vascular malformations,[152, 153] abscesses,[154] cysts,[147] and multiple sclerosis.[155–158]

Subarachnoid Processes

Uncal Herniation. A third nerve palsy accompanied by altered mental status should suggest uncal herniation.[159] Ipsilateral pupillary dilation may be the first sign of transtentorial uncal herniation before other signs of third nerve paresis develop. In this setting, mechanisms for third nerve dysfunction include direct compression by the herniating uncus beneath the tentorial edge (Kernohan's notch) (Fig. 15–21), compression by the posterior cerebral artery or hippocampal gyrus, compression of the oculomotor complex in the midbrain, or displacement and kinking of the nerve over the clivus.[160] As the syndrome progresses with a decrease in level of consciousness, the third nerve palsy may become complete along with signs of ipsilateral hemiplegia and extensor plantar response (due to contralateral compression of the cerebral peduncle). Further clinical progression may be monitored by examining the opposite pupil, which initially may be mid-position with a depressed light reaction, then slightly miotic, then finally dilated.[161] Transiently the pupils may acquire an oval shape.[162] Uncommonly in transtentorial herniation, the opposite pupil is paradoxically the first to dilate.[163]

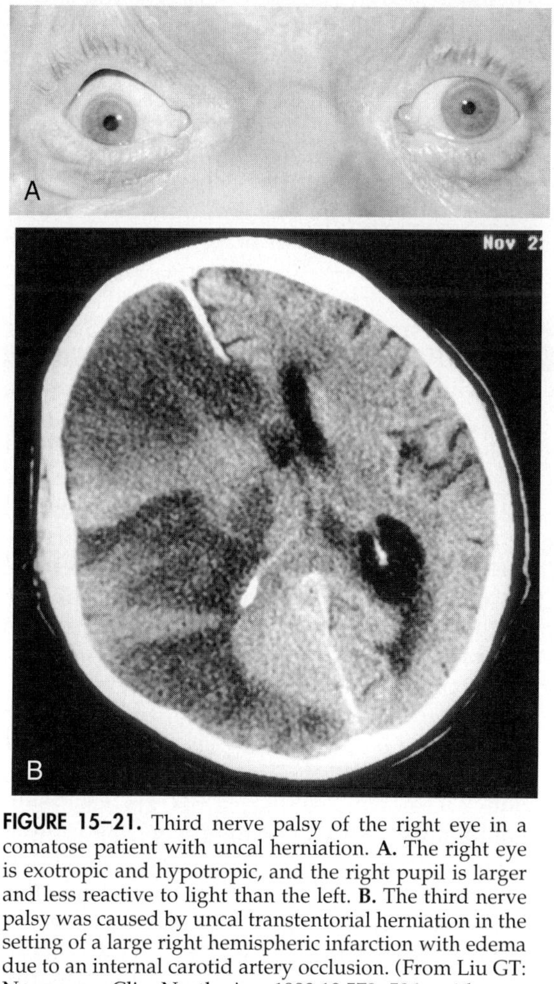

FIGURE 15–21. Third nerve palsy of the right eye in a comatose patient with uncal herniation. **A.** The right eye is exotropic and hypotropic, and the right pupil is larger and less reactive to light than the left. **B.** The third nerve palsy was caused by uncal transtentorial herniation in the setting of a large right hemispheric infarction with edema due to an internal carotid artery occlusion. (From Liu GT: Neurosurg Clin North Am 1999;10:579–586, with permission.)

Posterior Communicating Artery Aneurysms. Within the subarachnoid space, posterior communicating artery (PCoA) aneurysms may compress the third nerve (Fig. 15–22), almost always causing pupillary dilation. Aneurysms arising from the base of the PCoA as it emerges from the internal corotid artery are the second most common aneurysm in the anterior circle of Willis. In one study,[164] 34% of patients with a PCoA developed a third nerve palsy. However, greater than 90% of patients with PCoA aneurysms and subarachnoid hemorrhage present with symptoms of a third nerve palsy prior to rupture.[165–167] PCoA aneurysms and internal carotid artery aneurysms commonly project posterolaterally to compress the oculomotor nerve as it travels between the brain stem and cavernous sinus (Fig. 15–23).

The third nerve palsy resulting from aneurysmal compression is usually painful and complete.[168] Because of the dorsomedial location of the pupillomotor fibers in the oculomo-

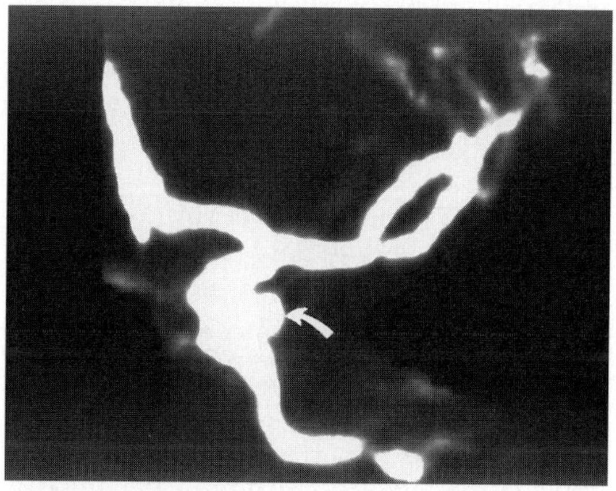

FIGURE 15–22. Posterior communicating artery aneurysm (*arrow*) demonstrated on MRI-angiography, lateral view. The patient presented with an acute, painful, pupil-involving complete third nerve palsy.

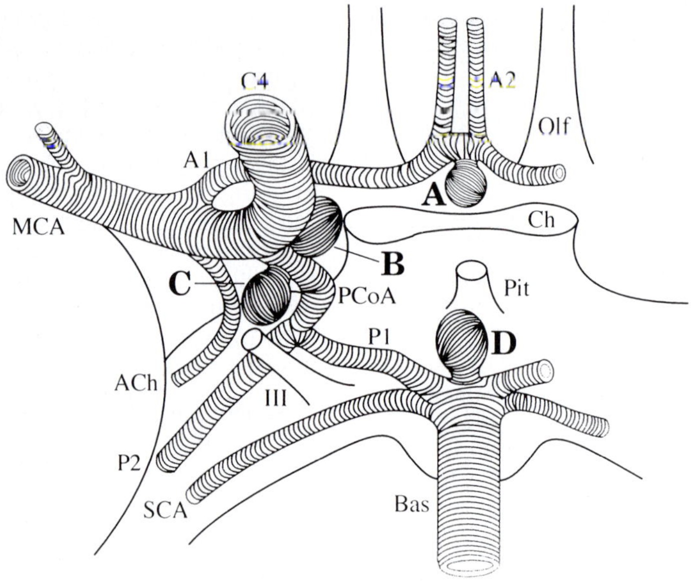

FIGURE 15–23. Drawing of the posterior communicating artery and other common aneurysms in the circle of Willis. **A.** Anterior communicating artery aneurysm. **B.** Internal carotid artery aneurysm. **C.** Posterior communicating artery aneurysm (PCoA, note its proximity to the third nerve (III)). **D.** Basilar artery tip aneurysm. A1, A2 = anterior cerebral artery segments; Ach = anterior choroidal artery; Bas = basilar artery; C4 = internal carotid artery, supraclinoid portion; MCA = middle cerebral artery; Olf = olfactory nerve; Pit = pituitary stalk; and P1, P2 = posterior cerebral artery segments. (Courtesy of Dr. Jeffrey Bennett.)

tor nerve bundle, aneurysmal compression often involves the pupil early, even before complete ophthalmoparesis. However, pupil sparing may occur,[169] and in one study,[170] 14% of third nerve palsies due to PCoA aneurysms presented with normal pupils and partial motility deficits, but pupillary mydriasis developed within days in most of those cases. Rare oculomotor presentations of PCoA aneurysms include isolated ptosis,[171] ptosis and mydriasis,[172] pupillary light-near dissociation,[173, 174] dorsal midbrain syndrome,[175] and transient third nerve palsies.[176] Visual loss[177, 178] may occur, and the pattern observed with PCoA aneurysms depends on the anterior pathway structure that is compressed: optic nerve, chiasm, or tract.[177, 179]

Treatment. Treatment of PCoA aneurysms should not be unduly delayed. After rupture, 60% of untreated PCoA aneurysms rebleed within 6 months. Treatment is generally surgical clipping.[180] Endovascular embolization and carotid occlusion offer alternatives to those patients unable to undergo surgical repair. Prior to surgery, it is important to assess fully the potential collateral circulation in the anterior circle of Willis and to examine the flow through the PCoA from the vertebrobasilar circulation.[181] The most significant complication of aneurysm surgery is ischemic stroke, due either to compromise of a dominant PCoA artery or to interruption of circulation through adjacent vessels. Third nerve palsies can worsen after surgical repair as a consequence of aneurysm thrombosis or iatrogenic manipulation. Recent advances in endovascular approaches, particularly coil embolization, have resulted in a higher success rate and lower frequency of acute bleeding in the treatment of ruptured and unruptured aneurysms of the anterior circulation. A lower success rate is still encountered with giant aneurysms, particularly those with broad necks.[182] While over half of the patients may have reduction in the size of the aneurysm, the risk of rupture 6 months after therapy remains equivalent to conservative management.[183]

After treatment of PCoA aneurysms, the recovery of the third nerve palsy is inconsistent and often slow.[164, 184] Diplopia, residual ptosis, and occasionally photophobia are the main complaints, and aberrant regeneration is often seen.[185] Some authors[164, 185] have suggested that patients who are treated within 10 days after onset of oculomotor dysfunction appear to have the best chance for recovery of third nerve function. Others[186] have reported that only the severity of the palsy was predictive, as those with incomplete palsies seem to have a better prognosis. The initial treatment for the diplopia is with patching until the oculomotor paresis stabilizes. Afterward, use of prisms or surgical correction can be entertained. Residual ptosis can be treated with lid tape, lid crutches, or eyelid surgery. Photophobia secondary to persistent pupillary dilation can be ameliorated with pharmacologic miosis or tinted lenses.

Basilar Artery Aneurysms. Aneurysms of the basilar artery, trunk, and bifurcation are the most common aneurysms in the posterior fossa (Fig. 15–23).[187] While the most frequent presentation is subarachnoid hemorrhage, neurologic dysfunction is present in 40% of cases.[165] Cranial nerve pareses are frequent, third and fourth nerve palsies being most common.[172,188,189] Patients with third or fourth nerve pareses may develop a concurrent crossed paralysis such as a Weber syndrome if the aneurysm injures the adjacent brain stem. Typically the third nerve palsies are pupil involving, but pupil sparing third nerve palsies in this setting have been reported.[190]

Other neurologic and neuro-ophthalmic signs may develop from basilar aneurysms due to brain stem compression or concurrent thromboembolic disease. Giant saccular or fusiform aneurysms may compress the adjacent midbrain or pons. Hemiparesis or other corticospinal tract signs may or may not be evident depending on the duration of the compression. Thrombus within the basilar aneurysm may obstruct flow or embolize to nearby perforating vessels, particularly at the basilar bifurcation.[139] Basilar artery insufficiency may result from midbasilar thrombosis. On rare occasions, giant fusiform aneurysms of the basilar artery may result in obstructive hydrocephalus due to aqueductal compression.

Other Aneurysms. Posterior cerebral artery aneurysms may result in third nerve palsies by compressing the oculomotor nerve as it travels between the posterior cerebral artery and superior cerebellar artery. Giant posterior cerebral artery aneurysms can compress the optic radiations or visual cortex, producing a contralateral homonymous hemianopsia.

Treatment. Therapy for posterior fossa aneurysms is either surgical or endovascular. Both treatments are complicated by significant morbidity and mortality due to occlusion of small perforating vessels or parent vessel thrombosis.[167] For instance, clipping of basilar tip aneurysms may cause infarction in paramedian mesencephalic–thalamic perforating territories. Surgical therapy is additionally complicated by cranial nerve palsies secondary to traction. The third nerve palsy is most common, occurring in more than 60% of patients.[187] Despite the significant risk, surgical treatment is often warranted because of the even greater morbidity and mortality associated with progressive brain stem dysfunction and posterior fossa subarachnoid hemorrhage. If vessel occlusion can be tolerated in the vertebral or basilar artery, then the endovascular approach is often the safest. In certain cases of basilar artery dolicoectasia, endovascular occlusion is the only feasible approach.

Vasculopathic Third Nerve Palsies. Ischemic (vasculopathic) third nerve palsies, associated with hypertension, diabetes, advanced age, atherosclerosis, smoking, and hypercholesterolemia,[191] are often preceded by orbital ache or pain and are characterized by pupillary sparing (Fig. 15–24).[192] In our experience, the pain can be rather severe, especially in younger patients. In fact, the presence or absence of pain cannot be used to distinguish aneurysmal from vasculopathic third nerve palsies. The symptoms and signs may progress over several days.[193]

Most cases are thought to have a peripheral lesion.[194] Presumably the third nerves develop ischemia and demyelination within the subarachnoid space[195] or cavernous sinus,[21] but there may also be a small infarction of the nerve within the mesencephalon.[196] The pupil sparing in peripheral cases is attributed to the location of the pupillary fibers on the outside of the third nerve in areas less vulnerable to vascular insufficiency. However, some studies have suggested that minor pupillary involvement (less than 2 mm of anisocoria) may occur in as many as 38% of patients.[197] The pupil is rarely dilated and unreactive. The pain may be due to ischemia of trigeminal fibers within or around the oculomotor nerve,[198] but this has

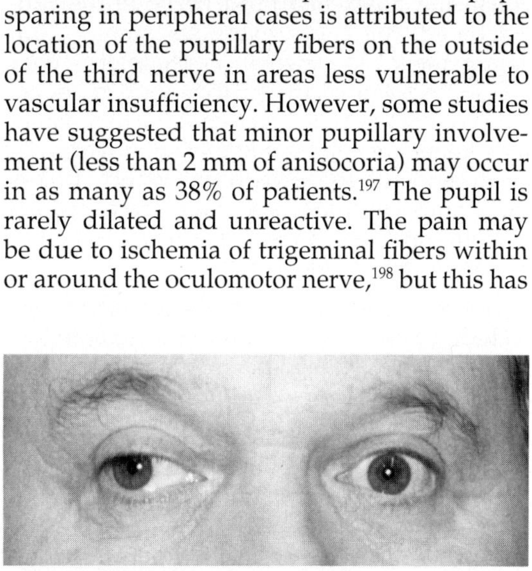

FIGURE 15–24. Right diabetic pupil-sparing third nerve palsy, which resolved spontaneously after 12 weeks.

not been confirmed. Most patients with vasculopathic oculomotor palsies recover spontaneously within 8 to 12 weeks.[199] Rarely, vasculopathic third nerve palsies may be seen in combination with fourth, sixth, and seventh nerve palsies.[200] Other causes include vasculitis due to giant cell arteritis,[201, 202] systemic lupus erythematosus,[203] and herpes zoster.

Trauma. Third nerve palsies due to trauma are typically caused by severe blows to the head,[64] often in a motor vehicle accident. The peripheral portion of the nerve may be damaged secondary to traction at the skull base or by an orbital or base of skull fracture. Alternatively, the nuclear complex or fascicle may be affected by brain stem shearing or hemorrhage.[204, 205] Alternative causes include penetrating orbital or intracranial trauma or iatrogenic trauma during removal of suprasellar or posterior fossa masses.[206, 207] Some oculomotor palsies from minor trauma are harbingers of an underlying aneurysm or mass lesion.[208, 209] The prognosis for recovery of function in most cases of traumatic third nerve palsies is very good, but often there is evidence of aberrant regeneration.

Primary Tumors of the Oculomotor Nerves.

Neurinomas and Schwannomas. Stable or slowly progressive oculomotor palsies may be caused by tumors derived from the Schwann cells surrounding the extra-axial portion of the third nerve.[210] Tumor types include neurinomas, neurofibromas, neurilemmomas, and schwanomas.[211,212] Neuroimaging typically reveals an enhancing, thickened third nerve in the subarachnoid space or cavernous sinus,[213] but enlargement to several centimeters with mass effect can occur.[214, 215] The best management of these cases is not certain. Because of their benign histology, complete removal is not necessary (although has been done)[216] unless the lesions become large enough to compress surrounding structures. It is unclear whether radiation therapy is useful.

Other Neoplasms. Uncommon considerations include primary neoplasms of the oculomotor nerve such as malignant meningioma[217] and primary glioblastoma multiforme.[218]

Other Causes of Third Nerve Palsies. Base of skull neoplasms, infectious disorders, and inflammatory disorders are discussed below in the section on combined oculomotor palsies. Less common causes include sinus mucoceles,[219–222] carotid insufficiency,[22, 223, 224] and intraneural cavernous hemangioma.[225]

Diagnostic Evaluation of Adults with Acquired Third Nerve Palsies

While many patients with acute third nerve palsies require neuroimaging or laboratory evaluation, some subgroups can be managed without further testing. General guidelines are given below, and some are based upon the age of the patient. The "rules" regarding acquired isolated (no other neurologic or ophthalmic signs) third nerve palsies are summarized in Table 15–4 and are primarily based upon the patient age and whether or not the pupil is spared.[226, 227]

In adults with acquired, isolated *pupil-involving complete or partial* third nerve palsies, a posterior communicating artery aneurysm should be excluded emergently. In this situation it is often useful to obtain an emergent computed tomography (CT) or magnetic resonance imaging (MRI) scan before proceeding with angiography since other compressive or infiltrative lesions may be found,[228] eliminating the need for an invasive procedure. However, if the scan cannot be obtained immediately, we would proceed directly to angiography. If the scan is negative, even if it includes MRI-angiography, conventional angiography is still necessary to exclude an aneurysm. Patients with third nerve palsy and PCoA aneurysms measuring 5 to 6 mm have been missed by MRI-angiography.[229] Although MRI-[227] and CT-angiographic techniques[230] continue to improve in their ability to detect small aneurysms, we are still reluctant to depend entirely on these noninvasive modalities.

Patients over 50 with vascular risk factors and isolated *complete pupil-sparing* third nerve palsies can be observed with an MRI performed only in those who worsen or fail to improve within 8 weeks.[199] Those without identified vascular risk factors should have their blood pressure and fasting glucose, lipids, and cholesterol levels measured. However, because isolated, *complete pupil-sparing* third nerve palsies can be caused by small infarcts in the mesencephalon and compressive lesions, we are gradually lowering our threshold to scan patients with isolated oculomotor palsies early in their course.

We also have a low threshold for imaging in patients with acquired, isolated, *pupil-sparing partial* third nerve palsies. However, it has also been accepted practice that such individuals can be observed serially for 1 week for evidence of pupillary involvement since most an-

TABLE 15–4. Recommendations for Neuroimaging in Adult Patients With Acquired, Isolated Third Nerve Palsies

Ophthalmoparesis	Pupil	Recommendations
Complete	Involved	CT or MRI, then angiography
Partial	Involved	CT or MRI, then angiography
Complete	Spared	Observation MRI if no improvement within 8 weeks
Partial	Spared	MRI for all such cases or: Serial observation of the pupil for 1 week MRI if no improvement within 8 weeks MRI for superior division paresis

eurysmal cases eventually develop pupillary mydriasis within days. Thus, if the pupil remains uninvolved after 1 week, an aneurysm can be considered less likely, and a vasculopathic cause can be assumed if the patient has appropriate risk factors. Patients with *superior division partial* third nerve paresis (levator and superior rectus weakness only), which is frequently associated with compressive lesions, are the exception and should undergo neuroimaging.

Processes that may mimic isolated *pupil-sparing* third nerve palsies in adults include myasthenia gravis, thyroid eye disease, and giant cell arteritis (due to muscle ischemia). When these disorders are considered, an edrophonium test, thyroid function tests, orbital neuroimaging, and erythrocyte sedimentation rate may be helpful.

We also have a low threshold for neuroimaging in patients with traumatic oculomotor palsies, even when isolated. These individuals may have a pseudo-aneurysm or posteriorly draining cavernous sinus fistula (see below). In the setting of minor trauma, an underlying aneurysm or mass lesion should be excluded.[209] Extraocular muscle entrapment resulting from orbital wall fracture may mimic an oculomotor palsy.

Meningeal processes also should be considered in patients with oculomotor palsies, especially when they occur bilaterally or in combination, and when other cranial nerves or nerve roots are involved. MRI with gadolinium may disclose meningeal enhancement. Cerebrospinal fluid (CSF) examination, including cultures and cytology, should be performed to exclude acute bacterial and chronic fungal meningitis, tuberculosis, syphilis, Lyme disease, sarcoidosis, and carcinomatous or lymphomatous meningitis. In oculomotor palsies due to Guillain–Barré syndrome, the Fisher variant, or chronic inflammatory demyelinating polyneuropathy, the CSF protein should be elevated.

Management of Third Nerve Palsy

The management of patients with third nerve dysfunction is the most complicated of all forms of paretic strabismus. This results from the potential involvement of four muscles and a complex pattern of extraocular muscle dysfunction. All decisions concerning the management of patients with third nerve palsy are divided into those that are recommended acutely and those recommended chronically when there is a fixed deficit. As with other patients with the acute onset of double vision, after a diagnosis has been established, monocular occlusion and prisms can be used. In certain cases botulinum toxin can be injected into the lateral rectus muscle, thereby eliminating the horizontal deviation and alleviating diplopia (occasionally with the aid of vertical prisms).[231, 232] Once the palsy has been determined to be chronic and measurements have been stable for at least 6 months (preferably 12 months), various surgical strategies can be used to attempt to achieve realignment in the primary position and occasionally a useful field of single binocular vision.[231–238]

For the purpose of treatment, patients with third nerve palsies may be separated into two broad categories. The first are those with total third nerve palsies, and the second are those with partial third nerve palsies. In the setting of complete third nerve palsy, only realignment in the primary position can be hoped for. This can be accomplished through a supramaximal lateral rectus recession. The goal here should be to abolish abduction completely by placing the lateral rectus muscle posterior to the equator. This procedure can be combined with a medial rectus resection, which may act as a tether, holding the eye in the primary position. When not combined with lateral rectus recession, medial rectus resection is ineffective in the long run. In the setting of a complete third nerve palsy, the surgeon must also consider the primary position ptosis. Many authorities believe that in the setting of complete ptosis, repair of the extraocular muscle alignment is not indicated.

The examiner should also look carefully for evidence of aberrant regeneration, resulting in anomalous eyelid movements, particularly with adduction. In this setting, eye muscle surgery may improve the variable ptosis. If functioning, the superior oblique muscle can also be resected and transposed to the area between the medial rectus and superior rectus to create an adducting force.[237,239] The placement of traction sutures attaching the eye to the medial eyelid (done in conjunction with recession/resection) may improve the long-range results and center the eye in some patients with complete third nerve palsy.[238] In patients with partial ptosis, correction of ptosis can allow for improved binocularity. If ptosis is complete and correction is attempted, the risk of corneal exposure is significant. Patients must be warned that although there may be significant cosmetic benefit from realignment of the eyes, the potential for more disabling diplopia exists as the images are brought closer together. At this point an occlusive contact lens can be used to achieve a reasonable cosmetic and functional result.

In patients with a partial third nerve palsy, further options exist, and surgery should be tailored to the particular patient problem. For instance, if there is isolated involvement of either elevation or depression, a resection of the involved vertical muscle combined with a weakening procedure of the contralateral yoke muscle (using adjustable sutures) may be successful in achieving a field of single binocular vision. In some patients in whom partial dysfunction of both the superior rectus and inferior rectus produces primary position alignment, a posterior fixation suture (which does not change the eye position in primary gaze but causes weakness in the muscle's field of action) may be performed on the contralateral eye. This matches the weakness and increases the field of single binocular vision. In patients with isolated adduction deficits, medial rectus resection may be combined with contralateral lateral rectus recession with or without a posterior fixation suture to increase the field of single binocular vision. Various combinations of these procedures (strengthening the partially paretic muscles and weakening the contralateral yoke muscles) may be used effectively in many patients with partial third nerve palsies. Occasionally in the absence of inferior rectus function, a horizontal recession/resection can be combined with transposition of the insertions inferiorly to provide downward movement of the eye.[232,240] In patients without medial rectus function but intact inferior and superior rectus function, a transposition procedure may be performed, moving the superior rectus and inferior rectus muscles to the insertion of the medial rectus muscle.

Considerations in Children With Third Nerve Palsies[241]

Third nerve palsies in childhood may be congenital or acquired (Table 15–5). Almost every pediatric series has shown that the most common cause of an acquired third nerve palsy in this age group is trauma.[33,241–247] Neoplasms, inflammatory disorders, and ophthalmoplegic migraine should also be considered. Isolated third nerve palsies due to PCoA aneurysms and vasculopathic causes are rare in children, so the management "rules" outlined above for adults are not applicable.[248]

Congenital Third Nerve Palsies. In Miller's series of isolated third nerve palsies in pediatric patients,[242] 43% were congenital in origin (Fig. 15–25). Most had pupillary involvement, aberrant regeneration, and amblyopia, and some went on to develop the phenomenon of oculomotor paresis with cyclic spasms. Forty percent of third nerve palsies in Harley's series[243] were also congenital, but in other studies[244,245] and in the Children's Hospital of Philadelphia (CHOP) series, they were seen less frequently. Monocular elevator palsies were grouped as congenital third nerve palsies in some series.[243]

Prior to the advent of modern neuroimaging, in most cases the responsible lesion was thought to be peripheral, due to birth trauma (skull molding) for instance, as suggested by the isolated nature of the third nerve palsy and the high frequency of aberrant regeneration.[249] However, Balkan and Hoyt[250] reported 10 patients with congenital third nerve palsies, of whom 4 had focal neurologic abnormalities (eg, hemiparesis) and 2 had developmental delay. They and subsequent authors[251–256] suggested that in some instances, congenital third nerve palsies may result from brain stem injury or reflect more widespread neurologic damage. Indeed, various autopsy studies have demonstrated aplasia of the ocular motor nuclei[257] or malformation of the mid-

TABLE 15–5. Causes of Third Nerve Palsies in Children

	Miller[242] 1977 (1951–76)	Harley[243] 1980 (1968–79)	Keith[244] 1987 (1974–85)	Ing[245] 1992 (1970–91)	Kodsi[246] 1992 (1966–88)	CHOP[241]† 1999 (1993–96)	Sch. Feer.[247] 1999 (1981–96)
Congenital	13	15	8	8/(3)*	not included	4	20
Trauma	6	4	7	20/(11)	14	5/(5)	15
Neoplasm	3	3	1	1/(1)	5	5/(2)	6
Inflammatory	4	3	6	6/(1)	1	3/(3)	3
Migraine	2	3	1	2	3	1	
Aneurysm	2	0	0	0	0	0/(1)	
Surgical	0	0	0	0	3	1	
Idiopathic	0	0	4	1	6	0	1
Other	2	4	1	0	3	1/(1)‡	4
Total	30	32	28	38/(16)	35	20/(12)	49

* When two figures are given, the first number refers to the number of isolated third nerve palsies in that category, while the number in parentheses refers to number of patients seen with a third nerve palsy combined with a fourth or sixth nerve palsy or both.
† The CHOP series represents third nerve palsies seen by the authors at the Children's Hospital of Philadelphia during one 3 year period.
‡ Mesencephalic arteriovenous malformation, hydrocephalus.

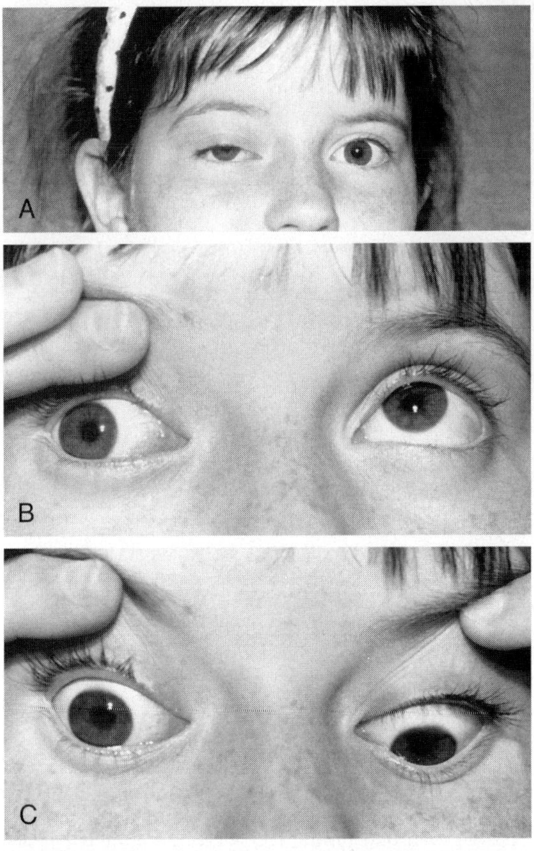

FIGURE 15–25. Pupil-sparing congenital right third nerve palsy. **A.** Primary gaze with right ptosis and head turn. Upgaze **(B)**, downgaze **(C)**, and adduction (not shown) were defective.

brain,[258] reflective of an in-utero insult to the central nervous system (CNS). MRI scans now readily confirm midbrain damage in many cases.[252, 259, 260]

Miscellaneous Common Acquired Causes

Inflammatory (Including Infections). Pneumococcal and *Haemophilus influenzae* meningitis have been associated with third nerve palsies in children.[242, 245] In addition, in the CHOP series an isolated third nerve palsy was caused by tuberculous meningitis, and combined palsies were seen in association with Lyme meningitis[261] and Miller Fisher syndrome. Rarely Tolosa–Hunt syndrome occurs in childhood[262] and can mimic ophthalmoplegic migraine (see below).[263]

Neoplasms. Posterior fossa tumors occur more frequently in children than in adults. However, these neoplasms tend to affect the pons and medulla, causing sixth nerve palsies more commonly (see below). When tumor-related third nerve palsies occur, lesions affecting the midbrain (eg, astrocytomas or higher-grade gliomas),[264] orbit, orbital apex (eg, rhabdomyosarcomas), and leptomeninges may be implicated.[242, 243] Schwannomas, neurinomas, and meningiomas of the oculomotor nerve may also be seen childhood.[265]

Ophthalmoplegic Migraine. In children, third nerve palsies can accompany vascular headaches in so-called ophthalmoplegic migraine. Any ocular motor nerve can be involved, but isolated third nerve paresis is by far the most common, occurring in approximately 95% of cases. Sixth nerve palsies are the next most common, but fourth nerve palsies are hardly ever seen.[266] The third nerve palsy in ophthalmoplegic migraine is usually pupil involving, and complete resolution over weeks is the rule. However, aberrant regeneration can occur in some instances,[119] and after multiple attacks, the motility deficits may heal only incompletely. We have seen a child who became progressively more exotropic with each attack, which occurred yearly for 3 years (Fig. 15–26).

Ophthalmoplegic migraine is a rare form of complicated migraine. The disorder was found in only 0.1% of children with migraine seen over an 18-year period in one institution,[267] and in only 8 of 5000 migraineurs in another study.[268] The first attack usually occurs before the child is 10 years of age, sometimes in infancy,[269, 270] and uncommonly after age 20. Ipsilateral headache or periorbital pain usually precedes the ophthalmoparesis, sometimes by days, and young children often exhibit irritability and pallor in addition to nausea and vomiting.[271] Attacks, usually separated by months or years, are almost always in the same eye and involve the same ocular motor nerve each time.

The diagnosis is one of exclusion, following normal neuroimaging, lumbar puncture, and blood studies, but is suggested by a personal or family history of migraine. Once the individual has had several recurrent, self-limited third nerve palsies over a period of years, with normal investigations and normal health be-

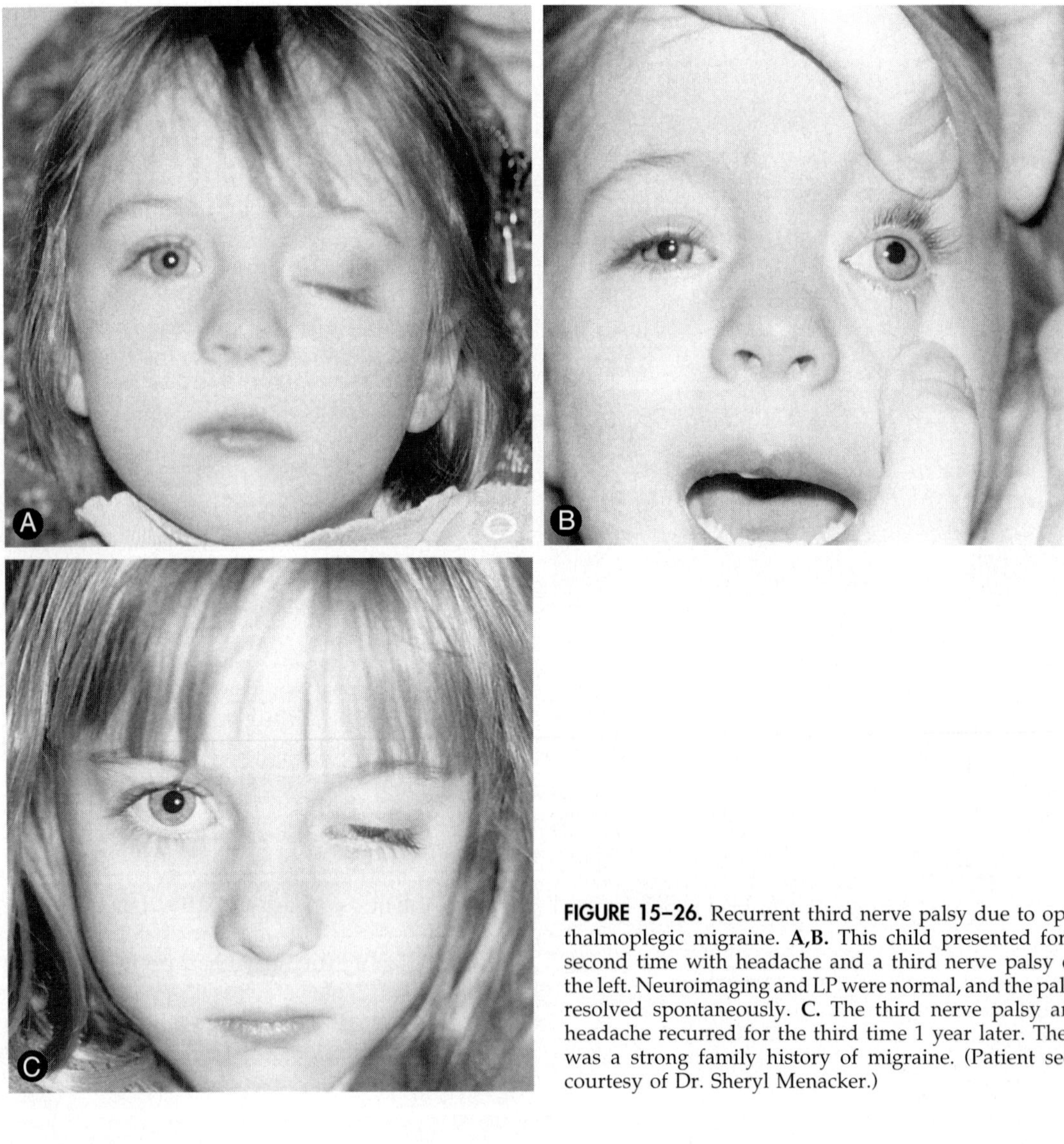

FIGURE 15–26. Recurrent third nerve palsy due to ophthalmoplegic migraine. **A,B.** This child presented for a second time with headache and a third nerve palsy on the left. Neuroimaging and LP were normal, and the palsy resolved spontaneously. **C.** The third nerve palsy and headache recurred for the third time 1 year later. There was a strong family history of migraine. (Patient seen courtesy of Dr. Sheryl Menacker.)

tween events, the diagnosis is more obvious. There have been reports of patients with migraine, a painful third nerve palsy, and gadolinium enhancement of the proximal portion of the nerve in the subarachnoid space.[272–275] Whether these cases might also be considered a variant of Tolosa–Hunt syndrome is unclear.

Etiology. Compression of the ocular motor nerves against the lateral wall of the cavernous sinus by an edematous or dilated cavernous carotid has been a popular although unproven explanation for ophthalmoplegia in migraine.[276] Arteriography is more frequently normal than abnormal. Alternatively, ischemia of the third nerve, due to insufficiency of one of the feeding arteries arising from the internal carotid, has been proposed.[277]

Treatment. Patients have been treated with ergotomines, corticosteroids, and propranolol, however, no abortive medication has actually been proven beneficial, as most patients' oculomotor palsies spontaneously resolve. Prophylaxis may not be ideal in young children in whom the attacks may be separated by months or years. There are too few cases to study any drug's efficacy formally. One approach is to treat the headache symptomatically, allow the motility deficit to improve spontaneously, and avoid prophylactic therapy.

Miscellaneous Uncommon Acquired Causes

Aneurysms. Intracranial aneurysms are uncommon in childhood. Of 5627 ruptured aneurysms reported in two large series,[278, 279] only 99 (2%) occurred in the pediatric age group (19 years of age or less).

Isolated third nerve palsies due to PCoA aneurysms are extraordinarily infrequent in childhood. In the pediatric series[242–246] only two such patients, ages 16 and 17 were reported by Miller.[242] Younger patients have been the subject of single case reports by Gabianelli et al (14 years old),[280] Wolin and Saunders (11 years old),[281] Mehkri et al (10 years old),[282] Branley (7 years old),[283] and Ebner (6 years old).[284] The first two had CT scans that missed the PCoA aneurysm, which was later confirmed on conventional angiography.

Fox,[285] in his editorial accompanying the article by Gabianelli et al, [280] mentioned a 6-year-old with a third nerve palsy due to a giant cavernous carotid aneurysm. A 4-year-old with bilateral third nerve palsies owing to bilateral giant saccular cavernous carotid artery aneurysms has been reported.[286] We have seen a 5-year-old boy who presented with a sudden third, fourth, and sixth nerve palsy and optic neuropathy (orbital apex syndrome) due to a similar aneurysm, which was embolized. A 10-month-old child developed an isolated adduction deficit 7 days prior to fatal rupture of a congenital distal basilar artery aneurysm.[189]

Diabetes. For unclear reasons, diabetic cranial mononeuropathies are very rare in children. Grunt et al.[287] reported three such patients, but each had features that were atypical. A 12-year-old boy had a purported sixth nerve palsy, but an ophthalmologist diagnosed hyperopia with accommodative esotropia, and this coincided with temporary hyperglycemia. The "left internal strabismus" in this patient improved when the refractive error and insulin requirement resolved. The second patient was a 13-year-old with a complete, pupil-sparing third nerve palsy, which did not resolve fully after 21 months of follow-up. The third patient was an 11-year-old with a partial, pupil-involving third nerve palsy which lasted 16 months until strabismus surgery was performed.

Diagnostic Evaluation in Children With Third Nerve Palsies. One suggested approach is outlined in Table 15–6. In children with congenital third nerve palsies present since birth, a careful neurologic examination should be performed, looking for other associated neurologic abnormalities. Then MRI of the brain should be ordered to exclude congenital brain malformations.

When the third nerve palsy is acquired, a history of trauma or migraine should be excluded. In all acquired cases, MRI and MRI-angiography should be performed, looking for mesencephalic, cavernous sinus, or orbital lesions, and to exclude an aneurysm. We dis-

TABLE 15–6. Pediatric Third Nerve Palsies: Suggested Workup

Congenital
Careful neurologic examination
MRI of the brain
Acquired
Exclude history of trauma or migraine
MRI and MRI-angiography
Consider LP if the neuroimaging is negative
If MRI and LP negative, consider ophthalmoplegic migraine
If MRI and LP are negative in a patient 10 years of age or older, consider conventional angiography

agree that some children with acquired, isolated third nerve palsies can be watched conservatively.[288] If the neuroimaging is negative and the child is ill appearing or has a fever or stiff neck, a lumbar puncture (LP) should be performed to exclude meningitis. If the MRI and LP are negative, a diagnosis of ophthalmoplegic migraine can be entertained. Finally, if the MRI and LP are negative in a patient 10 years of age or above, practitioners should consider conventional angiography to exclude a PCoA aneurysm.[241]

FOURTH NERVE PALSIES

Patients with superior oblique paresis complain of vertical diplopia, often with a torsional component, and they have an ipsilateral hypertropia worse on contraversive (contralateral conjugate) horizontal gaze and ipsilateral head tilt (Parks' three-step test, best demonstrated with alternate cover or Maddox Rod testing) (Fig. 15–27). In some instances the superior oblique weakness is evident on testing

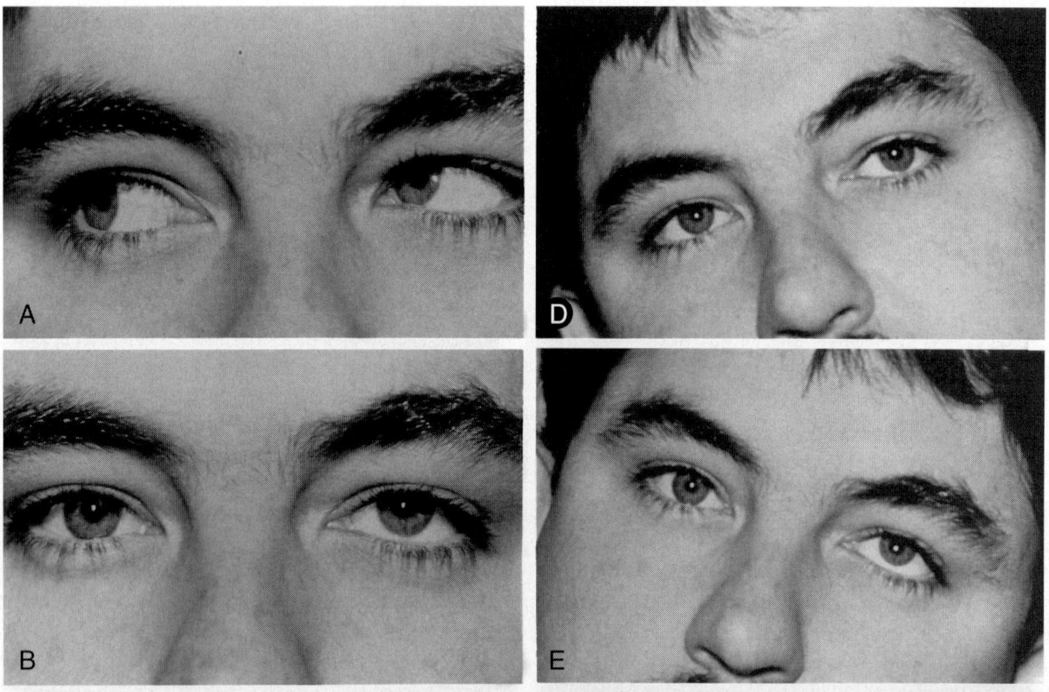

FIGURE 15–27. Traumatic left fourth nerve palsy, three-step test. **A.** Right gaze. **B.** Primary gaze. **C.** Left gaze. **D.** Right head tilt. **E.** Left head tilt. **F.** Preference for a right head turn (left gaze) and right head tilt, which minimizes the patient's vertical diplopia. *Step 1:* which eye is hypertropic (left—see B); *Step 2:* is the hypertropia worse in left or right gaze (right—see A vs. C); *Step 3:* is the hypertropia worse in left or right head tilt (left—see E vs. D). The *left* hypertropia, which is worse in *right* gaze and *left* head tilt, is consistent with weakness of the left superior oblique muscle. (From Liu GT: Disorders of the eyes and eyelids: Disorders of eye movements. In Samuels MA, Feske S (eds): The Office Practice of Neurology, p 54. New York, Churchill Livingstone, 1996, with permission.)

of ductions (Fig. 15–28), but more commonly alternate cover or Maddox rod testing is necessary to document the misalignment. In unilateral cases, excyclotorsion of the involved eye may be documented using double Maddox rods.[289] Head tilt toward the contralateral shoulder is usually seen (Fig. 15–28). One can occasionally elicit which fourth nerve is affected by asking the patient to look at a horizontal straight edge such as a door, projector screen, or pen. If the patient sees two images, he can be asked to describe how they intersect. A patient with a unilateral fourth nerve palsy will see a horizontal line and a tilted line below it, intersecting on the side of abnormal eye ("the arrow points to the affected fourth nerve").

Trauma is one of the most common causes of acquired fourth nerve palsies (Table 15–2).[30, 290–292] Traumatic fourth nerve palsies have been attributed to damage to the posterior decussation (anterior medullary vellum) due to its close anatomic relationship with the tentorium. Contusions in this area may be seen on neuroimaging. This is the likely explanation for the high incidence of bilateral fourth nerve palsies in trauma. Alternatively, skull base fractures may be responsible for traumatic fourth nerve palsies.

Decompensated congenital fourth nerve palsies are also common, and are discussed in more detail below. Ischemic fourth nerve palsies should be considered when an individual over 50 with vasculopathic risk factors develops vertical diplopia and periorbital ache. These patients may be observed, and the prognosis for spontaneous recovery is excellent. MR scanning can be performed if there is no improvement within 8 weeks. Aneurysmal causes of fourth nerve palsies[293] are much less common than in third nerve weakness. Other less frequent causes of fourth nerve palsies include neoplasms,[294] meningitis, multiple sclerosis,[158, 295] midbrain hemorrhages,[296, 297] vascular malformation,[298] giant cell arteritis,[299] schwannomas and neurinomas,[212, 214, 300] and anterior temporal lobectomy for epilepsy.[301]

Occasionally fourth nerve palsies are accompanied by other neurologic signs that aid in localization. For instance, a fourth nerve palsy accompanied by a contralateral Horner syndrome would localize to the dorsal pontomesencephalic junction (see Chapter 13).[302] A fourth nerve palsy with contralateral dysmetria suggests a lesion involving the superior cerebellar peduncle,[303] while one accompanied by contralateral internuclear ophthalmoplegia localizes to the proximal fascicle and MLF.[304]

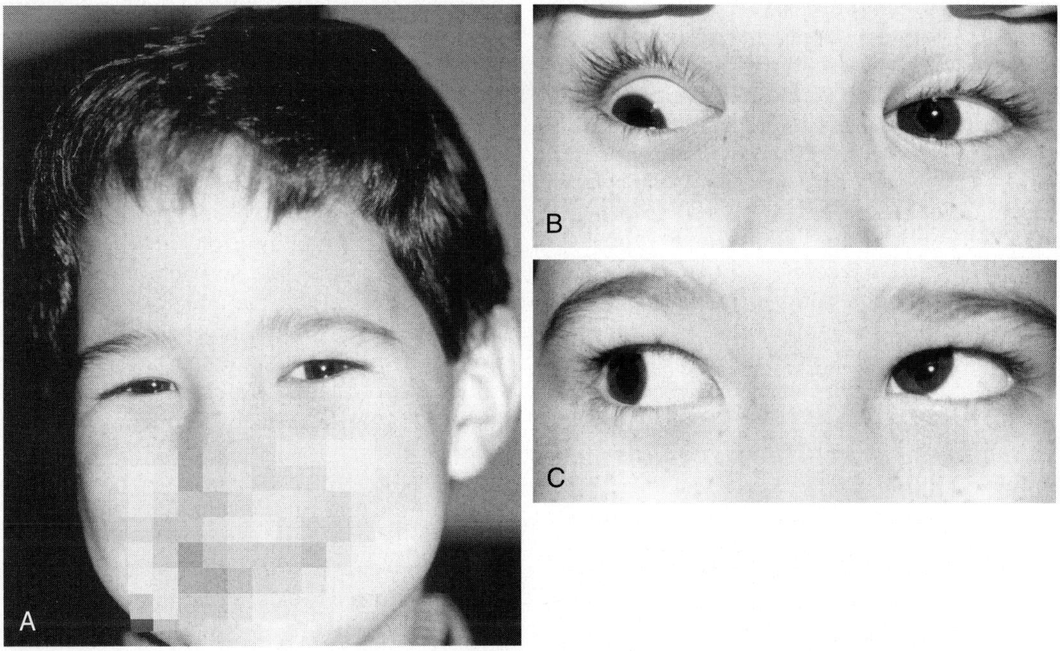

FIGURE 15–28. Congenital left fourth nerve palsy causing **(A)** spontaneous head tilt and turn to the right. **B.** The left eye had defective ductions in the inferomedial direction. Ductions down and to the right were normal (not shown). **C.** In horizontal gaze to the right, the left eye elevates, consistent with left inferior oblique overaction. This reflects the long-standing nature of the fourth nerve palsy.

When considering the diagnosis of fourth nerve palsy, mimickers such as myasthenia gravis, thyroid-associated ophthalmopathy, and skew deviation should be excluded.

Decompensated Congenital Fourth Nerve Palsies. Most of these patients present with head tilt or insidious onset of intermittent vertical double vision. Torsional complaints are less frequent than in cases of acquired fourth nerve palsy. Alternatively, a friend or family member may notice a vertical separation of the eyes. Additional overaction of the ipsilateral inferior oblique muscle in adduction is usually evident on examination (Fig. 15–28). Some authors[291] prefer to call these palsies "cryptogenic" or "idiopathic" because the cause is unclear. The congenital nature of the lesion is presumed, based upon the often-long-standing head tilt, as evidenced by review of old photographs and a family member's report, and the absence of an inciting event. Evidence of chronicity includes overaction of the ipsilateral inferior oblique muscle and a large vertical fusional amplitude. The latter refers to the patient's ability to fuse vertically separated images despite the placement of progressively larger amounts of vertical prism over one eye. Facial asymmetries are also frequently associated with the long-standing head tilt.[305]

Proposed causes for congenital fourth nerve palsies include hypoplasia or aplasia of the fourth nerve nucleus, birth trauma to the fourth nerve or superior oblique muscle, anomalous insertion of the muscle, muscle fibrosis, fibrous adhesions,[291] or structural abnormalities of the superior oblique tendon.[306] Usually congenital cases are sporadic. However, familial cases[307–309] and those associated with CNS abnormalities[310] have been reported. Decompensated congenital fourth nerve palsies are likely the result of progressive breakdown in vertical fusional capability rather than progression of fourth nerve weakness.[291]

Management of Fourth Nerve Palsy

Some patients can be treated with a base-down prism over the affected eye, and usually press-on Fresnel prisms are used before permanent ones are ground into the lenses. However the excyclotorsion and incomitancy of the deviation leave many patients unsatisfied with prisms. Others, particularly those with ischemic palsies, in whom recovery is expected, can occlude (with opaque or black tape, for instance), the lower half of the lens over the affected eye. This provides occlusion of the affected eye in the direction of action of the superior oblique muscle.

Persistent fourth nerve palsies may require surgery, and patients with hypertropia and double vision secondary to fourth nerve dysfunction represent the most heterogeneous group of the cranial nerve palsies that ultimately require surgical intervention. This heterogeneity largely results from the significant portion of patients within this group who have congenital fourth nerve palsies and therefore large fusional amplitudes, which greatly enhance the chance of successful surgery. As always, the decision to intervene surgically is based on the presence of increasing symptoms of double vision, and an inability to carry on normal activities combined with stable measurements over a several month period.

In the setting of congenital fourth nerve palsies, several options exist and have all been reported to have successful results.[311–317] Each strategy should be designed to identify and treat the variable hyperdeviation that is present in the different fields of gaze. In particular, the identification of associated superior rectus contracture, superior oblique tendon laxity, and inferior oblique overaction is critical to designing a successful surgical strategy. In our experience, superior oblique tendon tucking is rarely required in adult patients with symptomatic decompensation of the congenital fourth nerve palsy or acquired fourth nerve palsies. In cases in which inferior oblique overaction is identified, the inferior oblique muscle is weakened, and combined either with an ipsilateral superior rectus weakening procedure or a contralateral inferior rectus weakening procedure (adjustable sutures) depending on the presence or absence of superior rectus restriction. If there is no inferior oblique overaction, then ipsilateral superior rectus recession and/or contralateral inferior rectus recession (adjustable suture) can be performed to correct the hypertropia. We find this strategy, as outlined by Plager,[318] to be effective in the management of most adult patients with fourth nerve palsies. By avoiding superior oblique tucking procedures in the adult, the risk of an induced Brown syndrome (discussed later in this chapter) is eliminated.

In the setting of bilateral fourth nerve palsies, which are common after head injuries, the surgical strategy becomes more complicated. In this setting specific maneuvers may be needed to address torsional misalignment and associated esotropia. Most experts agree that in the setting of large amounts of excyclotorsion (greater than 10 to 15 degrees) surgery directly on the superior oblique muscle is required to eliminate the torsion.[314–316, 319] In this procedure (Harada–Ito), the anterior portion of the superior oblique tendon is advanced to the area of the lateral rectus insertion. This can be done with an adjustable suture. This is done in combination with surgery on the other vertical muscles.

Helveston reported on 190 patients undergoing surgery for superior oblique palsy,[311] and noted that 90% of the patients had an inferior oblique weakening as part of their operative procedure, and only 26 (13%) underwent superior oblique tucking. Fifteen patients (7%), required a Harada–Ito procedure. They reported a 92% success rate with resolution of symptoms of double vision. Seventy-six percent of their patients had no deviation in the primary position. Simons and associates[317] reported on their experience with 123 patients and found that approximately 90% could be corrected with a single muscle procedure on either the superior or inferior oblique. Brown syndrome was a common complication of superior oblique tucks. Sixty percent of their patients had a primary position deviation of less than three diopters of hypertropia.

Fourth Nerve Palsies in Children

Fourth nerve palsies are less common in childhood than third and sixth nerve palsies. This is perhaps in part due to the fact that minor superior oblique paresis is harder to detect in younger children, especially when the third nerve is already involved. In Harley's[243] and Kodsi and Younge's[246] series, trauma was the most common cause of an acquired fourth nerve palsy (Table 15–7). However, in Harley's[243] and the CHOP series, congenital or decompensated congenital fourth nerve palsies were the most common of all cases.

Diagnostic Evaluation in Children With Fourth Nerve Palsies. If the fourth nerve palsy is consistent with an isolated, decompensated congenital one, then no workup is necessary. Otherwise, head trauma and evidence for a posterior fossa mass should be excluded. If the cause is unclear, MRI can be performed, with attention to the posterior midbrain, cavernous sinus, and orbit. In children with a normal MRI scan but with a fever or stiff neck, LP should be performed to exclude meningitis.

SIXTH NERVE PALSIES

Patients with a lateral rectus palsy complain of binocular horizontal double vision worse on ipsiversive gaze and at distance. In many cases the limitation of abduction is evident (Fig. 15–29), but in more subtle instances, alternate cover or Maddox rod testing would confirm an esotropia largest on ipsiversive gaze.

Nuclear/Fascicular. A lesion in the region of the sixth nerve nucleus would result in an ipsiversive conjugate gaze palsy and ipsilateral facial weakness (facial colliculus syndrome—see Chapters 14 and 16).[320, 321] A lesion of the caudal ventral pons involving the abducens fascicle and corticospinal tract would result in a lateral rectus palsy and a contralateral hemiparesis (Raymond syndrome). However, isolated sixth nerve palsies due to pontine lesions may be seen in hypertension[322] or diabetes.[323] Embolic or thrombotic occlusion of par-

TABLE 15–7. Causes of Fourth Nerve Palsies in Children

	Harley[243] 1980 (1968–1979)	Kodsi[246] 1992 (1966–1988)	CHOP 1996 (1993–1996)
Congenital	12	not included	5
Trauma	5	7	0
Neoplasm	0	1	0/(1)*
Inflammatory	1	1	1/(2)
Surgical	0	1	0
Idiopathic	0	4	0
Other	0	5	1/(1)†
Total	18	19	7/(4)

* When two figures are given, the first number refers to the number of isolated fourth nerve palsies in that category, while the number in parentheses refers to the total of fourth nerve palsies combined with a third or sixth nerve palsy or both. The CHOP series represents fourth nerve palsies seen by the authors at the Children's Hospital of Philadelphia from 7/93 through 11/96.
† Elevated intracranial pressure, cavernous carotid aneurysm.

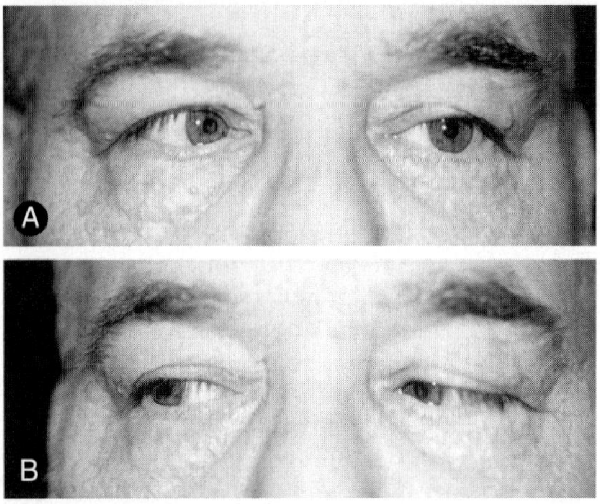

FIGURE 15–29. A. Diabetic left sixth nerve palsy causing left lateral rectus weakness and limitation of abduction **B.** Conjugate gaze to the right is normal.

amedian penetrating branches of the basilar artery is the usual cause for disturbances in these areas,[324] but multiple sclerosis,[158, 325, 326] vascular malformations, and metastases should also be considered.

Subarachnoid/Base of Skull. The sixth nerve, as it climbs along the clivus then over the petrous apex, is vulnerable to injury during downward brain stem shifts resulting from supratentorial masses ("false localizing sign"). Changes in intracranial pressure that occur in pseudotumor cerebri, supratentorial masses, or hydrocephalus (intracranial hypertension) or after lumbar puncture,[327] myelography,[328] or CSF leak[329] (intracranial hypotension) may also cause sixth nerve palsies. These tend to resolve within days or weeks after the intracranial pressure is normalized. Skull-base neoplasms such as meningiomas and chordomas (see below) are common causes of chronic isolated sixth nerve palsies.[330, 331] Sixth nerve palsies in this setting may sometimes improve spontaneously and therefore mimic inflammatory and ischemic palsies.[332] Since the parasympathetic fibers of the facial nerve travel along the floor of the middle cranial fossa on their way to supply the ipsilateral lacrimal gland, a patient with a sixth nerve palsy and ipsilateral dry eye may be harboring a mass in this region.

Otherwise, the same infectious and inflammatory processes in the subarachnoid space and that affect the third nerve can also cause a sixth nerve palsy. Similarly, trauma and ischemia can lead to sixth nerve palsies. As with other traumatic ocular motor palsies, the trauma tends to be severe. The prognosis for spontaneous improvement within weeks or months is good.[333] Ischemic sixth nerve palsies are typically painful, of relatively sudden onset, and resolve within 3 months. Guillain–Barré syndrome, Miller Fisher syndrome, and Gradenigo syndrome[334] should also be in the differential diagnosis of sixth nerve palsies. Other less common causes include giant cell arteritis.[299]

Diagnostic Evaluation in Adults With Acquired Sixth Nerve Palsies

Adults over 50 with vasculopathic risk factors with sixth nerve palsies may be observed. Indications for MRI would be lack of vasculopathic risk factors, progression of diplopia for more than 1 week, or lack of improvement after 8 weeks. Serologies, including those for syphilis and Lyme disease, as well as an erythrocyte sedimentation rate to exclude giant cell arteritis, may be performed. LP may be necessary when infectious, carcinomatous, or lymphomatous meningitis are suspected. Although vasculopathic sixth nerve palsies may occur in younger adults, neuroimaging should still be performed acutely in individuals in this age group because of their relatively higher risk for neoplasms.[335]

Management of Sixth Nerve Palsies

The management of patients with sixth nerve palsies is challenging both acutely and chronically. Once again, the options that exist acutely include occlusion and press-on Fresnel prisms. Base-out prisms can be used to significantly reduce head turns and improve head positioning while the patient is being followed for recovery. Alternatively, opaque tape can be placed over the temporal half of the lens over the affected eye. This occludes the affected eye in the direction of the lateral rectus palsy. In addition, botulinum injections to the ipsilateral medial rectus muscle can be very helpful in restoring a field of single binocular vision and potentially reducing the risk of medial rectus contracture.[232, 336–341] However, botulinum toxin injections may be limited by the side effect of ptosis and the need for repeated injections.

Once the sixth nerve palsy has been followed for 6 to 12 months without recovery, then patients can be offered surgery. Once again, the decision for the type of procedure is dependent on whether there is any residual function of the lateral rectus muscle. In the setting of partial sixth nerve dysfunction with some lateral rectus function remaining, we usually perform a medial rectus recession and lateral rectus resection. Surgery on the contralateral medial and lateral rectus muscles (weakening or posterior fixator suture) is often used to expand the field of single binocular vision. In the setting of total sixth nerve palsy, most experts agree that the lateral rectus muscle should be left alone and used to preserve anterior segment circulation. This allows the surgeon to potentially work on two or three of the other rectus muscles and attempt to correct the misalignment. Various types of vertical muscle transposition have been described, including split tendon transpositions, rectus muscle unions, where the lateral half of the inferior and superior rectus tendons are joined to the lateral rectus muscle belly, and finally the full tendon transposition. Full tendon transposition seems to be the most effective in our hands in reducing esotropia and providing an abducting force. We combine this with either an ipsilateral medial rectus weakening procedure or botulinum injection. As well, surgery to weaken the contralateral medial rectus muscle can be performed to increase the field of single vision toward the affected lateral rectus muscle.

Sixth Nerve Palsies in Children (Acquired)

In three pediatric series,[243, 246, 342] trauma was the most common cause of an acquired sixth nerve palsy. In Robertson et al's,[343] Aroichane and Repka's,[344] and the CHOP[345] series, neoplasms were the most frequent cause. Thus, accounting for the results from all series, the most common cause of acquired, nontraumatic sixth nerve palsy is a tumor (Table 15–8). Separating sixth nerve palsies by cause is often difficult because of the considerable overlap: trauma, neoplasms, and meningitis can be associated with elevated intracranial pressure or hydrocephalus, which by themselves are independent causes of sixth nerve palsies.

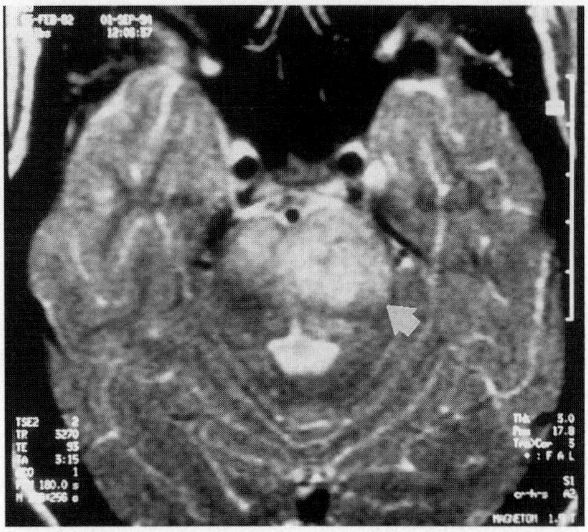

FIGURE 15–30. Pontine glioma. Axial MRI shows enlargement and enhancement of the pons (*arrow*). The patient presented with a left sixth nerve palsy, gait ataxia, bifacial palsies (left more than right), and a right hemiparesis.

Neoplasms. In contrast to adult brain tumors, the majority of which are supratentorial, 45% to 60% of childhood brain neoplasms occur in the posterior fossa.[346] These lesions, such as medulloblastomas, ependymomas, and pontine gliomas (Fig. 15–30), tend to compromise

TABLE 15–8. Causes of Sixth Nerve Palsies in Children

	Robertson[343] 1970 (1952–1964)	Harley[243] 1980 (1968–1979)	Afifi[342] 1992 (1966–1988)	Kodsi[246] 1992 (1966–1988)	Aroichane[344] 1995 (1985–1993) (age < 7)	CHOP[345]* 1999 (1993–1997)
Congenital	not included	5	17	not included	not included	8
Trauma	26	21	37	37	12	9
Neoplasm	52	17	25	18	21	34
Inflammatory	23	8	13	5	4	5
Increased ICP (nontumor)	15	3	17	2	15	11
Idiopathic	12	4	14	13	3	4
Other	5	4	9	13	9	4†
Total	133	62	132	88	64	75

* The CHOP series represents sixth nerve palsies seen by the authors at the Children's Hospital of Philadelphia from 7/93 through 3/97.[345]
† Basilar artery thrombosis, vertebral artery dissection, and cavernous carotid aneurysm. ICP = intracranial pressure.

midline structures in the dorsal pons and pontine tegmentum, resulting not infrequently in gaze palsies and sixth nerve palsies. Fourth ventricular compression, resulting in noncommunicating hydrocephalus, is also common and is another cause of sixth nerve palsies. Ataxia and nystagmus, due to cerebellar or cerebellar pathway interference, are also frequently seen.

Inflammatory. Several reports[347–355] have described a benign isolated sixth nerve palsy in childhood (Fig. 15–31). The patients tend to be otherwise healthy with an antecedent viral or febrile illness, or recent history of immunization. The sixth nerve palsy lasts for weeks or months, spontaneous resolves, and can recur. Many of these patients,[347–350] however, were seen prior to the widespread use of MRI, which might have detected demyelination (in acute disseminated encephalomyelitis (ADEM) or multiple sclerosis, for example). In addition, many reported patients did not have LPs to exclude meningitis.[349, 353, 355] Benign sixth nerve palsy in childhood is a diagnosis of exclusion following normal neuroimaging and CSF examination.

Acquired Comitant Esotropias. *Comitant esotropia does not exclude a neurologic process.* In comitant esotropias the angle of ocular misalignment is unchanged regardless of the direction of gaze.[356] Comitant esotropias may be mistaken for bilateral sixth nerve palsies. Some authors[357] suggested that comitant esotropias, in contrast to incomitant esodeviations, are benign and do not warrant further neurologic investigation. However, several other reports[358–362] have established that brain tumors and other intracranial processes in pediatric patients may in fact present with comitant esotropias. The topic has been discussed in recent reviews.[363, 364] Acquired comitant esotropias in childhood have been reported in association with cerebellar astrocytomas,[360–362] medulloblastomas,[360] pontine gliomas,[360] astrocytoma of the corpus callosum (with hydrocephalus),[358] and Arnold–Chiari malformation.[359, 365–368]

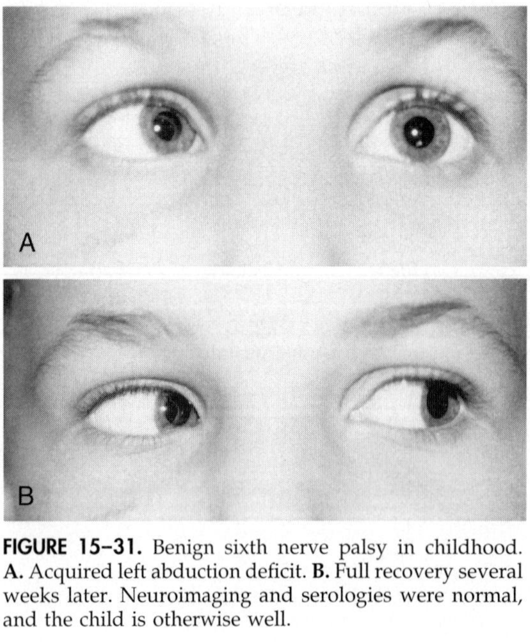

FIGURE 15–31. Benign sixth nerve palsy in childhood. **A.** Acquired left abduction deficit. **B.** Full recovery several weeks later. Neuroimaging and serologies were normal, and the child is otherwise well.

This finding appears to be primarily a pediatric phenomenon, and may not be as uncommon as previously suggested.[360] Of 30 children seen at CHOP with an acquired esodeviation associated with a neurologic insult, 12 (40%) had comitant measurements.[369] However, rarely is comitant esotropia the sole manifestation of an intracranial abnormality. Most patients will still have accompanying signs and symptoms of either elevated intracranial pressure (papilledema, headache, nausea or vomiting, or enlarging head size) or brain stem or cerebellar involvement (nystagmus, ataxia, hemiparesis, gait imbalance, dysarthria or Parinaud syndrome).

Several authors have reviewed the possible mechanisms for comitant esotropia in the setting of neurologic disease. Lennerstrand,[370] Hoyt and Good,[364] and Ciancia[363] reasoned that comitant strabismus might result from injury to supranuclear mesencephalic structures that control vergence eye movements. Others have ascribed infranuclear insults. Flynn[371] described a child who presented with an acute onset comitant esotropia who weeks later developed sixth and seventh nerve palsies as a manifestation of a pontine glioma. Jampolsky[372] and Kirkham et al[65] suggested that acquired esotropia and divergence paralysis may result from varying degrees of bilateral sixth nerve paresis. Spread of comitance is another proposed mechanism.[350]

Cyclic Esotropia. This rare ocular motility disorder is characterized by 48- to 96-hour cycles of esotropia and orthophoria or microstrabismus.[373] Usually idiopathic, cyclic esotropia may also be associated with intracranial tumors and epilepsy.[374] The cause is uncertain.

Suggested Workup in Pediatric Acquired Sixth Nerve Palsies. One suggested approach is

TABLE 15–9. Pediatric Sixth Nerve Palsies: Suggested Workup

Congenital
Consider Duane's retraction and Möbius syndromes
Acquired
Exclude history of trauma
MRI with and without gadolinium, looking particularly for a posterior fossa lesion
Consider LP, if the neuroimaging is negative, to exclude meningitis and to measure the CSF opening pressure
If MRI and LP negative, consider the diagnosis of a benign childhood sixth nerve palsy

given in Table 15–9. Because of the risk of an underlying neoplasm, even in isolated cases, in the absence of trauma MRI with and without gadolinium, looking particularly for a posterior fossa lesion is recommended. The diagnosis of a benign childhood sixth nerve palsy is one of exclusion.

Sixth Nerve Palsies in Children (Congenital)

Isolated congenital sixth nerve palsies are exceedingly rare. The vast majority have either Duane's retraction or Möbius syndromes.

Duane's Retraction Syndrome. This condition is characterized by the paradoxical co-contraction of the ipsilateral medial and lateral rectus muscles, which are normally antagonistic and customarily innervated by the third and sixth nerves, respectively.[375] Based on electromyographic recordings from the extraocular muscles of affected patients, Huber[376] classified cases into three types. *Narrowing of the palpebral fissure and retraction of the globe in attempted adduction are common to all.* Fissure narrowing is likely secondary to decreased levator firing in adduction.

1. Type I: *Abduction is impaired, but adduction is either normal or only slightly defective.* While the lateral rectus muscle does not contract during attempted abduction, both the medial and the lateral rectus muscles fire during adduction, thus producing the globe retraction (Fig. 15–32). Type I is the most common pattern of the three. Despite complete abduction deficits, most patients with type I are usually orthotropic in primary gaze. This feature distinguishes adults with Duane's retraction syndrome from those with acquired sixth nerve palsies, who are characteristically esotropic.
2. Type II: *Abduction is normal, but adduction is impaired.* Lateral rectus contraction in abduction is normal, but the muscle also inappropriately contracts in attempted adduction, producing defective adduction and globe retraction.
3. Type III: *Both abduction and adduction are defective.* The lateral and medial rectus muscles both contract in abduction and adduction, thus limiting motion of the eye in either direction (Fig. 15–33). Clinically this pattern may be hard to distinguish from type I.

Other common features include upshoot or downshoot of the eye in adduction, and A-, V-, or X-pattern ocular deviations. Many develop a compensatory head turn and preserve binocularity. In one meta-analysis,[377] there was a female preponderance (58%) and left eye (59%) predilection. Twenty-three percent of patients just had the right eye affected, while 18% had bilateral involvement. Other anomalous innervation phenomena, such as Marcus Gunn jaw wink and paradoxical–gustatory–lacrimal reflex ("crocodile tears"), have been

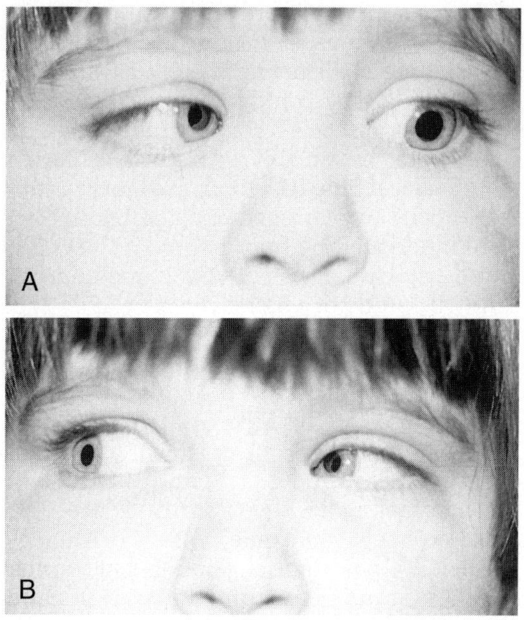

FIGURE 15–32. Duane's retraction syndrome type I. **A.** Left abduction deficit. **B.** In right gaze, globe retraction and fissure narrowing are seen.

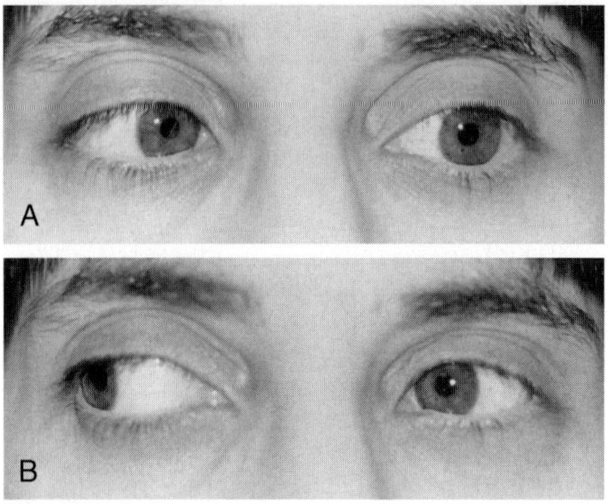

FIGURE 15–33. Duane's retraction syndrome type III. **A.** Left abduction deficit. **B.** In right gaze, a left adduction deficit, globe retraction, and fissure narrowing are seen.

reported in association with Duane's retraction syndrome.[377]

Pathologic studies published by Miller and colleagues[378, 379] have provided enormous insight into the neural substrate of Duane's retraction syndrome by confirming brain stem abnormalities and the anomalous innervation of the lateral rectus muscle. In their report of a patient with Duane's type I,[379] the sixth nerve was absent, the sixth nerve nucleus was hypoplastic, and branches of the inferior division of the oculomotor (third) nerve supplied the lateral rectus muscle. Within the hypoplastic nucleus, the sixth nerve interneurons, which connect with the contralateral medial rectus subnucleus via the MLF to mediate conjugate gaze, were presumably spared. In a patient with Duane's type III,[378] both sixth nerves and their nuclei were absent, and the lateral recti were innervated by branches from the oculomotor nerves. Consistent with these findings, in an MRI study of a patient with Duane's type I, the ipsilateral sixth nerve was absent.[380]

Duane's retraction syndrome usually occurs sporadically, but rarely cases are familial.[621] In one large family, linkage at chromosome 2q31 was obtained.[622] Occasionally Duane's retraction syndrome is associated with systemic anomalies.[377] Wildervanck (cervico-oculo-acoustic) syndrome consists of Duane's retraction syndrome, Klippel–Feil spinal anomaly, and sensorineural deafness.[381] Duane's retraction syndrome and congenital thenar hypoplasia comprise Okihiro syndrome. Duane's retraction syndrome may also be seen together with Goldenhar syndrome, which consists of epibulbar dermoids, conjunctival lipodermoids, upper lid colobomas, inner and external ear malformations (preauricular skin tags), facial hypoplasia, and cervical spine anomalies. Unusual associations with chromosomal abnormalities,[382] thalidomide embryopathy,[383] and intracranial lesions have also been reported.[384, 385] Orbital blow-out fractures with medial rectus entrapment or orbital metastases may mimic Duane's retraction syndrome.[386]

Treatment. Since most patients with Duane's retraction syndrome have no primary position misalignment, they usually do not require intervention. Strabismus surgery, the mainstay of treatment, is indicated in the minority of cases with ocular misalignment in the primary position, an abnormal head turn, cosmetically unacceptable globe retraction, or vertical deviation on adduction.[377, 387–389]

Möbius Syndrome. In addition to congenital facial diplegia, abducens palsy is the feature most commonly associated with Möbius syndrome, occurring in 82% of cases in the series reported by Henderson.[390] In addition, total external ophthalmoplegia was present in 25% of the cases in this series, oculomotor palsy in 21%, and bilateral ptosis in 10%. The abducens weakness is almost always bilateral, but of varying degree. When the lateral rectus palsy is severe, there is usually complete conjugate gaze paresis. Parents may not notice the facial weakness if it is subtle, and often the child is brought to medical attention solely because of an esotropia. Möbius syndrome is discussed in more detail in Chapter 14.

MISCELLANEOUS CAUSES OF COMBINED THIRD, FOURTH, AND SIXTH NERVE PALSIES

The differential diagnosis of any combination of third, fourth, and sixth nerve palsies is broad and includes brain stem, subarachnoid, base of skull, cavernous sinus, and orbital processes. Often the lesion can be localized and diagnosis made based upon the history and examination, but in many instances neuroimaging is required, especially to determine its cause.

Brain Stem

Motor Neuron Diseases. Amyotrophic lateral sclerosis (Lou Gehrig's disease) is a degenerative disorder of corticobulbar and spinal tracts (upper motor neurons) and lower cranial nerves in the brain stem and anterior horn cells in the spinal cord (lower motor neurons). Patients are easily recognized by their dysphagia, dysarthria, need for respiratory support, weakness, muscular atrophy, fasciculations, hyperreflexia, and extensor plantar responses. In most instances, clinically the eye movements are spared; however, pathologically minor changes in the ocular motor nuclei may be seen.[391] Rarely, supranuclear eye movement disorders may be observed, and in late-stage patients whose course is artificially prolonged by long-term respiratory support, some may develop complete external ophthalmoplegia (see also Chapter 16).

In other motor neuron diseases and spinal muscular atrophies, the eye movements and ocular motor nuclei are also usually spared. However, rare exceptions have been reported.[392–395]

Wernicke's Encephalopathy. Wernicke's disease may present with ophthalmoplegia, nystagmus, altered mental status, and ataxia. These findings result from localized hemorrhagic necrosis of the midbrain and thalamus. This diagnosis should be considered in all oculomotor palsies as administration of thiamine may rapidly reverse the ophthalmoplegia and be life saving. There is a more detailed discussion of this entity in Chapter 16.

Bickerstaff's Brain Stem Encephalitis. Elevated anti-GQ_1b antibody titers may be found in patients with isolated acute ophthalmoparesis, Miller Fisher syndrome, and Bickerstaff's brain stem encephalitis, and in patients with Guillian–Barré syndrome and ophthalmoparesis.[396] These antibodies may also be observed in some patients with chronic ophthalmoparesis of unknown cause.[623]

The anti-GQ_1b antibodies strongly stain the paranodal regions of the ocular motor nerves and has been found to inhibit acetylcholine release and neurite regrowth and may be cytotoxic to neurons.[397, 398] Bickerstaff's brain stem encephalitis is a monophasic disease process typically preceded by an infection or immunization. The disorder is characterized by stupor, ophthalmoparesis ataxia, brisk reflexes, and occasionally a CSF pleocytosis. There is growing consensus that Miller Fisher syndrome and Bickerstaff's brain stem encephalitis represent a spectrum of a similar disease process.[399] Both of these entities share the anti-GQ_1b antibodies and are self-limited disorders.

Subarachnoid Disturbances

Acute bacterial and chronic fungal, tuberculous, spirochetal (syphilitic and Lyme *Borrelia*),[400] and inflammatory (sarcoid) meningitic processes may affect the ocular motor nerves within the *subarachnoid space*, and other cranial nerves may be involved. Carcinomatous[401, 402] or lymphomatous[403, 404] meningitis may produce a similar clinical picture, sometimes accompanied by radicular signs and symptoms indicating more widespread meningeal involvement. Lymphoma may also directly invade the endoneurium of the cranial nerves.[405, 406] The ocular motor nerves can be involved in Guillain–Barré syndrome, the Fisher variant (ophthalmoparesis, ataxia, and areflexia), and chronic inflammatory demyelinating polyneuropathy,[407] usually in the setting of systemic weakness. These conditions are discussed in detail in Chapter 14. CSF examination with cytology is essential for diagnosing and sorting out these infectious, neoplastic, and inflammatory disorders.

Base of Skull Lesions

A combination of ocular motor nerve palsies may be due to skull base metastases[408] or primary skull base tumors such as sphenoid wing or clival meningiomas, chordomas, and chondrosarcomas. Metastatic tumors in this area typically derive from lung, breast, or prostate primary neoplasms.

Sphenoid Wing and Clival Meningiomas

Sphenoid Wing. The typical clinical presentation of a sphenoid wing meningioma is ipsilateral ophthalmoplegia, proptosis, and hyperostosis of the temporal bone. Frequently the anterior and middle cranial fossae as well as the zygomatic fossa are involved. Because of their relative lateral location, optic neuropathy is usually only a feature of large lesions. Surgical removal is often recommended.[409]

Clival Meningiomas. Meningiomas can develop primarily in the area of the clivus in the area of the sphenoid and occipital bones. These benign, slow-growing tumors can present with a variety of ophthalmic symptoms depending on whether their initial involvement is of the cranial nerves entering the cavernous sinus or compression of the brain stem or cerebellum. Patients can also present with signs and symptoms of increased intracranial pressure when

CSF outflow is affected. Thus, papilledema as well as cranial nerve abnormalities such as oculomotor palsies, facial palsy, and trigeminal nerve dysfunction can be seen.[410] The most common initial symptom is headache followed by visual symptoms, gait disturbances and trouble hearing. Dany[411] divided the clinical presentation of patients with clival meningioma into four stages. These stages include stage I tumors, which produce primarily cranial nerve dysfunction; stage II tumors, which in addition to cranial nerve dysfunction cause long tract signs; stage III tumors, which cause elevation of intracranial pressure; and finally, stage IV tumors, which produce compression of the basilar artery.

The diagnosis of a clival meningioma is suggested based on neuroimaging studies when patient presents with the syndrome outlined above. Meningiomas need to be differentiated radiographically from chordomas and chondrosarcomas also occurring in this region. The absence of extensive bony destruction (common in chordoma and chondrosarcoma) and diffuse and smooth gadolinium enhancement (present in meningioma and more irregular in chordoma and chondrosarcoma) are the features that best differentiate these tumors. The treatment involves surgical removal, which is rarely complete and can cause cranial nerve damage.[412] Depending on the clinical situation and the presence of residual tumor, adjunctive radiation therapy can be used.[413]

Chordomas. Chordomas are rare, CNS neoplasms that arise from the embryologic notochord, the foundation upon which the axial skeleton is formed. Ultimately, during embryology the notochord begins to involute and remains only in the intervertebral cartilaginous discs as the nucleus pulposus. It is from this tissue and/or remnants or ectopic fragments of notochord remaining in the bones of the base of the skull that chordomas arise. About 50% occur in the sacrococcygeal region and about 35% develop in the base of the skull, usually near the clivus.[414] Overall, they represent approximately 1% of intracranial tumors.[415] Intracranial chordomas can become symptomatic at any age. Although the tumors grow very slowly, they are locally invasive and destroy bone and infiltrate tissue. Histopathologically, the cytoplasm of chordomas has a physaliphorous or bubble-like appearance.

Because they tend to originate in clivus, chordomas most commonly present with either unilateral or bilateral sixth nerve palsies.[416] Other associated findings may include ipsilateral facial weakness and trigeminal nerve dysfunction. Patients also complain of headache. Rarely, they extend superiorly to effect the anterior visual pathways and cause optic neuropathy.[416] Chordomas should be considered in the differential diagnosis of any patient with chronic unilateral or bilateral sixth nerve palsy with or without remitting symptoms.[331, 416] Radiographically, a cystic, lobulated mass with evidence of bone erosion and destruction seen on CT or MRI is characteristic.[417] Biopsy can confirm the diagnosis. Some authors have recommended radical resection.[418] After tumor removal, most patients are treated with radiation therapy, but recurrences are common.[418–420]

Chondrosarcomas. Chondrosarcomas, which are also relatively rare tumors, arise from cartilage in bone. These generally are adult tumors and can occur both in the extremities and the base of the skull. These tumors represent far less than 1% of all intracranial neoplasms.[421] When they arise in the base of the skull, they tend to produce cranial nerve palsies in the cavernous sinus area. Sixth nerve palsies are common, although patients can present with third, fifth, and seventh nerve dysfunction as well, and multiple cranial nerve palsies are not uncommon.[416] Radiographically, they must be differentiated from nasopharyngeal carcinomas, chordomas, and meningiomas. When they arise around the tuberculum sella or the paranasal sinuses, they may invade the orbit, sometimes with optic neuropathy. The tumors are composed of undifferentiated mesenchymal cells surrounded by cartilage of varying levels of maturity with foci of immature chondrocytes. The most effective treatment is widespread surgical excision followed by radiation therapy.[422] Many of these tumors can demonstrate cellular atypia and behave aggressively, with recurrence and local invasion. Patients with Ollier disease (multiple skeletal enchondromas) and Maffucci syndrome (multiple enchondromas associated with subcutaneous hemangiomas) may develop skull base chondrosarcomas as a delayed consequence of these disorders. We have seen three such patients who presented with sixth nerve palsies.[423]

Cavernous Sinus Disturbances

Cavernous sinus involvement is suggested by any combination of unilateral third, fourth, or sixth nerve dysfunction accompanied by hypesthesia of the forehead, cornea, or cheek due to involvement of V_1 or V_2, or by a Horner syndrome, owing to oculosympathetic disruption. Complete interruption of all three ocular motor nerves would result in total ophthalmoplegia, ptosis, and mydriasis. Most cavernous sinus disturbances are due to mass lesions.

Symptoms of Cavernous Sinus Disease. Patients with cavernous sinus lesions may present with double vision, pupillary abnormalities, facial sensory loss, or orbital signs and symptoms.[11] Pain may be referred to the orbit or supraorbital region by direct involvement of the trigeminal nerve or structures innervated by this nerve.

Signs of Cavernous Sinus Disease. The features of a complete cavernous sinus syndrome were alluded to in the first paragraph of this section. Less prominent characteristics of incomplete lesions are:

1. *Isolated Cranial Nerve Palsies.* Commonly, only one or two of the nerves within the cavernous sinus are involved, and chronic isolated ocular motor palsies referable to this region are not rare.
2. *Alternating Anisocoria.* Simultaneous oculoparasympathetic and sympathetic disruption within the cavernous sinus may result in the unusual clinical syndrome of "alternating anisocoria." In the light, the pupil on the affected side is larger than its fellow normal eye, but in the dark the affected pupil may actually become smaller because of poor sympathetic tone.
3. *Pupillary Sparing.* Third nerve palsies of cavernous sinus origin often spare pupillary function. Pupil sparing in cavernous sinus lesions may be explained by the typically slow growth of tumors in this region. One must also consider the possibility of pseudopupillary sparing, which results when the pupillary signs of third nerve dysfunction are masked by a concurrent Horner syndrome or aberrant regeneration of the third nerve.
4. *Divisional Third Nerve Paresis.* Because the third nerve anatomically separates into superior and inferior divisions in the anterior cavernous sinus, a divisional paresis suggests a lesion in this region or anterior to it. However, this guideline has frequent exceptions, as a divisional third nerve palsy may occur anywhere posterior this region, including the brain stem.[104]
5. *Aberrant Regeneration of the Third Nerve.* Misdirection phenomena (see third nerve palsies, above) may occur with cavernous sinus masses such as a meningioma (Fig. 15–34).[111]
6. *Ipsilateral Horner Syndrome and Abducens Palsy.* This combination of findings results from a lesion involving both the sixth nerve and oculosympathetic fibers, where they comingle within the cavernous sinus.[424]
7. *Orbital Signs.* Proptosis, periorbital swelling, chemosis, and conjunctival injection may occur when cavernous sinus lesions block orbital drainage and venous return.

Neuroimaging. MRI, with thin-section coronal slices through the cavernous sinus region, with and without gadolinium, is the imaging procedure of choice in this setting. When aneurysms are suspected, an MRI-angiogram should also be ordered.

Differential Diagnosis. Pathologic processes in this region may arise from surrounding dural walls, contiguous sites, or remote foci.[425] The differential diagnosis of cavernous sinus lesions includes neoplasms, trauma, Tolosa–Hunt syndrome, infection, septic cavernous sinus thrombosis, carotid–cavernous sinus fistulas, and intracavernous aneurysms. In one large series,[426] neoplasms were the most common cause of a cavernous sinus syndrome.

Some cavernous sinus disturbances can be attributed to its anatomic features. Sellar

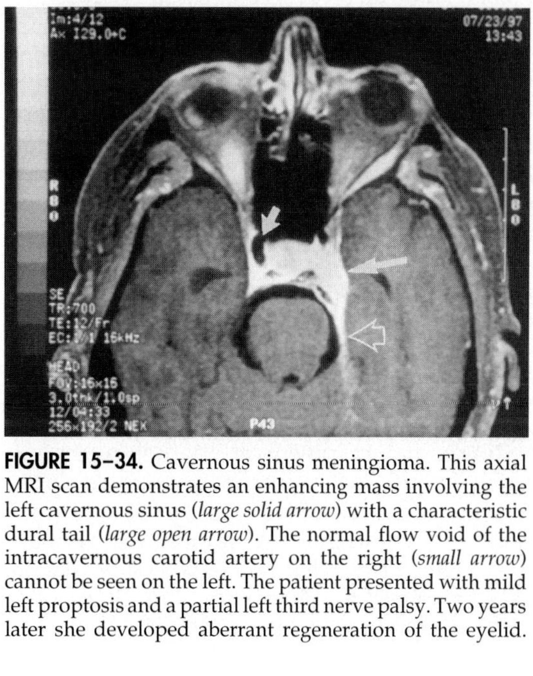

FIGURE 15–34. Cavernous sinus meningioma. This axial MRI scan demonstrates an enhancing mass involving the left cavernous sinus (*large solid arrow*) with a characteristic dural tail (*large open arrow*). The normal flow void of the intracavernous carotid artery on the right (*small arrow*) cannot be seen on the left. The patient presented with mild left proptosis and a partial left third nerve palsy. Two years later she developed aberrant regeneration of the eyelid.

masses (see Chapter 7), if large enough, may compress cavernous sinus structures, and the clinical scenario of acute headache, visual loss, and ophthalmoplegia should suggest pituitary apoplexy. The nerves within the cavernous sinus rarely give rise to primary tumors such as neuromas of the fifth nerve.[11] The trigeminal nerve may also serve as a conduit to the cavernous sinus for basal cell and squamous cell tumors arising from the face, head, and neck.[427] In a similar fashion, valveless veins of the face may spread infection from the skin to this region and ultimately lead to thrombosis of the cavernous sinus. The sphenoid sinus and nasopharynx lie inferiorly and medially to each cavernous sinus so that tumors and infections of these regions readily gain access to the cavernous sinus. The remainder of this section will discuss some of the common entities in this region.

Neoplasms. A variety of neoplasms may involve the cavernous sinus, including meningiomas, neuromas, chordomas, chondrosarcomas, nasopharyngeal carcinomas, lymphoma, plasmacytoma, pituitary adenoma, and metastatic disease.[428, 429] A complete discussion of these tumors is beyond the scope of this chapter, but some of the more important and common tumors will be reviewed. Some were discussed above.

Nasopharyngeal Tumors. Nasopharyngeal tumors may present as serous otitis media, nasal obstruction, atypical facial pain, or recurrent epistaxis, or as a chronic isolated sixth nerve palsy.[430] Careful examination of the nasopharynx is essential when evaluating the patient with unexplained ophthalmoplegia. MRI is often helpful in delineating a mass, but on rare occasions empiric biopsy of the nasopharynx is necessary for diagnosis. The tumors either erode the skull base or enter the cavernous sinus through the foramen ovale or lacerum.[431] Approximately 20% of nasopharyngeal tumors may present as a cavernous sinus syndrome. Fifth nerve dysfunction, followed closely by impairment of the ocular motor nerves is the major ophthalmic finding.[432]

Pituitary Tumors. Although there is frequent radiographic involvement of the cavernous sinus in pituitary adenomas, only rarely is there resultant chronic ocular motor dysfunction.[433, 434] Importantly, the rapid onset of bilateral complete ophthalmoplegia and headache should suggest the possibility of pituitary apoplexy, and neuroimaging studies should be obtained emergently.[435, 436] The clinical presentation of pituitary apoplexy may be confused with subarachnoid hemorrhage and bacterial meningitis. The administration of corticosteroids in this situation in order to prevent an addisonian crisis may be life saving.[437] Pituitary adenomas and apoplexy are discussed in more detail in Chapter 7.

Tumors Involving the Trigeminal Nerve. Trigeminal neuromas and schwannomas typically begin in the region of the gasserian ganglion and manifest clinically with complaints of altered facial sensation or facial pain.[438] Rarely, these tumors may present as a chronic isolated sixth nerve palsy without signs of fifth nerve dysfunction.[439] MRI is invaluable in the diagnosis of trigeminal neuroma and other tumors arising from the intrinsic structures of the cavernous sinus.

Occasionally, tumors of the skin such as basal cell carcinoma and squamous cell carcinoma travel perineurally along branches of the fifth nerve to gain access to the cavernous sinus and orbital apex, causing ophthalmoplegia.[427, 440] Facial nerve palsies are also frequent.[441] Remote tumor spread may present clinically years after the original skin lesion was removed.[442] Palliative radiation may be used, but the prognosis is poor.[443]

Cavernous Sinus Meningiomas. Meningiomas arising from the dural walls of the cavernous sinus represent one of the most frequent tumors of this area (Fig. 15–34). Cavernous sinus meningiomas typically present with painless, slowly progressive oculomotor palsies or a third nerve palsy with aberrant regeneration. Rarely, spontaneously resolving oculomotor palsies may occur.[444] Their MRI appearance is characteristic, as they are typically isointense with brain but enhance with gadolinium. A dural tail is often present. They may also encase the cavernous carotid, often leading to vascular narrowing.[445] Since these tumors may grow slowly, surgery or radiation therapy is usually not indicated until vital structures such as the brain stem or visual pathways are compromised.[112] Many patients with stable diplopia who can be treated with prisms may be followed clinically and radiographically.[446] Alternatively, some authors have recommended total[447, 448] or subtotal[445, 449] resection, but the morbidity, including internal carotid or middle cerebral artery infarction, oculomotor palsies, and trigeminal nerve dysfunction associated with neurosurgery of these tumors can be high. Perioperative deaths can also occur.[447, 450] Partial resection may be followed by adjunctive radiation therapy.[451–453]

Lymphoma. Lymphomatous involvement of the cavernous sinus may cause painful or painless ophthalmoplegia.[454]

Metastases. Breast, lung, and prostate cancer are well-recognized primary neoplasms that can metastasize to the cavernous sinus.[455] The ophthalmoplegia is frequently rapidly progressive.

Inflammatory Disorders. Idiopathic granulomatous inflammation of the superior orbital fissure or cavernous sinus is known as the Tolosa–Hunt syndrome. Painful ophthalmoplegia is the hallmark of this condition. The third nerve is the most commonly affected cranial nerve followed by the sixth, fifth, and fourth nerves.[456] Proptosis and optic nerve dysfunction is seen in approximately 20% to 30% of cases.[456] Based on limited anatomic studies, orbital pseudotumor and the Tolosa–Hunt syndrome appear to represent a similar pathologic process. Since there are many causes of painful ophthalmoplegia, diagnosis of this syndrome should be one of exclusion. MRI is helpful in delineating other disease processes in this region such as neoplasm and infection.[457] A rapid response to corticosteroids is characteristic but recurrence is not uncommon as steroids are tapered. Corticosteroids may have to be tapered over months, but steroid dependence should raise the suspicion of an alternative diagnosis such as lymphoma and a biopsy should be performed.[428] Systemic lupus erythematosus should also be excluded with serologic testing.[458, 459] Furthermore, a human immunodeficiency virus-positive patient with painful ophthalmoplegia was found to have an eosinophilic granuloma in the superior orbital fissure region.[460]

Herpes zoster ophthalmicus may also be associated with complete ophthalmoplegia or isolated oculomotor palsy resulting from a secondary vasculitis or direct inflammatory infiltration of the nerves and extraocular muscles. Although antiviral agents may be given to affected patients, most have resolution of the oculormotor palsy within 1 year.[461]

Cavernous Sinus Thrombosis. Prompt recognition of septic thrombosis of the cavernous sinus is essential because this condition represents a potentially life-threatening disorder. Patients present with fever, periorbital pain, swelling, and proptosis.[462] The abducens nerve is frequently affected first but complete ophthalmoplegia may rapidly ensue.[462] Vision may be impaired as the result of arterial occlusion or emboli, venous congestion, increased intraocular pressure, or corneal exposure.[463, 464] Staphylococcal and streptococcal organisms are the most frequent pathogens.[462] These organisms may gain entry through several routes, but most often invade the cavernous sinus by traversing the valveless veins of the face, teeth, middle ear, and neck. Direct spread of infection from the maxillary and sphenoid sinuses is an alternative route.[42] Within several days of onset, the infection may reach the contralateral cavernous sinus and further dispersal may lead to meningitis or cerebral infarction by compromising the cavernous carotid artery. Uncommonly, extension to other venous sinuses, such as the lateral, sigmoid, and inferior sagittal sinuses, may occur.[465]

Most patients will have an elevated white blood count and positive blood cultures. Thirty five percent of patients have changes in their CSF consistent with bacterial meningitis (ie, neutrophilic pleocytosis, elevated protein, and low glucose).[462] MRI is the preferred study to demonstrate thrombosis of the cavernous sinus.[466]

After cultures have been collected, intravenous antibiotics should be administered at once. Antibiotic coverage is dependent on the source of the infection but therapy against penicillinase-resistant staphylococci and anaerobes is essential.[462] Anticoagulation of patients with septic cavernous sinus thrombosis remains controversial, but a recent study suggests that early use of heparin reduces the morbidity but not mortality.[467]

Fungal Infections. Mucormycosis and rarely aspergillosis may rapidly spread from the sinuses to the cavernous sinus and orbit,[468] and immunocompromised individuals such as those with diabetes or the elderly are susceptible. Mucormycosis, which requires a rich source of iron to grow effectively, may occur in patients taking iron-chelating agents. These organisms have a propensity to invade blood vessels.[469] Visual loss from central retinal or ophthalmic artery occlusion is not uncommon. Spread of infection to the cavernous carotid is heralded by the acute onset of a contralateral hemiparesis. MRI is most useful in delineating the extent of the pathologic process. The diagnosis may be established by biopsy and drainage of infected areas. Treatment is with intravenous amphotericin and surgical débridement. The amount of débridement is often dependent on the degree of visual loss and the extent of the infectious process.[469] Those patients with preserved visual acuity and disease limited to the orbital structures and sinuses may be spared an exenteration without altering outcome.[470]

High-Flow (Direct) Carotid Cavernous Fistulas. Carotid cavernous fistulas (CCF) are communications between the intracavernous carotid artery and the surrounding cavernous sinus. Several different classification schemes have been proposed and generally divide these CCFs based on their cause, rate of flow, and source of feeder vessels. The most important of these is the high-flow, direct CCF. In the majority of cases (80%) direct CCFs result from trauma and much less commonly arise spontaneously.[167, 471] The neuro-ophthalmic presentation of these direct CCFs is generally dramatic and results from the reversal of blood flow in the orbital and ocular venous drainage. Usually there is an endothelized, single tear in the carotid wall.[472] These *direct,* high-flow fistulas are termed type A.[473] Types B, C and D fistulas are all low-flow, *indirect* communications between branches of the internal or external carotid artery within the dura of the cavernous sinus. These have also been grouped as dural CCFs or dural arteriovenous malformations (DAVMs). They generally arise spontaneously and have a lower flow and more insidious presentation compared to the direct CCFs. Type B fistulas are supplied by small branches of the cavernous carotid artery, type C by dural branches of the external carotid, and Type D by a combination of external and internal carotid artery branches. Accurate clinical diagnosis of CCFs (and DAVMs) is generally made based on the typical constellation of symptoms and signs (Table 15–10). Neuroradiologic confirmation of the diagnosis is based on orbital ultrasound, MRI, MRI-angiography, and conventional angiographic findings. Treatment generally involves embolization.

This section will detail the diagnosis and management of high-flow CCFs, while a review of low-flow CCFs follows in the next section.

Traumatic Direct CCFs. The majority of direct CCFs result from head trauma.[167, 471, 474] The trauma can take many different forms but most often is severe following motor vehicle accidents, sports injuries, and falls.[167, 471, 474] They can result from injuries involving skull fractures and bone fragments but also can be seen with relatively trivial injuries that otherwise have no associated signs of head injury. Traumatic CCFs can present at the time of the injury or may be delayed in onset for days or weeks. Penetrating injuries such as stab wounds that enter the cavernous sinus through the superior orbital fissure can also result in CCFs.[474] "Traumatic" CCFs can also result from iatrogenic injury to the carotid artery. This has been seen in the setting of carotid endarterectomy surgery, endovascular procedures, and as a complication of transsphenoidal pituitary surgery and otolaryngologic surgery, and in procedures directed at the gasserian ganglion for the treatment of trigeminal neuralgia.[475–477] In the setting of pituitary surgery or sphenoid ethmoidal otolaryngologic surgery, an anomalous position of the internal carotid artery may predispose to an iatrogenic CCF.[475, 477] These anatomic variants can be recognized by preoperative MRI.

TABLE 15–10. Ocular Signs and Symptoms in Carotid–Cavernous Fistulas and Dural AVMs of the Cavernous Sinus

Symptoms
Headache/orbital pain
Proptosis
Red eye
Blurred vision
Double vision
Bruit
Signs
Proptosis
Orbital congestions
Conjunctival chemosis
Arterialization of episcleral vessels
Increased intraocular pressure
Venous stasis retinopathy
Ophthalmoplegia
Bruit
Visual loss

From Bennett J, Volpe NJ, Liu GT, Galetta SL. Neurovascular neuro-ophthalmology. In: Albert D, Jakobiec FA (eds): Principles of Ophthalmology, pp 4238–4274. Philadelphia, WB Saunders, 2000, with permission.

Spontaneous Direct CCFs. Spontaneous, high-flow, direct CCFs arise in two different settings: (1) rupture of a pre-existing cavernous sinus aneurysm and (2) a defective vessel wall that may complicate a connective tissue disorder such as the Ehlers–Danlos syndrome. In Debrun's series of 100 patients with direct CCFs, only about 2% were spontaneous CCFs.[478] More recently, Lewis and associates found that 22 out of 100 direct CCFs resulted from rupture of a cavernous carotid aneurysm.[474] Moreover, Kupersmith and associates found that in about 60% of patients with spontaneous CCF, an underlying cause could not be found.[479] Therefore the entity probably also occurs idiopathically. Cavernous carotid aneurysm rupture may be heralded by CCF formation.[167] However, Kupersmith followed 78 patients with a cavernous sinus aneurysm, and none of these patients presented with rupture and CCF formation.[167] The systemic conditions associated with spontaneous CCFs include hypertension,[480] fibromuscular dysplasia,[481, 482] Ehlers–Danlos syndrome,[483, 484] and pseudoxanthoma elasticum.[485] Many of these patients presumably have a defect in the arterial wall as a result of their systemic disorder that presents after a tear from relatively minor trauma such as coughing or a Valsalva maneuver.

Clinical Presentation. Clinical findings in patients with high-flow direct CCFs result from arterialization of draining orbital veins by anterior blood flow from the cavernous carotid artery (Table 15–10). Usually this involves the eye and orbit ipsilateral to the fistula. However, the presentation can vary significantly and can include a silent orbital presentation, particularly when the CCF drains posteriorly. Bilateral orbital signs can also develop depending on the patency of the venous connections between the two cavernous sinuses. Recent advances of endovascular treatment techniques have made the chronic presentation of CCF a rarity.

Symptoms. Symptom onset is usually abrupt and may be rapidly progressive. Occasionally, the symptoms and signs that resulted from the traumatic injury (proptosis or cranial nerve palsy) may obscure the findings of the CCF. The most common complaints offered by patients with CCF include subjective bruit (80%), visual blur (59%), headache (53%), diplopia (53%), and ocular or orbital pain (35%).[167, 474] Patients may describe a whooshing or swishing that is synchronous with the pulse. The bruit is classically described as disappearing with ipsilateral carotid compression although this is not a commonly performed or recommended diagnostic maneuver. Proptosis and orbital congestion secondary to impaired orbital venous drainage is often readily apparent. Headache may result from distention of the dura or trigeminal nerve compression. Arterial blood flow in the venous system of the eye results in markedly dilated and tortuous episcleral veins and severe chemosis.

Signs. The clinical signs correlate with the symptoms and include pulsatile exophthalmos, arterialization of conjunctival vessels, elevated (often pulsatile) intraocular pressure, restrictive ocular motility disturbances and cranial neuropathies, optic disc swelling, and venous stasis retinopathy. The bruit audible to the patient is usually also audible to the examiner, although not always. The best method for listening is with the bell of the stethoscope over the closed eyelid. In posterior draining fistulas the bruit may be detected over the area of the mastoid. Proptosis results from congestion of tissue and displacement of the globe by the dilated superior ophthalmic vein. Exophthalmometry generally reveals between 3 and 10 mm of proptosis but even larger amounts have been reported.[167, 477] The proptosis generally progresses over several days and then stabilizes. It can be bilateral if blood flow is to the contralateral orbit as well and is frequently associated with eyelid swelling and conjunctival chemosis. Ocular pulsation may be visible as well as palpable and results from transmission of the arterial pulse to the dilated ophthalmic veins and globe. The absence of globe pulsation may reflect thrombosis of the ophthalmic veins. Abnormalities in the ocular pulse may be suggested by wide to and fro movements of the Myers rings during applanation tonometry. The wide pulse (up to 5 times normal) may also be documented with pneumotenometry.

Arterialization of conjunctival and episcleral vessels results from blood forced into the orbital veins and subsequently into the conjunctival veins. The arterialization pattern may be diffuse or can be localized to one or two vessels. The vessels have a corkscrew appearance and this tortuosity and dilation extends all the way to the limbus (Fig. 15–35; see Color Plates 48 and 49). These vessels can occasionally bleed profusely. Massive proptosis can lead to impaired corneal coverage and exposure. Exposure of the cornea (and conjunctiva) may lead to infectious ulceration if adequate lubrication is not used. This may be aggravated by corneal hypesthesia, which can occur secondary to trigeminal nerve dysfunction.

Increased intraocular pressure and glaucoma result from arterialization of episcleral vessels with elevation of episcleral venous pressure and forcing of blood into Schlemm's canal. This blood can be seen on gonioscopy. Ultimately intraocular pressure rises with this increase in episcleral venous pressure. Optic nerve damage ensues and glaucomatous optic neuropathy can occur in 20% of patients with

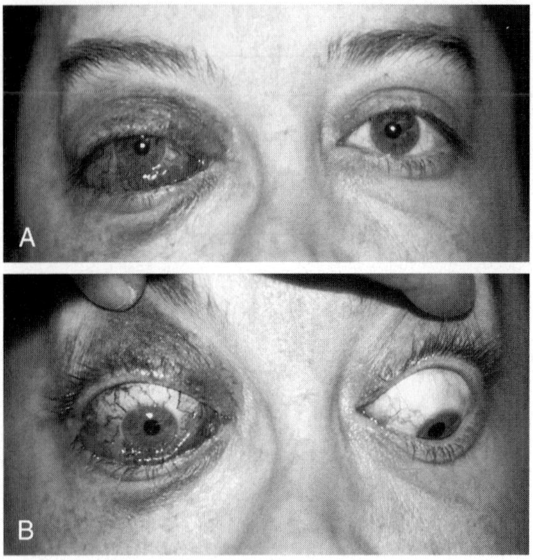

FIGURE 15–35. External appearance of a woman with a traumatic, high-flow, direct CCF on the right. **A.** Proptosis, chemosis, arterialization of scleral and eyelid vessels, and periorbital swelling are seen. **B.** She had almost complete ophthalmoplegia of the right eye, including defective infraduction. The corkscrew scleral vessels are seen. (See Color Plates 48 and 49.)

untreated CCFs.[167] Rarely intraocular pressure rise is precipitous and may result in central retinal artery occlusion.[167] Other mechanisms responsible for the development of glaucoma include elevation of orbital pressure secondary to venous stasis and edema, anterior segment neovascularization and secondary rubeotic glaucoma,[486] and secondary angle closure from congestion of the choroid and a forward shift of the lens iris diaphragm.

Double vision from ocular misalignment is very common. Isolated abduction deficits are quite common and presumably result from sixth nerve dysfunction in the majority of patients (50% to 85% of all patients with CCFs).[477] The sixth nerve is the most vulnerable because it floats freely adjacent to the lateral aspect of the carotid artery, while the third and fourth nerves are enveloped by dura in the lateral wall of the sinus. Despite this anatomic difference the third and fourth nerve are nevertheless frequently involved (67% and 49%, respectively, in Kupersmith's series).[477] However, oculor motor dysfunction from the initial head trauma may be difficult to distinguish from the deficit acquired with the CCF. The oculomotor palsies may result from compression by the fistula or from ischemia due to altered blood flow in the vasa nervorum. These cranial nerve palsies can develop at any time after the fistula forms. Many patients describe pain in the first or even second division of the trigeminal nerve, which can result from compression of the ophthalmic or maxillary divisions of the fifth nerve in the cavernous sinus.

Other patients develop double vision as a result of restrictive myopathy secondary to orbital congestion. The eye muscles are enlarged and double vision is coincident with the development of proptosis. In many patients a combination of neurogenic and myopathic eye movement dysfunction occurs. Forced duction testing with forceps should not be used because of the risk of bleeding from arterialized conjunctival and episcleral vessels.

Vision loss can result from a variety of trauma- or fistula-related causes (Table 15–11). In the era before routine, successful, endovascular treatment of CCFs, vision loss occurred in nearly every patient. In Kupersmith's series of 95 cases of traumatic CCFs, the most common causes of vision loss included traumatic optic neuropathy (5 patients), postsurgical optic neuropathy (2 patients), venous hypoxic retinopathy (3 patients), globe injury (3 patients), corneal ulceration and perforation (1 patient), and central retinal artery occlusion secondary to elevated intraocular pressure (1 patient).[167] In four patients he also recognized a reversible retrobulbar optic neuropathy, which was believed to result from either compression by the superior ophthalmic vein or a vascular steal phenomenon.[167] Other causes of vision loss include anterior ischemic optic neuropathy, compressive optic neuropathy from an extended cavernous sinus, and retrobulbar ischemia.[486, 487] Ophthalmoscopically, most patients show nonspecific findings of venous stasis retinopathy with distended retinal veins and intraretinal hemorrhages. Many patients have mild disc swelling as well. Choroidal detachment as an initial manifestation of direct CCF has also been noted.[488]

TABLE 15–11. Causes of Visual Loss Due to Carotid–Cavernous Fistulas

Venous stasis retinopathy
Ischemic optic neuropathy
Glaucoma
Choroidal effusions
Corneal ulcerations and perforation
Retinal vascular occlusion
Retrobulbar optic neuropathy (compressive versus vascular steal)
Retrobulbar ischemia

Rare manifestations of high-flow CCFs may result from unusual drainage patterns. If drainage occurs superiorly into the sphenoparietal sinus or deep sylvian veins into cerebral veins, spontaneous rupture can be associated with intracerebral or subarachnoid bleeding.[167, 489, 490] If drainage occurs inferiorly it can travel through the emissary veins at the base of the skull or through sphenoid sinus veins and end up in a dilated pterygomaxillary venous plexus with pseudoaneurysm formation. Rupture of this pseudoaneurysm can result in life-threatening epistaxis.[167]

Diagnostic Evaluation. The diagnosis of a high-flow, direct CCF is usually made on clinical grounds in patients with or without a recent history of trauma who suddenly develop a bruit, proptosis, and a red eye. The clinical suspicion should be confirmed by diagnostic testing, which can include pneumotonometry, orbital ultrasound, color Doppler ultrasound, and neuroimaging (including MRI, MRI-angiography, and conventional angiography). Pneumotonometry may be used to document wide pulse pressures.[491] Orbital ultrasonography can be used to document enlarged superior ophthalmic veins and extraocular muscles. A-scan ultrasonography can also demonstrate rapid echo spikes within the superior ophthalmic vein when done in real time.[492] Color Doppler ultrasonography can document reversal of flow in the superior ophthalmic vein with high-flow. CT and MRI can similarly document enlargement of the orbital veins, eye muscles, and cavernous sinus.

Although the diagnosis can be established by the clinical findings and noninvasive studies, formal cerebral angiography is usually required to document the extent and location of feeding vessels. Selected injections of both internal and external carotid arteries are necessary.[167, 474, 493, 494] Angiography will also help to define the other characteristics of the CCF, including the presence of pseudoaneurysms, venous drainage pattern, and whether cavernous sinus thrombosis is present. The presence of contributing dural collaterals, the presence of a patent trigeminal artery (embryologic artery connecting the carotid and basilar arteries), the patency of the circle of Willis, and the amount of crossflow from the contralateral carotid must also be evaluated and considered prior to treatment.[167, 495] In some patients flow is so rapid from the carotid artery into the cavernous sinus that it makes imaging the carotid distal to the cavernous sinus very difficult. This can be overcome using rapid-sequence imaging or imaging the carotid after filling the vertebral artery, which supplies the cavernous carotid through the posterior communicating artery.[495] These techniques help to rule out complete transections of the cavernous carotid prior to treatment.

Course and Treatment. Nearly all high-flow, direct CCFs require treatment. This is in contrast to the low-flow dural fistulas (types B–D DAVMs), which can often be followed and may close spontaneously (see below). In direct CCFs that are left untreated, there is significant risk for serious vision loss secondary to corneal exposure, glaucoma, and venous stasis.[496] Double vision may also linger as a chronic problem in untreated patients. Most authors agree that progressive vision loss, proptosis, ophthalmoplegia, elevated intracranial pressure, intracranial bleeding, and epistaxis are all indications for treatment.[478, 484, 495, 497] Prior to definitive therapy of the CCF, its secondary manifestations such as glaucoma and exposure should be treated. For glaucoma, topical medications, including beta-blockers or pilocarpine, may be administered. Topical or oral carbonic anhydrase inhibitors and any of the newer glaucoma therapies, such as prostaglandins and alpha-adrenergic agents, may also be used. None of these is directed at the primary cause of the elevated intraocular pressure and therefore only modest reductions in intraocular pressure may result. In general, surgical treatment of glaucoma in this setting should be avoided because in eyes with dilated choroidal vessels, lowering of the intraocular pressure could result in suprachoroidal hemorrhage. Exposure should be managed with aggressive lubrication and possibly tarsorrhaphy.

Approximately 20% of CCFs require emergency endovascular treatment because of vision compromise, rapid elevation of intraocular pressure, or bleeding (epistaxis or intracranial bleeding).[167] In the past, therapy for direct CCFs was surgical and largely consisted of ligating the common or internal carotid arteries. Cure rate with this method is about 40%.[498] Modifications included the ligation of the supraclinoid carotid artery and the ophthalmic artery. Surgical therapy of CCFs has been replaced by endovascular obliteration either transvenously or transarterially. Transarterial detachable balloon or platinum coil occlusion, first used by Serbenenko in 1974,[499] is the treatment of choice. Endovascular treatment preserves carotid artery patency and is successful in 59% to 88% of patients.[167,474,478,500] The remainder of the patients in these series were for the most part treated successfully with carotid occlusion. The technique entails introducing a flow-directed catheter through the femoral artery then floating it into the venous side of the CCF. Once in position, the balloon is inflated, occluding the shunt (not the carotid artery), and then the balloon is detached. Balloons are either silicone or latex and come in different sizes and shapes (up to 2 cm). They can be filled with contrast material, making them radio-opaque. They remain inflated for 6 weeks, which is long enough for the fistula to close.[495] Unique treatment considerations arise in patients with patent trigeminal arteries so that flow can be maintained in the basilar and carotid arteries.

Transvenous embolization can be performed through the femoral vein or through the orbit. The latter approach is generally reserved for cases in which the transarterial approach failed or is not possible because of carotid anatomy or occlusion from the previous trauma. Halbach and associates[501] treated 14 of 165 traumatic CCFs (8.5%) via the transvenous route. This method was successful in 11 patients but technically difficult because of multiple septations in the venous structures. In two patients perforation of the inferior petrosal sinus occurred. Miller and associates[502] also described a successful trans-superior ophthalmic vein technique of balloon occlusion in two patients with direct CCFs.

Complications of Treatment. Complications include pseudoaneurysm formation from cavernous sinus filling and oculomotor palsies that usually resolve and are presumably related to balloon stretching of the cavernous sinus. Stroke from errant embolic material or premature detachment of the balloon is very rare, occurring in 2% to 4% of patients.[167,474,501,503,504] Premature deflation of the balloon with recurrence of the fistula is seen in 5% of patients.[167]

Prognosis. With successful closure of a direct CCF, prognosis for virtual full recovery is excellent. The closure of the shunt is associated with immediate resolution of the bruit. Intraocular pressure elevation generally resolves within 2 days. Recurrence of the bruit or persistent elevated intraocular pressure strongly suggests that the fistula has recurred or was inadequately treated. Visual field defects that resulted from persistent elevated intraocular pressure would not be expected to improve. Orbital congestion and ophthalmoparesis generally take 1 to 4 weeks to resolve.[167,505]

Low-Flow Carotid–Cavernous Fistulas (Dural Arteriovenous Malformations). Dural arteriovenous malformations (DAVMs) are abnormal communications between the arteries that supply the dura mater and the intracranial venous sinuses (Fig. 15–36). Although most DAVMs are acquired arteriovenous shunts, some may represent congenital lesions.[506,507] They most likely develop from pre-existing microscopic communications between arteries and veins in the dura in the area near the venous sinuses. A second insult such as trauma or thrombosis then leads to conversion to a DAVM.[508,509]

In Kupersmith's series,[167] 68% of the patients seen with shunts in the area of the cavernous sinus had low-flow dural AVMs. There is considerable overlap in the symptomatology of DAVMs in the cavernous sinus region and direct CCFs since they both result in arterialization of the orbital venous drainage system (Ta-

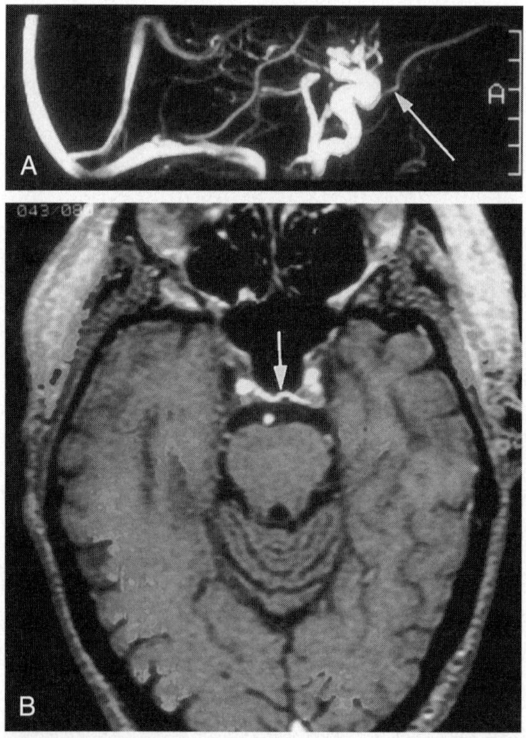

FIGURE 15–36. Dural, low-flow CCF. **A.** MRI-angiogram in lateral projection demonstrating abnormal flow in the left superior ophthalmic vein (*arrow*). **B.** Spoiled gradient-echo axial image illustrating high signal in the intercavernous region, indicating flow through the intercavernous sinuses (*arrow*). (From Standaert D, et al. J Neuroimag 1992;2:208–211, with permission.)

ble 15–10). In the region of the cavernous sinus, meningeal branches of the cavernous carotid artery contribute to the development of the shunt. The two most commonly involved arteries in DAVMs in the region of the cavernous sinus are the meningohypophyseal trunk and the artery of the inferior cavernous sinus.[473] Each of these arteries derives from the cavernous portion of the carotid artery and branches into three separate arteries. Arising from the meningohypophyseal trunk, the dorsal meningeal artery supplies the dura in the region of the clivus. The dorsal meningeal artery is the most commonly involved artery in the formation of DAVM. In this region branches off of the dorsal meningeal artery may anastomose with external carotid artery. The meningeal branches of the external carotid artery in this region include the internal maxillary, ascending pharyngeal, and occipital arteries. The middle meningeal artery arises from the internal maxillary artery and supplies the dura in the region of the foramen ovale and foramen spinosum. In this area, there may be anastomoses with branches from the artery of the inferior cavernous sinus.

Clinical Presentation. DAVMs in the region of the cavernous sinus are most often seen in woman over age 50 or in association with pregnancy, systemic hypertension, Ehlers Danlos syndrome and minor trauma. As with direct CCFs, DAVMs in the region of the cavernous sinus produce symptoms based on the rate of flow and pattern of venous drainage. Patients with posterior drainage into the petrosal sinus or basilar venous plexus would not be expected to have orbital symptoms. In fact, DAVMs draining posteriorly into the inferior petrosal sinus may cause no externally visible abnormalities (so-called white-eyed shunt). However, patients with posteriorly draining DAVMs in this region have also been reported to present with cranial nerve palsies including third, fourth, fifth, sixth, and seventh nerve palsies.[510–515]

Ocular and orbital symptoms in patients with anteriorly draining DAVMs include proptosis, arterialization of conjunctival vessels, elevated intraocular pressure, oculomotor palsies, ptosis, bruit, venous retinopathy, visual field defect, pain, chemosis, and lid swelling (Table 15–10). Because the onset of all of these symptoms is not explosive, there is often a delay in diagnosis with patients often treated for "nonspecific" red eye with antibiotics or steroids. In Kupersmith's series of 89 patients,[167] the most common findings were elevated intraocular pressure, arterialized conjunctival vessels, and proptosis. Eye movement abnormalities and lid swelling were seen next most commonly. Bruits are less commonly reported by patients and auscultated by examiners in patients with DAVM as opposed to direct CCFs. In one series, 25% of patients had audible bruits that were softer and harder to hear than with direct CCFs.[479] Pain is infrequent and usually mild. The arterialized loops of episcleral and conjunctival vessels have a characteristic appearance called "limbal loops" in which vessels have an acute angulation near the limbus.[516] Like CCFs, patients often develop intraocular pressure elevation and glaucomatous visual field defects as a result of episcleral venous pressure elevation.[517–520] Glaucoma is treated the same way as it is in the case of direct CCFs, temporarily with topical and oral medications and definitively with closure of the DAVM and correction of the abnormal venous congestion.[520]

Proptosis, chemosis and lid swelling are manifestations of elevated orbital venous pressure. These findings are milder than with direct CCFs and generally do not lead to sight-threatening complications such as exposure keratitis with ulceration. Common misdiagnoses in the setting of DAVM-induced orbital congestion include conjunctivitis, acute orbital inflammatory syndrome, and thyroid orbitopathy (see Chapter 18). Orbital congestion can paradoxically worsen (sometimes with treatment) as a result of thrombosis of the orbital veins with increased orbital venous stasis.[521] This worsening may be followed by improvement if the thrombosis propagates into the DAVM and closes the shunt.

Posterior segment complications include venous stasis retinopathy, vitreous hemorrhage, proliferative retinopathy, disc swelling, ischemic optic neuropathy, and exudative retinal detachments.[167, 521–525] Venous stasis retinopathy occurs in about 15% of patients and results most commonly in cases with ophthalmic vein thrombosis rather than from arterialization of the orbital vessels.[526] Vision loss occurs in about 20% to 30% of patients and is usually a sequela of venous stasis retinopathy, ischemic optic neuropathy, or uncontrolled glaucoma (Table 15–11).[479, 509, 527] Choroidal effusions may occur as well but are often small and peripheral. They can be recognized by ophthalmoscopy and by ultrasonography. Larger choroidal effusions can be associated with rotation of the ciliary body and movement of the lens iris diaphragm, resulting in angle closure glaucoma or anterior displacement of a posterior chamber lens.[167, 479, 509, 520, 523, 527, 528]

Eye movement abnormalities result from either congestion and hypoxia of the eye muscles or cranial nerve palsies. The sixth nerve is the most commonly affected, but third[511] and fourth nerve palsies[529] have been reported. After closure of the shunt, the prognosis for recovery of the eye movement abnormalities is good whether they are the result of myopathic or neuropathic processes. Patients rarely can develop cerebral dysfunction, including seizures, infarct, or hemorrhages, as a result of abnormal pial drainage into the cerebral hemispheres. This is more common when there is significant cavernous sinus thrombosis resulting from bilateral fistulas.[167]

Diagnostic Evaluation. The diagnostic modalities utilized in this setting are similar to those used in direct CCFs.[530–532] If symptoms are mild, the diagnosis may be established by clinical findings, ultrasonography, and neuroimaging. MRI can show thrombosis of the cavernous sinus and superior ophthalmic vein. This thrombosis usually appears as a white hyperintensity on T_1-weighted images.[167] MRI can also demonstrate signal decrease in the cavernous sinus on spin-echo imaging due to rapid blood flow.[533] If treatment is planned then angiography should be performed as it may be therapeutic and feeder vessels must be identified. Angiography must be performed on both the internal and external carotid arteries bilaterally.

Treatment. The morbidity of these DAVMs is primarily ocular, as hemorrhage and life-threatening complications are quite rare. Fortunately, between 20% and 50% of these lesions will close either spontaneously, after air travel, or after angiography.[167, 478, 479, 497, 509, 517] However, in Kupersmith's series,[167] 69 of 89 patients were considered for treatment based on progressive symptoms. Sixty of 66 patients were treated successfully treated by embolization, which in some patients had to be performed on more than one occasion. This resolution can occur over a period of days or years. Treatment by embolization is recommended for patients that have progressive or unacceptable symptoms. Ideally this is accomplished through the external carotid artery (external carotid artery only feeders) but occasionally transvenous[534, 535] or trans-internal carotid therapy, with or without detachable balloons is necessary. Rarely, direct surgery on the cavernous sinus with DAVM removal can be performed. Others have used radiation to treat extensive lesions not amenable to embolization or surgery.[479, 536–538] Complications of treatment are uncommon and include incomplete closure, venous thrombosis, cranial nerve palsies from nutrient vessel thrombosis, and cerebral infarctions. Ocular symptoms generally begin to improve within days of treatment and are usually completely resolved within 6 months. Pneumotonometry can be used prior to and after embolization to follow patients and be certain closure is complete without recanalization.

Intracavernous Aneurysm. Aneurysms of the cavernous carotid artery predominately present with orbital pain and diplopia due to oculomotor palsies. Cavernous carotid aneurysms are uncommon, accounting for only 2% of all intracranial aneurysms.[165] Among symptomatic, unruptured aneurysms, the proportion of cavernous carotid lesions increases to 15%.[165] Cavernous carotid aneurysms are rarely life threatening because their rupture is contained by rigid dural walls. Furthermore, due to their extradural location, cavernous carotid aneurysms rarely result in subarachnoid hemorrhage, as aneurysmal rupture instead produces a CCF (see above).

Symptoms and Signs. The frequency of involvement of the various cranial nerves with aneurysms in the cavernous sinus is dependent on their anatomic relationship to the carotid siphon. Cavernous aneurysms frequently involve the abducens nerve early due to its position lateral to the carotid artery within the cavernous sinus.[539] Oculomotor and ophthalmic (V_1) involvement may also occur, but isolated fourth nerve palsies are rare.[167] Unlike posterior communicating aneurysms in which the pupil is usually dilated, a cavernous carotid aneurysm may be associated with a pupil-sparing third nerve palsy. Pain in the distribution of V_1 is the most common manifestation of early trigeminal nerve involvement, complete anesthesia arising only after chronic compression. Neurotrophic keratopathy is a significant complication of V_1 compression, and patients complaining of visual blurring should receive a complete anterior segment examination. Additional causes of visual blurring include paralysis of accommodation from third nerve involvement and visual pathway impingement.

Visual loss secondary to anterior pathway compression is generally a late consequence of large aneurysmal expansion. The pattern of vision loss is dependent on the structure compressed. Anteromedial expansion results in optic nerve compression, while posteromedial expansion results in impingement on the optic chiasm. Proptosis, another late sequela of a cavernous aneurysm, occurs only after the enlarging mass has compromised venous drainage or compressed the globe by eroding through the posterior orbital wall.

Diagnostic Imaging. The lesion is usually detected using MRI (Fig. 15–37). MRI-angiography can be used to assess aneurysmal anatomy, luminal patency, and thrombus age. Cerebral angiography should be performed prior to treatment planning.

Treatment. Cavernous aneurysms in most patients, especially elderly ones, are not treated because of their relatively benign nature. However, treatment can be considered when oculomotor palsies or vision loss are progressive and debilitating or the orbital pain is intractable. With conservative therapy alone, 25% to 40% of patients will stabilize or improve.[167, 540] Treatment options include ipsilateral carotid occlusion, surgical clipping, or endovascular embolization. Due to the high morbidity and mortality of a surgical approach, treatment generally entails either carotid occlusion or endovascular therapy. A functional tolerance test can be performed prior to occlusion to test whether the patient can withstand permanent occlusion.[541] If neurologic symptoms result during a functional occlusion test, an extracranial–intracranial bypass may be indicated prior to definitive treatment.

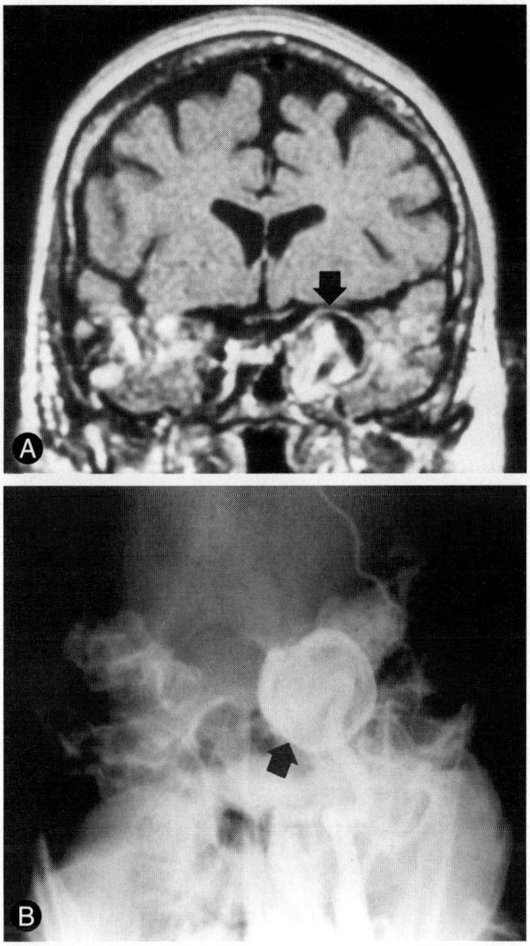

FIGURE 15–37. Cavernous carotid aneurysm. **A.** Coronal MRI demonstrates flow void (*arrow*) within left cavernous sinus. **B.** Angiography (coronal view) confirming large round aneurysm (*arrow*).

Reconstructive endovascular procedures of cavernous aneurysms are often difficult.[182] Recently, excellent results were reported in a series of patients with cavernous lesions treated with electrolytically detachable coils.[542] Since cavernous aneurysms often lack a definitive neck, successful endovascular therapy often requires deconstructive balloon embolization of the parent carotid artery. In this procedure, the cavernous aneurysm is trapped between proximal and distal occluding balloons, and the cervical carotid artery ligated to prevent thrombus from entering the external carotid circulation.[543]

Prognosis. Following embolization or carotid occlusion, the pain and ophthalmoplegia of cavernous aneurysms improve in most cases. The time course of improvement is generally weeks to months. If compression of the anterior visual pathway has occurred, visual function stabilizes but rarely improves. In some cases, there is temporary worsening of symptoms after therapy due to sudden thrombosis and expansion of the aneurysm sac. If signs of aberrant regeneration are present prior to treatment, abnormalities in oculomotor nerve function generally persist.

Superior Orbital Fissure Syndrome

Except for sparing of V_2, lesions of the *superior orbital fissure* are clinically difficult to distinguish from those of the cavernous sinus, and the differential diagnosis is similar. The *orbital apex syndrome* consists of third, fourth, and sixth nerve paresis, V_1 sensory loss, and optic neuropathy from cranial nerve II involvement (Fig. 15–38).

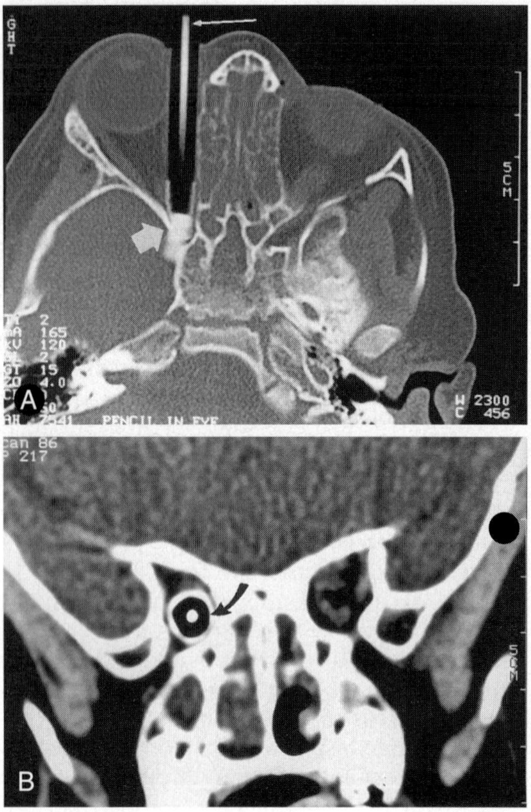

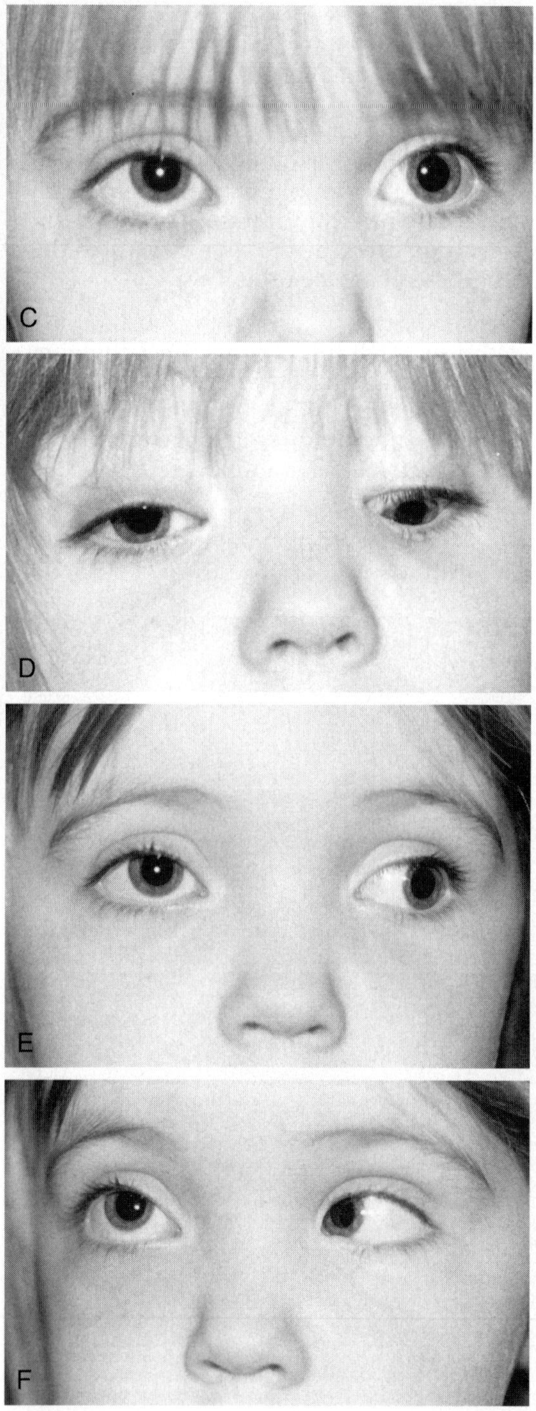

FIGURE 15–38. Orbital apex syndrome from a pencil in the orbit. This child had fallen, and a pencil (eraser end up) entered the orbit, medial to the medial rectus muscle. **A.** Orbital axial CT demonstrates the pencil eraser (*large arrow*) in the orbital apex and the rest of the pencil (*small arrow points to the pencil lead*) pushing the globe laterally. On funduscopic examination, indentation of the nasal retina was seen. **B.** Orbital coronal CT showing pencil (*arrow*) in orbital apex. The pencil was removed surgically without vascular complications. Postoperatively, the child had no light perception in the right eye from optic neuropathy; and ptosis and complete ophthalmoplegia of the right eye from third, fourth, and sixth nerve palsies (**C–F**). The ocular motor palsies resolved, but vision failed to recover.

Congenital Fibrosis Syndromes

Patients with congenital fibrosis syndromes are born with ptosis and restrictive ophthalmoparesis due to fibrosis of the extraocular muscles.[544–546] Because of severe strabismus or ptosis, binocular vision is usually compromised, and amblyopia is common. Associated ophthalmic findings may include Marcus Gunn jaw wink, nystagmus, exposure keratopathy, and synergistic divergence.[547] Typically, affected patients are otherwise neurologically normal.

The most common forms are the general fibrosis syndromes, which are familial disorders with diffuse bilateral ophthalmoparesis and ptosis. Engle and colleagues[548–550] have mapped the genetic defect in three forms (congenital fibrosis of the extraocular muscles types 1, 2, and 3 (CFEOM1, CFEOM2, CFEOM3)) to chromosomes 12p11-q12, 11q13, and 16q24, respectively. Several other variants have been described: primary involvement of the horizontal muscles; primary involvement of the vertically acting muscles[551]; and congenital unilateral fibrosis of the extraocular muscles with ptosis and enophthalmos.[552]

Neuroimaging may demonstrate atrophy or increased width of the extraocular muscles. Occasionally, diffusely infiltrating orbital masses can be seen. Pathologic examination of the extraocular muscles typically reveals replacement of striated muscle by dense fibrous tissue. It is still unclear if congenital fibrosis syndromes are neuropathic or myopathic in origin. However, in one reported case the superior division of the oculomotor nerve was absent, suggesting at least some of the abnormalities may result from defective congenital innervation of the extraocular muscles, analogous to Duane's retraction syndrome.[553] Treatment, consisting of strabismus and ptosis surgery, is aimed at improving cosmesis, ocular alignment, and head position.

CHILDHOOD STRABISMUS PATTERNS

This section will briefly review childhood strabismus patterns that may be mistaken for acquired ocular motility deficits. Long-standing eso- and exophorias can decompensate later in life, leading to chronic diplopia. The usual clues to the congenital onset of the ocular misalignment are their long-standing nature, full ductions, and the lack of diplopia. Other childhood strabismus patterns, such as congenital oculor motor nerve palsies and Duane's retraction syndrome, are discussed above, and Möbius syndrome is reviewed above and in Chapter 14.

Esotropia

The major categories of childhood esotropia include accommodative, infantile (congenital), acquired nonaccommodative, and esotropia associated with impaired sight (sensory esotropia).[356] Patients with these disturbances usually exhibit comitant esodeviations with full ductions. Esotropia is the most common type of ocular misalignment in childhood, comprising at least half of cases in this age group.[554] Comitant esotropia may also be acquired suddenly in older children. Neuroimaging, while required in such cases, is usually normal.[555]

Exotropia

Children with nonparalytic exotropia have a divergence of the eyes. Like in childhood esotropia, the deviation may be intermittent or constant, ductions are normal, and the child may alternately fixate with either eye. In infants, exotropias tend to be more constant, while in older children, intermittent exotropia with relatively good stereopsis is more commonly seen. When intermittent, fatigue or illness may worsen the exotropia.[554] Exotropia in childhood is associated with an increased prevalence of neurologic, ocular, and craniofacial abnormalities.[556]

Brown Syndrome

This motility abnormality, also known as the "superior oblique tendon sheath syndrome," is characterized by a restriction of elevation of the eye in adduction and normal or near normal elevation in abduction (Fig. 15–39). The disorder can be distinguished clinically from an inferior oblique palsy by the presence of positive forced duction testing, the absence of superior oblique overaction, and typically, normal alignment in primary gaze. Brown syndrome is attributed to a disturbance of free tendon movement through the trochlear pulley.[557] Patients may report an audible click, discomfort, or pain upon attempted upgaze.

Although usually congenital, acquired cases of Brown syndrome may occur in association

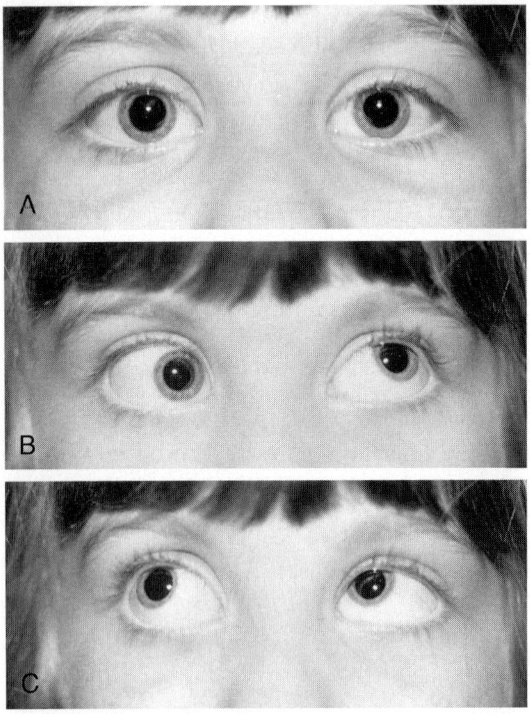

FIGURE 15–39. Congenital Brown syndrome. **A.** In primary gaze there is no ocular misalignment. **B.** Defective elevation of the right eye in adduction. **C.** Near normal elevation of the right eye in abduction. The child had no diplopia.

with trauma, paranasal sinusitis, or systemic inflammatory disease such as rheumatoid arthritis causing tenosynovitis of the trochlea.[558] Some of the acquired cases may respond to anti-inflammatory agents such as corticosteroids. Congenital cases are usually observed, and occasionally there is spontaneous resolution.[559] Strabismus surgery can be considered when there is a primary position hypotropia or abnormal head posture.

Dissociated Vertical Deviation

During cover testing, in dissociated vertical deviation (DVD) the covered eye deviates upward and excyclorotates, then refixates when the occlusion is removed. The fellow eye maintains fixation the entire time. The monocular upward drift may also occur spontaneously during periods of inattention. This dysmotility pattern contrasts to the vertical misalignment in skew or fourth nerve palsies, which is characterized by vertical drift and refixation movements of both eyes during cover testing.

DVD is usually associated with eso- or exotropias and nystagmus.[560–562] It may be mistaken for inferior oblique overaction. The mechanism is unknown, but is it is likely to be a supranuclear disturbance. Some authors have suggested that DVD is a disturbance or exaggeration of a normal vertical vergence eye movement.[563, 564]

Synergistic Divergence

In this miswiring phenomenon, both lateral rectus muscles contract when one eye is abducted.[565] This leads to a wall-eyed appearance. The exact anatomic substrate is unknown.

ORBITAL PROCESSES CAUSING DIPLOPIA

Thyroid-Associated Ophthalmopathy

Restrictive thyroid myopathy due to thyroid-associated ophthalmopathy is one of the most common causes of diplopia in adults. The double vision is typically insidious and painless, often accompanied by complaints of eye irritation due to reduced tear film and decreased blink rate. One or both eyes may be proptotic with eyelid edema, lid retraction, and lagophthalmos (see Chapter 14). Restriction of ocular elevation with a positive forced duction test is characteristic of the disorder, but any muscle or combination may be involved. Affected patients have either primary hyperthyroidism (Grave's disease), primary hypothyroidism (eg, Hashimoto's thyroiditis), or hypothyroidism due to treated hyperthyroidism. For unknown reasons, the extraocular muscles develop lymphocytic and plasmacytic infiltration with secondary production of acid mucopolysaccharides and fibrosis. CT and MRI of the orbits may demonstrate thickening of the extraocular muscles. The pathophysiology, diagnosis, and management of thyroid-associated ophthalmopathy are discussed in greater detail in Chapter 18.

Orbital Inflammatory Syndrome

Orbital myositis, with inflammation of muscles only, and *orbital pseudotumor,* with involvement of muscles and other contiguous structures, are characterized by painful double vision and restrictive ophthalmoplegia. Usually idiopathic but sometimes associated with systemic lupus erythematosus or Crohn's disease, they probably represent the orbital versions of the Tolosa–Hunt syndrome. The pain and diplopia are usually responsive to oral corticosteroids. This condition is also discussed in more detail in Chapter 18.

Muscle Infiltration

Isolated metastases to extraocular muscles are uncommon, but orbital metastasis from lung or breast carcinoma or lymphoma can involve the extraocular muscles.[566] CT or MRI usually reveals an orbital soft-tissue mass. The differential diagnosis of muscle infiltration is detailed in Chapter 18.

NEUROMUSCULAR JUNCTION

Myasthenia Gravis

The extraocular muscles are involved in over 90% of patients with myasthenia gravis. Fifty percent present with motility abnormalities or ptosis only, and of this group, half will remain "ocular myasthenics," while the other half will develop generalized symptoms, usually within 2 years. The diagnosis is supported by diurnal variation, fatigability, eyelid signs such as ptosis or Cogan's lid twitch (see Chapter 14), and the absence of pain. Any eye muscle can be affected, and the motility pattern may mimic a pupil-sparing third, fourth, or sixth nerve palsy, as well as supranuclear disturbances (see Chapter 16) such as a conjugate gaze palsy, internuclear ophthalmoplegia (Fig. 15–40), or one-and-a-half syndrome.[567–569] As a rule, the pupil is uninvolved. Resolution of appreciable ptosis or motility deficits following administration of intravenous edrophonium (Tensilon test) helps establish the diagnosis, but interpretation is more difficult with subtle ocular abnormalities. Acetylcholine receptor antibody levels, abnormal in half of patients with solely ocular myasthenia, and electromyography with repetitive stimulation and single fiber studies are important complementary tests. Acetylcholinesterases usually fail to control the diplopia, which often requires the addition of corticosteroids. Myasthenia gravis is discussed in detail in Chapter 14.

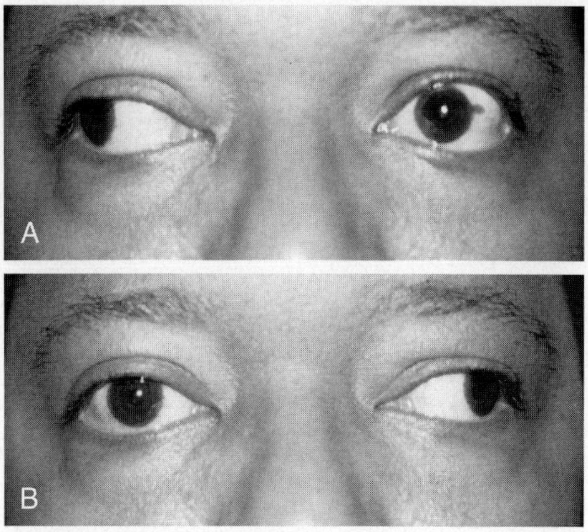

FIGURE 15–40. Pseudobilateral internuclear ophthalmoplegia in myasthenia gravis. The patient developed bilateral adduction weakness and abducting nystagmus. There was mild ptosis on the right. The motility disturbance and ptosis resolved with corticosteroids.

Others

Eye muscle involvement is unusual in Lambert–Eaton myasthenic syndrome, although rare patients may develop ptosis or minor transient motility disturbances. However, these patients do not show ocular misalignment on formal testing. Ocular motility and pupillary reactivity may be affected in botulism.

PRIMARY OCULAR MYOPATHIES

Chronic Progressive External Ophthalmoplegia and Kearns–Sayre Syndrome

Insidious, symmetric loss of eye movements, lack of diplopia, bilateral ptosis, and weakness of orbicularis oculi characterize *chronic progressive external ophthalmoplegia* (CPEO) due to mitochondrial dysfunction (*external* refers to extraocular muscles, internal refers to the pupillary sphincter). The Kearns–Sayre syndrome, typified by CPEO, pigmentary retinopathy, and cardiac conduction defects, is associated with mitochondrial DNA deletions. These conditions are reviewed in Chapter 14.

Other Ocular Myopathies

Patients with oculopharyngeal dystrophy and myotonic dystrophy, which are also discussed in Chapter 14, and myotubular myopathy, congenital fiber type disproportion, Bassen–Kornzweig syndrome (abetalipoproteinemia), Refsum's disease, and multicore myopathy[570] may develop slowly progressive ptosis and ophthalmoparesis. Abnormal eye movements in Duchenne, Becker, and nemaline muscular dystrophies are exceptional.[571, 572]

Extraocular Muscle Ischemia

Although uncommon, extraocular muscle ischemia due to giant cell arteritis (see Chapter 5) should be considered in any patient over 60 years of age with diplopia.[573] Ten to fifteen percent of patients with giant cell arteritis may have diplopia and unilateral ophthalmoplegia resulting from either ischemia of the extraocular muscles or oculor motor nerves.[574, 575] In elderly individuals, symptoms of jaw claudication, headache, weight loss, and fever should be sought, and a sedimentation rate and C-reactive protein obtained. The double vision associated with giant cell arteritis may remit following the administration of high-dose corticosteroids.

OTHER MISCELLANEOUS CAUSES OF DIPLOPIA

Diplopia After Cataract Surgery

Patients with diplopia after cataract surgery represent a heterogeneous group of patients with symptoms arising for a variety of reasons (Table 15–12).[576] One study estimated the incidence to be as high as 2% of patients undergoing cataract surgery.[577] In our experience it occurs less frequently. As in all cases of double vision, the examiner must first distinguish monocular diplopia from binocular diplopia. If the post-cataract surgery patient has monocular diplopia there is usually an abnormality in the cornea, intraocular lens, or posterior capsule. These should be apparent on examination, which should include keratometry and careful inspection of the lens and capsule through the dilated pupil.

Patients with binocular double vision after cataract surgery should be examined like all patients with diplopia. Examination should include careful assessment of ductions, cover testing, Maddox rod testing, and the three-step test for vertical misalignments. As well, prior to these measurements the examiner should carefully refract the patient and look for anisometropic refractive errors. The position of the intraocular lens should be noted through the dilated pupil. Decentration of smaller intraocular lenses (optical zone less than 6 mm) and the presence of positioning holes can lead to optical aberrations.[578] Usually patients have to have at least 2 mm of decentration (usually vertically) to induce significant prismatic effect and resultant diplopia. The group of patients with optical causes of double vision after cataract surgery can be hard to recognize and characterize. The changes, which may be subtle such as induced anisometropia or altered brightness sense between the eyes, may still be sufficient to hinder fusion and induce diplopia.

Another set of patients with binocular diplopia lost their ability to fuse when binocular function was disrupted by a unilateral cataract. Intractable diplopia results when the cataract is removed, as the patient is unable to fuse or suppress the images. This syndrome is termed *horror fusionis*, an acquired disruption of central fusion.[579, 580] Affected patients often resort to occlusion of one eye either by optical or mechanical means.

Most patients either have double vision from iatrogenic trauma (direct or secondary to anesthetic) to an extraocular muscle or nerve or had a pre-existing misalignment that was asymptomatic prior to cataract surgery because of reduced acuity in one eye. In our experience, the most common diagnoses made in

TABLE 15–12. Causes of Double Vision After Cataract Surgery

Monocular Diplopia
Decentered or tilted intraocular lens
Cracked foldable intraocular lens
Irregular or high astigmatism from wound closure
Posterior capsule opacity or irregular opening
Iridectomy creating multiple "pupils"
Binocular Diplopia
Iatrogenic anisophoria secondary to anisokonia or anisometropia from alteration of refractive error
Altered fusion secondary to surgical pupil changes
Extraocular muscle trauma from injection or bleeding:
Needle or surgical trauma and anesthetic toxicity
Fibrotic muscle with restrictive pattern
Dysfunctional muscle with paretic pattern
Trauma to an orbital nerve or extraocular muscle
Pre-existing sensory exotropia prior to cataract surgery
Unmasking of alternative preexisting cause of misalignment not previously symptomatic because of poor vision in the eye with the cataract
Decentered intraocular lens with induced prism
Horror fusionis

this setting include decompensated exotropia, decompensated congenital fourth nerve palsy, divergence insufficiency, and thyroid-associated ophthalmopathy. Some patients with poor vision from their cataract will develop a sensory exotropia. When the vision is cleared surgically the exotropia may persist and cause diplopia. This diplopia and sensory exotropia may spontaneously resolve over the next 6 months. Hence, we defer strabismus surgery for at least 6 months after cataract removal.

Other patients with pre-existing problems, such as thyroid-associated ophthalmopathy, will be recognized based on the characteristic exam findings such as proptosis and lid retraction and eye muscle enlargement on neuroimaging studies.[581] However, it often difficult to convince patients that their problem existed prior to the cataract surgery.

Patients with iatrogenic trauma to the extraocular muscles may have several different patterns of motility deficits and misalignment. Typically, the injury is produced by the periocular anesthetic injection. This type of strabismus appears to result from a toxic effect of the local anesthetic or from direct trauma to the extraocular muscle.[582] Occasionally the injection traumatizes the orbital nerves, ultimately producing strabismus. Previously it was thought that the bridle-suture used to hold the superior rectus muscle during cataract surgery was the culprit, but this seems to be less likely at this time. Carlson and associates,[583] were able to demonstrate that anesthetic injected directly into monkey extraocular muscles is capable of causing wide-spread damage to muscle fibers. This type of muscle injury can result in either contracture, overaction or paretic dysfunction, and therefore a variety of extraocular muscle dysfunction patterns have been reported.[584] The most vulnerable muscle is the inferior rectus muscle, which can develop contracture after cataract surgery.[576, 585–587] The resulting strabismus is very similar to that seen in patients with inferior rectus fibrosis from thyroid-associated ophthalmopathy. Patients develop a hypotropia with restriction of elevation in the affected eye. Similar contractures of the inferior oblique muscle have been described.[588] If the patient is seen acutely, a pattern of primary dysfunction or paresis may be evident before the muscle undergoes contractures.

Other patients may manifest with primary overaction of an extraocular muscle. This may result from myotoxicity of the antagonist muscle or may represent a component of the contracture phase of an injured muscle. A common scenario here again is primary inferior rectus dysfunction with superior rectus overaction.[589, 590] Most of these patients with overaction have patterns that simulate a mild contracture. These can be successfully repaired through procedures designed at weakening the overacting muscle. The final group of patients have a primary paresis (usually of the inferior rectus muscle). These patients are recognized by the inability to depress the affected eye.[591] In this setting, resection procedures as well as weakening of infraduction of the contralateral eye may be effective in correcting the strabismus.

Hemifield Slide Phenomenon

Individuals with bitemporal hemianopias due to chiasmal disturbances may develop double vision from misalignment of noncorresponding nasal hemifields. This diagnosis should be considered in any patient with double vision who states that the two images slide in relation to one another. They may also complain of visual areas in which they can not see. The hemifield slide phenomenon is discussed in detail in Chapter 7.

Spontaneous Extraocular Muscle Contractions

There are three conditions characterized by spontaneous extraocular muscle contractions: superior oblique myokymia, ocular neuromyotonia, and cyclic oculomotor spasms. The last was discussed above in the section on third nerve palsies.

Superior Oblique Myokymia. Intermittent, fine-amplitude oscillatory contractions of a superior oblique muscle characterize this unusual eye movement disorder.[592, 593] Patients are typically young adults, and they complain of monocular oscillopsia, often with vertical or torsional diplopia. The downward, intorting ocular oscillations are best seen with the slit lamp. Cover testing may reveal overaction of the affected superior oblique muscle. In the long-term follow-up in two series of patients,[594, 595] recurrent spontaneous remissions and relapses were observed.

Usually unprovoked, superior oblique myokymia occasionally is associated with recov-

TABLE 15–13. Common Causes of Acute Bilateral Ophthalmoparesis

Differential Diagnosis	Associated Symptoms and History	Signs	Ancillary Diagnostic Tests
Pituitary apoplexy	Severe headache, meningismus	Cranial nerve III, IV, VI, V_1 or V_2 involvement; visual loss may be present	MRI LP
Myasthenia gravis	Painless, fluctuates with fatigue, dysarthria	Pupil sparing, ptosis, with or without bulbar and generalized weakness	Edrophonium test, electrodiagnostic studies, anti-acetylcholine receptor antibody level
Botulism	May be associated with gastrointestinal symptoms: anorexia, nausea, vomiting	Dilated, unreactive pupils; bradycardia, constipation	Electrodiagnostic studies, serum bioassay
Wernicke's encephalopathy	History of alcohol abuse or malnutrition	Nystagmus, ataxia, confusional state, physical stigmata of long-term alcohol abuse	Improvement with thiamine
Guillain–Barré syndrome (Miller Fisher variant)	Preceding gastrointestinal or upper respiratory tract illness	Areflexia, ataxia, extremity weakness	LP, electrodiagnostic studies
Brain stem stroke	History of cardiac arrhythmia, vascular disease	Bilateral long tract signs, skew deviation	MRI

From Laskowitz D, Liu GT, Galetta SL: Acute visual loss and other disorders of the eyes. Neurol Clin North Am 1998:16:323–353, with permission.

ered fourth nerve palsies,[596] head trauma, and posterior fossa tumors.[597] As a result, some authors have attributed the myokymia to mild, usually subclinical fourth nerve injury, followed by axonal regeneration and spontaneous discharging of trochlear motor neurons.[598, 599] Defective supranuclear input to the fourth nerve nucleus has also been proposed.[595]

Frequently the symptoms are bothersome and uncomfortable enough to justify medical or surgical intervention. Initial treatment consists of medical therapy with carbamazepine[600] or propranolol.[601] We have also seen benefit with gabapentin. Patients refractory to medical treatment may undergo superior oblique tenotomy, sometimes combined with inferior oblique tenectomy.[595] One reported patient benefitted from microvascular decompression of the fourth nerve at the root exit zone.[602] Superior oblique myokymia is also discussed in Chapter 17.

Ocular Neuromyotonia. In ocular neuromyotonia, tonic spasms of the muscles of an ocular motor nerve occur following sustained eccentric gaze. Affected patients complain of paroxysms of sustained diplopia for seconds or minutes. Some feel a pulling sensation in their orbit. The disorder is a delayed one, usually months or years following radiation for a sellar or parasellar tumor[603–605] or some other intracranial neoplasm.[606–608] Cases without antecedent radiation have also been reported in patients with spontaneous ocular neuromyotonia[609, 610] and also individuals with thyroid-associated orbitopathy,[611] carotid artery aneurysm,[612] infectious cavernous sinus thrombosis,[613] and myelography with thorium dioxide.[608] The mechanism is thought to be related either to unstable axonal membranes, ephaptic neural transmission, reorganization of the oculor motor nuclei following peripheral injury, or changes in neural activity following denervation.[609] Treatment usually consists of carbamazepine, which has membrane-stabilizing properties.

Ocular Motility Deficits in High (Axial) Myopia

Adults with unilateral or bilateral high myopia may develop an esotropia, abduction deficit or, vertical misalignment. Various explanations, including an elongated globe, tightness of the medial recti, decompensated esotropia, a heavy globe, lateral rectus abnormalities, and defective orbital connective tissues and muscle paths, have been proposed.[614–616]

Fixation Switch Diplopia

In adults with a history of childhood strabismus (eso- or exotropia, for example), a change in refractive error of the dominant eye may cause fixation with the nondominant eye. This may lead to diplopia, but is managed by correcting the refractive error.[617]

ACUTE BILATERAL COMPLETE OPHTHALMOPLEGIA

The differential diagnosis of an acute inability to move both eyes is narrow, and consists primarily of pituitary apoplexy, myasthenia gravis, botulism, Wernicke's encephalopathy, Guillain–Barré syndrome and Miller Fisher variant, and brain stem stroke or hemorrhage.[618–620] Distinguishing historical, examination, and diagnostic features of each are listed in Table 15–13. Less common causes, such as meningitis, phenytoin toxicity, and bilateral cavernous sinus masses or infection, should also be considered.[619]

REFERENCES

1. Miller MJ, Mark LP, Ho KC, et al: Anatomic relationship of the oculomotor nuclear complex and medial longitudinal fasciculus in the midbrain. AJNR: Am J Neuroradiol 1997;18:111–113.
2. Warwick R: Representation of the extra-ocular muscles in the oculomotor nuclei of the monkey. J Comp Neurol 1953;98:449–495.
3. Donzelli R, Marinkovic S, Brigante L, et al: The oculomotor nuclear complex in humans. Microanatomy and clinical significance. Surg Radiol Anat 1998; 20:7–12.
4. Bienfang DC: Crossing axons in the third nerve nucleus. Invest Ophthalmol 1975;14:927–931.
5. Tubbs RS, Oakes WJ: Relationships of the cisternal segment of the trochlear nerve. J Neurosurg 1998;89:1015–1019.
6. Ziyal IM, Salas E, Wright DC, et al: The petrolingual ligament: the anatomy and surgical exposure of the posterolateral landmark of the cavernous sinus. Acta Neurochir 1998;140:201–204.
7. Spektor S, Piontek E, Umansky F: Orbital venous drainage into the anterior cavernous sinus space: microanatomic relationships. Neurosurgery 1997;40: 532–539.
8. Parkinson D: Anatomy of the cavernous sinus. In: Smith JL (ed): Neuro-ophthalmology, pp 73–101. St. Louis, CV Mosby, 1972.
9. Harris FS, Rhoton AL: Anatomy of the cavernous sinus, a microsurgical study. J Neurosurg 1976;45: 169–180.

10. Taptas TN: The so-called cavernous sinus: A review of the controversy and its implications for neurosurgeons. Neurosurgery 1982;11:712–717.
11. Bosley TM, Schatz NJ: Clinical diagnosis of cavernous sinus syndromes. Neurol Clin 1983;1:929–953.
12. Luco CF, Valenzuela RF: Diabetic complete external ophthalmoplegia. J Clin Neuro-ophthalmol 1990;10: 206–209.
13. Capo H, Kupersmith MJ, Berenstein A, et al: The clinical importance of the inferolateral trunk of the internal carotid artery. Neurosurgery 1991;28: 733–738.
14. Tran-Dinh H: Cavernous branches of the internal carotid artery: anatomy and nomenclature. Neurosurgery 1987;20:205–210.
15. Umansky F, Nathan H: The lateral wall of the cavernous sinus with special reference to the nerves related to it. J Neurosurg 1982;56:228–234.
16. Striph GG, Burde RM: Abducens palsy and Horner's syndrome revisited. J Clin Neuro-ophthalmol 1988;8:13–17.
17. Liu GT: Anatomy and physiology of the trigeminal nerve. In: Miller NR, Newman NJ (eds): Walsh and Hoyt's Clinical Neuro-ophthalmology, 4th edition, pp 1595–1648. Baltimore, Williams & Wilkins, 1998.
18. Porter JD, Baker RS, Ragusa RJ, et al: Extraocular muscles: basic and clinical aspects of structure and function. Surv Ophthalmol 1995;39:451–484.
19. Porter JD, Baker RS: Muscles of a different 'color': the unusual properties of the extraocular muscles may predispose or protect them in neurogenic and myogenic disease. Neurology 1996;46:30–37.
20. Porter JD, Poukens V, Baker RS, et al: Structure–function correlations in the human medial rectus extraocular muscle pulleys. Invest Ophthalmol Vis Sci 1996;37:468–472.
21. Asbury AK, Aldredge H, Hershberg R, et al: Oculomotor palsy in diabetes mellitus: a clinico-pathological study. Brain 1970;93:555–566.
22. Balcer LJ, Galetta SL, Yousem DM, et al: Pupil-involving third nerve palsy and carotid stenosis: rapid recovery following endarterectomy. Ann Neurol 1997;41:273–276.
23. Marinkovic S, Gibo H: The neurovascular relationships and the blood supply of the oculomotor nerve: the microsurgical anatomy of its cisternal segment. Surg Neurol 1994;42:505–516.
24. Parkinson D: A surgical approach to the cavernous portion of the carotid artery: anatomical studies and case report. J Neurosurg 1965;23:474–483.
25. Cahill M, Bannigan J, Eustace P: Anatomy of the extraneural blood supply to the intracranial oculomotor nerve. Br J Ophthalmol 1996;80:177–181.
26. Marinkovic S, Gibo H, Zelic O, et al: The neurovascular relationships and the blood supply of the trochlear nerve: surgical anatomy of its cisternal segment. Neurosurgery 1996;38:161–169.
27. Brazis PW, Lee AG: Acquired binocular horizontal diplopia. Mayo Clin Proc 1999;74:907–916.
28. Spector RH: Vertical diplopia. Surv Ophthalmol 1993;38:31–62.
29. Brazis PW, Lee AG: Binocular vertical diplopia. Mayo Clin Proc 1998;73:55–66.
30. Rush JA, Younge BR: Paralysis of cranial nerves III, IV, and VI. Arch Ophthalmol 1981;99:76–79.
31. Berlit P: Isolated and combined pareses of cranial nerves III, IV and VI. A retrospective study of 412 patients. J Neurol Sci 1991;103:10–15.
32. Richards DW, Jones FR, Younge BR: Causes and prognosis in 4,270 cases of paralysis of the oculomotor, trochlear, and abducens cranial nerves. Am J Ophthalmol 1992;113:489–496.
33. Holmes JM, Mutyala S, Maus TL, et al: Pediatric third, fourth, and sixth nerve palsies: a population-based study. Am J Ophthalmol 1999;127:388–392.
34. Newman NJ, Lambert SR: Botulinum toxin treatment of supranuclear ocular motility disorders. Neurology 1992;42:1391–1393.
35. Benegas NM, Egbert J, Engel WK, et al: Diplopia secondary to aniseikonia associated with macular disease. Arch Ophthalmol 1999;117:896–899.
36. Silverberg M, Schuler E, Veronneau-Troutman S, et al: Nonsurgical management of binocular diplopia induced by macular pathology. Arch Ophthalmol 1999;117:900–903.
37. Leigh RJ, Zee DS: The Neurology of Eye Movements, 3rd edition, pp 502–510. New York, Oxford University Press, 1999.
38. Smith JL, David NJ: Internuclear ophthalmoplegia. Two new clinical signs. Neurology 1964;14:307–309.
39. Zee DS: Internuclear ophthalmoplegia: pathophysiology and diagnosis. Baillière's Clin Neurol 1992;1: 455–470.
40. Marshall RS, Sacco RL, Kreuger R, et al: Dissociated vertical nystagmus and internuclear ophthalmoplegia from a midbrain infarction. Arch Neurol 1991;48:1304–1305.
41. Dehaene I, Casselman JW, D'Hooghe M, et al: Unilateral internuclear ophthalmoplegia and ipsiversive torsional nystagmus. J Neurol 1996;243:461–464.
42. Cremer PD, Migliaccio AA, Halmagyi GM, et al: Vestibulo-ocular reflex pathways in internuclear ophthalmoplegia. Ann Neurol 1999;45:529–533.
43. Smith JL, Cogan DG: Internuclear ophthalmoplegia. A review of fifty-eight cases. Arch Ophthalmol 1959;61:687–694.
44. Gonyea EF: Bilateral internuclear ophthalmoplegia. Association with occlusive cerebrovascular disease. Arch Neurol 1974;31:168–173.
45. Strauss C, Ganslandt O, Huk WJ, et al: Isolated unilateral internuclear ophthalmoplegia following head injury. Findings in magnetic resonance imaging. Neuro-ophthalmology 1995;15:15–19.
46. Constantoyannis C, Tzortzidis F, Papadakis N: Internuclear ophthalmoplegia following minor head injury: a case report. Br J Neurosurg 1998;12:377–379.
47. Hamed LF, Schatz NJ, Galetta SL: Brainstem ocular motility defects and AIDS. Am J Ophthalmol 1988;106:437–442.
48. Keane JR: Eye movement abnormalities in systemic lupus erythematosus. Arch Neurol 1995;52:1145–1149.
49. Yigit A, Bingol A, Mutluer N, et al: The one-and-a-half syndrome in systemic lupus erythematosus. J Neuro-ophthalmol 1996;16:274–276.
50. Galindo M, Pablos JL, Gomez-Reino JJ: Internuclear ophthalmoplegia in systemic lupus erythematosus. Semin Arthritis Rheum 1998;28:179–186.
51. Masai H, Kashii S, Kimura H, et al: Neuro-Behçet disease presenting with internuclear ophthalmoplegia. Am J Ophthalmol 1996;122:897–898.
52. Hughes TAT, Wiles CM, Hourihan M: Cervical radculopathy and bilateral internuclear ophthalmoplegia caused by temporal arteritis. J Neurol Neurosurg Psychiatry 1994;57:764–765.
53. Arnold AC, Baloh RW, Yee RD, et al: Internuclear ophthalmoplegia in the Chiari type II malformation. Neurology 1990;40:1850–1854.

54. Hunnewell J, Miller NR: Bilateral internuclear ophthalmoplegia related to chronic toluene abuse. J Neuro-ophthalmol 1998;18:277–280.
55. Silverman IE, Liu GT, Volpe NJ, et al: The crossed paralyses: the original brainstem syndromes of Millard–Gubler, Foville, Weber, and Raymond–Cestan. Arch Neurol 1995;52:635–638.
56. Thömke F, Hopf HC, Krämer G: Internuclear ophthalmoplegia of abduction: clinical and electrophysiological data on the existence of an abduction paresis of prenuclear origin. J Neurol Neurosurg Psychiatry 1992;55:105–111.
57. Griffin JF, Wray SH, Anderson DP: Misdiagnosis of spasm of the near reflex. Neurology 1976;26:1018–1020.
58. Keane JR: Neuro-ophthalmic signs and symptoms of hysteria. Neurology 1982;32:757–762.
59. Goldstein JH, Schneekloth BB: Spasm of the near reflex: a spectrum of anomalies. Surv Ophthalmol 1996;40:269–278.
60. Newman NJ, Lessell S: Pupillary dilatation with monocular occlusion as a sign of nonorganic oculomotor dysfunction. Am J Ophthalmol 1989;108:461–462.
61. Moster ML, Hoenig EM: Spasm of the near reflex associated with metabolic encephalopathy. Neurology 1989;38:150.
62. Dagi LR, Chrousos GA, Cogan DG: Spasm of the near reflex associated with organic disease. Am J Ophthalmol 1987;103:582–585.
63. Manor RS: Use of special glasses in treatment of spasm of near reflex. Ann Ophthalmol 1979;11:903–905.
64. Lepore FE: Disorders of ocular motility following head trauma. Arch Neurol 1995;52:924–926.
65. Kirkham TH, Bird AC, Sanders MD: Divergence paralysis with raised intracranial pressure. Br J Ophthalmol 1972;56:776–782.
66. Schanzer B, Bordaberry M, Jeffery AR, et al: The child with divergence paresis. Surv Ophthalmol 1998;42:571–576.
67. Brown SM, Iacuone JJ: Intact sensory fusion in a child with divergence paresis caused by a pontine glioma. Am J Ophthalmol 1999;128:528–530.
68. Wiggins RE, Baumgartner S: Diagnosis and management of divergence weakness in adults. Ophthalmology 1999;106:1353–1356.
69. Keane JR: Ocular skew deviation. Arch Neurol 1975;32:185–190.
70. Dieterich M, Brandt T: Wallenberg's syndrome: lateralpulsion, cyclorotation, and subjective visual vertical in thirty-six patients. Ann Neurol 1992;31:399–408.
71. Brandt T, Dieterich M: Skew deviation with ocular torsion: a vestibular brainstem sign of topographic diagnostic value. Ann Neurol 1993;33:528–534.
72. Brandt T, Dieterich M: Vestibular syndromes in the roll plane: topographic diagnosis from brainstem to cortex. Ann Neurol 1994;36:337–347.
73. Halmagyi GM, Gresty MA, Gibson WPR: Ocular tilt reaction with peripheral vestibular lesion. Ann Neurol 1979;6:80–83.
74. Wolfe GI, Taylor CL, Flamm ES, et al: Ocular tilt reaction resulting from vestibuloacoustic nerve surgery. Neurosurgery 1993;32:417–421.
75. Safran AB, Vibert D, Issoua D, et al: Skew deviation after vestibular neuritis. Am J Ophthalmol 1994;118:238–245.
76. Zee DS: Considerations on the mechanisms of alternating skew deviation in patients with cerebellar lesions. J Vestib Res 1996;6:395–401.
77. Riordan-Eva P, Harcourt JP, Faldon M, et al: Skew deviation following vestibular nerve surgery. Ann Neurol 1997;41:94–99.
78. Galetta SL, Liu GT, Raps EC, et al: Cyclodeviation in skew deviation. Am J Ophthalmol 1994;118:509–514.
79. Moster ML, Schatz NJ, Savino PJ, et al: Alternating skew on lateral gaze (bilateral abducting hypertropia). Ann Neurol 1988;23:190–192.
80. Keane JR: Alternating skew deviation: 47 patients. Neurology 1985;35:725–728.
81. Merikangas JR: Skew deviation in pseudotumor cerebri. Ann Neurol 1978;4:583.
82. Frohman LP, Kupersmith MJ: Reversible vertical ocular deviations associated with raised intracranial pressure. J Neuro-ophthalmol 1986;5:158–163.
83. Donahue SP, Lavin PJ, Hamed LM: Tonic ocular tilt reaction simulating a superior oblique palsy: diagnostic confusion with the 3-step test. Arch Ophthalmol 1999;117:347–352.
84. Trobe JD: Cyclodeviation in acquired vertical strabismus. Arch Ophthalmol 1984;102:717–720.
85. Donohue SP, Lavin PJ, Hamed L: Tonic ocular tilt reaction simulating a superior oblique palsy: diagnostic confusion with the 3 step test. Arch Ophthalmol 1999;117:347–352.
86. Brandt T, Dieterich M: Pathological eye-head coordination in roll: tonic ocular tilt reaction in mesencephalic and medullary lesions. Brain 1987;110:649–666.
87. Halmagyi GM, Brandt T, Dieterich M, et al: Tonic contraversive ocular tilt reaction due to unilateral meso-diencephalic lesion. Neurology 1990;40:1503–1509.
88. Ohashi T, Fukushima K, Chin S, et al: Ocular tilt reaction with vertical eye movement palsy caused by localized unilateral midbrain lesion. J Neuro-ophthalmol 1998;18:40–42.
89. Westheimer G, Blair SM: The ocular tilt reaction—a brainstem oculomotor routine. Invest Ophthalmol 1975;14:833–839.
90. Rabinovitch HE, Shape JA, Sylvester TO: The ocular tilt reaction. A paroxysmal dyskinesia associated with elliptical nystagmus. Arch Ophthalmol 1977;95:1395–1398.
91. Hedges TR, Hoyt WF: Ocular tilt reaction due to an upper brain stem lesion: paroxysmal skew deviation, torsion, and oscillation of the eyes with head tilt. Ann Neurol 1982;11:537–540.
92. Lueck CJ, Hamlyn P, Crawford TJ, et al: A case of ocular tilt reaction and torsional nystagmus due to direct stimulation of the midbrain in man. Brain 1991;114:2069–2079.
93. Galimberti CA, Versino M, Sartori I, et al: Epileptic skew deviation. Neurology 1998;50:1469–1472.
94. Corbett JJ, Schatz NJ, Shults WT, et al: Slowly alternating skew deviation: description of a pretectal syndrome in three patients. Ann Neurol 1981;10:540–546.
95. Mitchell JM, Smith JL, Quencer RM: Periodic alternating skew deviation. J Clin Neuro-ophthalmol 1981;1:5–8.
96. Jampel RS, Fells P: Monocular elevation paresis caused by a central nervous system lesion. Arch Ophthalmol 1968;80:45–57.
97. Lessell S: Supranuclear paralysis of monocular elevation. Neurology 1975;25:1134–1136.
98. Ford CS, Schwartze GM, Weaver RG, et al: Monocular elevation paresis caused by an ipsilateral lesion. Neurology 1984;34:1264–1267.

99. Muñoz M, Page LK: Acquired double elevator palsy in a child with a pineocytoma. Am J Ophthalmol 1994;118:810–811.
100. Wiest G, Baumgartner C, Schnider P, et al: Monocular elevation paresis and contralateral downgaze paresis from unilateral mesodiencephalic infarction. J Neurol Neurosurg Psychiatry 1996;60:579–581.
101. Pollard ZF: Diagnosis and treatment of inferior oblique palsy. J Pediatr Ophthalmol Strabismus 1993;30:15–18.
102. Harrison AR, Wirtshafter JD: Isolated inferior rectus paresis secondary to mesencephalic cavernous angioma. Am J Ophthalmol 1999;127:617–619.
103. Guy JR, Savino PJ, Schatz NJ, et al: Superior division paresis of the oculomotor nerve. Ophthalmology 1985;92:777–784.
104. Ksiazek SM, Repka MX, Maguire A, et al: Divisional oculomotor nerve paresis caused by intrinsic brainstem disease. Ann Neurol 1989;26:714–718.
105. Guy JR, Day AL: Intracranial aneurysms with superior division paresis of the oculomotor nerve. Ophthalmology 1989;96:1071–1076.
106. Czarnecki JSC, Thompson HS: The iris sphincter in aberrant regeneration of the third nerve. Arch Ophthalmol 1978;96:1606–1610.
107. Spector RH, Faria MA: Aberrant regeneration of the inferior division of the oculomotor nerve. Arch Neurol 1981;38:460–461.
108. Landau K: Discovering a dys-covering lid. Surv Ophthalmol 1997;42:87–91.
109. Sibony PA, Lessell S: Transient oculomotor synkinesis in temporal arteritis. Arch Neurol 1984;41: 87–88.
110. Johnson LN, Pack WL: Transient oculomotor nerve misdirection in a case of pituitary tumor with hemorrhage (letter). Arch Ophthalmol 1988;106:584–585.
111. Schatz NJ, Savino PJ, Corbett JJ: Primary aberrant oculomotor regeneration. A sign of intracavernous meningioma. Arch Neurol 1977;34:29–32.
112. Trobe JD, Glaser JS, Post JD: Meningiomas and aneurysms of the cavernous sinus. Neuro-ophthalmologic features. Arch Ophthalmol 1978;96:457–467.
113. Boghen D, Chartrand J-P, Laflamme P, et al: Primary aberrant third nerve regeneration. Ann Neurol 1979; 6:415–418.
114. Lepore FE, Glaser JS: Misdirection revisited. A critical appraisal of acquired oculomotor nerve synkinesis. Arch Ophthalmol 1980;98:2206–2209.
115. Cox TA, Wurster JB, Godfrey WA: Primary aberrant oculomotor regeneration due to intracranial aneurysm. Arch Neurol 1979;36:570–571.
116. Johnson LN, Kamper CA, Hepler RS, et al: Primary aberrant regeneration of the oculomotor nerve from presumed extracavernous neurilemmoma, meningioma, and asymmetric mammillary body. Neuro-ophthalmology 1989;9:227–232.
117. Varma R, Miller NR: Primary oculomotor nerve synkinesis caused by an extracavernous intradural aneurysm. Am J Ophthalmol 1994;118:83–87.
118. Keane JR: Bilateral aberrant regeneration of the third cranial nerve following trauma. J Neurosurg 1975;43: 95–97.
119. O'Day J, Billson F, King J: Ophthalmoplegic migraine and aberrant regeneration of the oculomotor nerve. Br J Ophthalmol 1980;64:534–536.
120. Laguna JF, Smith MS: Aberrant regeneration in idiopathic oculomotor nerve palsy. J Neurosurg 1980;52: 854–856.
121. Sibony PA, Lessell S, Gittinger JW, Jr: Acquired oculomotor synkinesis. Surv Ophthalmol 1984;28: 382–390.
122. Loewenfeld IE, Thompson HS: Oculomotor paresis with cyclic spasms. A critical review of the literature and a new case. Surv Ophthalmol 1975;20:81–124.
123. Susac JO, Smith JL: Cyclic oculomotor paralysis. Neurology 1974;24:24–27.
124. Bateman DE, Saunders M: Cyclic oculomotor palsy: description of a case and hypothesis of the mechanism. J Neurol Neurosurg Psychiatry 1983;46: 451–453.
125. Growdon JH, Winkler GF, Wray SH: Midbrain ptosis. A case with clinicopathologic correlation. Arch Neurol 1974;30:179–181.
126. Bogousslavsky J, Regli F, Ghika J, et al: Internuclear ophthalmoplegia, prenuclear paresis of contralateral superior rectus, and bilateral ptosis. J Neurol 1983; 230:197–203.
127. Bogousslavsky J, Regli F: Nuclear and prenuclear syndromes of the oculomotor nerve. Neuro-ophthalmology 1983;3:211–216.
128. Stevenson GC, Hoyt WF: Metastasis to midbrain from mammillary carcinoma. JAMA 1963;186:514–516.
129. Biller J, Shapiro R, Evans LS, et al: Oculomotor nuclear complex infarction. Clinical and radiological correlation. Arch Neurol 1984;41:985–987.
130. Liu GT, Carrazana EJ, Charness ME: Unilateral oculomotor palsy and bilateral ptosis from paramedian midbrain infarction. Arch Neurol 1991;48:983–986.
131. Bengel D, Huffmann G: Oculomotor nuclear complex syndrome as a single sign of midbrain haemorrhage. Neuro-ophthalmology 1994;14:279–282.
132. Pratt DV, Orengo-Nania S, Horowitz BL, et al: Magnetic resonance imaging findings in a patient with nuclear oculomotor palsy. Arch Ophthalmol 1995; 113:141–142.
133. Martin TJ, Corbett JJ, Babikian PV, et al: Bilateral ptosis due to mesencephalic lesions with relative preservation of ocular motility. J Neuro-ophthalmol 1996;16:258–263.
134. Keane JR, Zaias B, Itabashi HH: Levator sparing oculomotor nerve palsy caused by a solitary midbrain metastasis. Arch Neurol 1984;41:210–212.
135. Bryan JS, Hamed LM: Levator-sparing nuclear oculomotor palsy. J Clin Neuro-ophthalmol 1992;12:26–30.
136. Pusateri TJ, Sedwick LA, Margo CE: Isolated inferior rectus muscle palsy from solitary metastasis to the oculomotor nucleus. Arch Ophthalmol 1987;105: 675–677.
137. Chou TM, Demer JM: Isolated inferior rectus palsy caused by a metastasis to the oculomotor nucleus. Am J Ophthalmol 1998;126:737–740.
138. Liu GT, Crenner CW, Logigian EL, et al: Midbrain syndromes of Benedikt, Claude, and Nothnagel: setting the record straight. Neurology 1992;42:1820–1822.
139. Caplan LR: "Top of the basilar" syndrome. Neurology 1980;30:72–79.
140. Kim JS, Kang JK, Lee SA, et al: Isolated or predominant ocular motor nerve palsy as a manifestation of brain stem stroke. Stroke 1993;24:581–586.
141. Nadeau SE, Trobe JD: Pupil sparing in oculomotor palsy: a brief review. Ann Neurol 1983;13:143–148.
142. Breen LA, Hopf HC, Farris BK, et al: Pupil-sparing oculomotor nerve palsy due to midbrain infarction. Arch Neurol 1991;48:105–106.
143. Kumar P, Ahmed I: Pupil-sparing oculomotor palsy due to midbrain infarction [letter]. Arch Neurol 1992;49:348.

144. Gauntt CD, Kashii S, Nagata I: Monocular elevation paresis caused by an oculomotor fascicular impairment. J Neuro-ophthalmol 1995;15:11–14.
145. Ksiazek SM, Slamovitz TL, Rosen CE, et al: Fascicular arrangement in partial oculomotor paresis. Am J Ophthalmol 1994;118:97–103.
146. Saeki N, Murai N, Sunami K: Midbrain tegmental lesions affecting or sparing the pupillary fibres. J Neurol Neurosurg Psychiatry 1996;61:401–406.
147. Eggenberger ER, Miller NR, Hoffman PN, et al: Mesencephalic ependymal cyst causing an inferior divisional paresis of the oculormotor nerve. Neurology 1993;43:2419–2420.
148. Castro O, Johnson LN, Mamourian AC: Isolated inferior oblique paresis from brain-stem infarction. Perspective on oculomotor fascicular organization in the ventral midbrain tegmentum. Arch Neurol 1990;47:235–237.
149. Bogousslavsky J, Meienberg O: Eye-movement disorders in brainstem and cerebellar stroke. Arch Neurol 1987;44:141–148.
150. Bogousslavsky J, Maeder P, Regli F, et al: Pure midbrain infarction: clinical syndromes, MRI, and etiologic patterns. Neurology 1994;44:2032–2040.
151. Ishikawa H, Satoh H, Fujiwara M, et al: Oculomotor nerve palsy caused by lung cancer metastasis. Intern Med 1997;36:301–303.
152. Keane JR: Isolated brain-stem third nerve palsy. Arch Neurol 1988;45:813–814.
153. Getenet J-C, Vighetto A, Nighoghossian N, et al: Isolated bilateral third nerve palsy caused by a mesencephalic hematoma. Neurology 1994;44:981–982.
154. Traboulsi EI, Azar DT, Achram M, et al: Brainstem tuberculoma and isolated third nerve palsy. Neuro-ophthalmology 1985;5:43–45.
155. Uitti RJ, Rajput AH: Multiple sclerosis presenting as isolated oculomotor nerve palsy. Can J Neurol Sci 1986;13:270–272.
156. Galer BS, Lipton RB, Weinstein S, et al: Apoplectic headache and oculomotor nerve palsy: an unusual presentation of multiple sclerosis. Neurology 1990;40:1465–1466.
157. Newman NJ, Lessell SL: Isolated pupil-sparing third-nerve palsy as the presenting sign of multiple sclerosis. Arch Neurol 1990;47:817–818.
158. Thömke F, Lensch E, Ringel K, et al: Isolated cranial nerve palsies in multiple sclerosis. J Neurol Neurosurg Psychiatry 1997;63:682–685.
159. Liu GT: Coma. Neurosurg Clin North Am 1999;10:579–586.
160. Ropper AH, Cole D, Louis DN: Clinicopathologic correlation in a case of pupillary dilation from cerebral hemorrhage. Arch Neurol 1991;48:1166–1169.
161. Ropper AH: The opposite pupil in herniation. Neurology 1990;40:1707–1709.
162. Fisher CM: Oval pupils. Arch Neurol 1980;37:502–503.
163. Chen R, Sahjpaul R, Del Maestro RF, et al: Initial enlargement of the opposite pupil as a false localising sign in intraparenchymal frontal haemorrhage. J Neurol Neurosurg Psychiatry 1994;57:1126–1128.
164. Soni SR: Aneurysms of the posterior communicating artery and oculomotor paresis. J Neurol Neurosurg Psychiatry 1974;37:475–484.
165. Locksley HB: Natural history of subarachnoid hemorrhage, intracranial aneurysm and arteriovenous malformations. J Neurosurg 1966;25:219–239.
166. Okawara S: Warning signs prior to rupture or an intracranial aneurysm. J Neurosurg 1973;38:575–580.
167. Kupersmith MJ: Neuro-vascular Neuro-ophthalmology. Berlin, Springer-Verlag, 1993.
168. Green WR, Hackett ER, Schlezinger NS: Neuro-ophthalmologic evaluation of oculomotor nerve paralysis. Arch Ophthalmol 1964;72:154–167.
169. Kasoff I, Kelly DL: Pupillary sparing oculomotor palsies with internal carotid-posterior communicating artery aneurysms. J Neurosurg 1975;42:713–717.
170. Kissel JT, Burde RM, Klingele TG, et al: Pupil-sparing oculomotor palsies with internal carotid-posterior communicating artery aneurysms. Ann Neurol 1983;13:149–154.
171. Good EF: Ptosis as the sole manifestation of compression of the oculomotor nerve by an aneurysm of the posterior communicating artery. J Clin Neuro-ophthalmol 1990;10:59–61.
172. Bartleson JD, Trautmann JC, Sundt TM: Minimal oculomotor nerve paresis secondary to unruptured intracranial aneurysm. Arch Neurol 1986;43:1015–1020.
173. Payne JW, Adamkiewicz J: Unilateral ophthalmoplegia with intracranial aneurysm. Report of a case. Am J Ophthalmol 1969;68:349–352.
174. Cromptom JL, Moore CE: Painful third nerve palsy: how not to miss an intra-cranial aneurysm. Aust NZ J Ophthalmol 1981;9:113–115.
175. Coppeto JR, Lessell S: Dorsal midbrain syndrome from giant aneurysm of the posterior fossa: report of two cases. Neurology 1983;33:732–736.
176. Greenspan BN, Reeves AG: Transient partial oculomotor nerve paresis with posterior communicating artery aneurysm. A case report. J Clin Neuro-ophthalmol 1990;10:56–58.
177. Peiris JB, Russel WR: Giant aneurysms of the carotid system presenting as visual field defect. J Neurol Neurosurg Psychiatry 1980;43:1053–1064.
178. Takahashi T, Kanatani I, Isayama Y, et al: Visual disturbance due to internal carotid aneurysm. Ann Ophthalmol 1983;13:1014–1024.
179. Pia HW, Fontana H: Aneurysms of the posterior cerebral artery. Acta Neurochir 1977;39:13–35.
180. Pikus HJ, Heros RC: Surgical treatment of internal carotid and posterior communicating artery aneurysms. Neurosurg Clin North Am 1998;9:785–795.
181. Day J, Levy M, Gianotta S: Surgery of internal carotid artery aneurysms. In: Tindall GT, Cooper PR, Barrow DL, (eds): The Practice of Neurosurgery, pp 2033–2045. Baltimore, Williams & Wilkins, 1996.
182. Nelson PK, Levy D, Masters LT, et al: Neuroendovascular management of intracranial aneurysms. Neuroimag Clin North Am 1997;7:739–762.
183. Winn HR, Richardson AE, Jane JA: Late morbidity and mortality of common carotid ligation of posterior communicating aneurysms (a comparison to conservative therapy). J Neurosurg 1977;47:727–736.
184. Fujiwara S, Fujii K, Nishio S, et al: Oculomotor nerve palsy in patients with cerebral aneurysms. Neurosurg Rev 1989;12:123–132.
185. Grayson MC, Soni SR, Spooner VA: Analysis of the recovery of third nerve function after direct surgical intervention for posterior communicating aneurysms. Br J Ophthalmol 1974;58:118–125.
186. Kyriakides T, Aziz TZ, Torrens MJ: Postoperative recovery of third nerve palsy due to posterior communicating aneurysms. Br J Neurosurg 1989;3:109–111.
187. McKinna AJ: Eye signs in 61 cases of posterior fossa aneurysms: their diagnostic and prognostic value. Can J Ophthalmol 1983;18:3–6.

188. Boccardo M, Ruelle A, Banchero MA: Isolated oculomotor palsy caused by aneurysm of the basilar artery bifurcation. J Neurol 1986;233:61–62.
189. DiMario FJ, Rorke LB: Transient oculomotor nerve paresis in congenital distal basilar artery aneurysm. Pediatr Neurol 1992;8:303–306.
190. Lustbader JM, Miller NR: Painless, pupil-sparing but otherwise complete oculomotor nerve paresis caused by basilar artery aneurysm. Arch Ophthalmol 1988; 106:583–584.
191. Jacobson DM, McCanna TD, Layde PM: Risk factors for ischemic ocular motor nerve palsies. Arch Ophthalmol 1994;112:961–966.
192. Teuscher AU, Meienberg O: Ischaemic oculomotor nerve palsy. Clinical features and vascular risk factors in 23 patients. J Neurol 1985;232:144–149.
193. Jacobson DM, Broste SK: Early progression of ophthalmoplegia in patients with ischemic oculomotor nerve palsies. Arch Ophthalmol 1995;113:1535–1537.
194. Keane JR, Ahmadi J: Most diabetic third nerve palsies are peripheral. Neurology 1998;51:1510.
195. Weber RB, Daroff RB, Mackey EA: Pathology of oculomotor nerve palsy in diabetics. Neurology 1970;20:835–838.
196. Hopf HC, Gutmann L: Diabetic 3rd nerve palsy: evidence for a mesencephalic lesion. Neurology 1990;40:1041–1045.
197. Jacobson DM: Pupil involvement in patients with diabetes-associated oculomotor nerve palsy. Arch Ophthalmol 1998;116:723–727.
198. Bortolami R, D'Alessandro R, Manni E: The origin of pain in 'ischemic–diabetic' third nerve palsy (letter). Arch Neurol 1993;50:795.
199. Capó H, Warren F, Kupersmith MJ: Evolution of oculomotor nerve palsies. J Clin Neuro-ophthalmol 1992;12:21–25.
200. Eshbaugh CG, Siatkowski RM, Smith JL, et al: Simultaneous, multiple cranial neuropathies in diabetes mellitus. J Neuro-ophthalmol 1995;15:219–224.
201. Davies GE, Shakir RA: Giant cell arteritis presenting as oculomotor nerve palsy with pupillary dilation. Postgrad Med J 1994;70:298–299.
202. Bondenson J, Asman P: Giant cell arteritis presenting with oculomotor nerve palsy. Scand J Rheumatol 1997;26:327–328.
203. Rosenstein ED, Sobelman J, Kramer N: Isolated, pupil-sparing third nerve palsy as initial manifestation of systemic lupus erythematosus. J Clin Neuro-ophthalmol 1989;9:285–288.
204. Tognetti F, Godano U, Galassi E: Bilateral traumatic third nerve palsy. Surg Neurol 1988;29:120–124.
205. Balcer LJ, Galetta SL, Bagley LJ, et al: Localization of traumatic oculomotor nerve palsy to the midbrain exit site by magnetic resonance imaging. Am J Ophthalmol 1996;122:437–439.
206. Yoss RE, Rucker CW, Miller RH: Neurosurgical complications affecting oculomotor, trochlear, and abducent nerves. Neurology 1968;18:594–600.
207. Keane JR: Third-nerve palsy due to penetrating trauma. Neurology 1993;43:1523–1527.
208. Eyster EF, Hoyt WF, Wilson CB: Oculomotor palsy from minor head trauma. An initial sign of basal intracranial tumor. JAMA 1972;220:1083–1086.
209. Walter KA, Newman NJ, Lessell S: Oculomotor palsy from minor head trauma: initial sign of intracranial aneurysm. Neurology 1994;44:148–150.
210. Kansu T, Özcan OE, Ösdirim E, et al: Neurinoma of the oculomotor nerve. Case report. J Clin Neuro-ophthalmol 1982;2:271–272.
211. Hiscott P, Symon L: An unusual presentation of neurofibroma of the oculomotor nerve. Case report. J Neurosurg 1982;56:854–856.
212. Celli P, Ferrante L, Acqui M, et al: Neurinoma of the third, fourth, and sixth cranial nerves: a survey and report of a new fourth nerve case. Surg Neurol 1992;38:216–224.
213. Kadota T, Miyawaki Y, Nakagawa H, et al: MR imaging of oculomotor nerve neurilemmoma. Magn Reson Imaging 1993;11:1071–1075.
214. Leunda G, Vaquero J, Cabezydo J, et al: Schwannoma of the oculomotor nerves. Report of four cases. J Neurosurg 1982;1982:57.
215. Mehta VS, Singh RVP, Misra NK, et al: Schwannoma of the oculomotor nerve. Br J Neurosurg 1990;4: 69–72.
216. Kaye-Wilson LG, Gibson R, Bell JE, et al: Oculomotor nerve neurinoma. Neuro-ophthalmology 1994;14: 37–41.
217. Hart AJ, Allibone J, Casey AT, et al: Malignant meningioma of the oculomotor nerve without dural attachment. Case report and review of the literature. J Neurosurg 1998;88:1104–1106.
218. Reifenberger G, Bostrom J, Bettag M, et al: Primary glioblastoma multiforme of the oculomotor nerve. Case report. J Neurosurg 1996;84:1062–1066.
219. Johnson LN, Hepler SS, Yee RD, et al: Sphenoid sinus mucocele (anterior clinoid variant) mimicking diabetic ophthalmoplegia and retrobulbar neuritis. Am J Ophthalmol 1986;102:111–115.
220. Ehrenpreis SJ, Biedlingmaier JF: Isolated third-nerve palsy associated with frontal sinus mucocele. J Neuro-ophthalmol 1995;15:105–108.
221. Legge RH: Isolated third-nerve palsy associated with frontal sinus mucocele [letter]. J Neuro-ophthalmol 1996;16:231–232.
222. Sethi DS, Lau DP, Chan C: Sphenoid sinus mucocoele presenting with isolated oculomotor nerve palsy. J Laryngol Otol 1997;111:471–473.
223. Wilson WB, Leavengood JM, Ringel SP, et al: Transient ocular motor paresis associated with acute internal carotid artery occlusion. Ann Neurol 1989;25:286–290.
224. Schievink WI, Mokri B, Garrity JA, et al: Ocular motor nerve palsies in spontaneous dissections of the cervical internal carotid artery. Neurology 1993;43:1938–1941.
225. Yamada T, Nishio S, Matsunaga M, et al: Cavernous haemangioma in the oculomotor nerve. A case report. J Neurol 1986;233:63–64.
226. Trobe JD: Third nerve palsy and the pupil. Footnotes to the rule. Arch Ophthalmol 1988;106:601–602.
227. Jacobson DM, Trobe JD: The emerging role of magnetic resonance angiography in the management of patients with third cranial nerve palsy. Am J Ophthalmol 1999;128:94–96.
228. Blake PY, Mark AS, Kattah J, et al: MR of oculomotor nerve palsy. AJNR: Am J Neuroradiol 1995;16:1665–1672.
229. Keane JR, Ahmadi J: Third-nerve palsies and angiography. Arch Neurol 1991;48:470.
230. McFadzean RM, Teasdale EM: Computerized tomography angiography in isolated third nerve palsies. J Neurosurg 1998;88:679–684.
231. Saad N, Lee J: The role of botulinum toxin in third nerve palsy. Aust N Z J Ophthalmol 1992;20:121–127.
232. Metz HS, Mazow M: Botulinum toxin treatment of acute sixth and third nerve palsy. Graefes Arch Clin Exp Ophthalmol 1988;226:141–144.

233. Kattleman B, Flanders M, Wise J: Supramaximal horizontal rectus surgery in the management of third and sixth nerve palsy. Can J Ophthalmol 1986;21:227–230.
234. Mudgil AV, Repka MX: Ophthalmologic outcome after third cranial nerve palsy or paresis in childhood. J AAPOS 1999;3:2–8.
235. Noonan CP, O'Connor M: Surgical management of third nerve palsy. Br J Ophthalmol 1995;79:431–434.
236. Salazar Leon JA, Ramirez Ortiz MA, Salas Vargas M: The surgical correction of paralytic strabismus using fascia lata. J Pediatr Ophthalmol Strabismus 1998;35:27–32.
237. Saunders RA, Rogers GL: Superior oblique transposition for third nerve palsy. Ophthalmology 1982;89:310–316.
238. Daniell MD, Gregson RM, Lee JP: Management of fixed divergent squint in third nerve palsy using traction sutures. Aust N Z J Ophthalmol 1996;24:261–265.
239. Maruo T, Iwashige H, Kubota N, et al: Results of surgery for paralytic exotropia due to oculomotor palsy. Ophthalmologica 1996;210:163–167.
240. Metz HS: The use of vertical offsets with horizontal strabismus surgery. Ophthalmology 1988;95:1094–1097.
241. Liu GT: Discussion of Mehkri IA, Awner S, Olitsky SE, et al: "Double vision in a child." Surv Ophthalmol 1999;44:45–52.
242. Miller NR: Solitary oculomotor nerve palsy in childhood. Am J Ophthalmol 1977;83:106–111.
243. Harley RD: Paralytic strabismus in children. Etiologic incidence and management of the third, fourth, and sixth nerve palsies. Ophthalmology 1980;87:24–43.
244. Keith CG: Oculomotor nerve palsy in childhood. Aust N Z J Ophthalmol 1987;15:181–184.
245. Ing EB, Sullivan TJ, Clarke MP, et al: Oculomotor nerve palsies in children. J Pediatr Ophthalmol Strabismus 1992;29:331–336.
246. Kodsi SR, Younge BR: Acquired oculomotor, trochlear, and abducent cranial nerve palsies in pediatric patients. Am J Ophthalmol 1992;114:568–574.
247. Schumacher-Feero LA, Yoo KW, Solari FM, et al: Third cranial nerve palsy in children. Am J Ophthalmol 1999;128:216–221.
248. Yang YC, Laws DE, Chandna A: The rules of third nerve palsy in children [letter]. Eye 1996;10:646–647.
249. Victor DI: The diagnosis of congenital unilateral third nerve palsy. Brain 1976;99:711–718.
250. Balkan R, Hoyt CS: Associated neurologic abnormalities in congenital third nerve palsies. Am J Ophthalmol 1984;97:315–319.
251. Good WV, Barkovich AJ, Nickel BL, et al: Bilateral congenital oculomotor nerve palsy in a child with brain anomalies. Am J Ophthalmol 1991;111:555–558.
252. Hamed LM: Associated neurologic and ophthalmologic findings in congenital oculomotor nerve palsy. Ophthalmology 1991;98:708–714.
253. White WL, Mumma JV, Tomasovic JJ: Congenital oculomotor nerve palsy, cerebellar hypoplasia, and facial capillary hemangiomas. Am J Ophthalmol 1992;113:497–500.
254. Parmeggiani A, Posar A, Leonardi M, et al: Neurological impairment in congenital bilateral ptosis with ophthalmoplegia. Brain Dev 1992;14:107–109.
255. Patel CK, Taylor DS, Russell-Eggitt IM, et al: Congenital third nerve palsy associated with mid-trimester amniocentesis. Br J Ophthalmol 1993;77:530–533.
256. Tsaloumas MD, Willshaw HE: Congenital oculomotor palsy: associated neurological and ophthalmological findings. Eye 1997;11:500–503.
257. Norman MG: Unilateral encephalomalacia in cranial nerve nuclei in neonates. Neurology 1974;24:378–380.
258. Routon MC, Expert-Bezançon MC, Bursztyn J, et al: Polymicrogyrie bioperculaire associée a une ophtalmoplégie congénitale par atteinte du noyau du nerf moteur oculaire commun. Rev Neurol 1994;150:363–369.
259. Prats JM, Monzon MJ, Zuazo E, et al: Congenital nuclear syndrome of oculomotor nerve. Pediatr Neurol 1993;9:476–478.
260. Lagrèze W-DA, Warner JEA, Zamani AA, et al: Mesencephalic clefts with associated eye movement disorders. Arch Ophthalmol 1996;114:429–432.
261. Savas R, Sommer A, Gueckel F, et al: Isolated oculomotor nerve paralysis in Lyme disease: MRI. Neuroradiology 1997;39:139–141.
262. Gordon N: Ophthalmoplegia in childhood. Dev Med Child Neurol 1994;36:370–374.
263. Kandt RS, Goldstein GW: Steroid-responsive ophthalmoplegia in a child. Diagnostic considerations. Arch Neurol 1985;42:589–591.
264. Barbas NR, Hedges TR, Schwenn M: Isolated oculomotor nerve palsy due to neoplasm in infancy. Neuro-ophthalmology 1995;15:157–160.
265. Piatt JH, Campbell GA, Oakes WJ: Papillary meningioma involving the oculomotor nerve in an infant. J Neurosurg 1986;64:808–812.
266. Troost BT: Ophthalmoplegic migraine. Biomed Pharmacother 1996;50:49–51.
267. Rust RS, Schutta HS: Ophthalmoplegic migraine [abstract]. Ann Neurol 1994;36:521.
268. Friedman AP, Harter DH, Merritt HH: Ophthalmoplegic migraine. Arch Neurol 1962;7:320–327.
269. Raymond LA, Tew J, Fogelson MH: Ophthalmoplegic migraine of early onset. J Pediatr 1977;90:1035–1036.
270. Robertson WC, Schnitzler ER: Ophthalmoplegic migraine in infancy. Pediatrics 1978;61:886–888.
271. Elser JM, Woody RC: Migraine headache in infant and young child. Headache 1990;30:366–368.
272. Mark AS, Blake P, Atlas SW, et al: Gd-DTPA enhancement of the cisternal portion of the oculomotor nerve on MR imaging. AJNR Am J Neuroradiol 1992;13:1463–1470.
273. Stommel EW, Ward TN, Harris RD: MRI findings in a case of ophthalmoplegic migraine. Headache 1993;33:234–237.
274. Østergaard JR, Moller HU, Christensen T: Recurrent ophthalmoplegia in childhood: diagnostic and etiologic considerations. Cephalalgia 1996;16:276–279.
275. Wong V, Wong WC: Enhancement of oculomotor nerve: a diagnostic criterion for ophthalmoplegic migraine? Pediatr Neurol 1997;17:70–73.
276. Walsh JP, O'Doherty DS: A possible explanation of the mechanism of ophthalmoplegic migraine. Neurology 1960;10:1079–1084.
277. van Pelt W, Andermann F: On the early onset of ophthalmoplegic migraine. Am J Dis Child 1964;107:628–630.
278. Locksley HB: Report on the cooperative study of intracranial aneurysms and subarachnoid hemorrhage. Section V, Part I. Natural history of subarachnoid hemorrhage, intracranial aneurysms and arteriovenous malformations. Based on 6368 cases in the cooperative study. J Neurosurg 1966;25:219–239.
279. Patel AN, Richardson AE: Ruptured intracranial aneurysms in the first two decades of life. J Neurosurg 1971;35:571–576.
280. Gabianelli EB, Klingele TG, Burde RM: Acute oculomotor palsy in childhood. Is arteriography necessary? J Clin Neuro-ophthalmol 1989;9:33–36.

281. Wolin MJ, Saunders RA: Aneurysmal oculomotor nerve palsy in an 11-year-old boy. J Clin Neuro-ophthalmol 1992;12:178–180.
282. Mehkri IA, Awner S, Olitsky SE, et al: Double vision in a child. Surv Ophthalmol 1999;44:45–52.
283. Branley MG, Wright KW, Borchert MS: Third nerve palsy due to cerebral artery aneurysm in a child. Aust NZ J Ophthalmol 1992;20:137–140.
284. Ebner R: Angiography for IIIrd nerve palsy in children (letter). J Clin Neuro-ophthalmol 1990;10: 154–155.
285. Fox R: Angiography for third nerve palsy in children [editorial]. J Clin Neuro-ophthalmol 1989;9:37–38.
286. Cekirge S, Saatci I, Firat MM, et al: Bilateral cavernous carotid artery aneurysms in a 4-year-old child: endovascular treatment with mechanically detachable coils. Neuroradiology 1997;39:367–370.
287. Grunt JA, Destro RL, Hamtil LW, et al: Ocular palsies in children with diabetes mellitus. Diabetes 1976;25:459–462.
288. Mizen TR, Burde RM, Klingele PG: Cryptogenic oculomotor nerve palsies in children. Am J Ophthalmol 1985;100:65–67.
289. Kraft SP, O'Reilly C, Quigley PL, et al: Cyclotorsion in unilateral and bilateral superior oblique paresis. J Pediatr Ophthalmol Strabismus 1993;30:361–367.
290. von Noorden GK, Murray E, Wong SY: Superior oblique paralysis: a review of 270 cases. Arch Ophthalmol 1986;104:1771–1776.
291. Mansour AM, Reinecke RD: Central trochlear palsy. Surv Ophthalmol 1986;30:279–297.
292. Keane JR: Fourth nerve palsy: historical review and study of 215 inpatients. Neurology 1993;43:2439–2443.
293. Agostinis C, Caverni L, Moschini L, et al: Paralysis of fourth cranial nerve due to superior-cerebellar artery aneurysm. Neurology 1992;42:457–458.
294. Astle WF, Miller SJ: Bilateral fluctuating trochlear nerve palsy secondary to cerebellar astrocytoma. Can J Ophthalmol 1994;29:34–38.
295. Jacobson DM, Moster ML, Eggenberger ER, et al: Isolated trochlear nerve palsy in patients with multiple sclerosis. Neurology 1999;53:877–880.
296. Galetta SL, Balcer LJ: Isolated fourth nerve palsy from midbrain hemorrhage. Case report. J Neuro-ophthalmol 1998;18:204–205.
297. Thömke F, Ringel K: Isolated superior oblique palsies with brainstem lesions. Neurology 1999;53:682–685.
298. Gonyea EF: Superior oblique palsy due to a midbrain vascular malformation. Neurology 1990;40:554–555.
299. Lotery A, Best J, Houston S: Occult giant cell (temporal) arteritis presenting with bilateral sixth and unilateral fourth nerve palsies [letter]. Eye 1998;12:1014–1016.
300. Santoreneos S, Hanieh A, Jorgensen RE: Trochlear nerve schwannomas occurring in patients without neurofibromatosis: case report and review of the literature. Neurosurgery 1997;41:282–287.
301. Jacobson DM, Warner JJ, Ruggles KH: Transient trochlear nerve palsy following anterior temporal lobectomy for epilepsy. Neurology 1995;45:1465–1468.
302. Guy J, Day AL, Mickle JP, et al: Contralateral trochlear nerve paresis and ipsilateral Horner's syndrome. Am J Ophthalmol 1989;107:73–76.
303. Brazis PW: Localization of lesions of the trochlear nerve: diagnosis and localization—recent concepts. Mayo Clin Proc 1993;68:501–509.
304. Vanooteghem P, Dehaene I, Van Zandycke M, et al: Combined trochlear nerve palsy and internuclear ophthalmoplegia. Arch Neurol 1992;49:108–109.
305. Greenberg MF, Pollard ZF: Ocular plagiocephaly: ocular torticollis with skull and facial asymmetry. Ophthalmology 2000;107:173–179.
306. Helveston EM, Krach D, Plager DA, et al: A new classification of superior oblique palsy based on congenital variations in the tendon. Ophthalmology 1992;99:1609–1615.
307. Astle WF, Rosenbaum AL: Familial congenital fourth cranial nerve palsy. Arch Ophthalmol 1985;103: 532–535.
308. Harris DJ, Memmen JE, Katz NNK, et al: Familial congenital superior oblique palsy. Ophthalmology 1986;93:88–90.
309. Botelho PJ, Giangiacomo JG: Autosomal-dominant inheritance of congenital superior oblique palsy. Ophthalmology 1996;103:1508–1511.
310. Bale JF, Scott WE, Yuh W, et al: Congenital fourth nerve palsy and occult cranium bifidum. Pediatr Neurol 1988;4:320–321.
311. Helveston EM, Mora JS, Lipsky SN, et al: Surgical treatment of superior oblique palsy. Trans Am Ophthalmol Soc 1996;94:315–328.
312. Aseff AJ, Muñoz M: Outcome of surgery for superior oblique palsy with contracture of ipsilateral superior rectus treated by superior rectus recession. Binocul Vis Strabismus Q 1998;13:177–180.
313. Maruo T, Iwashige H, Kubota N, et al: Long-term results of surgery for superior oblique palsy. Jpn J Ophthalmol 1996;40:235–238.
314. Kushner BJ: The diagnosis and treatment of bilateral masked superior oblique palsy. Am J Ophthalmol 1988;105:186–194.
315. Metz HS, Lerner H: The adjustable Harada–Ito procedure. Arch Ophthalmol 1981;99:624–626.
316. Mitchell PR, Parks MM: Surgery of bilateral superior oblique palsy. Ophthalmology 1982;89:484–488.
317. Simons BD, Saunders TG, Siatkowski RM, et al: Outcome of surgical management of superior oblique palsy: a study of 123 cases. Binoc Vis Strabis Q 1998;13:273–282.
318. Plager DA: Superior oblique palsy and superior oblique myokymia. In: Rosenbaum AL, Santiago AP (eds): Clinical Strabismus Management: Principles and Surgical Techniques, pp 219–229. Philadelphia, WB Saunders, 1999.
319. Ohtsuki H, Hasebe S, Hanabusa K, et al: Intraoperative adjustable suture surgery for bilateral superior oblique palsy. Ophthalmology 1994;101:188–193.
320. Pierrot-Deseilligny C, Goasguen J: Isolated abducens nucleus damage due to histiocytosis X. Electro-oculographic analysis and physiological deductions. Brain 1984;107:1019–1032.
321. Müri RM, Chermann JF, Cohen L, et al: Ocular motor consequences of damage to the abducens nucleus area in humans. J Neuro-ophthalmol 1996;16: 191–195.
322. Donaldson D, Rosenberg NL: Infarction of abducens nerve fascicle as cause of isolated sixth nerve palsy related to hypertension. Neurology 1988;38:1654.
323. Fukutake T, Hirayama K: Isolated abducens nerve palsy from pontine infarction in a diabetic patient. Neurology 1992;42:2226.
324. Kataoka S, Hori A, Shirakawa T, et al: Paramedian pontine infarction. Neurological/topographical correlation. Stroke 1997;28:809–815.
325. Rose JW, Digre KB, Lynch SG, et al: Acute VIth cranial nerve dysfunction in multiple sclerosis. J Clin Neuro-ophthalmol 1992;12:17–20.

326. Sturzenegger M: Isolated sixth-nerve palsy as the presenting sign of multiple sclerosis. Neuro-ophthalmology 1994;14:43–48.
327. Thömke F, Mika-Grüttner A, Visbeck A, et al: The risk of abducens palsy after diagnostic lumbar puncture. Neurology 2000;54:768–769.
328. Bell JA, McIllwaine GG, O'Neill D: Iatrogenic lateral rectus palsies. A series of five postmyelographic cases. J Clin Neuro-ophthalmol 1994;14:205–209.
329. Berlit P, Berg-Dammer E, Kuehne D: Abducens nerve palsy in spontaneous intracranial hypotension. Neurology 1994;44:1552.
330. Currie J, Lubin JH, Lessell S: Chronic isolated abducens paresis from tumors at the base of the brain. Arch Neurol 1983;40:226–229.
331. Galetta SL, Smith JL: Chronic isolated sixth nerve palsies. Arch Neurol 1989;46:79–82.
332. Volpe NJ, Lessell S: Remitting sixth nerve palsy in skull base tumors. Arch Ophthalmol 1993;111:1391–1395.
333. Mutyala S, Holmes JM, Hodge DO, et al: Spontaneous recovery rate in traumatic sixth-nerve palsy. Am J Ophthalmol 1996;122:898–899.
334. Davé AV, Diaz-Marchan PJ, Lee AG: Clinical and magnetic resonance imaging features of Gradenigo syndrome. Am J Ophthalmol 1997;124:568–570.
335. Moster ML, Savino PJ, Sergott RC, et al: Isolated sixth-nerve palsies in younger adults. Arch Ophthalmol 1984;102:1328–1330.
336. Fitzsimons R, Lee JP, Elston J: Treatment of sixth nerve palsy in adults with combined botulinum toxin chemodenervation and surgery. Ophthalmology 1988;95:1535–1542.
337. Fitzsimons R, Lee JP, Elston J: The role of botulinum toxin in the management of sixth nerve palsy. Eye 1989;3:391–400.
338. Lee J: Modern management of sixth nerve palsy. Aust NZ J Ophthalmol 1992;20:41–46.
339. McManaway JW, Buckley EG, Brodsky MC: Vertical rectus muscle transposition with intraoperative botulinum injection for treatment of chronic sixth nerve palsy. Graefes Arch Clin Exp Ophthalmol 1990;228:401–406.
340. Rosenbaum AL, Kushner BJ, Kirschen D: Vertical rectus muscle transposition and botulinum toxin (Oculinum) to medial rectus for abducens palsy. Arch Ophthalmol 1989;107:820–823.
341. Metz HS, Dickey CF: Treatment of unilateral acute sixth-nerve palsy with botulinum toxin. Am J Ophthalmol 1991;112:381–384.
342. Afifi AK, Bell WE, Menezes AH: Etiology of lateral rectus palsy in infancy and childhood. J Child Neurol 1992;7:295–299.
343. Robertson DM, Hines JD, Rucker CW: Acquired sixth-nerve paresis in children. Arch Ophthalmol 1970;83:574–579.
344. Aroichane M, Repka MX: Outcome of sixth nerve palsy or paresis in young children. J Pediatr Ophthalmol Strabismus 1995;32:152–156.
345. Lee MS, Galetta SL, Volpe NJ, et al: Sixth nerve palsies in children. Pediatr Neurol 1999;20:49–52.
346. Pollack IF: Brain tumors in children. N Engl J Med 1994;331:1500–1507.
347. Knox DL, Clark DB, Schuster FF: Benign VI nerve palsies in children. Pediatrics 1967;40:560–564.
348. Barnett AM: Benign recurrent abducens palsy in children. S Afr Med J 1972;46:1662–1663.
349. Sternberg I, Ronen S, Arnon N: Recurrent isolated post febrile abducens nerve palsy. J Pediatr Ophthalmol Strabismus 1980;17:323–324.
350. Bixenman WW, von Noorden GK: Benign/recurrent VI nerve palsy in childhood. J Pediatr Ophthalmol Strabismus 1981;18:29–34.
351. Werner DB, Savino PJ, Schatz NJ: Benign recurrent sixth nerve palsies in childhood secondary to immunization or viral illness. Arch Ophthalmol 1983; 101:607–608.
352. Boger WP, Puliafito CA, Magoon EH, et al: Recurrent isolated sixth nerve palsy in children. Ann Ophthalmol 1984;237–238, 240–244:
353. Sullivan SC: Benign recurrent isolated VI nerve palsy of childhood. Clin Pediatr 1985;24:160–161.
354. Cohen HA, Nussinovitich M, Ashkenazi A, et al: Benign abducens nerve palsy of childhood. Pediatr Neurol 1993;9:
355. Straussberg R, Cohen AH, Amir J, et al: Benign abducens palsy associted with EBV infection. J Pediatr Ophthalmol Strabismus 1993;30:60.
356. Parks MM, Wheeler MB: Concomitant esodeviations. In: Tasman W, Jaeger EA (eds): Duane's Clinical Ophthalmology, pp 1–14. Philadelphia, JB Lippincott, 1992.
357. Watson AP, Fielder AR: Sudden-onset squint. Dev Med Child Neurol 1987;29:207–211.
358. Anderson WD, Lubow M: Astrocytoma of the corpus callosum presenting with acute comitant esotropia. Am J Ophthalmol 1970;69:594–598.
359. Bixenman WW, Laguna JF: Acquired esotropia as initial manifestation of Arnold–Chiari malformation. J Pediatr Ophthalmol Strab 1987;24:83–86.
360. Williams AS, Hoyt CS: Acute comitant esotropia in children with brain tumors. Arch Ophthalmol 1989;107:376–378.
361. Astle WF, Miller SJ: Acute comitant esotropia: a sign of intracranial disease. Can J Ophthalmol 1994;29: 151–154.
362. Jaafar MS, Collins MLZ, Rabinowitz AI: Cerebellar astrocytoma presenting as acquired comitant esotropia at age 18 and 27 months [abstract]. J Pediatr Ophthalmol Strabismus 1995;32:63.
363. Ciancia AO: On infantile esotropia with nystagmus in abduction. J Pediatr Ophthalmol Strab 1995;32: 280–288.
364. Hoyt CS, Good WV: Acute comitant esotropia: when is it a sign of serious neurologic disease? Br J Ophthalmol 1995;79:498–501.
365. Passo M, Shults WT, Talbot T, et al: Acquired esotropia. A manifestation of Chiari I malformation. J Clin Neuro-ophthalmol 1984;4:151–154.
366. Lewis AR, Kline LB, Sharpe JA: Acquired esotropia due to Arnold–Chiari I malformation. J Neuro-ophthalmol 1996;16:49–54.
367. Simon JW, Waldman JB, Couture KC: Cerebellar astrocytoma manifesting as isolated, comitant esotropia in childhood. Am J Ophthalmol 1996;121:584–586.
368. Weeks CL, Hamed LM: Treatment of acute comitant esotropia in Chiari I malformation. Ophthalmology 1999;106:2368–2371.
369. Liu GT, Hertle RW, Quinn GE, et al: Comitant esodeviation due to neurologic insult in children. J Am Assoc Pediatr Ophthalmol Strabismus 1997; 1:143–146.
370. Lennerstrand G: Central motor control in concomitant strabismus. Graefes Arch Clin Exp Ophthalmol 1988;226:172–174.
371. Flynn JT: Problems in strabismus management. In: Transactions New Orleans Academy of Ophthalmology, p 456. New York, Raven Press, 1986.

372. Jampolski A: Ocular divergence mechanisms. Trans Am Ophthalmol Soc 1970;68:756–762.
373. Parlato CJ, Nelson LB, Harley RD: Cyclic strabismus. Ann Ophthalmol 1983;15:1126–1129.
374. Pillai P, Dhand UK: Cyclic esotropia with central nervous system disease: report of two cases. J Pediatr Ophthalmol Strabismus 1987;24:237–241.
375. Duane A: Congenital deficiency of abduction, associated with impairment of adduction, retraction movements, contraction of the palpebral fissure and oblique movements of the eye. [Reprinted in abridged form in Arch Ophthalmol 1996 114:1255–1257]. Arch Ophthalmol 1905;34:133–159.
376. Huber A: Electrophysiology of the retraction syndromes. Br J Ophthalmol 1974;58:293–300.
377. DeRespinis PA, Caputo AR, Wagner RS, et al: Duane's retraction syndrome. Surv Ophthalmol 1993;38:257–288.
378. Hotchkiss MG, Miller NR, Clark AW, et al: Bilateral Duane's retraction syndrome. A clinical-pathologic case report. Arch Ophthalmol 1980;98:870–874.
379. Miller NR, Kiel SM, Green WR, et al: Unilateral Duane's retraction syndrome (Type 1). Arch Ophthalmol 1982;100:1468–1472.
380. Parsa CF, Grant PE, Dillon WP, et al: Absence of the abducens nerve in Duane syndrome verified by magnetic resonance imaging. Am J Ophthalmol 1998;125:399–401.
381. Brodsky MC, Fray KJ: Brainstem hypoplasia in the Wildervanck (cervico-oculo-acoustic) syndrome. Arch Ophthalmol 1998;116:383–385.
382. Chew CKS, Foster P, Hurst JA, et al: Duane's retraction syndrome associated with chromosome 4q27-31 segment deletion. Am J Ophthalmol 1995;119: 807–809.
383. Miller MT, Strömland K: Ocular motility in thalidomide embryopathy. J Pediatr Ophthalmol Strabismus 1991;28:47–54.
384. Yamanouchi H, Iwasaki Y, Sugai K, et al: Duane retraction syndrome associated with Chiari I malformation. Pediatr Neurol 1993;9:327–329.
385. Brodsky MC, Boop FA: Fourth ventricular ependymoma in a child with Duane retraction syndrome. Pediatr Neurosurg 1997;26:157–159.
386. Duane TD, Schatz NJ, Caputo AR: Pseudo-Duane's retraction syndrome. Trans Am Ophthalmol Soc 1976;74:122–129.
387. Rogers GL, Bremer DL: Surgical treatment of the upshoot and downshoot in Duane's retraction syndrome. Ophthalmology 1984;91:1380–1383.
388. Pressman SH, Scott WE: Surgical treatment of Duane's syndrome. Ophthalmology 1986;93:29–38.
389. Molarte AB, Rosenbaum AL: Vertical rectus muscle transposition surgery for Duane's syndrome. J Pediatr Ophthalmol Strabismus 1990;27:171–177.
390. Henderson JL: The congenital facial diplegia syndrome: clinical features, pathology, and etiology. Brain 1939;62:381–403.
391. Okamoto K, Hirai S, Amari M, et al: Oculomotor nuclear pathology in amyotrophic lateral sclerosis. Acta Neuropathol 1993;85:458–462.
392. Aberfeld DC, Namba T: Progressive ophthalmoplegia in Kugelberg–Welander disease. Report of a case. Arch Neurol 1969;20:253–256.
393. Gruber H, Zeitlhofer J, Prager J, et al: Complex oculomotor dysfunctions in Kugelberg–Welander disease. Neuro-ophthalmology 1983;3:125–128.
394. Sima AAF, Caplan M, D'Amato CJ, et al: Fulminant multiple system atrophy in a young adult presenting as motor neuron disease. Neurology 1993;43:2031–2035.
395. Hamano K, Tsukamoto H, Yazawa T, et al: Infantile progressive spinal muscular atrophy with ophthalmoplegia and pyramidal symptoms. Pediatr Neurol 1994;10:320–324.
396. Yuki N: Acute paresis of extraocular muscles associated with anti IgG anti GQ_1b antibody. Ann Neurol 1996;39:668–672.
397. Yuki N: Successful plasmapheresis in Bickerstaff's brainstem encephalitis associated with anti GQ_1b antibody. J Neurol Sci 1995;131:108–110.
398. Chiba A, Kusunoki S, Obata H, et al: Serum anti-GQ_{1b} antibody is associated with ophthalmoplegia in Miller Fisher syndrome and Guillain–Barré syndrome. Clinical and immunohistochemical studies. Neurology 1993;43:1911–1917.
399. Al-Din ASN: The nosological position of the ophthalmoplegia ataxia and areflexia syndrome: "The spectrum hypothesis." Acta Neurol Scand 1987; 75:287–294.
400. Jordan K, Marino J, Damast M, et al: Bilateral oculomotor paralysis due to neurosyphilis. Ann Neurol 1978;3:90–93.
401. Balm M, Hammack J: Leptomeningeal carcinomatosis. Presenting features and prognostic factors. Arch Neurol 1996;53:626–632.
402. Oostenbrugge v, Twijnstra A: Presenting features and value of diagnostic procedures in leptomeningeal metastases. Neurology 1999;53:382–385.
403. Galetta SL, Sergott RC, Wells GB, et al: Spontaneous remission of a third-nerve palsy in meningeal lymphoma. Ann Neurol 1992;32:100–102.
404. Liu GT, Kay MD, Byrne GE, et al: Ophthalmoparesis due to Burkitt's lymphoma following cardiac transplantation. Neurology 1993;43:2147–2149.
405. Newman NJ: Multiple cranial neuropathies: presenting signs of systemic lymphoma. Surv Ophthalmol 1992;37:125–129.
406. Diaz-Arrastia R, Younger DS, Hair L, et al: Neurolymphomatosis: A clinicopathologic syndrome re-emerges. Neurology 1992;42:1136–1141.
407. Arroyo JG, Horton JC: Acute, painful, pupil-sparing third nerve palsy in chronic inflammatory demyelinating polyneuropathy. Neurology 1995;45:846–847.
408. Cullom ME, Savino PJ: Adenocarcinoma of the prostate presenting as a third nerve palsy. Neurology 1993;43:2146–2147.
409. Carrizo A, Basso A: Current surgical treatment for sphenoorbital meningiomas. Surg Neurol 1998; 50:574–578.
410. Mayberg MR, Symon L: Meningiomas of the clivus and apical petrous bone. J Neurosurg 1986; 65:160–167.
411. Dany A, Delcour J, Laine E: Les meningiomes du clivus: Etudes clinique, radiologique et therapeutique. Neurochiurige 1963;9:249–277.
412. Spallone A, Makhmudov UB, Mukhamedjanov DJ, et al: Petroclival meningioma. An attempt to define the role of skull base approaches in their surgical management. Surg Neurol 1999;51:412–419.
413. Subach BR, Lunsford LD, Kondziolka D, et al: Management of petroclival meningiomas by stereotactic radiosurgery. Neurosurgery 1998;42:437–443.
414. Mindell ER: Current concept review: Chordoma. J Bone Joint Surg 1981;63:501–505.
415. Kendall BE, Lee BC: Cranial chordomas. Br J Radiol 1977;50:687–698.

416. Volpe NJ, Liebsch NJ, Munzenrider JE, et al: Neuro-ophthalmologic findings in chordoma and chondrosarcoma of the skull base. Am J Ophthalmol 1993;115:97–104.
417. Sze G, Uichanco LS, Brant-Zawadzki MN, et al: Chordomas: MR imaging. Radiology 1988;166:187–191.
418. al-Mefty O, Borba LAB: Skull base chordomas: a management challenge. J Neurosurg 1997;86:182–189.
419. Suit HD, Goitein M, Munzenrider J, et al: Increased efficacy of radiation therapy by use of proton beam. Strahlenther Onkol 1990;166:40–44.
420. Austin Seymour M, Munzenrider J, Goitein M, et al: Fractionated proton radiation therapy of chordoma and low-grade chondrosarcoma of the base of the skull. J Neurosurg 1989;70:13–17.
421. Kveton JF, Brackmann DE, Glasscock ME, et al: Chondrosarcoma of the skull base. Otolaryngol Head Neck Surg 1986;94:23–32.
422. Korten AGGC, ter Berg HJ, Spincemaille GH, et al: Intracranial chondrosarcoma: review of the literature and report of 15 cases. J Neurol Neurosurg Psychiatry 1998;65:88–92.
423. Balcer LJ, Galetta SL, Cornblath WT, et al: Neuro-ophthalmologic manifestations of Maffucci's syndrome and Ollier's disease. J Neuro-ophthalmol 1999;19:62–66.
424. Myles WM, Maxner CE: Localizing value of concurrent sixth nerve paresis and postganglionic Horner's syndrome. Can J Ophthalmol 1994;29:39–42.
425. Sheldon JJ, Tobias J, Soila K: MRI of the cavernous sinus. In: Smith JL, Katz R (eds): Neuro-ophthalmology Enters the Nineties, pp 67–90. Hialeah, Dutton Press, 1988.
426. Keane JR: Cavernous sinus syndrome. Analysis of 151 cases. Arch Neurol 1996;53:967–971.
427. Trobe JD, Hood I, Parsons JT, et al: Intracranial spread of squamous carcinoma along the trigeminal nerve. Arch Ophthalmol 1982;100:608–611.
428. Thomas JE, Yoss RE: The parasellar syndrome; problems in determining etiology. Mayo Clin Proc 1970;45:617–623.
429. Unsold R, Safran AB, Safran E, et al: Metastatic infiltration of nerves in the cavernous sinus. Arch Neurol 1980;37:59–61.
430. Neel HB: Nasopharyngeal carcinoma. Otolaryngol Clin North Am 1985;18:479–490.
431. Chong VF, Fan YF, Khoo JB: Nasopharyngeal carcinoma with intracranial spread: CT and MR characteristics. J Comput Assist Tomogr 1996;20:563–569.
432. Godtfredsen F, Lederman M: Diagnostic and prognostic roles of ophthalmoneurologic signs and symptoms in malignant nasopharyngeal tumors. Am J Ophthalmol 1965;59:1063–1069.
433. Trautmann JC, Laws ER: Visual status after transsphenoidal surgery at the Mayo Clinic, 1971–1982. Am J Ophthalmol 1983;96:200–208.
434. Wykes WN: Prolactinoma presenting with intermittent third nerve palsy. Br J Ophthalmol 1986;70:706–707.
435. Robinson R, Toland J, Eustace P: Pituitary apoplexy. A cause for painful third nerve palsy. Neuro-ophthalmology 1990;10:257–260.
436. Seyer H, Kompf D, Fahlbusch R: Optomotor palsies in pituitary apoplexy. Neuro-ophthalmology 1992;12:217–224.
437. Reid RL, Quigley ME, Yen SSC: Pituitary apoplexy: A review. Arch Neurol 1985;40:712–719.
438. Turgut M, Palaoglu S, Akpinar G, et al: Giant schwannoma of the trigeminal nerve misdiagnosed as maxillary sinusitis. A case report. S Afr J Surg 1997;35:131–133.
439. Del Priore LV, Miller NR: Trigeminal schwannoma as a cause of chronic, isolated sixth nerve palsy. Am J Ophthalmol 1989;108:726–729.
440. Alonso PE, Bescansa E, Salas J, et al: Perineural spread of cutaneous squamous cell carcinoma manifesting as ptosis and ophthalmoplegia (orbital apex syndrome). Br J Plast Surg 1995;48:564–568.
441. Clouston PD, Sharpe DM, Corbett AJ, et al: Perineural spread of cutaneous head and neck cancer. Its orbital and central neurologic complications. Arch Neurol 1990;47:73–77.
442. Catalano PJ, Sen C, Biller HF: Cranial neuropathy secondary to perineural spread of cutaneous malignancies. Am J Otol 1995;16:772–777.
443. McNab AA, Francis IC, Berger R, et al: Perineural spread of cutaneous squamous cell carcinoma via the orbit. Ophthalmology 1997;104:1457–1462.
444. Phillips PH, Newman NJ: Here today . . . gone tomorrow. Surv Ophthalmol 1997;41:354–356.
445. O'Sullivan MG, van Loveren HR, Tew JM: The surgical resectability of meningiomas of the cavernous sinus. Neurosurgery 1997;40:238–245.
446. Braunstein JB, Vick NA: Meningiomas: the decision not to operate. Neurology 1997;48:1459–1462.
447. DeMonte F, Smith HK, Al-Mefty O: Outcome of aggressive removal of cavernous sinus meningiomas. J Neurosurg 1994;81:245–251.
448. De Jesús O, Sekhar LN, Parikh HK, et al: Long-term follow-up of patients with meningiomas involving the cavernous sinus: recurrence, progression, and quality of life. Neurosurgery 1996;39:915–919.
449. Knosp E, Perneczky A, Koos WT, et al: Meningiomas of the space of the cavernous sinus. Neurosurgery 1996;38:434–442.
450. Kim DK, Grieve J, Archer DJ, et al: Meningiomas in the region of the cavernous sinus: a review of 21 patients. Br J Neurosurg 1996;10:439–444.
451. Kurita H, Sasaki T, Kawamoto S, et al: Role of radiosurgery in the management of cavernous sinus meningiomas. Acta Neurol Scand 1997;96:297–304.
452. Pendl G, Schrottner O, Eustacchio S, et al: Cavernous sinus meningiomas—what is the strategy: upfront or adjuvant gamma knife surgery? Stereotact Funct Neurosurg 1998;70:33–40.
453. Chang SD, Adler JR, Jr., Martin DP: LINAC radiosurgery for cavernous sinus meningiomas. Stereotact Funct Neurosurg 1998;71:43–50.
454. Case records of the Massachusetts General Hospital: Case 4-1993. N Engl J Med 1993;328:266–275.
455. Agarwal P, Sharma K, Gupta RK, et al: Acute bilateral ophthalmoplegia secondary to metastatic prostatic carcinoma. J Neuro-ophthalmol 1995;15:45–47.
456. Kline LB: The Tolosa–Hunt syndrome. Surv Ophthalmol 1982;27:79–95.
457. Odabasi Z, Gokcil Z, Atilla S, et al: The value of MRI in a case of Tolosa–Hunt syndrome. Clin Neurol Neurosurg 1997;99:151–154.
458. Evans OB, Lexow SS: Painful ophthalmoplegia in systemic lupus erythematosus. Ann Neurol 1978;4:584–585.
459. Dávalos A, Matías-Guiu J, Codina A: Painful ophthalmoplegia in systemic lupus erythematosus [letter]. J Neurol Neurosurg Psychiatry 1984;47:323–324.
460. Gross FJ, Waxman JS, Rosenblatt MA, et al: Eosinophilic granuloma of the cavernous sinus and orbital

apex in an HIV positive patient. Ophthalmology 1989;96:462–467.
461. Marsh RJ, Dulley B, Kelly V: External ocular motor palsies in ophthalmic zoster: a review. Br J Ophthalmol 1977;61:677–682.
462. Dinubile MJ: Septic thrombosis of the cavernous sinus. Arch Neurol 1988;45:567–572.
463. Geggel HS, Isenberg SJ: Cavernous sinus thrombosis as a cause of unilateral blindness. Ann Ophthalmol 1982;14:569–574.
464. Gupta A, Jalali S, Bansal RV, et al: Anterior ischemic optic neuropathy and branch retinal artery occlusion in cavernous sinus thrombosis. J Clin Neuro-ophthalmol 1990;10:193–196.
465. Southwick FS, Richardson EP, Jr, Swartz MN: Septic thrombosis of the dural venous sinuses. Medicine 1986;65:82–106.
466. Igarashi H, Igarashi S, Fujio N, et al: Magnetic resonance imaging in the early diagnosis of cavernous sinus thrombosis. Ophthalmologica 1995;209: 292–296.
467. Levine SR, Twyman RE, Gilman S: The role of anticoagulation in cavernous sinus thrombosis. Neurology 1988;38:517–522.
468. Case records of the Massachusetts General Hospital: Case 33-1991. N Engl J Med 1991;325:494–504.
469. Galetta SL, Wulc AE, Goldberg H, et al: Rhinocerebral mucormycosis: management and survival after carotid occlusion. Ann Neurol 1990;28:103–107.
470. Kohn R, Helper R: Management of limited rhino-orbital mucormycosis without exenteration. Ophthalmology 1985;92:1440–1444.
471. Fleishman JA, Garfinkel RA, Beck RW: Advances in the treatment of carotid cavernous fistula. Int Ophthalmol Clin 1986;26:301–311.
472. Parkinson D: Carotid cavernous fistulas. Direct repair with preservation of the carotid artery: Technical note. J Neurosurg 1973;38:99–106.
473. Barrow DL, Spector RH, Braun IF, et al: Classification and treatment of spontaneous carotid–cavornous sinus fistulas. J Neurosurg 1985;62:248–256.
474. Lewis AI, Tomsick TA, Tew JM, Jr: Management of 100 consecutive direct carotid-cavernous fistulas: results of treatment with detachable balloons. Neurosurgery 1995;36:239–245.
475. Takahashi M, Killeffer F, Wilson G: Iatrogenic carotid cavernous fistulas: case report. J Neurosurg 1969; 30:498–500.
476. Pedersen RA, Troost TB, Schramm VL: Carotid-cavernous sinus fistula after external ethmoid-sphenoid surgery. Arch Otolaryngol 1981;107: 307–309.
477. Kupersmith MJ, Berenstein A, Flamm E, et al: Neuro-ophthalmologic abnormalities and intravascular therapy of traumatic carotid cavernous fistulas. Ophthalmology 1986;93:906–912.
478. Debrun GM, Vinuela F, Fox AJ, et al: Indications for treatment and classification of 132 carotid–cavernous fistulas. Neurosurgery 1988;22:285–289.
479. Kupersmith MJ, Berenstein A, Choi IS, et al: Management of nontraumatic vascular shunts involving the cavernous sinus. Ophthalmology 1988;95:121–130.
480. Rwiza HT, Vliet AM, Keyser A, et al: Bilateral spontaneous carotid–cavernous fistulas associated with systemic hypertension and generalized arteriosclerosis: A case report. J Neurol Neurosurg Psychiatry 1988;51:1003–1005.
481. Kaufman HH, Lind TA, Mullan S: Spontaneous carotid-cavernous fistula with fibromuscular dysplasia. Acta Neurochir 1978;40:123–129.
482. Hieshima GB, Cahan LD, Mehringer CM, et al: Spontaneous arteriovenous fistulas of cerebral vessels in association with fibromuscular dysplasia. Neurosurgery 1986;18:454–458.
483. Farley MK, Clark RD, Fallor MK, et al: Spontaneous carotid–cavernous fistula and the Ehlers–Danlos syndromes. Ophthalmology 1983;90:1337–1342.
484. Halbach VV, Higashida RT, Dowd CF, et al: Treatment of carotid–cavernous fistulas associated with Ehlers–Danlos syndrome. Neurosurgery 1990;26: 1021–1027.
485. Koo AH, Newton TH: Pseudoxanthoma elasticum associated with carotid rate mirable. Am J Roentgenol Radium Ther Nucl Med 1972;116:16–22.
486. Spencer WH, Thompson HS, Hoyt WF: Ischaemic ocular necrosis from carotid-cavernous fistula: pathology of stagnant anoxic "inflammation" in orbital and ocular tissues. Br J Ophthalmol 1973;57:145–152.
487. Hedges TR, Debrun G, Sokol S: Reversible optic neuropathy from carotid cavernous fistula. J Clin Neuro-ophthalmol 1985;5:37–40.
488. Berk AT, Ada E, Kir E, et al: Choroidal detachent associated with direct spontaneous carotid–cavernous sinus fistula. Ophthalmologica 1997;211: 53–55.
489. Turner DM, vanGilder JC, Mojthedi S, et al: Spontaneous intracerebral hematoma in carotid cavernous fistula. J Neurosurg 1983;1983:680–686.
490. d'Angelo VA, Monte V, Scialfa G, et al: Intracerebral venous hemorrhage in "high risk" carotid–cavernous fistula. Surg Neurol 1988;30:387–390.
491. Golnik KC, Miller NR: Diagnosis of cavernous sinus arteriovenous fistula by measurement of ocular pulse amplitude. Ophthalmology 1992;99:1146–1152.
492. Moster MR, Kennerdell JS: B-scan ultrasonic evaluation of dilated superior ophthalmic vein in orbital and retro-orbital arteriovenous anomalies. J Clin Neuro-ophthalmol 1983;3:105–198.
493. Debrun GM, Nauta HJ, Miller NR, et al: Combining the detachable balloon technique and surgery in imaging carotid cavernous fistulae. Surg Neurol 1989;32:3–10.
494. Wilms G, Peene P, Nowe G, et al: Angiographic diagnosis and treatment of posttraumatic carotid-cavernous sinus fistulas. Bull Soc Belge Ophthalmol 1989;23:83–89.
495. Barnwell SL, O'Neill OR: Endovascular therapy of carotid cavernous fistulas. Neurosurg Clin North Am 1994;5:485–495.
496. Palestine AG, Younge BR, Piepgras DG: Visual prognosis in carotid–cavernous fistulas. Arch Ophthalmol 1981;99:1600–1603.
497. Vinuela F, Fox AJ, Debrun GM, et al: Spontaneous carotid cavernous fistulas: clinical, radiological and therapeutic considerations. J Neurosurg 1984;60: 976–984.
498. Ismat F, Ferrer E, Twose J: Direct intracavernous obliteration of high-flow fistulas. J Neurosurg 1986;65:770–775.
499. Serbinenko FA: Balloon catheterization and occlusion of major cerebral vessels. J Neurosurg 1974;41: 125–145.
500. Kwan E, Heishima GB, Higashida RT, et al: Interventional neuroradiology in neuro-ophthalmology. J Clin Neuro-ophthalmol 1989;9:83–97.
501. Halbach VV, Higashida RT, Hieshima GB, et al: Transvenous embolization of direct carotid cavernous fistulas. AJNR Am J Neuroradiol 1988;9:741–746.

502. Miller NR, Monsein LH, Debrun GM, et al: Treatment of carotid-cavernous sinus fistulas using a superior ophthalmic vein approach. J Neurosurg 1995;83: 838–842.
503. Debrun G, Lacour P, Vinuela F, et al: Treatment of 54 traumatic carotid-cavernous fistulas. J Neurosurg 1981;55:678–692.
504. Higashida R, Halbach VV, Tsai F: Interventional neurovascular treatment of traumatic carotid and vertebral artery lesions. AJR Am J Roentgerol 1989;153:577.
505. Leonard TJ, Moseley IF, Sanders MD: Ophthalmoplegia in carotid cavernous sinus fistula. Br J Ophthalmol 1984;68:128–134.
506. Awad IA, Little JR, Akrawi WP, et al: Intracranial dural arteriovenous malformations: factors predisposing to an aggressive neurological course. J Neurosurg 1990;72:839–850.
507. Houser OW, Campbell JK, Campbell RJ, et al: Arteriovenous malformation affecting the transverse dural sinus—an acquired lesion. Mayo Clin Proc 1979;54:651–661.
508. Houser OW, Baker HL, Rhonton AL, et al: Intracranial dural arteriovenous malformations. Radiology 1972;105:55–64.
509. Newton TH, Hoyt WF: Dural arteriovenous shunts in the region of the cavernous sinus. Neuroradiology 1970;1:71–81.
510. Rizzo M, Bosch EP, Gross CE: Trigeminal sensory neuropathy due to dural external carotid–cavernous sinus fistula. Neurology 1982;32:89–91.
511. Hawke SHB, Mullie MA, Hoyt WF, et al: Painful oculomotor palsy due to dural–cavernous sinus shunt. Arch Neurol 1989;46:1252–1255.
512. Miyachi S, Negoro M, Handa T, et al: Dural carotid cavernous sinus fistula presenting as isolated oculomotor nerve palsy. Surg Neurol 1993;39:105–109.
513. Brazis PW, Capobianco DJ, Chang FLF, et al: Low flow dural arteriovenous shunt: another cause of "sinister" Tolosa–Hunt syndrome. Headache 1994; 34:523–525.
514. Acierno MD, Trobe JD, Cornblath WT, et al: Painful oculomotor palsy caused by posterior-draining dural carotid cavernous fistulas. Arch Ophthalmol 1995;113:1045–1049.
515. Uehara T, Tabuchi M, Kawaguchi T, et al: Spontaneous dural carotid cavernous sinus fistula presenting isolated ophthalmoplegia: evaluation with MR angiography. Neurology 1998;50:814–816.
516. DeKeizer RJW: Spontaneous carotid-cavernous fistulas. The importance of the typical limbal vascular loops for the diagnosis, the recognition of glaucoma and the uses of conservative therapy in this condition. Doc Ophthalmol 1979;46:403–412.
517. Phelps CD, Thompson HS, Ossoinig KC: The diagnosis and prognosis of atypical carotid–cavernous fistula (red-eyed shunt syndrome). Am J Ophthalmol 1982;93:423–426.
518. Keltner JL, Gittinger JW, Miller NR, et al: A red eye and high intraocular pressure. Surv Ophthalmol 1986;31:328–336.
519. Keltner JL, Satterfield D, Dublin AB, et al: Dural and carotid cavernous sinus fistulas: diagnosis, management and complications. Ophthalmology 1987;94: 1585–1600.
520. Fiore PM, Latina MA, Shingleton BJ, et al: The dural shunt syndrome. I. Management of glaucoma. Ophthalmology 1990;97:56–62.
521. Sergott RC, Grossman RI, Savino PJ, et al: The syndrome of paradoxical worsening of dural–cavernous sinus arteriovenous malformations. Ophthalmology 1987;94:205–212.
522. Harbison JW, Guerry D, Weisinger H: Dural arteriovenous fistula and spontaneous choroidal detachment: New cause of an old disease. Br J Ophthalmol 1978;62:483–490.
523. Harris GJ, Rice PR: Angle closure in carotid–cavernous fistula. Ophthalmology 1979;86:1521–1529.
524. Jorgensen JS, Gutthoff RF: 24 cases of carotid cavernous fistulas: frequency, symptoms, diagnosis and treatment. Acta Ophthalmologica 1985;63:67–71.
525. Brunette I, Boghen D: Central retinal vein occlusion complicating spontaneous carotid–cavernous fistula. Arch Ophthalmol 1987;105:464–465.
526. Kupersmith MJ, Vargas EM, Warren F, et al: Venous obstruction as the cause of retinal/choroidal dysfunction associated with arteriovenous shunts in the cavernous sinus. J Neuro-ophthalmol 1996;16:1–6.
527. DeKeizer RJW: Spontaneous carotid cavernous fistulas. Neuro-ophthalmol 1981;2:35–46.
528. Fourman S: Acute closed-angle glaucoma after arteriovenous fistulas. Am J Ophthalmol 1989;107: 156–159.
529. Selky AK, Purvin VA: Isolated trochlear nerve palsy secondary to dural carotid–cavernous sinus fistula. J Neuro-ophthalmol 1994;14:52–54.
530. Spector RH: Echographic diagnosis of dural carotid cavernous sinus fistulas. Am J Ophthalmol 1991;111: 77–83.
531. Flaharty PM, Lieb WE, Sergott RC, et al: Color Doppler imaging. A new noninvasive technique to diagnose and monitor carotid cavernous sinus fistulas. Arch Ophthalmol 1991;109:522–526.
532. Munk P, Downey D, Nicolle D, et al: The role of colour flow Doppler ultrasonography in the investigation of disease in the eye and orbit. Can J Ophthalmol 1993;28:171–176.
533. Hirabuki N, Miura T, Mitomo M, et al: MR imaging of dural arteriovenous malformations with ocular signs. Neuroradiology 1988;30:390–394.
534. Goldberg RA, Goldey SH, Duckwiler G, et al: Management of cavernous sinus–dural fistulas. Indications and techniques for primary embolization via the superior ophthalmic vein. Arch Ophthalmol 1996;114:707–714.
535. Krisht AF, Burson T: Combined pretemporal and endovascular approach to the cavernous sinus for the treatment of carotid–cavernous dural fistulae: technical case report. Neurosurgery 1999;44:415–418.
536. Bito S, Hasegawa H, Fujiwara M, et al: Irradiation of spontaneous carotid–cavernous fistulas. Surg Neurol 1982;17:282–286.
537. Kobayashi H, Hayashi M, Noguchi Y, et al: Dural arteriovenous malformations in the anterior cranial fossa. Surg Neurol 1988;30:396–401.
538. Guo WY, Pan DH, Wu HM, et al: Radiosurgery as a treatment alternative for dural arteriovenous fistulas of the cavernous sinus. AJNR: Am J Neuroradiol 1998;19:1081–1087.
539. Barr HWR, Blackwood W, Meadows SP: Intracavernous carotid aneurysms a clinical pathological report. Brain 1971;94:607–622.
540. Linskey ME, Sekhar LN, Hirsch WL, Jr., et al: Aneurysms of the intracavernous carotid artery: natural history and indications for treatment. Neurosurgery 1990;26:933–937.
541. Berenstein A, Ransohoff J, Kupersmith M, et al: Endovascular treatment of giant aneurysms of the carotid

and vertebral arteries. Functional investigation and embolization. Surg Neurol 1984;21:3–12.
542. Halbach VV, Higashida RT, Dowd CF, et al: Cavernous internal carotid artery aneurysms treated with electrolytically detachable coils. J Neuro-ophthalmol 1997;17:231–239.
543. Kupersmith MT, Berenstein A, Choi IS, et al: Percutaneous transvascular treatment of giant carotid aneurysms: Neuro-ophthalmologic findings. Neurology 1984;34:328–335.
544. Harley RD, Rodrigues MM, Crawford JS: Congenital fibrosis of the extraocular muscles. J Pediatr Ophthalmol Strabismus 1978;15:346–358.
545. Apt L, Axelrod RN: Generalized fibrosis of the extraocular muscles. Am J Ophthalmol 1978;85:822–829.
546. Hiatt RL, Halle AA: General fibrosis syndrome. Ann Ophthalmol 1983;15:1103–1109.
547. Brodsky MC: Hereditary external ophthalmoplegia, synergistic divergence, jaw winking, and oculocutaneous hypopigmentation. Ophthalmology 1998;105: 717–725.
548. Engle EC, Marondel I, Houtman WA, et al: Congenital fibrosis of the extraocular muscles (autosomal dominant congenital external ophthalmoplegia): genetic homogeneity, linkage refinement, and physical mapping on chromosome 12. Am J Hum Genet 1995;57:1086–1094.
549. Wang SM, Zwaan J, Mullaney PB, et al: Congenital fibrosis of the extraocular muscles type 2, an inherited exotropic strabismus fixus, maps to distal 11q13. Am J Hum Genet 1998;63:517–525.
550. Doherty EJ, Macy ME, Wang WM, et al: CFEOM3: a new extraocular congenital fibrosis syndrome that maps to 16q24.2-q24.3. Invest Ophthalmol Vis Sci 1999;40:1687–1694.
551. Gillies WE, Harris AJ, Brooks AMV, et al: Congenital fibrosis of the vertically acting extraocular muscles. Ophthalmology 1995;102:607–612.
552. Hertle RW, Katowitz JA, Young TL, et al: Congenital unilateral fibrosis, blepharoptosis, and enophthalmos syndrome. Ophthalmology 1992;99:347–355.
553. Engle EC, Goumnerov BC, McKeown CA, et al: Oculomotor nerve and muscle abnormalities in congenital fibrosis of the extraocular muscles. Ann Neurol 1997;41:314–325.
554. Nelson LB: Diagnosis and management of strabismus and amblyopia. Ped Clin N Am 1983;30:1003–1014.
555. Simon AL, Borchert M: Etiology and prognosis of acute, late-onset esotropia. Ophthalmology 1997;104: 1348–1352.
556. Hunter DG, Ellis FJ: Prevalence of systemic and ocular disease in infantile exotropia. Comparison with infantile esotropia. Ophthalmology 1999;106:1951–1956.
557. Wilson ME, Eustis HS, Parks MM: Brown's syndrome. Surv Ophthalmol 1989;34:153–172.
558. Thorne JE, Volpe NJ, Liu GT: Magnetic resonance imaging of acquired Brown syndrome in a patient with psoriasis. Am J Ophthalmol 1999;127:233–234.
559. Gregersen E, Rindziunski E: Brown's syndrome. A longitudinal study of spontaneous course. Acta Ophthalmol 1993;71:371–376.
560. Helveston E: Dissociated vertical deviation: a clinical and laboratory study. Trans Am Ophthalmol Soc 1980;78:734–779.
561. Harcourt B, Mein J, Johnson F: Natural history and associations of dissociated vertical divergence. Trans Ophthal Soc UK 1980;100:495–497.
562. Noel LP, Parks MM: Dissociated vertical deviation: associated findings and results of surgical treatment. Can J Ophthalmol 1982;17:10–12.
563. Cheeseman EW, Guyton DL: Vertical fusional vergence. The key to dissociated vertical deviation. Arch Ophthalmol 1999;117:1188–1191.
564. Brodsky MC: Dissociated vertical divergence. A righting reflex gone wrong. Arch Ophthalmol 1999;117:1216 1222.
565. Freedman HL, Kushner BJ: Congenital ocular aberrant innervation—new concepts. J Pediatr Ophthalmol Strabismus 1997;34:10–16.
566. Lacey B, Chang W, Rootman J: Nonthyroid causes of extraocular muscle disease. Surv Ophthalmol 1999;44:187–213.
567. Glaser JS: Myasthenic pseudo-internuclear ophthalmoplegia. Arch Ophthalmol 1966;75:363–366.
568. Weinberg DA, Lesser RL, Vollmer TL: Ocular myasthenia: a protean disorder. Surv Ophthalmol 1994;39:169–210.
569. Schmidt D: Signs in ocular myasthenia and pseudomyasthenia. Differential diagnostic criteria. A clinical review. Neuro-ophthalmology 1995;15:21–58.
570. Tein I, Haslam RHA, Rhead WJ, et al: Short-chain acyl-CoA dehydrogenase deficiency. A cause of ophthalmoplegia and multicore myopathy. Neurology 1999;52:366–372.
571. Scelsa SN, Simpson DM, Reichler BD, et al: Extraocular muscle involvement in Becker muscular dystrophy. Neurology 1996;46:564–566.
572. Wright RA, Plant GT, Landon DN, et al: Nemaline myopathy: an unusual cause of ophthalmoparesis. J Neuro-ophthalmol 1997;17:39–43.
573. Barricks ME, Traviesa DB, Glaser JS, et al: Ophthalmoplegia in cranial arteritis. Brain 1977;100: 209–221.
574. Mehler MF, Rabinowich L: The clinical neuro-ophthalmologic spectrum of temporal arteritis. Am J Med 1988;85:839–843.
575. Hayreh SS, Podhajsky PA, Zimmerman B: Ocular manifestations of giant cell arteritis. Am J Ophthalmol 1998;125:509–520.
576. Hamed LM: Strabismus presenting after cataract surgery. Ophthalmology 1991;98:247–252.
577. Wylie J, Henderson M, Doyle M, et al: Persistent binocular diplopia following cataract surgery: aetiology and management. Eye 1994;8:543–546.
578. McDonnell PJ, Spalton DJ, Falcon MG: Decentration of the posterior chamber lens implant: the effect of optic size on the incidence of visual aberrations. Eye 1990;4:132–137.
579. Pratt-Johnson JA, Tillson G: Intractable diplopia after vision restoration in unilateral cataract. Am J Ophthalmol 1989;107:23–26.
580. Sharkey JA, Sellar PW: Acquired central fusion disruption following cataract extraction. J Pediatr Ophthalmol Strabismus 1994;31:391–393.
581. Hamed LM, Lingua RW: Thyroid eye disease presenting after cataract surgery. J Pediatr Ophthalmol Strabismus 1990;27:10–15.
582. Rainin EA, Carlson BM: Postoperative diplopia and ptosis. A clinical hypothesis based on the myotoxicity of local anesthetics. Arch Ophthalmol 1985;103:1337–1339.
583. Carlson BM, Emerick S, Komorowski TE, et al: Extraocular muscle regeneration in primates. Local anesthetic-induced lesions. Ophthalmology 1992;99: 582–589.

584. Spierer A, Schwalb E: Superior oblique muscle paresis after sub-Tenon's anesthesia for cataract surgery. J Cataract Refract Surg 1999;25:144–145.
585. Hamed LM, Mancuso A: Inferior rectus muscle contracture syndrome after retrobulbar anesthesia. Ophthalmology 1991;98:1506–1512.
586. Muñoz M: Inferior rectus muscle overaction after cataract extraction. Am J Ophthalmol 1994;118: 664–666.
587. Ong Tone L, Pearce WG: Inferior rectus muscle restriction after retrobulbar anesthesia for cataract extraction. Can J Ophthalmol 1989;24:162–165.
588. Hunter DG, Lam GC, Guyton DL: Inferior oblique muscle injury from local anesthesia for cataract surgery. Ophthalmology 1995;102:501–509.
589. Capó H, Guyton DL: Ipsilateral hypertropia after cataract surgery. Ophthalmology 1996;103:721–730.
590. Capó H, Roth E, Johnson T, et al: Vertical strabismus after cataract surgery. Ophthalmology 1996;103: 918–921.
591. Esswein MB, von Noorden GK: Paresis of a vertical rectus muscle after cataract extraction. Am J Ophthalmol 1993;116:424–430.
592. Hoyt WF, Keane JR: Superior oblique myokymia. Report and discussion on five cases of benign intermittent uniocular microtremor. Arch Ophthalmol 1970;84:461–467.
593. Thurston SE, Saul RF: Superior oblique myokymia: quantitative description of the eye movement. Neurology 1991;41:1679–1681.
594. Rosenberg ML, Glaser JS: Superior oblique myokymia. Ann Neurol 1983;13:667–669.
595. Brazis PW, Miller NR, Henderer JD, et al: The natural history and results of treatment of superior oblique myokymia. Arch Ophthalmol 1994;112:1063–1067.
596. Lee JP: Superior oblique myokymia. A possible etiologic factor. Arch Ophthalmol 1984;102:1178–1179.
597. Morrow M, Sharpe JA, Ranalli PJ: Superior oblique myokymia associated with a posterior fossa tumor: oculographic correlation with an idiopathic case. Neurology 1990;40:367–370.
598. Leigh RJ, Tomsak RL, Seidman SH, et al: Superior oblique myokymia: quantitative characteristics of the eye movements in three patients. Arch Ophthalmol 1991;109:1710–1713.
599. Mehta AM, Demer JL: Magnetic resonance imaging of the superior oblique muscle in superior oblique myokymia. J Pediatr Ophthalmol Strabismus 1994;31:378–383.
600. Susac JO, Smith JL, Schatz NJ: Superior oblique myokymia. Arch Neurol 1973;29:432–434.
601. Tyler TD, Ruiz RS: Propranolol in the treatment of superior oblique myokymia. Arch Ophthalmol 1990;108:175–186.
602. Samii M, Rosahl SK, Carvalho GA, et al: Microvascular decompression for superior oblique myokymia: first experience. Case report. J Neurosurg 1998; 89:1020–1024.
603. Shults WT, Hoyt WF, Behrens M, et al: Ocular neuromyotonia: a clinical description of six patients. Arch Ophthalmol 1986;104:1028–1034.
604. Lessell S, Lessell I, Rizzo JF: Ocular neuromyotonia after radiation therapy. Am J Ophthalmol 1986; 102:766–770.
605. Morrow MJ, Kao GW, Arnold AC: Bilateral ocular neuromyotonia: oculographic correlations. Neurology 1996;46:264–266.
606. Barroso L, Hoyt WF: Episodic exotropia from lateral rectus neuromyotonia—appearance and remission after radiation therapy for a thalamic glioma. J Pediatr Ophthalmol Strabismus 1993;30:56–57.
607. Haupert CL, Newman NJ: Ocular neuromyotonia 18 years after radiation therapy. Arch Ophthalmol 1997;115:1331–1332.
608. Yee RD, Purvin VA: Ocular neuromyotonia: three case reports with eye movement recordings. J Neuro-ophthalmol 1998;18:1–8.
609. Frohman EM, Zee DS: Ocular neuromyotonia: clinical features, physiological mechanisms, and response to therapy. Ann Neurol 1995;37:620–626.
610. Safran AB, Magistris M: Terminating attacks of ocular neuromyotonia. J Neuro-ophthalmol 1998;18:47–48.
611. Chung SM, Lee AG, Holds JB, et al: Ocular neuromyotonia in Graves dysthyroid orbitopathy. Arch Ophthalmol 1997;115:365–370.
612. Ezra E, Spalton D, Sanders MD, et al: Ocular neuromyotonia. Br J Ophthalmol 1996;80:350–355.
613. Harrison AR, Wirtshafter JD: Ocular neuromyotonia in a patient with cavernous sinus thrombosis secondary to mucormycosis. Am J Ophthalmol 1997; 124:122–123.
614. Aydin P, Kansu T, Sanac AS: High myopia causing bilateral abduction deficiency. J Clin Neuro-ophthalmol 1992;12:163–165.
615. Krzizok TH, Kaufman H, Traupe H: Elucidation of restrictive motility in high myopia by magnetic resonance imaging. Arch Ophthalmol 1997;115:1019–1027.
616. Krzizok TH, Schroeder BU: Measurement of recti eye muscle paths by magnetic resonance imaging in highly myopic and normal subjects. Invest Ophthalmol Vis Sci 1999;40:2554–2560.
617. Kushner BJ: Fixation switch diplopia. Arch Ophthalmol 1995;113:896–899.
618. Worthington JM, Halmagyi GM: Bilateral total ophthalmoplegia due to midbrain hematoma. Neurology 1996;46:1176.
619. Keane JR: Acute bilateral ophthalmoplegia: 60 cases. Neurology 1986;36:279–281.
620. Laskowitz D, Liu GT, Galetta SL: Acute visual loss and other disorders of the eyes. Neurol Clin North Am 1998;16:323–353.
621. Chung M, Stout JT, Borchert MS: Clinical diversity of hereditary Duane's retraction syndrome. Ophthalmology 2000;107:500–503.
622. Appukuttan B, Gillanders E, Juo SH, et al: Localization of a gene for Duane retraction syndrome to chromosome 2q31. Am J Hum Genet 1999;65: 1639–1646.
623. Reddel SW, Barnett MH, Yan WX, et al: Chronic ophthalmoplegia with anti-GQ1b antibody. Neurology 2000;54:1000–1002.

CHAPTER 16

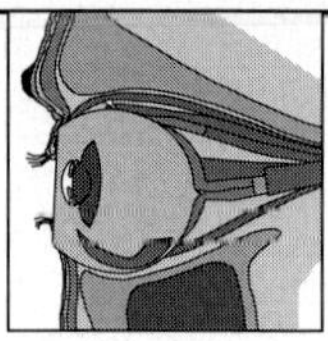

Eye Movement Disorders: Conjugate Gaze Abnormalities

This chapter will cover eye movement disorders that are characterized by intact alignment, but the eyes either have restricted motility, move too slowly, or are misdirected. In neuro-ophthalmic terminology, these include horizontal and vertical conjugate gaze limitations, voluntary smooth pursuit and saccadic deficits, and involuntary conjugate gaze deviations.

These conditions tend to result from impaired supranuclear input upon the ocular motor nuclei. Thus, for the most part, third, fourth, and sixth nerve function, as well the oculocephalic and oculovestibular reflexes, are intact except in the situations where noted. Disorders in which the eyes tend to be misaligned are covered in Chapters 15 and 18. In Chapter 17, conditions characterized by excessive or inaccurate saccades are reviewed.

TYPES OF CONJUGATE EYE MOVEMENTS: DEFINITIONS

The four major types of conjugate eye movements include saccades, pursuit, the vestibulo-ocular reflex, and optokinetic nystagmus (Table 16–1).[1] Because saccadic and pursuit abnormalities make up the majority of the voluntary conjugate gaze abnormalities, they will be emphasized in this chapter, and their anatomy and physiology will be discussed in great detail. The vestibulo-ocular reflex and optokinetic nystagmus, deficits of which are typically not considered conjugate gaze abnormalities, will be alluded to throughout this chapter because of their close relationship with saccadic and pursuit function. However, they are discussed in more detail elsewhere (Chapter 17).

Saccades

Saccades are fast conjugate eye movements designed to refixate both foveas on a novel target (see Fig. 2–26). They have a peak velocity of up to 700 degrees per second.[2] There are several subtypes of saccades.[3] *Voluntary* saccades are intended eye movements towards a remembered target or during a search. *Reflexive* saccades occur in response to the sudden appearance of a new target in the retinal periphery or to a sudden noise. *Spontaneous* saccades, which may occur during speech or at rest during the darkness, have no particular goal. The saccadic system also supplements smooth pursuit by compensating for differences in target and foveal positions.[4]

Pursuit

On the other hand, smooth *pursuit* eye movements maintain both foveas conjugately on a slowly moving visual target (see Fig. 2–25). The goal of the pursuit system is to generate eye velocities that are similar to the target speed. Accurate pursuit can be achieved if the target is moving at less than 50 degrees per second.[2]

TABLE 16–1. The Five Different Types of Eye Movements and Their Supranuclear Control

Eye Movement Type	Purpose	Important Supranuclear Structure(s)	Important Supranuclear Structure Receives Major Input From
Saccades	Rapid gaze shift	Parapontine reticular formation (PPRF); rostral interstitial nucleus of the medial longitudinal fasciculus (riMLF); interstitial nucleus of Cajal (inC)	Cortical eye fields Superior colliculus
Pursuit	Follow slowly moving object	Vestibular nuclei; inC	Parietal pursuit area; pontine nuclei; cerebellum
Vestibulo-ocular reflex	Coordinate eye position during head movements	Vestibular nuclei; inC	Semicircular canals
Optokinetic nystagmus	Coordinate eye movements when environment moves	Vestibular nuclei	Parietal pursuit area and accessory optic nuclei
Vergence	Foveation	Pretectum; pons	? Cortex

Saccades, pursuit, the vestibulo-ocular reflex, and optokinetic nystagmus are conjugate eye movements, while vergences are dysconjugate (eg, convergence and divergence). All five types have as their final common output signals to the extraocular muscles from the third, fourth, and sixth nerve nuclei.

Vestibulo-Ocular Reflex

These eye movements stabilize a retinal image during head movement. The oculocephalic maneuver (see Fig. 2–27), elicited by moving the patient's head while asking him or her to maintain fixation, utilizes this reflex. Ice-water irrigation of the ears (cold caloric testing) directly tests the vestibulo-ocular reflex (see Fig. 2–41).

Optokinetic Nystagmus

A slow pursuit eye movement followed by a fast corrective saccade occurs when the surrounding visual field moves over the retina. Optokinetic nystagmus is readily seen at the bedside when small targets are moved in front of the patient's eyes (see Fig. 2–29).

SYMPTOMS

Most patients with conjugate gaze abnormalities offer only vague visual complaints such as blurriness or dizziness.[5] Those with downgaze palsies may complain that they are unable to read or go down steps, but such patients are usually unaware that the problem stems from an inability to look down. Similarly, those with conjugate upgaze pareses might say they have trouble seeing bookshelves or other objects above eye level. We have seen a patient whose hydrocephalus manifested with difficulty playing basketball because he had trouble looking at the basket. Few actually complain that they are unable to look sideways or vertically, although exceptions occur. Some are visually asymptomatic, and the ocular motility deficit is detected on examination.

EXAMINATION

Smooth pursuit can be tested at the bedside by having the patient follow a slowly moving target with both eyes. Optokinetic testing and suppression of the vestibulo-ocular reflex by visual fixation are two other ocular motor functions related to smooth pursuit eye movements. The relative speed and accuracy of saccades can be evaluated during refixation from eccentric gaze to a central target. Spontaneous saccades during the history taking should also be observed. Chapter 2 also reviews these examination techniques, with figures, for testing conjugate gaze.

When pursuit is defective, it can either be slow, interrupted by saccades as in "saccadic pursuit," or limited. In such patients, pursuit of optokinetic targets may be slow and refixa-

TABLE 16–2. Etiology of Horizontal Conjugate Gaze Deficits

Cortical lesions
- Frontal eye fields: saccades
- Occipitoparietal junction: pursuit
- Acquired ocular motor apraxia

Pontine lesions
- Paramedian pontine reticular formation
- Sixth nerve nucleus
- One-and-a-half syndrome

Other brain stem lesions
Congenital ocular motor apraxia
Other neurological diseases
- Ataxia-telangiectasia*
- Inherited spinocerebellar ataxias*
- Multisystem atrophy
- Huntington's disease
- Parkinson's disease
- Corticobasal ganglionic degeneration
- Gaucher's disease*
- Wernicke's encephalopathy and Leigh's disease

Drugs

* = disorders whose ocular motility abnormality may mimic congenital ocular motor apraxia.

tion saccades are absent. Failure of suppressing the vestibulo-ocular response may be evident when slippage of the eyes with corrective saccades occurs.

Defective saccades are often characterized by slow velocities that cannot be mimicked by individuals with normal ocular motor systems. In striking cases the eyes appear to moving through molasses. Some patients with defective saccades will use a compensatory head thrust in an attempt to shift gaze (see ocular motor apraxia, below). When saccades are completely absent, a conjugate gaze palsy results. Sometimes the fast phase of optokinetic nystagmus is noted to be defective. The supranuclear nature of some pursuit and saccadic deficits can be proven by enhancing the ocular excursions with oculocephalic and vestibulo-ocular maneuvers.

The remainder of the neuro-ophthalmic and neurologic examinations should be used to screen for cortical deficits such as aphasia or hemianopia, and brain stem and cerebellar abnormalities such as facial palsies or incoordination. Finally, evidence of a degenerative process such as bradykinesia, tremor, or chorea, should be excluded.

TABLE 16–3. Etiology of Abnormal Horizontal Conjugate Gaze Deviations

Hemispheric lesions
- Frontal eye field
- Neglect, hemianopia

Seizures
Thalamic lesions
Brainstem lesions
- Pontine
- Medullary

Periodic alternating gaze deviation
- "Ping-pong" gaze

TABLE 16–4. Etiology of Vertical Conjugate Gaze Deficits

Pretectal syndrome
- Paramedian midbrain–thalamic stroke
- Pineal region and thalamic masses
- Hydrocephalus

Midbrain downgaze paresis
Limitation of upgaze in elderly
Other neurologic disorders
- Progressive supranuclear palsy
- Niemann–Pick disease*
- Whipple's disease
- Amyotrophic lateral sclerosis

* =disorders whose ocular motility abnormality may mimic congenital ocular motor apraxia.

APPROACH

One method for distinguishing supranuclear conjugate gaze disorders is to divide them into those that cause primarily horizontal versus vertical defects, although there is considerable overlap (Tables 16–2 through 16–5). Those that are in the horizontal plane tend to localize to cerebral cortex or pontine lesions, while those that are in the vertical plane usually localize to midbrain disturbances. Then the type of disorder, such as a conjugate gaze limitation, smooth pursuit and saccadic deficit, or conjugate gaze deviation, should be determined. Since conjugate gaze limitations and smooth pursuit and saccadic abnormalities are related, they will be discussed below under the heading of "gaze deficits." When supranuclear gaze defects in all directions are present, the cause is often a degenerative neurologic disorder.

TABLE 16–5. Etiology of Abnormal Vertical Conjugate Gaze Deviations

Oculogyric crises
Ocular tics
Benign, tonic form in infancy
- Upward
- Downward

Pretectal syndrome

HORIZONTAL CONJUGATE GAZE: NEUROANATOMY

Saccades

The major cortical control of horizontal saccadic eye movements, especially intentional ones, lies in the frontal eye fields (Brodmann's area 8).[6] Each hemisphere has a frontal eye field located in the posterior portion of the second frontal gyrus and the adjacent part of the precentral gyrus and sulcus (Fig. 16–1). In one study[7] of awake patients evaluated with subdural electrodes for epilepsy surgery, electrical stimulation of the frontal eye fields caused contralateral horizontal conjugate eye movements in all patients. The ocular deviation was usually saccadic and accompanied by head versions. Two other cortical areas (Fig. 16-1) are capable of triggering other types of saccades: (1) the supplementary eye field in the supplementary motor area of the frontal lobe is important for generating saccades coordinated with head or body movements[8, 9]; and (2) the parietal eye field, located in the posterior parietal cortex, is instrumental in producing reflexive saccades.[3] Saccades are likely controlled by a neural network connecting these areas.[10, 11]

These cortical areas mediating saccades send supranuclear fibers that decussate at the level of the oculomotor and trochlear nuclei before reaching the contralateral paramedian pontine reticular formation (PPRF) (Fig. 16–2).[12] Each PPRF also receives connections from the deep layer of the contralateral superior colliculus,[13] which can independently trigger saccades. Located near the midline just ventral and rostral to each sixth nerve nucleus (see Chapter 15),

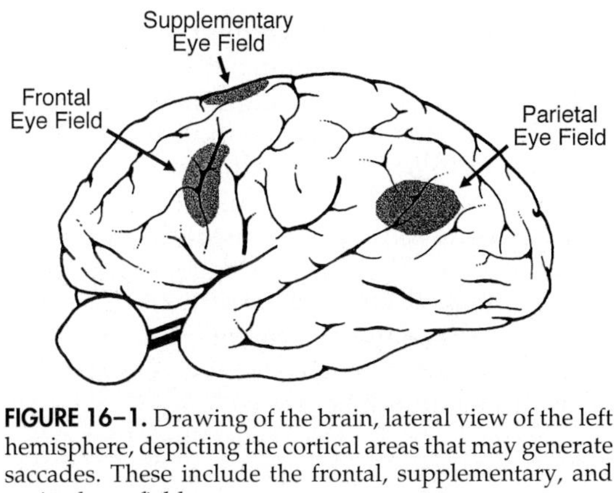

FIGURE 16–1. Drawing of the brain, lateral view of the left hemisphere, depicting the cortical areas that may generate saccades. These include the frontal, supplementary, and parietal eye fields.

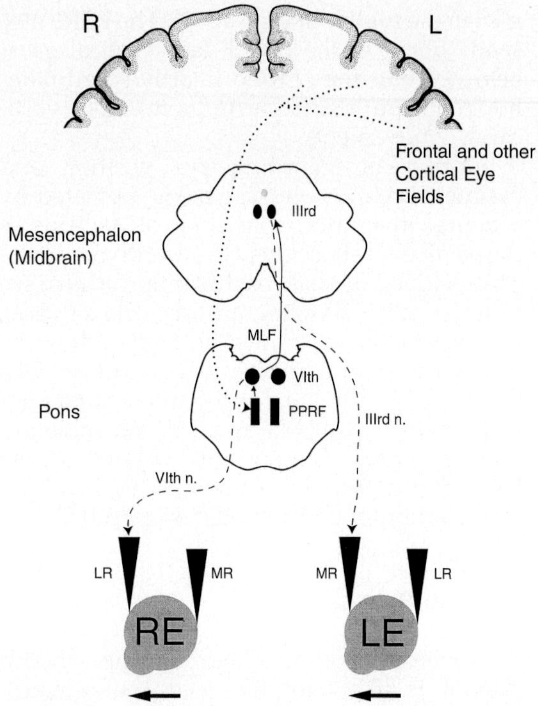

FIGURE 16–2. Generation of horizontal saccades. In this schematic drawing (ventral view), the pathways for a rightward saccade are depicted. The frontal and other cortical eye fields (see Fig. 16–1) from the left (L) hemisphere send fibers that decussate then reach the (R) paramedian pontine reticular formation (PPRF). Burst neurons in the right PPRF excite cell bodies in the right sixth nerve (VIth) nucleus, which in turn innervates the ipsilateral lateral rectus (LR) muscle, which abducts the right eye (RE). Another set of neurons from the right sixth nerve nucleus cross the midline then ascend within the left medial longitudinal fasciculus (MLF). These reach the left medial rectus (MR) subnucleus in the oculomotor complex (IIIrd) in the midbrain, which issues third nerve neurons (IIIrd n.) that supply the left medial rectus muscle to adduct the left eye (LE).

each PPRF is the premotor center for generating horizontal saccadic eye movements. Each PPRF contains burst cell neurons that fire immediately before an ipsilateral saccade.[14] Between saccades, omnipause neurons in the nucleus raphe interpositus of the pons inhibit the burst neurons in the PPRF and rostral interstitial nucleus of the medial longitudinal fasciculus (riMLF).[15, 16]

Each PPRF innervates the ipsilateral sixth nerve nucleus, which in turn innervates the ipsilateral lateral rectus muscle. The sixth nerve nucleus also supplies the interneurons that immediately cross the midline and then climb within the medial longitudinal fasciculus (MLF) to reach the contralateral medial rectus subnucleus within the oculomotor complex in the midbrain (Fig. 16–2). The PPRF also sends fibers to the riMLF (see vertical gaze, below). Thus, the PPRF primarily coordinates horizontal but also has an influence upon vertical eye movements.[5]

Information regarding eye position and maintenance of eccentric gaze is mediated by a neural integrator, consisting of neurons in the cerebellar flocculus, the perihypoglossal complex, and medial vestibular nuclei (also see Chapter 17). Following an eccentric saccade, viscoelastic forces in the orbit tend to drag the eye back into primary position. To counter this, neural integrator neurons modulate burst neuron activity in the PPRF and riMLF to maintain eccentric gaze.[17] The posterior vermis and the fastigial nuclei of the cerebellum are involved in the calibration of saccadic amplitude.[18]

Smooth Pursuit

The main cortical area that controls smooth pursuit is likely located near the occipito-temporal-parietal junction in Brodmann's areas 19, 37, and 39 (area V5, see Fig. 9–6), which are homologous to monkey areas MT (middle temporal) and MST (medial superior temporal).[19] Although areas 19, 37, and 39 are part of the dorsal stream, or magnocellular pathway, responsible for motion and spatial analysis of visual information (see Chapter 9), smooth pursuit is independent of motion detection and spatial attention.[20] The frontal eye fields, supplementary motor area, and posterior parietal cortex are other cortical areas involved in smooth pursuit,[21] but their roles in this regard are less well understood.[22]

The descending pathway for smooth pursuit likely follows a double decussation in a parieto-occipito-ponto-cerebellar system (Fig. 16–3).[23] Fibers from Brodmann's areas 19, 37, and 39 descend ipsilaterally through the posterior limb of the internal capsule before reaching the dorsal pons. The exact region in the pons that is important for smooth pursuit is unclear, but the dorsal pontine nuclei in the basis pontis have been implicated. From there, axons project to the contralateral flocculus and posterior vermis of the cerebellum. Floccular basket and stellate cells inhibit floccular Purkinje cells, which in turn send inhibitory fibers via the inferior cerebellar peduncle to the medial vestibular nucleus, which then excites the contralateral sixth nerve nucleus.[24] Note the smooth pursuit system is independent of the PPRF.

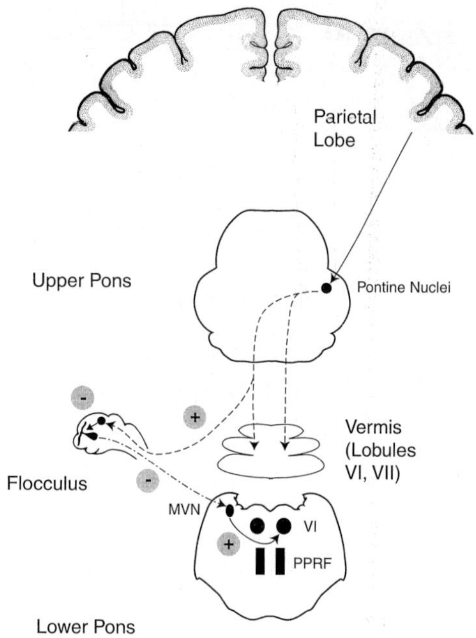

FIGURE 16–3. Horizontal pursuit pathways. Neurons from the parietal lobe descend ipsilaterally to the pontine nuclei. A postulated double decussation of pursuit pathways in the brain stem and cerebellum then occurs. The first decussation consists of excitatory mossy fiber projections from the pontine nuclei to granule cells, which excite basket cells and stellate cells in the contralateral cerebellar flocculus. The basket and stellate cells inhibit Purkinje cells, which in turn inhibit neurons in the medial vestibular nucleus (MVN). The second decussation consists of excitatory projections from the MVN to the opposite abducens nucleus (VI), leading to ipsilateral gaze deviation (see Fig. 16–2). (Adapted from Johnston JL et al: Paresis of contralateral smooth pursuit and normal vestibular smooth eye movements after unilateral brainstem lesions. Ann Neurol 1992;31:495–502, with permission.)

Vestibulo-Ocular Reflex and Optokinetic Nystagmus

Fibers mediating the vestibulo-ocular reflex arise from the vestibular nuclei, travel rostrally via the medial longitudinal fasiculus, pass through but do not synapse in the caudal portion of the PPRF, then finally arrive and synapse at the sixth nerve nucleus. The cerebellum is involved in the suppression of the vestibulo-ocular reflex. The generation of optokinetic nystagmus relies first on cortical and subcortical areas that mediate smooth pursuit, then on structures responsible for the generation of saccades as described above.[25]

The pathways for the vestibulo-ocular reflex and optokinetic nystagmus are discussed in more detail in Chapter 17.

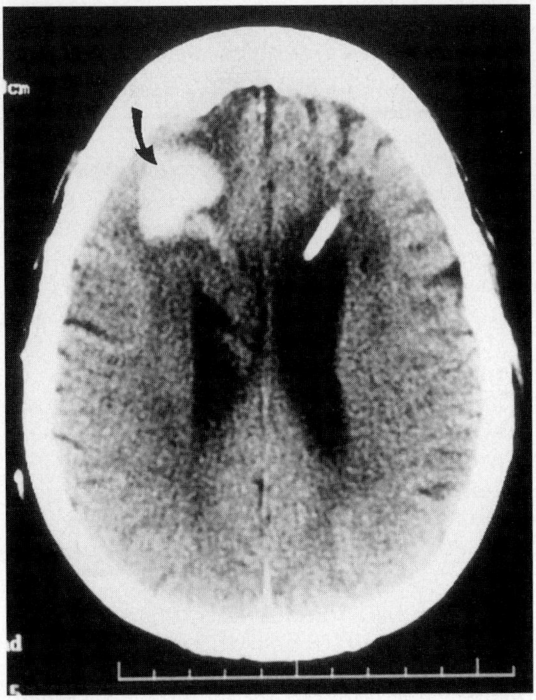

FIGURE 16–4. Axial CT scan of right frontal lobe hemorrhage (*arrow*), which caused difficulty with leftward saccades.

HORIZONTAL CONJUGATE GAZE DEFICITS

Deficits Caused by Cortical Lesions

Saccades. Unilateral frontal eye field lesions tend to cause contralateral saccade eye movement impairment (Fig. 16–4).[26, 27] Patients with lesions large enough to involve the adjoining motor cortex have a hemiparesis on the same side as the direction of the gaze paresis. Acutely, the eyes may be deviated ipsilaterally toward the lesion (see gaze deviations, below), but this is usually only temporary.

Pursuit. Unilateral lesions within the occipito-temporal-parietal junction or the frontal eye fields can cause a *directional* pursuit deficit, in which smooth pursuit of targets moving ipsilaterally toward the lesion is affected.[4, 22] Directional deficits are independent of target position in space.[28] Less commonly, unilateral lesions in the occipito-temporo-parietal junction and in striate cortex may also cause *retinotopic* pursuit abnormalities of targets in the contralateral hemifield.[29, 30] Retinotopic defects are location dependent and uninfluenced by the direction of the target motion. Thus, in this situation, pursuit is abnormal in both directions in the contralateral hemifield. In a third type pursuit defect, *craniotopic*, the patient cannot generate contralaterally directed pursuit eye movements past the midline of the head.[31] For instance, a patient with such a defect due to a left parietal lesion can pursue a rightward-moving target only until the eyes reach midline.

In practice, cortical ipsilateral directional pursuit defects are most commonly associated with lesions at the occipito-parietal-temporal junction (Fig. 16–5). Reflecting this, optokinetic responses can be defective in patients with parietal lobe lesions with contralateral

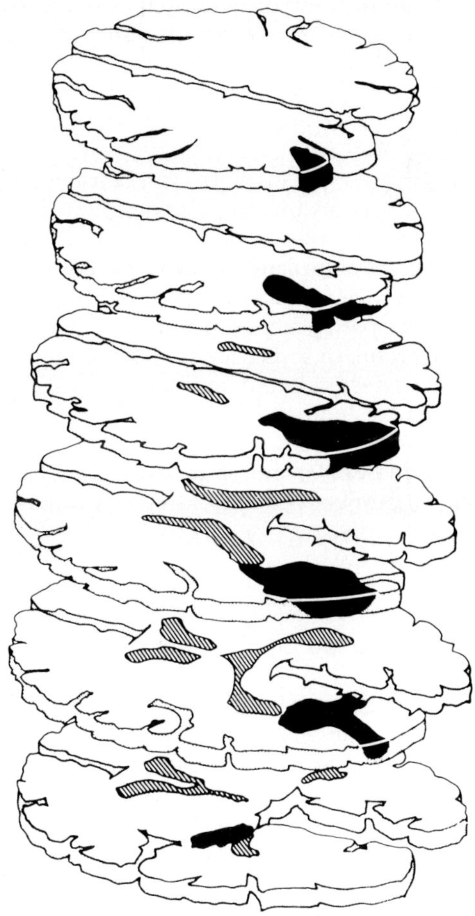

FIGURE 16–5. Computer-generated three-dimensional reconstruction of the cortical area common to a group of patients with asymmetric horizontal pursuit; ipsilateral pursuit velocities were consistently lower than contralateral velocities. The region likely includes area V5 in the lateral parieto-occipito-temporal region (see Chapter 9). Top of figure is dorsal, bottom is ventral. Left is rostral, right is caudal. (From Morrow MJ, Sharpe JA: Cerebral hemispheric localization of smooth pursuit asymmetry. Neurology 1990;40:284–292, with permission.)

hemianopia.[32] When the optokinetic targets move toward the side of the lesion, either the pursuit component is broken up, the amplitudes of the pursuit and saccades are smaller, or there is no corrective saccade.

Acquired Ocular Motor Apraxia. Bilateral parieto-occipital lesions may lead to an acquired ocular motor apraxia, characterized by an absence or severe impairment of smooth pursuit, optokinetic responses, and visually guided saccades.[27] Because the eyes appear not to move, the term *spasm of fixation* has also been used. However, reflexive saccades may be preserved, justifying the use of the term *apraxia.* When ocular motor apraxia is combined with optic ataxia and simultanagnosia, the symptom complex is known as Balint syndrome, which is discussed in detail in Chapter 9 (see Fig. 9–8).

The combination of bilateral parieto-occipital injury combined with bilateral lesions affecting both frontal eye fields, as in watershed ischemia, for instance, can cause a more severe form of acquired ocular motor apraxia.[33] Voluntary saccades and pursuit in all directions may be completely paralyzed. The ocular motility deficit mimics the congenital type (see below), as patients may use a head thrust to aid refixation. In some cases reflexive saccades are also affected,[34] and in such instances the term ocular motor *paresis* may be preferred over *apraxia.*[35]

Acquired ocular motor apraxia may also be seen in a number of progressive and inherited neurologic diseases (see Table 16–2 and discussion below).

Deficits Caused by Pontine Lesions

A lesion in the pons is the most common location for a brain stem disturbance that causes a horizontal gaze deficit, and there are frequently other accompanying signs. Pontine lesions are suggested when a conjugate gaze paresis is bilateral or accompanied by an internuclear ophthalmoplegia, ipsilateral facial paresis, contralateral hemiparesis, or skew deviation and when convergence and vertical eye movements are preserved.[36]

Conjugate Gaze Paresis. Two types of pontine lesions may result in a conjugate gaze paresis:

1. *Paramedian pontine reticular formation (PPRF).* Lesions restricted to the PPRF cause loss of all ipsilateral horizontal rapid eye movements such as voluntary and involuntary saccades and quick phases of nystagmus. Smooth pursuit and vestibulo-ocular reflexes may spared in selective lesions of the rostral portion of the PPRF.[37]
2. *Sixth nerve nucleus.* A lesion of the sixth nerve nucleus, by damaging neurons innervating the ipsilateral lateral rectus muscle and the interneurons for the contralateral medial rectus, will cause an ipsilateral conjugate gaze palsy.[38] Because of the anatomic proximity of the genu of the facial nerve to the sixth nerve nucleus (see Chapters 14 and 15), a nuclear sixth nerve palsy is often accompanied by ipsilateral facial weakness as in the facial colliculus syndrome (Fig. 16–6).[39] All voluntary and reflexive ipsilateral conjugate eye movements are eliminated.[40]

Any combination of bilateral lesions affecting either the PPRF or sixth nerve nuclei will cause a bilateral conjugate gaze palsy (Fig. 16–7).

In patients with pontine horizontal gaze palsies who attempt to look in the direction of the palsy, an upward vertical or oblique movement of both eyes is often seen (Fig. 16–6). The misdirection or substitution movement may be explained by compensatory contraction or overaction of the obliquely acting extraocular muscles, but this is uncertain. In addition, some observers have documented abnormal oblique misdirection and slowing of vertical saccades in patients with lesions of the PPRF.[41,42] This finding, which is an inconsistent one,[37] has been attributed to disruption of the caudal PPRF's influence on the riMLF.[43]

One-and-a-Half-Syndrome. This highly localizing ocular motility disorder is characterized by a conjugate gaze palsy to one side accompanied by an ipsilateral internuclear ophthalmoplegia when the patient looks to the other side (Fig. 16–8). The name of the syndrome derives from the absence of conjugate eye movements in one direction and only preservation of abduction in the other direction.[44] In primary gaze the eyes may be exotropic, with lateral deviation of the eye with intact abduction. The association of one-and-a-half syndrome and exotropia has been termed *paralytic pontine exotropia.*[45] Convergence is often preserved.[46]

The one-and-a-half syndrome is caused by involvement of the PPRF or sixth nerve nucleus, causing the conjugate gaze paresis, com-

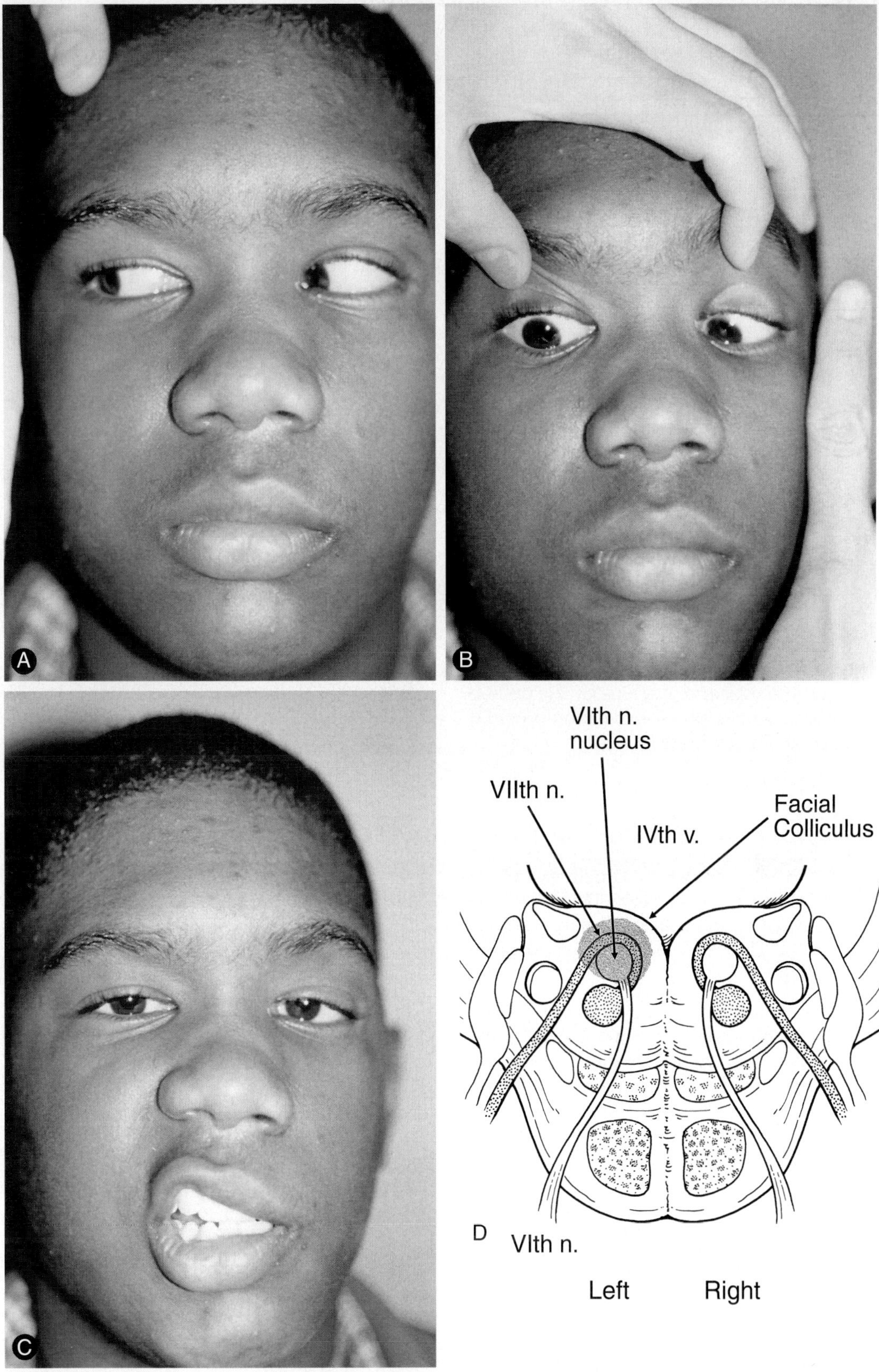

FIGURE 16–6. Left facial colliculus syndrome (peripheral VIIth n. palsy and nuclear VIth n. palsy causing ipsilateral facial and gaze paresis) due to radiation necrosis following treatment of a brain stem arteriovascular malformation. **A**. Normal gaze to the right. **B**. Defective gaze to the left. Note the eyes move downward in attempted leftward gaze. **C**. Left peripheral facial weakness. **D**. Drawing of location of the critical lesion (*grey area*) in the left dorsal midpons (n. = nerve, v. = ventricle).

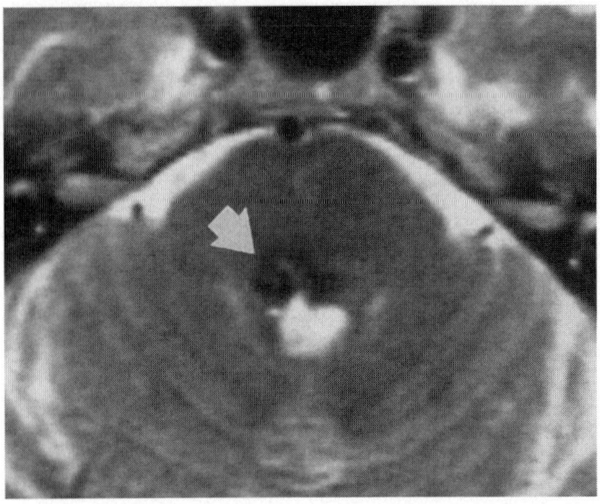

FIGURE 16–7. Dorsal pontine hemorrhage (*arrow*) associated with cocaine use, leading to bilateral horizontal conjugate gaze palsies. The patients subsequently developed oculopalatal myoclonus.

bined with a lesion affecting the just-crossed MLF (Fig. 16–9), which causes the internuclear ophthalmoplegia (see Chapter 15).[47, 48] A lesion of the PPRF can be distinguished from one affecting the sixth nerve nucleus by the preservation of the oculocephalic or vestibulo-ocular responses in the former.[49]

Foville Syndrome. A lesion in the caudal tegmental pons may cause a facial paralysis, conjugate gaze paresis, and contralateral hemiparesis by disrupting the fascicle of the seventh nerve, the PPRF or sixth nerve nucleus, and the corticospinal tract, respectively. This localizing combination of findings, described by Foville,[50] is one of the crossed brain stem syndromes (see Chapter 15).[51]

Locked-In Syndrome. Large bilateral lesions almost transecting the pons may cause a neurologic state characterized by quadriplegia, absence of horizontal eye movements, and mutism, but preservation of vertical eye movements, blinking, and consciousness. Patients in this "locked-in" state use these preserved functions to communicate, but they are often mistakenly diagnosed with coma. The area of the pons most commonly affected is the basis pontis, at the level of the sixth nerve nuclei.[52]

Defective Smooth Pursuit. Unilateral lesions of the dorsolateral pons have been associated with ipsilateral smooth pursuit deficits, without considerable abnormalities in saccades or the vestibulo-ocular reflex.[23, 53] These findings confirm the notion of a parieto-occipito-ponto-cerebellar pathway for smooth pursuit described above (Fig. 16–3).

Etiology. In older adults the most frequent cause of a pontine horizontal gaze palsy is ischemia in the distribution of one of the pontine paramedian penetrating arteries arising from the basilar artery.[54] Atherosclerosis is by far the most common cause, but vasculitis due to giant cell arteritis,[55, 56] for example, may be responsible. In younger adults, demyelinating processes such as multiple sclerosis are the most common cause.[57] Other considerations in

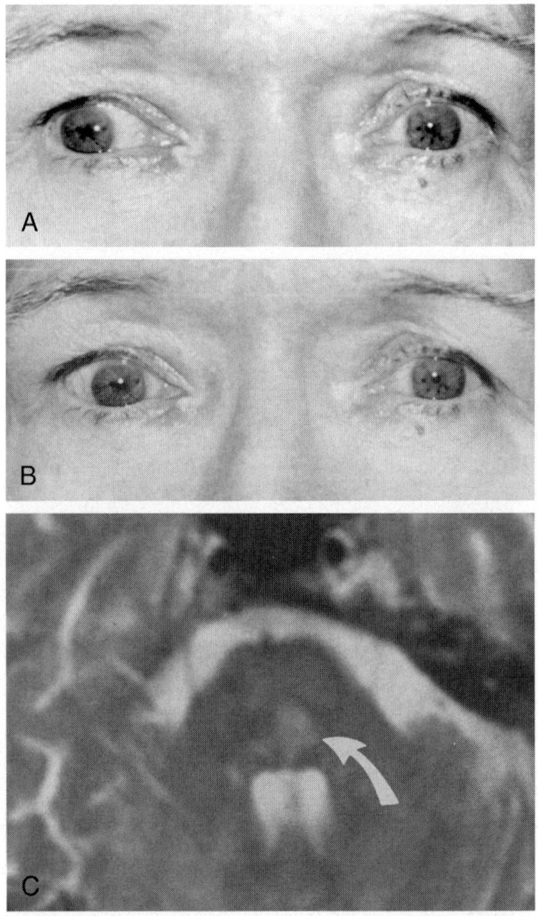

FIGURE 16–8. Left one-and-a-half syndrome due to pontine infarction associated with giant cell arteritis. **A**. On attempted right gaze, the patient has a left internuclear ophthalmoplegia (defective adduction of the left eye and abducting nystagmus of the right eye). **B**. There is a conjugate gaze paresis on attempted left gaze, and neither eye can move past midline. **C**. Axial MRI through the pons demostrates dorsal pontine infarctions, large on the left (*arrow*). (From Galetta SL, et al: Giant cell arteritis with unusual flow-related neuro-ophthalmologic manifestations. Neurology 1997;49:1463–1465, with permission.)

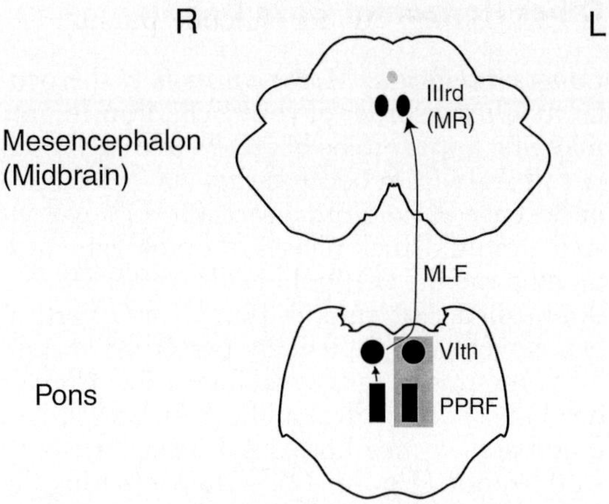

FIGURE 16–9. Schematic drawing of lesions responsible for a left one-and-a-half syndrome (as in Fig. 16–8). This is caused by a lesion affecting the just crossed medial longitudinal fasciculus (MLF)—which contains fibers connecting the right VIth n. nucleus with the left medial rectus (MR) subnucleus in the IIIrd n. nuclear complex—leading to a left internuclear ophthalmoplegia (defecting adduction of the left eye), and both the left paramedian pontine reticular formation (PPRF) and the left VIth n. nucleus, either of which could cause defective conjugate gaze paresis to the left. Usually, because the VIth n. nucleus and the PPRF are in anatomic proximity, lesions that cause the one-and-a-half syndrome usually involve both.

adults include hemorrhages due to hypertension, cavernous angiomas (Fig. 16–10), or trauma, as well as opportunistic infections.[58] Overly rapid correction of hyponatremia may result in central pontine myelinolysis.[59, 60]

In contrast, mid- and lower brain stem neoplasms such as pontine gliomas or medulloblastomas are the most common cause in children. Möbius syndrome (see Chapter 14), when it affects the sixth nerve nucleus, may cause horizontal conjugate gaze palsies.

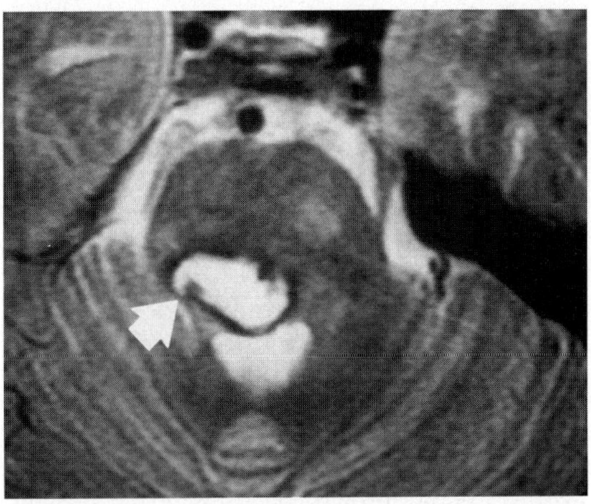

FIGURE 16–10. Cavernous angioma (*arrow*) of the pons associated with conjugate gaze deficits, demonstrated by high-resolution 4.0 Tesla MRI (TR = 5000, TE = 30, FOV = 22 cm, matrix = 512 × 256).

Caution should be applied when diagnosing pontine lesions in this setting, because pontine horizontal gaze palsies can be mimicked by the Fisher variant of Guillain–Barré syndrome, myasthenia gravis, and thyroid eye disease. Thus, if neuroimaging is normal, these peripheral nerve, neuromuscular junction, and myopathic disorders should be excluded (see Chapters 14 and 18).

Horizontal Gaze Deficits Caused by Other Posterior Fossa Lesions

Midbrain. Rarely conjugate horizontal saccades and pursuit may be abnormal following damage to the midbrain tegmentum. Presumably the lesions affect descending horizontal gaze fibers destined for the PPRF. Zackon and Sharpe[61] reported two such patients, each with adduction paresis of the eye ipsilateral to the lesion accompanied by paresis of contralateral saccades in the fellow eye. These patients also exhibited conjugate paresis of ipsilateral smooth pursuit. Isolated lesions of the superior colliculi, which are also rare, may cause defective reflexive saccades.[62]

Medullary. Lateropulsion of saccades, characterized by overshoot of ipsilaterally directed saccades, undershoot of contralaterally directed saccades, and ipsilateral oblique trajectories during vertical refixation, is often a prominent ocular finding in lateral medullary lesions (see discussion of other neuro-ophthalmic complications of Wallenberg syndrome in Chapter 13).[63–66] Such patients also complain of body ipsipulsion, a sensation of the entire body being pulled toward the side of the lesion. Ipsilateral horizontal conjugate eye deviation may also occur, and is usually most obvious upon removal of visual fixation.[67–69] In other words, if the patient is asked to fixate straight ahead and close the eyes momentarily, the eyes may drift ipsilaterally.[70] As a result of this, upon eyelid opening a contralaterally directed refixation movement back to midline will then be seen (Fig. 16–11). Less commonly, an ipsilateral conjugate eye deviation is seen with eyelids open.[71, 72]

Separate mechanisms may account for ipsipulsion of saccades and the conjugate eye deviation. However, each could result from damage to the inferior cerebellar peduncle and

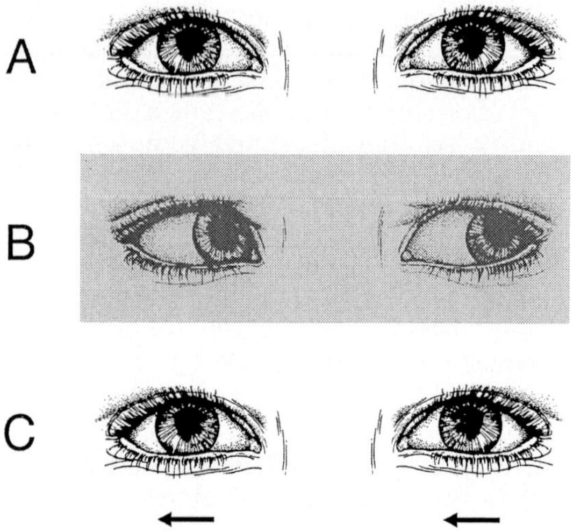

FIGURE 16–11. Ipsilateral conjugate gaze deviation in left Wallenberg syndrome. At rest the eyes may be straight (**A**); but with removal of fixation or with the eyes closed, the eyes deviate toward the side of the lesion (**B**); upon refixation or with the eyelids reopened, the eyes move back to the midline (**C**).

interruption of climbing fibers: (1) ipsipulsion of saccades from increased inhibition of the ipsilateral fastigial nucleus in the cerebellum and ultimately the contralateral PPRF, and (2) conjugate gaze deviation either from increased inhibition of the ipsilateral vestibular nucleus or possibly from decreased tonic excitation of the contralateral PPRF.[72]

Lateral medullary lesions are also infrequently associated with difficulty pursuing contralaterally moving targets.[73] This deficit likely reflects damage to the vestibular nucleus.

Cerebellar. Lesions in the cerebellum can cause saccadic overshoot and undershoot (dysmetria) as well as unsustained eccentric gaze with gaze-evoked nystagmus.[74] This results from damage to structures in the cerebellum responsible for the calibration of saccadic amplitude and gaze-holding, respectively (see above). Cerebellar hemispheric lesions tend to cause ipsilateral saccadic hypermetria (overshoot) and contralateral saccadic hypometria (undershoot). During attempted vertical saccades, there may be a contralaterally directed oblique drift (contrapulsion).[75] This is particularly true of lesions in the region of the superior cerebellar peduncle. Cerebellopontine angle tumors may cause an ipsilateral smooth pursuit defect if the vestibular nucleus, flocculus, or inferior cerebellar peduncle is involved.[73, 76]

Other Horizontal Gaze Deficits

Congenital Ocular Motor Apraxia. In this ocular motility disorder of young children, infants may first appear to be blind or have decreased peripheral vision because they have defective or absence of horizontal saccades to novel visual stimuli. Quick phases of optokinetic nystagmus and the vestibulo-ocular reflex are also diminished, but smooth pursuit and vertical eye movements are usually preserved. At age 5 or 6 months of age, when they achieve better head and neck control and can sit unassisted, they begin to use horizontal head thrusts to shift fixation (Fig. 16–12).[77] Often initiating the sequence with an eyelid blink, patients move their heads rapidly toward a new visual target.[78] Then the eyes slowly refixate. A final correction in head position sometimes then occurs, as the eyes are maintained on target using the vestibulo-ocular reflex.[79] Congenital ocular motor apraxia is almost always symmetric and bidirectional in the horizontal plane, but there have been exceptional asymmetric and vertical cases.[80, 81] In many instances the head thrusting and defective saccades spontaneously improve as the child gets older,[82] but the ocular motility disturbance may persist.[83] Because there are many causes (see below), the exact pathologic substrate is unclear although usually a defect in the saccadic system is implicated.

Two caveats regarding the use of the term *congenital ocular motor apraxia* should be made:

1. Because in some instances both voluntary and some reflexive saccades are defective, the term *apraxia,* implying only voluntary saccades are affected, has been criticized. Other terms, such as *congenital saccadic palsy*[84] and *intermittent horizontal saccade failure,*[85] have been proposed. However, the term that Cogan[86] originally coined is unlikely to be supplanted, having already been heavily imbedded in the neuro-ophthalmic vernacular.
2. Although some authors[82, 87] have applied the term *congenital* ocular motor apraxia in children of any age, we feel the term should be used only in those instances when the motility disorder is present in infancy.

Congenital ocular motor apraxia is observed in three main clinical situations:

1. In the "benign" or "idiopathic" variety of congenital ocular motor apraxia, neuro-

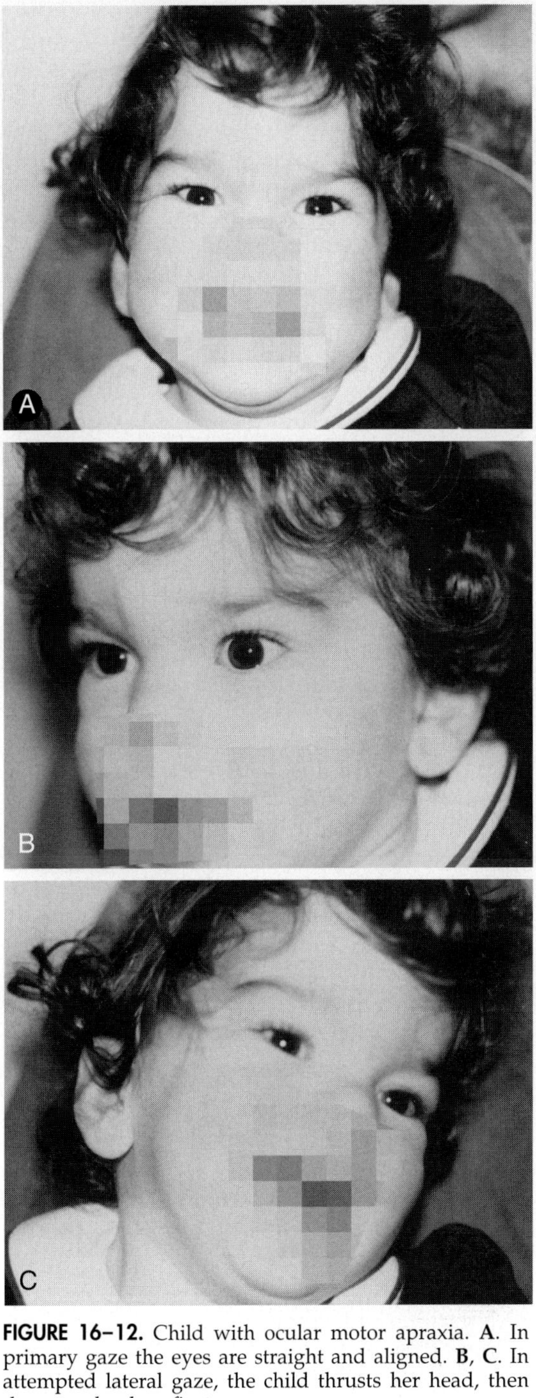

FIGURE 16–12. Child with ocular motor apraxia. **A.** In primary gaze the eyes are straight and aligned. **B, C.** In attempted lateral gaze, the child thrusts her head, then the eyes slowly refixate.

imaging is normal and there is no readily identifiable explanation for the disorder. Although the neurologic examination and intellect are usually normal, occasionally associated neurologic defects include hypotonia, motor and speech delay, and ataxia.[85] Many have infantile esotropia.[77] Familial cases have also been reported.[82, 88]

2. Some patients with congenital ocular motor apraxia have a nonprogressive, noninherited structural abnormality of the brain, caused either by a developmental anomaly or prenatal or perinatal insult. These include dysgenesis of the cerebellar vermis[89] or corpus callosum,[90, 91] cerebellar hypoplasia, Dandy–Walker syndrome, grey matter heterotopias,[85] and perinatal ischemia.[80, 81]
3. A variety of genetic disorders with multisystem involvement may present in infancy with congenital ocular motor apraxia.[79] These include Joubert syndrome (see Chapter 17),[92] Jeune syndrome (nephronophthisis, asphyxiating thoracic dystrophy, retinal degeneration, and ataxia),[93] and a subset of patients with Leber's congenital amaurosis, a retinal dystrophy.[94]

In contrast, we think the term *acquired* ocular motor apraxia is more appropriate when a similar disorder of head and eye coordination is seen in older children presenting with progressive, degenerative, or inherited metabolic neurologic diseases (see next section), for instance. The distinction may be difficult when children present with ocular motor apraxia at 6 to 12 months of age, at which time mild "congenital" and early "acquired" neurologic diseases may be confused.[95] However, some diagnostic guidelines include: (1) the voluntary ophthalmoparesis and head thrusts are almost always limited to the horizontal plane in congenital ocular motor apraxia and the acquired form due to Gaucher's disease; (2) in contrast, the eye movement abnormalities and compensatory head movements are often in both the horizontal and vertical planes in ataxia–telangiectasia and spinocerebellar ataxias; (3) they are primarily in the vertical plane in Niemann–Pick type C.

Other Neurologic Disorders Associated With Horizontal Gaze Deficits

Ataxia Telangiectasia (Louis–Bar) Syndrome. The cardinal clinical features of this childhood autosomal recessive phakomatosis are oculocutaneous nonhemorrhagic telangiectasias, cerebellar ataxia and dysarthria, multidirectional supranuclear ophthalmoparesis, and recurrent sinopulmonary infections.[96] The telangiectasias are seen most commonly on the conjunctivae. These can become more prominent with age and can also be observed on the earlobes, limbs, and trunk. Other skin lesions in this condition include follicular keratosis, seborrheic dermatitis, pigmentary disturbances, and secondary skin infections. Additionally, there are often dry, coarse hair, vitiligo, and café au lait spots.[97]

Other neurologic features such as mental retardation, impassive facies, chorea, dystonia, and peripheral neuropathy can be observed.[98] Additional features include growth retardation, lymphoid hyperplasia, abnormally high rates of malignancy such as leukemia or breast cancer,[99, 100] and elevated alpha-fetoprotein levels. The predisposition to infections and malignancy has been attributed to a high frequency of breaks in the loci on chromosome 11 containing a gene necessary for proper T- and B-cell function.[101, 102] The gene codes for a putative DNA binding protein kinase called ATM.[103]

Most patients also have a supranuclear deficit in horizontal and vertical voluntary saccades and pursuit.[104, 105] Reflexive saccades and the optokinetic quick phases may also be defective.[106] However, the oculocephalic and the slow phase of the vestibulo-ocular reflex are often preserved, so patients often exhibit head thrusts during attempted shifts of gaze similar to those seen in congenital ocular motor apraxia.[107] Fixation is sometimes also affected, as patients with ataxia-telangiectasia may exhibit abnormal saccadic intrusions such as square wave jerks or ocular flutter (see Chapter 17).[106]

Imaging studies reveal diffuse cerebellar atrophy with marked involvement of the vermis and atrophy of the superior aspect of the cerebellar hemispheres.[108] The neuropathology of ataxia-telagiectasia consists of atrophy of the cerebellar cortex, particularly of the Purkinje cells. This is associated with the reduction in various neurotransmitters including glutamate and gamma-aminobutyric acid (GABA).

Treatment of patients with ataxia-telangiectasia is difficult. The prognosis for both quality and length of life is poor. Because of the risk of infections and lymphoreticular malignancies, patients must be aware of the need for careful periodic examinations and the potential consequences of even minor infections.

Inherited Spinocerebellar Ataxias. These inherited diseases are divided into autosomal dominant and recessive types. Diseases with slow saccades or ophthalmoparesis in the dominantly inherited category include the spinocerebellar ataxias (SCA) types 1 (inherited olivo-ponto-cerebellar atrophy), 2, and 3 (Machado–Joseph disease), and 7.[109] A CAG trinucleotide repeat is responsible for each. Recessively inherited diseases with slow saccades include Friedreich's ataxia. The identification of the molecular basis of many of these disorders has allowed a genetic[110-113] rather than a phenomenologic[114] or pathologic classification. Table 16–6 highlights these disorders, including the localization of their genetic defect, and their major neuro-ophthalmic and neurologic features.

Patients with spinocerebellar ataxia usually exhibit dysmetria and gait ataxia, with some combination of absent tendon reflexes, defective proprioception, pyramidal (eg, spasticity, hyperreflexia, and extensor plantar responses), and extrapyramidal (eg, dystonia, parkinsonism,) signs. Eye movement abnormalities are frequent and include gaze-evoked nystagmus, saccadic dysmetria, square-wave jerks, abnormal smooth pursuit, and inability to suppress the vestibulo-ocular response.[109, 115, 116] Saccades may be slow, and in severe cases patients lack voluntary saccades, use head thrusts, and have only preserved reflexive eye movements.[117, 118] The slow eye movements and defective saccades have been attributed to degeneration of neurons in the PPRF.[119, 120] Some subtypes have optic atrophy associated with progressive acuity, field, and color vision loss,[121] while others have macular or pigmentary retinal degeneration (see Chapter 4).[110, 122] Magnetic resonance imaging (MRI) scans typically show some combination of cerebellar, pontine, and spinal cord atrophy.[123]

Multiple-System Atrophy. Diseases in this category are sporadic and nonhereditary. They are characterized clinically by parkinsonism which is usually levodopa unresponsive, autonomic failure, ataxia, and pyramidal signs. Three subtypes can be identified:

1. Noninherited olivo-ponto-cerebellar atrophy (OPCA), in which cerebellar signs predominate. Patients with this disorder may also have slow eye movements or an inability to initiate saccades in any direction.[124]
2. Striatonigral deneration, which is highlighted by parkinsonism, and sometimes by slow saccades and ophthalmoplegia. The pathologic hallmarks are loss of neurons and degeneration of the caudate nucleus and putamen, cerebellum, dentate nucleus, substantia nigra, inferior olivary nucleus,

TABLE 16–6. Dominantly and Recessively Inherited Cerebellar Ataxias With Slow Saccades or Ophthalmoparesis: Genetic Loci, and Neuro-ophthalmic and Neurologic Features

Name	Genetic Locus	Slow Saccades/ Ophthalm. Oparesis	Nystagmus	Optic Atrophy	Retinal/ Macular Degeneration	Ataxia	Pyramidal Signs	Extrapyramidal Signs	Posterior Column Dysfunction	Other	References
Autosomal Dominant											
SCA 1 inherited OPCA, (formerly ADCA type I)	6p22-p23 with CAG repeats (ataxin 1 gene)	+	+	+	+/−	+	+	+/−	+		109,117, 120–122, 375,376
SCA 2 (formerly ADCA type I)	12q23-24 with CAG repeats (ataxin 2 gene)	+	−	−	−	+	+	−	+		109,118,376, 377
SCA 3 (Machado–Joseph disease)	14q24.3-q32 with CAG repeats (ataxin 3 gene)	+ Vertical more than horizontal	+	−	−	+	+	+	−	Dystonia Amyotrophy Parkinsonism Facial fasciculations Lid retraction	109,376, 378-382
SCA 7 (formerly ADCA type II)	3p14-21.1 with CAG repeats (ataxin 7 gene)	+	−	−	++ (Defining feature—see Chapter 4 and Figure 4–20)	+	+	−	−		110,383,384
Autosomal Recessive											
Friedreich's ataxia	9q13-q21.113 with GAA repeats (frataxan gene)	+/−	+/−	+/−	−	+	+	−	+	Areflexia in lower limbs Cardiomyopathy Diabetes mellitus	385,386

+ = often present, +/− = occasionally present, − = often absent, ADCA = autosomal dominant cerebellar ataxia, CAG = CAG trinucleotide, GAA = GAA trinucleotide, OPCA = olivopontocerebellar atrophy, SCA = spinocerebellar ataxia. The ADCA types derive from Harding's[114] previous classification.

Note: Patients with other autosomal dominant cerebellar ataxias, such as SCA 4, 5, and 6, and dentatorubropallidoluysian atrophy (DRPLA) usually have normal saccadic velocities, although scaccades may be dysmetric.[111,387] However, one kindred with DRPLA has been described with opsoclonus and nystagmus as prominent features.[388]

and intermediolateral columns of the spinal cord.[125]

3. Shy–Drager syndrome, which has no prominent eye movement features and has autonomic insufficiency as the primary abnormality.

Huntington's Disease. Principal clinical features of this neurodegenerative disease include progressive choreoathetosis, rigidity, and dystonia. The pathologic hallmark is atrophy of the caudate nucleus and putamen. The genetic basis is an abnormal CAG trinucleotide repeat expansion on chromosome 4p16.3.

Defective saccades in both horizontal and vertical directions have been documented in Huntington's disease.[126] Slow saccades and difficulty in initiating saccades appear to be the most prominent eye movement deficits.[127, 128] Patients also have increased distractability and unwanted saccades during attempted fixation as well as square-wave jerks (see Chapter 17).[129, 130] Smooth pursuit can also be affected, but to a lesser extent.[131]

Parkinson's Disease. Parkinson's disease is the second most common neurodegenerative disorder following Alzheimer's disease. It is characterized by parkinsonism (tremor, bradykinesia, rigidity, and postural instability) and is due to dopamine deficiency in striatonigral pathways. First-line treatment primarily consists of levodopa therapy sometimes in combination with a neuroprotective agent such as selegiline. Clinically, some patients exhibit saccadic pursuit in all directions of gaze. However, most patients with Parkinson's disease do not exhibit any prominent eye movement abnormalities, distinguishing them from those with progressive supranuclear palsy. Abnormalities in saccades and pursuits may be found under experimental conditions.[132, 133] Some of the ocular motility abnormalities are thought to reflect basal ganglia dysfunction and dopamine deficiency, as many[134, 135] but not all[136] of these deficits have been shown to improve with levodopa therapy.

Because the ocular motor findings in Parkinson's disease are usually not a prominent feature, the reader is referred elsewhere[137-139] for the details of the pathophysiology and treatment of this condition.

Corticobasal Ganglionic Degeneration. Corticobasal ganglionic degeneration is a rare, sporadic progressive neurodegenerative disease of the middle aged and elderly.[140] It is characterized by clinical features that suggest both cortical and basal ganglionic dysfunction. These include dementia, levodopa-unresponsive parkinsonism, limb dystonia, ideomotor apraxia, hyper-reflexia, cortical sensory loss, focal reflex myoclonus, and the "alien limb" phenomenon.[141, 142] In the late stages of this disease, a supranuclear gaze paresis in all directions and eyelid opening apraxia (see Chapter 14) may be seen.[141, 143, 144] Although the clinical presentation may be confused with progressive supranuclear palsy (PSP), corticobasal ganglionic degeneration more commonly has asymmetric frontoparietal atrophy on neuroimaging, whereas patients with PSP more typically have midbrain atrophy.[145]

Pharmacologic therapies are largely ineffective.[146] The diagnosis can be confirmed only at autopsy, which typically demonstrates swollen, poorly staining (achromatic) neurons and degeneration of the cortex and substantia nigra.[141]

Gaucher's Disease. A lysosomal storage disorder, Gaucher's disease is caused by decreased enzyme activity of glucocerebrosidase with resulting accumulation of a glyocolipid, glucocerebroside, in macrophages. The glucocerebrosidase gene has been mapped to chromosome 1q21–31.[147] Anemia, thrombocytopenia, hepatosplenomegaly, infiltration of bone marrow with abnormal histiocytes, and fracture or aseptic necrosis of bone are common systemic features. In the infantile acute GD2 and later onset subacute GD3 forms, neurologic involvement is also seen, with a supranuclear horizontal gaze paresis as the most predominant feature.[148, 389] Vertical eye movements are typically spared. Eye movements and head thrusts may mimic congenital ocular motor apraxia, but lateral movements of the eyes may be accompanied by an upward arcuate or looping excursion.[107]

Others. Horizontal saccadic failure has also been documented in association with other childhood neurodegenerative diseases such as Krabbe leukodystrophy, Pelizaeus–Merzbacher disease, GM_1 gangliosidosis, Refsum disease, and propionic acidemia.[149]

Ocular Motor Abnormalities as Biological Markers. Interest has grown in the detection of abnormal eye movements, which are often subtle, as biological markers in neuropsychiatric diseases in which abnormal ocular motility is not usually a prominent finding.[17, 150, 151] For instance, patients with Alzheimer's disease[152, 153] and schizophrenia[17] many have abnormal antisaccades. These are saccades made in the direction opposite to that of a new visual stimulus, and they require the suppression of reflexive saccades. Smooth pursuit may also be abnormal in these patients[154, 155] and their relatives.[156] These ocular motor abnormalities may offer insight into the abnormal neuronal circuitry and pharmacology of these disorders. However, their detection often requires eye movement recordings, they are rarely tested at the bedside, and are frequently too nonspecific to offer any diagnostic utility. Furthermore, in some cases they may be the result of neuropsychotropic medications.

Wernicke's Encephalopathy. This disorder, due to a vitamin B_1 (thiamine) deficiency, is characterized clinically by a triad of eye movement abnormalities, gait ataxia, and encephalopathy. The full triad is present only in a minority of cases.[157]

In a large series of patients with Wernicke's encephalopathy,[158] 44% had conjugate gaze palsies. Typically the gaze palsy was horizontal, but sometimes vertical gaze was also affected. Vertical gaze abnormalities, which were usually upward, were rarely seen alone. Other prominent neuro-ophthalmic findings included nystagmus in 85%, lateral rectus palsies in 54%, and pupillary abnormalities in 19%.[158] Less frequent neuro-ophthalmic abnormalities include retinal hemorrhages, ptosis, and optic neuropathy.

Wernicke's encephalopathy is seen primarily in alcoholics and other malnourished individuals such as prisoners of war or women with hyperemesis gravidarum. Forced or involuntary starvation, cancer, gastric plication, and chronic renal dialysis are other associated conditions. Because thiamine is required for carbohydrate metabolism, Wernicke's encephalopathy can also be caused inadvertently in individuals with marginal thiamine stores who are given a carbohydrate (eg, IV glucose) load.[159]

Characteristic neuropathogic findings include necrosis of nerves and myelin, hypertrophy and hyperplasia of small blood vessels, and pinpoint hemorrhages. These are typically located symmetrically in the mamillary bodies, superior cerebellar vermis, hypothalamus, thalamus, midbrain, and ocular motor and vestibular nuclei.[159] The gaze abnormalities may be attributed to pathologic lesions affecting the sixth nerve nuclei, pretectal area, and periaqueductal grey matter. The nystagmus can be related to the damage to cerebellar and vestibular structures.[160] Neuroimaging typically reveals mamillary body and midline cerebellar atrophy.[161, 162]

Following parenteral administration of 50 to 100 mg of thiamine in addition to receiving a balanced, high-caloric diet, patients often begin recovering from sixth nerve palsies and gaze deficits within 1 to 24 hours, and almost always within 1 week.[158] By 1 month these deficits usually resolve. However, many require several weeks for nystagmus, ataxia, and confusion to resolve. Improvement in the cognitive changes and ataxia is predictable. In addition, some patients develop Korsakoff's psychosis, characterized by retrograde and anterograde amnesia and confabulation, as a long-term sequela.

Leigh Syndrome (Subacute Necrotizing Encephalomyelopathy). Abnormal conjugate and dysconjugate eye movements may be seen in this rare, invariably fatal disorder of young children. Psychomotor delay and hypotonia are typically the first manifestations, usually in the first year of life. Subsequent symptoms include abnormal eye movements, vision loss related to optic atrophy, ataxia, peripheral neuropathy, somnolence, deafness, movement disorders, spasticity, and respiratory difficulties. Spasmus nutans has also been reported in association with Leigh syndrome.[163]

MRI characteristically demonstrates high-signal lesions in the basal ganglia. Pathologically, bilaterally symmetric necrotic lesions extend from the thalamus to the pons, but they also involve the inferior olives and posterior columns.[164] These abnormalities resemble those in Wernicke's encephalopathy and infantile beriberi.

Several biochemical and genetic defects affecting energy metabolism can lead to Leigh syndrome.[164] The more commonly identified ones are a defect involving the pyruvate dehydrogenase complex, cytochrome oxidase deficiency, a T-to-G mutation at nucleotide 8993 in the mtDNA gene encoding ATPase 6 (the same mutation as in NARP syndrome; see Chapter 4),[165, 166] and complex I deficiency.[167] Treatment in most cases is unsatisfactory.

Vitamin E Deficiency. There are three major causes of vitamin E (alpha-tocopherol) deficiency: (1) abetalipoproteinemia (Bassen–Kornzweig disease), in which patients lack apolipoprotein B, which is essential for transporting fat-soluble vitamins; (2) malabsorption, due either to cholestatic liver disease with resultant failure to secrete bile, cystic fibrosis, or bowel resection; and (3) familial isolated (autosomal recessive) vitamin E deficiency.[168] Slow saccades may be a feature of the first two causes, but not usually of the familial type.[169] Some exhibit dissociated eye movements, with slow but full abduction of one eye and fast but limited adduction of the other in attempted lateral gaze. Ocular motor palsies may occur, and we have seen aberrant regeneration of the third nerve in this condition. A pigmentary retinopathy may also be observed. Neurologically, patients with vitamin E deficiency may develop ataxia, long-tract signs, proprioceptive loss, and areflexia, mimicking Friedreich's ataxia.[170]

In suspected cases, serum vitamin E levels should be tested. In many instances vitamin E supplementation may halt or reverse the progression of ocular motor and neurologic symptoms.

Drugs. A number of drugs may impair smooth pursuit. These include phenytoin, barbiturates, carbamazepine, and lithium. Most drugs in toxic doses may cause a variety of ocular motor abnormalities when consciousness is decreased. At toxic levels the drugs mentioned above may cause complete ophthalmoplegia.

ABNORMAL HORIZONTAL CONJUGATE GAZE DEVIATIONS

Stroke

Supratentorial. Acutely following a supratentorial infarction or hemorrhage, the eyes may be conjugately deviated ipsilaterally toward the lesion (Figs. 16–13 and 16–14).[171] This gaze deviation usually results either from impairment or neglect of the contralateral visual field or from damage to ipsilateral frontopontine fibers descending from the frontal eye field to the PPRF. The oculocephalic response is typically normal, but in the first few days it may be difficult to elicit.

Rarely, thalamic (see below) or frontoparietal hemorrhages may result in contralateral conjugate eye deviations.[172, 173] Possible mechanisms include involvement or mass effect in the mesencephalon upon frontopontine fibers after they have crossed, irritative effects on the descending fibers (see below), or an interhemispheric smooth pursuit imbalance.[174]

Infratentorial. Unilateral pontine disturbances affecting the PPRF or sixth nerve nucleus may result in a contralateral gaze preference and ipsilateral gaze paresis (Fig. 16–13). As alluded to earlier, medullary lesions may produce an ipsilateral gaze deviation. However, patients with medullary lesions usually have full contralateral gaze but with hypometric saccadic eye movements.

Seizures

Ictal head and eye deviations are usually contralateral to a cortical seizure focus (Figs. 16–13 and 16–15).[175] The diagnosis is usually obvious when there is hemibody twitching or loss of consciousness if the seizure activity generalizes. The gaze deviation may be nystagmoid, with a contralateral fast component followed by a slow drift of the eyes back toward midline.

Thalamic Hemorrhages

Thalamic hemorrhages, which are usually the result of long-standing hypertension, are suggested by the sudden onset of headache and contralateral hemisensory loss and hemiparesis.[176] Large hemorrhages may cause a contralateral hemianopia (see Fig. 8–27). Depressed consciousness to the point of stupor or coma can occur, particularly when there is intraventricular extension. Stupor or coma at presentation is associated with a high mortality.[177]

Large hemorrhages in this area can cause both horizontal and vertical eye deviations (see below). Patients with severe hemianopia or neglect may exhibit an ipsilateral gaze preference. Contralateral saccades may be hypometric, and ipsilateral pursuit may be defective.[178] Occasionally the eyes may deviate away from the hemorrhage and toward the hemiparesis in so-called wrong-way eyes.[44, 179] This pattern mimics that of a paramedian pontine hemorrhage. Possible mechanisms were discussed above in the section on supratentorial lesions.

Periodic Alternating Gaze

This disorder is related to periodic alternating nystagmus (see Chapter 17), and consists of cycles of conjugate horizontal gaze deviation with compensatory contralateral head turning for 1 to 2 minutes, followed by a 10- to 15-second transition period with the eyes and head straight ahead, then subsequent gaze de-

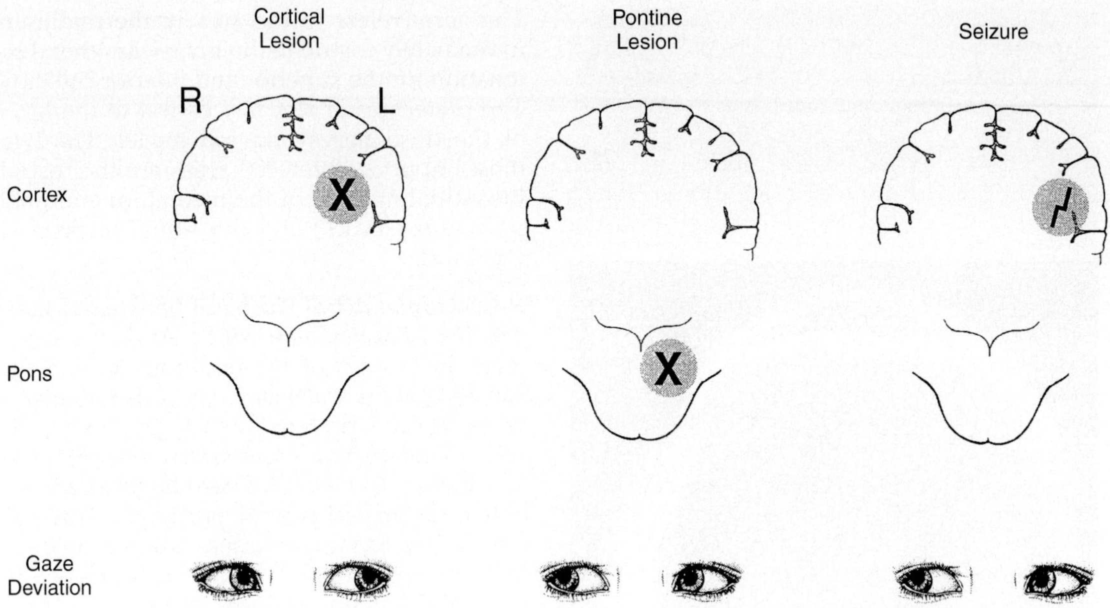

FIGURE 16–13. Common ipsilateral gaze deviations due to cerebral and pontine lesions and seizures. The eyes may deviate horizontally toward a cortical lesion, away from a pontine lesion, and away from a cortical seizure focus.

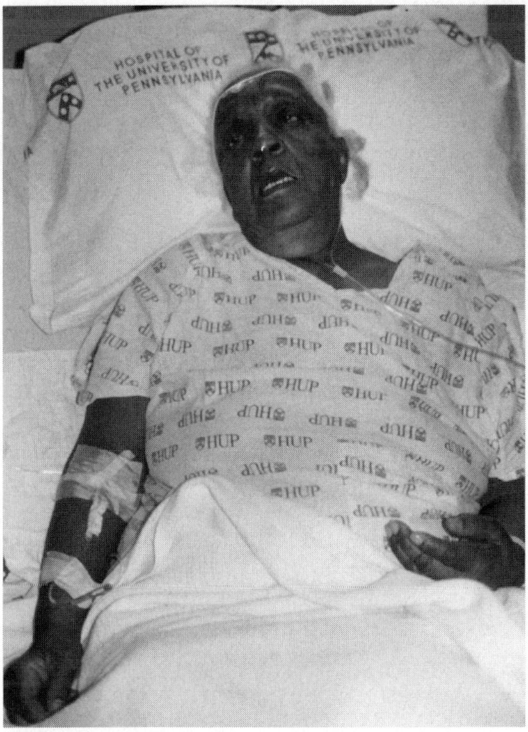

FIGURE 16–14. Right gaze preference in a patient with a right middle cerebral artery stroke, left homonymous hemianopia, left neglect, and left hemiparesis.

viation to the opposite side with compensatory head turning for another 1 to 2 minutes. The eye deviation may be overcome by oculocephalic maneuvers. Nystagmus may be seen but is intermittent and not a major feature. Patients are typically awake although the pattern may be seen in comatose patients.[180]

In general, this motility pattern localizes to the posterior fossa. Reported underlying congenital conditions include hypoplasia of the cerebellar vermis (as in Dandy–Walker malformation and Joubert syndrome (see Chapter 17)), Arnold–Chiari malformations (downward cerebellar tonsillar herniation), occipital encephalocele, and spinocerebellar degeneration.[181] Acquired causes such as pontine damage, a medulloblastoma, and hepatic encephalopathy have been described.[180]

Like periodic alternating nystagmus, period alternating gaze may reflect damage to the cerebellar inferior vermis, including the uvula and nodulus.[181]

Ping-Pong Gaze. Also called *short-cycle periodic alternating gaze deviation,* this ocular motility pattern has horizontal oscillation cycles of only 2.5 to 8 seconds.[182] Patients appear as if they are watching a ping-pong match. The side to side movements are usually smooth and sinusoidal, but a saccadic form has also been described.[183]

Ping-pong gaze is almost always seen in comatose or stuporous patients but implies the

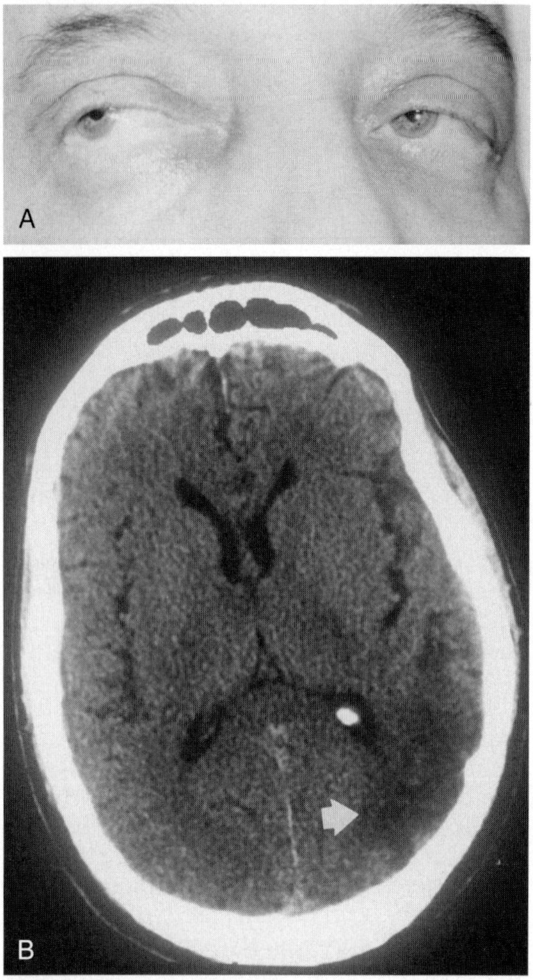

FIGURE 16–15. **A**. Right gaze deviation in a patient with seizures. **B**. CT scan reveals an old left middle cerebral infarction (*arrow*), which acted as a seizure focus.

brain stem, especially the pons, is relatively intact. The responsible lesions are thought to disconnect the brain stem from cortical influences, which may hypothetically release oculovestibular generators. They are typically rostral midbrain–thalamic, bilateral basal ganglia, or bilateral hemispheric.[184-186] Cases associated with a cerebellar vermis hemorrhage[187] and bilateral cerebral peduncle infarctions have been reported.[188]

VERTICAL CONJUGATE GAZE: NEUROANATOMY

Crucial supranuclear structures mediating vertical gaze are located in the midbrain at the level of the *pretectum* (Figs. 16–16 and 16–17). This term refers to the area in the midbrain immediately rostral to the *tectum*, another designation for the superior and inferior colliculi. The pretectum is also just rostral to the level of the third nerve and red nuclei. The two most important pretectal areas are the rostral interstitial nucleus of the medial longitudinal fasciculus (riMLF) and interstitial nucleus of Cajal (inC).

Rostral Interstitial Nuclei of the Medial Longitudinal Fasciculus (riMLF). At the pretectal level, in an area of the midbrain termed the *mesencephalic reticular formation*, up- and downward saccades are mediated by burst neurons within the paired paramedian riMLF (Figs. 16–16 and 16–17).[189–192] These lie immediately above the rostral-medial portions of the red nuclei. The topographic separation of upgaze and downgaze burst and tonic neurons within each riMLF is uncertain in man.[193]

In the current view of vertical gaze control,[194, 195] saccadic innervation is bilateral to the elevator muscles (the superior rectus and inferior oblique) (Fig. 16–17A), but only ipsilateral for downgaze (inferior rectus subnucleus and fourth nerve nucleus) (Fig. 16–17B). Projections for upgaze arising from the riMLF are no longer thought to cross in the posterior commissure, but rather bifurcate at the level of the third nerve nucleus. Each riMLF also contains neurons for ipsilateral torsional saccades.

The major clinicoanatomic implications of this arrangement are:

1. Unilateral lesions of an riMLF or its descending fibers will affect downward saccades more than upward saccades. This is due to the duplication of riMLF input into the oculomotor subnuclei for upgaze but not downgaze.
2. Bilateral lesions of an riMLF or its descending fibers will result in a more severe defect of vertical saccades than that due to unilateral lesions. Again, downward saccades may be affected more than upward saccades.
3. A unilateral riMLF lesion may cause defective ipsitorsional quick phases with ipsilateral head tilting. For instance, in a left riMLF lesion there would be no quick extorsion of the left eye or intorsion of the right eye upon leftward head tilting. Therefore, torsional nystagmus may be evident in the opposite direction.

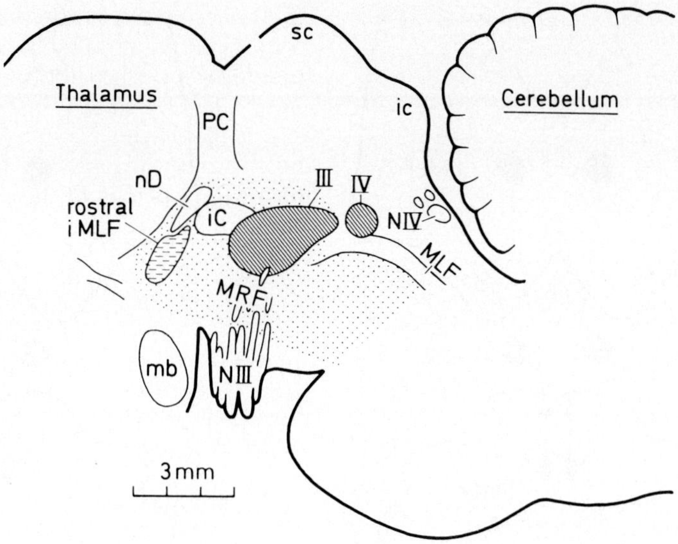

FIGURE 16–16. A schematic sagittal view of the upper brain stem, to demonstrate the anatomic localization of some structures involved in the generation of vertical eye movements. (III = oculomotor nucleus; IV = trochlear nucleus; iC = interstitial nucleus of Cajal; ic = inferior colliculus; iMLF = (rostral) interstitial nucleus of the MLF; mb = mamillary body; MLF = medial longitudinal fasciculus; MRF = mesencephalic reticular formation; NIII = oculomotor nerve; NIV = trochlear nerve; NVII = facial nerve; nD = nucleus Darkschewitsch; PC = posterior commissure; sc = superior colliculus. (Adapted from Büttner-Ennever JA: Anatomy of the ocular motor nuclei. In Kennard C, Rose FC (eds): Physiological Aspects of Clinical Neuro-ophthalmology, p. 203. Chicago, Year Book, 1988, with permission.)

Interstitial Nucleus of Cajal (inC). By coordinating signals from the saccadic burst neurons in the riMLF, vestibular projections (from the vestibular nuclei via the MLF), and descending pursuit fibers, the paired inC act as the neural integrator for vertical gaze and torsion.[194, 195] They lie adjacent but dorsal and caudal to the riMLF (Fig. 16–16).[196] For upgaze, fibers from the inC cross via the posterior commissure, then connect to the contralateral superior rectus and inferior oblique subnuclei. For downgaze, fibers again travel across the posterior commissure, then innervate the contralateral inferior rectus subnucleus and fourth nerve nucleus (Fig. 16–17).

The major clinicoanatomic implications of this arrangement are:

1. Lesions to the inC or its afferents tend to abolish the vertical vestibulo-ocular response,[1] while in contrast, lesions solely of the riMLF tend not to affect it.
2. Because the inC is considered a vertical and torsional integrator, lesions of the inC are thought to be responsible for the ocular torsion and skew deviation seen in midbrain lesions (see Chapter 15).
3. Lesions involving the projections of the inC in the posterior commissure are thought to produce vertical gaze abnormalities for all classes of eye movements. This is particularly true for upgaze.
4. Interestingly, the vertical saccades may be limited in their range of movement but their velocities will be normal with inC lesions.

Other Supranuclear Structures. The nucleus of the posterior commissure (nPC) likely aids in coordinating eyelid and vertical eye position (see Chapter 14) and also may play an important role in mediating upgaze. The role of the nucleus of Darkschewitsch in vertical eye movements is unclear.

There is considerable evidence in animals that the superior colliculus has a role in rapid gaze shifts, such as facilitating and inhibiting reflexive visually guided saccades. The function of the superior colliculus with regard to eye movements in humans is probably similar but is less well understood, as isolated lesions of the superior colliculus are only rarely reported in humans.[62]

The cortical control of vertical eye movements is poorly understood. Fibers from the frontal and supplementary eye fields may pass

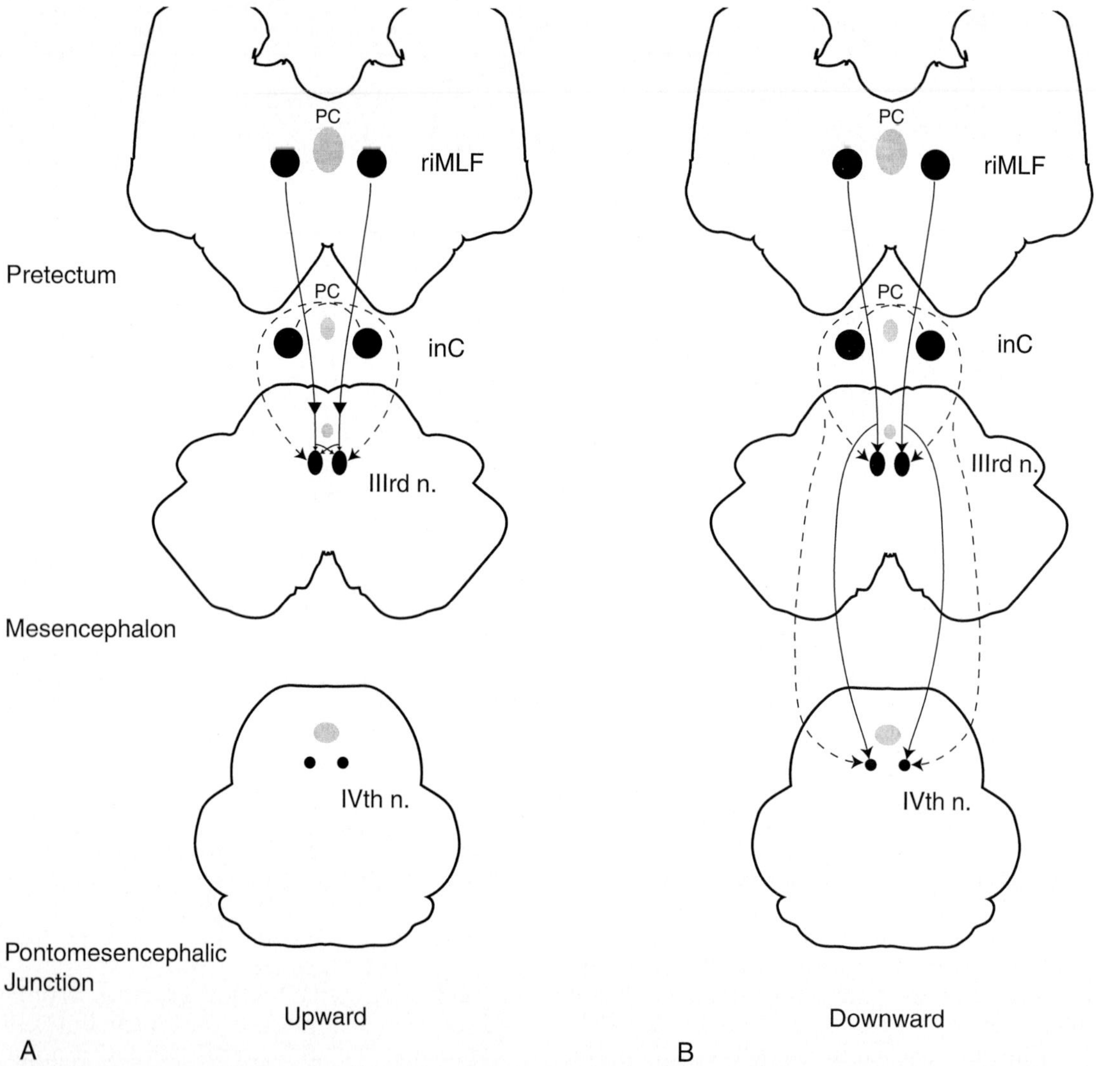

FIGURE 16–17. Major pathways subserving vertical eye movements.[194, 195] **A**. Upward eye movements. Neurons from the rostral interstitial nucleus of the medial longitudinal fasciculus (riMLF), which contain burst neurons for vertical saccades, project ipsilaterally to the oculomotor nuclear complex. There fibers divide, with some crossing at this level, to innervate the superior rectus (SR) and inferior oblique (IO) subnuclei bilaterally. On the other hand, fibers from the interstitial nucleus of Cajal (inC), the neural integrator for vetical gaze, cross within the posterior commissure (PC) before reaching the oculomotor complex and the SR and IO subnuclei. **B**. Downgaze eye movements. For downgaze, each riMLF supplies the ipsilateral inferior rectus subnucleus and the fourth nerve nucleus (IVth n.), which innervates the contralateral superior oblique muscle. Axons from the inC cross via the posterior commissure then innervate the contralateral inferior rectus subnucleus and fourth nerve nucleus.

through the thalamus before reaching the pretectum.[197]

VERTICAL GAZE LIMITATIONS

Pretectal (Parinaud, Dorsal Midbrain) Syndrome

This syndrome, the elements of which are listed in Table 16–7, is highlighted by supranuclear vertical upgaze paresis due to a dorsal midbrain disturbance (Fig. 16–18). The eponym is attributed to Henri Parinaud, an ophthalmologist who worked under Charcot at the Salpêtrière in Paris in the late 19th century[198] and wrote two landmark articles describing various types of conjugate gaze palsies and paralyses of convergence.[199, 200]

More modern definitions of the syndrome have included pupillary and eyelid abnormalities, as well as convergence retraction nystag-

TABLE 16–7. Elements of the Pretectal (Parinaud) Syndrome

Major Components
Supranuclear vertical gaze paresis
Pupillary light–near dissociation
Lid retraction (Collier's sign)
Convergence–retraction nystagmus
Minor Components
Pseudoabducens palsy (thalamic esotropia)
Convergence insufficiency
Accommodative insufficiency
Associated Ocular Motility Deficits
Skew deviation,
Third nerve palsy
Internuclear ophthalmoplegia
See-saw nystagmus

mus. For this reason, authors such as Keane[201] have recommended using the anatomic term *pretectal syndrome*, but the term *dorsal midbrain syndrome* is also popular. Other names, such as Koeber–Salus–Elschnig sylvian aqueduct syndrome[202] and Nothnagel syndrome[203, 204] have been used but are less familiar.

A lesion in the posterior commissure appears to be the one critical to producing the pretectal syndrome and all of the major elements.[205] The follow sections describe the major and minor elements and some of the important disorders that commonly cause the pretectal syndrome.

Symptoms. Common neuro-ophthalmic complaints associated with the pretectal syndrome are difficulty looking up, diplopia, and blurred vision at near. Accompanying neurologic symptoms such as headache, nausea, and vomiting are suggestive of obstructive hydrocephalus. Acute pretectal neuro-ophthalmic symptoms in addition to ataxia or alteration in consciousness can occur in a midbrain infarction or thalamic hemorrhage.

Vertical Upgaze Paresis in the Pretectal Syndrome. The supranuclear vertical gaze restriction in this syndrome results from involvement of the posterior commissure, inC, or riMLF (Figs. 16–16 and 16–17). Although vertical saccades and pursuit are both affected, the deficit of saccades is usually more prominent. Upgaze deficits may be seen alone or in combination with downgaze paresis, depending on the location of the involvement: lesions affecting the posterior commissure usually produce greater involvement of upgaze while those located more ventrally are usually associated with greater downgaze paresis.[190] Oculocephalic and oculovestibular maneuvers and attempted eye closure usually improve the vertical gaze limitation.[206] Lack of improvement by these measures frequently indicates coinvolvment of the third nerve nuclei or fascicles.

Other Major Elements of the Pretectal Syndrome

Pupillary Light-Near Dissociation. The pupils are typically midposition (see Fig. 13–9), and they are poorly reactive to light but more reactive to near. The pathophysiology is discussed in Chapter 13.

Eyelid Retraction (Collier's Sign). The eyelids may be elevated above the limbus in primary gaze. Sometimes there is also lid lag in downgaze. The involved pathways and mechanism are discussed in Chapter 14.

Convergence Retraction Nystagmus. Especially in attempted upward saccades, the eyes may jerk inward and into the globe. This type of nystagmus, which is reviewed in Chapter 17, is highly localizing to the pretectum.

Minor Elements of the Pretectal Syndrome

Pseudo-Sixth Nerve Palsy. Although the pons and sixth nerve may be spared, the eyes in patients with pretectal lesions may be esotropic (Figs. 16–18 and Fig. 16–19).[207] One or both eyes may have an abduction deficit which is variable and easily overcome by horizontal oculocephalic movements. The "thalamic esotropia"[208, 209] associated with thalamic strokes and hemorrhages is likely explained by pretectal involvement.[210] Like convergence retraction nystagmus, this ocular motility finding may in part reflect excess convergence tone as the pupils can be miotic. Other explanations include disruption in supranuclear fibers governing horizontal gaze, and fixation with the contralateral eye, which may have an adduction deficit due to an oculomotor palsy.[211]

Convergence and Accommodative Insufficiency. The critical structures for convergence (bilateral adduction) and accommodation lie in the midbrain and are reviewed in Chapter 13. Both functions are required for binocular viewing of near targets. Convergence insufficiency (see Chapter 15) causes horizontal binocular vision at near. Patients with accommodative insufficiency are unable to focus on near targets and may require the aid of plus lenses. We have seen young children with pineal region masses whose first complaints were diplopia and blurred vision at near.

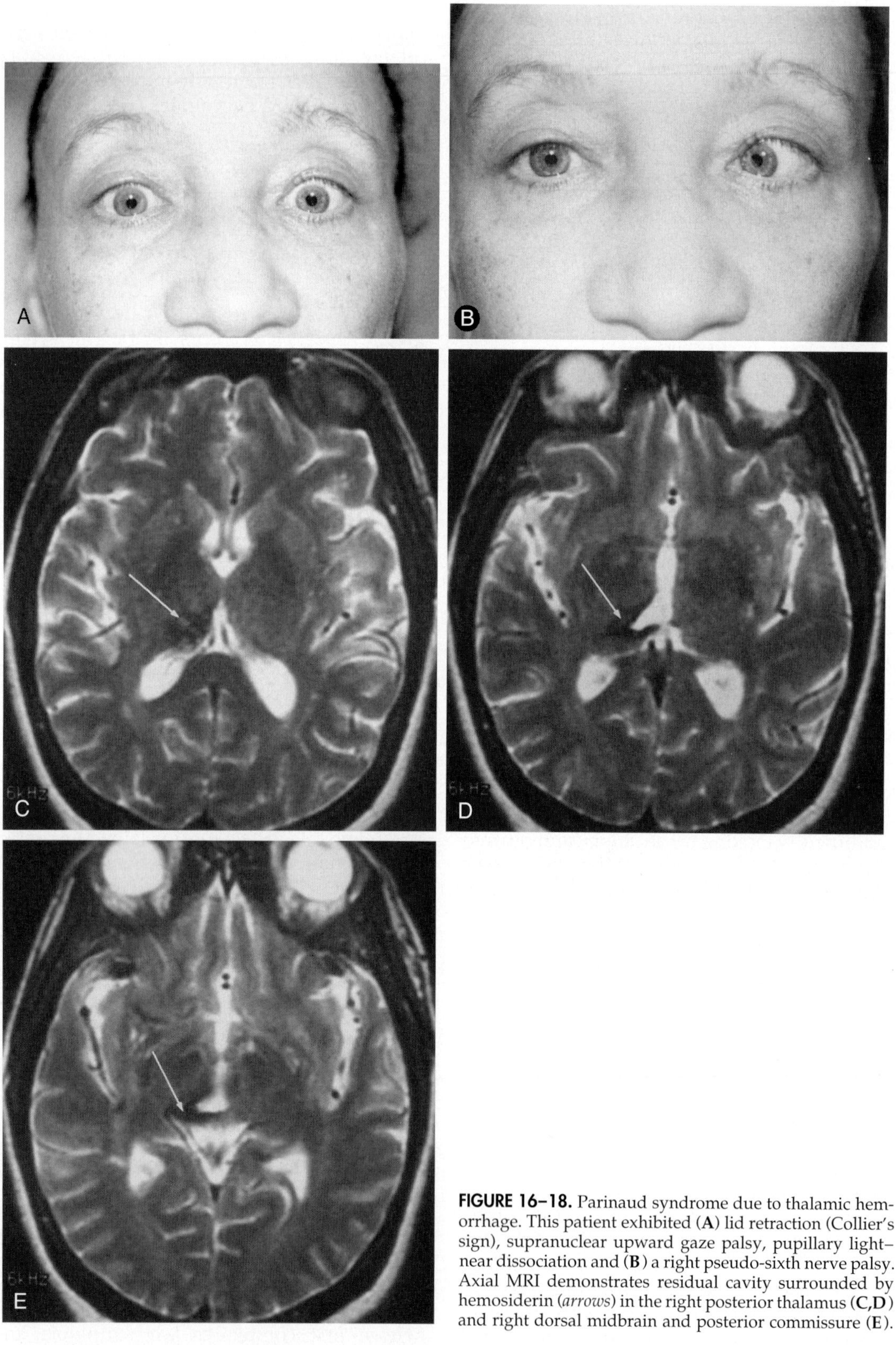

FIGURE 16–18. Parinaud syndrome due to thalamic hemorrhage. This patient exhibited (**A**) lid retraction (Collier's sign), supranuclear upward gaze palsy, pupillary light–near dissociation and (**B**) a right pseudo-sixth nerve palsy. Axial MRI demonstrates residual cavity surrounded by hemosiderin (*arrows*) in the right posterior thalamus (**C,D**) and right dorsal midbrain and posterior commissure (**E**).

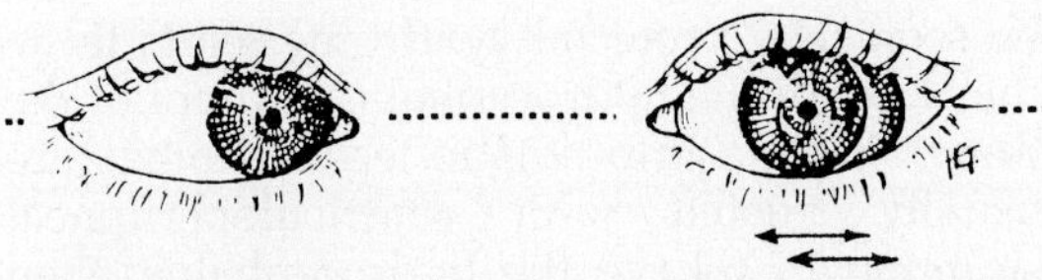

FIGURE 16–19. Pseudo-sixth nerve palsy. In attempted conjugate gaze to the left, the right eye converges strongly, but the left fails to abject fully and adducting jerks are visible. (From Caplan LR: "Top of the basilar" syndrome. Neurology 1980;30:72–79, with permission.)

Other Associated Ocular Motility Deficits

Skew Deviation, See-Saw Nystagmus, Third Nerve Palsy, and Internuclear Ophthalmoplegia. These ocular motility deficits may occur when the inC, the oculomotor nerve nucleus or fascicle, or medial longitudinal fasciculus, respectively, are disrupted by dorsal midbrain lesions that are large enough to affect the midbrain tegmentum. The skew may alternate sides,[212] or be part of an ocular tilt reaction.[213] They are discussed in great detail in Chapter 15. See-saw nystagmus, which may also be seen in this setting, is reviewed in Chapter 17.

Causes of the Pretectal Syndrome. Diagnostic considerations should be made in the context of the patient's age. In infants, obstructive hydrocephalus is the most common cause. In toddlers and other young children, pineal region masses are more common. In contrast, in adults, strokes and hemorrhages are the most frequent causes.

Hydrocephalus. Pretectal signs and symptoms are frequently the first manifestations of obstructive (noncommunicating) hydrocephalus. The forced downward eye position in infants with hydrocephalus is said to mimic two setting suns. The mechanism is likely dilation of the third ventricle and of the rostral aqueduct, causing compression of pretectal structures.[214] Aqueductal dilation may also increase periaqueductal tissue water, which may decrease blood flow to structures in this area.[215] Ocular motor deficits usually resolve within days or weeks following ventricular decompression, but some patients are left with subtle permanent findings. Typical causes include congenital aqueductal stenosis or posterior fossa tumors causing fourth ventricular or aqueductal compression.

Pineal Region Tumors. Neoplasms in this region, when large enough, may compress the superior colliculi posteriorly and present with the pretectal syndrome. In most series,[216, 217] about 90% of pineal region tumors presented with signs and symptoms due to increased intracranial pressure, such as papilledema, while about half presented with the pretectal syndrome.

One of the common neoplasms occurring in this region is a *germinoma* (Fig. 16–20, and see Fig. 13–9), which when isolated is associated with an excellent long-term outcome following radiation therapy. Treatment and presentation of germinomas, which also occur commonly in the sellar region, are discussed in Chapter 7. Less common germ cell tumor types occurring in the pineal region include embryonal cell, endodermal sinus, choriocarcinoma, and mature and immature teratomas.[218]

The other common tumor type in this area is a *pinealblastoma,* which is more highly malignant. It is also termed *pineal primitive neuroectodermal tumor* (PNET), similar in pathologic characteristics with medulloblastomas and supratentorial PNETs. These require surgical removal, exclusion of subarachnoid seeding, and in most instances radiation and chemotherapy. Pinealcytomas tend to occur in older individuals and are usually more benign. Occasionally aggressive atypical rhabdoid tumors are seen in this region as well.

Following surgical or radiotherapeutic decompression of pineal region tumors, most of the elements of Parinaud syndrome tend to resolve. The vertical gaze paresis usually resolves first, followed by improvement in the pupillary and eyelid abnormalities. Subtle convergence retraction nystagmus, provoked only

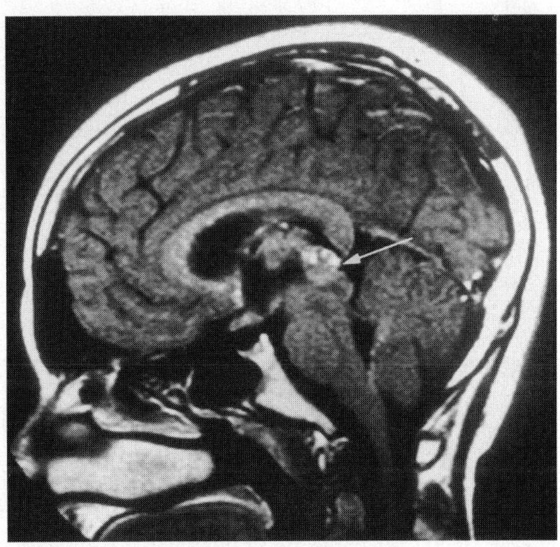

FIGURE 16–20. Pineal region germinoma (*arrow*) that presented with Parinaud syndrome.

by upward saccades, may be evident chronically in some patients. More prominent and persistent findings are typically the result of peritumoral radiation necrosis.

Pineal Region Cysts. Fluid-filled structures abutting the superior colliculi are usually asymptomatic.[219] They are often discovered incidentally in patients undergoing neuroimaging for other reasons such as headache. On MRI the cyst fluid, contained by a thin wall, is isointense or slightly hyperintense compared with cerebrospinal fluid (CSF). On CT, the cyst rim may contrast enhance. They usually can be followed conservatively with serial examinations and neuroimaging. In only unusual instances the cysts are large enough to cause aqueductal compression and hydrocephalus. A case of hemorrhage into a pineal cyst associated with anticoagulation has been reported as a cause of "pineal apoplexy."[220]

Tectal Gliomas. These relatively benign tumors usually surround the sylvian aqueduct and involve the superior collicular plate.[221] They are characterized pathologically as low-grade astrocytomas and radiographically on MRI by hyperintensity on T_2-weighted images and gadolinium enhancement. Despite their location, they tend to be asymptomatic unless aqueductal compression and noncommunicating hydrocephalus occur. Consequently, the pretectal syndrome and signs and symptoms of elevated intracranial pressure such as headache, nausea, vomiting, and papilledema may be seen. The pretectal syndrome tends to be the result of the hydrocephalus and not of the tumor itself. Symptomatic tectal gliomas are usually treated with ventriculoperitoneal shunting to relieve the hydrocephalus, then serial examinations and radiographic observation of the neoplasm.[222] Surgery is usually not performed unless the lesions are exophytic or progressive, or appear to be higher grade,[223] when radiation or chemotherapy are also considered.

Paramedian Midbrain/Thalamic Infarction. "Top of the basilar" strokes are associated with various combinations of oculomotor, behavioral, and motor findings.[207, 224] The infarctions occur in the distribution of paramedian penetrating arteries arising from the proximal posterior cerebral arteries at the basilar bifurcation (P_1 segments, or Percheron's basilar communicating arteries[225]) (see Fig. 8–1). The strokes can be unilateral, but because one paramedian artery may bifurcate and supply both sides of the mesencephalon and both thalami, often bilateral infarction at the two levels is seen (Fig. 16–21).[226] The infarctions sometimes take on "butterfly" shape when viewed coronally. The cause is typically vertebrobasilar atherosclerosis,[227] but emboli to the basilar bifurcation and proximal posterior cerebral arteries may also be responsible.[228]

When the lesions are ventral in the mesencephalon, fascicular third nerve palsies accompanied by contralateral weakness or ataxia are

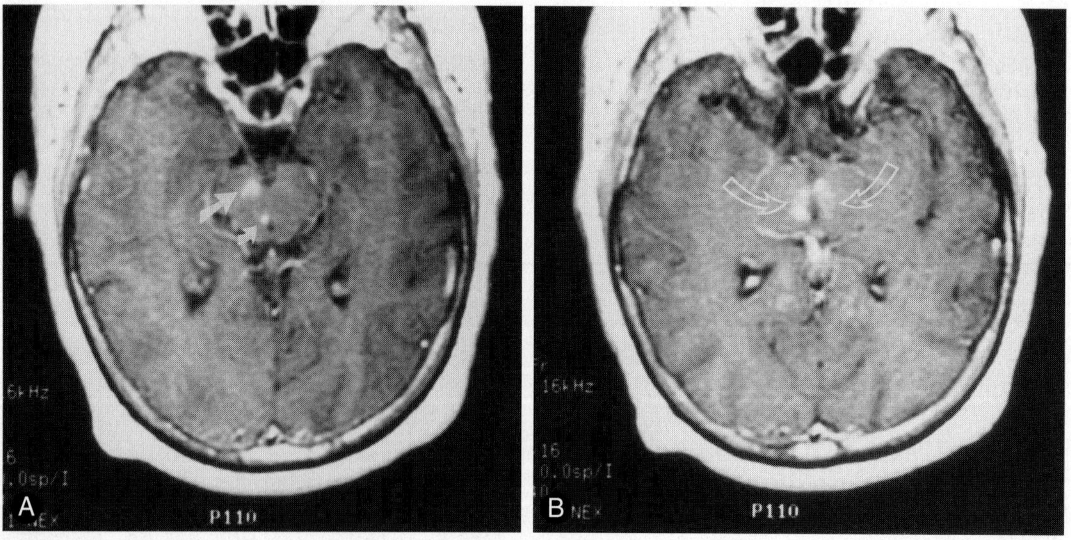

FIGURE 16–21. Top of the basilar infarction presenting with upgaze paresis and lethargy. **A.** Axial MRI with gadolinium through the midbrain demonstrating paramedian infarction of the ventral (*large arrow*) and dorsal (*small arrow*) mesencephalon. **B.** In the same patient, more rostral axial MRI showing bilateral mesial thalamic infarctions (*arrows*).

seen (see Chapter 15). Rarely, peduncular hallucinations (Chapter 12) may also develop in ventral lesions. More dorsal infarction may affect the midbrain tegmentum and pretectum (Fig. 16–22).[229] These patients often exhibit nuclear and supranuclear vertical ocular motor disturbances and hypersomnolence due to disruption of the ascending reticular activating fibers and thalamic structures governing nonrapid eye movement (NREM) sleep.[230, 231] Sensory deficits, aphasia, akinetic mutism, amnesia, and coma may also result from thalamic involvement.[232] If the proximal cerebral artery is occluded, occipital lobe infarction leading to visual field defects (Chapter 8) and higher cortical visual disturbances (Chapter 9) may be seen.[207]

Thalamic Hemorrhages. These lesions were discussed above in the section on horizontal gaze deviation. However, downward extension or hydrocephalus due to intraventricular extension of a thalamic hemorrhage may cause a pretectal syndrome (see Fig. 16–18).[178] In more severe cases the eyes may be esotropic and pointed downward, as if they were peering at the nose (Fig. 16–23).[233] The pupils tend to be small and sluggish or unreactive to light. The combination of a hemiparesis, sensory loss, hemianopia or aphasia, and pretectal syndrome is highly suggestive of a thalamic hemorrhage.

Thalamic Tumors. The pretectal syndrome may result from thalamic tumors, usually gliomas, which extend below the tentorium to involve the upper midbrain.[234] Third ventricular compression may also lead to hydrocephalus and pretectal signs and symptoms on that basis.

Infections. Tuberculomas and toxoplasmosis abcesses in the dorsal midbrain region should be considered, especially in immunocompromised patients such as those with acquired immunodeficiency syndrome (AIDS).[235, 236] In Keane's series,[201] cysticercosis was one of the

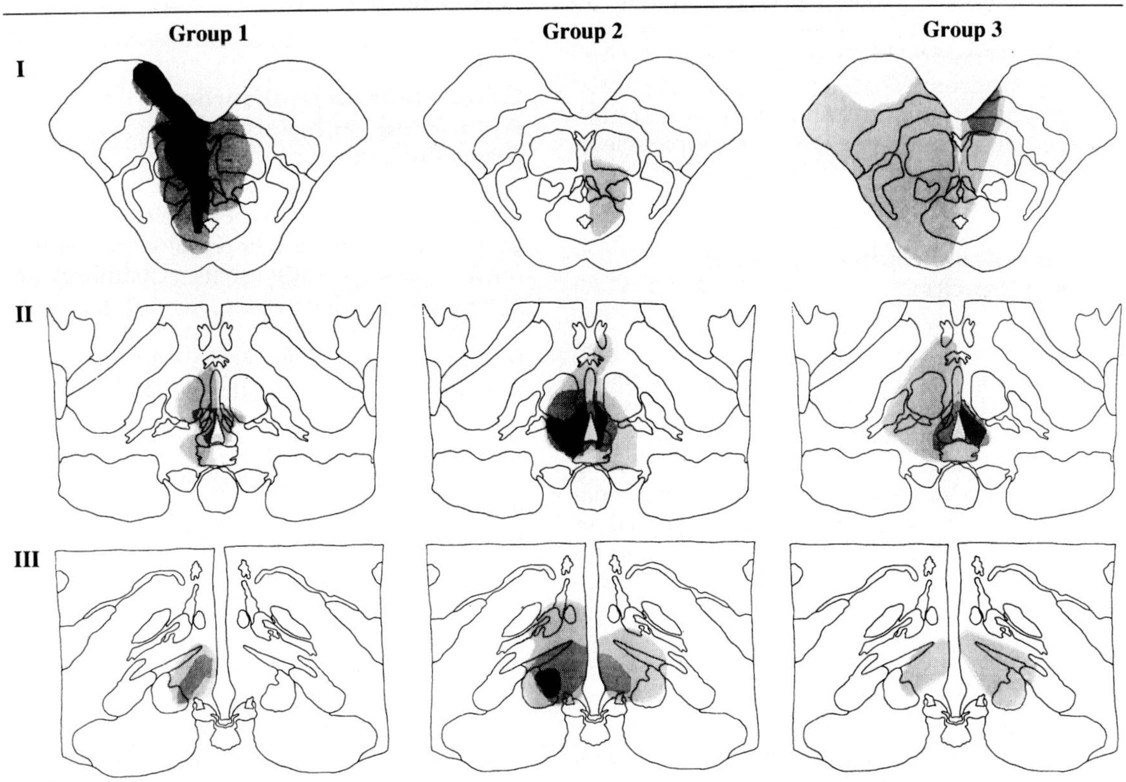

FIGURE 16–22. Templates showing infarct topography for patients with thalamopeduncular infarcts. The anatomic levels include level I (upper midbrain), level II (midbrain–thalamic junction), and level III (ventral thalamus). The clinical groups are comprised of patients with nuclear or infranuclear third nerve palsy (Group 1), patients with supranuclear gaze palsy (Group 2), and patients with combined nuclear and supranuclear palsies (Group 3). The degree of "shading" indicates the areas most frequently involved by infarction. (From Tatemichi TK, et al: Paramedian thalamopeduncular infarction: clinical syndromes and magnetic resonance imaging. Ann Neurol 1992;32:162-171, with permission).

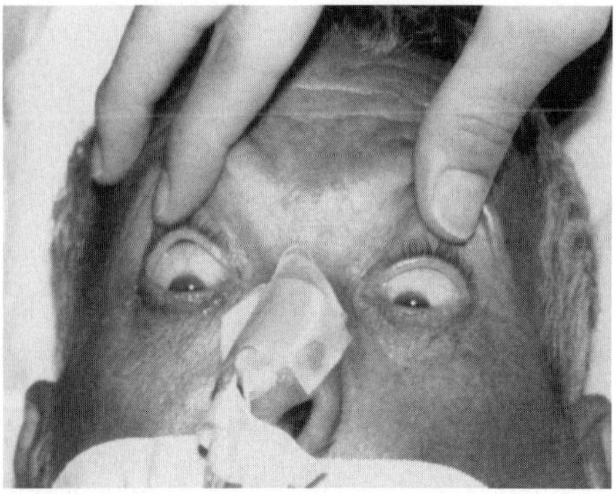

FIGURE 16–23. Severe downgaze deviation and stupor due to thalamic hemorrhage with intraventricular extension and hydrocephalus.

most frequent causes of dorsal midbrain syndrome. However, this likely reflected the prevalence of this infection in his patient population.

Other Causes. A large variety of vascular, inflammatory, and compressive lesions have also been reported in association with the pretectal syndrome. These include transtentorial herniation,[237] arteriovenous malformations,[201] cavernous hemangiomas,[238, 239] multiple sclerosis,[240-242] and posterior fossa aneurysms.[243]

Other Mesencephalic Vertical Gaze Deficits

Supranuclear Downgaze Paresis. Isolated downgaze paresis due to a midbrain lesion is much less common than isolated upgaze paresis or combined up- and downgaze paresis. Downgaze paresis may occur following damage in the mesencephalic reticular formation just dorsal and medial to the upper halves of the red nuclei.[190, 244, 245] Such lesions disrupt the efferents that emerge from the caudal-medial portions of the riMLF and head caudally toward the third and fourth nerve nuclei (see Fig. 16–17). As alluded to earlier, lesions producing prominent downgaze palsy are almost always bilateral.[234, 244, 246-248]

The most common cause is a vascular insult involving a paramedian artery of the mesencephalon and thalamus.[249] However, degenerative disorders such as progressive supranuclear palsy (see below) and, less commonly, Huntington's disease and Hallervorden–Spatz disease, should be considered.[250]

Vertical "One-and-a-Half" Syndrome. There are two variations of this ocular motility disorder, which borrow their label from their horizontal counterpart. In one of these vertical types, a monocular paresis of downgaze accompanied by a bilateral symmetric upgaze deficit can be caused by a unilateral thalamomesencephalic lesion.[251] This condition results from disruption of the ipsilateral inferior rectus portion of the oculomotor fascicle and either (1) the posterior commissure, resulting in a supranuclear vertical gaze paresis, or (2) the oculomotor nucleus, which would lead to bilateral superior rectus weakness (see Chapter 15).

In another variation, there is a bilateral symmetric downgaze deficit accompanied by a monocular upgaze palsy. This results from bilateral lesions in the mesencephalon affecting the downgaze efferents from the riMLF along with concomitant disruption of the supranuclear fibers for upgaze of one eye (see supranuclear monocular elevator palsy, Chapter 15) or the fascicular fibers for the superior rectus and inferior oblique.[252]

Other Neurologic Disorders Associated With Vertical Gaze Deficits

Limited Upgaze in Elderly Patients. Conjugate upgaze may be limited or reduced in otherwise normal elderly individuals. Chamberlain[253] measured eye elevation in 367 normal volunteers 5 to 94 years of age. Those who were 5 to 14 years of age averaged 40.1 degrees of upward rotation, while those between 45 and 54 years averaged 30.4 degrees, and those 85 to 94 averaged 16.1 degrees. Downward rotations did not vary between age groups. The mechanism is unclear, but the deficits in many instances appear to be supranuclear.

Progressive Supranuclear Palsy. In 1963 and 1964, Steele, Richardson, and Olszewski[254-256] reported the clinical and pathologic findings of a neurodegenerative disorder to which there had previously been only vague reference in the literature. Clinically, their patients had progressive supranuclear ophthalmoparesis, pseudobulbar palsy, dysarthria, and rigidity of the neck and upper trunk. Pathologically, there were globose neurofibrillary tangles, neuronal loss, granulovacuolar degeneration, and gliosis in the basal ganglia, cerebellum, and mesencephalon. Richardson called the disorder *progressive supranuclear palsy* (PSP), although it is often referred to as the Steele–Richardson–Olszewski syndrome in honor of the individuals who crystallized the current understanding of its distinctive clinical and pathologic features. Previous cases with similar clinical findings had been reported before their seminal reports, but in retrospect many of these had other diseases.[257, 258] Today PSP is considered highly in the differential diagnosis of "parkinsonism plus."

Because neuro-ophthalmic signs and symptoms are so prominent in PSP, it is appropriate here to review the disorder in more detail.

Demographics. PSP is most common in elderly men. In a study from Olmsted County,[259] no cases were seen before age 50, while the incidence rate (new cases per 100,000 person years) for ages 50 to 99 years was 6.9 for men, 4.1 for women, and 5.3 combined. Patients with PSP are less likely to have completed at least 12 years of school, suggesting either poor early-life nutrition or occupational or residential toxic exposure is partly responsible.[260] Familial cases have been reported but are uncommon.[261, 262] The exact cause is unknown.

Neuro-Ophthalmic Features. Eye movement abnormalities are seen in a majority of patients with PSP. Affected patients may complain of blurred vision, trouble focusing, difficulty reading or looking down steps, eye pain, irritation, photophobia, or diplopia.[263] Because of their inability to look downward, patients with PSP can be "messy eaters."[264]

The clinical hallmark of PSP is a supranuclear vertical gaze paresis (Fig. 16–24), typically downward more than upward, which is usually evident within 3 years of symptom onset.[264] Often the oculocephalic maneuver is difficult to perform because of the nuchal rigidity. At first volitional vertical saccades are hypometric or slow,[265, 266] but later they may become absent. In contrast to other saccadic disorders, head thrusting is generally not observed. Convergence is often impaired, and pursuit may be saccadic or "cogwheel."[267] As the disease progresses, horizontal gaze may become affected. The amplitude of quick phases of vestibular and optokinetic nystagmus may be diminished.[268] In late, severe cases, some patients with PSP develop an internuclear[269] or complete nuclear ophthalmoparesis.[270] However, autopsy-proven cases without eye movement deficits are well recognized.[271]

Other neuro-ophthalmic findings include horizontal square-wave jerks,[267] nystagmus, in-

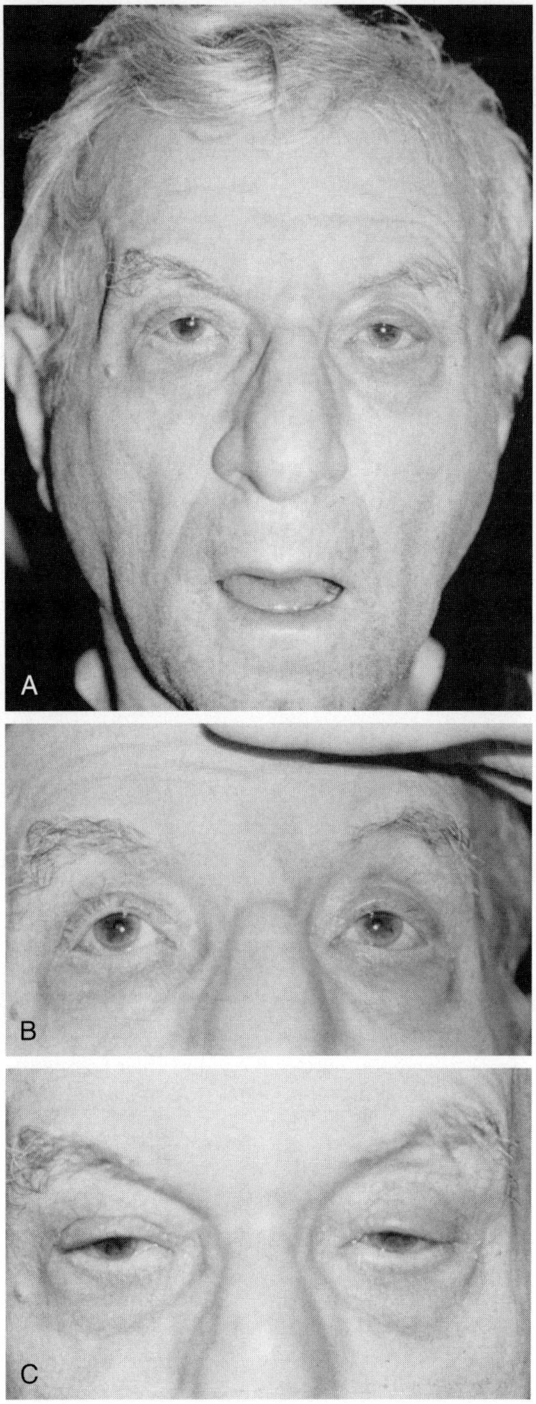

FIGURE 16–24. Patient with progressive supranuclear palsy. **A**. Characteristic stare. Defective (**B**) upgaze and (**C**) downgaze were also present.

ability to suppress the vestibulo-ocular response (especially vertically), blepharospasm, and eyelid opening apraxia.[271-273] Many have a characteristic facies with eyelid retraction, slow blink rate, and staring (Fig. 16–24).[274, 275] The results from one study that analyzed the neuro-ophthalmic features of PSP and their frequency are summarized in Table 16–8.

Neurologic Features. The most common initial neurologic complaints are postural instability and falling (often backwards), gait difficulty, dysarthria, and memory problems. Common behavioral features include apathy, disinhibition, depression or withdrawal, but not irritability or agitation.[276]

On examination, parkinsonism is the most conspicuous finding and is characterized by bradykinesia and rigidity. Until patients with PSP develop the characteristic ocular motility findings, many are mistakenly given the diagnosis of Parkinson's disease. However, in PSP, tremor is usually absent, and the rigidity is typically axial, affecting the neck and trunk, more than appendicular. Patients with PSP typically stand more upright than those with Parkinson's disease, who often have a flexed posture. In PSP, limb dystonia may also be observed.[277] Cognitive impairment is most evident in tests sensitive to frontal lobe dysfunction, such as verbal fluency and motor sequencing.[278]

TABLE 16–9. Criteria for a Clinical Diagnosis of Progressive Supranuclear Palsy

Mandatory Inclusionary Criteria
- Onset at age 40 or later
- Progressive disease course
- Vertical supranuclear gaze palsy with downward gaze abnormalities
- Severe postural instability with unexplained falls

Supportive Criteria
- Symmetric akinesia or rigidity, proximal more than distal
- Abnormal neck posture, especially retrocollis
- Poor or absent response of parkinsonism to levodopa therapy
- Early dysphagia and dysarthria
- Early onset of cognitive impairment including at least two of the following: apathy, impairment in abstract throught, decreased verbal fluency, utilization or imitation behavior, or frontal release signs.

Mandatory Exclusionary Criteria (and the Disease for Which the Feature Is More Typical)
- History of encephalitis (Postencephalitic parkinsonism)
- Hallucinations (Dementia with Lewy bodies)
- Early or prominent cerebellar signs (multisystem atrophy)
- Noniatrogenic dysautonomia (multisystem atrophy)
- Alien hand syndrome (corticobasal ganglionic degeneration)
- Early cortical dementia characterized by amnesia, aphasia, or agnosia (Alzheimer's disease)
- Focal lesion on neurologic examination or neuroimaging (multi-infarct state)

Note these criteria are specific but not sensitive; they have a high positive predictive value. The diagnosis can be established with certainty only at autopsy, and even in retrospect some cases diagnosed postmortem will not have satisfied these criteria.

TABLE 16–8. Neuro-ophthalmic Features of Progressive Supranuclear Palsy and Their Frequency in a Retrospective Series of 38 Patients

	%
Eye Movement Abnormalities	
Downgaze palsy	97
Upgaze palsy	97
Abnormal smooth pursuit	74
Lateral gaze palsy	61
Hypometric saccades	50
Internuclear ophthalmoplegia	29
Square-wave jerks	21
Slow saccades	16
Nystagmus	13
Ocular flutter	5
Eyelid Abnormalities	
Lid retraction	100
Apraxia of eyelid opening	37
Blepharospasm	29
Apraxia of eyelid closure	10

Adapted from Friedman DI, Jankovic J, McCrary JA: Neuro-ophthalmic findings in progressive supranuclear palsy. J Clin Neuro-ophthalmol 1992;12:104–109, with permission.

Table 16–9 summarizes criteria for the clinical diagnosis of PSP.[279, 280] The combination of a supranuclear vertical gaze paresis plus postural instability and falling is highly suggestive of the diagnosis of PSP.[274, 281] The median survival time in PSP is approximately 6 years following symptom onset, but it can range from 1 to 17 years.[282]

Pathologic Features. The diagnosis of PSP can be established with certainty only at autopsy. PSP is characterized pathologically by atrophy predominantly of the subthalamic nucleus, the substantia nigra, and the globus pallidus.[283] Microscopically, gliosis, neuronal loss, and globose neurofibrillary tangles or neuropil threads are seen in these areas.[284] Other regions also involved include the striatum, periaqueductal grey matter, superior colliculi, oculomotor nuclei, red nuclei, locus ceruleus, pontine tegmentum, pontine nuclei, medulla, and cerebellar dentate nuclei.[274, 284, 285] Although the cerebral cortex may also be involved, the damage is typically less prominent.[286]

Within the neurofibrillary tangles, intraneuronal inclusions formed by aggregated tau protein are observed. Abnormal tau, a microtubule-associated protein, also accumulates in other neurodegenerative disorders such as Alzheimer's and Pick's diseases. Although the tau gene A0/A0 genotype has been strongly associated with PSP,[287-289] a responsible genetic defect has yet to be elucidated.[290, 291]

The supranuclear vertical gaze paresis can be explained by the presence of neurofibrillary tangles and neuronal damage in the riMLF.[275] The inC may also be involved.[292] Defective horizontal saccades may result from cell loss in the PPRF,[293] while horizontal smooth pursuit impairment may owe to damage in nuclei of the basis pontis.[294] Damage to omnipause neurons in the PPRF, leading to disinhibition of saccadic burst neurons, may be responsible for square-wave jerks and other saccadic intrusions.[295]

Neuroimaging. MRI early in the course of the disease may be normal. However, patients who have had PSP for years may exhibit putaminal hypointensity on T_2-weighted images, representing iron deposition, and brain stem atrophy.[296, 297] Focal midbrain atrophy, particularly of the superior colliculus, and blurring ("smudging") of the margins of the substantia nigra are often striking features.[145, 298] Increased signal in the periaqueductal area may also be seen. MRI is also helpful in distinguishing patients with true PSP from those with PSP-like states due to multiple infarcts.[299]

Treatment. Although dopaminergic drugs such as levodopa, amantadine, bromocriptine, and pergolide are generally unhelpful, a minority of patients may experience a transient mild to moderate benefit with these drugs.[270, 300] However, the improvement is usually seen in the parkinsonism and bulbar signs, but not in ocular motility. Idazoxan, which increases norepinephrine transmission, was shown in a double-blind study to improve some aspects of motor function.[301]

Difficulty reading is a major complaint of patients with PSP because of their inability to look downward at their reading material and through their bifocal segment. Instructing such patients to bring reading materials to eye level may be the most practical advice, along with prescribing full-frame single-vision reading glasses for near.[263] Reading may also be complicated by convergence insufficiency, which can be ameliorated with base-in prisms. Base-up prisms may be tried in patients with downgaze paresis to improve their awareness of objects below their eyes, but most find this too confusing.

Niemann–Pick Disease. The Niemann–Pick disorders are autosomal recessive lysosomal storage conditions characterized by hepatosplenomegaly and progressive neurologic deterioration. The type C chronic neuronopathic form, one of the type II disorders in the more modern classification, typically presents with supranuclear vertical gaze paresis, mental and motor deterioration, ataxia, and visceromegaly.[302] The disorder has been mapped to chromosome 18q11–12 in most studied families. It is caused by a defect in intracellular mobilization and esterification of LDL-derived cholesterol. Three subtypes of Niemann–Pick type C can be identified: (1) a rapidly progressive infantile form, (2) a juvenile form, which occurs in previously healthy children, and (3) a slowly progressive form in adolescents and adults.[303, 304] The bone marrow typically exhibits sea-blue histiocytes and foam cells. Cytochemical staining of cultured fibroblasts with filipine, which fluoresces after binding with unesterified cholesterol, may also be performed. Treatment, which is usually aimed at reducing cholesterol intake and administering cholesterol-lowering agents, is relatively ineffective.

The ocular motor disturbance, which occurs in about two thirds of cases,[305] typically presents as a supranuclear downgaze saccadic paresis. This is followed by upgaze involvement, then results in extreme cases in a total vertical saccadic palsy.[306] Vertical pursuit movements as well as horizontal eye movements are usually preserved. Because of the characteristic phenotype, the designation DAF syndrome, for *d*owngaze paresis, *a*taxia, and *f*oam cells, has also been used.[107] A macular cherry-red spot, secondary to opacification of the nerve fiber layer, may also be seen.

Whipple's Disease. Central nervous system (CNS) involvement is a well-recognized complication of a multisystem chronic infection called Whipple's disease, which is caused by the bacillus *Tropheryma whippelii.* In the brain there is a predilection for involvement of the periaqueductal grey matter, hypothalamus, hippocampus, cerebral cortex, basal ganglia, and cerebellum.[307]

A supranuclear vertical gaze paresis, in either up- or downgaze, is observed in approximately one third of patients with CNS involvement.[308] When the vertical supranuclear gaze palsy is accompanied by dementia and a gait disturbance, Whipple's disease may be mimic progressive supranuclear palsy.[309] In a smaller proportion of patients, the supranuclear gaze paresis is both vertical and horizontal.[257] An isolated horizontal gaze paresis is usually not seen.

Oculomasticatory myorhythmia, characterized by pendular convergent–divergent nystagmus associated with rhythmic movements of the muscles of mastication, face, and extremities, is considered virtually pathognomonic (also see Chapter 17).[307, 310] In a large meta-analysis of reported patients with Whipple's disease,[308] oculomasticatory myorhythmia was found always to occur with a supranuclear gaze paresis. Hypothalamic involvement may result in the syndrome of inappropriate antidiuretic hormone secretion (SIADH), insomnia, hypersomnia, and hyperphagia. Cognitive and psychiatric symptoms are also observed frequently.[308]

The most common symptoms in Whipple's disease are gastrointestinal and include malabsorption, abdominal pain, weight loss, and diarrhea. Other systemic symptoms, such as pleuritis, lymphadenopathy, cardiac valvular lesions, fever, and arthritis, are often present.[311] CNS complications usually occur in association with systemic symptoms, but the latter may be absent in up to one fifth of cases of CNS Whipple's disease.[308] Rarely ocular involvement can occur and is characterized by uveitis, keratitis, vitreous hemorrhage, retinitis, or optic disc edema.[312, 313]

The diagnosis is best established by small-bowel biopsy or other sample of involved tissue and demonstration of *T. whippeli* DNA by polymerase chain reaction (PCR) testing.[311, 314] Staining for period acid-Schiff (PAS) positivity in macrophages, which can also be used, is not as sensitive or specific. Electron micrographic demonstration of the organism can be performed. *T. whippeli* is difficult to culture. Midbrain, hypothalamic, and temporal lobe hyperintensities may be seen on MRI,[315] and the CSF analysis may reveal a pleocytosis and elevated protein. However, both neuroimaging and spinal fluid may also be normal.

Treatment with antibiotics such as intravenous trimethoprim-sulfamethoxazole or ceftriaxone[316] for 2 weeks followed by oral trimethoprim-sulfamethoxazole twice daily for 1 year is often effective. Tetracycline and chloramphenicol have also been used.

Miscellaneous

Amyotrophic Lateral Sclerosis. Some reports[317-321] have suggested that supranuclear conjugate gaze rarely may be affected in amyotrophic lateral sclerosis (Lou Gehrig's disease), even very early in its course. Slow saccades and pursuit in all directions, as well as vertical gaze palsies, were documented in one study.[319] In another,[321] neuropathologic examination in two patients with supranuclear upgaze paresis confirmed neuronal loss in the riMLF and periaqueductal grey matter and sparing of the third and fourth nerve nuclei. Amyotrophic lateral sclerosis, including third, fourth, and sixth cranial nerve involvement in this disorder, is also discussed in Chapter 15.

Other Neuromuscular Conditions. Subclinical defective saccades have been documented in myotonic dystrophy. It has been controversial whether the saccadic abnormalities in myotonic dystrophy are peripheral or central in origin.[322-326] Saccades may also be defective in myasthenia gravis. These disorders are discussed in more detail in Chapters 14. Rare patients with mitochondrial disorders such as MELAS (mitochondrial encephalomyopathy, lactic acidosis, and stroke-like episodes—see Chapter 8) have been reported with slow horizontal saccades.[327]

Other Basal Ganglia Disorders. Slow or limited saccades, particularly in upgaze, have been reported in Wilson's disease.[328] We have also seen a patient with idiopathic calcification of the basal ganglia and dentate nuclei (Fahr's disease) presenting with supranuclear ophthalmoparesis and parkinsonism, mimicking progressive supranuclear palsy.[329]

Paraneoplastic Brain Stem Encephalitis. Ophthalmoparesis, both of nuclear and supranuclear origin, may be a manifestation of a paraneoplastic brain stem encephalitis. The anti-Hu antibody is most commonly associated antibody and lung cancer is the most frequently found tumor.[330] Recently, an antibody known as anti-Ta has been associated with testicular cancer and ophthalmoparesis.[331, 332]

ABNORMAL VERTICAL CONJUGATE GAZE DEVIATIONS

Oculogyric Crises

Oculogyric crises are a dystonia of ocular muscles[333] characterized by dramatic involuntary conjugate deviation of the eyes.[334] The eyes usually inadvertently move straight upward or up and to the left or right, and the position can change from crisis to crisis. Oculogyric crises are often associated with thought or emotional disturbances, are preceded by a brief stare, and last for hours.[335] However, they can occur without these features and last only a few seconds. Frequently they are accompanied by other dystonic or dyskinetic movements such as tongue protrusion, lip smacking, blepharospasm, choreoathetosis, anterocollis, and retrocollis.[336-338]

In the 1920's the French described crises (*crises oculogyres*) as complications of postencephalitic Parkinsonism,[334, 339] but today are they are usually acute or tardive extrapyramidal reactions to neuroleptics.[335-338, 340-342] In addition to postencephalitic parkinsonism, oculogyric crises have been associated with other neurologic disorders such as Parkinson's disease,[343] familial Parkinson-dementia syndrome,[344] dopa-responsive dystonia,[345] neurosyphilis, multiple sclerosis, ataxia-telangiectasia,[346] Rett syndrome,[347] Wilson's disease,[348] cerebellar disease, trauma,[349] acute herpetic brainstem encephalitis,[350] a third ventricular cystic glioma,[351] paraneoplastic disease,[331] and striatocapsular infarction.[352, 353] Besides neuroleptics, carbemazepine,[354, 355] tetrabenazine,[356] gabapentin,[357] and several other drugs[349] can also cause oculogyric crises.

The etiology of oculogyric crises is not certain. In postencephalitic patients, some authors believed they resulted from a release of supranuclear control of oculomotor centers due to injury to the corpus striatum or subthalamic nucleus.[334] Onuaguluchi[339] hypothesized they were due to an abnormal vestibulo-ocular reflex in the setting of brain stem lesions involving vestibular pathways. Leigh et al[335] attributed the deviations to an incorrect efference copy of eye position. Based on the response to anticholinergic agents in neuroleptic-induced crises, they alternatively invoked a defect in mesencephalic vertical gaze-holding mechanisms normally dependent on balanced cholinergic and dopaminergic systems.[335] Another hypothesis explains oculogyric crises as a limbic-motor disorder.[349]

Treatment. Severe or painful oculogyric crises can be treated acutely with benztropine 2 mg IM or IV or diphenhydramine 50 mg IM or IV.[349] A dose can be repeated in 30 minutes if there is no response. If these are unsuccessful, then diazepam 5 to 10 mg IV or lorazepam 1 mg IM or IV can be used. The underlying condition should be treated, or the offending drug removed or dosage lowered. Some patients with oculogyric crises due to neuroleptic use may require short-term treatment with oral benztropine 2 to 6 mg qd or oral trihexyphenidyl 4 to 15 mg qd for 2 weeks following the acute episode.[349] One reported patient improved with vagus nerve stimulation.[358] Seizures should be excluded with electroencephalography (EEG).

Ocular Tics

Brief dystonic eye rolling and torticollis, mimicking unsustained oculogyric crises, have also been described in tic disorders.[359, 360] Tourette syndrome is one that is inherited, and children with this disorder have vocal tics and behavioral disturbances in addition to motor tics.[361] Typically an irresistible urge and an ability to suppress the eye movements precedes them. Ninety percent of Tourette patients develop their first motor tic by age 10.[362] Isolated motor tics can be idiopathic or secondary to drugs or basal ganglia injury ("acquired tourettism").[361] When bothersome, the tics may be treated with dopamine antagonists. Eyelid tics are discussed in Chapter 14.

Benign Tonic Vertical Gaze in Infancy

Tonic up- or downward gaze in infants, lasting weeks to months, is well recognized (Fig. 16–25).[363-365] The finding was seen in 5 of 242 healthy neonates in one study.[366] The gaze deviation is typically intermittent, lasting minutes, hours, or days.[367] Children can appear to have either a supranuclear gaze deficit or jerk nystagmus in the direction opposite to the gaze preference.[368] The eyes can easily be moved into a normal position by the oculocephalic maneuver. There are usually no CNS abnormalities. The course is usually benign with a gradual decrease in the frequency and duration of the episodes, and ultimately the children are normal within the first few months of age.[369, 370] The mechanism is usually attributed to immaturity of either an ocular motor or visual pathway: the vertical gaze centers in the midbrain, the vestibulo-ocular reflexes, or the afferent visual system.[365]

All patients should undergo a careful pediatric neurologic examination and neuroimag-

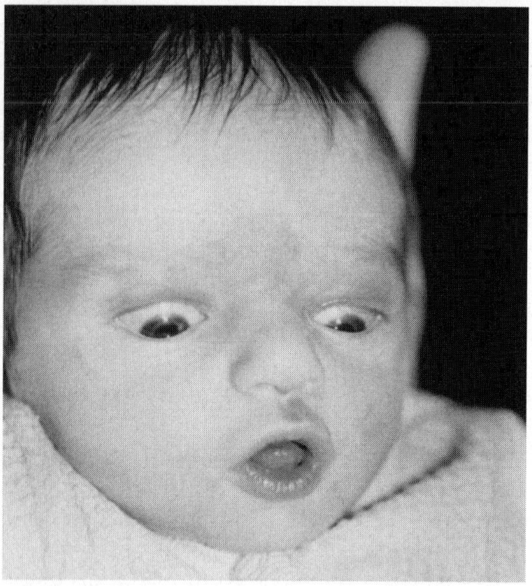

FIGURE 16–25. Ten-day-old infant exhibiting episodic tonic downward gaze, which was easily overcome by vertical oculocephalic movements. The workup was negative and the disorder spontaneously resolved by 4 months of age.

ing. This is particularly important in those with tonic downgaze, in whom a pretectal syndrome due to hydrocephalus or a pineal region mass needs to be considered. EEG should be performed to exclude seizure activity. Improvement with levodopa/carbidopa preparations has been reported. However, in most instances pharmacologic manipulations are not helpful and are usually unneccessary because of the self-limited nature of the disorder.

Acquired Cases. A variation of this condition has been described, in which some patients are normal at birth, but develop the ocular motility disorder later in infancy.[371] The onset of the tonic gaze in some instances follows an intercurrent illness or vaccination. Some patients have similarly affected family members. The outcome in these acquired cases may be less sanguine, with some patients later exhibiting developmental delay, intellectual disability, language delay, and either persistent tonic vertical gaze or other eye movement disorder.[372] The guarded prognosis may reflect the presence of a more widespread neurologic disorder.

COMPLETE OPHTHALMOPLEGIA

Most of the disorders that cause complete absence of eye movements are nuclear or infranuclear, affecting the oculomotor nerves, neuromuscular junction, or extraocular muscles. However, some supranuclear disorders discussed in this chapter, when severe or in their end stages, may affect the ocular motor nuclei and therefore disrupt all voluntary and involuntary eye movements. These include Wernicke's encephalopathy, spinocerebellar ataxias, and progressive supranuclear palsy. A list of disorders that cause complete ophthalmoplegia is in Chapter 15.

COMA

Conjugate gaze deviations and paresis during oculocephalic or vestibulo-ocular testing may be highly localizing in patients with coma.

Conjugate Gaze Deviations

The guidelines for considering causes according to those that cause horizontal versus vertical gaze deviations apply here as well. For instance, a horizontal conjugate gaze deviation may be caused by an ipsilateral hemispheric lesion (Figs. 16–13 and 16–14), contralateral pontine lesion, or contralateral hemispheric epileptic focus (Figs. 16–13 and 16–15). Occasionally "wrong-way" eyes due to a contralateral hemispheric or thalamic hemorrhage should be considered. Fast-cycle horizontal periodic alternating gaze, or "ping-pong" gaze, indicates an intact pons that is disconnected from bilateral hemispheric influences.

Eyes that are deviated downward suggest a dorsal midbrain or thalamic lesion such as an infarction, hemorrhage, or hydrocephalus. However, persistent downgaze has also been reported in patients with subarachnoid hemorrhage and hypoxic encephalopathy without pretectal lesions.[373] Tonic upgaze may be observed in anoxia, presumably due to diffuse injury to the cortex and cerebellum.[374] Inhibitory fibers from the cerebellum to the anterior semicircular canal projections are removed, resulting in tonic elevation of the eyes. Several weeks following the initial injury, downbeat nystamus may evolve as the cortical inputs begin to recover. In general, the appearance of tonic upgaze after anoxic arrest is a poor prognostic sign.

Conjugate Gaze Paresis

An inability to move the eyes conjugately either by the oculocephalic maneuver or by cold caloric stimulation (see Chapter 2) is highly suggestive of an ipsilateral sixth nerve nucleus lesion in the pons, but a vestibular nerve or nucleus lesion should also be excluded. Defective vertical gaze during reflex testing implies a midbrain lesion involving the inC or oculomotor nuclei, fascicles, or nerves. Voluntary saccadic and pursuit function is obviously untestable in comatose patients.

Localization in coma is discussed further in Chapter 2.

REFERENCES

1. Büttner-Ennever JA, Büttner U: Neuroanatomy of the ocular motor pathways. Baillière's Clin Neurol 1992;1:263–287.
2. Sharpe JA: Neural control of ocular motor systems. In: Miller NR, Newman NJ (eds): Walsh and Hoyt's Clinical Neuro-ophthalmology, 4th edition, pp 1101–1167. Baltimore, Williams & Wilkins, 1998.
3. Pierrot-Deseilligny C, Rivaud S, Gaymard B, et al: Cortical control of saccades. Ann Neurol 1995; 37:557–567.
4. Morrow MJ, Sharpe JA: Deficits of smooth-pursuit eye movement after unilateral frontal lobe lesions. Ann Neurol 1995;37:443–451.
5. Henn V: Pathophysiology of rapid eye movements in the horizontal, vertical and torsional directions. Bailliére's Clin Neurol 1992;1:373–391.
6. Pierrot-Deseilligny C, Gaymard B, Müri R, et al: Cerebral ocular motor signs. J Neurol 1997;244:65–70.
7. Godoy J, Lüders H, Dinner DS, et al: Versive eye movement elicited by cortical stimulation of the human brain. Neurology 1990;40:296–299.
8. Gaymard B, Pierrot-Deseilligny C, Rivaud S: Impairment of sequences of memory-guided saccades after supplementary motor area lesions. Ann Neurol 1990;28:622–626.
9. Gaymard B, Rivaud S, Pierrot-Deseilligny C: Role of the left and right supplementary motor areas in memory-guided saccade sequences. Ann Neurol 1993;34:404–406.
10. Schall JD: Neural basis of saccade target selection. Rev Neurosci 1995;6:63–85.
11. Sharpe JA: Cortical control of eye movements. Curr Opin Neurol 1998;11:31–38.
12. Bender MB: Brain control of conjugate horizontal and vertical eye movements. A survey of the structural and functional correlates. Brain 1980;103:23–69.
13. Pierrot-Deseilligny C, Rivaud S, Penet C, et al: Latencies of visually guided saccades in unilateral hemispheric cerebral lesions. Ann Neurol 1987;21: 138–148.
14. Leigh RJ, Rottach KG, Das VE: Transforming sensory perceptions into motor commands: evidence from programming of eye movements. Ann NY Acad Sci 1997;835:353–362.
15. Horn AKE, Büttner-Ennever JA, Büttner U: Saccadic premotor neurons in the brainstem: functional neuroanatomy and clinical implications. Neuro-ophthalmol 1996;16:229–240.
16. Büttner-Ennever JA, Horn AKE: Anatomical substrates of oculomotor control. Curr Opin Neurobiol 1997;7:872–879.
17. Kennard C, Crawford TJ, Henderson L: A pathophysiological approach to saccadic eye movements in neurological and psychiatric disease (editorial). J Neurol Neurosurg Psychiatry 1994;57:881–885.
18. Gaymard B, Rivaud S, Amarenco P, et al: Influence of visual information on cerebellar saccadic dysmetria. Ann Neurol 1994;35:108–112.
19. Morrow MJ, Sharpe JA: Cerebral hemispheric localization of smooth pursuit asymmetry. Neurology 1990;40:284–292.
20. Barton JJS, Sharpe JA, Raymond JE: Directional defects in pursuit and motion perception in humans with unilateral cerebral lesions. Brain 1996;119:1535–1550.
21. Petit L, Haxby JV: Functional anatomy of pursuit eye movements in humans as revealed by fMRI. J Neurophysiol 1999;81:463–471.
22. Heide W, Kurzidim K, Kömpf D: Deficits of smooth pursuit eye movements after frontal and parietal lesions. Brain 1996;119:1951–1969.
23. Johnston JL, Sharpe JA, Morrow MJ: Paresis of contralateral smooth pursuit and normal vestibular smooth eye movements after unilateral brainstem lesions. Ann Neurol 1992;31:495–502.
24. Ohtsuka K, Enoki T: Transcranial magnetic stimulation over the posterior cerebellum during smooth pursuit eye movements in man. Brain 1998; 121:429–435.
25. Bucher SF, Dieterich M, Seelos KC, et al: Sensorimotor cerebral activation during optokinetic nystagmus. Neurology 1997;49:1370–1377.
26. Rivaud S, Müri RM, Gaymard B, et al: Eye movement disorders after frontal eye field lesions in humans. Exp Brain Res 1994;102:110–120.
27. Pierrot-Deseilligny C: Saccade and smooth-pursuit impairment after cerebral hemispheric lesions. Eur Neurol 1994;34:121–134.
28. Thurston SE, Leigh RJ, Crawford T, et al: Two distinct deficits of visual tracking caused by unilateral lesions of cerebral cortex in humans. Ann Neurol 1988; 23:266–273.
29. Sharpe JA, Morrow MJ: Cerebral hemispheric smooth pursuit disorders. Acta Neurol Belg 1991;91:81–96.
30. Morrow MJ, Sharpe JA: Retinotopic and directional deficits of smooth pursuit initiation after posterior cerebral hemispheric lesions. Neurology 1993;43: 595–603.
31. Morrow MJ: Craniotopic defects of smooth pursuit and saccadic eye movements. Neurology 1996;46: 514–521.
32. Baloh RW, Yee RD, Honrubia V: Optokinetic nystagmus and parietal lobe lesions. Ann Neurol 1980; 7:269–276.
33. Dehaene I, Lammens M: Paralysis of saccades and pursuit: clinicopathologic study. Neurology 1991;41: 414–415.
34. Pierrot-Deseilligny C, Gautier J-C, Loron P: Acquired ocular motor apraxia due to bilateral frontoparietal infarcts. Ann Neurol 1988;23:65–70.
35. Sharpe JA, Johnston JL: Ocular motor paresis versus apraxia (letter). Ann Neurol 1989;25:209–210.
36. Pierrot-Deseilligny C, Goasguen J, Chain F, et al: Pontine metastasis with dissociated bilateral horizontal gaze paresis. J Neurol Neurosurg Psychiatry 1984; 47:159–164.
37. Baloh RW, Furman JM, Yee RD: Eye movements in patients with absent voluntary horizontal gaze. Ann Neurol 1985;17:283–286.

38. Hirose G, Furui K, Yoshioka A, et al: Unilateral conjugate gaze palsy due to a lesion of the abducens nucleus. J Clin Neuro-ophthalmol 1993;3:54–58.
39. Pierrot-Deseilligny C, Goasguen J: Isolated abducens nucleus damage due to histiocytosis X. Brain 1984;107:1019–1032.
40. Müri RM, Chermann JF, Cohen L, et al: Ocular motor consequences of damage to the abducens nucleus area in humans. J Neuro-ophthalmol 1996;16:191–195.
41. Larmande P, Hénin D, Jan M, et al: Abnormal vertical eye movements in the locked-in syndrome. Ann Neurol 1982;11:100–102.
42. Johnston JL, Sharpe JA, Ranalli PJ, et al: Oblique misdirection and slowing of vertical saccades after unilateral lesions of the pontine tegmentum. Neurology 1993;43:2238–2244.
43. Hanson MR, Hamid MA, Tomsak RL, et al: Selective saccadic palsy caused by pontine lesions: clinical, physiological and pathological correlations. Ann Neurol 1986;20:209–217.
44. Fisher CM: Some neuro-ophthalmological observations. J Neurol Neurosurg Psychiatry 1967;30:383–392.
45. Sharpe JA, Rosenberg MA, Hoyt WF, et al: Paralytic pontine exotropia. A sign of acute unilateral pontine gaze palsy and internuclear ophthalmoplegia. Neurology 1974;24:1076–1081.
46. Pierrot-Deseilligny C, Chain F, Serdaru M, et al: The 'one-and-a-half' syndrome. Electro-oculographic analyses of five cases with deductions about the physiological mechanisms of lateral gaze. Brain 1981; 104:665–699.
47. Wall M, Wray SH: The one-and-a-half syndrome—a unilateral disorder of the pontine tegmentum: a study of 20 cases and review of the literature. Neurology 1983;33:971–980.
48. Bogousslavsky J, Miklossy J, Regli F, et al: One-and-a-half syndrome in ischaemic locked-in state: a clinicopathological study. J Neurol Neurosurg Psychiatry 1984;47:927–935.
49. Deleu D, Solheid C, Michotte A, et al: Dissociated ipsilateral horizontal gaze palsy in one-and-a-half syndrome. Neurology 1988;38:1278–1280.
50. Foville A: Note sur une paralysie peu connue de certains muscles de l'oeil, et sa liaison avec quelques poins de l'anatomie et la physiologie de la protubérance annulaire. Bull Soc Anat Paris 1858;33:393–414.
51. Silverman IE, Liu GT, Volpe NJ, et al: The crossed paralyses: the original brainstem syndromes of Millard–Gubler, Foville, Weber, and Raymond–Cestan. Arch Neurol 1995;52:635–638.
52. Nordgren RE, Markesbery WR, Fukuda K, et al: Seven cases of cerebromedullospinal disconnection. The "locked in" syndrome. Neurology 1971;21:1140–1148.
53. Thier P, Bachor A, Faiss J, et al: Selective impairment of smooth-pursuit eye movements due to an ischemic lesion of the basal pons. Ann Neurol 1991;29:443–448.
54. Bassetti C, Bogousslavsky J, Barth A, et al: Isolated infarcts of the pons. Neurology 1996;46:165–175.
55. Galetta SL, Balcer LJ, Liu GT: Giant cell arteritis with unusual flow-related neuro-ophthalmologic manifestations. Neurology 1997;49:1463–1465.
56. Eggenberger E: Eight-and-a-half syndrome: one-and-a-half syndrome plus cranial nerve VII palsy. J Neuro-ophthalmol 1998;18:114–116.
57. Tan E, Kansu T: Bilateral horizontal gaze palsy in multiple sclerosis. J Clin Neuro-ophthalmol 1990;10: 124–127.
58. Hamed LF, Schatz NJ, Galetta SL: Brainstem ocular motility defects and AIDS. Am J Ophthalmol 1988;106:437–442.
59. Ayus JC, Krothapalli RK, Arieff AI: Treatment of symptomatic hyponatreia and its relation to brain damage. A prospective study. N Engl J Med 1987;317:1190–1195.
60. Brunner JE, Redmond JM, Haggar AM, et al.: Central pontine myelinolysis and pontine lesions after rapid correction of hyponatremia: a prospective magnetic resonance imaging study. Ann Neurol 1990;27:61–66.
61. Zackon DH, Sharpe JA: Midbrain paresis of horizontal gaze. Ann Neurol 1984;16:495–504.
62. Pierrot-Deseilligny C, Rosa A, Masmoudi K, et al: Saccadic deficits after a unilateral lesion affecting the superior colliculus. J Neurol Neurosurg Psychiatry 1991;54:1106–1109.
63. Kommerell G, Hoyt WF: Lateropulsion of saccadic eye movements: electro-oculographic studies in a patient with Wallenberg's syndrome. Arch Neurol 1973;28:313–318.
64. Meyer KT, Baloh RW, Krohel GB, et al: Ocular lateropulsion. A sign of lateral medullary disease. Arch Ophthalmol 1980;98:1614–1616.
65. Kirkham TH, Guitton D, Gans M: Task dependent variations of ocular lateropulsion in Wallenberg's syndrome. Can J Neurol Sci 1981;8:21–26.
66. Waespe W, Wichmann W: Oculomotor disturbances during visual-vestibular interaction in Wallenberg's lateral medullary syndrome. Brain 1990;113:821–846.
67. Baloh RW, Yee RD, Honrubia V: Eye movements in patients with Wallenberg's syndrome. Ann NY Acad Sci 1981;600–613.
68. Crevits L, vander Eecken H: Ocular lateropulsion in Wallenberg's syndrome: A prospective clinical study. Acta Neurol Scand 1982;65:219–222.
69. Estañol B, Lopez-Rios G: Neuro-otology of the lateral medullary infarct syndrome. Arch Neurol 1982;39:176–179.
70. Brazis PW: Ocular motor abnormalities in Wallenberg's lateral medullary syndrome. Mayo Clin Proc 1992;67:365–368.
71. Hörnsten G: Wallenberg's syndrome. Part I. General symptomology, with special reference to visual disturbances and imbalance. Part II. Oculomotor and oculostatic disturbances. Acta Neurol Scand 1974;50:434–468.
72. Solomon D, Galetta SL, Liu GT: Possible mechanisms for horizontal gaze deviation and lateropulsion in the lateral medullary syndrome. J Neuro-ophthalmol 1995;15:26–30.
73. Furman JMR, Hurtt MR, Hirsch WL: Asymmetrical ocular pursuit with posterior fossa tumors. Ann Neurol 1991;30:208–211.
74. Zee DS, Leigh RJ, Mathieu-Millaire F: Cerebellar control of ocular gaze stability. Ann Neurol 1980;7:37–40.
75. Ranalli PJ, Sharpe JA: Contrapulsion of saccades and ipsilateral ataxia: a unilateral disorder of the rostral cerebellum. Ann Neurol 1986;20:311–316.
76. Baloh RW, Konrad HR, Dirks D, et al: Cerebellar-pontine angle tumors. Results of quantitative vestibulo-ocular testing. Arch Neurol 1976;33: 507–512.
77. Tychsen L: Pediatric ocular motility disorders of neuro-ophthalmic significance. Ophthalmol Clin North Am 1991;4:615–643.
78. Zee DS, Yee RD, Singer HS: Congenital ocular motor apraxia. Brain 1977;100:581–599.

79. Gresty MA: Disorders of head–eye coordination. Baillire's Clin Neurol 1992;1:317–343.
80. Hughes JL, O'Connor PS, Larsen PD, et al: Congenital vertical ocular motor apraxia. J Clin Neuro-ophthalmol 1985;5:153–157.
81. Ebner RB, Lopez L, Ochoa S, et al: Vertical ocular motor apraxia. Neurology 1990;40:712–713.
82. Prasad P, Nair S: Congenital ocular motor apraxia: sporadic and familial. Support for natural resolution. J Clin Neuro-ophthalmol 1994;14:102–104.
83. Cogan DG, Chu FU, Reingold RD, et al: A long-term follow up of congenital ocular motor apraxia: a case report. Neuro-ophthalmology 1980;1:145–147.
84. Daroff RB, Troost BT, Leigh RJ: Supranuclear disorders of eye movements. Clin Ophthalmol 1988;10: 8–9.
85. Harris CM, Shawkat F, Russell-Eggitt I, et al: Intermittent horizontal saccade failure ('ocular motor apraxia') in children. Br J Ophthalmol 1996; 80:151–158.
86. Cogan DG: A type of congenital ocular motor apraxia presenting with jerky head movements. Trans Am Acad Ophthalmol Otol 1952;56:853–862.
87. Eustace P, Beigi B, Bowell R, et al: Congenital ocular motor apraxia. Neuro-ophthalmology 1994;14:167–174.
88. Narbona J, Crisci CD, Villa I: Familial congenital ocular motor apraxia and immune deficiency (letter). Arch Neurol 1980;37:325.
89. Whitsel EA, Castillo M, D'Cruz O: Cerebellar vermis and midbrain dysgenesis in oculomotor apraxia: MR findings. AJNR Am J Neuroradiol 1995;16 (Suppl 4):831–834.
90. Fielder AR, Gresty MA, Dodd KL, et al: Congenital ocular motor apraxia. Trans Ophthalmol Soc U K 1986;105:589–598.
91. Borchert MS, Sadun AA, Sommers JD, et al: Congenital ocular motor apraxia in twins. J Clin Neuro-ophthalmol 1987;7:104–107.
92. Lambert SR, Kriss A, Gresty M, et al: Joubert syndrome. Arch Ophthalmol 1989;107:709–713.
93. Donaldson MDC, Werner AA, Trompeter RS, et al: Familial juvenile nephronophthisis, Jeune's syndrome, and associated disorders. Arch Dis Child 1985;60:426–434.
94. Moore AT, Taylor SI: A syndrome of congenital retinal dystrophy and saccade palsy—a subset of Leber's amaurosis. Br J Ophthalmol 1984;68:421–431.
95. Zaret CR, Behrens MM, Eggers HM: Congenital ocular motor apraxia and brainstem tumor. Arch Ophthalmol 1980;98:328–330.
96. Bundey S: Clinical and genetic features of ataxia-telangiectasia. Int J Radiat Biol 1994;66:S23–29.
97. Cohen LE, Tanner DJ, Schaefer HG, et al: Common and uncommon cutaneous findings in patients with ataxia-telangiectasia. J Am Acad Dermatol 1984;10:431–438.
98. Woods CG, Taylor AM: Ataxia telangiectasia in the British Isles: the clinical and laboratory features of 70 affected individuals. Q J Med 1992;82:169–179.
99. Swift M, Morrell D, Massey RB, et al: Incidence of cancer in 161 families affected by ataxia-telangiectasia. N Engl J Med 1991;32:1831–1836.
100. Bebb G, Glickman B, Gelmon K, et al: "At risk" for breast cancer. Lancet 1997;349:1784–1785.
101. Case records of the Massachusetts General Hospital: Case 2-1987. N Engl J Med 1987;316:91–100.
102. Carbonari M, Cherchi M, Paganelli R, et al: Relative increase of T cells expressing the gamma/delta rather than the alpha/beta receptor in ataxia-telangiectasia. N Engl J Med 1990;322:73–76.
103. Hurko O: Recent advances in heritable ataxias (editorial). Ann Neurol 1997;41:4–6.
104. Baloh RW, Yee RD, Boder E: Eye movements in ataxia telangiectasia. Neurology 1978;28:1099–1104.
105. Stell R, Bronstein AM, Plant GT, et al: Ataxia telangiectasia: a reappraisal of the ocular motor features and their value in the diagnosis of atypical cases. Mov Disord 1989;4:320–329.
106. Lewis RF, Lederman HM, Crawford TO: Ocular motor abnormalities in ataxia telangiectasia. Ann Neurol 1999;46:287–295.
107. Cogan DG, Chu FC, Reingold D, et al: Ocular motor signs in some metabolic diseases. Arch Ophthalmol 1981;99:1802–1808.
108. Farina L, Uggetti C, Ottolini A, et al: Ataxia-telangiectasia: MR and CT findings. J Comput Assist Tomogr 1994;18:724–727.
109. Rivaud-Pechoux S, Durr A, Gaymard B, et al: Eye movement abnormalities correlate with genotype in autosomal dominant cerebellar ataxia type I. Ann Neurol 1998;43:297–302.
110. Gouw LG, Digre KB, Harris CP, et al: Autosomal dominant cerebellar ataxia with retinal degeneration: clinical, neuropathic, and genetic analysis of a large kindred. Neurology 1994;44:1441–1447.
111. Rosenberg RN: Autosomal dominant cerebellar phenotypes: the genotype has settled the issue (editorial). Neurology 1995;45:1–5.
112. Moseley MI, Benzow KA, Schut LJ, et al: Incidence of dominant spinocerebellar and Friedreich triplet repeats among 361 ataxia families. Neurology 1998;51:1666–1671.
113. Martin JB: Molecular basis of the neurodegenerative disorders. N Engl J Med 1999;340:1970–1980.
114. Harding AE: Clinical feature and classification of inherited ataxias. Adv Neurol 1993;61:1–14.
115. Baloh RW, Konrad HR, Honrubia V: Vestibulo-ocular function in patients with cerebellar atrophy. Neurology 1975;25:160–168.
116. Zee DS, Yee RD, Cogan DG, et al: Ocular motor abnormalities in hereditary cerebellar ataxia. Brain 1976;99:207–234.
117. Koeppen AH, Hans MB: Supranuclear ophthalmoplegia in olivopontocerebellar degeneration. Neurology 1976;26:764–768.
118. Wadia N, Pang J, Desai J, et al: A clinicogenetic analysis of six Indian spinocerebellar ataxia (SCA2) pedigrees. The significance of slow saccades in diagnosis. Brain 1998;121:2341–2355.
119. Zee DS, Optican LM, Cook JD, et al: Slow saccades in spinocerebellar degeneration. Arch Neurol 1976; 33:243–251.
120. Murphy MJ, Goldblatt D: Slow eye movements with absent saccades, in a patient with hereditary ataxia. Arch Neurol 1977;34:191–195.
121. Abe T, Abe K, Aoki M, et al: Ocular changes in patients with spinocerebellar degeneration and repeated trinucleotide expansion of spinocerebellar ataxia type 1 gene. Arch Ophthalmol 1997;115:231–236.
122. Colan RV, Snead OC, Ceballos R: Olivopontocerebellar atrophy in children: a report of seven cases in two families. Ann Neurol 1981;10:355–363.
123. Wüllner U, Klockgether T, Petersen D, et al: Magnetic resonance imaging in hereditary and idiopathic ataxia. Neurology 1993;43:318–325.

124. Lepore FE: Disorders of ocular motility in the olivopontocerebellar atrophies. Adv Neurol 1984;41:97–103.
125. Case records of the Massachusetts General Hospital: Case 30-1992. N Engl J Med 1992;327:261–268.
126. Starr A: A disorder of rapid eye movements in Huntington's chorea. Brain 1967;90:545–564.
127. Leigh RJ, Newman SA, Folstein SE, et al: Abnormal ocular motor control in Huntington's disease. Neurology 1983;33:1268–1275.
128. Lasker AG, Zee DS, Hain TC, et al: Saccades in Huntington's disease: slowing and dysmetria. Neurology 1988;38:427–431.
129. Lasker AG, Zee DS, Hain TC, et al: Saccades in Huntington's disease: initiation defects and distractibility. Neurology 1987;37:364–370.
130. Tian JR, Zee DS, Lasker AG, et al: Saccades in Huntington's disease: predictive tracking and interaction between release of fixation and initiation of saccades. Neurology 1991;41:875–881.
131. Lasker AG, Zee DS: Ocular motor abnormalities in Huntington's disease. Vision Res 1997;37:3639–3645.
132. White OB, Saint-Cyr JA, Tomlinson RD, et al: Ocular motor deficits in Parkinson's disease. II. Control of the saccadic and smooth pursuit systems. Brain 1983;106:571–587.
133. Crawford TJ, Henderson L, Kennard C: Abnormalities of nonvisually guided eye movements in Parkinson's disease. Brain 1989;112:1573–1586.
134. Gibson JM, Pimlott RM, Kennard C: Oculomotor and manual tracking in Parkinson's disease and the effect of treatment. J Neurol Neurosurg Psychiatr 1987;50:853–860.
135. Rascol O, Clanet M, Montastruc JL, et al: Abnormal ocular movements in Parkinson's disease: evidence for involvement of dopaminergic systems. Brain 1989;112:1193–1214.
136. Sharpe JA, Fletcher WA, Lang AE, et al: Smooth pursuit during dose related on–off fluctuations in Parkinson's disease. Neurology 1987;37:1389–1392.
137. Stern MB: Contemporary approaches to the pharmacotherapeutic management of Parkinson's disease: an overview. Neurology 1997;49(Suppl 1):S2–S9.
138. Olanow CW, Koller WC: An algorithm (decision tree) for the management of Parkinson's disease: treatment guidelines. Neurology 1998;50(Suppl 3):S1–S57.
139. Lang AE, Lozano AM: Parkinson's disease. N Engl J Med 1998;339:1044–1053, 1130–1143.
140. Schneider JA, Watts RL, Gearing M: Corticobasal degeneration: neuropathologic and clinical heterogeneity. Neurology 1997;48:959–969.
141. Riley DE, Lang AE, Lewis A, et al: Cortical-basal ganglionic degeneration. Neurology 1990;40:1203–1212.
142. Grimes DA, Lang AE, Bergeron CB: Dementia as the most common presentation of cortical-basal ganglionic degeneration. Neurology 1999;53:1969–1974.
143. Gibb WRG, Luthert PJ, Marsden CD: Corticobasal degeneration. Brain 1989;112:1171–1192.
144. Vidailhet M, Rivaud S, Gouider-Khouja N, et al: Eye movements in Parkinsonian syndromes. Ann Neurol 1994;35:420–426.
145. Soliveri P, Monza D, Paridi D, et al: Cognitive and magnetic resonance imaging aspects of corticobasal degeneration and progressive supranuclear palsy. Neurology 1999;53:502–507.
146. Kompoliti K, Goetz CG, Boeve BF, et al: Clinical presentation and pharmacological therapy in corticobasal degeneration. Arch Neurol 1998;55:957–961.
147. Tsuji S, Choudary PV, Martin BM, et al: A mutation in the human glucocerebrosidase gene in neuronopathic Gaucher's disease. N Engl J Med 1987;316:570–575.
148. Patterson MC, Horowitz M, Abel RB, et al: Isolated horizontal supranuclear gaze palsy as a marker of severe systemic involvement in Gaucher's disease. Neurology 1993;43:1993–1997.
149. Shawkat FS, Kingsley D, Kendall B, et al: Neuroradiological and eye movement correlates in children with intermittent saccade failure: "ocular motor apraxia." Neuropediatrics 1995;26:298–305.
150. Abel LA, Levin S, Holzman PS: Abnormalities of smooth pursuit and saccadic control in schizophrenia and affective disorders. Vision Res 1992;32:1009–1014.
151. Clementz BA, Sweeney JA: Is eye movement dysfunction a biological marker for schizophrenia? A methodological review. Psychol Bull 1990;108:77–92.
152. Fletcher WA, Sharpe JA: Saccadic eye movement dysfunction in Alzheimer's disease. Ann Neurol 1986; 20:464–471.
153. Currie J, Ramsden B, McArthur C, et al: Validation of a clinical antisaccadic eye movement test in the assessment of dementia. Arch Neurol 1991;48: 644–648.
154. Hutton S, Kennard C: Oculomotor abnormalities in schizophrenia. A critical review. Neurology 1998; 50:604–609.
155. Fletcher WA, Sharpe JA: Smooth pursuit dysfunction in Alzheimer's disease. Neurology 1988;38:272–277.
156. Thaker GK, Ross DE, Cassady SL, et al: Smooth pursuit eye movements to extraretinal motion signals: deficits in relative of patients with schizophrenia. Arch Gen Psychiatry 1998;55:830–836.
157. Charness ME, Simon RP, Greenberg DA: Ethanol and the nervous system. N Engl J Med 1989;321:442–454.
158. Victor M, Adams RD, Collins GH: The Wernicke–Korsakoff Syndrome and Related Neurologic Disorders due to Alcoholism and Malnutrition, 2nd edition, pp 17–21,31–34,114–116. Philadelphia, FA Davis, 1989.
159. Reuler JB, Girard DE, Cooney TG: Wernicke's encephalopathy. N Engl J Med 1985;312:1035–1039.
160. Furman JMR, Becker JT: Vestibular responses in Wernicke's encephalopathy. Ann Neurol 1989;26: 669–674.
161. Charness ME, DeLaPaz RL: Mamillary body atrophy in Wernicke's encephalopathy: antemortem identification using magnetic resonance imaging. Ann Neurol 1987;22:595–600.
162. Antunez E, Estruch R, Cardenal C, et al: Usefulness of CT and MRI imaging in the diagnosis of acute Wernicke's encephalopathy. AJR, Am J Roentgenol 1998;171:1131–1137.
163. Sedwick LA, Burde RM, Hodges FJ: Leigh's subacute necrotizing encephalomyelopathy manifesting as spasmus nutans. Arch Ophthalmol 1984;102:1046–1048.
164. DiMauro S, De Vivo DC: Genetic heterogeneity in Leigh syndrome. Ann Neurol 1996;40:5–7.
165. Shoffner JM, Fernhoff PM, Krawiecki NS, et al: Subacute necrotizing encephalopathy: oxidative phosphorylation defects and the ATPase 6 point mutation. Neurology 1992;42:2168–2174.
166. Santorelli FM, Shanske S, Macaya A, et al: The mutation at nt 8993 of mitochondrial DNA is a common cause of Leigh's syndrome. Ann Neurol 1993; 34:827–834.

167. Morris AAM, Leonard JV, Brown GK, et al: Deficiency of respiratory chain complex I is a common cause of Leigh disease. Ann Neurol 1996;40:25–30.
168. Kayden HJ: The neurologic syndorme of vitamin E deficiency: a significant cause of ataxia (editorial). Neurology 1993;43:2167–2169.
169. Hamida MB, Belal S, Sirugo G, et al: Friedreich's ataxia phenotype not linked to chromosome 9 and associated with selective autosomal recessive vitamin E deficiency in two inbred Tunisian families. Neurology 1993;43:2179–2183.
170. Perkin GD, Murray-Lyon I: Neurology and the gastrointestinal system. J Neurol Neurosurg Psychiatry 1998;65:291–300.
171. Tijssen CC, van Gisbergen JAM, Schulte BPM: Conjugate eye deviation: side, site, and size of the hemispheric lesion. Neurology 1991;41:846–850.
172. Pessin MS, Adelman LS, Prager RJ, et al: 'Wrong-way eyes' in supratentorial hemorrhage. Ann Neurol 1981;9:79-81.
173. Tijssen CC: Contralateral conjugate eye deviation in acute supratentorial lesions. Stroke 1994;25:1516–1519.
174. Sharpe JA, Bondar RL, Fletcher WA: Contralateral gaze deviation after frontal lobe haemorrhage. J Neurol Neurosurg Psychiatry 1985;48:86–88.
175. Kernan JC, Devinsky O, Luciano DJ, et al: Lateralizing significance of head and eye deviation in secondary generalized tonic–clonic seizures. Neurology 1993;43:1308–1310.
176. Kumral E, Kocaer T, Ertübey NÖ, et al: Thalamic hemorrhage. A prospective study of 100 patients. Stroke 1995;26:964–970.
177. Steinke W, Sacco RL, Mohr JP, et al: Thalamic stroke. Presentation and prognosis of infarcts and hemorrhages. Arch Neurol 1992;49:703–710.
178. Chung CS, Caplan LR, Han W, et al: Thalamic haemorrhage. Brain 1996;119:1873–1886.
179. Keane JR: Contralateral gaze deviation with supratentorial hemorrhage: three pathologically verified cases. Arch Neurol 1975;32:119–122.
180. Averbuch-Heller L, Meiner Z: Reversible periodic alternating gaze deviation in hepatic encephalopathy. Neurology 1995;45:191–192.
181. Legge RH, Weiss HS, Hedges TR, et al: Periodic alternating gaze deviation in infancy. Neurology 1992;42:1740–1743.
182. Ishikawa H, Ishikawa S, Mukuno K: Short-cycle periodic alternating (ping-pong) gaze. Neurology 1993;43:1067–1070.
183. Johkura K, Komiyama A, Tobita M, et al: Saccadic ping-pong gaze. J Neuro-ophthalmol 1998;18:43–46.
184. Stewart JD, Kirkham TH, Mathieson G: Periodic alternating gaze. Neurology 1979;29:222–224.
185. Masucci EF, Fabara JA, Saini N, et al: Periodic alternating ping-pong gaze. Ann Ophthalmol 1981;13: 1123–1127.
186. Larmande P, Henin D, Jan M, et al: Periodic alternating gaze: electro-oculographic and anatomical observation of a new case. Neurosurgery 1982;10:263–265.
187. Senelick RC: "Ping-pong" gaze: periodic alternating gaze deviation. Neurology 1976;26:532–535.
188. Larmande P, Dongmo L, Limodin J, et al: Periodic alternating gaze: a case without any hemispheric lesion. Neurosurgery 1987;20:481–483.
189. Pasik P, Pasik T, Bender MB: The pretectal syndrome in monkeys. I. Disturbances of gaze and body posture. Brain 1969;92:521–534.
190. Pierrot-Deseilligny C, Chain F, Gray F, et al: Parinaud's syndrome. Electro-oculographic and anatomical analyses of six vascular cases with deductions about vertical gaze organization in the premotor structures. Brain 1982;105:667–696.
191. Büttner-Ennever JA, Büttner U, Cohen B, et al: Vertical gaze paralysis and the rostral interstitial nucleus of the medial longitudinal fasciculus. Brain 1982; 105:125–149.
192. Hommel M, Bogousslavsky J: The spectrum of vertical gaze palsy following unilateral brainstem stroke. Neurology 1991;41:1229–1234.
193. Büttner U, Büttner-Ennever JA, Henn V: Vertical eye movement related unit activity in the rostral mesecephalic reticular formation of the alert monkey. Brain Res 1977;130:239–252.
194. Leigh RJ, Zee DS: The Neurology of Eye Movements, 3rd edition, pp 511–520. New York, Oxford University Press, 1999.
195. Bhidayasiri R, Plant GT, Leigh RJ: New concepts of mechanisms for vertical gaze. Development of a scheme to interpret the effects of brain stem lesions. Neurology 2000;54:1985–1993.
196. Horn AKE, Büttner-Ennever JA: Premotor neurons for vertical eye movements in the rostral mesencephalon of monkey and human: histologic identification by parvalbumin immunostaining. J Comp Neurol 1998;392:413–427.
197. Clark JM, Albers GW: Vertical gaze palsies from medial thalamic infarctions without midbrain involvement. Stroke 1995;26:1467–1470.
198. Ouvrier R: Henri Parinaud and his syndrome. Med J Aust 1993;158:711–714.
199. Parinaud H: Paralysie des mouvements associés des yeux. Arch Neurol 1883;5:145–172.
200. Parinaud H: Paralysis of the movement of convergence of the eyes. Brain 1886;9:330–341.
201. Keane JR: The pretectal syndrome: 206 patients. Neurology 1990;40:684–690.
202. Hatcher MA, Klintworth GK: The sylvian aqueduct syndrome. A clinicopathologic study. Arch Neurol 1966;15:215–222.
203. Nothnagel H: On the diagnosis of diseases of the corpora quadrigemina. Brain 1889;12:21–35.
204. Liu GT, Crenner CW, Logigian EL, et al: Midbrain syndromes of Benedikt, Claude, and Nothnagel: setting the record straight. Neurology 1992;42:1820–1822.
205. Keane JR, Davis RL: Pretectal syndrome with metastatic malignant melanoma to the posterior commissure. Am J Ophthalmol 1976;82:910–914.
206. Baloh RW, Furman JM, Yee RD: Dorsal midbrain syndrome: clinical and oculographic findings. Neurology 1985;35:54–60.
207. Caplan LR: "Top of the basilar" syndrome. Neurology 1980;30:72–79.
208. Hertle RW, Bienfang DC: Oculographic analysis of acute esotropia secondary to a thalamic hemorrhage. J Clin Neuro-ophthalmol 1990;10:21–26.
209. Gomez CR, Gomez SM, Selhorst JB: Acute thalamic esotropia. Neurology 1988;38:1759–1762.
210. Siatkowski RM, Schatz NJ, Sellitti TP, et al: Do thalamic lesions really cause vertical gaze palsies? J Clin Neuro-ophthalmol 1993;13:190–193.
211. Masdeu J, Brannegan R, Rosenberg M, et al: Pseudoabducens palsy with midbrain lesions (abstract). Ann Neurol 1980;8:103.
212. Corbett JJ, Schatz NJ, Shults WT, et al: Slowly alternating skew deviation: description of a pretectal syndrome in three patients. Ann Neurol 1981;10:540–546.

213. Hedges TR, Hoyt WF: Ocular tilt reaction due to an upper brainstem lesion: paroxysmal skew deviation, torsion, and oscillation of the eyes with head tilt. Ann Neurol 1982;11:537–540.
214. Swash M: Periaqueductal dysfunction (the Sylvian aqueduct syndrome): a sign of hydrocephalus? J Neurol Neurosurg Psychiatry 1974;37:21–26.
215. Corbett JJ: Neuro-ophthalmologic complications of hydrocephalus and shunting procedures. Semin Neurol 1986;6:111–123.
216. Donat JF, Okazaki H, Gomez MR, et al: Pineal tumors: a 53-year experience. Arch Neurol 1978;35:736–740.
217. Cho B-K, Wang K-C, Nam D-H, et al: Pineal tumors: experience with 48 cases over 10 years. Child's Nerv Syst 1998;14:53–58.
218. Halperin EC, Constine LS, Tarbell NJ, et al: Supratentorial brain tumors except ependymoma; brain tumors in babies and very young children. In: Pediatric Radiation Oncology, 2nd edition, pp 40–89. New York, Raven Press, 1994.
219. Fetell MR, Bruce JN, Burke AM, et al: Non-neoplastic pineal cysts. Neurology 1991;41:1034–1040.
220. Apuzzo MLJ, Davey LM, Manuelidis EE: Pineal apoplexy associated with anticoagulant therapy. J Neurosurg 1976;45:223–226.
221. Squires LA, Allen JC, Abbott R, et al: Focal tectal tumors: management and prognosis. Neurology 1994;44:953–956.
222. May PL, Blaser SI, Hoffman HJ, et al: Benign intrinsic tectal "tumors" in children. J Neurosurg 1991;74: 867–871.
223. Vandertop WP, Hoffman HJ, Drake JM, et al: Focal midbrain tumors in children. Neurosurgery 1992; 31:186–194.
224. Segarra JM: Cerebral vascular disease and behavior. I: The syndrome of the mesencephalic artery (basilar artery bifurcation). Arch Neurol 1970;22:408–418.
225. Percheron G: Les artères du thalamus humain, II: Artères et territoires thalmiques paramédians de l'artère basilaire communicante. Rev Neurol (Paris) 1976;132:309–324.
226. Castaigne P, Lhermitte F, Buge A, et al: Paramedian thalamic and midbrain infarcts: clinical and neuropathological study. Ann Neurol 1981;10:127–148.
227. Sieben G, De Reuck J, Vander Eecken H: Thrombosis of the mesencephalic artery. A clinico-pathological study of two cases and its correlation with the arterial vascularisation. Acta Neurol Belg 1977;77:151–162.
228. Bogousslavsky J, Regli F, Uske A: Thalamic infarcts: clinical syndormes, etiology, and prognosis. Neurology 1988;38:837–848.
229. Tatemichi TK, Steinke W, Duncan C, et al: Paramedian thalamopeduncular infarction: clinical syndromes and magnetic resonance imaging. Ann Neurol 1992;32:162–171.
230. Beversdorf DQ, Jenkyn LR, Petrowski JT, et al: Vertical gaze paralysis and intermittent unresponsiveness in a patient with a thalamomesencephalic stroke. J Neuro-ophthalmol 1995;15:230–235.
231. Bassetti C, Mathis J, Gugger M, et al: Hypersomnia following paramedian thalamic stroke. Ann Neurol 1996;39:471–480.
232. Bogousslavsky J, Miklossy J, Deruaz JP, et al: Unilateral left paramedian infarction of the thalamus and midbrain: a clinico-pathological study. J Neurol Neurosurg Psychiatry 1986;49:686–694.
233. Walshe TM, Davis KR, Fisher CM: Thalamic hemorrhage: a computed tomographic-clinical correlation. Neurology 1977;27:217–222.
234. Christoff N: A clinicopathological study of vertical eye movements. Arch Neurol 1974;31:1–8.
235. Keane JR: Neuro-ophthalmologic signs of AIDS: 50 patients. Neurology 1991;41:841–845.
236. Hedges TR, Katz B, Slavin M: Ophthalmoplegia associated with AIDS. Surv Ophthalmol 1994;39:43–51.
237. Keane JR: Bilateral ocular motor signs after tentorial herniation in 25 patients. Arch Neurol 1986;43: 806–807.
238. Sand JJ, Biller J, Corbett JJ, et al: Partial dorsal mesencephalic hemorrhages. Report of three cases. Neurology 1986;36:529–533.
239. Lee AG, Brown DG, Diaz PJ: Dorsal midbrain syndrome due to mesencephalic hemorrhage. Case report with serial imaging. J Neuro-ophthalmol 1996; 16:281–285.
240. Slyman JF, Kline LB: Dorsal midbrain syndrome in multiple sclerosis. Neurology 1981;31:196–198.
241. Trend P, Youl BD, Sanders MD, et al: Vertical gaze palsy due to a resolving midbrain lesion (letter). J Neurol Neurosurg Psychiatry 1990;53:708.
242. Quint DJ, Cornblath WT, Trobe JD: Multiple sclerosis presenting as Parinaud syndrome. AJNR Am J Neuroradiol 1993;14:1200–1202.
243. Coppeto JR, Lessell S: Dorsal midbrain syndrome from giant aneurysm of the posterior fossa: report of two cases. Neurology 1983;33:732–736.
244. Trojanowski JQ, Wray SH: Vertical gaze ophthalmoplegia: selective paralysis of downgaze. Neurology 1980;30:605–610.
245. Jacobs L, Anderson PJ, Bender MB: The lesions producing paralysis of downward but not upward gaze. Arch Neurol 1973;28:319–323.
246. Halmagyi GM, Evans WA, Hallinan JM: Failure of downward gaze. The site and nature of the lesion. Arch Neurol 1978;35:22–26.
247. Trojanowski JQ, Lafontaine MH: Neuroanatomical correlates of selective downgaze paralysis. J Neurol Sci 1981;52:91–101.
248. Jacobs L, Heffner RR, Newman RP: Selective paralysis of downward gaze caused by bilateral lesions of the mesencephalic periaqueductal gray matter. Neurology 1985;35:516–521.
249. Green JP, Newman NJ, Winterkorn JS: Paralysis of downgaze in two patients with clinical-radiologic correlation. Arch Ophthalmol 1993;111:219–222.
250. Cogan DC: Paralysis of down-gaze. Arch Ophthalmol 1974;91:192–199.
251. Bogousslavsky J, Regli F: Upgaze palsy and monocular paresis of downward gaze from ipsilateral thalamo-mesencephalic infarction: a vertical "one-and-a-half" syndrome. J Neurol 1984;231:43–45.
252. Deleu D, Buisseret T, Ebinger G: Vertical one-and-a-half syndrome. Supranuclear downgaze paralysis with monocular elevation palsy. Arch Neurol 1989;46:1361–1363.
253. Chamberlain W: Restriction in upward gaze with advancing age. Trans Am Ophthalmol Soc 1970;68:234–244.
254. Richardson JC, Steele J, Olszewski J: Supranuclear ophthalmoplegia, pseudobulbar palsy, nuchal dystonia and dementia: a clinical report on eight cases of 'heterogeneous system degeneration'. Trans Am Neurol Assoc 1963;88:25–29.
255. Olszewski J, Steele J, Richardson JC: Pathological report on six cases of 'heterogeneous system degeneration'. J Neuropathol Exp Neurol 1963;23:187–188.
256. Steele JC, Richardson JC, Olszewski J: Progressive supranuclear palsy. Arch Neurol 1964;10:333–359.

257. Knox DL, Green WR, Troncoso JC, et al: Cerebral ocular Whipple's disease: a 62-year odyssey from death to diagnosis. Neurology 1995;45:617–625.
258. Siderowf AD, Galetta SL, Hurtig H, et al: Posey and Spiller and progressive supranuclear palsy: An incorrect attribution. Mov Disord 1998;13:170–174.
259. Bower JH, Maraganore DM, McDonnell SK, et al: Incidence of progressive supranuclear palsy and multiple system atrophy in Olmsted County, Minnesota, 1976 to 1990. Neurology 1997;49:1284–1288.
260. Golbe LI, Rubin RS, Cody RP, et al: Follow-up study of risk factors in progressive supranuclear palsy. Neurology 1996;47:148–154.
261. David NJ, Mackey EA, Smith JL: Further observations in progressive supranuclear palsy. Neurology 1968; 18:349–356.
262. Tetrud JW, Golbe LI, Forno LS, et al: Autopsy-proven progressive supranuclear palsy in two siblings. Neurology 1996;46:931–934.
263. Friedman DI, Jankovic J, McCrary JA: Neuro-ophthalmic findings in progressive supranuclear palsy. J Clin Neuro-ophthalmol 1992;12:104–109.
264. Jankovic J: Progressive supranuclear palsy. Clinical and pharmacologic update. Neurol Clin 1984;2: 473–486.
265. Newman N, Gay AJ, Stroud MH, et al: Defective rapid eye movements in progressive supranuclear palsy—an ocular electromyographic study. Brain 1970;93:775–784.
266. Chu FC, Reingold DB, Cogan DG, et al: The eye movement disorders of progressive supranuclear palsy. Ophthalmology 1979;86:422–428.
267. Troost BT, Daroff RB: The ocular motor defects in progressive supranuclear palsy. Ann Neurol 1977;2:397–403.
268. Dix MR, Harrison MJG, Lewis PD: Progressive supranuclear palsy (the Steele–Richardson–Olszewski syndrome): a report of 9 cases with particular reference to the mechanism of the oculomotor disorder. J Neurol Sci 1971;13:237–256.
269. Mastaglia FL, Grainger MR: Internuclear ophthalmoplegia in progressive supranuclear palsy. J Neurol Sci 1975;25:303–308.
270. Jackson JA, Jankovic J, Ford J: Progressive supranuclear palsy: clinical features and response to treatment in 16 patients. Ann Neurol 1983;13:273–278.
271. Duvoisin RC, Golbe LI, Lepore FE: Progressive supranuclear palsy. Can J Neurol Sci 1987;14:547–554.
272. Dehaene I: Apraxia of eyelid opening in progressive supranuclear palsy (letter). Ann Neurol 1984;15: 115–116.
273. Golbe LI, Davis PA, Lepore FE: Eyelid movement abnormalities in progressive supranuclear palsy. Mov Disord 1989;4:297–302.
274. Collins SJ, Ahlskog JE, Parisi JE, et al: Progressive supranuclear palsy: neuropathologically based diagnostic clinical criteria. J Neurol Neurosurg Psychiatry 1995;58:167–173.
275. Daniel SE, de Bruin VMS, Lees AJ, et al: The clinical and pathological spectrum of Steele–Richardson–Olszewski syndrome (progressive supranuclear palsy): a reappraisal. Brain 1995;118:759–770.
276. Litvan I, Mega MS, Cummings JL, et al: Neuropsychiatric aspects of progressive supranuclear palsy. Neurology 1996;47:1184–1189.
277. Rafal RD, Friedman JH: Limb dystonia in progressive supranuclear palsy. Neurology 1987;37:1546–1549.
278. Pillon B, Dubois B, Lhermitte F, et al: Heterogeneity of cognitive impairment in progressive supranuclear palsy, Parkinson's disease, and Alzheimer's disease. Neurology 1986;36:1179–1185.
279. Litvan I, Agid Y, Calne D, et al: Clinical research criteria for the diagnosis of progressive supranuclear palsy (Steele–Richardson–Olszewski syndrome): Report of the NINDS-SPSP International Workshop. Neurology 1996;47:1–9.
280. Litvan I, Agid Y, Jankovic J, et al: Accuracy of clinical criteria for the diagnosis of progressive supranuclear palsy (Steele–Richardson–Olszewski syndrome). Neurology 1996;46:922–930.
281. Litvan I, Campbell G, Mangone CA, et al: Which clinical features differentiate progressive supranuclear palsy (Steele–Richardson–Olszewski syndrome) from related disorders? A clinicopathological study. Brain 1997;120:65–74.
282. Santacruz P, Uttl B, Litvan I, et al: Progressive supranuclear palsy. A survey of the disease course. Neurology 1998;50:1637–1647.
283. Case records of the Massachusetts General Hospital: Case 26–1997. N Engl J Med 1997;337:549–556.
284. Hauw J-J, Daniel SE, Dickson D, et al: Preliminary NINDS neuropathologic criteria for Steele–Richardson–Olszewski syndrome (progressive supranuclear palsy). Neurology 1994;44:2015–2019.
285. Kida M, Koo H, Grossniklaus HE, et al: Neuropathologic findings in progressive supranuclear palsy. A brief review with two additional case reports. J Clin Neuro-ophthalmol 1988;8:161–170.
286. Verny M, Duyckaerts C, Agid Y, et al: The significance of cortical pathology in progressive supranuclear palsy. Clinico-pathological data in 10 cases. Brain 1996;119:1123–1136.
287. Bennett P, Bonifati V, Bonuccelli U, et al: Direct genetic evidence for involvement of tau in progressive supranuclear palsy. Neurology 1998;51:982–985.
288. Oliva R, Tolosa E, Ezquerra M, et al: Significant changes in the Tau A0 and A3 alleles in progressive supranuclear palsy and improved genotyping by silver detection. Arch Neurol 1998;55:1122–1124.
289. Hoenicka J, Pérez M, Pérez-Tur J, et al: The tau gene A0 allele and progressive supranuclear palsy. Neurology 1999;53:1219–1225.
290. Higgins JJ, Litvan I, Nee LE, et al: A lack of the *R406W tau* mutation in progressive supranuclear palsy and corticobasal degeneration. Neurology 1999;52:404–406.
291. Litvan I, Saunders AM: Apolipoprotein E4 (epsilon) allele does not affect the onset or symptom severity in progressive supranuclear palsy (letter). Arch Neurol 1998;55:752–753.
292. Juncos JL, Hirsch EC, Malessa S, et al: Mesencephalic cholinergic nuclei in progressive supranuclear palsy. Neurology 1991;41:25–30.
293. Malessa S, Hirsch EC, Cervera P, et al: Progressive supranuclear palsy: loss of choline-acetyltransferase-like immunoreactive neurons in the pontine reticular formation. Neurology 1991;41:1593–1597.
294. Malessa S, Gaymard B, Rivaud S, et al: Role of pontine nuclei damage in smooth pursuit impairment of progressive supranuclear palsy: a clinical-pathologic study. Neurology 1994;44:716–721.
295. Revesz T, Sangha H, Daniel SE: The nucleus raphe interpositus in the Steele–Richardson–Olszewski syndrome (progressive supranuclear palsy). Brain 1996;119:1137–1143.
296. Stern MB, Braffman BH, Skolnick BE, et al: Magnetic resonance imaging in Parkinson's disease and parkinsonian syndromes. Neurology 1989;39:1524–1526.

297. Case records of the Massachusetts General Hospital: Case 46–1993. N Engl J Med 1993;329:1560–1567.
298. Savoiardo M, Strada L, Girotti F, et al: MR imaging in progressive supranuclear palsy and Shy–Drager syndrome. J Comput Assist Tomogr 1989;13:555–560.
299. Dubinsky RM, Jankovic J: Progressive supranuclear palsy and a multi-infarct state. Neurology 1987; 37:570–576.
300. Kompoliti K, Goetz CG, Litvan I, et al: Pharmacological therapy in progressive supranuclear palsy. Arch Neurol 1998;55:1099–1102.
301. Ghika J, Tennis M, Hoffman E, et al: Idazoxan treatment in progressive supranuclear palsy. Neurology 1991;41:986–991.
302. Higgins JJ, Patterson MC, Dambrosia JM, et al: A clinical staging classification for type C Niemann–Pick disease. Neurology 1992;42:2286–2290.
303. Hulette CM, Earl NL, Anthony DC, et al: Adult onset Niemann–Pick disease type C presenting with dementia and absent organomegaly. Clin Neuropathol 1992;11:293–297.
304. Lossos A, Schlesinger H, Okon E, et al: Adult-onset Niemann–Pick type C disease. Arch Neurol 1997; 54:1536–1541.
305. van de Vlasakker CJW, Gabreëls FJM, Wijburg HC, et al: Clinical features of Niemann-Pick disease type C. An example of the delayed onset, slowly progressive phenotype and an overview of recent literature. Clin Neurol Neurosurg 1994;96:119–123.
306. Neville BGR, Lake BD, Stephens R, et al: A neurovisceral storage disease with vertical nuclear ophthalmoplegia and its relationship to Niemann–Pick disease: a report of nine patients. Brain 1973;96:97–120.
307. Simpson DA, Winslow R, Gargulinski RB, et al: Oculofacial-skeletal myorhythmia in central nervous system Whipple's disease: additional case and review of the literature. Mov Disord 1995;10:195–200.
308. Louis ED, Lynch T, Kaufmann P, et al: Diagnostic guidelines in central nervous system Whipple's disease. Ann Neurol 1996;40:561–568.
309. Amarenco P, Roullet E, Hannoun L, et al: Progressive supranuclear palsy as the sole manifestation of system Whipple's disease treated with perfloxacine (letter). J Neurol Neurosurg Psychiatry 1991;54:1121–1122.
310. Schwartz MA, Selhorst JB, Ochs AL, et al: Oculomasticatory myorhythmia: a unique movement disorder occurring in Whipple's disease. Ann Neurol 1986;20:677–683.
311. Ramzan NN, Loftus E, Burgart LJ, et al: Diagnosis and monitoring of Whipple disease by polymerase chain reaction. Ann Intern Med 1997;126:520–527.
312. Rickman LS, Freeman WR, Green WR, et al: Brief report: uveitis caused by *Tropheryma whippelii* (Whipple's disease). N Engl J Med 1995;332:363–366.
313. Williams JG, Edward DP, Tessler HH, et al: Ocular manifestations of Whipple disease. An atypical presentation. Arch Ophthalmol 1998;116:1232–1234.
314. Lynch T, Odel J, Fredericks DN, et al: Polymerase chain reaction-based detection of *Tropheryma whippelii* in central nervous system Whipple's disease. Ann Neurol 1997;42:120–124.
315. Verhagen WIM, Huygen PLM, Dalman JE, et al: Whipple's disease and the central nervous system. A case report and a review of the literature. Clin Neurol Neurosurg 1996;98:299–304.
316. Adler CH, Galetta SL: Oculo-facial-skeletal myorhythmia in Whipple's disease: treatment with ceftriaxone. Ann Intern Med 1990;112:467–469.
317. Kushner MJ, Parrish M, Burke A, et al: Nystagmus in motor neuron disease. Ann Neurol 1984;16:71–77.
318. Mizutani T, Sakamaki S, Tsuchiya N, et al: Amyotrophic lateral sclerosis with ophthalmoplegia and multisystem degeneration in patients on long-term use of respirators. Acta Neuropathol 1992;84: 372–377.
319. Okuda B, Yamamoto T, Yamasaki M, et al: Motor neuron disease with slow eye movements and vertical gaze palsy. Acta Neurol Scand 1992;85:71–76.
320. Shaunak S, Orrell RW, O'Sullivan E, et al: Oculomotor function in amyotrophic lateral sclerosis: evidence for frontal impairment. Ann Neurol 1995;38:38–44.
321. Averbuch-Heller L, Helmchen C, Horn AKE, et al: Slow vertical saccades in motor neuron disease: correlation of structure and function. Ann Neurol 1998;44:641–648.
322. Verhagen WIM, ter Bruggen JP, Huygen PLM: Oculomotor, auditory, and vestibular responses in myotonic dystrophy. Arch Neurol 1992;49:954–960.
323. Anastasopoulos D, Kimmig H, Mergner T, et al: Abnormalities of ocular motility in myotonic dystrophy. Brain 1996;119:1923–1932.
324. Verhagen WI, Huygen PL: Abnormalities of ocular motility in myotonic dystrophy [letter]. Brain 1997;120:1907–1909.
325. Osanai R, Kinoshita M, Hirose K: Saccadic slowing in myotonic dystrophy and CTG repeat expansion. J Neurol 1998;245:674–680.
326. Versino M, Romani A, Bergamaschi R, et al: Eye movement abnormalities in myotonic dystrophy. Electroencephalogr Clin Neurophysiol 1998;109: 184–190.
327. Gupta SR, Brigell M, Gujrati M, et al: Supranuclear eye mvoement dysfunction in mitochondrial myopathy with $tRNA^{LEU}$ mutation. J Neuro-ophthalmol 1995;15:20–25.
328. Kirkham TH, Kamin DF: Slow saccadic eye movements in Wilson's disease. J Neurol Neurosurg Psychiatry 1974;37:191–194.
329. Saver JL, Liu GT, Charness ME: Idiopathic striopallidodentate calcification with prominent abnormality of eye movement. J Neuro-ophthalmol 1994;14: 29–33.
330. Crino PB, Galetta SL, Sater RA, et al: Clinicopathologic study of paraneoplastic brainstem encephalitis and ophthalmoparesis. J Neuro-ophthalmol 1996; 16:44–48.
331. Bennett JL, Galetta SL, Frohman LP, et al: Neuro-ophthalmologic manifestations of a paraneoplastic syndrome and testicular carcinoma. Neurology 1999;52:864–867.
332. Voltz R, Gultekin SH, Rosenfeld MR, et al: A serologic marker of paraneoplastic limbic and brain-stem encephalitis in patients with testicular cancer. N Engl J Med 1999;340:1788–1795.
333. Fahn S, Marsden CD, Calne DB: Classification and investigation of dystonia. In: Marsden CD, Fahn S (eds): Movement Disorders, 2nd edition, pp 332–358. London, Butterworths, 1987.
334. McCowan PK, Cook LC, Cantab BA: Oculogyric crises in chronic epidemic encephalitis. Brain 1928; 51:285–309.
335. Leigh RJ, Foley JM, Remler BF, et al: Oculogyric crises: a syndrome of thought disorder and ocular deviation. Ann Neurol 1987;22:13–17.
336. Munetz MR: Oculogyric crises and tardive dyskinesia. Am J Psychiatry 1980;137:1628.

337. Nasrallah HA, Pappas NJ, Crowe RR: Oculogyric dystonia in tardive dyskinesia. Am J Psychiatry 1980;137:850–851.
338. FitzGerald PM, Jankovic J: Tardive oculogyric crises. Neurology 1989;39:1434–1437.
339. Onuaguluchi G: Crises in post-encephalitic parkinsonism. Brain 1961;84:395–414.
340. Dorevitch A: Neuroleptics as causes of oculogyric crises. Arch Neurol 1984;41:15–16.
341. Sachdev P: Tardive and chronically recurrent oculogyric crises. Mov Disord 1993;8:93–97.
342. Dave M: Tardive oculogyric crises with clozapine (letter). J Clin Psychiatry 1994;55:264–265.
343. Smith JL: Ocular signs of parkinsonism. J Neurosurg 1966;24:284–285.
344. Mata M, Dorovini-Zis K, Wilson M, et al: New form of familial Parkinson-dementia syndrome: clinical and pathologic findings. Neurology 1983;33:1439–1443.
345. Lamberti P, de Mari M, Iliceto G, et al: Effect of L-dopa on oculogyric crises in a case of dopa-responsive dystonia (letter). Mov Disord 1993;8: 236–237.
346. Urra DG, Campos J, Ruiz PG, et al: Movement disorders in ataxia–telangiectasia: review of six patients. Neurology 1989;39(Suppl 1):321.
347. FitzGerald PM, Jankovic J, Glaze DG, et al: Extrapyramidal involvement in Rett's syndrome. Neurology 1990;40:293–295.
348. Lee MS, Kim YD, Lyoo CH: Oculogyric crisis as an initial manifestation of Wilson's disease. Neurology 1999;52:1714–1715.
349. Benjamin S: Oculogyric crisis. In: Joseph AB, Young RR, (eds): Movement Disorders in Neurology and Neuropsychiatry, pp 111–122. Oxford, Blackwell, 1992.
350. Mastumura K, Sakuta M: Oculogyric crisis in acute herpetic brainstem encephalitis. J Neurol Neurosurg Psychiatry 1987;50:365–366.
351. Heimburger RF: Positional oculogyric crises. Case report. J Neurosurg 1988;69:951–953.
352. Liu GT, Carrazana EJ, Macklis JD, et al: Delayed oculogyric crises associated with striatocapsular infarction. J Clin Neuro-ophthalmol 1991;11:208–211.
353. Kim JS, Kim HK, Im JH, et al: Oculogyric crisis and abnormal magnetic resonance imaging signals in bilateral lentiform nuclei. Mov Disord 1996;11:756–758.
354. Berchou RC, Rodin EA: Carbamazepine-induce oculogyric crisis. Arch Neurol 1979;36:522–523.
355. Gorman M, Barkley GL: Oculogyric crisis induced by carbamazepine. Epilepsia 1995;36:1158–1160.
356. Burke RE, Reches A, Traub MM, et al: Tetrabenazine induces acute dystonic reactions. Ann Neurol 1998;17:200–202.
357. Reeves AL, So EL, Sharbrough FW, et al: Movement disorders associated with the use of gabapentin. Epilepsia 1996;37:988–990.
358. Gatzonis SD, Georgaculias N, Singounas E, et al: Elimination of oxcarbazepine-induced oculogyric crisis following vagus nerve stimulation. Neurology 1999;52:1918–1919.
359. Frankel M, Cummings JL: Neuro-ophthalmic abnormalities in Tourette's syndrome: functional and anatomic implications. Neurology 1984;34:359–361.
360. Jankovic J, Stone L: Dystonic tics in patients with Tourette's syndrome. Mov Disord 1991;6:248–252.
361. Jankovic J, Rohaidy H: Motor, behavioral and pharmacologic findings in Tourette's syndrome. Can J Neurol Sci 1987;14:541–546.
362. Shapiro AK, Shapiro ES, Young JG, et al: Gilles de la Tourette Syndrome, 2nd edition, pp 129. New York, Raven Press, 1988.
363. Ahn JC, Hoyt WF, Hoyt CS: Tonic upgaze in infancy. A report of three cases. Arch Ophthalmol 1989; 107:57–58.
364. Echenne B, Rivier R: Benign paroxysmal tonic upward gaze. Pediatr Neurol 1992;8:154–155.
365. Kleiman MD, DiMario FJ, Jr., Leconche DA, et al: Benign transient downward gaze in preterm infants. Pediatr Neurol 1994;10:313–316.
366. Hoyt CS, Mousel DK, Weber AA: Transient supranuclear disturbances of gaze in healthy neonates. Am J Ophthalmol 1980;89:708–713.
367. Daroff RB, Hoyt WF: Supranuclear disorders of ocular control systems in man. In: Bach-y-Rita P, Collins CC, Hyde JE (eds): The Control of Eye Movements, pp 198–199. New York, Academic Press, 1971.
368. Goldblum TA, Effron LA: Upbeat nystagmus associated with tonic downward deviation in healthy neonates. J Pediatr Ophthalmol Strabismus 1994;31:334–335.
369. Miller VS, Packard AM: Paroxysmal downgaze in term newborn infants. J Child Neurol 1998;13: 294–295.
370. Deonna T, Roulet E, Meyer HU: Benign paroxysmal tonic upgaze of childhood. Neuropediatrics 1990; 21:213–214.
371. Campistol J, Prats JM, Garaizar C: Benign paroxysmal tonic upgaze of childhood with ataxia. A neuro-ophthalmological syndrome of familial origin? Dev Med Child Neurol 1993;35:436–439.
372. Hayman M, Harvey AS, Hopkins IJ, et al: Paroxysmal tonic upgaze: a reappraisal of outcome. Ann Neurol 1998;43:514–520.
373. Keane JR, Rawlinson DG, Lu AT: Sustained downgaze deviation: two cases without structural pretectal lesions. Neurology 1976;26:594–595.
374. Keane JR: Sustained upgaze in coma. Ann Neurol 1981;9:409–412.
375. Klostermann W, Zuhlke C, Heide W, et al: Slow saccades and other eye movement disorders in spinocerebellar atrophy type 1. J Neurol 1997;244:105–111.
376. Buttner N, Geschwind D, Jen JC, et al: Oculomotor phenotypes in autosomal dominant ataxias. Arch Neurol 1998;55:1353–1357.
377. Storey E, Forrest SM, Shaw JH, et al: Spinocerebellar ataxia type 2. Clinical features of a pedigree displaying prominent frontal-executive dysfunction. Arch Neurol 1999;56:43–60.
378. Nakano KK, Dawson DM, Spence A: Machado disease: a hereditary ataxia in Portuguese emigrants to Massachusetts. Neurology 1972;22:49–55.
379. Woods BT, Schaumburg HH: Nigro-spino-dentatal degeneration with nuclear ophthalmoplegia: a unique and partially treatable clinicopathological entity. J Neurol Sci 1972;17:149–166.
380. Rosenberg RN, Nyhan WL, Bay C, et al: Autosomal dominant striatonigral degeneration. Neurology 1976;26:703–714.
381. Dawson DM, Feudo P, Zubick HH, et al: Electro-oculographic findings in Machado–Joseph disease. Neurology 1982;32:1272–1276.
382. Sudarsky L, Coutinho P: Machado-Joseph disease. Clin Neurosci 1995;3:17–22.
383. Benomar A, Le Guern E, Dürr A, et al: Autosomal-dominant cerebellar ataxia with retinal degeneration (ADCA type II) is genetically different from ADCA type II. Ann Neurol 1994;35:439–444.

384. Morrow MJ, Zinn AB, Tucker T, et al: Maculopathy in spinocerebellar ataxia type 7. Neurology 1999;53:244.
385. Dürr A, Cossee M, Agid Y, et al: Clinical and genetic abnormalities in patients with Friedreich's ataxia. N Engl J Med 1996;335:1169–1175.
386. Rosenberg RN: DNA-triplet repeats and neurologic disease (editorial). N Engl J Med 1996;335:1222–1224.
387. Gomez CM, Thompson RM, Gammack JT, et al: Spinocerebellar ataxia type 6: gaze-evoked and vertical nystagmus, Purkinje cell degeneration, and variable age of onset. Ann Neurol 1997;42:933–950.
388. Naito H, Oyanagi S: Familial myoclonus epilepsy and choreoathetosis: hereditary dentatorubral-pallidoluysian atrophy. Neurology 1982;32:798–807.
389. Bohlega S, Kambouris M, Shahid M, et al: Gaucher disease with oculomotor apraxia and cardiovascular calcification (Gaucher type IIIC). Neurology 2000;54:261–263.

CHAPTER 17

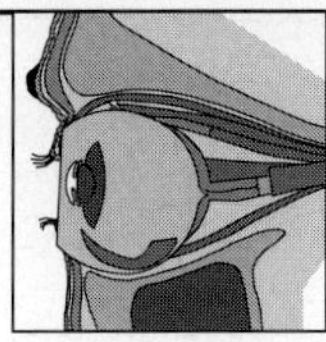

Eye Movement Disorders: Nystagmus and Nystagmoid Eye Movements

Nystagmus is a rhythmic biphasic oscillation of the eyes. Since nystagmus results from a defect in the slow eye movement system, nystagmus always has a slow phase that initiates the ocular oscillation. Nystagmus should also be distinguished from other ocular oscillations or nystagmoid eye movements. These other ocular oscillations usually do not have a slow phase and often represent disorders of saccades. Characteristically, they interrupt foveal fixation and although they can be distinguished clinically, some may be best characterized by eye movement recordings.[1]

This chapter will review the symptoms and examination of patients with nystagmus, and detail each of the important types of nystagmus and nystagmoid eye movements and their pathophysiology.

NYSTAGMUS

Nystagmus may occur physiologically in response to environmental stimuli or from rotation of the body. More importantly, it may be a sign of central nervous system (CNS) dysfunction, peripheral vestibular disease, or visual loss. One method to organize the different types of nystagmus is to distinguish those cases with jerk properties from those with pendular waveforms and to consider the various types according to the patient's age (Table 17–1). In pendular nystagmus, the slow phases are of equal velocity and there are no corrective saccades. Jerk nystagmus has a slow phase followed by a rapid corrective phase in the opposite direction. Entities such as congenital nystagmus and spasmus nutans will more likely present in childhood.

By convention, the direction of jerk nystagmus is defined by its fast phase. Patients who have a slow phase to the left and a corrective phase to the right are said to have right-beating nystagmus. Frequently, jerk nystagmus will have a torsional or rotary component. This type of nystagmus is usually defined as clockwise or counter-clockwise from the examiner's perspective. Alternatively, torsional nystagmus may be described by whether it beats to the patient's right or left shoulder (Fig. 17–1). Pendular nystagmus has no fast phase, so it is described as either vertical or horizontal. Occasionally, nystagmus results from a combination of vertical and horizontal phases to produce a circular, elliptical, or oblique waveform.

Most forms of nystagmus can be interpreted at the bedside. However, eye movement recordings can more accurately characterize the slow phases of nystagmus and define its underlying pathophysiologic substrate. For example, the slow phase velocity of vestibular nystagmus is linear, while congenital nystagmus displays an increasing slow phase velocity. Gaze paretic nystagmus usually has a declining slow phase.[1]

TABLE 17–1. Grouping of Nystagmus Types by Waveform and Typical Age at Presentation

	Childhood	Any Age
Jerk	Latent	Vestibular Peripheral and central Gaze-evoked Physiologic Pathologic Brun's Dissociated Periodic alternating (PAN) Downbeat Upbeat Convergence retraction Epileptic Drug-induced Optokinetic See-saw
Pendular	Spasmus nutans Monocular nystagmus due to visual deprivation/loss	Oculopalatal Oculomasticatory myorhythmia See-saw
Either pendular and/or jerk in the same patient	Congenital	

Symptoms Associated With Nystagmus

The accompanying symptoms may be extremely helpful in discerning the various forms of nystagmus. Nystagmus may be asymptomatic or produce a jumping of the visual environment called *oscillopsia.* The patient with nystagmus often sees the visual environment moving in the direction of the fast phase. In contrast, patients with congenital nystagmus typically have a reduction in visual acuity without oscillopsia. The reason for the lack of oscillopsia is unclear, but it may be due to an elevated motion detection threshold.[1] Nausea and vomiting may accompany nystagmus and it can be a prominent complaint of patients with peripheral vestibular disease. Symptoms such as diplopia, dysarthria, facial numbness, and dysphagia indicate a brain stem origin for the nystagmus. In contrast, hearing loss and tinnitus suggest a peripheral vestibular cause. Some patients with chronic complaints of dizziness have no identifiable cause and suffer from a psychological condition such as anxiety. These patients may describe their dizziness as lightheadedness or as a floating, swimming, or rocking sensation.[2] Occasionally, hyperventilation will reproduce their symptoms.

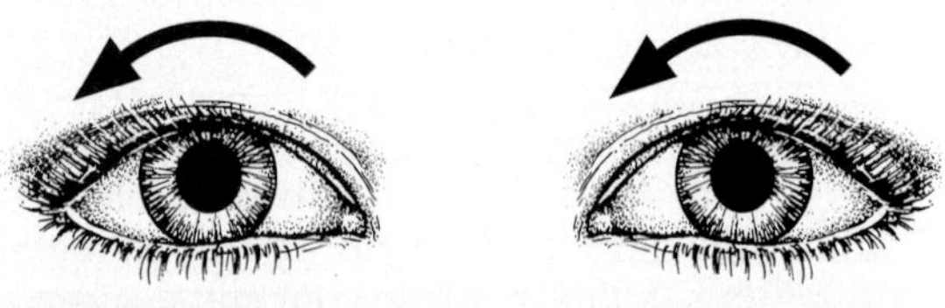

FIGURE 17–1. Diagram of torsional nystagmus. Nystagmus as demonstrated in this figure may be described as counter-clockwise or alternatively, it is described as beating toward the patient's right shoulder.

Examination

The examination begins by observing the patient's eyes while they look straight ahead. The eyes are then observed in all positions of gaze. Smooth pursuit and saccadic eye movements are then checked (see Chapter 16). An abnormality of either the saccadic or the pursuit system suggests a central cause for the nystagmus. The vestibular ocular reflex may be tested by having the patient focus on a distant object as the head is moved from side to side at 2 Hz. Alternatively, the patient focuses on the examiner's nose or finger as the examiner moves the patient's head quickly over very short distances (Fig. 17–2).[3] The appearance of nystagmus with this maneuver suggests a vestibular disorder.

Another useful bedside test is cancellation of the vestibular ocular reflex (see Fig. 2–28). In this test, patients focus on their outstretched thumb as they are rotated in a chair at low frequency. It is normal to observe no movement of the eyes. If the reflex is defective, the eyes fall off the thumb and nystagmus is gener-

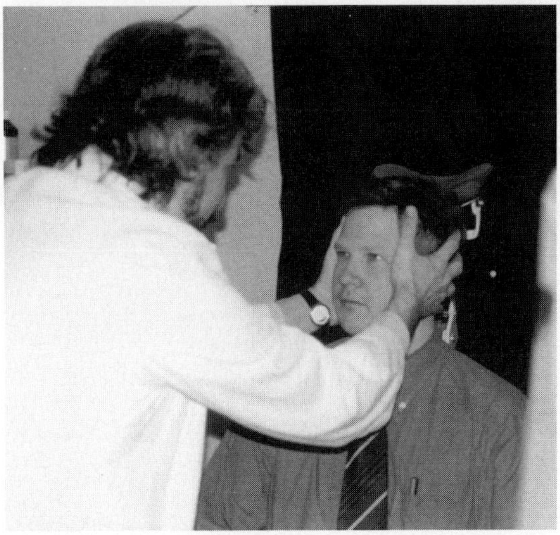

FIGURE 17–2. Testing of the vestibulo-ocular reflex. The patient's head is rotated quickly over short distances to check for nystagmus.

ated. This is usually a sign of cerebellar or central vestibular dysfunction.

Occasionally, nystagmus is difficult to discern or is suppressed by fixation. Under these conditions, one eye is viewed with an ophthalmoscope. Simultaneously, the other eye is covered manually (Fig. 17–3). This procedure removes fixation, and the eye being viewed by the ophthalmoscope may be now checked for nystagmus. It is helpful to remember that the disc moves in the opposite direction from the movement generated by the front of the eye. Therefore, if the disc is moving rapidly upward, the nystagmus direction is downbeat. Frenzel goggles, which contain high-plus lenses, also eliminate fixation and may provide magnification to help detect subtle forms of nystagmus (Fig. 17–4). Patients with perilymph fistulas may have nystagmus induced by a Valsalva maneuver or by replicating nose blowing.

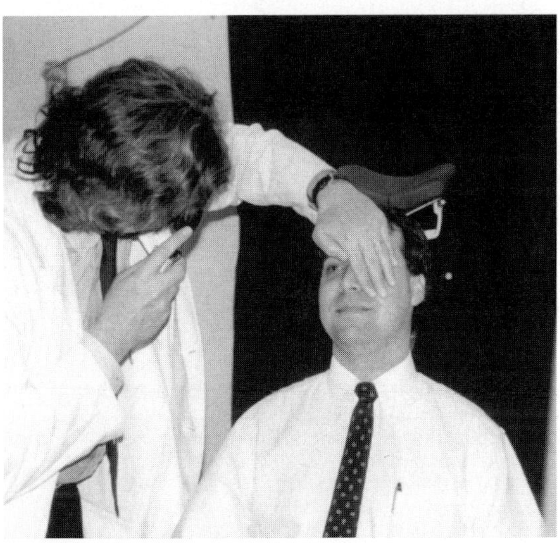

FIGURE 17–3. The examiner checks for nystagmus by viewing the eye with an ophthalmoscope and covering the other eye with his hand. This removes fixation.

In many patients, nystagmus may be evident only with provocative maneuvers. In the Dix–Hallpike maneuver (Fig. 17–5 A,B), which is used in patients with positional vertigo, the patient sits on a table lengthwise. The patient is then brought backward and the head is rotated 45 degrees to one side. The characteristics of the nystagmus, if present, may be helpful in differentiating central and peripheral forms of positional nystagmus. The examiner is interested in the nature of the nystagmus, its direction, its latency, and whether or not it fatigues (Table 17–2).

The optokinetic flag (see Fig. 2–29) may be helpful in the diagnosis of congenital nystagmus and convergence retraction nystagmus. Patients with congenital nystagmus may have a reversal of the normal response. For instance, the eyes usually beat away from the direction of the moving tape. In some patients with congenital nystagmus, the eyes beat in the direc-

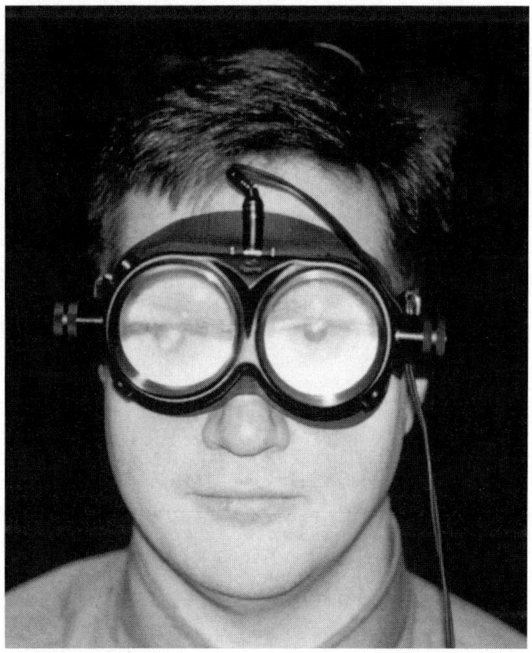

FIGURE 17–4. Frenzel goggles are lenses of high magnification that remove the patient's fixation and provide the examiner a large view of the patient's eyes.

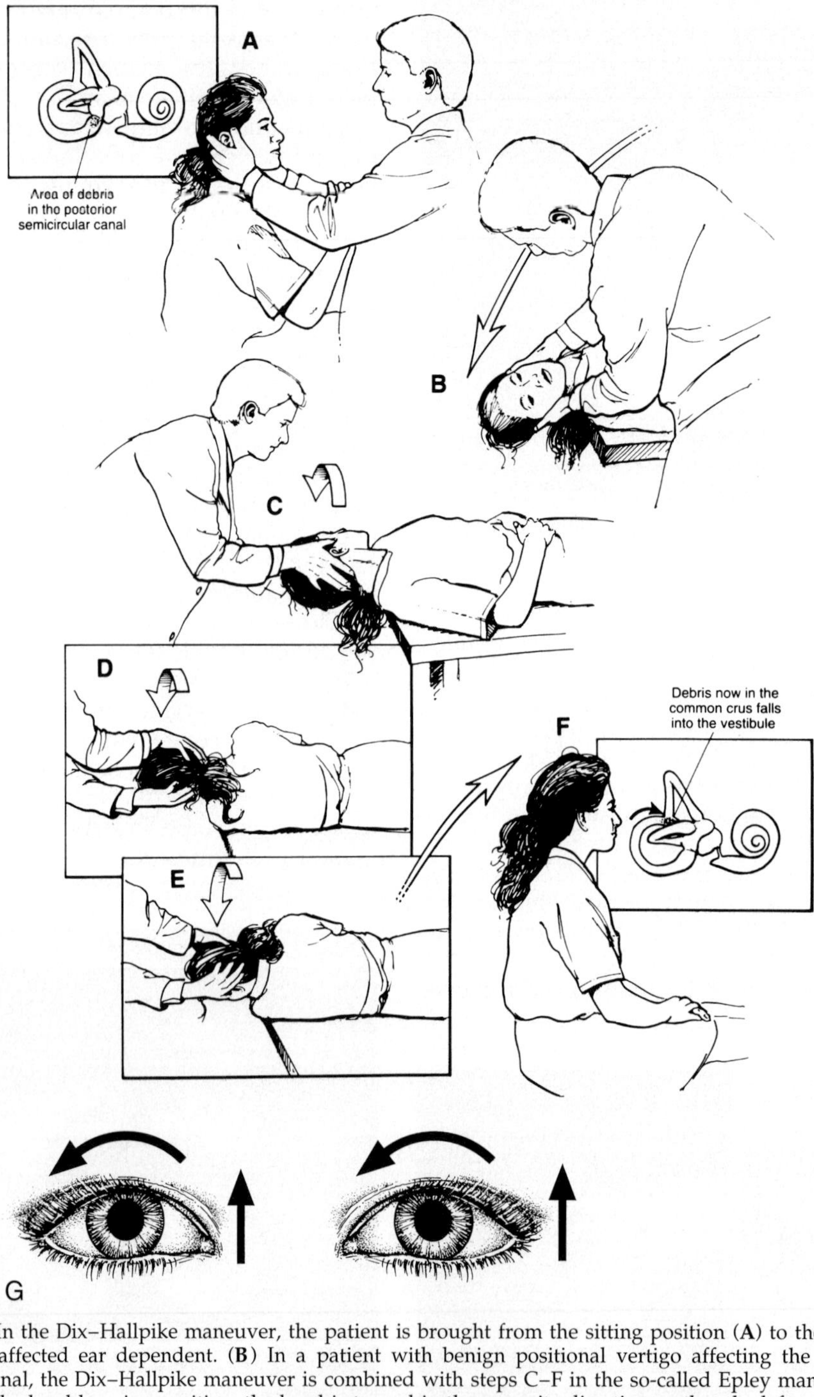

FIGURE 17–5. In the Dix–Hallpike maneuver, the patient is brought from the sitting position (**A**) to the head-hanging position with affected ear dependent. (**B**) In a patient with benign positional vertigo affecting the right posterior semicircular canal, the Dix–Hallpike maneuver is combined with steps C–F in the so-called Epley maneuver. **C.** After 30 seconds in the head-hanging position, the head is turned in the opposite direction so that the left ear is dependent. **D.** The patient is then placed on her left shoulder. **E.** The patient's head is moved to the face down position. **F.** The patient is brought upright again. (A–F from Fife TD: Barrow Neurol Instit Q 1994;10:2-8, with permission). **G.** In a patient with benign positional vertigo, the eyes show a torsional upbeating nystagmus. The nystagmus may be more torsional in the dependent eye and more vertical in the upright eye (not shown).

TABLE 17–2. Characteristics of Nystagmus During the Hallpike Maneuver in Peripheral Versus Central Positional Vertigo

Findings	Peripheral	Central
Latency	Present	Absent
Duration	<1 minute	>1 minute
Fatigability	Yes	No
Nystagmus waveform	Upbeating, variable	Torsional

tion of the moving tape. Patients with a dorsal midbrain syndrome often display a characteristic eye movement abnormality, particularly in attempted upgaze, known as convergence retraction nystagmus. This nystagmus may be enhanced by moving the optokinetic nystagmus (OKN) tape downward, which induces upward saccades.

Caloric stimulation is another method for provoking nystagmus. The test procedure itself is discussed in detail in Chapter 2 (see Fig. 2–41). Cold water injected into one ear produces a slow movement of the eyes toward the irrigated ear. There is a corrective phase toward the opposite direction in the awake and normal patient. By convention, nystagmus is named by its fast phase. Therefore, the consequence of canal irrigation with cold water may be remembered by the term "cows," which stands for cold–opposite and warm–same. This means when the right ear is irrigated with cold water, the fast phase of nystagmus should be to the left in a normal patient. In a comatose patient, just a slow phase or no response at all may be seen. Vertical eye movements in the comatose patient may be assessed by bilateral caloric stimulation. Cold water simultaneously injected into both ears produces a slow down phase and a corrective up phase. This might be remembered by the term "cuwd," which stands for cold–up and warm–down. One can elicit some forms of nystagmus by asking patients to shake their head from side to side for 15 seconds. The appearance of nystagmus with this maneuver usually signifies a peripheral vestibular process.[4] Other patients with peripheral vestibular disease may march in the direction of the affected ear with their eyes closed.

Pathophysiology of Nystagmus

Nystagmus usually results from a defect in the slow eye movement system. The slow eye movement systems includes visual fixation, the vestibular system, smooth pursuit, vergence, and the optokinetic and neural integrator pathways.

The vestibular system allows images to remain steady on the fovea while the head is moving. Under normal conditions, the vestibular ocular reflex generates slow eye movements that are equal and in the opposite direction of the head movement. The vestibular ocular reflex pathway originates in the semicircular canals and synapses in the vestibular nuclei, ultimately connecting to the ocular motor nuclei and cerebellum. Peripheral vestibular nystagmus results from an imbalance of input from the semicircular canals. On the other hand, central vestibular nystagmus results from injury to the vestibular nuclei or cerebellovestibular pathways, or possibly from otolith input.[1] The otoliths respond to linear acceleration of the head. Imbalance of this system will produce torsional eye movements and skew deviation.

The neural integrator is a network of cells responsible for maintaining the eyes in eccentric gaze. When the system is defective, the eyes will drift back to the midline with a corrective fast phase. The cerebellar flocculus, the nucleus prepositus hypoglossi, and medial vestibular nucleus make up the neural integrator. A defect in this system is implicated in pathologic gaze-evoked nystagmus.

Some forms of nystagmus, like the dissociated nystagmus seen in internuclear ophthalmoparesis, may represent an adaptive phenomenon, while other forms of nystagmus may result from muscle fatigue and the inability to overcome the viscoelastic forces of the orbit. For instance, patients with myasthenia gravis may demonstrate a fatigue-induced type of gaze-evoked nystagmus.[1] Some forms of nystagmus, such as congenital nystagmus, latent nystagmus, and acquired pendular nystagmus, have poorly understood mechanisms.

Types of Nystagmus

In the following discussion of the various entities, those presenting predominantly in childhood will be reviewed first, then those without any particular age predilection will be detailed afterwards (Table 17–3).

Congenital Nystagmus. Congenital nystagmus may be recognized at birth but much more commonly arises in the second through fourth

TABLE 17–3. Pendular Nystagmus in Early Life

Nystagmus Features	Spasmus Nutans	Congenital	Acquired
Waveform	Horizontal; monocular or asymmetric	Mixed waveform (pendular and jerk)	Pendular, ellipitical
Amplitude	Low	Low	Medium
Frequency	High	Low	Low
Neurologic signs	No	No	Diencephalic syndrome
Onset	4 to 12 months	2 to 4 months	age > 6 months
Other visual signs	Amblyopia, anisometropia	Amblyopia, strabismus	Afferent pupillary defect, optic atrophy

months of life as visual fixation develops.[5, 6] Classically, it is a horizontal nystagmus with a pendular waveform, but it may be rotatory or rarely vertical in nature. Patients with congenital nystagmus may demonstrate jerk properties, particularly in endgaze. It is this mixed waveform containing both pendular and jerk properties that suggests the presence of congenital nystagmus.[7] Congenital nystagmus also is one of the few types of nystagmus that remains horizontal in vertical gaze. It is this property that helps distinguish congenital nystagmus from gaze-evoked nystagmus. Other forms of nystagmus that remain horizontal in vertical gaze include peripheral vestibular nystagmus and periodic alternating nystagmus. Patients with congenital nystagmus usually have a null point. The null point is the position of the eyes where the nystagmus is quiet or markedly dampened. Affected patients often have a head turn to position their eyes at the null point. Although oscillopsia is not a concern of the patient with congenital nystagmus, the ocular oscillations may reduce visual acuity.

Convergence usually dampens congenital nystagmus while fixation may exacerbate it. In the most common example of the *nystagmus blockage syndrome,* an individual with congenital nystagmus, attempting to suppress it by converging, develops an esotropia with a head turn. A reverse optokinetic response may be seen in which the fast phase of the response abnormally moves in the same direction of the moving OKN tape.[5, 8] The OKN tape should be moved vertically before the patient since superimposed vertical eye movements upon the horizontal nystagmus suggests that the infant still has the potential to see well.[9, 10]

Etiology. Congenital nystagmus may occur in isolation with relatively normal vision, fundus, and afferent visual pathways. In this situation, which some have termed *congenital motor nystagmus,* it may be considered to be an efferent pathway disorder, perhaps involving the ocular motor systems involved in visual fixation. Although usually sporadic, congenital motor nystagmus can be inherited in an autosomal dominant, autosomal recessive, or X-linked fashion.[11]

However, most patients with congenital nystagmus have a component of sensory or afferent pathway dysfunction. Common causes include optic nerve hypoplasia, ocular albinism, congenital stationary night blindness, Leber's congenital amaurosis, and other childhood optic nerve and retinal conditions.[12] High refractive error, including astigmatism, is frequently associated with congenital nystagmus.

Evaluation. Workup of the patient with congenital nystagmus requires a careful assessment of visual function and fundus appearance. Paradoxic constriction of the pupils when the lights are turned off (see Chapter 13) suggests a retinal disorder. Children with congenital nystagmus require a refraction by a pediatric ophthalmologist. When the examination alone is not conclusive, magnetic resonance imaging (MRI), visual evoked responses, and electroretinography (ERG) are the laboratory tests that are most likely to provide useful diagnostic information.

Treatment. Treatment of congenital nystagmus first involves correction of any refractive error. Prism therapy may be used to shift the null point to the primary position or to induce convergence. In such cases, base-out prisms are used to induce convergence. If prism therapy fails, eye muscle surgery (Kestenbaum procedure) may be performed to move the null point into the straight ahead position.[13, 14] Botulinum toxin has also been used in the therapy of congenital nystagmus, but its effect remains limited by its side effects of ptosis and double vision.[15, 16]

Latent Nystagmus. Latent nystagmus is a form of congenital nystagmus produced by covering one eye. The slow phase of this jerk nystagmus always beats toward the nose, while the fast phase beats in the direction of the uncovered eye (Fig. 17–6). These patients may fail routine eye tests because of the oscillopsia induced by the nystagmus during monocular testing. However, with both eyes open these patients may have much better vision. Latent nystagmus is often a benign condition and not necessarily associated with other neurologic abnormalities. However, ophthalmologic abnormalities may be associated findings and include (1) congenital esotropia, (2) congenital nystagmus, and (3) dissociated vertical deviation.[17] Latent nystagmus has a declining slow phase waveform in distinction to the increasing slow phase velocity characteristic of congenital nystagmus.[1] In *manifest* latent nystagmus, a process that reduces acuity in one eye, such as a cataract, uncorrected refractive error, or amblyopia, may cause latent nystagmus in the fellow eye.

Spasmus Nutans. Spasmus nutans is characterized by the triad of (1) torticollis, (2) head nodding (2 to 3 Hz), and (3) monocular or asymmetric nystagmus.[18] The nystagmus is the hallmark, but both of the other features are not always present. The disorder usually starts between ages 4 and 14 months. Nystagmus may last between 1 to 2 years and almost always resolves clinically by 5 years. The nystagmus of spasmus nutans shows a pendular waveform of low amplitude and high frequency (up to 15 Hz).[19] However, the amplitude and frequency of the nystagmus may vary with gaze position. The nystagmus is often described as shimmering and may be horizontal, vertical, or rotary in nature. Rarely,[20] the nystagmus may be convergent. Some patients may have subclinical nystagmus detected by eye movement recordings only.

Spasmus nutans is usually a benign condition. However, there are a number of reports that document a similar nystagmus with parasellar and hypothalamic tumors.[21–24] The nystagmus and head movements may be indistinguishable from idiopathic spasmus nutans, despite eye and head movement recordings.[25] The most common associated neoplasm is an optic pathway glioma. Patients who harbor tumors usually have other signs of afferent pathway dysfunction such as acuity loss, field defects or optic disc atrophy, or endocrinologic abnormalities including poor feeding or diencephalic syndrome (see Chapter 7). Spasmus nutans-like nystagmus and head movements have also been described in association with retinal diseases such as congential stationary night blindness[26, 27] and in spinocerebellar degenerations.[28]

Evaluation and Treatment. Patients with findings suggesting spasmus nutans should have brain MRI to exclude a mass lesion. Some authors have suggested a more conservative ap-

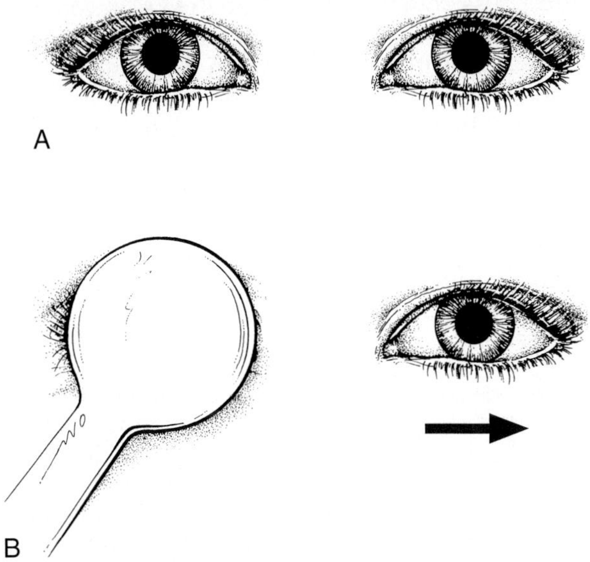

FIGURE 17–6. In latent nystagmus, with both eyes open (**A**) no abnormal eye movements may be evident. When one eye is covered (**B**), the uncovered eye has a slow phase that beats toward the nose with a fast phase outward.

proach,[29] but we believe that relying on an abnormal endocrinologic history or the presence of decreased vision or optic atrophy is problematic in young children, in whom the examination may be difficult. ERG to should be considered when a paradoxic pupillary reaction, severe myopia, or photophobia suggest a retinal disorder.

Idiopathic spasmus nutans requires no specific treatment as the disorder usually spontaneously remits. However, careful follow-up by a pediatric ophthalmologist is mandatory as many children with idiopathic spasmus nutans will have amblyopia or strabismus in the eye with the nystagmus of greater amplitude.[30] Refractive errors are also common. In some patients, subclinical nystagmus may persist up to the age of 12.[18]

Monocular Nystagmus and Visual Deprivation (Heimann–Bielschowsky Phenomenon). Children who develop visual loss in one eye may develop a slow vertical oscillation of the eye known as the Heimann–Bielschowsky phenomenon.[31] It may appear years after visual loss and can resolve if vision is restored in the affected eye. Most cases do not have any significant neurologic implications.[32] However, monocular pendular nystagmus has been reported as result of visual loss associated with a chiasmal glioma.[1, 33] Therefore, acquired monocular pendular nystagmus in childhood should be evaluated with MRI.

Some adult patients with severe monocular visual loss can develop a similar slow (1 to 5 Hz) vertical pendular nystagmus in the affected eye, but this is much less common in this age group. Although the waveform is classically vertical, we have seen horizontal and elliptical oscillations in this situation. We would recommend neuroimaging in such patients.

Vestibular Nystagmus. Vestibular nystagmus may result from dysfunction of the peripheral or central vestibular pathway. Unilateral peripheral vestibular lesions are quite common and usually produce a horizontal rotary nystagmus. The horizontal direction of vestibular nystagmus does not change with gaze position. This is Alexander's law, which describes the observation that the amplitude of the nystagmus usually increases when the eyes are moved in the direction of their fast phase.[34] In a peripheral vestibular lesion, the fast phase of the lesion is usually directed away from the side of a destructive lesion. For instance, a patient with left vestibular neuronitis will have a fast component to the right. Patients with peripheral vestibular lesions typically fall toward the side of their lesion or opposite the direction of their nystagmus.

The various *peripheral* vestibular lesions are usually distinguished by the duration of the vertigo and the accompanying signs:

Labyrinthitis causes vertigo associated with hearing loss that lasts for days. The vertigo may recur weeks or months later.

Vestibular neuronitis is a similar condition but without the hearing loss. Both vestibular neuronitis and labyrinthitis may be caused by a variety of viruses, including Epstein–Barr, mumps, measles, and herpes.

Meniere's syndrome is characterized by attacks of vertigo that lasts hours. Patients often describe a fullness in their ear, tinnitus, and hearing loss. This disorder usually begins between the ages of 30 and 50. It may lead to progressive hearing loss. Patients who have a severe attack may suddenly fall to the ground. This event occurs without loss of consciousness and is known as *Tumarkin's crisis.*

Migraine is another common cause of vertigo, but it remains underrecognized. Approximately 20% of patients with migraine associated vertigo will have an abnormal electronystagmogram. The most common abnormality is unilateral hypoexcitability to caloric stimulation, consistent with a peripheral vestibular lesion.[35]

Benign positional vertigo (BPV) produces symptoms with changes in body position. This vertigo is short-lived and usually lasts no more that 30 to 60 seconds.[36] It is very common for patients to experience this type of vertigo when they first lie down to go to bed or arise in the morning.

In BPV the nystagmus becomes mainly vertical when looking away from the affected ear and more rotatory when looking toward the involved ear. The pathophysiology of BPV is best explained by the canalolithiasis theory.[36] This theory suggests that canal debris gravitates toward the cupula of the posterior semicircular canal to stimulate it.[37] For instance, stimulation of the right semicircular canal produces contraction of the right superior oblique and left inferior rectus muscles. This produces a slow phase down phase of both eyes with a corrective upbeat phase. The fast corrective phase has a torsional component beating toward the stimulated or dependent ear. There also is a horizontal canal variant of BPV.[38, 39] In these patients rotation to the affected ear produces an intense horizontal nystagmus beating toward the undermost ear. Occasionally the nystagmus will beat toward the uppermost ear. Some patients experience a change of their horizontal nystagmus with a change of position. Treatment of this form of BPV involves rotating the patient 270° in rapid steps of 90° (Fig. 17–7).[40, 41]

It is important to distinguish peripheral causes of positional vertigo from those of central nervous system origin (Table 17–2). This may be best accomplished by recording the findings after placing the patient in the Dix–Hallpike or the head-hanging position (Fig. 17–5A,B). This routine may be extended in the Epley maneuver to treat the patient for BPV (Fig. 17–5A–F).[42, 43]

Central Causes. It is the distinction between peripheral vestibular disease and CNS dysfunction that is essential in evaluating the patient with acute vertigo and nystagmus. Occasionally, CNS vestibular dysfunction will mimic the findings observed with peripheral vestibular disease. Features that strongly suggest a central cause include (1) pure torsional nystagmus, particularly when fixation is removed, (2) asymmetric nystagmus between the two eyes, (3) vertical nystagmus in the primary position, and (4) nystagmus that changes direction in different gaze positions.

Evaluation. When the diagnosis of vestibular disease remains poorly localized or defined, a battery of tests should be performed. Brain MRI, electronystagmography, and audiometry are the most useful diagnostic tests in this situation.

Treatment. A variety of positioning techniques have been developed to treat BPV (Figs. 17–5A–F and 17–7).[44,45] Both the Epley and the Semont maneuvers have a high degree of success, in the 80% range.[43,46] In the Epley maneuver, the patient is brought to the head-hanging position with the affected ear down at a 45° angle for 30 seconds. The head is then rotated 90° in the opposite direction for 30 seconds to place the unaffected ear in the dependent position. The patient is then brought onto the shoulder of the nonaffected side. Finally, the head is turned so that the patient is looking toward the floor for approximately 30 seconds. The patient is then rapidly brought to the sitting position. The patient should remain upright for the next 48 hours, usually sleeping in a lounge chair.[46]

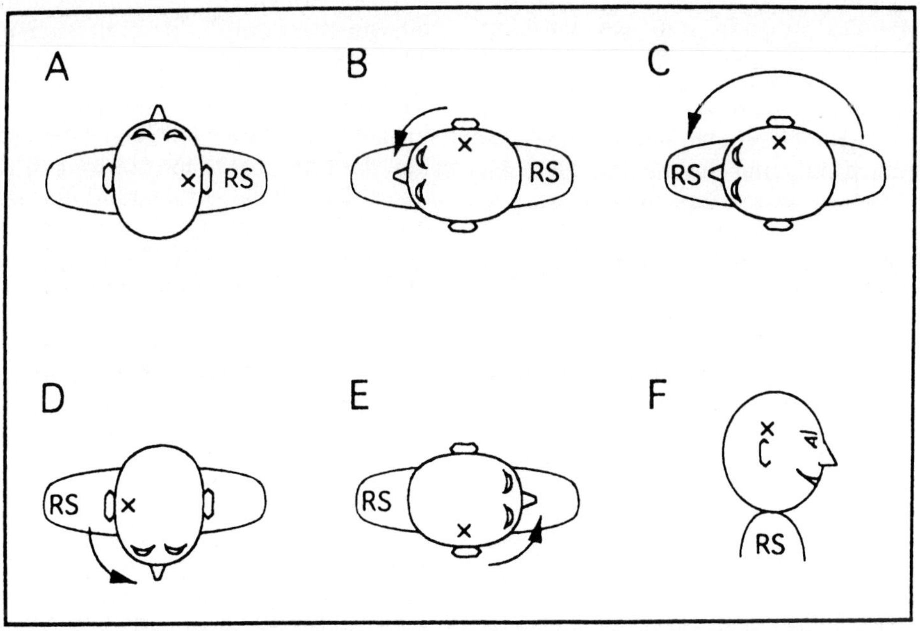

FIGURE 17–7. Positional maneuver for treatment of horizontal canal–benign positional vertigo. In contrast to the Dix–Hallpike and Epley maneuvers illustrated in Fig. 17–5, the patient starts in the supine position in this maneuver. Each 90-degree head rotation is performed rapidly within a half second. Head positions are maintained for between 30 and 60 seconds until all nystagmus has subsided. **A.** Starting position. **B.** Supine position. Head rotation toward the unaffected ear. **C.** Body turn from supine to prone while head position is maintained. **D.** Head rotation to nose-down position. **E.** Final head turn to affected ear-down position. **F.** Sitting-up position. X = affected ear (right side), RS = right shoulder. (From Lempert T, Tiel-Wilck K: A positional maneuver for treatment of horizontal canal benign positional vertigo. Laryngoscope 1996;106:476–478, with permission.)

If the patient does not have BPV, then treatment depends on whether the patient suffers from acute or chronic vertigo. In patients with acute vertigo, it is reasonable to prescribe a vestibular suppressant such as diazepam for several days. Thereafter, vestibular adaptation exercises are prescribed for patients with chronic vertigo. Vestibular rehabilitation is the mainstay of therapy for those patients with chronic vertigo. Chronic use of vestibular suppressants is strongly discouraged as they will delay adaptation and recovery.

Physiologic Gaze-Evoked Nystagmus. Most normal individuals will have jerk nystagmus that fatigues with prolonged lateral gaze of about 30°. In extreme lateral gaze of 40 °, some normal patients will develop sustained physiologic nystagmus.[47] However, the amplitude of this nystagmus is less than 3° and it is symmetric in right and left gaze. Occasionally, physiologic nystagmus may be asymmetric between the two eyes. In this situation, it may be confused with the dissociated nystagmus that accompanies internuclear ophthalmoparesis.

Pathologic Gaze-Evoked Nystagmus. End gaze jerk nystagmus is pathologic when there is (1) an amplitude of greater than 4 degrees, (2) asymmetry in right and left gaze, or (3) exponential slow phase velocity when the gaze angle is less than 40 degrees (Table 17–4).[47] Unilateral gaze-evoked nystagmus may indicate ipsilateral cerebellar or brain stem disease. Lesions involving the medial vestibular nucleus, nucleus prepositus hypoglossi, and flocculus have been implicated in gaze-evoked nystagmus of CNS origin. Gaze-evoked nystagmus may also be observed *contralateral* to peripheral vestibular pathway damage.

When present in both horizontal and upgaze, gaze-evoked nystagmus usually signifies a toxic metabolic process. When gaze-evoked nystagmus is asymmetric or present in only one direction, a structural lesion is suggested (ie, stroke, demyelinating disease). Gaze-evoked upbeat nystagmus commonly accompanies bilateral internuclear ophthalmoparesis.

A special form of gaze-evoked nystagmus known as *Brun's nystagmus* may be seen with cerebellopontine angle lesions.[48, 49] Pathologic horizontal gaze-evoked nystagmus is typically observed when the patient gazes toward the side of the lesion and is probably produced by impaired connections from the cerebellar flocculus. Gaze away from the lesion is associated with the appearance of a high-frequency, low-amplitude horizontal–torsional nystagmus with fast phase in the direction of gaze reflective of vestibular dysfunction.

Dissociated Nystagmus. The prototypical example of dissociated nystagmus occurs with internuclear ophthalmoparesis, which is discussed in greater detail in Chapter 15. In this disorder, the abducting eye shows nystagmus with impaired adduction of the contralateral eye. The cause of the abducting nystagmus is uncertain, but most evidence favors an adaptive mechanism that drives the paretic eye toward the intended position.[1] As will be discussed below, dissociated nystagmus may also be observed with the pendular nystagmus that occasionally complicates brain stem infarction and multiple sclerosis.

Rebound Nystagmus. After the eyes have returned from eccentric gaze to the primary position the eyes beat in the opposite direction for up to 30 seconds.[50] In rebound nystagmus, the eyes will occasionally change their fast phase direction with prolonged eccentric gaze. This finding usually indicates cerebellar disease.[47] Rebound nystagmus usually beats in the direction opposite the lesioned side. For instance, a patient with a right cerebellar lesion will have rebound nystagmus to the left when the eyes are brought back to the midline from eccentric right gaze.[165]

TABLE 17–4. Gaze-Evoked Nystagmus

Nystagmus Features	Physiologic	Peripheral Vestibular	Gaze Paretic
Waveform	Horizontal rotary	Horizontal rotary	Horizontal and/or vertical
Amplitude	Low	Medium	High
Frequency	High	High	Low
Symmetry in gaze positions	Yes	No	Yes/no
Rebound nystagmus	No	No	Yes
Other neurologic signs	No	Hearing loss	Yes
Fatigue	Yes	No	No

Periodic Alternating Nystagmus. This is a rare nystagmus that may be acquired or congenital.[51] It is a nystagmus that changes directions every 90 seconds with a rest period of 5 to 10 seconds. The hallmark of periodic alternating nystagmus (PAN) is a shifting null (quiet) point. PAN may be seen with downbeat nystagmus and usually indicates a lesion of the cervicomedullary junction.[52] PAN may also occur in degenerative processes involving the cerebellum. Experimentally, removal of the nodulus and uvula produce periodic alternating nystagmus in the dark.[53] PAN may persist in sleep and remain horizontal even in vertical gaze. PAN may be associated with a skew deviation similar to that seen with downbeat nystagmus. Even periodic skew deviation has been observed with PAN.[54] As an adaptive phenomenon the patient may demonstrate alternating head turning and gaze deviation.[55] One patient with PAN and visual loss related to vitreous hemorrhage had resolution of the nystagmus after vitrectomy.[56] Presumably this improvement was related to enhanced visual fixation.

Baclofen (Lioresal) may ameliorate the acquired form of PAN (Table 17–5).[57, 58] For patients with congenital periodic alternating nystagmus, surgical therapy may be appropriate.[59] Large horizontal recti resections have been effective.[51]

Downbeat Nystagmus. This typically signifies a lesion of the craniocervical junction (Table 17–6). Common causes are Arnold–Chiari type I malformations (Fig. 17–8), foramen magnum mass lesions, and spinocerebellar degenerations.[52, 60, 61] Occasionally, downbeat nystagmus will be observed with midbrain lesions. Other important causes to consider include hypomagnesemia,[62, 63] thiamine deficiency, and B_{12} deficiency, along with phenytoin, carbamazepine, alcohol, and lithium toxicity.[52, 64–68] Congenital downbeat nystagmus

TABLE 17–6. Localizing Value of Nystagmus Patterns and Nystagmoid Eye Movements

Type	Localization
Downbeat	Cervicomedullary junction
Periodic alternating	Cervicomedullary junction
Upbeat	Cerebellum, pontomesencephalic, pontomedullary
Convergence retraction	Dorsal midbrain
See-saw	Parasellar, midbrain
Oculopalatal myoclonus	Central tegmental tract
Oculomasticatory myorhythmia	Whipple's disease
Rebound	Cerebellum
Spasmus nutans	Exclude chiasmal glioma and craniopharyngioma
Brun's nystagmus[a]	Cerebellopontine angle

[a] Refers to ipsilateral gaze-evoked nystagmus and contralateral high-frequency, low-amplitude nystagmus of vestibular origin.

TABLE 17–5. Pharmacologic Treatment of Nystagmus and Nystagmoid Eye Movements

Nystagmus Type	Effective Medications
Periodic alternating nystagmus	Baclofen, phenytoin
Downbeat	Clonazepam, baclofen, scopolamine, gabapentin
See-saw nystagmus	Baclofen, clonazepam
Oculopalatal myoclonus	Valproic acid, trihexyphenidyl, scopolamine, clonazepam, gabapentin
Opsoclonus	Corticosteroids, IVIG, clonazepam
Superior oblique myokymia	Carbamazepine, gabapentin propranolol
Oculomasticatory myorhythmia	Ceftriaxone

IVIG = intravenous immunoglobin

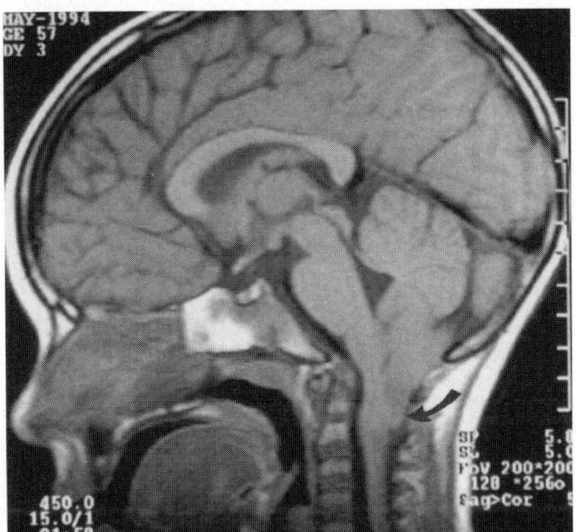

FIGURE 17–8. Arnold-Chiari malformation. Sagittal T_1-weighted MRI scan in a patient with downbeat nystagmus due to low-lying cerebellar tonsils (*arrow*).

has also been reported and these patients may experience a spontaneous remission.[69] In about one quarter of cases of acquired downbeat nystagmus, no cause is found despite MRI of the cervicomedullary junction.[70]

Downbeat nystagmus is often seen best in down and lateral gaze. Patients with downbeat nystagmus usually demonstrate downward pursuit abnormalities.[71]

The mechanism for downbeat nystagmus appears to be an imbalance of the vertical semicircular canal pathways favoring the anterior canal (Fig. 17–9).[1] Unopposed input from the anterior semicircular canal will drive the eyes slowly upward. As such, lesions involving the dorsal medulla may selectively damage crossing information from the posterior semicircular canals. Alternatively, lesions of cerebellar flocculus may damage inhibitory projections to the anterior semicircular canal pathways.

Treatment. Management of persistent downbeat nystagmus is difficult but clonazepam, gabapentin, and baclofen (Lioresal) may be used.[72, 73] A small number of patients respond to prism therapy either to induce convergence or to deflect the perceived image upward.[1, 74] The latter technique keeps the eyes out of downgaze, where downbeat nystagmus is usually maximal.

Upbeat Nystagmus. In the primary position, upbeat nystagmus does not have the localizing value of downbeat nystagmus (Table 17–6). Lesions producing upbeat nystagmus presumably damage connections of the anterior semicircular canal crossing in the ventral medulla and traveling through the brachium conjunctivum (Fig. 17–10).[75–78] However, upbeat nystagmus may also occur with lesions of the midbrain and cerebellum. Upbeat nystagmus that increases in downgaze usually signifies a medullary lesion. A recent clinicopathologic study of a patient with upbeat nystagmus worse in downgaze revealed damage to the intercalatus nuclei in the medulla.[79] Other patients with upbeat nystagmus have had a similar lesion in the dorsal paramedian medullary region.[80, 81]

Daroff and Troost[82] have divided upbeat nystagmus into two types, each having localizing value: (1) a coarse, large-amplitude nystagmus that increases in upgaze and that usually signifies a lesion in anterior vermis of the cerebellar; and (2) a small-amplitude (1 to 2 degrees) upbeat nystagmus in the primary position, which is usually caused by a medullary lesion. In addition to increasing in downgaze, this later type may become oblique in prolonged upgaze.

Tobacco smoking has also been observed to produce upbeat nystagmus in normal subjects

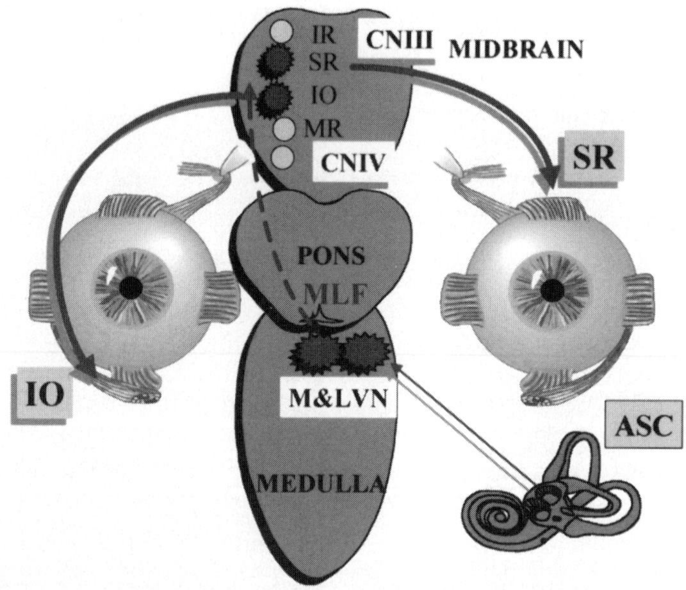

FIGURE 17–9. Mechanism of downbeat nystagmus. Unopposed input from anterior semicircular canal (ASC) pathways leads to a slow upward movement of eyes by activating the contralateral superior rectus (SR) and inferior oblique nuclei. M and LVN = medial and lateral vestibular nuclei. MLF = medial longitudinal fasciculus. (Figure courtesy of Lawrence Gray, O.D.)

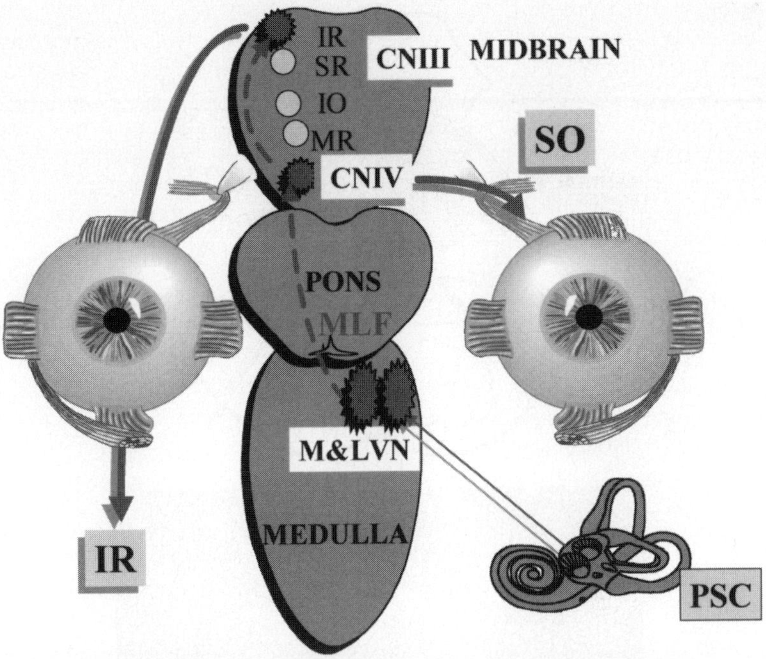

FIGURE 17–10. Mechanism of upbeat nystagmus. Unopposed input from posterior semicircular canal (PSC) pathways leads to slow downward movement of eyes by activating the contralateral inferior rectus (IR) and superior oblique (SO) nuclei. M + LVN = medial and lateral vestibular nuclei. MLF = medial longitudinal fasciculus. (Figure courtesy of Lawrence Gray, O.D.)

when visual fixation is removed. Persumably, nicotine acts as a CNS excitatory neurotransmitter in this situation.[83] Multiple sclerosis, infarction, cerebellar degeneration, and tumors are among the most common causes of upbeat nystagmus.[52]

Pendular Nystagmus/Other Types. Pendular nystagmus occurs when the eyes move back and forth with equal velocity. There are only slow phases without a jerk or fast component. This type of nystagmus may be horizontal or vertical. Oblique, elliptical or circular pendular nystagmus may occur depending on how the vertical phase of nystagmus relates to the horizontal phase. Pendular nystagmus may also be dissociated, and this tends to occur when one eye has impaired visual function. One MRI study suggested that dysconjugate pendular nystagmus was produced by asymmetric brain stem damage.[84] Acquired pendular nystagmus in adults is most often caused by multiple sclerosis and brain stem infarctions. Patterns of pendular nystagmus more commonly seen in childhood, such as spasmus nutans and monocular nystagmus associated with visual loss, were discussed earlier in this chapter.

Oculopalatal Myoclonus. When pendular nystagmus occurs in combination with palatal myoclonus, the term *oculopalatal myoclonus* is used. There may also be rhythmic movements of the facial muscles, larynx, and diaphragm. Oculopalatal myoclonus usually beats at a rate of 1 to 3 Hz. The entity most often follows a brain stem infarction by several months. The pathologic hallmark is olivary hypertrophy. Interruption of connections between the red nucleus, inferior olive, and dentate nucleus (so-called Mollaret's triangle) have been implicated as the cause of oculopalatal myoclonus. Most cases involve the *central tegmental tract* connecting the red nucleus and inferior olive. Since the parapontine reticular formation lies near the central tegmental tract, oculopalatal myoclonus may subsequently develop in those patients who have a horizontal one-and-a-half syndrome (Fig. 17–11).[85] Valproic acid, gabapentin, and clonazepam may lessen the nystagmus.[86]

Oculomasticatory Myorhythmia. A rare pendular slow (1 Hz) convergence nystagmus may occur in association with slow rhythmic movements of the jaw and other muscles. This has been

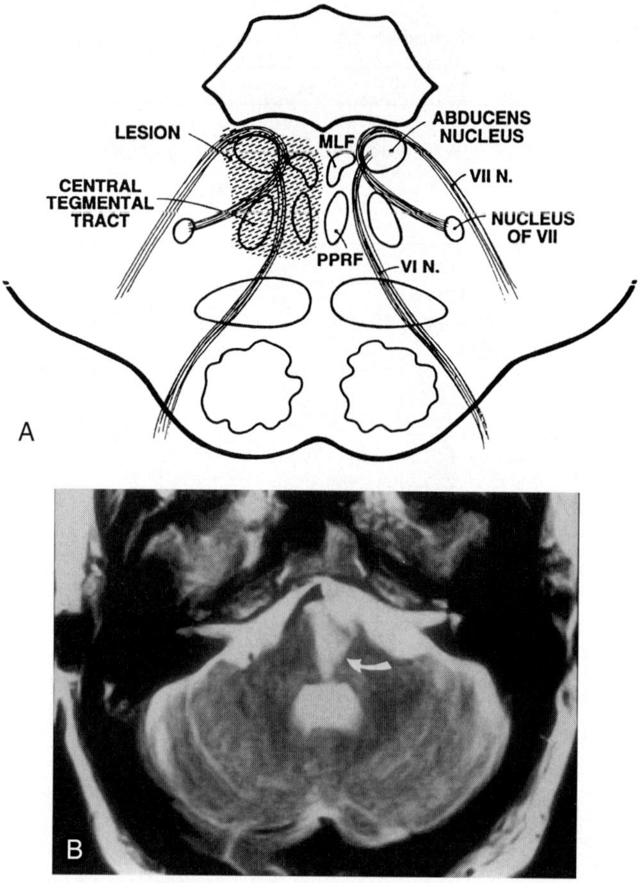

FIGURE 17–11. A. Cross-section of pons demonstrating relationship of the central tegmental tract and parapontine reticular formation. Hatched lines represent a lesion producing horizontal one-and-a-half syndrome. (From Wolin MJ, Trent RG, Lavin PJM: Oculopalatal myoclonus after the one-and-a-half syndrome with facial nerve palsy. Ophthalmology 1996;103:177–180, with permission). **B.** MRI scan from a patient with oculopalatal myoclonus and horizontal one-and-a-half syndrome. Note high-signal wedge-shaped-abnormality (*arrow*) involving paramedian pontine structures.

called *oculomasticatory myorhythmia* and it strongly suggests the diagnosis of Whipple's disease (see Chapter 16).[87, 88]

Other Types. Pendular convergent divergent nystagmus at higher frequences may be seen in patients with multiple sclerosis and brain stem stroke.[89] Elliptical pendular nystagmus together with upbeat nystagmus may also occur in Pelizaeus–Merzbacher disease,[90] a rare X-linked neurodegenerative condition in young children caused by a deficiency in the proteolipid apoprotein PLP.[91–94] The disease primarily affects the CNS white matter, and pendular nystagmus accompanied by vision loss and optic atrophy may be the initial manifestations. Other childhood white matter disorders with a similar presentation include adrenoleukodystrophy (see Chapter 8) and Cockayne syndrome.[95]

Joubert Syndrome. Pendular torsional, see-saw, and gaze-evoked nystagmus may be prominent features of Joubert syndrome.[96] This congenital, structural disorder is characterized by the symptom complex of developmental delay, hypotonia, truncal ataxia, episodic hypernea, and apnea in infancy,[97–99] and eye movement abnormalities such as nystagmus, impaired smooth pursuit and saccades, ocular motor apraxia, an inability to cancel the vestibulo-ocular reflex, and strabismus.[100] Other neuro-ophthalmic abnormalities include retinal dystrophy, chorioretinal coloboma,[101] and ptosis.[102] The unifying structural abnormality is dysgenesis or absence of the cerebellar vermis, creating the characteristic "molar tooth" sign with a deep interpeduncular fossa and thickened cerebellar peduncles seen radiographically (Fig. 17–12). The genetic basis is unknown.

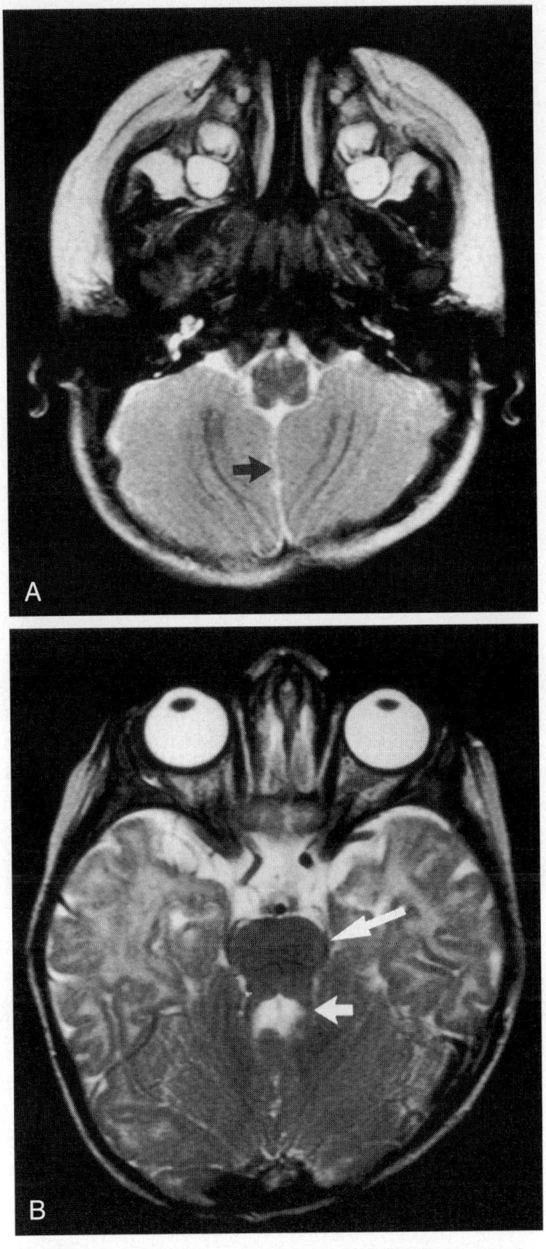

FIGURE 17–12. Joubert syndrome. Axial MRI scans of a child with pendular torsional nystagmus who was found to have (**A**) absence of the cerebellar vermis (*arrow*) and (**B**) stretching and thickening of the cerebellar peduncles (*small arrow*), producing a "molar tooth" appearance of the pontomesencephalon (*large arrow*).

Treatment. The major drugs to treat pendular nystagmus include anticholinergics, baclofen (Lioresal), valproic acid, clonazepam, and carbamazepine. In a randomized control trial of three muscarinic antagonists, scopolamine was found to be superior to benztropine and glycopyrrolate. Both visual acuity and oscillopsia improved significantly with scopolomine.[103] Recent experience also suggests gabapentin may be helpful to treat acquired pendular nystagmus.[104, 105] The glutamate antagonist memantine holds promise in the treatment of acquired pendular nystagmus (see treatment overview, below). In one report, canabis suppressed pendular nystagmus in a patient with multiple sclerosis.[166]

Prisms and other devices, such as a plus-sphere spectacle lens combined with a minus-sphere contact lens, may also be used.[1, 74, 104, 106–108] Invasive procedures may include muscle surgery and botulinum toxin injections. Eye muscle surgery attempts to move the eyes from their eccentric null point to the primary position. This will shift the null point to a more cosmetically acceptable position. Injecting botulinum toxin into the extraocular muscles may help a small number of patients but it is limited by the ptosis and double vision it produces. Typically, patients will have to patch the worse-seeing eye for comfort.[16, 109] The need for repetitive injections is another detracting factor.

Convergence Retraction Nystagmus. This is a sign of pretectal dysfunction and may in part reflect excess convergence tone. It is not a true nystagmus because there is no slow phase, just opposing adducting saccades. Retraction results from cofiring of horizontally and vertically acting extraocular muscles. Convergence retraction saccades are elicited by having the patient look upward or by running an OKN tape downward. Accompanying neurologic signs are usually present, including upgaze palsy, pupillary light–near dissociation, and eyelid retraction (see discussion on the Parinaud or pretectal syndrome in Chapter 16).

Thyroid-associated ophthalmopathy may also produce eyelid retraction, and decreased upgaze. In rare instances, the globes may also retract, mimicking convergence retraction nystagmus. The absence of any pupillary abnormalities and the presence of exophthalmos, conjunctival injection, eyelid edema and forced ductions all should make the distinction relatively clear. Unfortunately, eyelid lag cannot be used as distinguishing feature since it may occur in both disorders (see Chapter 14).

See-Saw Nystagmus. This unusual nystagmus is highly localizing to the midbrain or parasellar region (Table 17–6), although there are many exceptions. See-saw nystagmus is characterized by the simultaneous pendular elevation and intorsion of one eye with the depression and extorsion of the other eye (see Fig. 7–15).[110, 111] To complete the see-saw cycle, the eye that was depressed and extorted will elevate and intort and the eye that was elevated will fall and extort. Patients with *congenital see-saw nystagmus* may show no torsional component and the elevating eye may extort while the falling eye intorts. Some patients will display half of a see-saw cycle with a corrective quick phase. This has been called *hemi-* or *jerk see-saw nystagmus.*[112] It typically occurs from a unilateral mesodiencephalic lesion involving the interstitial nucleus of Cajal. The torsional nystagmus seen in midbrain lesions may beat either to the right or left shoulder. Lesions affecting the interstitial nucleus of Cajal, but sparing the rostral interstitial nucleus of the medial longitudinal fasciculus (riMLF) produce a torsional nystagmus that beats towards the ipsilateral shoulder. If the riMLF is involved, the nystagmus may beat contralesionally.[113] Patients with visual loss alone may also have see-saw nystagmus.[114]

Pendular see-saw nystagmus is usually caused by a sellar mass lesion (eg, pituitary tumor, craniopharyngioma) (Fig. 17–13). It may abolished by removal of the offending sellar mass lesion. The relationship between see-saw nystagmus and chiasmal visual loss is discussed in Chapter 7. Joubert syndrome (see above) is also a cause of this eye movement disorder. Baclofen (Lioresal) and clonazepam may help lessen see-saw nystagmus.[72, 74]

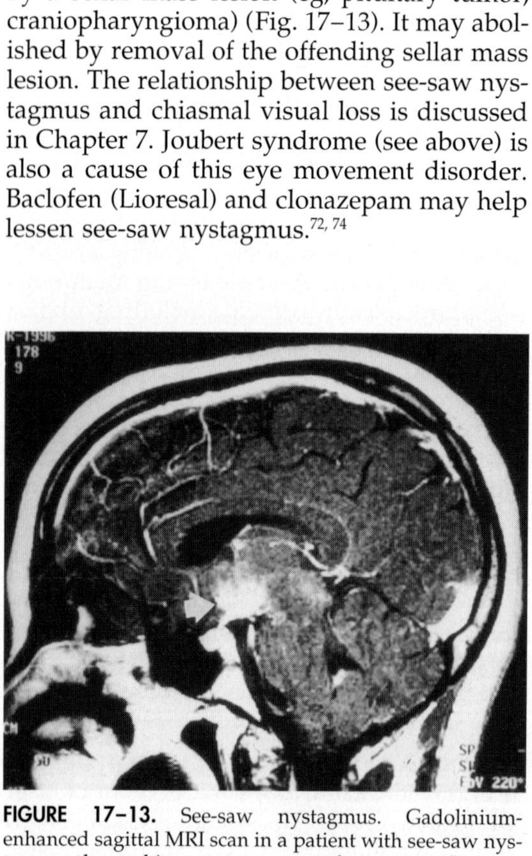

FIGURE 17–13. See-saw nystagmus. Gadolinium-enhanced sagittal MRI scan in a patient with see-saw nystagmus due to biopsy-proven granulomatous inflammation of the hypothalamus and chiasm (*arrow*), presumed to be sarcoidosis.

Voluntary Nystagmus. Voluntary nystagmus is usually produced by patients seeking secondary gain,[115–118] but this nystagmus may also be seen in families.[119, 120] Most patients complain of decreased vision and oscillopsia.[121] The nystagmus is recognized as a high-frequency, low-amplitude pendular oscillation that cannot be sustained. Eye movement recordings show the oscillations to be a series of rapidly alternating saccades, usually horizontal, with a frequency of 3 to 42 Hz.[122] Voluntary nystagmus usually occurs in bursts that last 5 to 10 seconds. Lid fluttering and squinting may accompany the ocular oscillation. Occasionally one may observe the strain in the patient's face as he or she tries to maintain the eye movements. One can often interrupt the voluntary oscillations by having the patient pursue a target. Also, voluntary nystagmus disappears when the patient is distracted since significant concentration is required to generate it.

Convergence-Evoked Nystagmus. Convergence usually dampens nystagmus. However, in rare instances it may precipitate it. Both congenital and acquired nystagmus may be enhanced by convergence.[123] The congenital form may have conjugate oscillations, while the acquired form has disjunctive eye movements. Occasionally, upbeat nystagmus changes to downbeat with convergence. The pendular convergent nystagmus of Whipple's disease may be increased by convergence, and an acquired convergence-evoked pendular nystagmus in multiple sclerosis has been described.[124]

Lid Nystagmus. The lids normally beat upward in patients with upbeat nystagmus. However, in some patients the amplitude of the lid movements is greater than that of the eye movements. Convergence may also precipitate lid nystagmus.[125] Both of these forms of lid nystagmus have poor localizing value.[47] However, lid nystagmus initiated by lateral gaze has been associated with lateral medullary lesions.[126]

Epileptic Nystagmus. Nystagmus may be induced by epileptic activity. Occasionally, nystagmus may be the only manifestation of a seizure. In most cases, the jerk horizontal nystagmus is directed away from the seizure focus.[127] There is a tendency for the epileptic focus to be located in the temporoparietol-occipital junction. The discharge frequency tends to be high, with a rate of approximately 10 per second. Rarely, ictal nystagmus may be vertical or ipsilateral to the seizure focus, and an epileptic periodic alternating nystamus has been described.[128]

Drug-Induced Nystagmus. Drug-induced nystagmus is one one of the most common forms of nystagmus. A variety of medications may produce nystagmus in the therapeutic range, including anticonvulsants, sedatives, barbituates, and the phenothiazines. Typically the nystagmus is present in horizontal endgaze and upgaze, but not downgaze. The nystagmus is symmetrical and usually does not fatigue. Rarely, drug-induced nystagmus is present in downgaze. In contrast, some medications, such as carbamazepine, phenytoin, and lithium, may produce a pure downbeat nystagmus.

Acute alcohol intoxication may produce a horizontal endgaze nystagmus known as positional alcohol nystagmus. Peripheral vestibular dysfunction resulting from the alcohol entering the cupula, rendering it lighter than the endolymph, is the purported "buoyancy" mechanism.[129] However, we cannot advocate the presence of nystagmus alone to assess intoxication.[130] Clearly, the presence of physiologic nystagmus, congenital nystagmus, and the effects of other medications may fool the unwary observer.

Optokinetic Nystagmus. When rotation of the head is sustained for more than a few seconds, the optokinetic system becomes active to permit fixation on stationary objects. It is an involuntary reflex, but may be suppressed if the stimulus is not full field and the patient decides to look above or below the moving target. At the bedside, the optokinetic response may be elicited by moving a striped tape in front of the patient (see Fig. 2–29). Optokinetic nystagmus (OKN) is generated by pursuit of an object and a corrective saccade in the opposite direction to detect the next target.[131] Both retinal and cerebral projections contribute to the optokinetic response, but it is the cerebral connections that are the most important in the adult patient.[132] The cerebral projections begin in the middle temporal (MT), medial superior temporal (MST), and parietal areas (PP) and connect to the accessory optic tract system and dorsolateral pontine nuclei. Ultimately these projections will reach the medial vestibular nucleus and from this area to the ocular motor nuclei.[1]

OKN may be helpful as a diagnostic tool to detect (1) intact vision in infants with congenital nystagmus and preserved vertical OKN; (2) a reverse OKN response characteristic of congenital nystagmus; (3) a deep parietal lesion (a reduced response is observed when the OKN tape is moved in the direction of a parietal lesion); (4) residual vision in a patient who claims complete blindness (an intact OKN response suggests vision is at least count fingers); (5) a subtle ocular motor palsy such as the adduction weakness seen in internuclear ophthalmoparesis; and (6) convergence retraction nystagmus (the OKN tape is taken downward to elicit this pretectal sign).

NYSTAGMOID EYE MOVEMENTS

The eye movements discussed in this section are not pure forms of nystagmus. They are usually saccades that interrupt fixation. Alternatively, the ocular oscillations in this group have a fast phase followed by a slow phase. Ocular bobbing is an example of this type of eye movement.

Saccadic Intrusions

Neurons in the pons and midbrain help generate the saccadic eye movements that allow the eyes to overcome the viscoelastic forces of the orbit. These neurons are called *burst neurons* and they reside in the paramedian pontine reticular formation for horizontal saccades and in the rostral interstitial nucleus of the medial longitudinal fasciculus for vertical saccades (see Chapter 16). The burst neurons are kept silent by a group of neurons called *pause cells* that reside in the paramedian pontine region. When a saccade is made, the pause cells are turned off by an inhibiting input from supranuclear structures. Thus, many of the saccadic disorders described below are thought to be caused by pause cell dysfunction. However, pathologic confirmation of this theory is lacking.[133] Inappropriate saccades (intrusions) may also result from disordered input to the burst neurons from other structures such as the superior colliculus, basal ganglia, or cerebellum.[1]

In order of increasing severity, square wave jerks, ocular dysmetria, macrosaccadic oscillations, and ocular flutter and opsoclonus represent the spectrum of saccadic intrusions.

Square Wave Jerks. These are horizontal back-to-back saccades that interrupt fixation (Fig.

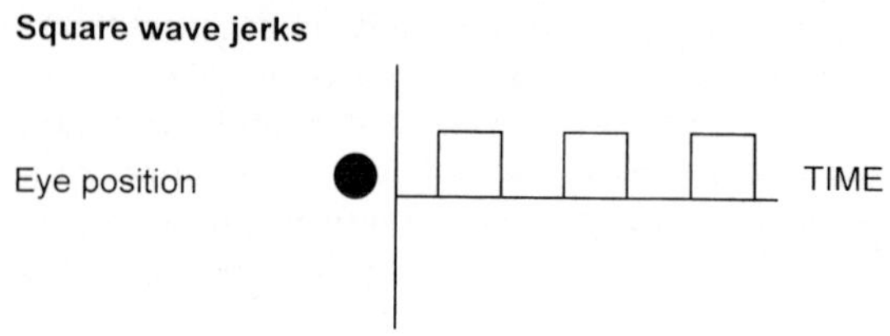

FIGURE 17–14. Square wave jerks. Eye movement recording (x-axis = time, y-axis = horizontal eye position) demonstrating back-to-back horizontal saccades separated by a 200-msec interval.

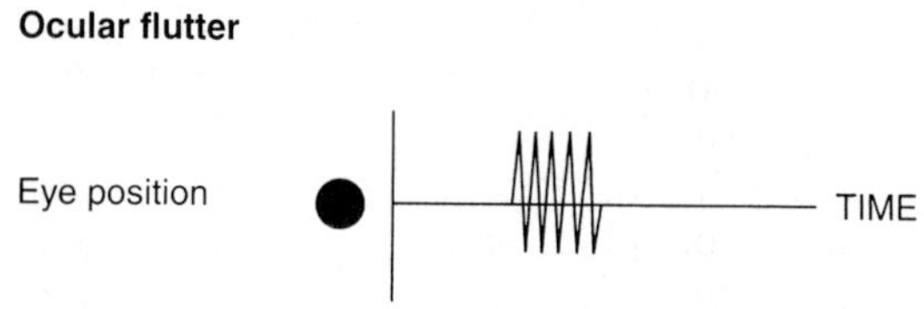

FIGURE 17–16. Ocular flutter. Eye movement recording (x-axis = time, y-axis = horizontal eye position) demonstrating spontaneous back-to-back horizontal saccades without an intersaccadic interval.

17–14).[47] There is an intersaccadic interval to help distinguish this saccadic disorder from ocular flutter. If the amplitude is greater than 5 degrees, the term *macrosquare wave jerk* is used. Square wave jerks may be seen in normal individuals but more than 9 per minute is considered abnormal. Common causes of square wave jerks include cerebellar disease, schizophrenia, Parkinson's disease, and progressive supranuclear palsy.

Ocular Dysmetria. This is a sign of cerebellar dysfunction similar to limb dysmetria. If upon refixation, the eyes overshoot the target and then saccade back to the intended fixation point, this is termed *saccadic hypermetria.* In saccadic hypometria, the eyes undershoot the target.

Macrosaccadic Oscillations. These are horizontal saccades that occur across the intended fixation point in a crescendo–decrescendo pattern (Fig. 17–15). They may have a large amplitude of 15 to 30 degrees. Unlike square wave jerks, macrosaccadic oscillations are not evident in the dark. Again, this a cerebellar eye sign that is most commonly observed in patients with multiple sclerosis.[47]

Opsoclonus and Ocular Flutter. Opsoclonus describes the dramatic occurrence of involuntary conjugate multidirectional saccades (saccadomania) that occur without an intersaccadic interval.[134] The eye movement abnormality is often associated with eye blinking, facial twitching, myoclonus, and ataxia (Kinsbourne's "dancing eyes and dancing feet"). Ocular flutter, a related disorder, refers to back-to-back horizontal saccades without an intersaccadic interval (Fig. 17–16). There is no vertical component. The lack of an interval between the saccades distinguishes ocular flutter from square wave jerks. Ocular flutter has the same localizing value and differential diagnosis as opsoclonus. Reflecting saccadic dysfunction, ocular dysmetria is an associated finding of both opsoclonus and ocular flutter. Saccadic oscillations very similar to ocular flutter and opsoclonus can rarely occur on a nonorganic basis.[135]

Relationship With Neuroblastoma. Fifty percent of children with opsoclonus harbor a neuroblastoma, thus it is essential to exclude this tumor in any child with saccadomania. Conversely, only 2% with neuroblastoma have opsoclonus.[136] Screening tests include urine vanillymandelic acid (VMA) and homovanillic acid (HVA) levels and MRI of the thorax and abdomen. There may be a pleocytosis in the cerebrospinal fluid, and somatostatin receptor (octreotide) imaging may also be used.[137] This

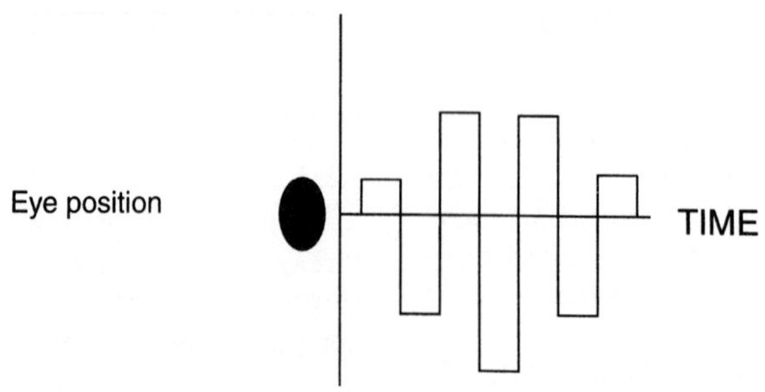

FIGURE 17–15. Macrosaccadic oscillations. Eye movement recording (x-axis = time, y-axis = horizontal eye position) demonstrating a crescendo–decrescendo pattern of saccades after the eyes attempt to return to fixation from eccentric gaze.

condition often responds to tumor removal and adrenocorticotropic hormone (ACTH) or prednisone, but may also require other immunomodulatory therapy such as gammaglobulin or plasmapheresis. The response to these modalities suggests the pathogenesis of opsoclonus associated with neuroblastoma is autoimmune.[138] However, this is unconfirmed because only a few patients with circulating antibodies, such as anti-Hu,[139] antineurofilament, and anti-Purkinje cell[140] have been identified.[141] Pathologic brain specimens have also either been normal or have shown Purkinje cell and granular cell loss with gliosis.[136]

Children with neuroblastoma and opsoclonus have a more favorable prognosis than those without opsoclonus. This may be due to immune surveillance, earlier tumor detection, or favorable tumor biology. Neuroblastomas associated with a poor prognosis often demonstrate amplification of the N-*myc* protooncogene, a feature almost always absent in patients with opsoclonus.[141] Furthermore, hyperdiploid neuroblastomas tend to have a lower-stage disease and longer survival than diploid tumors.[141]

Relapses and corticosteroid dependence are common in opsoclonus associated with neuroblastoma, and some children have long-term neurologic deficits.[142]

Other Forms of Opsoclonus in Childhood. These include a benign, self-limited opsoclonus in neonates,[143] and opsoclonus associated with severe visual disturbances,[144] parainfectious cerebellitis, and encephalitis.[136] Like the paraneoplastic type, parainfectious opsoclonus myoclonus sometimes requires either ACTH or prednisone, and some children may still be left with some permanent neurologic abnormalities, including ataxia and defective cognition.[142]

Opsoclonus in Adults. In adults, opsoclonus may be postinfectious or drug induced (eg, amitriptyline, lithium, phenytoin, cocaine),[136] or occur as the remote effect of cancers or encephalitis.[1, 145] Associated tumors include lung (one case with anti-Hu antibodies[146]), breast (with anti-Ri antibodies[147]), and gynecologic neoplasms. Stroke, trauma, tumors, or hyperosmolar nonketotic coma are other associations. Opsoclonus may also occur from cerebellar, brain stem, or diffuse cerebral injury. Postinfectious opsoclonus usually slowly improves spontaneously, but may be dampened in the recovery phase by clonazepam and corticosteroids.

Other Nystagmoid Eye Movements

Superior Oblique Myokymia. Superior oblique myokymia, or microtremor, is a high-frequency monocular oscillation produced by spontaneous firing of one superior oblique muscle.[148, 149] Patients often complain of monocular vertical oscillopsia. The diagnosis is made by asking the patient to look into the field of action of the superior oblique muscle while the eye is observed with a slit lamp or the fundus with an ophthalmoscope.[150] This condition is usually idiopathic, but neuroimaging should be performed to exclude a midbrain lesion.[151] The mechanism of superior oblique myokymia is thought to result from phasic activity of the fourth nerve fascicles with resultant periodic contraction of the superior oblique muscle.[148]

Treatment. This disorder may spontaneously remit but carbamazepine, baclofen (Lioresal), or propranolol may be tried in resistant cases.[150] If symptoms persist and are disabling, one could consider tenotomy of the superior oblique muscle, in combination with resection of the inferior oblique muscle. A more recent surgical approach involves weakening of the anterior portion of the superior oblique tendon only. This procedure may eliminate the superior oblique myokymia without affecting the ocular motility balance.[152]

Ocular Bobbing. Ocular bobbing signifies brain stem dysfunction, and in many instances it reflects a pontine process.[153] It is an asynchronous eye movement disorder that begins with a quick conjugate down movement followed by a slow drift back to the midline. This sequence and its asynchronous pattern serve to distinguish ocular bobbing from nystagmus.[154] Since ocular bobbing is commonly associated with pontine lesions, horizontal gaze palsies often coexist. A variety of lesions may produce ocular bobbing, including stroke, tumors, toxic–metabolic conditions, and inflammatory processes.[155, 156] Ocular bobbing is usually associated with intra-axial brain stem disease, however, extra-axial brain stem compression may also produce this eye movement disorder.[157]

Variants of bobbing exist in which the eyes quickly move upward and then drift slowly downward (reverse bobbing). Some patients show a downward slow phase with a quick upward correction (ocular dipping or inverse bobbing).[158, 159] This sequence of eye movement disturbance may be seen in patients who suffered from status epilepticus or anoxic injury. Clearly, it is difficult to remember all the variants of bobbing and their names. Sometimes, it is more practical just to describe the bobbing phenomena and recognize its significance as a brain stem sign.

NYSTAGMUS AND NYSTAGMOID EYE MOVEMENT TREATMENT OVERVIEW

No medicine or device can provide consistent relief from nystagmus or nystagmoid eye movements.[160] However, in certain patients, pharmacologic therapy can have a dramatic beneficial effect. For instance, acquired periodic alternating nystagmus can be eliminated by baclofen (Lioresal).[57] Clonazepam, valproic acid, or baclofen may be tried in the treatment of almost any ocular oscillation.[72–74] Clonazepam tends to be our first choice when attempting to eliminate the oscillopsia from nystagmus. Recently, gabapentin (up to 900 mg a day) was compared to baclofen (up to 30 mg a day) as a treatment for acquired nystagmus. Gabapentin was found to be superior to baclofen in the treatment of acquired pendular nystagmus.[161] Unfortunately, both gabapentin and baclofen have a less predictable effect on downbeat nystagmus.

A variety of anticholinergic drugs have been used to treat nystagmus. In a randomized control of three intravenous preparations, scopolamine was superior to both benztropine and glycopyrrolate.[103] In another study of anticholinergics, trihexyphenidyl was not effective and tridihexethyl only showed partial benefit.[108]

Further delineation of the pharmacologic pathways of the vestibular system should provide new avenues for the treatment of nystagmus (Fig. 17–17).[162] For instance, hair cell sensitivity appears to be modulated by CNS efferent pathways utilizing gamma-aminobutyric acid (GABA), acetylcholine, and other peptide molecules as transmitters. The glutamate antagonist memantine in daily doses ranging from 15 to 60 mg had dramatic beneficial effect on pendular nystagmus in one study.[163]

Botulinum toxin has been used to treat both acquired and congenital nystagmus. Botulinum may be injected into the extraocular muscles or into the retrobulbar space.[160] Although botulinum may reduce oscillopsia, its overall effect has been limited by its side effects of double vision and ptosis. Repetitive injections of botulinum are usually necessary every 2 to 3 months, and this creates another deterrent to its long-term use.

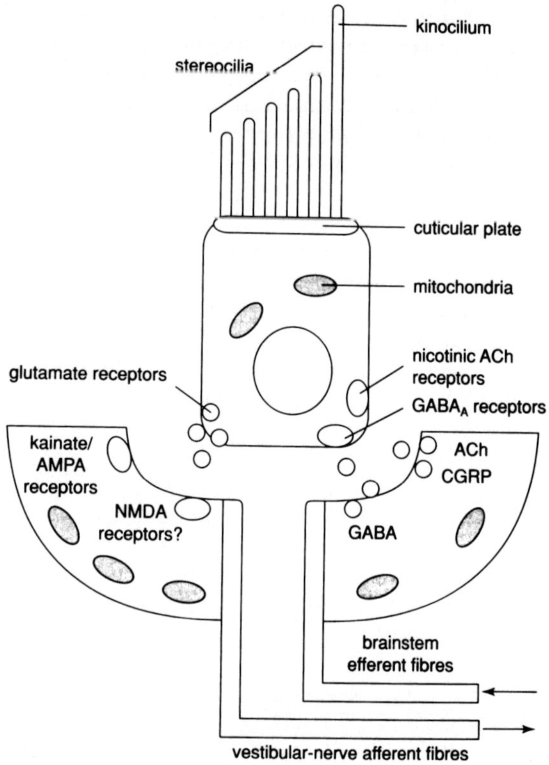

FIGURE 17–17. Diagram illustrating the transmitters and receptors involved in the afferent synapse between the vestibular receptor hair cells and the the vestibular nerve and the efferent synapse between the brain stem efferent neurones and the hair cells. Ach = acetylcholine, CGRP = calcitonin gene-related peptide. (From Smith PF, Darlington CL: Recent advances in the pharmacology of the vestibulo-ocular reflex system. Trends Pharmacol Sci 1996;17:421–427, with permission.)

We treat saccadic intrusions like nystagmus. Clonazepam and gabapentin tend to be our first-line agents. Paraneoplastic or parainfectious opsoclonus may respond to ACTH and steroids. This effect tends to be more evident in children than in adults.[160] Plasma exchange using a protein A column to remove immunoglobins may be effective in treating paraneoplastic opsoclonus.[164]

Prisms and other optical devices may also lessen ocular oscillations. For instance, a high positive spectacle lens can be combined with a negative contact lens to improve oscillopsia. Unfortunately, such devices have limited use because they cannot correct for refractive change associated with convergence or the oscillopsia created by head and eye movement.[160] Devices such as base-out prisms to induce convergence may be helpful, particularly in congenital nystagmus. Base-down prisms over both eyes have been used to treat downbeat nystagmus. However, we have had limited success with this technique.

Surgical therapy is primarily reserved for the patient with congenital oscillations. Most surgical interventions aim to move the eyes so their null point is in the primary position.

REFERENCES

1. Leigh RJ, Zee DS: The Neurology of Eye Movements, 3rd edition, pp 405–610. New York, Oxford University Press, 1999.
2. Tusa RJ, Herdman SJ: Diagnosis and treatment of the dizzy patient. Hosp Phys 1997;33:22–37.
3. Hain TC, Fetter M, Zee DS: Head-shaking nystagmus in patients with unilateral peripheral vestibular lesions. Am J Otolaryngol 1987;8:36–47.
4. Halmagyi GM, Curthoys IS: A clinical sign of canal paresis. Arch Neurol 1988;45:737–739.
5. Gresty M, Page N, Barratt H: The differential diagnosis of congenital nystagmus. J Neurol Neurosurg Psychiatry 1984;47:936–942.
6. Gottlob I: Infantile nystagmus. Development documented by eye movement recordings. Invest Ophthalmol Vis Sci 1997;38:767–773.
7. Dell'Osso LF, Daroff RB: Congenital nystagmus waveforms and foveation strategy. Doc Ophthalmol 1975;39:155–182.
8. Halmagyi GM, Gresty MA, Leech J: Reversed optokinetic nystagmus (OKN): mechanism and clinical significance. Ann Neurol 1980;7:429–435.
9. Cogan DG: Congenital nystagmus. Can J Ophthalmol 1967;2:4–10.
10. O'Connor PS: Making sense of nystagmus—can it be done? Otolaryngol Clin 1987;20:35–49.
11. Kerrison JB, Vagefi MR, Barmada MM, et al: Congenital motor nystagmus linked to Xq26–q27. Am J Hum Genet 1999;64:600–607.
12. Gelbart SS, Hoyt CS: Congenital nystagmus: a clinical perspective in infancy. Graefes Arch Klin Exp Ophthalmol 1988;226:178–180.
13. Sigal MB, Diamond GR: Survey of management strategies for nystamus patients with vertical or torsional head posture. Ann Ophthalmol 1990;22:134–138.
14. Zubcov AA, Stärk N, Weber A, et al: Improvement of visual acuity after surgery for nystagmus. Ophthalmology 1993;100:1488–1497.
15. Carruthers J: The treatment of congenital nystagmus with Botox. J Pediatr Ophthalmol Strabismus 1995;32:306–308.
16. Tomsak RL, Remler BF, Averbuch-Heller L, et al: Unsatisfactory treatment of acquired nystagmus with retrobulbar injection of botulinum toxin. Am J Ophthalmol 1995;119:489–496.
17. Gresty MA, Metcalfe T, Timms C, et al: Neurology of latent nystagmus. Brain 1992;115:1303–1321.
18. Gottlob I, Wizov SS, Reinecke RD: Spasmus nutans. A long-term follow-up. Invest Ophthalmol Vis Sci 1995;36:2768–2771.
19. Weissman RM, Dell'Osso LF, Abel LA, et al: Spasmus nutans. A quantitative prospective study. Arch Ophthalmol 1987;105:525–528.
20. Massry GG, Bloom JN, Cruz OA: Convergence nystagmus associated with spasmus nutans. J Neuroophthalmol 1996;16:196–198.
21. Antony JH, Ouvrier RA, Wise G: Spasmus nutans. A mistaken identity. Arch Neurol 1980;37:373–375.
22. Lavery MA, O'Neill JF, Chu FC, et al: Acquired nystagmus in early childhood: A presenting sign of intracranial tumor. Ophthalmology 1984;91:425–435.
23. Farmer J, Hoyt CS: Monocular nystagmus in infancy and early childhood. Am J Ophthalmol 1984;98: 504–509.
24. Schulman JA, Shults WT, Jones JM: Monocular vertical nystagmus as an initial sign of chiasmal glioma. Am J Ophthalmol 1979;87:87–90.
25. Gottlob I, Zubcov A, Catalano RA, et al: Signs distinguishing spasmus nutans (with and without central nervous system lesions) from infantile nystagmus. Ophthalmology 1990;97:1166–1175.
26. Lambert SR, Newman NJ: Retinal disease masquerading as spasmus nutans. Neurology 1993;43:1607–1609.
27. Gottlob I, Wizov SS, Reinecke RD: Quantitative eye and head movement recordings of retinal disease mimicking spasmus nutans. Am J Ophthalmol 1995;119:374–376.
28. Kalyanaraman K, Jagannathan K, Ramanujam RA, et al: Congenital head nodding and nystagmus with cerebellar degeneration. J Pediatr 1973;83:1023–1026.
29. Arnoldi KA, Tychsen L: Prevalence of intracranial lesions in children initially diagnosed with disconjugate nystagmus (spasmus nutans). J Pediatr Ophthalmol Strabismus 1995;32:296–301.
30. Young TL, Weis JR, Summers CG, et al: The association of strabismus, amblyopia, and refractive errors in spasmus nutans. Ophthalmology 1997;104:112–117.
31. Yee RD, Jelks GW, Baloh RW, et al: Uniocular nystagmus in monocular visual loss. Ophthalmology 1979;86:511–518.
32. Davey K, Kowal L, Friling R, et al: The Heimann–Bielscholwsky phenomenon: dissociated vertical nystagmus. Aust NZ J Ophthalmol 1998;26:237–240.
33. King RA, Nelson LB, Wagner RS: Spasmus nutans. A benign clinical entity? Arch Ophthalmol 1986; 104:1501–1504.
34. Doslak MJ, Dell'Osso LF, Daroff RB: Alexander's law: a model and resulting study. Ann Otol Rhinol Laryngol 1982;91:316–322.
35. Cutrer FM, Baloh RW: Migraine-associated dizziness. Headache 1992;32:300–304.
36. Lanska DJ, Remler B: Benign paroxysmal positioning vertigo: classic descriptions, origins of the provocative positioning technique, and conceptual developments. Neurology 1997;48:1167–1177.
37. Furman JM, Cass SP: Benign paroxysmal positional vertigo. N Engl J Med 1999;341:1590–1596.
38. Baloh RW, Yue Q, Jacobson KM, et al: Persistent direction-changing positional nystagmus: Another variant of benign positional nystagmus? Neurology 1995;45:1297–1301.
39. Casani A, Giovanni V, Bruno F, et al: Positional vertigo and ageotropic bidirectional nystagmus. Laryngoscope 1997;107:807–813.

40. Lempert T, Wilck KT: A positional maneuver for treatment of horizontal canal benign positional vertigo. Laryngoscope 1996;106:476–478
41. Nuti D, Agus G, Barbieri MT, et al: The managment of horizontal canal paryoxysmal positional vertigo. Acta Otolaryngol 1998;118:455–460.
42. Katsarkas A: Paroxysmal positional vertigo: an overview and the deposits repositioning maneuver. Am J Otol 1995;16:725–730.
43. Serafini G, Palmieri AMR, Simoncelli C: Benign paroxysmal positional vertigo of posterior semicircular canal: results in 160 cases treated with Semont's maneuver. Ann Otol Rhinol Laryngol 1996;105:770–775.
44. Troost BT, Patton JM: Exercise therapy for positional vertigo. Neurology 1992;42:1441–1444.
45. Brandt T, Steddin S, Daroff RB: Therapy for benign paroxysmal positioning vertigo, revisited. Neurology 1994;44:796–800.
46. Epley JM: The canalith repositioning procedure: For treatment of benign paroxysmal positional vertigo. Otolaryngol Head Neck Surg 1992;107:399–404.
47. Dell'Osso LF, Daroff RB: Nystagmus and saccadic intrusions and oscillations. In: Glaser JS (ed): Neuro-ophthalmology, 3rd edition, pp 369–401. Philadelphia, Lippincott, Williams & Wilkins, 1999.
48. Ash PR, Keltner JL: Neuro-ophthalmic signs in pontine lesions. Medicine 1979;58:304–320.
49. Baloh RW, Konrad HR, Dirks D, et al: Cerebellar–pontine angle tumors. Results of quantitative vestibulo-ocular testing. Arch Neurol 1976;33:507–512.
50. Hood JD, Kayan A, Leech J: Rebound nystagmus. Brain 1973;96:507–526.
51. Gradstein L, Reinecke RD, Wizov SS, et al: Congenital periodic alternating nystagmus. Diagnosis and management. Ophthalmology 1997;104:918–929.
52. Fletcher WA: Nystagmus: an overview. In: Sharpe JA, Barber HO (eds): The Vestibular–Ocular Reflex and Vertigo, pp 195–215. New York, Raven Press, 1993.
53. Waespe W, Cohen B, Raphan T: Dynamic modification of the vestibulo-ocular reflex by the nodulus and uvula. Science 1985;228:199–202.
54. Lewis JM, Kline LB: Periodic alternating nystagmus associated with periodic alternating skew deviation. J Clin Neuro-ophthalmol 1983;3:115–117.
55. Kennard C, Barger G, Hoyt WF: The association of periodic alternating nystagmus with periodic alternating gaze. A case report. J Clin Neuro-ophthalmol 1981;1:191–193.
56. Cross SA, Smith JL, Norton EWD: Periodic alternating nystagmus clearing after vitrectomy. J Clin Neuro-ophthalmol 1982;2:5–11.
57. Halmagyi GM, Rudge P, Gresty MA, et al: Treatment of periodic alternating nystagmus. Ann Neurol 1980;8:609–611.
58. Larmande P: Baclofen as a treatment for nystagmus (letter). Ann Neurol 1982;11:213.
59. Shallo-Hoffmann J, Faldon M, Tusa RJ: The incidence and waveform characteristics of periodic alternating nystagmus in congenital nystagmus. Invest Ophthalmol Vis Sci 1999;40:2546–2553.
60. Halmagyi GM, Rudge P, Gresty M, et al: Downbeating nystagmus. A review of sixty-two cases. Arch Neurol 1983;40:777–784.
61. Büttner U, Helmchen CH, Büttner-Ennever JA: The localizing value of nystagmus in brainstem disorders. Neuro-ophthalmology 1995;15:283–290.
62. Saul RF, Selhorst JB: Downbeat nystagmus with magnesium depletion. Arch Neurol 1981;38:650–652.
63. Du Pasquier R, Vingerhoets F, Safran AB, et al: Periodic downbeat nystagmus. Neurology 1998;51:1478–1480.
64. Alpert JN: Downbeat nystagmus due to anticonvulsant toxicity. Ann Neurol 1978;4:471–473.
65. Wheeler SD, Ramsay RE, Weiss J: Drug-induced downbeat nystagmus. Ann Neurol 1982;12:227–228.
66. Chrousos GA, Cowdry R, Schuelin M, et al: Two cases of downbeat nystagmus and oscillopsia associated with carbamazepine. Am J Ophthalmol 1987;103:221–224.
67. Halmagyi GM, Lessell I, Curthoys IS, et al: Lithium induced downbeat nystagmus. Am J Ophthalmol 1989;107:664–670.
68. Corbett JJ, Jacobson DM, Thompson HS, et al: Downbeating nystagmus and other ocular motor defects caused by lithium toxicity. Neurology 1989;39:481–487.
69. Brodsky MC: Congenital downbeat nystagmus. J Pediatr Ophthalmol Strabismus 1996;33:191–193.
70. Bronstein AM, Miller DH, Rudge P, et al: Downbeating nystagmus: case report with magnetic resonance imaging and neuro-otological findings. J Neurol Sci 1987;81:173–184.
71. Zee DS, Friendlich AR, Robinson DA, et al: The mechanism of downbeat nystagmus. Arch Neurol 1974;30:227–237.
72. Currie JN, Matsuo V: The use of clonazepam in the treatment of nystamus induced oscillopsia. Ophthalmology 1986;93:924–932.
73. Dieterich M, Straube A, Brandt T, et al: The effects of baclofen and cholinergic drugs in upbeat and downbeat nystagmus. J Neurol Neurosurg Psychiatry 1991;54:627–632.
74. Carlow TJ: Medical treatment of nystagmus and ocular motor disorders. Int Ophthalmol Clin 1986;26:251–264.
75. Keane JR, Itabashi HH: Upbeat nystagmus: clinicopathologic study of two patients. Neurology 1987;37:491–494.
76. Traccis S, Rosati G, Aiello I, et al: Upbeat nystagmus as an early sign of cerebellar astrocytoma. J Neurol 1989;1989:359–360.
77. Hirose G, Kawada J, Tsukada K, et al: Primary position upbeat nystagmus. J Neurol Sci 1991;105:159–167.
78. Hirose G, Ogasawara T, Shirakawa T, et al: Primary position upbeat nystagmus due to unilateral medial medullary infarction. Ann Neurol 1998;43:403–406.
79. Ohkoshi N, Komatsu Y, Mizusawa H, et al: Primary position upbeat nystagmus increased on downward gaze: clinicopathologic study of a patient with multiple sclerosis. Neurology 1998;50:551–553.
80. Janssen JC, Larner AJ, Morris H, et al: Upbeat nystagmus: clinicoanatomical correlation. J Neurol Neurosurg Psychiatry 1998;65:380–381.
81. Munro NAR: The role of the nucleus intercalatus in vertical gaze holding (letter). J Neurol Neurosurg Psychiatry 1999;66:552.
82. Daroff RB, Troost BT: Upbeat nystagmus (letter). JAMA 1973;225:312.
83. Sibony PA, Evinger C, Manning KA: Tobacco-induced primary-position upbeat nystagmus. Ann Neurol 1987;21:53–58.
84. Lopez LI, Bronstein AM, Gresty MA: Clinical and MRI correlates in 27 patients with acquired pendular nystagmus. Brain 1996;119:465–472.

85. Wolin MJ, Trent RG, Lavin PJM: Oculopalatal myoclonus after the one-and-a-half syndrome with facial nerve palsy. Ophthalmology 1996;103:177–180.
86. Lefkowitz D, Harpold G: Treatment of ocular myoclonus with valproic acid. Ann Neurol 1985; 17:103–104.
87. Schwartz MA, Selhorst JB, Ochs AL, et al: Oculomasticatory myorhythmia: a unique movement disorder occurring in Whipple's disease. Ann Neurol 1986;20:677–683.
88. Louis ED, Lynch T, Kaufmann P, et al: Diagnostic guidelines in central nervous system Whipple's disease. Ann Neurol 1996;40:561–568.
89. Averbuch-Heller L, Zivotofsky AZ, Remler BF, et al: Convergent–divergent pendular nystagmus: possible role of the vergence system. Neurology 1995; 45:509–515.
90. Trobe JD, Sharpe JA, Hirsh DK, et al: Nystagmus of Pelizaeus–Merzbacher disease. A magnetic searchcoil study. Arch Neurol 1991;48:87–91.
91. Pratt VM, Naidu S, Dlouhy SR, et al: A novel mutation in exon 3 of the proteolipid protein gene in Pelizaeus–Merzbacher disease. Neurology 1995;45:394–395.
92. Osaka H, Kawanishi C, Inoue K, et al: Pelizaeus–Merzbacher disease: three novel mutations and implication for locus heterogeneity. Ann Neurol 1999; 45:59–64.
93. Garbern J, Cambi F, Shy M, et al: The molecular pathogenesis of Pelizaeus–Merzbacher disease. Arch Neurol 1999;56:1210–1214.
94. Inoue K, Osaka H, Imaizumi K, et al: Proteolipid protein gene duplications causing Pelizaeus–Merzbacher disease: molecular mechanisms and phenotypic manifestations. Ann Neurol 1999;45:624–632.
95. Kori AA, Robin NH, Jacobs JB, et al: Pendular nystagmus in patients with peroxisomal assembly disorder. Arch Neurol 1998;55:554–558.
96. Lambert SR, Kriss A, Gresty M, et al: Joubert syndrome. Arch Ophthalmol 1989;107:709–713.
97. Joubert M, Eisenring J-J, Robb JP, et al: Familial agnesis of the cerebellar vermis. A syndrome of episodic hyperpnea, abnormal eye movements, ataxia, and retardation. Neurology 1969;19:813–825.
98. Saraiva JM, Baraitser M: Joubert syndrome: a review. Am J Med Genet 1992;43:726–731.
99. Steinlin M, Schmid M, Landau K, et al: Follow-up in children with Joubert syndrome. Neuropediatrics 1997;28:204–211.
100. Maria BL, Hoang KB, Tusa RJ, et al: "Joubert syndrome" revisited: key ocular motor signs with magnetic resonance imaging correlation. J Child Neurol 1997;12:423–430.
101. Laverda AM, Saia OS, Drigo P, et al: Chorioretinal coloboma and Joubert syndrome: a nonrandom association. J Pediatr 1984;105:282–284.
102. Houdou S, Ohno K, Takashima S, et al: Joubert syndrome associated with unilateral ptosis and Leber congenital amaurosis. Pediatr Neurol 1986;2:102–105.
103. Barton JJ, Huaman AG, Sharpe JA: Muscarinic antagonists in the treatment of acquired pendular and downbeat nystagmus: a double-blind, randomized trial of three intravenous drugs. Ann Neurol 1994;35:319–325.
104. Leigh RJ, Averbuch-Heller L, Tomsak RL, et al: Treatment of abnormal eye movements that impair vision: strategies based on current concepts of physiology and pharmacology. Ann Neurol 1994;36:129–141.
105. Stahl JS, Rottach KG, Averbuch-Heller L, et al: A pilot study of gabapentin as treatment for acquired nystagmus. Neuro-ophthalmology 1996;16:107–113.
106. Herishanu Y, Louzoun Z: Trihexyphenidyl: treatment of vertical pendular nystagmus. Neurology 1986;36:82–84.
107. Leigh RJ, Rushton DN, Thurston SE, et al: Effects of retinal image stabilization in acquired nystagmus due to neurologic disease. Neurology 1988;38: 122–127.
108. Leigh RJ, Burnstine TH, Ruff RW, et al: Effect of anticholinergic agents upon acquired nystagmus: a double blind study of trihexyphenidyl and tridihexethyl chloride. Neurology 1991;41:1737–1741.
109. Repka MX, Savino PJ, Reinecke RD: Treatment of acquired nystagmus with botulinum neurotoxin A. Arch Ophthalmol 1994;112:1320–1324.
110. Daroff RB: See-saw nystagmus. Neurology 1965; 15:874–877.
111. Nakada T, Kwee IL: Seesaw nystagmus. Role of visuovestibular interaction in its pathogenesis. J Clin Neuro-ophthalmol 1988;8:171–177.
112. Halmagyi GM, Aw ST, Dehaene I: Jerk-waveform see-saw nystamus due to a unilateral meso-diencephalic lesion. Brain 1994;117:789–803.
113. Helmchen C, Glasauer S, Bartl K, et al: Contralesionally beating torsional nystagmus in a unilateral rostral midbrain lesion. Neurology 1996;47:482–486.
114. May EF, Truxal AR: Loss of vision alone may result in seesaw nystagmus. J Neuro-ophthalmol 1997; 17:84–85.
115. Blair CJ, Goldberg MF, von Noorden GK: Voluntary nystagmus. Arch Ophthalmol 1967;77:349–354.
116. Coren S, Komada MK: Eye movement control in voluntary nystagmus. Am J Ophthalmol 1972;74:1161–1165.
117. Blumenthal H: Voluntary nystagmus. Neurology 1973;23:223–225.
118. Zahn JR: Incidence and characterization of voluntary nystagmus. J Neurol Neurosurg Psychiatry 1978;41: 617–623.
119. Keyes MJ: Voluntary nystagmus in two generations. Arch Neurol 1973;29:63–64.
120. Aschoff JC, Becker W, Rettelbach R: Voluntary nystagmus in five generations. J Neurol Neurosurg Psychiatry 1976;39:300–304.
121. Rosenblum JA, Shafer N: Voluntary nystagmus associated with oscillopsia. Arch Neurol 1966;15:560–562.
122. Shults WT, Stark L, Hoyt WF, et al: Normal saccadic structure of voluntary nystagmus. Arch Ophthalmol 1977;95:1399–1404.
123. Sharpe JA, Hoyt WF, Rosenberg MA: Convergence-evoked nystagmus. Arch Neurol 1975;32:191–194.
124. Barton JJS, Cox TA, Digre KB: Acquired convergence-evoked pendular nystagmus in multiple sclerosis. J Neuro-ophthalmol 1999;19:34–38.
125. Sanders MD, Hoyt WF, Daroff RB: Lid nystagmus evoked by ocular convergence: an ocular electromyographic study. J Neurol Neurosurg Psychiatry 1968;31:368–371.
126. Daroff RB, Hoyt WF, Sanders MD, et al: Gaze-evoked eyelid and ocular nystagmus inhibited by the near reflex: unusual ocular motor phenomena in a lateral medullary syndrome. J Neurol Neurosurg Psychiatry 1968;31:362–367.
127. Kaplan PW, Tusa RJ: Neurophysiologic and clinical correlations of epileptic nystagmus. Neurology 1993;43:2508–2514.
128. Moster ML, Schnayder E: Epileptic periodic alternating nystagmus. J Neuro-ophthalmol 1998;18:292–293.
129. Fetter M, Haslwanter T, Bork M, et al: New insights into positional alcohol nystagmus using three-

dimensional eye-movement analysis. Ann Neurol 1999;45:216–223.
130. O'Connor PS. Nystagmus. In: Farris BK (ed): The Basics of Neuro-ophthalmology, pp 35–49. St. Louis, Mosby–Year Book, 1991.
131. Dell'Osso LF: Nystagmus and other ocular motor oscillations. In: Van Dalen JTW, Lessell S (eds): Neuro-ophthalmology, pp 146–170. Amsterdam, Excerpta Medica, 1980.
132. Dieterich M, Bucher SF, Seelos KC, et al: Horizontal or vertical optokinetic stimulation activates visual motion-sensitive, ocular motor and vestibular cortex areas with right hemispheric dominance. An fMRI study. Brain 1998;121:1479–1495.
133. Ridley A, Kennard C, Scholtz CL, et al: Omnipause neurons in two cases of opsoclonus associated oat cell carcinoma of the lung. Brain 1987;110:1699–1709.
134. Digre KB: Opsoclonus in adults. Report of three cases and review of the literature. Arch Neurol 1986;43: 1165–1175.
135. Yee RD, Spiegel PH, Yamada T, et al: Voluntary saccadic oscillations, resembling ocular flutter and opsoclonus. J Neuro-ophthalmol 1994;14:95–101.
136. Pranzatelli MR: The neurobiology of the opsoclonus–myoclonus syndrome. Clin Neuropharmacol 1992; 15:186–228.
137. Posada JC, Tardo C: Neuroblastoma detected by somatostatin receptor scintigraphy in a case of opsoclonus–myoclonus–ataxia syndrome. J Child Neurol 1998;13:345–346.
138. Pranzatelli MR: The immunopharmacology of the opsoclonus–myoclonus syndrome. Clin Neuropharmacol 1996;19:1–47.
139. Fisher PG, Wechsler PG, Singer HS: Anti-Hu antibody in a neuroblastoma-associated paraneoplastic syndrome. Pediatr Neurol 1994;10:309–312.
140. Connolly AM, Pestronk A, Mehta S, et al: Serum autoantibodies in childhood opsoclonus–mycolonus syndrome: an analysis of antigenic targets in neural tissues. J Pediatr 1997;130:878–884.
141. Case records of the Massachusetts General Hospital: Case 27–1995. N Engl J Med 1995;333:579–586.
142. Hammer MS, Larsen MB, Stack CV: Outcome of children with opsoclonus–myoclonus regardless of etiology. Pediatr Neurol 1995;13:21–24.
143. Hoyt CS, Mousel DK, Weber AA: Transient supranuclear disturbances of gaze in healthy neonates. Am J Ophthalmol 1980;89:708–713.
144. Bienfang DC: Opsoclonus in infancy. Arch Ophthalmol 1974;91:203–205.
145. Scharf D: Opsoclonus–myoclonus following the intranasal usage of cocaine. J Neurol Neurosurg Psychiatry 1989;52:1447–1448.
146. Hersh B, Dalmau J, Dangond F, et al: Paraneoplastic opsoclonus–myoclonus associated with anti-Hu antibody. Neurology 1994;44:1754–1755.
147. Luque FA, Furneaux HM, Ferziger R, et al: Anti-Ri: An antibody associated with paraneoplastic opsoclonus and breast cancer. Ann Neurol 1991;29:241–251.
148. Hoyt WF, Keane JR: Superior oblique myokymia. Report and discussion on five cases of benign intermittent uniocular microtremor. Arch Ophthalmol 1970;84:461–467.
149. Susac JO, Smith JL, Schatz NJ: Superior oblique myokymia. Arch Neurol 1973;29:432–434.
150. Rosenberg ML, Glaser JS: Superior oblique myokymia. Ann Neurol 1983;13:667–669.
151. Morrow M, Sharpe JA, Ranalli PJ: Superior oblique myokymia associated with a posterior fossa tumor: oculographic correlation with an idiopathic case. Neurology 1990;40:367–370.
152. Kosmorsky GS, Ellis BD, Fogt N, et al: Treatment of superior oblique myokymia utilizing the Harado–Ito procedure. J Neuro-ophthalmol 1995;15:142–146.
153. Daroff RB, Waldman AL: Ocular bobbing. J Neurol Neurosurg Psychiatry 1965;28:375–377.
154. Susac JO, Hoyt WF, Daroff RB, et al: Clinical spectrum of ocular bobbing. J Neurol Neurosurg Psychiatry 1970;33:771–775.
155. Rai GS, Buxton-Thomas M, Scanlon M: Ocular bobbing in hepatic encephalopathy. Br J Clin Prac 1976;30:202–205.
156. Rudick R, Satran R, Eskin TA: Ocular bobbing in encephalitis. J Neurol Neurosurg Psychiatry 1981; 44:441–443.
157. Finelli PF, McEntee WJ: Ocular bobbing with extra-axial haematoma of posterior fossa. J Neurol Neurosurg Psychiatry 1977;40:386–388.
158. Knobler RL, Somasundaram M, Schutta HS: Inverse ocular bobbing. Ann Neurol 1981;9:194–197.
159. Ropper AH: Ocular dipping in anoxic coma. Arch Neurol 1981;38:297–299.
160. Averbuch-Heller L, Leigh RJ: Medical treatments for abnormal eye movements: pharmacological, optical and immunological strategies. Aust NZ J Ophthalmol 1997;25:7–13.
161. Averbuch-Heller L, Tusa RJ, Fuhry L, et al: A double-blind controlled study of gabapentin and baclofen as treatment for acquired nystagmus. Ann Neurol 1997;41:818–825.
162. Smith PF, Darlington CL: Recent advances in the pharmacology of the vestibulo-ocular reflex system. Trends Pharmacol Sci 1996;17:421–427.
163. Starck M, Albrecht H, Pöllmann W: Drug therapy for acquired pendular nystagmus in multiple sclerosis. J Neurol 1997;244:9–16.
164. Cher LM, Hochberg FH, Teruya J: Therapy for paraneoplastic neurologic syndromes in six patients with protein column immunoabsorption. Cancer 1995;75: 1678–1683.
165. Lin C-Y, Young Y-H: Clinical significance of rebound nystagmus. Laryngoscope 1999;109:1803–1805.
166. Schon F, Hart PE, Hodgson TL, et al: Suppression of pendular nystagmus by smoking cannabis in a patients with multiple sclerosis. Neurology 1999;53:2209–2210.

CHAPTER 18

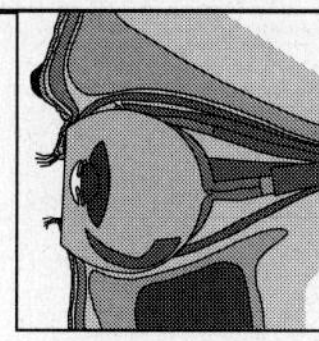

Orbital Disease in Neuro-Ophthalmology

Orbital disorders usually manifest with a unifying constellation of symptoms and signs that include proptosis, periocular swelling, blurred vision, and double vision. The presence of proptosis distinguishes disease of the orbit from other neuro-ophthalmic conditions with similar symptomatology. The discussion below describes the relevant orbital anatomy and the typical signs and symptoms encountered in orbital disease. A review of orbital imaging techniques follows and emphasizes the advantages and disadvantages of each modality. Finally, the orbital entities frequently encountered in neuro-ophthalmic practice are analyzed.

ORBITAL ANATOMY

Familiarity with orbital anatomy is critical to understanding and recognizing the various conditions that are encountered. Several excellent texts and atlases are available.[1–3] The orbit contains a wide variety of tissue types, including bone; periorbita; fibroadipose tissue; striated and smooth muscle; epithelial tissue of the lacrimal gland; the optic nerve; peripheral autonomic, sensory, and motor nerves; the ciliary ganglion; arteries and veins; and finally cartilage in the trochlear of the superior oblique muscle. The orbit contains no known lymphatics.

A "functional" understanding of orbital anatomy and the interaction of all of these structures is grounded in the relationship of the various spaces within the 25 to 30 cc of the bony orbit.[4] These spaces include the globe and the space immediately around it (Tenon's space), the intraconal portion of the orbit (formed by the cone of the rectus muscles and containing the optic nerve), and the extraconal space (Fig. 18–1). There is also a potential space between the bone and the periorbita that is a common site for orbital involvement by paranasal sinus infections and tumors. Further division into the superior and inferior extraconal spaces is helpful as many conditions, such as lymphoma and idiopathic orbital inflammatory syndrome, have a predilection for affecting the superior and temporal orbit.

Bones of the Orbit

The orbit is bound by portions of seven different bones (frontal, sphenoidal, zygomatic, lacrimal, maxillary, palatine, and ethmoidal), and they contribute variably to form the walls of the orbit (Fig. 18–2, Table 18–1). The ethmoidal bone contains the medially located thin lamina papyracea, which is vulnerable both to fractures and to the passage of infection from the paranasal sinuses. The posterior border of the orbit is the optic canal, and the anterior extent is the orbital septum, which originates in the periorbita and blends into the connective tissue of the upper and lower eyelids.

There are three major bony openings into the orbit. The first is the optic canal through which passes the optic nerve, oculosympathetic nerves, and the ophthalmic artery. The second is the superior orbital fissure, formed by the greater and lesser wings of the sphenoid bone. The superior ophthalmic vein and the

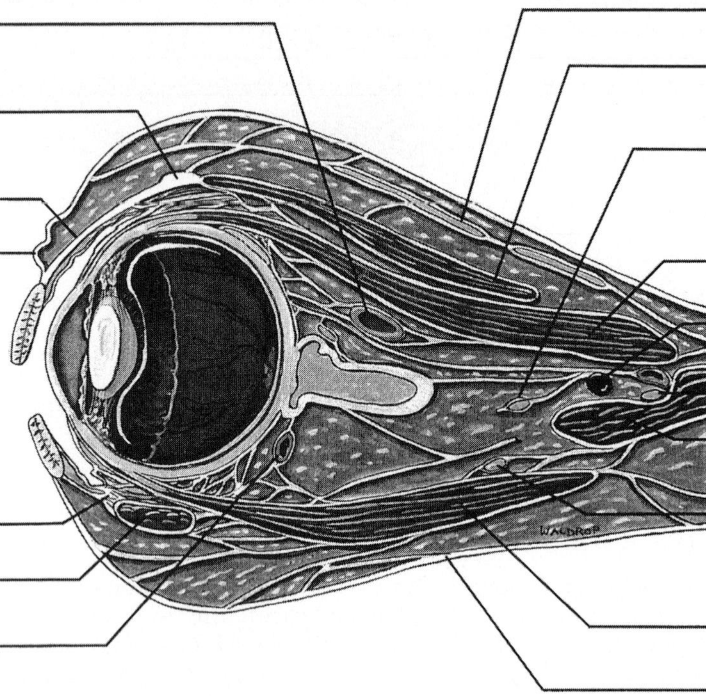

FIGURE 18–1. Sagittal section of the orbit demonstrating the various anatomic spaces and the orbital fascial system. The extraocular muscles and the intermuscular septae define the intraconal space. The extraconal space is outside of the muscle cone. Tenon's space is between the Tenon's fascia (which surrounds the globe) and the globe. These spaces are often considered when developing a differential diagnosis of orbital lesions. (From Dutton JJ: Atlas of Clinical and Surgical Orbital Anatomy. Philadelphia, WB Saunders, 1994, with permission.)

third, fourth, first (ophthalmic) division of the fifth, and sixth cranial nerves as well as some sympathetic nerves pass through the superior orbital fissure. Finally, the inferior orbital fissure is in the floor of the orbit, and through it passes the second (maxillary) branch of the fifth nerve, the inferior ophthalmic vein, heading into the pterygoid plexus, and branches of the sphenopalatine ganglion.

There are other important vascular foramina, including openings in the medial orbital wall for the anterior and posterior ethmoidal arteries. The ethmoidal arteries are branches of the ophthalmic artery and supply the dura in the anterior cranial fossa and the nose. The anterior ethmoidal nerve, a branch of the nasociliary nerve, also passes through the anterior ethmoidal canal and supplies sensation to the tip of the nose and upper lip. This sensory branch of the first division of the fifth cranial nerve is the reason why the tip of the nose is often involved in herpes zoster ophthalmicus (Hutchinson's sign).

The bones of the orbit also contain important grooves and fossae. The infraorbital groove contains the infraorbital nerve, the terminal branch of the maxillary nerve, which exits the floor of the orbit through the infraorbital foramen to supply sensation to the cheek and upper part of the jaw. The supraorbital nerve (a branch of the frontal nerve, which derives from the ophthalmic division of the fifth nerve) similarly reaches the skin of the forehead and frontal sinus through the supraorbital foramen or notch.[5] The trochlear fossa is located superomedially 5 mm from the anterior orbital rim. Here the cartilaginous trochlear (through which the tendon of the superior oblique passes) is attached. The lacrimal fossa is located superotemporally in the frontal bone.

The lateral wall of the orbit is thickest anteriorly and is the strongest of the orbital walls. In the most anterior portion of the lateral wall about 10 to 11 mm below the frontozygomatic suture is found the lateral orbital (Whitnall's) tubercle. This bony tubercle serves as the point of attachment of the levator aponeurosis, the suspensory (Lockwood's) ligament of the globe, the lateral palpebral ligament, and the check ligament of the lateral rectus muscle.

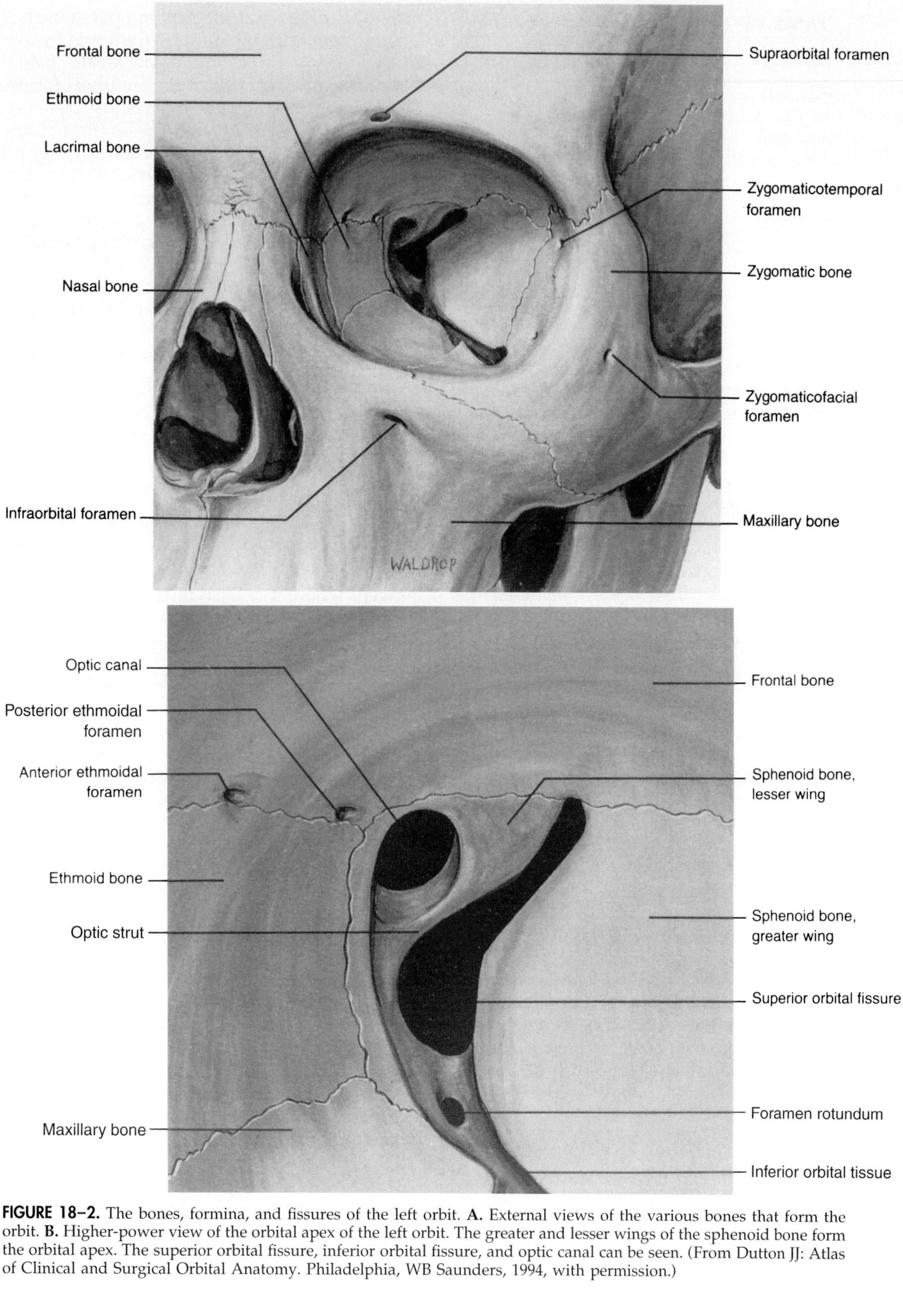

FIGURE 18–2. The bones, formina, and fissures of the left orbit. **A.** External views of the various bones that form the orbit. **B.** Higher-power view of the orbital apex of the left orbit. The greater and lesser wings of the sphenoid bone form the orbital apex. The superior orbital fissure, inferior orbital fissure, and optic canal can be seen. (From Dutton JJ: Atlas of Clinical and Surgical Orbital Anatomy. Philadelphia, WB Saunders, 1994, with permission.)

TABLE 18–1. Bones of the Walls of the Orbit

Orbital roof	Frontal bone Lesser wing of sphenoid
Lateral wall	Greater wing of sphenoid bone Zygomatic bone
Medial wall	Ethmoid bone Lacrimal bone Lesser wing of sphenoid Tip of maxilla
Orbital floor	Maxilla Zygomatic Palatine

The zygomatic canal is posterior to the tubercle, and through it passes the zygomatic nerve, a proximal branch of the maxillary nerve. It divides in the orbit into the zygomaticotemporal and zygomaticofacial nerves, which supply the skin on the lateral portion of the forehead and cheek.

Vascular Structures

The blood supply to the orbit derives from the ophthalmic artery, which is the first branch of the internal carotid artery after it pierces the dura of the cavernous sinus.[6,7] The artery enters the orbit inferiorly through the optic canal and then moves laterally between the optic nerve and lateral rectus, then superiorly, and finally medially. Its terminal branches are the supratrochlear and dorsal nasal arteries. Some blood reaches the orbit through the facial, maxillary, and temporal branches of the external carotid artery. The branches of the ophthalmic artery, the structures they supply, and their important external carotid artery anastomoses are summarized in Table 18–2 and are pictured in Figure 4–1.

The orbital veins are valveless. The superior ophthalmic vein and central retinal vein drain into the cavernous sinus. The inferior orbital vein drains into the pterygoid plexus. Anterior venous drainage can also occur into the facial veins via the angular and inferior ophthalmic veins.

Extraocular Muscles

The six extraocular muscles are striated with unique properties.[8] The four rectus muscles (each about 3 to 4 cm long) originate from the annulus of Zinn at the orbital apex, which is contiguous with the dura surrounding the optic nerve and the periorbita. The levator palpebrae also originates from the annulus of Zinn. The superior oblique originates just posterior to the annulus of Zinn and passes through the trochlear before turning posterolateral to insert on the globe under and posterior to the insertion of the superior rectus. The inferior oblique originates from the bone just posterolateral to the nasolacrimal fossa and travels posterolaterally under the inferior rectus (attached to inferior rectus by Lockwood's ligament) to insert posteriorly on the globe in the region of the macula. The nerves innervating the rectus muscles enter them at the junction of the posterior and middle third of their bellies. These structures are discussed in more detail in Chapter 15.

Periorbita and Septae

The periorbita is the periosteum of the orbital bones. It is only loosely adherent to the bones except where it is fixed at the anterior orbital rim, margins of fissures and canals, and the lacrimal crest. Posteriorly it is contiguous with the dura at the superior orbital fissure and optic nerve. The intraconal space is defined by the extraocular muscles and the intermuscular septa, which are denser anteriorly and may be absent posteriorly.[9] Koornneef[10] has demonstrated that the anatomic distinction of the intraconal and extraconal spaces is more complex and that this division results from radial fibrovascular connective tissue septae, which also attach the muscles to the periorbita. These septae separate the orbital fat into lobules. The orbital septum is the anterior border of the orbit. It originates at the anterior orbital rim and superiorly fuses with the levator aponeurosis and inferiorly with the capsulopalpebral fascia.

Tenon's capsule is a layer of delicate connective tissue attached to the globe near the limbus. The capsule envelopes the globe, has fine posterior attachments to it, and separates it from the orbital fat. The extraocular muscles pierce the capsule anterior to the equator of the globe and are enveloped in a sleevelike extension of the capsule. The muscles travel in the capsule for 7 to 10 mm, and the capsule gives off lateral extensions, forming the intermuscular membrane between the rectus muscles.

TABLE 18–2. Branches of the Ophthalmic Artery, Structures They Supply, and Important Anastomoses

Branch of Ophthalmic Artery	Structure(s) Supplied	Important Anastomoses With External Carotid Artery
Central retinal a.	Retina, optic nerve	
Lateral posterior ciliary a.	Choroid, optic nerve (20 short branches) Ciliary muscle, iris, anterior choroid (two long branches)	
Lacrimal a.	Lacrimal gland	With transverse facial, zygomatic, and frontal branches of superficial temporal aa. With middle meningeal a. from maxillary a.
Lateral muscular a.	Superior rectus, superior oblique, lateral rectus, and levator muscles Rectus muscles give off anterior ciliary aa. to anterior segment of eye	With orbital branches of infraorbital a., a branch of maxillary a.
Posterior ethmoid a.	Posterior ethmoid air cells	With lateral nasal a. from maxillary a.
Supraorbital a. (together or separately)	Eyebrow, forehead Levator muscle	
Medial posterior ciliary a.	See lateral posterior ciliary a., above	
Muscular a.	Inferior rectus inferior oblique, and medial rectus muscles	
To areolar tissue	Areolar tissue	
Anterior ethmoid a.	Anterior ethmoid cells Frontal sinus Dura in anterior fossa Nose	With sphenopalatine a. from maxillary a.
Medial, inferior medial, and superior medial palpebral aa.	Eyelids	
Dorsal nasal (terminal) a.	Nose	With angular branch of facial a.
Supratrochlear a.	Superomedial orbit	

a = artery, aa = arteries.

Ciliary Ganglion

The ciliary ganglion, which is also discussed in Chapter 13 (see Fig. 13–3), lies in the posterior orbit between optic nerve and the lateral rectus muscle. The ganglion contains the synapses of the preganglionic parasympathetic fibers from the Edinger–Westphal nucleus of the third nerve and provides the postganglionic neurons destined for the ciliary body and pupillary sphincter. These fibers reach the ciliary ganglion with the oculomotor branch to the inferior oblique muscle. Postganglionic fibers reach the anterior portion of the globe via short posterior ciliary nerves. Sensory fibers from the ophthalmic division of the trigeminal nerve and postganglionic sympathetic fibers pass through the ciliary ganglion on their way to the globe but do not synapse there.

Lacrimal Gland

The lacrimal gland sits in the lacrimal fossa and is separated from the globe by Tenon's capsule and orbital fat. The most lateral portion of the levator aponeurosis separates the lacrimal gland into the smaller palpebral and larger orbital lobes. Small portions of the palpebral lobe can be seen superolaterally upon eversion of the eyelid. The blood supply to the lacrimal gland derives from the lacrimal artery, a branch of the ophthalmic artery. Sensory innervation is from the ophthalmic division of the trigeminal nerve. Autonomic innervation is from parasympathetic fibers, which synapse in the pterygopalatine ganglion and travel with the zygomatic branches of the maxillary division of the trigeminal nerve before reaching the lacrimal gland.

NEURO-OPHTHALMOLOGY OF ORBITAL DISEASE

Symptoms

Patients with orbital disease present with a variety of symptoms, including blurring, double vision, swelling, ptosis, and proptosis. Most orbital disease is space occupying, and therefore the hallmark of orbital disease is proptosis or exophthalmos due to axial or forward displacement of the globe. Although many patients may notice prominence of one eye or a widening of the palpebral fissure, others may have unrecognized moderate to severe proptosis. Lid retraction (sclera visible between superior limbus and upper eyelid) is the hallmark of thyroid eye disease. Other causes of proptosis are generally not associated with lid retraction. In fact, superior orbital disease might also be associated with ptosis. Patients with orbital disease (particularly thyroid-associated ophthalmopathy and idiopathic orbital inflammatory syndrome) also present with eyelid soft tissue swelling or conjunctival injection.

Double vision secondary to impaired eye movements is a frequent complaint. Double vision is binocular and results from misalignment of the two eyes. Strabismus in this setting is usually noncomitant and results from a mechanical effect. The mass lesion or inflammatory process interferes with the movement of the eye directly or indirectly. Double vision can also result when the mass inhibits normal extraocular muscle function by restricting the movement of the globe as in thyroid-associated ophthalmopathy. Lastly, diplopia can also result from cranial nerve (third, fourth, or sixth) dysfunction within the orbit or through invasion of the tumor into the cavernous sinus. Facial hypoesthesia can result from involvement of the fifth cranial nerve or its branches in the orbit.

Slowly expanding benign orbital neoplasms may not cause any visual symptoms. However, optic nerve tumors (gliomas and meningiomas) frequently present with proptosis and decreased vision. Patients may describe a blur or recognize loss of visual field (see Chapter 5). A peculiar variation of transient monocular vision loss occurs in patients with orbital mass lesions, and is termed *gaze evoked amaurosis*.[11] Vision darkens as the eye is moved and the optic nerve or central retinal artery is compressed by the mass lesion. Vision clears upon moving the eye back to the central position. Decreased vision can also result from direct compression of the optic nerve or from indentation of the globe by a mass lesion, compression of the optic nerve by enlarged eye muscles in thyroid-associated ophthalmopathy, or from an inflammatory perineuritis associated with idiopathic orbital inflammation.

Examination Overview

The details of formal neuro-ophthalmic examination have been described in Chapter 2. As with all patients, examination of patients with orbital disease begins with careful assessment of visual function, including visual acuity, color vision, and visual fields. Beyond this, certain features of the examination of patients with orbital disease are unique and deserve review.

Examination. External examination begins by assessing the appearance of the eye, looking for asymmetry, globe position, swelling, and abnormal eyelid position. Since lid retraction is often associated with lid lag, the patient is asked to look down. The lid is then observed to see if it "hangs up" abnormally. Since mass lesions can be often felt around the eye, particularly if they primarily involve the lacrimal gland, the orbit and globe should be palpated. At the same time the globe is retrodisplaced into the orbit and the presence of abnormal resistance or firmness, typical of most orbital disease, can be noted. Careful examination should be performed of the preauricular area and neck to look for evidence of abnormal adenopathy. The orbit should be auscultated since bruits are present in some patients with arteriovenous malformations.

Proptosis can often be better appreciated if the patients are asked to tilt their head backward. Then the examiner looks from below, comparing the position of the eyes in relation to the brow or anterior orbital rim. Formal measurements of proptosis can be accomplished with various devices. The Hertel exophthalmometer, a combination of a scale and mirror (see Chapter 2), is placed on the lateral orbital rims of the patient. The examiner can then determine the relative position of each globe compared to the lateral orbital rim. Generally, the eyes are within 1 to 2 mm of each other, and any difference greater than that suggests either enophthalmos or exophthalmos. Serial measurements of proptosis with exophthalmometry are important in patients with active orbital disease to assess progression.

Optic Disc Findings. The optic nerve usually appears normal in patients presenting with orbital disease. Subsequently chronic low-grade compression of the intraorbital optic nerve can lead to atrophy of the optic nerve and disc pallor. Some patients with optic nerve tumors and, rarely, patients with other orbital tumors may present with optic nerve head swelling. Swelling usually results from compression of the first half of the optic nerve, leading to impaired axonal transport. Lesions around the orbital apex usually do not cause optic disc swelling. As a rule, optic disc swelling is not associated with intracanalicular or intracranial tumors unless there is associated mass effect, elevated intracranial pressure, and resulting papilledema. Disc swelling secondary to a chronic compressive lesion is sometimes further characterized by the presence of collateral or shunt vessels. These abnormal vessels develop to shunt blood flow from the retinal to choroidal circulation, bypassing the chronically obstructed central retinal vein. Collateral vessels are a common feature of optic nerve sheath meningiomas and gliomas and are less commonly encountered with other causes of orbital disease.

Retinal Findings. Retinal vascular changes are sometimes observed in patients with orbital disease. Venous engorgement or impending venous occlusion may be seen with optic nerve tumors, but is very rare in patients with neoplastic or inflammatory disease of the orbit. The most common fundus abnormality in patients with orbital mass lesions is choroidal (chorioretinal) folding. This has also been described in patients with thyroid-associated ophthalmopathy, inflammatory diseases of the orbit, and mucoceles.[12] The folding (Fig. 18–3) is the result of extrinsic compression of the globe, leading to flattening of the sclera and subsequent wrinkling or folding of the retina. The outer retina is thrown into folds that follow corrugations in the choroid, Bruch's membrane, and retinal pigment epithelium.[13] This creates a highly characteristic funduscopic finding of parallel, alternating lines or folds most often seen in the posterior pole. The fluorescein angiographic pattern was first described by Norton[14] and has a diagnostic appearance of alternating light and dark lines (Fig. 18–4). The recognition of choroidal folds demands investigation for orbital disease and globe compression, although they may also be secondary to hyperopia, hypotony, choroidal or retinal detachments, raised intracranial pressure, scleral buckles, subretinal neovascular membranes, and choroidal tumors. In many patients, and particularly in bilateral cases, choroidal folds are idiopathic.

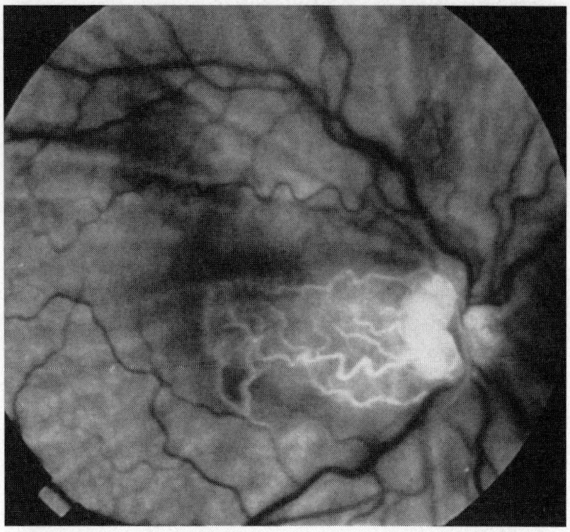

FIGURE 18–4. Late-phase fluorescein angiogram of a patient with an inflammatory mass lesion that produced obstruction of the central retinal artery. Choroidal and cilioretinal circulations are preserved and choroidal folds are seen as alternating light and dark lines.

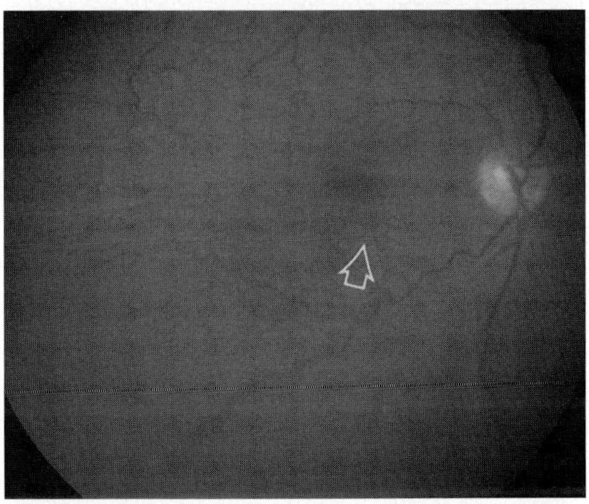

FIGURE 18–3. Fundus photograph of the right eye of a patient with a metastatic carcinoid tumor to the orbit. Chorioretinal or choroidal folds are seen as linear lines in the fundus (*arrow*).

Retinal arterial abnormalities are uncommon. Rarely occlusions of the retinal arteries can occur in association with acute trauma and retrobulbar hemorrhage or secondary to angioinvasive forms of mucormycosis or aspergillosis. Exudative retinal detachments can be seen in patients with idiopathic orbital inflammatory syndrome.

Eye Movement Abnormalities. A mixed pattern of eye movement impairment is the hallmark of orbital disease and may reflect both muscle restriction and cranial nerve dysfunction. The speed of ocular ductions should be noted. For instance, if an eye moves quickly but abruptly stops, a restrictive process or mass lesion is suggested. When the movement is slow for the entire excursion it suggests a cranial nerve palsy rather than a restrictive process. Neurogenic and mechanical eye movement limitation may also be distinguished by performing forced duction and forced generation testing (see Chapter 2). In general, patients with orbital tumors will have a mixed pattern of eye movement limitation that does not fit clearly into the pattern of a single cranial nerve. For instance, if a patient can neither elevate nor abduct an eye, it is more likely the result of mass effect or restrictive myopathy than a combined partial third and sixth nerve palsy.

DIAGNOSTIC ORBITAL IMAGING

The diagnostic evaluation of orbital disease includes noninvasive imaging of the orbit either by echography (orbital ultrasound), computed tomography (CT), or magnetic resonance imaging (MRI). Each modality has advantages and disadvantages (Table 18–3), but the techniques are often complementary. Imaging studies may be nondiagnostic except for the unique patterns seen with thyroid eye disease and paraorbital sinus disease. However, taken in conjunction with the history and examination, a tentative diagnosis can usually be made.

Echography

Two types of analysis are used in orbital echography: amplitude mode (A scan) and brightness mode (B scan). Many different orbital disorders can be diagnosed and followed echographically.[15, 16] An A scan provides one-dimensional images and displays echoes as spikes. Elevated spike height implies increased echogenicity. The length between the transducer and the tissue is represented by the distance between spikes. An A scan is commonly used to look for calcifications in the setting of optic nerve head drusen, to measure the size of lesions or of the extraocular muscles, and to determine the reflectivity (echogenicity) of a lesion or abnormal tissue. B scan produces two-dimensional images of tissue sections, and images of the orbit are obtained along several different planes. An increase in the acoustic density of a tissue results in an increase in the brightness of the image. Fluid-filled structures (blood vessels, the globe, and cysts, for example) appear dark.

Echography is generally not used as the definitive study for orbital disease, although it has some particularly useful roles.[17] One example is in the diagnosis of posterior scleritis, a form of idiopathic orbital inflammatory syn-

TABLE 18–3. Advantages and Disadvantages of Various Imaging Modalities of the Orbit

Modality	Advantages	Disadvantages
Echography	Instant results Readily available Echogenicity helps determine lesion type Images globe 30 degree test Images eye muscles well	Requires skilled operator Dose not image posterior orbit
CT scan	Available Affordable Evaluates bony changes Demonstrates calcification	Radiation exposure Inferior to MRI for soft tissue of the brain Poor imaging of cavernous sinus Lacks multiplanar reformatting capabilities of MRI
MRI scan	Most machines surpass resolution of CT Exquisite soft tissue detail Demonstrates optic nerve enhancement Images cavernous sinus and orbital apex well No radiation Possible to perform MRI–angiography Images wood foreign body Uniquely images melanin and hemosiderin	Does not image bone Expensive (cost of unit, slower, more technician time) Thicker sections Unwanted nonspecific data (white matter changes) Longer scan time Claustrophobia is prohibitive for some patients Incompatible with magnetic materials or pacemakers

drome, where a very typical finding of fluid in Tenon's space can be seen on echography. Similarly, enlarged extraocular muscles of thyroid disease are easily demonstrated, and ultrasound can be also be used to quantify extraocular muscle thickness.[18] In the evaluation of mass lesions, the nature of the mass lesion and its relation to the globe can be characterized. In addition, the internal reflectivity of a lesion, suggestive of a vascular or cystic nature, may be ascertained. Echography has been combined with color Doppler imaging to assess blood flow in the eye and orbit, particularly with vascular lesions.[19]

Computed Tomography

Since bone, calcification, fat, and blood all have unique x-ray absorption patterns, CT is a very effective technique for orbital imaging. In fact, the contrast of the surrounding orbital fat allows for excellent imaging of the soft tissues (muscles and optic nerve) of the orbit by CT. Specific absorption patterns can be highlighted ("windows") to emphasize bone, soft tissue, or blood.

CT images can be obtained in the axial, coronal, and sagittal planes and generally are done at 3-mm intervals. If necessary, CT scans of the orbit can have a 1-mm slice interval with good resolution. Axial and coronal images are obtained directly, and sagittal images are usually obtained by computer reformatting. Coronal images are often not included in regular studies and should be requested whenever ordering orbital CT. Occasionally patients will be unable to position for these images and reformatted views are necessary. Bone windows and blood windows are usually viewed as well and contrast is reserved for evaluation of mass lesions or to evaluate for intracranial extension of orbital disease (MRI preferred, see below). Routine facial bone imaging is done with 5-mm axial and coronal cuts, and when optic canal fractures are suspected, 1- to 3-mm coronal images should be obtained. In these cases, contrast is not utilized if bone and soft tissue windows are viewed. Images are reformatted to produce three-dimensional, reconstructed views of the bony surface or deeper soft tissue areas. These three-dimensional reconstructions are used for presurgical evaluation of facial fractures and for evaluation of the skull in children with craniosynostoses and are not necessary in routine orbital imaging.

Magnetic Resonance Imaging

MRI is considered noninvasive because it does not utilize radiation. Instead, a powerful magnetic field and radio frequency (RF) pulses are used to create images. The images are created when the nuclei of atoms found within the various tissues align with the magnetic field and a RF pulse is applied. Most of the signals produced are from mobile protons of hydrogen atoms found within the water and lipids of tissues; protons that are immobile (as in bone) give no appreciable signal. Signals are received by RF receiver coils, and can be reconstructed in axial, coronal, or sagittal planes.

Prior to the advent of surface coils (receiver coils that wrap around the patient's face and eyes) and fat suppression techniques, CT was the preferred procedure for orbital imaging, even for the evaluation of soft tissue. However, MRI now offers many advantages over CT. MRI provides excellent images of the globe, orbit, and visual pathways and has become an invaluable tool in the diagnosis of pathologic lesions in the orbit and cavernous sinus. MRI provides excellent contrast resolution between soft tissues, and multiplanar imaging can be done without repositioning the patient. As with CT, contrast agents are used (gadolinium complexes) to highlight normal anatomy, show breakdown of the normal blood–brain barrier, distinguish mass from inflammation, and demonstrate vascularity. MRI gives very little information about bones and fractures. CT should always be used when evaluating bony changes from tumors and in trauma. MRI scan times are considerably longer than those of CT. MRI is very sensitive to movement artifact (especially with surface coils), which can become significant when imaging the globe and orbit in uncooperative patients. MRI is contraindicated in patients with metallic objects in their eyes or head, cardiac pacemakers, or non-MR-compatible surgical clips.

APPROACH TO THE DIAGNOSIS OF ORBITAL DISEASE

Clinical History

The time course over which pain, proptosis, blurred vision, and double vision develops often helps distinguish neoplastic disease from infectious and inflammatory disease. Patients with infectious or non-thyroid-associated inflammatory disease of the orbit generally have an acute course with symptom development over hours or days. In contrast, neoplastic conditions, including primary optic nerve tumors, usually evolve insidiously. The exceptions are with malignant tumors such as adenoid cystic carcinoma of the lacrimal gland, some metastatic tumors, and secondary orbital tumors extending from the paranasal sinuses.

Age

The patient's age group helps in the differential diagnosis of orbital disease. In the pediatric age group, congenital, developmental, and infectious lesions predominate. Fortunately, the majority of children with orbital disease will have a benign process.[20–25] Rhabdomyosarcoma is the most common malignant tumor of the orbit in children, while neuroblastoma and Ewing's sarcoma may both metastasize to the orbit. Both idiopathic inflammatory disease of the orbit and thyroid-associated ophthalmopathy may occur in children, but are relatively infrequent entities. In adults, orbital cellulitis is less common, and thyroid eye disease becomes the most frequent cause of orbital dysfunction. Tumors of several different types may occur, with lymphoma being the most common.[26] In older adults, metastatic and secondary orbital tumors and dural sinus fistulas increase in frequency.

General Physical Findings

General physical findings are particularly important in several instances. In suspected thyroid-associated ophthalmopathy, the physical examination might show vital signs suggesting hyperthyroidism or hypothyroidism. Other patients may have a goiter. Any patient with an orbital mass lesion should have a careful examination to search for other signs of malignancy such as adenopathy that might be associated with systemic lymphoma or metastatic disease.

Imaging

Imaging will help localize the process and will often define a cause. Although thyroid-associated ophthalmopathy may be diagnosed on clinical grounds, imaging is confirmatory and helps in staging and in determining whether the patient is at risk for vision loss. Patients with idiopathic orbital inflammatory disease should be imaged (echography, CT, or MRI) to aid in the differential diagnosis and determine disease extent at presentation. The vast majority of patients with orbital tumors undergo neuroimaging with either CT or MRI. CT is the preferred modality in patients with a recent history of trauma and in patients in whom evaluation of bony changes is important. Both lytic lesions (malignant tumors) and hyperostosis (meningiomas) can be best demonstrated on a CT scan. MRI has a distinct advantage over CT in terms of the details of soft tissue anatomy and abnormalities around the orbital apex and cavernous sinus. Both CT and MRI will provide the necessary information to determine the relationship of an orbital mass lesion to the optic nerves, extraocular muscles, paranasal sinuses, and intracranial structures. Specific radiologic features for each of the various lesions are discussed below.

Neuro-ophthalmic Examination

Although there is significant overlap in the examination findings of patients with each of the different forms of orbital disease and most cases are best qualified by diagnostic imaging studies, there are certain neuro-ophthalmologic examination features that help establish specific diagnoses (see examination section above). In general, the examiner must focus attention on identifying orbital disease. Externally the presence of chemosis and hyperemia of the skin suggests an infectious or inflammatory process. Preseptal and orbital cellulitis commonly are associated with significant enough swelling to close the eye and create pseudoptosis. Idiopathic orbital inflammatory syndrome characteristically causes redness and swelling. The swelling of thyroid-associated ophthalmopathy is usually less acute but can be significant (Fig. 18–5). Rarely, metastatic tumors and vascular lesions (with recent bleeding) can present with acute swelling of the eyelid and periocular skin. The eyelid findings of lid retraction and lid lag are virtually diagnostic of thyroid-associated ophthalmopathy. Characteristic S-shaped deformity of the eyelid is present in patients with masses in and around the lacrimal gland (Fig. 18–6). A mixed-pattern eye movement abnormality with positive forced ductions is generally found on examination. Slowly expanding neoplasms can cause significant proptosis without motility restriction as opposed to

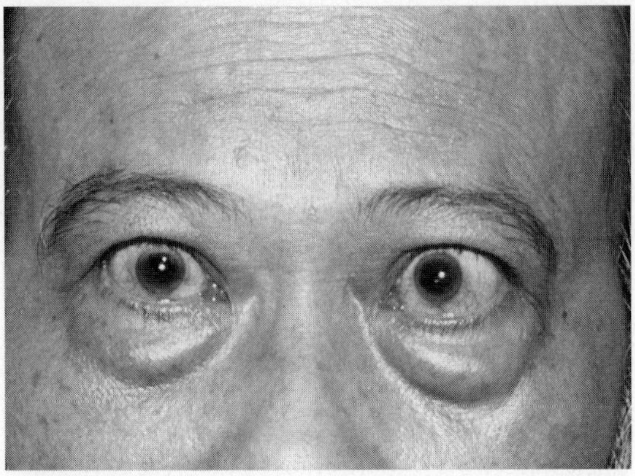

FIGURE 18–5. Acute presentation of thyroid-associated ophthalmopathy. Note proptosis as well as significant soft tissue swelling around the eyes and lid retraction.

thyroid-associated ophthalmopathy and myositis, which tend to restrict eye movements. The presence of optic nerve dysfunction with orbital signs suggests a primary optic nerve tumor, thyroid-associated ophthalmopathy, idiopathic orbital inflammation disease, or a tumor of the sphenoid bone such as a meningioma. Other mass lesions and inflammatory diseases infrequently cause optic neuropathy.

THYROID-ASSOCIATED OPHTHALMOPATHY

Thyroid-associated ophthalmopathy (TAO) is a self-limited, autoimmune condition usually occurring in association with hyperthyroidism. Historically a number of different terms have been used to label this condition, including *Graves' orbitopathy, Graves' ophthalmopathy, thyroid eye disease, thyroid orbitopathy, endocrine exophthalmos, malignant exophthalmos,* and *infiltrative ophthalmopathy.* It is the most common orbital disorder in adults. In two separate series by orbital specialists, TAO composed 32% to 47% of orbital disorders.[27,28] This percentage is different from the frequency of TAO in biopsy series,[29,30] since it rarely requires tissue confirmation to establish this clinical diagnosis. TAO should be considered in the neuro-ophthalmic differential diagnosis of double vision and in any patient with orbital signs and symptoms.

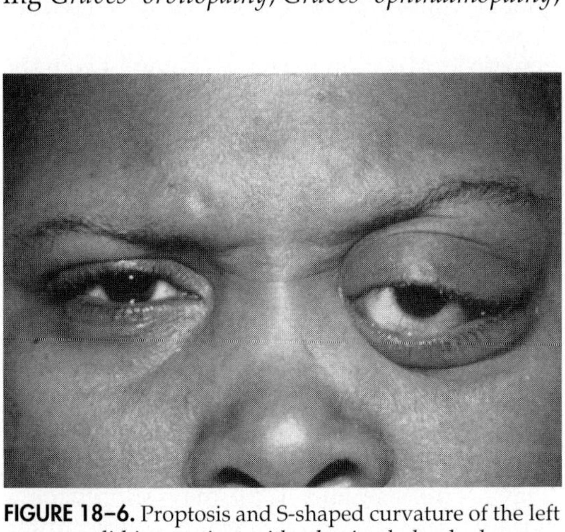

FIGURE 18–6. Proptosis and S-shaped curvature of the left upper eyelid in a patient with a lacrimal gland adenocystic carcinoma.

Endocrine Aspects of Graves' Disease

A negative feedback loop between the hypothalamus–anterior pituitary gland and the thyroid gland modulates thyroid function (see Chapter 7). The gland is composed of numerous tightly packed follicles invested in a rich capillary network. These follicles contain a rich proteinaceous colloid whose major component is thyroglobulin. Thyroglobulin is the matrix protein in which thyroid hormones are synthesized. The hypothalamus secretes thyrotropin releasing hormone (TRH), which in turn releases thyroid stimulating hormone (TSH), a glycoprotein whose actions are mediated by cyclic adenosine monophosphate (cAMP). The TSH receptor on thyroid follicles is the site of action of autoantibodies that cause hyperthyroidism in Graves' disease.[31–33] These antibodies are believed to be produced in the thyroid gland by clonally restricted B cells.[34] As well, there may be an alteration in the organ specific T-suppressor cells.[31–33] There is an extensive literature, recently summarized by Char,[35] describing various environmentally triggered, immunogenetic events that lead to the development of Graves' disease.

Hormone production in the thyroid gland is followed by secretion of iodothyronines (T_3 and T_4). Most thyroid hormone is secreted as T_4 and converted peripherally to T_3. T_4 is highly bound to thyroxin binding globulin (TBG) and thyroxin binding prealbumin (TBPa). Thyrotoxicosis can result from overproduction of the hormone (true hyperthyroidism) or from inflammation-induced glandular hormone leakage.[35] *Graves' disease* (or *diffuse toxic goiter*) is the term used to describe a number of different conditions associated with elevated levels of thyroid hormones and associated ophthalmopathy and infiltrative dermatopathy.

Patients who develop hyperthyroidism present with a classic constellation of symptoms, including nervousness, fatigue, weight loss, palpitations, heat intolerance, increased appetite, increased bowel movements, and sweating. Examination findings include tachycardia and a palpable goiter over which a thrill can often be felt. The laboratory abnormalities that accompany the presentation of Graves' disease include elevated T_3 and T_4 levels, increased T_3 to T_4 ratio, low TSH levels, thyrotropin receptor antibodies, antithyroid antibodies, and abnormal T_3 suppression tests. Char[36] has recently proposed that thyroid function tests be obained sequentially starting with a TSH level (serum thyrotropin). Next a free T_3 and T_4 index are ordered followed by tests for thyroid stimulating immunoglobulins and antithyroid antibodies. Finally a serum T_3 can be checked if none of the above tests confirm the presence of thyroid dysfunction. A low TSH level is believed to be the most sensitive indicator of thyroid dysfunction.[37, 38]

Incidence and Relationship of TAO to Thyroid Disease

Bartley[39] reviewed the Mayo Clinic series within the Rochester Epidemiology project and identified 120 patients (103 women) with TAO over 15 years in Olmsted County. The age adjusted incidence rate for men was 3 cases per year per 100,000 people and for women 16 cases per year per 100,000 people. A bimodal age peak occurred in both sexes in the forties and sixties, with the peak in men occurring 5 years later than the peak in women. Endocrine dysfunction (most commonly Graves' disease–autoimmune-induced hyperplasia of the thyroid gland associated with goiter and hyperthyroidism) developed in approximately 80% to 90% of patients found to have TAO. This endocrine dysfunction may manifest before, after, or concurrently with the ophthalmic bindings.[40–42] However, many patients (35%) are diagnosed with TAO more than 6 months after the diagnosis of hyperthyroidism. In the least common scenario, TAO precedes the endocrine dysfunction by more than 6 months (7%). Of all patients with hyperthyroidism, about 40% will develop TAO at some time.[43]

Risk Factors

The most potent risk factor for the development of TAO is hyperthyroidism, although there is a subset of patients who remain euthyroid. There may be other risk factors for the development of TAO. These risk factors include age, gender, smoking, and treatment of the hyperthyroid state with radioactive iodine. In several studies, smoking was shown to be a risk factor for the development and progression of TAO.[44–47] There is sufficient evidence to suggest that patients with hyperthyroidism or early TAO should be urged to stop smoking.

TAO may also be more common and more severe in women with hyperthyroidism and in patients (particularly men) as they get older.[48] Although it remains a controversial issue, it appears that treatment of the hyperthyroid state with radioactive iodine is associated with exacerbations of TAO, perhaps associated with a sudden increase in autoantibodies.[46, 49, 50] This risk factor appears to be modified by the use of oral corticosteroids, which seem to reduce the risk of developing TAO and its progression to more severe stages in patients treated with radioactive iodine.[50] Some have recommended that radioactive iodine treatment be avoided in patients with active or severe TAO, and that medical therapy with antithyroid drugs be used instead.[49, 51]

Genetic Predisposition

Graves' disease and TAO occur in a population that is likely to be genetically at risk for an environmentally triggered autoimmune disease. An immunogenetic predisposition is likely based on the increased incidence in certain HLA (DR, B8, and DW) types and recent genetic mapping of loci for Graves' disease in some patients to chromosome 14.[52–61] This genetic localization to chromosome 14 is in the area of the gene for the TSH receptor, but to date no mapping to the area of the HLA region has been found.[58]

Pathophysiology

There is an extensive literature concerning the actual autoimmune mechanism of Graves' disease and TAO. It appears to be mediated by both humoral and cell-mediated immunity although the cause and precise immunopathology are unknown.[62] The relationship between Graves' disease and TAO may simply be a closely related organ-specific autoimmune condition with an antigenic similarity between orbital tissue and thyroid tissue. Graves' disease is likely to be mediated by an autoimmune process directed against a portion of the thyrotropin receptor.[63] These antibodies bind to the TSH receptor sites and increase the gland's activity. These thyrotropin receptor antibodies may stimulate the development of intracellular matrix proteins (glycosaminoglycans) in orbital fat and eye muscles. This subsequently leads to swelling of the orbital tissue and inflammation, which results in scarring. Activation of orbital fibroblasts seems also to play a role.[64] Abnormal binding of the sera of patients with TAO to extraocular muscles in culture has been demonstrated.[65] However, the exact nature of the cross-reactive antigen in the orbital tissue is less clear and controversial, but it may be the thyrotropin receptor or a 64-kDa membrane antigen, tropomodulin.[66,67] Most recently a novel protein, G2s (a portion of mitochondrial succinate dehydrogenase), has been cloned and characterized and may be the best candidate for the cross-reactive antigen in eye muscle.[68] Wall and associates[69–72] have postulated a two-stage process in which autoantibodies and CD4 (helper) T cells first cross-react with eye muscle proteins leading to inflammation and swelling. In the second, more cytotoxic, stage there is inflammation and scarring of the muscles and orbital connective tissue secondary to release of muscle membrane antigens during stage one.

Pathology

The pathology of TAO reflects the above autoimmune inflammation. Infiltrating plasma cells, lymphocytes, and mast cells are seen. In addition there is deposition of hydrophilic glycosaminoglycans and collagen that are part of the scarring process. In acute stages, the changes are largely inflammatory. As the disease progresses there is more deposition of collagen and muscle degeneration. In the chronic inactive stage there is often fatty infiltration of the muscles.

Neuro-ophthalmic Features of TAO

The clinical presentation of TAO is highly variable and has been divided and grouped in many different ways. Most classifications are artificial and do not reflect the stepwise progression that often characterizes TAO.

Symptoms. These include periocular soft tissue swelling (Fig. 18–5), lid retraction, and bulging of the eyes. Some patients recognize and present with binocular double vision in upgaze or downgaze. Bartley and associates[73] reviewed their 120 patients and noted that 36 complained of pain, 20 patients had double vision, 25 patients had tearing, 19 patients had photophobia, and 9 had "blurred vision." Only two patients complained of decreased vision attributed to optic nerve dysfunction at presentation.[73] Thus, vision loss secondary to optic neuropathy is usually recognized while the patient is being monitored.

While discomfort, corneal irritation, foreign-body sensation, and "burning" are common complaints in patients with TAO, significant pain and pain on eye movements are unusual. In fact, this is an important historical point to clarify in a patient with an acute orbital syndrome. The presence of significant pain should point the examiner away from TAO and toward idiopathic orbital inflammation, infections, and tumors. Similarly, the tempo of presentation is usually gradual as symptoms develop over weeks. Orbital symptoms developing over hours or even a few days are more consistent with other acute conditions, including infections and nonthyroid inflammatory conditions. The majority of patients with TAO will have bilateral signs and symptoms although asymmetric and even unilateral disease does occur.

Eyelid Signs. The eyelid manifestations of TAO are virtually pathognomonic. Lid retraction, which is present if the upper eyelid rests above the superior corneal limbus, is evident in most patients with TAO (Figs. 18–5, 18–7,

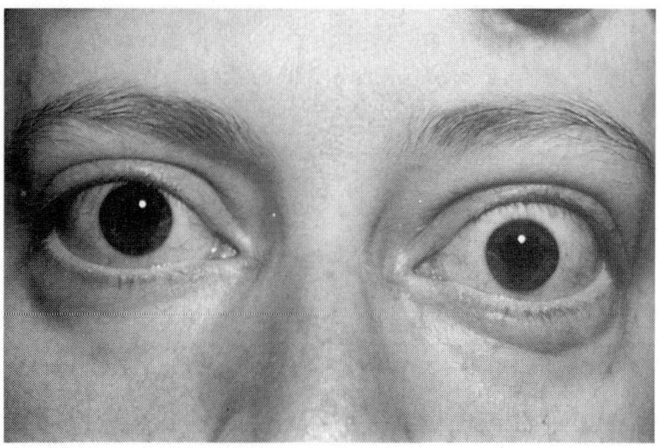

FIGURE 18–7. Proptosis and lid retraction in TAO. In this patient lid retraction is asymmetric. Sclera is visible between the superior limbus and upper eyelid of the left eye. Inferior scleral show is demonstrated on the right side.

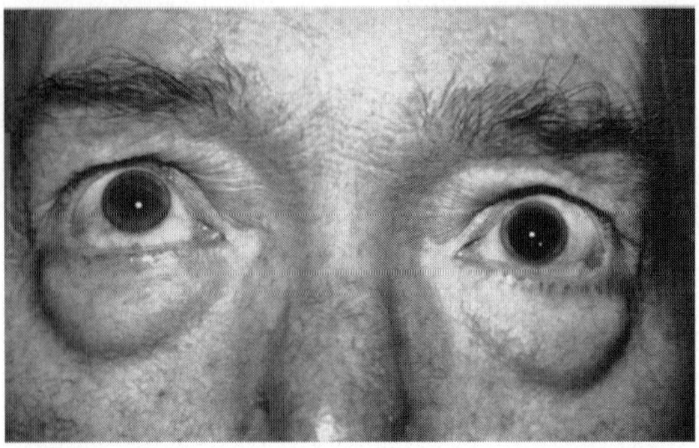

FIGURE 18–8. Thyroid associated ophthalmopathy with lid retraction, impaired upgaze in the left eye, and inferior orbital fat herniation in both eyes.

and 18–8).[73] This likely results from local adhesion of the levator muscle to fixed orbital tissue.[74] Other postulated mechanisms include superior rectus overaction, secondary inferior rectus scarring, increased circulating sympathomimetics, and muscle hypertrophy. Lid retraction can also be seen in patients with dorsal midbrain dysfunction, ptosis of the contralateral eyelid, use of sympathomimetic drugs, aberrant regeneration of the third nerve, previous retinal detachment surgery, and Guillain–Barré syndrome (see Chapter 14). Lid lag (persistent elevation of the upper eyelid in downgaze) and lagophthalmos (inferior corneal exposure (Fig. 18–7)) are other common eyelid manifestations of TAO. Swelling and edema of the eyelids and periocular skin, dermatochalasis, and orbital fat herniation are also common (Fig. 18–8). Periorbital swelling is typically worse in the morning after the patient sleeps, during which the eye is in a gravity-dependent position. Conjunctival chemosis and injection (particularly over the rectus muscle insertions) is often present.

Proptosis. Proptosis is recognized in about two thirds of patients with TAO.[73] The average normal measurement for the exophthalmometer in each eye is 17 mm, and in most patients is less than 22 mm. Any interocular difference greater than 2 mm is considered abnormal. The base used should be the same from exam to exam so that measurements from each visit can be compared.

Myopathy. The presentation of TAO-associated myopathy may be symptomatic (double vision or eye movement limitation) or asymptomatic (recognized on imaging studies). Muscle dysfunction usually begins gradually, may be intermittent, and can occur without other evidence of significant inflammation. The inflammatory process has a peculiar predilection for the inferior and medial rectus muscles, and the restrictive myopathy results in the characteristic hypertropia and esotropia, respectively (Figs. 18–8 and 18–9). Involvement of the superior rectus is less frequent, while lateral rectus involvement is rare.

Ocular Ductions and Alignment. Efforts have been made to measure eye movements in TAO, particularly for the purpose of classification within a grading system. Mourits and associates[75] suggested using a hand perimeter to measure the extent of ocular ductions. Although their method proved to be precise and reproducible, it is not widely available, and in our opinion does not aid in the management of TAO-associated myopathy. Our preference is to grade eye movement limitations on a scale from −4 to +4 or in percentages (see Chapter 2) and to quantify ocular misalignments in all fields of gaze with prisms. "Diplopia visual fields" are also an effective method that can be use to "quantify" and follow patients with TAO-associated ocular misalignments. To perform this test a Goldmann perimeter is used, with both eyes left uncovered and the head positioned in the center. The patient is asked to follow the stimulus and report when it becomes double. A field of single binocular vision is then charted (Fig. 18–10). Photographic documentation of the ocular ductions may also be helpful in following patients (Fig. 18–11).

Ocular cyclodeviations have also been described in TAO both spontaneously and as a complication of surgical treatment.[76, 77] Infiltrative TAO with restrictive myopathy is also associated with elevation of intraocular pressure on upgaze.[78, 79] The significance of the

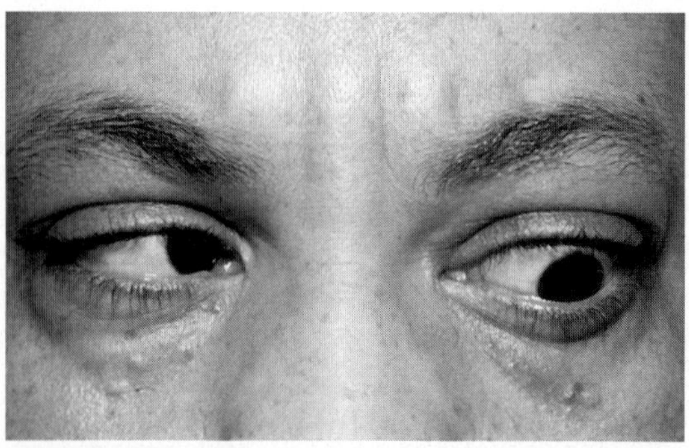

FIGURE 18–9. TAO with restrictive myopathy. The most common misalignment pattern is an hypotropia and esotropia. As demonstrated in this patient, the left eye has incomplete abduction and is hypotropic.

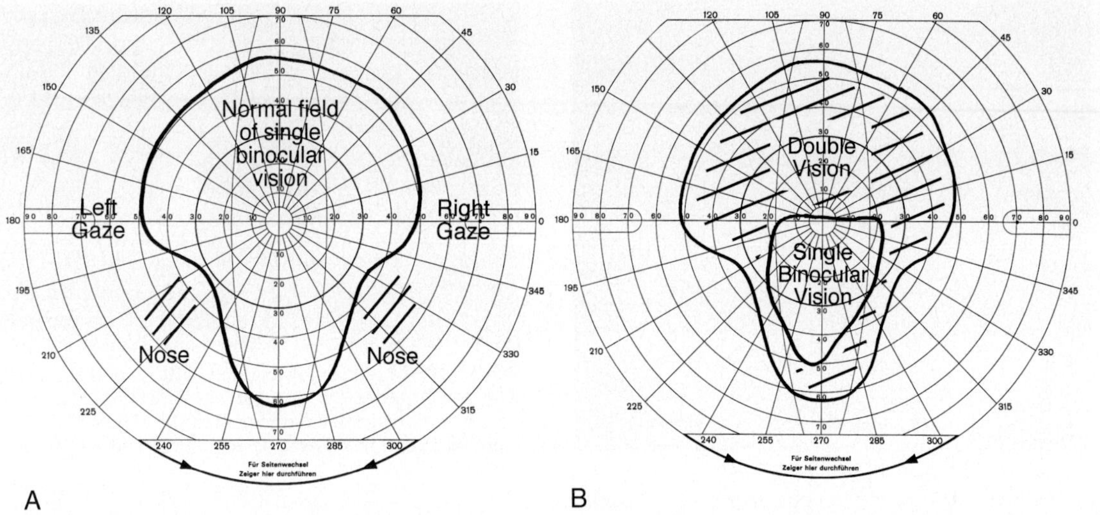

FIGURE 18–10. Diplopia visual fields are charted on the Goldmann perimeter and may be used to follow patients with double vision. The patient is tested with both eyes open and asked to track the V4e stimulus and signal the perimetrist when diplopia develops. **A.** The normal field of single binocular vision is "skull" shaped and limited in down and lateral gaze by the nose. **B.** A patient with TAO demonstrating a reduced field of single binocular vision particularly in upgaze and lateral gaze.

pressure elevation is uncertain and is rarely used to make a diagnosis. Other causes of extraocular muscle dysfunction in patients with TAO include ocular neuromyotonia[80] and concurrent myasthenia gravis.[73, 81, 82]

Optic Neuropathy. Optic neuropathy is the most feared complication of TAO. The incidence of visual loss is between 2% and 9% of all patients with TAO.[73, 83, 84] However, in patients with "severe" TAO requiring orbital decompression, optic neuropathy occurs in up to 50% of patients.[85] Vision loss from optic nerve dysfunction requires immediate management.

Neigel et al[83] reported on the clinical profile of dysthyroid optic neuropathy in 58 (8.6%) of 675 patients with TAO. About 20% of the patients presented unilaterally. At the time of presentation roughly half the patients had normal-appearing nerves, one quarter showed pallor, and another quarter had mild swelling and hyperemia (Fig. 18–12). About half the patients had acuity better than 20/40, but half were worse. In this and other studies, many patients were 20/20 but were still found to have other evidence of optic nerve dysfunction.[86, 87] Visual field defects were measured in two thirds of patients, and the most common defect types included paracentral scotomas, in-

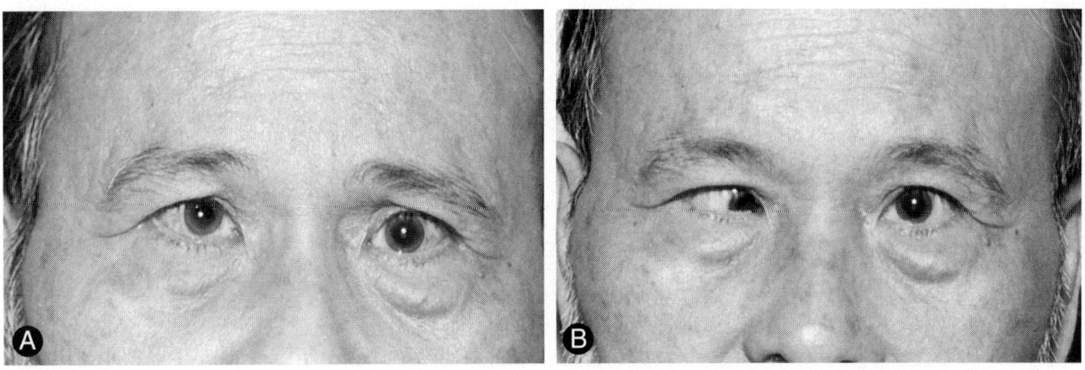

FIGURE 18–11. Photographic record of ocular deviation in TAO. **A.** This is the same patient 3 months after presentation pictured in Figure 18–5. **B.** Increasing esotropia 6 months later with resolution of the acute swelling.

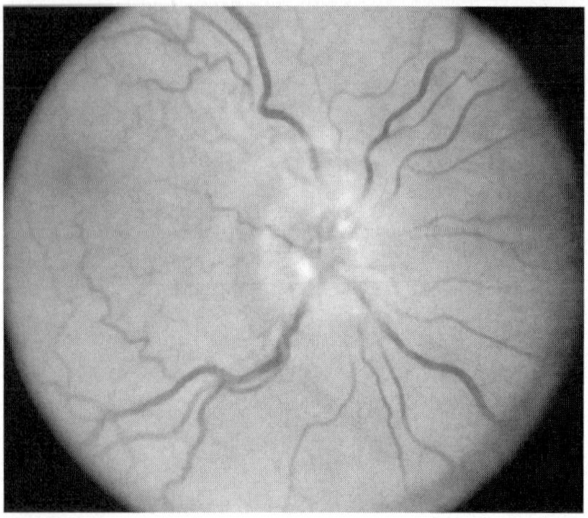

FIGURE 18–12. Fundus photograph of the right eye of a patient with TAO-associated optic neuropathy. Note the presence of diffuse disc swelling and choroidal folds.

creased blind spots, nerve fiber defects, central or centrocecal defects, and generalized constriction.[83] Persistent elevation of the intraocular pressure in patients with TAO may be associated with glaucomatous optic neuropathy, and this should be considered in the differential diagnosis of visual field defects in these patients.[88]

Apical crowding of the optic nerve by the enlarged extraocular muscles is the main mechanism of vision loss (Fig. 18–13).[86, 87] Men with TAO seem to be at greater risk for the development of optic neuropathy. Advancing age, diabetes, the amount of restrictive strabismus, as well as total volume of the extraocular muscles have all been reported as risk factors.[83, 89, 90]

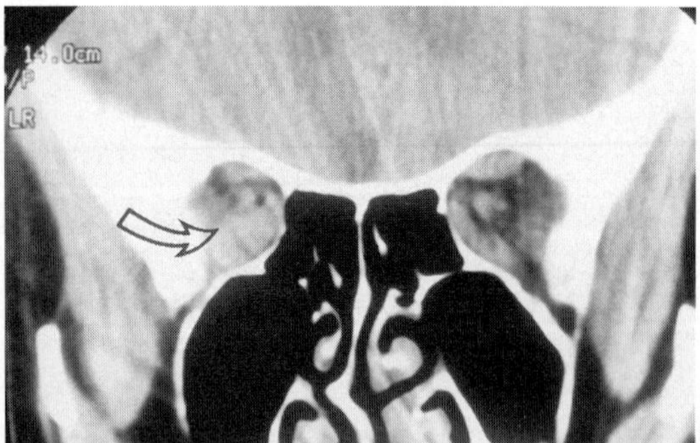

FIGURE 18–13. Coronal CT scan in a patient with TAO-associated optic neuropathy. Note the crowding of the right orbital apex (*arrow*) by enlarged extraocular muscles.

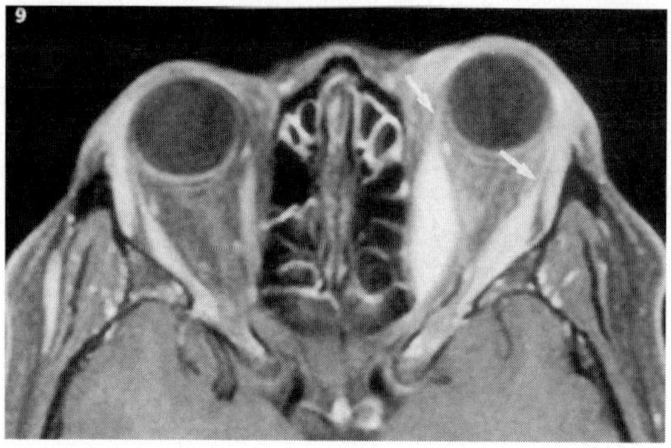

FIGURE 18–14. Axial T_1-weighted MRI scan of the orbits with fat suppression in a patient with TAO. Note the presence of fusiform enlargement of the bellies of the medial and lateral recti with sparing of the tendons (*arrows*).

Imaging in TAO

Noninvasive imaging of the orbit is the gold standard for the diagnosis of TAO. Echography, CT and MRI may be used to confirm the diagnosis of TAO. The classic finding is enlargement of the extraocular muscle belly with relative sparing of the tendon (Fig. 18–14). Proptosis may also be recognized without extraocular muscle enlargement and presumably results from increased swelling and volume of the intraorbital fat. In addition to the extraocular enlargement with tendon sparing, CT frequently demonstrates proptosis, enlargement of the lacrimal gland, and eyelid soft tissue swelling.[91–94] As expected, enlargement is most commonly seen in the inferior rectus and medial rectus (Fig. 18–15). CT, unlike echography, provides excellent images of the orbital apex and usually documents enlarged muscles surrounding and in contact with the optic nerve in patients with optic neuropathy. Low-density areas may be noted in the muscle bellies and may represent collections of lymphocytes or glycosaminoglycan deposition (Figs. 18–15 and 18–16). With chronic inactive disease larger low-density lesions can be seen within the muscles, owing to fatty infiltration. Occasionally chronic medial rectus muscle enlargement can be associated with bone molding and bowing into the ethmoid sinus. CT can be used to monitor treatment.

More recently MRI of the orbit has been shown to be effective in imaging the orbital soft tissues, including enlarged extraocular muscles[95–97] and the orbital apex (Figs. 18–14 and 18–17). The recommended sequence is STIR (short tau inversion recovery), which highlights the extraocular muscles. High water

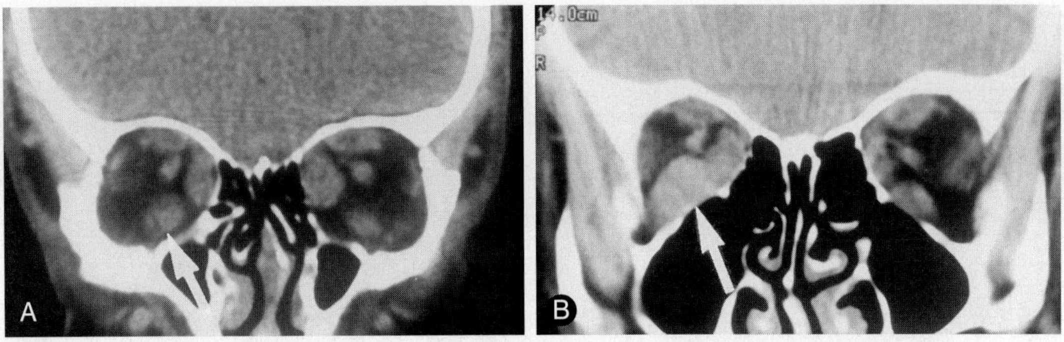

FIGURE 18–15. Coronal CT scans of two different patients with TAO. Note the presence of enlarged extraocular muscles (particularly the inferior recti (*arrows*)). The medial and superior recti are also enlarged. **A.** Significant asymmetry between the right and left orbit is not uncommon. **B.** The muscles often have a granular or irregular appearance from low-density areas.

content can be detected with this sequence, presumably reflecting disease activity. This may be a way to follow patients for radiographic evidence of persistent inflammation.[95–97] Studies measuring eye movements during cine MRI have demonstrated normal movements early in the disease but confirmed the presence of restricted eye movements later in the course of the disease.[95]

Echography has proven valuable in the office diagnosis of TAO.[15,16,18,98,99] Abnormal muscle size (A and B scan) and internal reflectivity (A scan) can be compared to normative data, and enlargement can be documented (Fig. 18–18).[100,101] In two separate studies, echography was shown to be more sensitive than CT in detecting extraocular muscle enlargement and abnormal internal reflectivity secondary to separation of the muscle fibers.[17,98] However, echography may not be as efficacious as other modalities for diagnosing orbital tumors and for distinguishing the different causes of extraocular muscle enlargement.

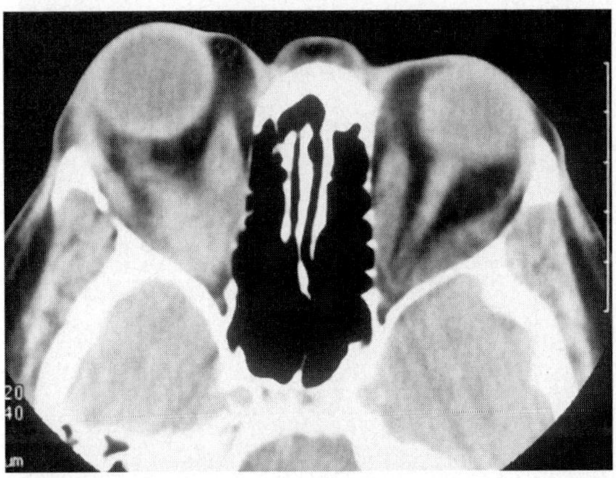

FIGURE 18–16. Axial CT scan in a patient with TAO demonstrating enlargement of the inferior and medial rectus of the right eye and to a lesser extent of the medial rectus of the left orbit. Note the irregular low densities in the enlarged muscles secondary to fatty infiltration or glycosaminoglycan deposition.

Classification

Several different classification systems have been proposed for descriptive and clinical research studies of TAO. The most popular is the so-called NOSPECS classification system initially described by Werner (Table 18–4).[102,103] This classification system is widely used in clinical research studies. Not all patients progress through the seven classes as listed, and some have prominent features in the higher-numbered classes without some of the milder signs. The NOSPECS classification system has been recently criticized because (1) its characterization of the condition is poor, with no indication of disease activity, marked underrepresentation of eyelid position, and overrepresentation of corneal problems; (2) it implies a continuous or stepladder progression of disease as a numbered classification system would suggest; (3) parts of it are subjective; and (4) the gradings within classes 3, 5, and 6 are poor.[104–106]

From a practical clinical and management standpoint it is often unnecessary to use such a formal classification system. We recommend considering patients as having mild, moderate, or severe periorbital swelling, extraocular muscle dysfunction, or visual dysfunction secondary to compressive optic neuropathy. In this system patients with only mild or moderate symptoms (presumably noninfiltrative disease) are treated conservatively. Patients with

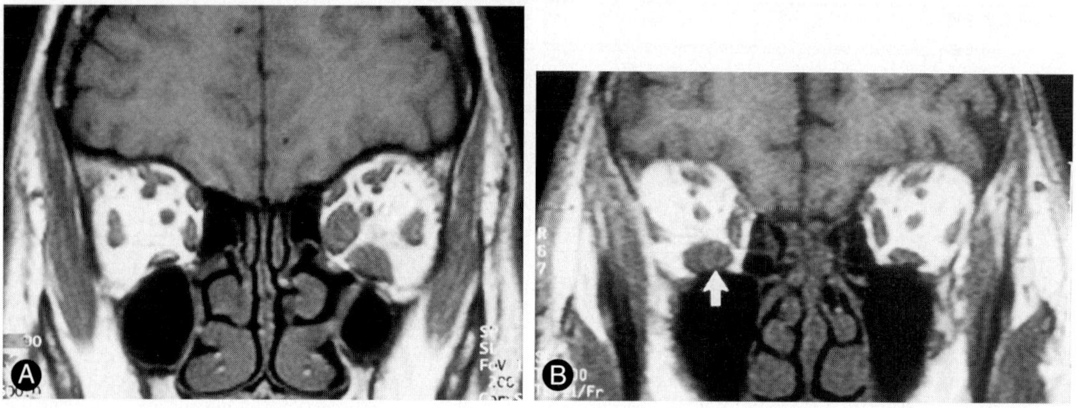

FIGURE 18–17. MRI scans of the orbits in two patients with TAO. **A.** Coronal T_1-weighted image without fat suppression or contrast demonstrating enlargement of the inferior and lateral rectus muscles on the left. **B.** Coronal T_1-weighted image without fat suppression or contrast of a different patient demonstrating enlargement of the right inferior rectus muscle with fatty infiltration seen as a brighter circle within the muscle (*arrow*; also see Fig. 18–14).

more debilitating symptoms of swelling and eye muscle involvement (infiltrative disease) are considered for more aggressive treatment, including systemic corticosteroids and radiation therapy. Finally patients with vision-threatening disease are treated emergently both medically (intravenous steroids) and with orbital decompression if necessary.

Treatment of TAO

The treatment of TAO is complex, often requiring a multidisciplinary approach that includes a neuro-ophthalmologist, orbital specialist and surgeon, radiation therapist, and endocrinologist. Fortunately most patients do well, and in fact three quarters of patients require no or only supportive therapy. Most patients do not develop sight-threatening complications of double vision or optic neuropathy.[107] The disease usually runs a self-limited course of 18 to 36 months, and up to two thirds of patients with TAO will improve spontaneously.[108]

Appropriate management is dependent on accurate assessment of the clinical findings at the time of presentation, including careful evaluation of visual function, eye movements,

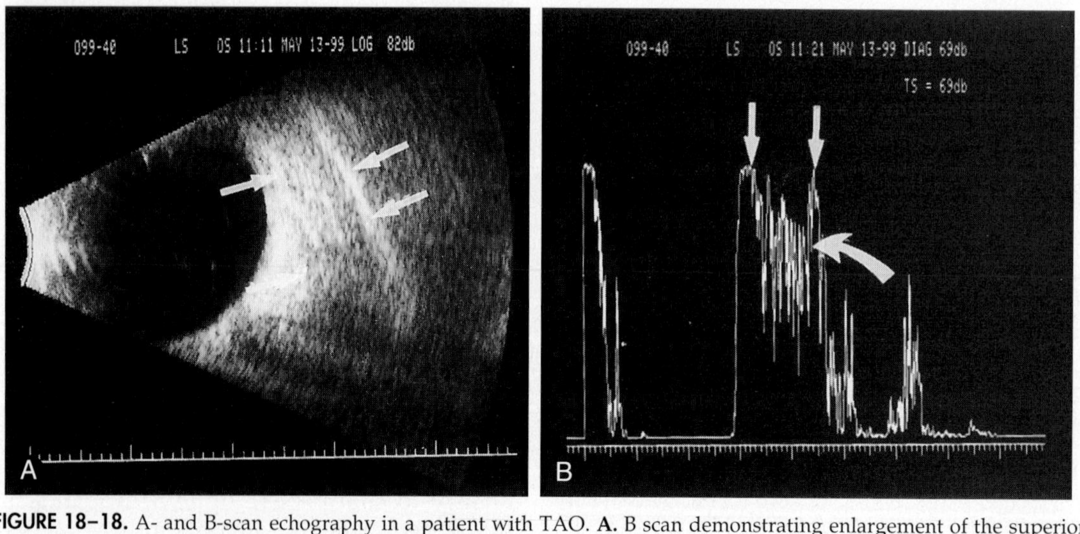

FIGURE 18–18. A- and B-scan echography in a patient with TAO. **A.** B scan demonstrating enlargement of the superior rectus/levator complex (*arrows*). **B.** A scan showing a widened superior rectus/levator complex measuring approximately 10 mm (*small arrows*; the normal median width is 5.4 mm[18]). High spikes (*curved arrow*) indicate high internal reflectivity typical of TAO. (Photo courtesy of E. Kym Gendron.)

TABLE 18–4. The NOSPECS Classification of Thyroid-Associated Ophthalmopathy

Class	Clinical Features
0	No signs or symptoms
1	Only signs such as lid retraction
2	Soft tissue periorbital swelling A–C: minimal to marked
3	Proptosis of the eyes A = 3–4 mm, B = 5–7mm, C ≥ 8mm
4	Extraocular muscle involvement A = limitation B = evidence of restriction C = fixation of globe
5	Corneal involvement with exposure A = stippling B = ulceration C = clouding, necrosis, perforation
6	Sight loss secondary to optic neuropathy A = disc pale or swollen, 20/20–20/60, field defect, B = same but vision 20/70–20/200, C = same but vision < 20/200

and orbital imaging. In patients with lid retraction and proptosis only (noninfiltrative disease), reassurance and ocular lubrication when exposure or ocular discomfort is present are the only treatments recommended. Here it is important to emphasize to the patient that the condition does remit, and that ultimately cosmetic aspects of the disease can be addressed. These patients tend to be young and when the disease is quiescent may choose to have orbital decompression or eyelid surgery to improve their appearance.

Infiltrative disease with myopathy and increased orbital congestion is an indication for more aggressive forms of therapy to reduce symptoms and the likelihood of developing permanent dysfunction. The two major options are systemic corticosteroids and orbital radiation.

Steroids and Other Medical Therapies. As signs and symptoms of severe congestive orbitopathy increase, treatment should first consist of oral prednisone at a dose of 1 to 1.5 mg/kg daily.[109] This dose is arbitrary and not based on any prospective data. About two thirds of patients will have reduction in their symptoms and swelling in about 1 week.[110] This dose is continued and then slowly tapered by 10 mg per daily dose each week. If symptoms worsen then reinstituting the original successful dose and radiation therapy should be considered. In patients with more severe orbitopathy, or significant vision loss from compressive optic neuropathy, intravenous methylprednisolone has been shown to be effective.[111–113] Although symptoms of congestion improve on steroids, only about one third of patients show improvement of the eye movements. Rootman[109] concluded that that the long-term use of steroids in these patients (3 to 12 months) is associated with significant side effects and therefore should be avoided.

Other medical therapies, including plasmapheresis,[109, 114] intravenous immunoglobulin,[115–117] and intravenous somatostatin,[118] have been shown to be effective but have not assumed primary roles in the medical management of TAO. While not effective on its own, cyclosporine has been shown to be effective as a combined therapy with prednisone in patients who do not respond to either drug alone.[119]

Special medical treatment issues arise in patients with TAO who plan radioactive iodine therapy for their thyroid disease. Although it remains a controversial issue, there is evidence to suggest that treatment of hyperthyroidism with radioactive iodine is associated with worsening of TAO. Furthermore this worsening may be lessened by the use of oral corticosteroids before and after the radioactive iodine treatment.[46, 49, 50, 120] Bartalena and associates[50] found that 15% of patients treated with radioactive iodine alone developed or had worsening of TAO. In contrast, none of the patients treated with radioactive iodine and prednisone had progression of disease. We advocate the use of prednisone in all patients with active TAO who are going to be treated with radioactive iodine for hyperthyroidism.

Radiation Therapy. Radiotherapy for TAO is effective in 70% of patients,[109, 110, 121] but can take several weeks (often with transient worsening requiring steroids) to take effect. Several series have demonstrated favorable responses in patients treated either with radiation or with steroids and radiation.[110, 113, 121–126] There is increasing evidence to suggest that radiation should not be considered as a last resort, but more appropriately should be part of the early discussions the physician has with the patient. However, some centers use radiotherapy infrequently; in the Olmstead County cohort of 120 patients, only one was treated with radiotherapy.[107]

The technique generally involves the use of 1500 to 2000 cGy in divided fractions over 10 days. Care is taken to irradiate only the posterior two thirds of the orbit, thereby avoiding the globe. Radiation has been shown to be more effective than steroids in the treatment of optic neuropathy. In one study, only 1 of 29 patients treated with radiation for optic neuropathy went on to require surgical decompression, while 6 of 16 treated with steroids needed surgery.[127] Improvement in soft tissue swelling almost always occurs. MRI has been used to monitor the positive affects of radiation treatment, as reduced signal in the eye muscles presumable correlates with lower water content.[125] Careful, quantitative measurements of eye movements often demonstrate some improvement, although this does not correlate with improvement in double vision.[128] Rootman found that only 14% of his patients had recurrence of symptoms after radiotherapy.[109] Complications of radiation therapy are rare, although radiation retinopathy has been reported.[129]

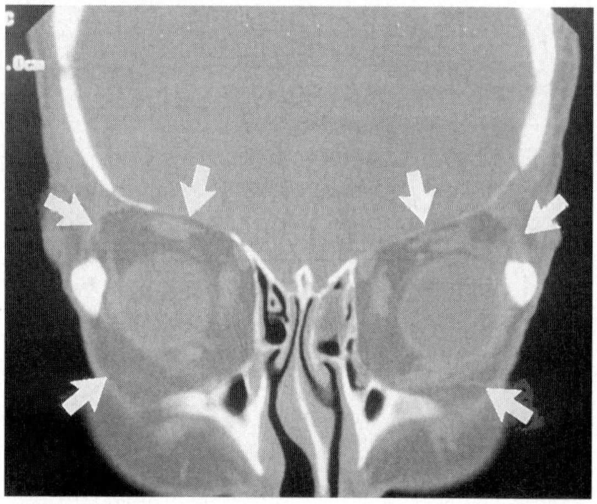

FIGURE 18–19. Coronal CT scan of the orbits (bone windows) in a patient who had undergone four-wall orbital decompression for proptosis and optic neuropathy. In this section portions of the superior and lateral walls of the orbit are missing (*arrows*).

Surgery. Surgical treatment of TAO is indicated in two separate situations. The first is orbital decompression for sight-threatening disease secondary to orbital apex crowding. The second is the use of orbital decompression, eye muscle surgery, and eyelid surgery in the patient with quiescent disease who has double vision, exposure, or a significant cosmetic problem. Orbital decompression should not be used in the acute treatment of proptosis and swelling from TAO unless there is sight-threatening disease. Mechanical decompression of the orbit has been described in several large series and is safe and effective in improving visual function in patients with apex crowding secondary to TAO-associated myopathy.[85, 127, 130–140] Removal of the orbital floor and medial wall using various approaches is the most common surgery performed.[141] Mourits and associates[142] compared the coronal method to the inferomedial and the inferomedial plus lateral approach and found each to be equally effective in treating vision loss. Recently, endoscopic approaches have become popular as they appear to be equally effective and avoid external scarring.[139, 143–145] Regardless of the technique employed, successful treatment requires decompression of the orbital apex through removal of the apical portions of the orbital walls and opening or removing the periorbita (Fig 18–19). Visual improvement should be prompt and if vision fails to improve, the decompression was likely incomplete at the orbital apex. Severe vision loss preoperatively is associated with a worse prognosis postoperatively as only 4 of 7 patients with less than 20/200 vision preoperatively attained visual acuity of 20/40 postoperatively in one series.[130] Significant improvement in nearly all parameters of the optic neuropathy, including visual fields and optic disc swelling, occurs in most patients.[85] Patients also notice improvement in their congestive symptoms since the orbit is no longer under pressure. Most patients who undergo orbital decompression do so within 1 year from the onset of eye symptoms.[85] Double vision is present postoperatively in 33% to 63% of patients and may be worsened because of associated postoperative scarring.[130, 146, 147] Up to 70% of patients require one or two eye muscle surgeries to correct their double vision after orbital decompression.[85] Interestingly approximately 5% of patients experience improvement in their double vision after orbital decompression.[130, 138, 147]

Other indications for orbital decompression include severe orbital inflammation, the reduction of proptosis prior to eye muscle surgery, exposure, and steroid intolerance.[85] With increasing surgeon experience and successful results, orbital decompression is being performed more commonly for cosmetic reasons.[85, 131, 148, 149] Reductions in proptosis of 4 to 5 mm may be achieved with good patient satisfaction. Further surgery may be performed for eyelid (many patients experience worsening of lid retraction) and eye muscle abnormalities. In one series of 15 patients with no preoperative double vision who underwent transantral orbital decompression primarily for cosmetic reasons, 11 (73%) developed double vision postoperatively although no patients were dissatisfied with their surgical result.[131] A modified approach to orbital decompression involves only removing orbital fat without bone removal.[150]

Eye muscle surgery for dysthyroid myopathy is often required to correct double vision. The goal is to establish a field of single vision as large as possible, including the primary postion and downgaze. Rootman[109] found that 9% of his patients ultimately required eye muscle surgery. The most common misalignment is a combined esotropia and hypertropia, for which inferior rectus recession and/or medial rectus recessions either unilaterally or bilaterally are required (Fig. 18–20 see Color Plate 50). Resections should be avoided. Adjustable sutures are particularly helpful and should be used whenever possible. We use the rule of thumb that three prism diopters are corrected for every millimeter of muscle recessed. The amount of correction increases when the disease only affects one muscle, which is more likely to be tethered. Surgery should not be performed until measurements have been stable for 6 months and a similar time has elapsed since the last intervention (radiation or decompression).[151] Intraoperative decision making is always based on the results of forced duction testing, and the surgeon should be prepared to alter the plan, particularly if the superior rectus is found to be tight. In cases with severe scarring, surgery of the muscle may be difficult. The initial surgical goal should be a slight undercorrection as a drift toward overcorrection occurs postoperatively.[151, 152] About two thirds of patients achieve a successful result of single vision in the primary position and downgaze after a single operation.[78, 153] Greater than 90% of patients may be corrected with a second surgery, and it is not uncommon for patients to require multiple procedures.[85]

One common complication of strabismus surgery is lower eyelid retraction, and this is one reason why eyelid surgery should be deferred to after strabismus surgery. A detailed discussion of eyelid surgery is beyond the scope of this text. Eyelid surgery is reserved as the last procedure performed (after decompression and muscle surgery), and usually entails lowering the upper eyelid and raising the lower eyelid. Procedures on the lower eyelid usually require detaching the capsulopalpebral fascia from the tarsus and inserting some type of spacer (sclera, hard palate, cartilage, or fascia). The upper eyelid can be lowered by müllerectomy or levator recession, and in many instances because of chronic swelling and fat herniation, this is combined with blepharoplasty.

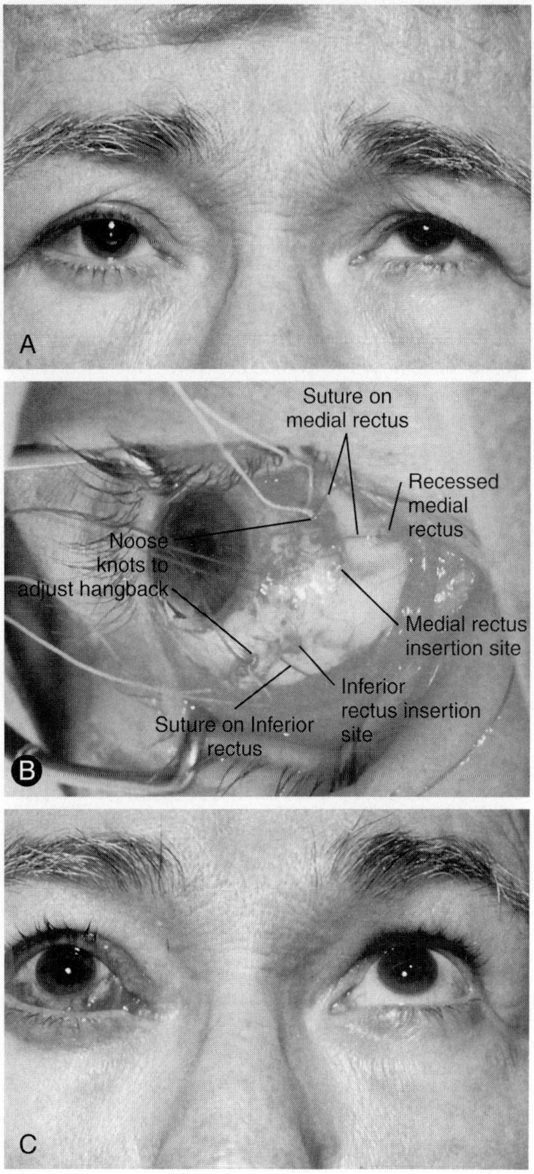

FIGURE 18–20. **A.** Patient with TAO with associated right hypotropia and esotropia. **B.** Intraoperative photograph demonstrating adjustable-suture, hangback recession of the right inferior and medial rectus muscles. A suture is attached to the medial and inferior rectus muscles. The suture is passed back through the original insertion. A noose suture is placed so that during the adjustment the recessed muscle can either be advanced or recessed further to obtain the appropriate alignment. (See Color Plate 50). **C.** Immediate postoperative result showing improved upgaze and correction of the hypotropia.

Course and Outcome. The disease usually runs a course of 18 months to 3 years. The symptoms may vary on a diurnal basis depending on the amount of venous and lymphatic drainage. Careful monitoring of the patient's endocrine status must be performed by an endocrinologist. We believe it is inadequate for the ophthalmologist or neurologist to order simply "thyroid function tests" and not involve the expertise of an endocrinologist. Bartley and associates[84] followed their cohort of 120 patients in Olmstead County for a median time of 10 years. Only two eyes had persistent vision loss from optic neuropathy (20/30 and 20/60). Seven patients had intermittent double vision and two other patients had constant double vision that was correctable by prisms. Twenty percent of the patients underwent at least one surgical procedure.[107] Many patients complained of persistent ocular discomfort that in most cases was the result of dry eyes. Although many patients (one third) were unhappy with their appearance, with successful treatment functional impairment seems to be uncommon.[84]

Pediatric Thyroid Eye Disease. Pediatric Graves' disease or hyperthyroidism is not uncommon, and rarely may be associated with the development of TAO. Orbital signs and symptoms occur in about one half of the patients,[154] and the proptosis may be dramatic.[155] Fortunately restrictive myopathy, exposure, and optic neuropathy are rare in children.[155] Echography, CT and MRI have all demonstrated enlargement of the extraocular muscles in children, although motility for the most part remains normal.[154, 155] The majority of children can be treated conservatively,[154] and orbital fat decompression has been reported to be helpful in reducing proptosis.

IDIOPATHIC ORBITAL INFLAMMATORY SYNDROME (ORBITAL PSEUDOTUMOR)

Patients with idiopathic orbital inflammatory syndrome (IOIS) are typified by their acute onset of proptosis and eyelid swelling associated with pain and double vision. There is usually conjunctival swelling (chemosis) and injection, and there may be a violaceous injection over the muscle insertions (Fig. 18–21; see Color Plate 51). IOIS is usually distinguished from other causes of orbital disease (except infections and hemorrhages) by the rapidity of onset and discomfort. Symptoms result from a non-thyroid-related, noninfectious inflammation of the orbit characterized by polymorphous orbital infiltration of lymphocytes and plasma cells with varying amounts of fibrosis and mass effect.

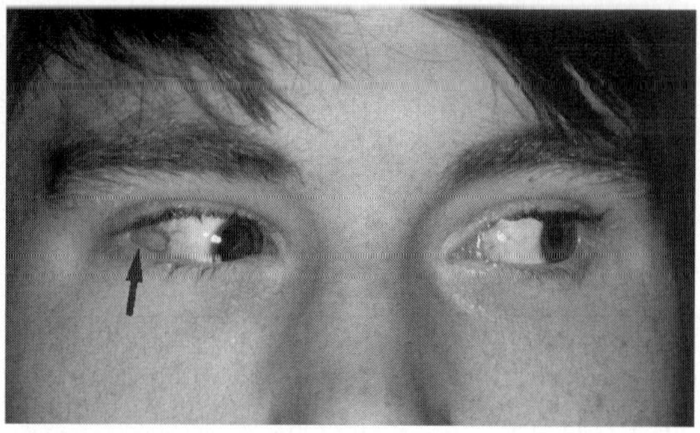

FIGURE 18–21. Photograph of a patient with idiopathic orbital inflammatory syndrome and myositis involving the right lateral rectus. Violaceous injection is seen over the area of the right lateral rectus insertion (*arrow*). (See Color Plate 51).

IOIS is an umbrella term that applies to a heterogeneous group of presentations. It may be further subclassed according to the location of the inflammation within the orbit. In this section, the pathogenesis and pathology of IOIS will be discussed, followed by a review of its classification, imaging, and treatment.

Pathogenesis

The cause of IOIS is unknown, and theories concerning pathogenesis include viral, allergic, and autoimmune mechanisms. Based on the lymphocytic nature of the infiltration, it is assumed to be an immune-mediated condition mediated by both B and T lymphocytes.[156] Whether it is a genetically predetermined autoimmune condition or an environmentally triggered immune event is unclear. Other theories include aberrant wound healing and infection.[157] Several observations have been made to support an autoimmune inflammatory condition, although the significance of each is unclear. These include the identification of antibodies to eye muscle surface antigens in patients with IOIS[158]; reports of patients with upper respiratory tract infections prior to developing IOIS[159–161]; and the occasional association of IOIS with similar nonspecific inflammation of the paranasal sinuses.[162, 163]

Differential Diagnosis

IOIS-like presentations may occur with orbital inflammation as a result of systemic inflammatory conditions or vasculitis such as Wegener's granulomatosis, polyarteritis nodosa, systemic lupus eythematosis, gout, psoriatic and rheumatoid arthritis, syphilis, tuberculosis, sarcoidosis, ulcerative colitis, and Crohn's disease. Contrary to old theories concerning IOIS, it is no longer believed to be related to orbital reactive lymphoid hyperplasia (pseudolymphoma), or a lymphoid tumor. There is no apparent potential for malignant transformation.[157]

Pathology

Histologically, IOIS is characterized by lymphocyte, plasma cell, macrophage, and polymorphonuclear cell infiltration associated with a fibrovascular stroma. This inflammation eventually leads to fibrosis, but there should be no vasculitic features. More chronic forms of the disease are characterized by insidious development of fibrosis or desmoplasia leading to an apparent soft tissue mass, without an acute phase of cellular infiltration. Although there is significant overlap, some have suggested subgrouping IOIS pathologically into lymphoid, granulomatous, and sclerosing varieties.[164] However, usually a more clinical and anatomic classification is preferred (see below).

Prevalence

IOIS is a relatively uncommon condition. In clinical series of patients presenting with orbital disease, patients with IOIS compose between 6% and 8%.[27, 28] It can occur at any age with most patients presenting in middle life. There is no sex or race predilection.

Classification

Several different classifications schemes for IOIS have been described. Rootman[165] has proposed a classification system that groups patients depending on the location of orbital involvement. Categories include *anterior, diffuse, apical, lacrimal gland,* and *myositis.* This system is helpful in understanding the highly variable clinical presentations of IOIS. For the purposes of neuro-ophthalmic differential diagnosis we find another related system helpful and consider patients with IOIS in six different categories: *posterior scleritis, diffuse, myositis, dacryoadenitis, perineuritis,* and finally *sclerosing inflammation.* This classification system allows for separating patients into categories that are unique with regards to their differential diagnosis, evaluation, and treatment.

Posterior Scleritis. This group of patients has inflammation focused on the eye wall and surrounding Tenon's capsule. Patients develop pain, proptosis, ptosis, lid swelling, chemosis and injection of the conjunctiva, and decreased vision (Fig. 18–22). This form of IOIS may be characterized by funduscopic abnormalities including choroidal folds, exudative retinal detachment (Fig. 18–22), papillitis, and uveitis. It occurs in all age groups but seems to be the most common form of IOIS to affect children.[166] Imaging reveals anterior ragged orbital inflammation, which involves the globe and is associated with retinochoroidal thickening.[165, 167] Ultrasound may demonstrate sclerotenonitis with edema or widening of Tenon's space (Fig. 18–22). This effusion at the neuroocular junction and doubling of the optic nerve shadow creates a specific echographic sign called the T sign. Fluorescein angiographic abnormalities may include patchy choroidal infiltrates, exudative retinal detachments, and macular edema.[168] Treatment is with oral steroids, and their effect is usually prompt and dramatic. Glaucoma may complicate anterior IOIS. Mechanisms include choroidal effusion with anterior rotation of the lens iris diaphragm and uveitic glaucoma.

Diffuse Inflammation. In the diffuse presentation, inflammation involves the entire orbit. Clinically patients have proptosis, eyelid swelling, ptosis, and occasionally extraocular muscle involvement and double vision. Papillitis and exudative retinal detachments may be present in this subgroup of patients as well. On imaging studies, the entire orbit is involved by the irregular infiltrate that often obscures normal orbital anatomy (Fig. 18–23). When orbital inflammation primarily involves the orbital apex (often subcategorized as "posterior IOIS") there may be a disproportionate amount of visual and eye movement dysfunction.[165] Pupillary defects (internal ophthalmoplegia) have also been described with posterior orbital involvement, presumably due to disruption of the ciliary ganglion or third nerve.[169]

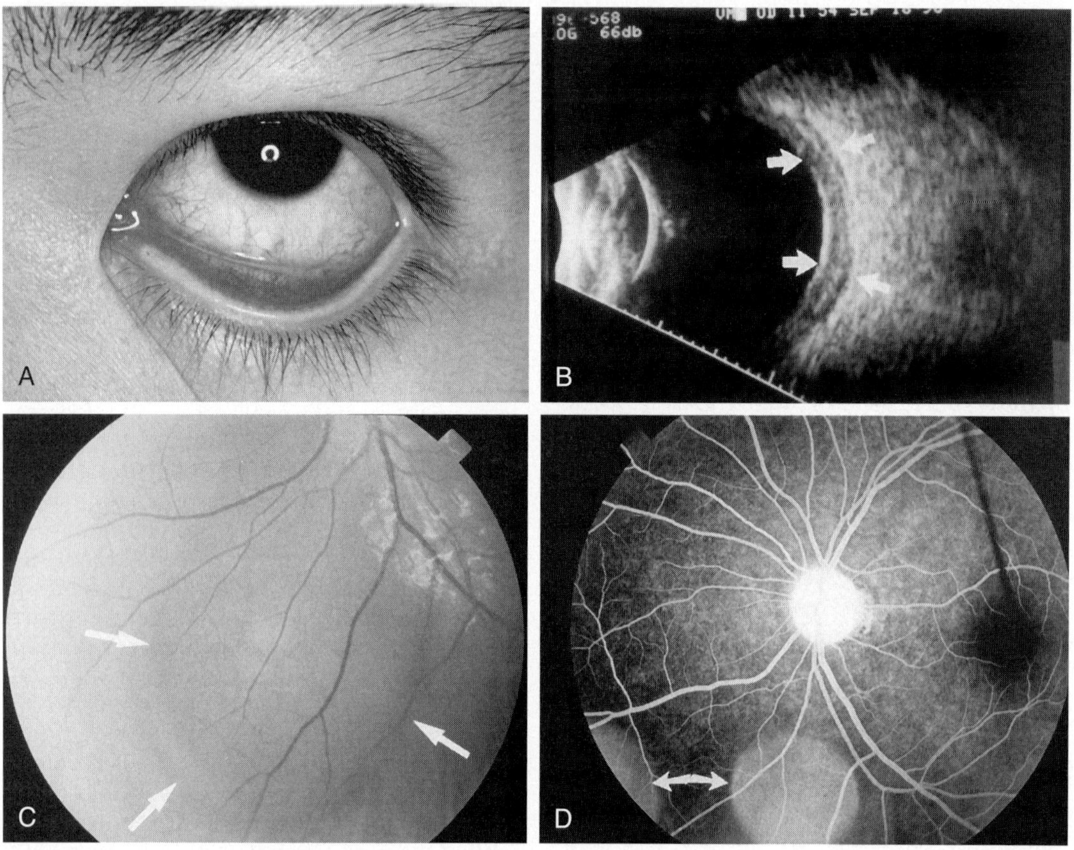

FIGURE 18–22. **A.** Posterior scleritis presenting with diffuse conjunctival injection and chemosis. **B.** B-scan echography demonstrates thickening or widening of the sclera and Tenon's space (*arrows*). **C.** Fundus examination showed exudative retinal detachment with rounded area of retinal elevation secondary to subretinal fluid (*arrows*). **D.** Late-phase fluorescein angiography confirms subretinal fluid (*arrows*) in the area of the exudative retinal detachments.

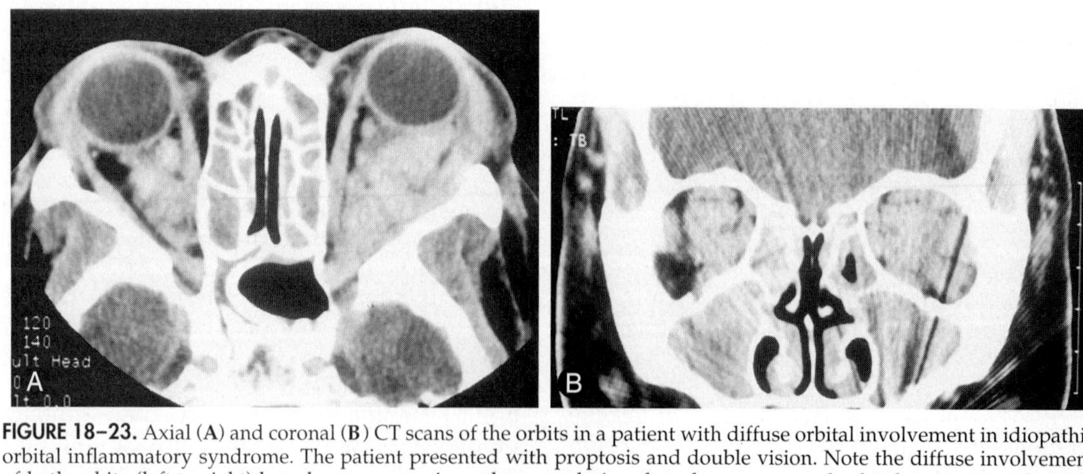

FIGURE 18–23. Axial (**A**) and coronal (**B**) CT scans of the orbits in a patient with diffuse orbital involvement in idiopathic orbital inflammatory syndrome. The patient presented with proptosis and double vision. Note the diffuse involvement of both orbits (left > right) by a homogenous, irregular mass lesion that obscures normal orbital anatomy and molds the globe.

Myositis. Patients with myositis have a clinical presentation dominated by symptoms of double vision and pain on eye movements. Ptosis and eyelid swelling are common, and chemosis and conjunctival injection in the area overlying the inflamed muscle are prominent (Fig. 18–21).

Clinical distinction from TAO can usually be made based on the rapid development of myositis and its characteristic pain, eyelid findings, and diffuse involvement of the muscle and tendon on imaging (Figs. 18–24 and 18–25; see Table 18–5 and discussion of other causes of enlarged eye muscles below). The most common muscles involved in Rootman's series were the superior rectus/levator complex (Fig. 18–26) and the medical rectus, but any or multiple muscles may be involved.[170] Involvement of the superior oblique with point tenderness over the superomedial aspect of the orbit has been described.[171]

Dacryoadenitis. Inflammation of the lacrimal gland occurs in a variety of circumstances, including infection, infiltration by neoplasm, systemic inflammatory conditions, and finally nonspecific inflammation. Pathologically these can be divided into categories that are specific (ie, lymphoma, sarcoidosis) and nonspecific (IOIS, dacryoadenitis). Therefore biopsy of these lesions is often recommended.[170] In addition to the more typical acute and subacute varieties, there is a unique chronic (sometimes painless) presentation of IOIS involving the lacrimal gland.

Patients with dacryoadenitis typically develop pain and swelling and redness of the temporal portion of the eyelid (Fig. 18–27; see Color Plate 52). The lid acquires a characteristic S-shaped deformity. The globe may be displaced downward and inferiorly.[170] Bilateral presentation occurs occasionally. Elevation of the eyelid and inspection of the superotemporal area of the conjunctiva shows prominence of the secretory ducts and injection of the visible portions of the lacrimal gland. The superotemporal portion of the orbit may be exquisitely tender. Patients rarely have double vision or complain of decreased vision. Imaging studies document the presence of an inflammatory mass lesion in the superotemporal orbit that is contiguous with the globe and generally does not involve other orbital tissues.

Perineuritis. The presence of optic neuropathy in association with nonspecific orbital inflammation is well recognized and is termed *perineuritis*.[167] Vision loss results from either optic nerve sheath inflammation or mass effect on the optic nerve. Patients often develop optic disc edema and mild retinal venous obstruction (Fig. 18–28; see Color Plate 53). Sarcoid

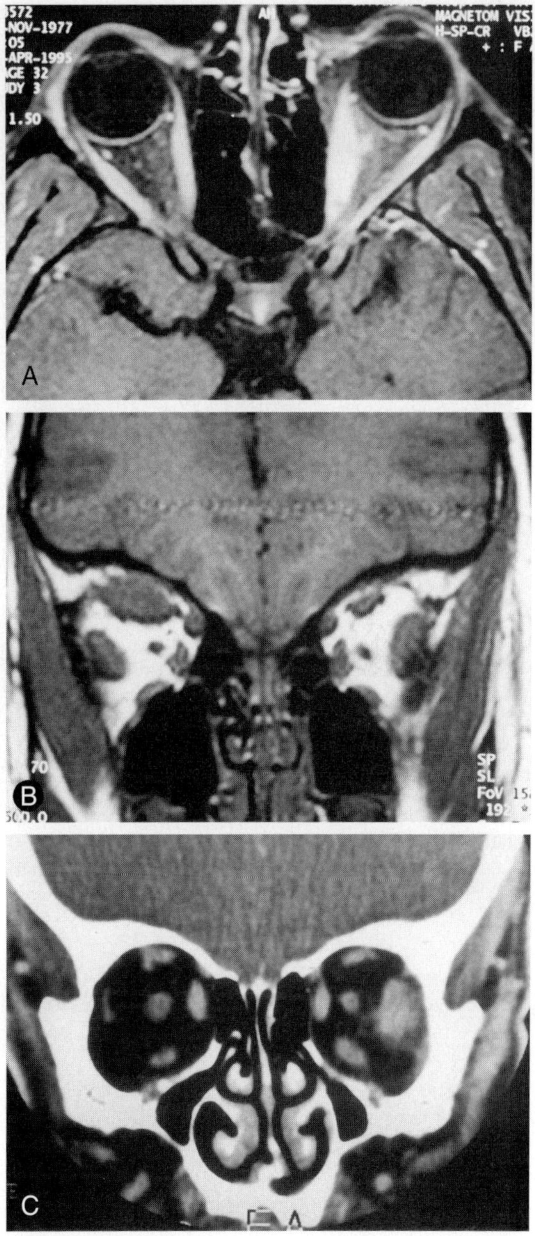

FIGURE 18–24. Imaging of the orbit in myositis. **A.** Axial T_1 weighted MRI scan of the orbits with contrast (fat suppression) in an 18-year-old with acute onset of pain, proptosis, and abduction deficit. Left-sided medial rectus muscle enlargement is noted. **B.** Coronal T_1-weighted MRI scan of the orbits in an 8-year-old with diffuse myositis and multiple (bilateral) muscle involvement. **C.** Coronal CT scan of the orbits demonstrating left lateral rectus enlargement secondary to myositis.

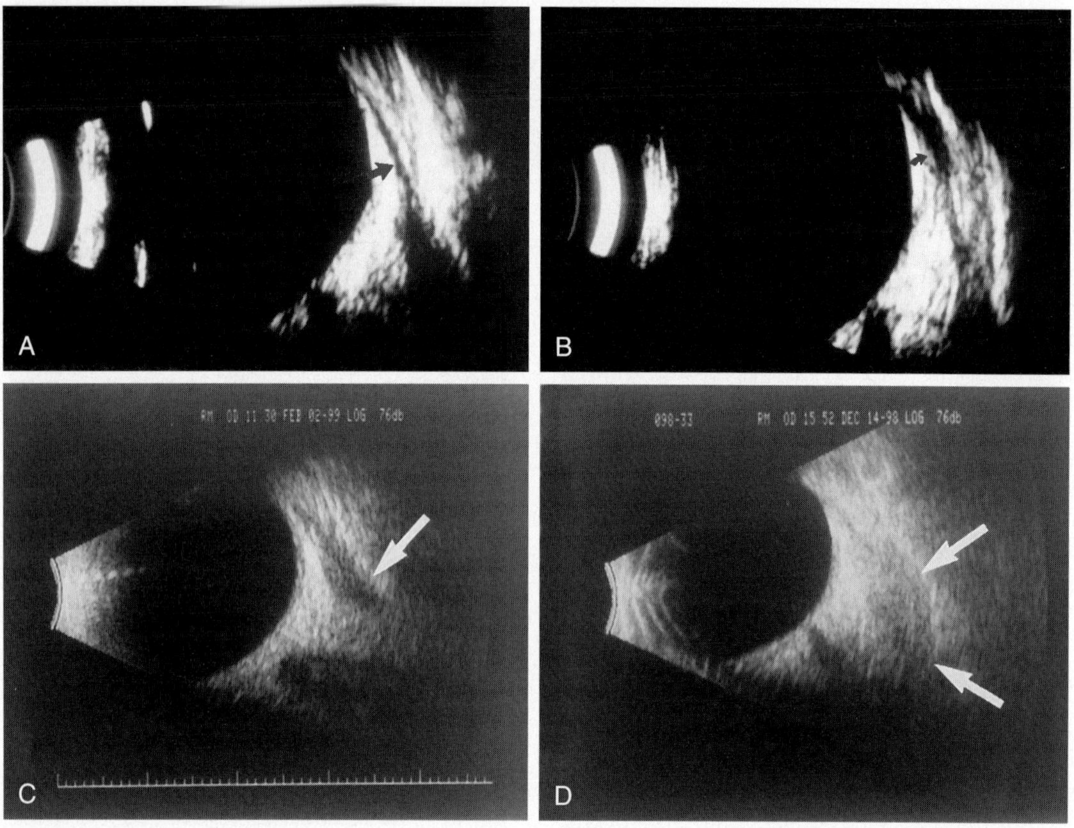

FIGURE 18–25. B-scan echography of orbital myositis in two patients. Normal tendinous insertion **A,** (*arrow*) and enlarged **B,** (*arrow*) tendinous insertion of rectus muscle in a patient with myositis. In another patient the normal muscle belly **C,** (*arrow*) is seen compared to an enlarged muscle belly **D,** (*arrows*) in the inflamed muscle.

and syphilis are important alternative causes of perineuritis to consider. These must be excluded in patients with optic neuropathy and abnormal appearing optic nerve sheaths with enlargement and enhancement on neuroimaging.[172–174]

Sclerosing Orbital Inflammation. Some patients with IOIS-like conditions develop a chronic scarring orbitopathy with exuberant desmoplastic reaction (fibroblastic proliferation with formation of dense fibrous connective tissue) and severe orbital dysfunction.

TABLE 18–5. Clinical Distinction of Thyroid-Associated Orbitopathy From Idiopathic Orbital Inflammation

Feature	Thyroid	Idiopathic Orbital Inflammation
Pain	Mild	More severe; worse on eye movement
Laterality	Most commonly bilateral Some asymmetry	Almost always unilateral
Onset	Gradual, subacute	Acute (hours or days)
Vision	May be impaired	Usually good
Eye movement	Restrictive	Impaired in field of inflamed muscle
Eyelid	Retraction	Ptosis
Imaging	Multiple muscles enlarged; regular borders and tendon sparing; does not extend to fat	Mutiple muscles enlarged with irregular borders and extension to the orbial fat, enhancement around globe
Response to steroids	Slow and moderate	Immediate and often complete

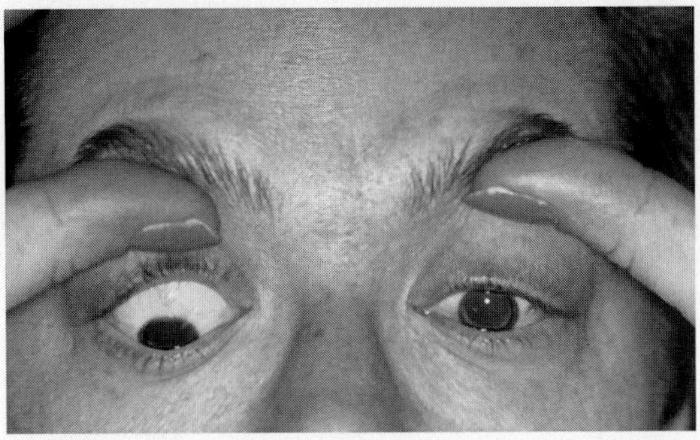

FIGURE 18–26. Impaired left eye downgaze and eyelid swelling in a patient with myositis involving the superior rectus/levator complex.

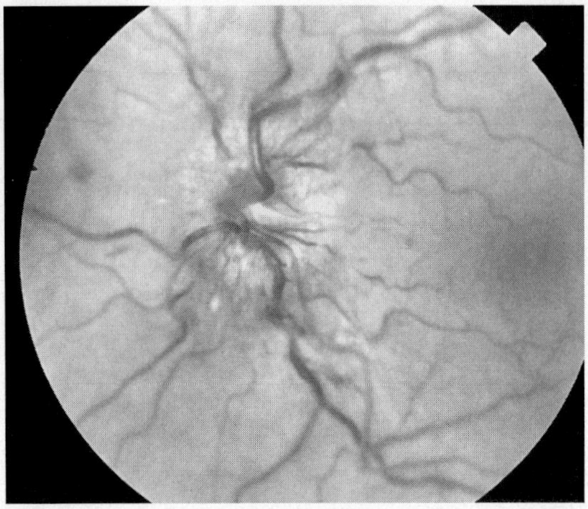

FIGURE 18–28. Fundus photograph of a patient with the perineuritis form of idiopathic orbital inflammatory syndrome. The optic nerve is diffusely swollen and hyperemic. Mild retinal venous obstruction with dilated retinal veins and intraretinal blot hemorrhages are seen (See Color Plate 53).

This condition has been termed *idiopathic sclerosing inflammation* or *sclerosing orbital pseudotumor*.[164, 175–181] This chronic sclerosing variant is characterized by relentless loss of vision from optic nerve dysfunction and entrapment of the extraocular muscles, leading to double vision. The onset is more insidious and often simulates a tumor. Patients develop pain and double vision along with proptosis. Desmoplastic reaction around the optic nerve or elsewhere in the orbit can mimic a primary optic nerve tumor radiographically because of its density, regularity, and smooth enhancement. This may result in a venous obstructive appearance on funduscopy.

The defining feature histopathologically is the dense desmoplastic reaction with scarring (collagen deposition) and only scant inflammatory infiltrates. These cases may respond poorly to treatment and may be the most common subtype of idiopathic orbital inflammation to erode bone and extend intracranially.[182–186] Patients may respond early to steroids but often have a relentless course regardless of treatment. Five of six patients in Rootman's[170] series experienced permanent damage in the form of either optic neuropathy or muscle restriction. Since this type of chronic scarring is unusual in other cases of appropriately treated IOIS, it is likely that orbital idiopathic sclerosing inflammation is a distinct clinical entity.[180] It is possible that this is a manifestation of a multifocal fibrosclerotic process, as patients who simultaneously developed retroperitoneal or mediastinal fibrosis have been described.[187–189]

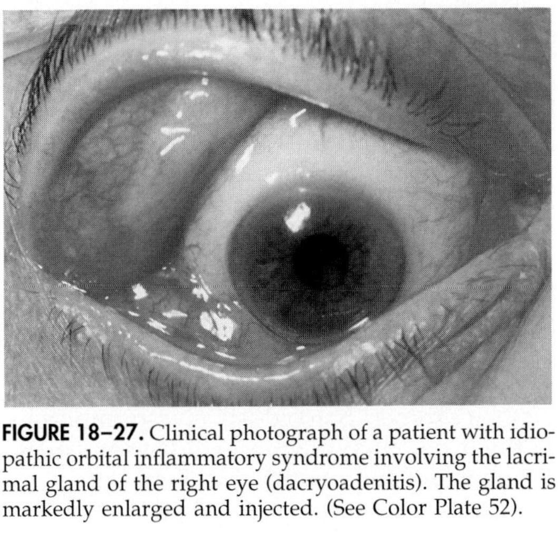

FIGURE 18–27. Clinical photograph of a patient with idiopathic orbital inflammatory syndrome involving the lacrimal gland of the right eye (dacryoadenitis). The gland is markedly enlarged and injected. (See Color Plate 52).

Pediatric IOIS

IOIS occurs at any age. In Rootman's[28] series 1OIS was the cause of orbital disease in 13 of 241 (5%) pediatric patients seen. Pediatric patients may have the diffuse or anterior forms of IOIS, posterior scleritis, uveitis, and disc swelling. In the pediatric population, the disorder is frequently bilateral even without a predisposing systemic condition. However, we have also seen several instances of isolated myositis. Diagnostic testing may show an elevated erythrocyte sedimentation rate, eosinophilia and cerebrospinal fluid (CSF) pleocytosis.[166]

Imaging

The diagnosis of IOIS is a clinical one but is usually confirmed by imaging studies of the orbit. These typically reveal an area of primary inflammation surrounded by an irregular margin. This irregular infiltrate may involve all of the soft tissues of the orbit, including Tenon's capsule, the optic nerve, the orbital fat, and the extraocular muscles. In one series of 21 patients, the most commonly identified CT features were contrast enhancement, fat infiltration, proptosis, and muscle enlargement.[190] MRI has also been shown to be helpful in the diagnosis of IOIS. In one series of 10 patients, IOIS lesions were found to be hypointense to fat and isointense to muscle on T_1-weighted images. On T_2-weighted images the lesions were isointense or only minimally hyperintense to fat in 9 of 10 cases; in 1 case, the enlarged muscle was markedly hyperintense to fat.[191] This pattern was thought to distinguish IOIS from orbital metastases, infections, and hematomas. Therefore it appears that MRI adds significantly to the diagnostic evaluation of patients with IOIS.

Other Diagnostic Studies

Biopsy is generally deferred unless the inflammation is recurrent or atypical in appearance, or primarily involves the lacrimal gland. It is reasonable to perform a systemic workup to screen for other systemic inflammatory conditions, although this is almost always negative. Blood work should include syphilis serologies and antineutrophilic cytoplasmic antibody (ANCA), antinuclear antibody, and angiotensin converting enzyme (ACE) levels, and chest roentgenography should be performed. In patients with a history of malignancy, the possibility of metastatic disease to the orbit must be carefully considered, and the threshold for biopsy should be low.

Treatment

Treatment is initiated immediately after the clinical diagnosis is suspected and imaging studies support the diagnosis of IOIS. Treatment with corticosteroids (60 to 100 mg prednisone) is usually both therapeutic and diagnostic. Most patients with IOIS will have a dramatic response within days of treatment, although recurrences are common.[192] The course of steroids and a slow taper usually needs to be extended for several months. Nonsteroidal anti-inflammatory drugs may be helpful during the steroid taper but occasionally are useful as a primary treatment. Nonsteroidals may be most effective when the inflammatory burden is low and in patients, such as those with diabetes, who tolerate steroids poorly.

A poor response to steroids should lead to consideration of alternative diagnoses, and then biopsy is often required.[193] Similarly, if the disease recurs, then biopsy is also recommended. Cytotoxic agents, including cyclophosphamide[179] and cyclosporine,[194, 195] have been successfully used as adjunctive therapies to prednisone.

In patients with refractory inflammation, recurrences, contraindications to systemic steroids, or the sclerosing variety of IOIS, radiation therapy to the orbit is an excellent alternative treatment.[164, 180, 182, 196–198] The dosage is between 1000 and 3000 cGy in 10 divided fractions, and complications are rare. Lanciano and associates[197] report their experience with 23 patients who had either relapsed on steroids or had poor initial response and found nearly 90% of patients had an initial response to 2000 cGy. Two thirds of the patients remained in complete remission, and three others were controlled with short courses of oral steroids after radiation. Three of five patients with decreased vision from optic neuropathy improved with radiation treatment.

OTHER INFLAMMATORY ORBITAL CONDITIONS

Granulomatous Orbital Inflammation

A unique subset of patients have a noninfectious, granulomatous inflammation of the orbit. These patients often present with mild (compared to the more painful and acute IOIS) inflammatory symptoms with a palpable mass lesion.[170] In such cases, an extensive systemic evaluation for granulomatous disease is indicated. However, in some cases the orbital disease is the sole location of involvement.

Sarcoidosis

Sarcoidosis is a well-characterized systemic granulomatous disorder affecting multiple organ syndromes. Sarcoidosis is also important in the differential diagnosis of lacrimal gland enlargement and perineuritis. Fortunately, orbital involvement is uncommon in sarcoidosis.

However, sarcoidosis may manifest as extraocular muscle enlargement, a soft tissue mass lesion, or as a lesion arising from contiguous bony involvement. Sarcoidosis is discussed in further detail in Chapters 5 and 7.

Wegener's Granulomatosis

The classic clinical triad of this systemic inflammatory condition includes necrotizing granulomas of the upper and lower respiratory tract, necrotizing vasculitis of the lung, and glomerulonephritis. Wegener's is believed to be a T-cell-mediated condition and is characterized pathologically by granulomatous inflammation and necrotizing vasculitis. Patients usually present in the fifth decade with pneumonitis, sinusitis, and renal involvement.

Wegener's granulomatosis may involve the orbit in nearly 20% of patients, however, some patients will have a limited form in which the orbital and sinus involvement predominates. Adjacent bony destruction may complicate the sinus disease and produce a saddle-nose deformity, fistulas, and orbital extension. Approximately 40% of patients develop ocular manifestations, including scleritis and episcleritis, uveitis, peripheral corneal ulceration, and occasionally conjunctival or retinal involvement.[170] The clinical presentation is variable, ranging from mild indolent inflammation to a more explosive inflammatory picture with proptosis, chemosis, optic nerve swelling, and decreased vision. These findings may necessitate orbital decompression. The diagnosis of Wegener's may be established by biopsy of the affected area. In some patients is reasonable to treat the patient on the basis of a positive ANCA titer and appropriate clinical findings.

Neurologic involvement in Wegener's occurs in about one third of patients.[199] The most common findings include peripheral neuropathy, cranial neuropathy, ophthalmoplegia, stroke, seizure, and cerebritis.[199] Treatment of Wegener's usually requires long-term therapy with corticosteroids and immunosuppressant drugs such as methotrexate or cyclophosphamide.

Polyarteritis Nodosa

Patients with polyarteritis nodosa may occasionally present with orbital involvement. This condition results from a vasculitis of medium and small arteries. The disorder may be segmental, and is characterized by inflammation and fibrinoid necrosis. The major sites of involvement are the kidney, heart, liver, and gastrointestinal tract. The condition shows a predilection for males in the second and fourth decades. Ophthalmic manifestations include retinal and choroidal ischemia related to vasculitis changes. On occasion, patients may present with a nonspecific orbital inflammatory syndrome in the absence of systemic symptoms.

Histiocytic Disorders

A distinct group of histiocytic orbital inflammation is well recognized and includes eosinophilic granuloma (histiocytosis X), juvenile xanthogranuloma, Erdheim–Chester disease, and necrobiotic xanthogranuloma. Erdheim–Chester disease is a systemic xanthogranulomatous disorder that affects bones and viscera, and bilateral diffuse orbital involvement has been described. The classic histologic features include Touton giant cells and a mixture of lymphocytes and plasma cells. Some of these entities are discussed further in Chapter 7.

OTHER CAUSES OF ENLARGED EXTRAOCULAR MUSCLES

The vast majority of patients with enlarged extraocular muscles have either TAO or IOIS. However, there are several other causes of enlarged extraocular muscles (Table 18–6). The clinical presentation often provides enough information to distinguish the various entities, however, significant overlap does exist. Radiographic features of the various causes of extraocular muscle enlargement have been reviewed.[93, 200]

TABLE 18–6. Differential Diagnosis of Enlarged Extraocular Muscles

Thyroid-associated ophthalmopathy
Idiopathic orbital inflammatory syndrome with myositis
Lymphoma
Metastatic tumors
Acromegaly
Trichinosis
Carotid-cavernous fistula
Sarcoidosis
Wegener's granulomatosis
Rhabdomyosarcoma
Amyloidosis

Patients with dural arteriovenous fistulas may have a clinical presentation very similar to that of IOIS, with acute proptosis, conjunctival injection, chemosis, and enlarged muscles. These patients generally have less pain than IOIS patients and have the characteristic arteriolized conjunctival vessels with elevation of intraocular pressure. An enlarged superior ophthalmic vein is diagnostic of blood flow reversal in the orbit and muscle enlargement is usually fusiform. These fistulas are discussed in more detail in Chapter 15.

Metastatic tumors to the extraocular muscles may present with an acute onset of proptosis, double vision, and enlarged muscles on neuroimaging studies. The pain is usually less severe than in IOIS, and only one muscle may be enlarged. The involved muscle may appear lumpy or irregular on neuroimaging studies.[201, 202] Orbital lymphoid tumors usually involve the orbit diffusely but may be confined to a single extraocular muscle.[203]

Trichinosis may produce a myositis with enlarged extraocular muscles. The infection results from the ingestion of *Trichinella spiralis* found in uncooked meat. Patients typically manifest with gastrointestinal complaints followed by myalgias, fever, periorbital pain, and chemosis of the conjunctiva.[204–206] Patients may develop proptosis and double vision.[204–206]

Amyloid deposition in the orbit and acromegaly may also result in diffuse fusiform enlargement of the extraocular muscles.[93, 200, 207, 208] In addition, sarcoidosis may present with either focal or diffuse extraocular muscle enlargement along with proptosis and pain.[209–211]

ORBITAL TUMORS AND OTHER ORBITAL MASSES

Frequency of Various Orbital Tumors

The proportion of orbital lesions that are neoplastic depends on the type of study (eg, clinical, pathologic, or radiographic) and whether the patients are children or adults.[20, 24, 27–30, 212] In most series, inflammatory diseases (thyroid and idiopathic orbital inflammatory syndrome) make up about one third to one half of patients. This fraction is lower in pathologic studies since TAO is rarely biopsied. In Rootman's series of 1409 patients,[28] 22.3% had neoplastic lesions.

The most common orbital mass lesions are neurogenic tumors (gliomas, meningiomas, and schwannomas), cystic lesions (dermoids), vascular lesions (cavernous hemangiomas), lymphoproliferative lesions (lymphomas), and finally secondary tumors (metastatic and contiguous spread). A recent survey of a cancer registry found lymphoma to be the most common malignancy.[26] In children, congenital and development lesions with cysts and vascular lesions make up 40% of the cases.[20] A familiarity with the most common causes of orbital space-occupying mass lesions is helpful when considering differential diagnoses.

Orbital Lymphoma

Orbital lymphomas have been increasingly recognized, and in one series represented 55% of the orbital tumors.[26] Orbital lymphoma may be primary, in which it arises and is localized to the orbit, or secondary as a manifestation of a systemic lymphoma. The clinical and radiographic presentations are the same in both situations. The orbital lesions tend to grow slowly and conform to the orbital tissues (Fig. 18–29). The lesions are painless and may be recognized only after producing noticeable proptosis, double vision, or a palpable mass. A visible subconjunctival component, or "salmon patch," may be present (Fig. 18–30; see Color Plates 54 and 55). On orbital imaging, lymphoma lesions are generally well defined and almost always demonstrate a characteristic "molding" to the orbital tissue and globe (Fig. 18–29). Idiopathic orbital inflammation may also have a similar appearance (Fig. 18–23A). There are usually no bony changes.

When neuroimaging suggests a lymphoma, a systemic evaluation is indicated. The orbital

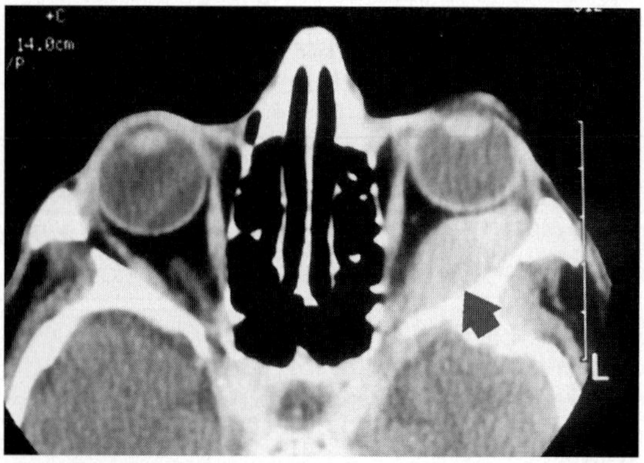

FIGURE 18–29. Axial CT scan of a patient with left-sided orbital lymphoma. A homogeneous mass is seen that conforms to the globe contour (*arrow*).

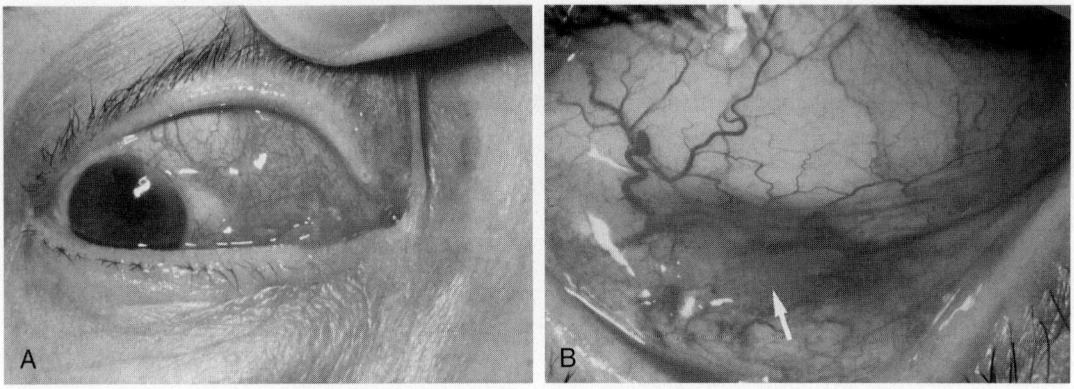

FIGURE 18–30. Subconjunctival lesions of orbital lymphoma. **A.** Nasal subconjunctival mass with elevation and injection. **B.** "Salmon" patch lesion (*arrow*). (See Color Plates 54 and 55).

mass may be biopsied, as it is often in an accessible anterior lesion. The biopsy tissue should then be examined using light microscopy and immunohistochemistry. If the orbital lesion is isolated, it is treated with local irradiation.[213, 214] If there is evidence of multiorgan involvement with lymphoma then systemic protocols using chemotherapy are used. A small percentage of patients with localized orbital disease will develop systemic lymphoma.

Plasma cell tumors may manifest lymphoproliferative lesions. The presenting manifestation of multiple myeloma is proptosis or double vision. The infiltrate usually affects the lacrimal gland, orbital fat, and muscles, and unlike lymphoma it is often associated with pain. Systemic workup for multiple myeloma is necessary, and if negative patients must be monitored closely for its development.

Neurogenic Tumors

Most orbital peripheral nerve sheath tumors, such as schwannomas and neurofibromas, originate from the sensory branches of the first division of the trigeminal nerve. Unlike the optic nerve, the peripheral nerves contain an outer sheath called an *epineurium,* and are further divided into bundles by perineural cells possessing both contractile and undulating properties. Within each of the perineural compartments are located supportive Schwann cells. These Schwann cells give rise to the most common (peripheral) nerve tumors of the orbit, called *schwannomas* or *neurilemomas.* In all, schwannomas represent about 1% of all orbital tumors.[28–30]

Schwannomas most commonly present in the second to fourth decades, with a history of proptosis that extends over a period of several months or years.[215–218] Rarely, patients manifest with vision loss because of crowding of the orbital apex and optic nerve compression. In this setting, their presentation is not unlike other benign, well-circumscribed, rounded, slow-growing, orbital masses. In fact, schwannomas are very similar to cavernous hemangiomas in their presentation, with the insidious onset of well-tolerated proptosis. On CT and MRI scans, schwannomas may be difficult to distinguish from primary optic nerve tumors, and this distinction should be made prior to surgical excision. Neuroradiographic features include a well-defined lesion that is isointense with the brain and enhances with gadolinium. They appear radiographically similar to cavernous hemangiomas, fibrous histiocytomas, and hemangiopericytomas.

Patients with an orbital plexiform neurofibroma due to neurofibromatosis type 1 (NF-1) may manifest with proptosis and massive overgrowth of the eyelid skin. A characteristic S-shaped deformity of the upper eyelid may be seen. Multiple isolated neurofibromas, café-au-lait spots, iris Lisch nodules, optic pathway gliomas (see Chapters 5 and 7), or a family history of neurofibromatosis should suggest the diagnosis of NF-1. The plexiform neurofibroma has a diagnostic appearance of infiltrating cords of cells that are nonencapsulated. Whether neurofibromas are truly schwannomas is a matter of debate as they often contain histologic features of perineural cells and fibroblasts.

Lacrimal Tumors

Lacrimal tumors are relatively rare. Tumors may be primary or secondarily involve the lacrimal gland from other sites. About one half of lacrimal gland masses are ultimately proven to be inflammatory (see discussion above on dacryoadenitis). About half of the tumors of the lacrimal gland are epithelial in nature; of these, approximately half are benign and half are malignant.[28, 219–221] The typical clinical presentation is characterized by deformity of the upper eyelid contour (S-shaped), fullness of the upper eyelid, and downward and nasal displacement of the globe (Fig. 18–6). Mass lesions may be palpated in the superior sulcus at the lateral portion of the upper eyelid. Radiographically, CT and MRI are helpful. Both studies may help to determine whether one or both lobes of the lacrimal gland are involved and whether extension of the lesion has gone beyond the lacrimal gland. CT is important to evaluate bony changes. Excavation of the lacrimal fossa or erosion is characteristic of a pleomorphic adenoma, while lytic lesions of the bone characterize adenocystic carcinoma. Clinical and radiographic distinction of benign and malignant lacrimal tumors is critical so that incisional (removing a piece of the tumor) versus excisional (complete removal of the gland) surgical therapy may be planned.

Pleomorphic adenomas (or benign mixed tumors) of the lacrimal gland represent benign epithelial proliferations with a myxoid fibrous stroma that is believed to result from metaplasia of the outer layers of the epithelium. The tumor is characterized by pseudocapsule formation resulting from compression of the surrounding tissue. This tumor usually manifests in middle age and symptoms include proptosis and lid deformity evolving over 1 year. Many patients do not experience pain. With accurate preoperative identification, the goal of surgical therapy (usually via lateral orbitotomy) is complete excisional biopsy. Incomplete removal or incisional biopsy will invariably lead to recurrences with orbital dysfunction and will increase the risk of malignant transformation.[222]

Adenoid cystic carcinoma of the lacrimal gland is the most common malignant lesion to arise in this area. The clinical presentation is characterized by a mass lesion and neuropathic pain from perineural invasion. Unlike inflammatory lesions of the lacrimal gland, the eye is usually white and quiet, and the pain is not exacerbated by eye movements. The lesions usually arise in the orbital lobe of the lacrimal gland and therefore can reach a significant size before producing symptoms. The tumor is characterized by five different histologic subtypes, and the dominant subtype determines the tumor prognosis. The most aggressive type is the basaloid pattern, with a 5-year survival of only 21%. Unfortunately, only 71% of all patients with adenoid cystic carcinoma are alive at 5 years.[223] The major cause of morbidity and mortality is intracranial invasion, which is facilitated by the perineural spread of the tumor. The perineural spread may extend for centimeters beyond the apparent borders of the soft tissue mass and is the main feature that ultimately affects the prognosis. Hematogenous metastases to the lung can also occur.

Surgical exenteration, or removal of all orbital contents, with or without postoperative radiation, is the recommended therapy for this type of tumor. Even with the most radical surgery and radiation the disease-free survival rate does not improve. Some recent success has been described with local orbital radiation in the form of brachytherapy. In this technique, radiation is delivered by surgically implanted radioactive iridium-192 wires after gross total tumor resection.[224]

Metastatic and Secondary Tumors

The orbit is the second most common site for metastatic disease to the eye and its adnexa, with the uveal tract involved most frequently. The incidence of metastatic tumors as the cause of orbital disease ranges in various series from 1% to 3%.[28, 29] The prognosis for survival in patients with metastatic orbital tumors is uniformly poor, and few patients survive for more than 1 year. Using modern combined modalities of therapy, patient survival may be prolonged. However, most treatment is only palliative. Prompt recognition of this condition may help in the detection of an unrecognized primary systemic malignancy and allow for early treatment.

The clinical presentation of metastatic tumors is variable, but there are certain recurrent themes. Patients frequently complain of diplopia, ptosis, proptosis, eyelid swelling, and pain.[225–227] Most important is the relative abruptness and disproportionate amount of symptoms that these lesions cause compared with other space-occupying orbital lesions. Double vision is often an early manifestation of metastatic disease. This compares with primary orbital tumors, which are generally better compensated for because of their more insidious evolution. Other commonly reported symptoms include a palpable mass and decreased vision. The most common signs include exophthalmos, noncomitant eye deviation, conjunctival injection, palpable mass, subnormal visual acuity, disc edema, choroidal folds, and enophthalmos. Metastatic breast carcinoma often causes enophthalmos secondary to contraction induced by the scirrhous nature of the tumor.[228]

At the time of diagnosis, metastatic tumors are usually characterized by unencapsulated tumor growth with diffuse involvement of the orbital structures Fig 18–31. Tumor emboli may lodge in muscle, fat, or bone. In clinical studies in which tumor localization can be accomplished by high-resolution CT, the bone and fat are involved twice as often as the muscle.[225, 226] Breast carcinoma most frequently involves the fat initially, and prostate carcinoma has a strong predilection for bone. Capone and Slamovits[202] found that 16 cases arose from the breast, and that 6 cases arose from melanoma in their literature review of 31 cases of metastatic tumors to the extraocular muscles. Healy[229] reviewed 22 cases of orbital metastases evaluated by CT; two thirds of these patients had some evidence of adjacent bone destruction; 60% of lesions were extraconal, 20% were intraconal, and 20% were both. Enhancement was seen in all cases examined with contrast. Interestingly, two thirds of patients had evidence of intracranial disease, either by direct extension or discrete metastases.[229] Goldberg and associates[226] examined the spectrum of CT scan features reported in the literature

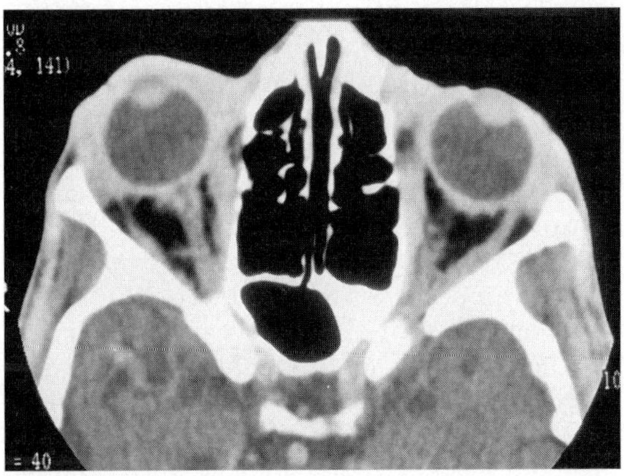

FIGURE 18–31. Axial CT scan of a patient with metastatic breast carcinoma to the orbits. Bilateral, homogeneous infiltration of the anterior orbits by the mass is present. The right medial rectus is irregular and "bumpy" secondary to tumor infiltration.

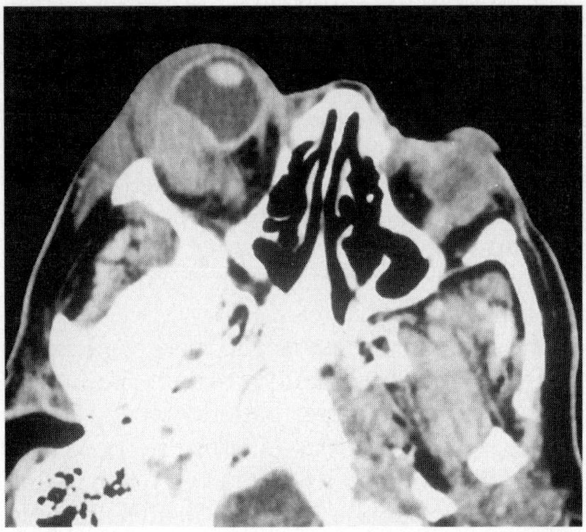

FIGURE 18–32. Axial T_1-weighted MRI scan of the orbits demonstrating a focal mass lesion in the right orbit from carcinoid metastases. The metastatic lesion indents the globe.

and found that a mass lesion Fig 18–32 followed by bone involvement was the most common CT scan feature.

The mainstay of treatment for metastatic tumors is radiotherapy. Most patients do not have radiation sequelae, which normally occur in a time frame beyond the average survival of these patients.

Secondary Orbital Tumors

Secondary orbital tumors involve the orbit by direct extension. They arise in any of the adjacent structures, including the sinuses and nasopharynx, the meninges and brain, the eye, the conjunctiva and lids, and the lacrimal sac. Secondary tumors are a common cause of orbital disease and, unfortunately, the most common setting in which patients require exenteration.

The majority of secondary neoplasms arise from the paranasal sinus cavities.[28] Many patients with sinus tumors have signs and symptoms related to the eye or orbit. The primary mode of extension of sinus tumors to the orbit is direct extension. This may occur by bone erosion, extension through pre-existing bone canals, or extension along normal neurovascular bundles.[230] The maxillary sinus is the most common origin of these secondary orbital tumors. Only thin bone separates the inferior orbital fissure from the mucosa of the sinus.[230] The sinus tumors invading the orbit can be benign or malignant. Benign lesions include inverting papilloma, osteomas, juvenile angiofibroma, and unusual neuroectodermal tumors. Mucoceles of the paranasal sinuses are benign lesions that are capable of invading the orbit and causing orbital disease. Although mucoceles are typically unassociated with malignancy, Weaver and Bartley reported[231] seven patients in whom a malignancy was found incidentally in association with the mucocele at the time of surgery.

The overall prognosis for these patients is poor, and the treatment is usually palliative. In general, sinus tumor patients have a 5-year survival rate as high as 74%, but in those with orbital involvement it is 25% even when a combination of radiation and radical surgery is used.[230] This difference in survival reflects a more advanced disease state when the orbit is involved. In many cases, these tumors, may be partially excised at initial surgery, producing persistent morbidity through local invasion. These tumors metastasize only at a very late stage. Distant spread to lymph nodes and the lung is most common. Disease that is limited to regional nodes may be curable in certain cases with combined surgery and radiation therapy.

Orbital Extension of Intracranial Tumors

Orbital involvement by intracranial tumors is rare. This mainly occurs with meningiomas, particularly those involving the sphenoid bone. Meningiomas may extend along the lateral orbital wall and posterior orbit, causing proptosis and lid swelling. If the tumor grows medially or along the lesser wing of the sphenoid, these tumors may involve the posterior orbit structures, producing ophthalmoplegia and visual loss with only minimal proptosis.

High-grade astrocytomas of the frontal lobe may invade the orbital roof. Clivus tumors, including chordoma, have also been reported to extend into the orbit.[232, 233] Typically, proptosis occurs late and is a manifestation of advanced disease. Other tumors occurring in the region of the sella and the base of the skull may also invade the orbit. Pituitary tumors and craniopharyngiomas very rarely invade the orbit and cause proptosis. Orbital involvement may also occur, with the extension of meningeal tumors, through the subarachnoid space, and along the optic nerve sheath.

Vascular Tumors

Cavernous hemanigiomas are the most common vascular tumors of the orbit. They are also being recognized with increasing frequency in the central nervous system based on the more widespread use of CT and MRI. They manifest insidiously in the orbit with proptosis and double vision. Blurred vision can result from an hyperopic shift from compression and shortening of the globe. Most patients become symptomatic in the second to fourth decades.[234] The lesions are usually solitary and arise in the intraconal space. Imaging studies reveal a well-circumscribed, nonenhancing lesion.[235] They are usually well defined, lobulated purplish lesions composed of a large number of spaces of variable size containing blood. Lesions can contain thrombus or be calcified. Like intracranial cavernous hemangiomas, there usually is no large feeding vessel. The lesions are relatively easily excised via a lateral orbitotomy, do not recur, and have no potential to extend intracranially.

Venous angiomas may occur in the orbit and are often called *varices*. The clinical syndrome is usually characterized by intermittent filling and emptying of the varix, resulting in variable proptosis. Eye bulging in a crying infant, proptosis during Valsalva maneuver, or orbital ecchymoses should raise this diagnostic possibility. Lesions can be identified by CT or MRI, with and without raising intravenous pressure, and may be followed by orbital venography. Surgical intervention is recommended only for sight-threatening lesions or progressive proptosis causing cosmetic disfiguration.

Hemangioblastomas in the orbit usually arise in or adjacent to the optic nerve sheath in patients with von Hippel–Lindau disease.[236–238] Patients may manifest with vision loss and proptosis from the effects of an orbital mass lesion. However, hemangioblastomas arising in the cerebellum more commonly result in neuro-ophthalmic symptoms.

Because *hemangiopericytomas* are tumors that arise from pericytes of blood vessels, they can arise anywhere in the body where blood vessels are located, including the orbit. Rarely, they arise in the area of the occipital lobe and may present with homonymous hemianopia. In the orbit they may manifest with diplopia, proptosis, and choroidal folds.[239, 240] These tumors usually arise outside of the muscle cone, and patients develop vision loss as a manifestation of compression of the optic nerve. The diagnosis is rarely made preoperatively. Up to one third of these lesions recur and some metastasize, therefore successful treatment is greatly enhanced by the completeness of the excision.[239, 240]

PEDIATRIC ORBITAL TUMORS

Congenital tumors and infectious processes are the most common causes of orbital disease in children. However, the types of orbital lesions in children vary among reported series.[20, 24, 28, 29] Certain patterns are clear in a meta-analysis of these reports. Most children with proptosis have benign conditions that are either infectious, inflammatory, or neoplastic. The benign tumors are commonly dermoids and vascular tumors (particularly capillary hemangiomas). The most common malignant tumors to involve the orbit in children are rhabdomyosarcoma and metastatic tumors, including neuroblastoma and Ewing's sarcoma. The orbit is also occasionally involved by extension of intraocular retinoblastoma, leukemia, or lymphoma. The benign congenital cystic lesions, such as dermoid tumors, as well as the common congenital vascular tumors (capillary hemangioma) often present with isolated orbital findings and rarely manifest with intracranial abnormalities.

Rhabdomyosarcoma is the most common orbital malignancy in children and is also the most common soft tissue tumor of childhood. Dramatic improvement in the survival of patients treated promptly with appropriate chemotherapy and radiotherapy has made the early diagnosis of rhabdomyosarcoma of the orbit critical. Patients with localized orbital disease enjoy a 90% chance for survival after successful chemo- and radiotherapy. Extension of rhabdomyosarcoma into the paranasal sinuses is not uncommon, although intracranial extension is quite rare. Nevertheless, staging of patients with rhabdomyosarcoma should include lumbar puncture to rule out central nervous system metastases.

Metastatic orbital tumors in children are distinct from those seen in adults. In children, tumors almost exclusively travel to the bony orbit. Soft tissue and ocular metastases as seen in adults are extremely rare. Neuroblastoma arises from primitive neuroblastic tissue and is the most common tumor to metastasize to the orbit in children. This tumor is second only to rhabdomyosarcoma as the most frequent malignant tumor of the orbit. The adrenal medulla is the most common primary site. Musarella and co-workers[241] found that 20% of children with neuroblastoma developed orbital metastases and typically present with either proptosis or ecchymoses. This occurs because these tumors grow so rapidly and outstrip their blood supply. On CT, the temporal orbit (zygomatic bone) frequently demonstrates lytic bone destruction. Disc swelling may be evident because of optic nerve compression or from simultaneous intracranial involvement and elevated intracranial pressure. Diagnosis is established through a series of noninvasive tests, including imaging studies of the head and orbit, chest, and abdomen and analysis of urinary catecholamines. Treatment consists of removal of the primary tumor followed by radiation and chemotherapy.

Fibrous Dysplasia

Fibrous dysplasia is a benign bone condition in which normal bone is replaced by immature bone and osteoid in a cellular fibrous matrix. In Rootman's series[28] of 1409 patients, 33 had bone tumors and 9 of these patients had fibrous dysplasia. The associated expansion of the bone may be associated with swelling, disfigurement, and pain. When the orbital bones are involved, proptosis, decreased vision, and double vision may occur. In some patients, the abnormal bone growth occurs in one site and is termed *monostotic*. In other patients, multiple sites are involved (polyostotic). The McCune–Albright syndrome is characterized by polyostotic fibrous dysplasia, skin rash, and endocrine abnormalities. Fibrous dysplasia involves the craniofacial bones in about 20% of patients and is usually thought to be a disease of children and adolescents. However, it may also present in adults.[242, 243]

The clinical syndrome of fibrous dysplasia evolves as the bones enlarge and the globe is displaced (dystopia). If the bones of the optic canal are involved and narrowed, vision loss from optic neuropathy can ensue. Rootman[244] found that pain, proptosis, and globe displacement were the most common manifestations. In Rootman's series,[244] the frontal bone was the most frequently involved orbital bone, although in Katz and Nerad's series[242] the maxilla was the most commonly involved. Fibrous dysplasia has a virtually diagnostic appearance on CT, with the bone taking on a homongenous, dense, ground-glass appearance

(Fig. 18–33). Many patients show a more pagetoid appearance, with alternating areas of lucency and increased density.[242] Features on MRI include low to intermediate signal intensity on spin-echo sequences, and most lesions demonstrate moderate enhancement.[245] Distinction of fibrous dysplasia from meningioma may occasionally be difficult on a CT scan, but MRI will usually discriminate the two entities.[242]

Management of patients is directed at improving the craniofacial abnormality and resulting facial deformity through surgical debulking (complete surgical resection is impossible). Radiation is not usually employed because of the potential increased risk of malignant degeneration. Craniofacial surgical teams have been increasingly successful, with more than 60% of patients having a good cosmetic result at one year.[246]

Vision loss is a frequent complication of fibrous dysplasia involving the skull. Osguthorpe and Gudeman[247] identified 30 cases of monocular or binocular vision loss in the literature between 1965 and 1987. In Katz and Nerad's series[242] of 20 patients, 4 were identified with vision loss and they emphasized that conditions associated with the bony abnormality such as mucoceles, hemorrhage, and aneurysmal bone cysts were the cause for the vision loss as opposed to actual bony narrowing of the optic canal by the fibrous dysplasia. Patients with vision loss from compressive optic neuropathy have been successfully treated with steroids[248] and surgical decompression of the orbital apex and optic canal.[249–251] Blindness has also been described as a complication of prophylactic canal decompression in fibrous dysplasia.[252] Usually the process spontaneously arrests with no further bone growth. Thus, conservative therapy and observation are often employed, particularly when there is no or minimal visual impairment.

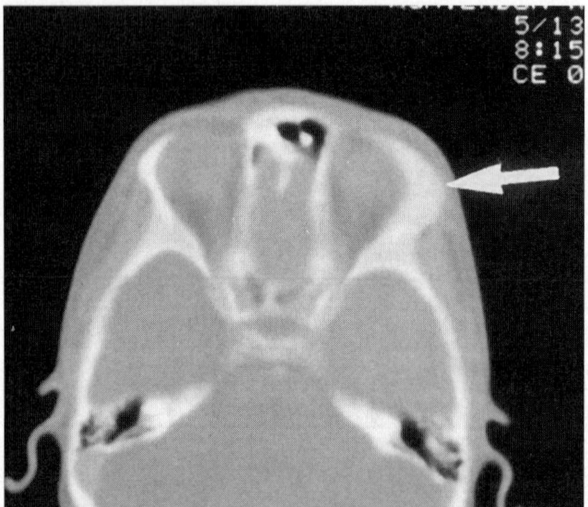

FIGURE 18–33. Axial CT scan of the orbits (bone window) in a patient with fibrous dysplasia. The zygomatic bone in the left lateral orbit (*arrow*) is seen to have a thickened, homogeneous, ground-glass appearance.

ORBITAL INFECTIONS

Infections of the orbit are both potentially sight- and life-threatening conditions that demand prompt recognition and therapeutic intervention. The spectrum of orbital infectious disease is wide and ranges from acute, bacterial infections to more insidious processes due to fungi. Various bacteria have been reported to cause infectious orbital cellulitis, and the clinical setting may help determine the etiologic agent (pediatric, history of trauma, recent surgery). Anatomy also plays an important role in the genesis of orbital infection. Since the paranasal sinuses structurally represent walls of the orbit, infectious processes in the sinuses are frequent causes of orbital cellulitis. Organisms may also gain entry into the orbit by traveling through the valveless veins of the face, teeth, and neck. The orbital septum is an effective barrier to spread the infection. Thus, it is unusual for infections involving the eyelids (without penetrating trauma) to extend into the orbit.

Orbital infections may be characterized as being preseptal or postseptal. Preseptal cellulitis is usually characterized by isolated eyelid swelling, tenderness, and induration, but the patient remains free of any inflammatory changes in the orbit or eye movement limitations (Fig. 18–34). Postseptal infections and orbital cellulitis are characterized by similar external eyelid changes, in association with proptosis, eye movement limitations, and occasionally vision loss (Fig. 18–34). Patients with a subperiosteal abscess may have a relatively benign orbital examination with eyelid edema as sole manifestation of the infectious process.[253]

Clinical Presentation

Presentation in children with an orbital infection is relatively common and characterized by pain, redness, fever, and an elevation of the white blood cell count. Sinus disease is

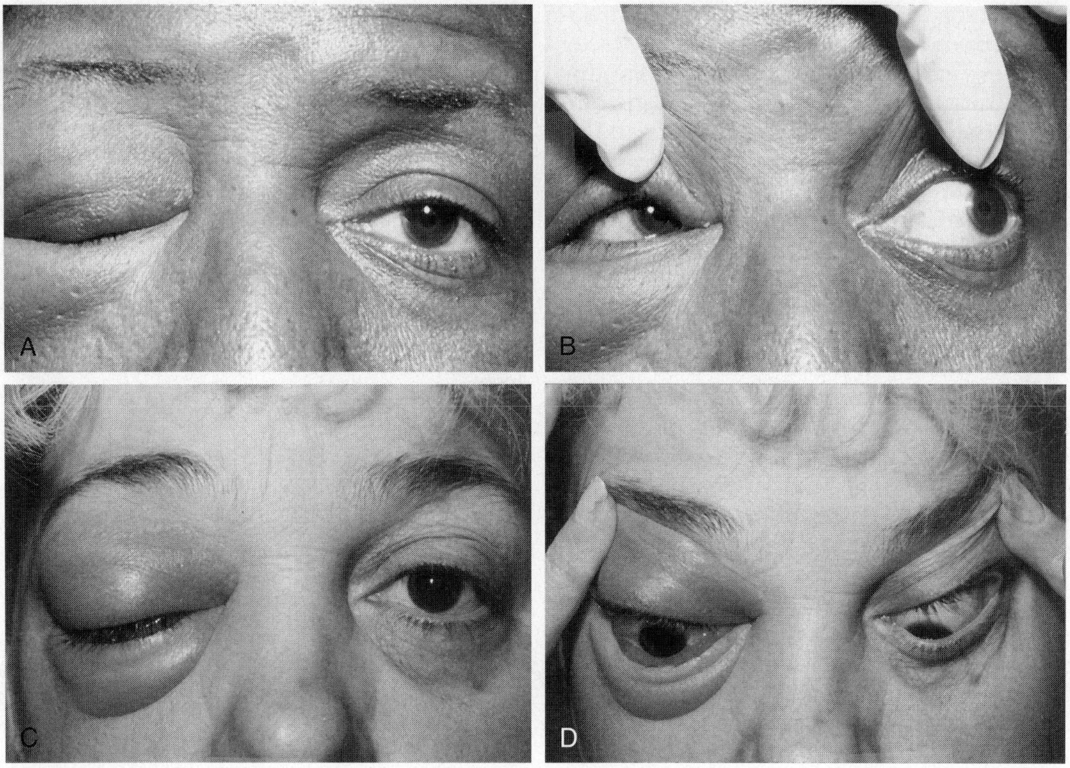

FIGURE 18–34. Preseptal cellulitis (**A, B**) and orbital cellulitis (**C, D**). **A.** In this patient with preseptal cellulitis, the right eye is swollen shut by periocular soft tissue swelling. The skin was mildly erythematous. **B.** Despite the significant external swelling the conjunctiva is only minimally injected and the eye movements are intact. **C.** Marked swelling and eryethema of the right eyelid soft tissues in orbital cellulitis. **D.** Significant chemosis and injection of the conjunctiva are present with limitation of eye movements.

common and the ethmoid sinus is the most frequently involved.[254] A purple-colored hue to the skin is sometimes seen in *Haemophilus* infections. In children, *Staphylococcus aureus, Streptococcus* sp., and *Haemophilus influenzae* are the most commonly encountered pathogenic organisms.[255, 256] Evaluation of patients with suspected orbital cellulitis begins with imaging studies (usually CT), measurement of body temperature, blood cultures, and a white blood cell count. Therapy is directed at the infection and includes intravenous antibiotics in addition to surgical drainage when necessary. Antibiotic coverage should include therapy against penicillinase-resistant staphylococci and anaerobes. Ominous signs include loss of vision or worsening of proptosis, which could indicate either abscess compression of the optic nerve or extension of the infection into the cavernous sinus with resulting cavernous sinus thrombosis. Such cases with posterior orbital extension or cavernous sinus involvement may require more aggressive therapy.[257]

Fungal Infections

Unlike patients with bacterial infections, fungal infections tend to occur in patients who are debilitated or immunocompromised. Both mucormycosis and asperigillosis may spread from the sinus to the orbit. Isolated examples of even more obscure fungi such as *Blastomyces* and *Sporothorix* may be occasionally be encountered in the orbit.[258]

Phycomycosis (Mucormycosis). Infections with the phycomycetes may involve the lungs, gastrointestinal tract, or the rhino-orbital structures. The rhino-orbital infection typically begins in the nose and spreads through the maxillary and ethmoid sinuses into the orbit.[259, 260] However, occasionally there will be no obvious sinus lesion. The organism spreads by invading blood vessel walls and may produce necrosis, thrombosis, and ultimately infarction of the involved orbital tissues.[261] Most patients who develop mucormycosis have a predisposing risk factor such diabetes, leukemia, lymphoma, septicema, or burns.

Symptoms may include pain, fever, headache, reduced acuity, double vision, facial numbness, and sometimes a seropurulent discharge from the nose.[262] On examination of involved tissues, a black eschar characterized by necrosis and dark discoloration is frequently noted. However, the eschar is usually a late finding, and its absence does exclude the diagnosis of mucormycosis. Many affected patients have both internal and external ophthalmoplegia, ptosis, and sensory loss in the trigeminal distribution. Most cases are unilateral, but bilateral cases are well recognized.

Neuroimaging studies typically reveal inflammatory disease in the sinuses and the orbits. Both blood and CSF cultures are seldom positive. The diagnosis of mucormycosis is best established by a biopsy demonstration of nonseptate hyphae branching at 90-degree angles.

Treatment must be initiated promptly and usually requires both surgical and medical approaches. Complete excision of necrotic tissue is necessary and antifungal agents are started. However, many patients may be treated without orbital exenteration, particularly those with preserved visual acuity.[260] Amphotericin is the first-line drug but supplemental use of ketoconazole has also been suggested. Simultaneously, the medical team must correct any metabolic acidosis or underlying bacterial infection. Ultimately, the extensive and aggressive debridement may require reconstructive efforts in the future. Mortality rates are in the range of 15% to 35%[261] and the prognosis seems to be dependent on prompt recognition. Those individuals treated successfully have usually been diagnosed within 4 days of symptom onset.[260]

Aspergillosis is another ubiquitous fungal organism that spreads to the orbits from the paranasal sinuses. Occasionally the organism affects immunocompetent hosts, but in general, patients are immunocompromised to some extent at the time of diagnosis.[263] Orbital involvement in aspergillosis occurs as a manifestation of a disseminated infection with widespread necrotizing angiitis from microscopic fungal invasion of small vessels. Endophthalmitis may occasionally occur in this setting. Infections tend to be more indolent than those in patents with mucormycosis. Despite this slower course, patients with orbital aspergillus may still lose vision or die from their infection. A recent patient with a steroid-responsive optic neuropathy was ultimately found to have aspergillosis as the primary cause of the problem and succumbed to the illness.[264]

Patients usually present with orbital signs of progressive exophthalmos and a chronic inflammation of the sinuses. Occasionally patients manifest with vision loss and the diagnosis is dependent on a biopsy that reflects dichotomously branching septated hyphae. Treatment, as with mucormycosis, requires wide surgical debridement in conjunction with systemic amphotericin alone or in combination with other antifungal agents. Mortality, unfortunately, is high and successful treatment again requires prompt recognition of the condition.

Allergic Fungal Sinusitis. Allergic fungal sinusitis (AFS) is a type of paranasal sinus mycosis encountered in patients with chronic sinusitis.[265–271] Unlike other forms of paranasal mycosis, AFS is a noninvasive form of sinusitis, and therefore requires a different approach to treatment. AFS typically occurs in immunocompetent hosts with a history of nasal polyposis and chronic sinusitis. Patients are frequently atopic and may have peripheral eosinophilia. Presenting symptoms include nasal obstruction, pain, rhinorrhea, visual loss, diplopia, proptosis, cranial nerve palsy, facial deformity, and production of thick green or brown mucus.[265–271] In one series, 17% of patients presented with orbital symptoms.[272] Radiographic studies typically show multiple sinus of involvement with bone erosion or remodeling. The inflamed mucosa exhibits increased signal intensity on T_2-weighted MRI (Fig. 18–35). Histopathologically there are embedded eosinophils, Charcot–Leyden crystals, and extramucosal fungal hyphae. The offending organisms are the dematiaceous fungi such as *Bipolaris, Exserohilum, Curvularia, Alternaria,* and *Aspergillus* species.[265] Unlike treatment of invasive sino-orbital mycoses that require more aggressive debridement, treatment in AFS includes debridement of just fungal debris, aeration of the involved sinuses, and systemic and topical steroids.[265] The role of topical antifungal agents has not yet been clarified.

ORBITAL TRAUMA

Patients with craniofacial trauma commonly present for ophthalmic or neuro-ophthalmic evaluation, in both the acute and resolution phases. Patients usually are evaluated in a

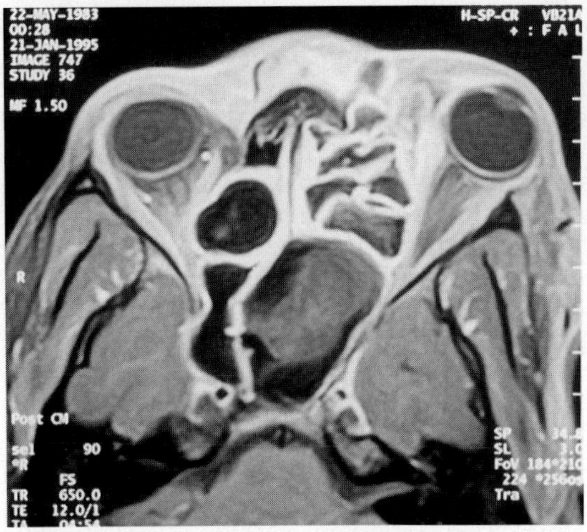

FIGURE 18–35. T_1 weighted axial MRI scan of a patient with allergic fungal sinusitis. Extensive involvement of the ethmoid and sphenoid sinuses is seen with bone remodeling with proptosis and lateral displacement of the globe.

compromised state, secondary to associated cranial injuries. Therefore, historical and examination information may be limited. Patients may also have significant proptosis and orbital soft tissue swelling that limit the initial evaluation. Exclusion of a ruptured globe or a significant retrobulbar hemorrhage (Fig. 18–36; see Color Plate 56) requiring decompression is critical in the early phases of evaluation. Recognition and treatrnent of traumatic optic nerve injuries may improve the ultimate prognosis in this condition (see Chapter 5). Radiographic imaging in the acute setting is critical to determine the extent of orbital injury and involvement of the extraocular muscles. Important features to evaluate include bony fractures, the degree and direction of bone displacement, soft tissue injury or abnormal globe contour, retrobulbar hemorrhage (Fig. 18–37), and the presence of air or foreign body in the orbit. CT is the imaging modality of choice and should include bony windows in both the axial and coronal planes. Occasionally MRI is helpful in the identification of traumatic optic nerve sheath hemorrhages or in the characterization of soft tissue swelling.

Orbital "blowout" or floor fractures are common after facial trauma. Palpation of the bony orbital rim is necessary to rule out step-off fractures and to identify areas of reduced sensation. Exophthalmometry of the globe position should be performed to rule out enophthalmos or proptosis. Limited eye movements from entrapment should be distinguished from cranial nerve palsies through the use of forced duction testing. Other facial fractures important in craniofacial trauma include those involving the frontal bone since their presence may suggest brain involvement or optic nerve injury. Nasal ethmoidal fractures can present with telecanthus and lacrimal injury. Zygomatic fractures are important as they may involve the lateral rectus muscle and impair eye movements.

The appropriate management of orbital blowout fractures remains a controversial issue, particularly in the early stages. Some favor early surgical intervention to restore orbital volume and anatomic relationships. Most agree that early surgical intervention for blowout fractures is indicated in patients with symptomatic diplopia and positive forced ductions, particularly when there is CT scan evidence of soft tissue or muscle entrapment and no improvement over the first 7 to 14 days.

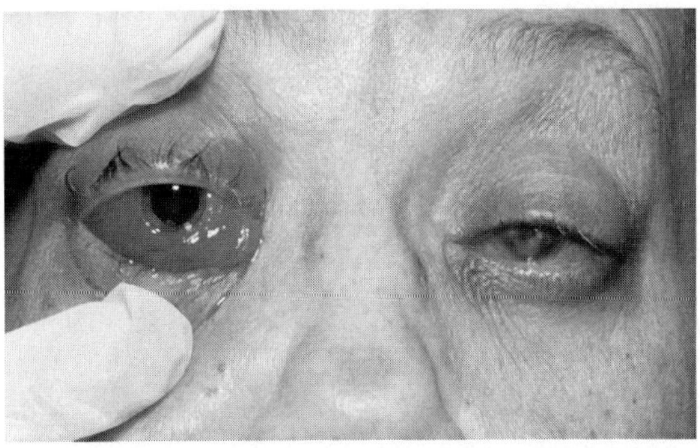

FIGURE 18–36. Acute presentation of traumatic retrobulbar hemorrhage. The right globe is proptotic and immobile, and there is extensive subconjunctival hemorrhage. (See Color Plate 56).

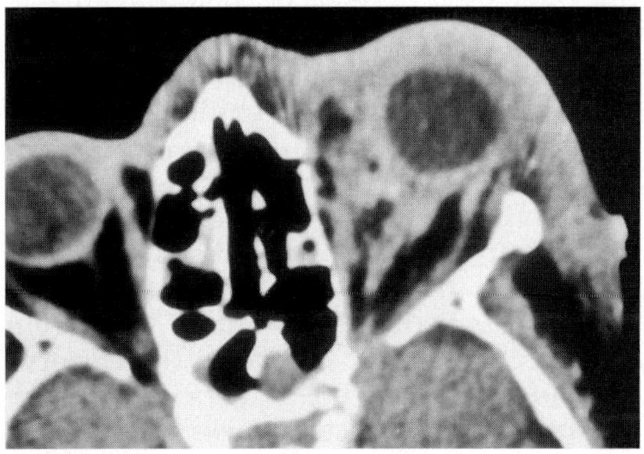

FIGURE 18–37. Axial CT scan of a patient with blunt trauma to the left orbit with proptosis and retrobulbar hemorrhage.

Similarly, early enophthalmos of greater than 3 mm and significant globe ptosis or inferior displacement are important indications for orbital surgery. Early surgery is indicated in patients with extensive fractures in whom subsequent enophthalmos is almost certain.

However, it is clear that conservative management in patients with normal eye movements, no soft tissue entrapment on CT scan, only small fractures, and minimal enophthalmos is a reasonable course. Such patients require no further surgery and will not develop more significant cosmetic or eye muscle abnormality.

The repair of orbital fractures usually involves surgery on the floor of the orbit, either through the eyelid or transconjunctivally. The fractures are identified under the periorbita and soft tissue is released. Some type of material is then used to bridge the orbital floor defect and to allow for restoration of normal soft tissue position. Both autogenous tissue, such as harvested graft material in the form of bone, and alloplastic materials may be used. Most favor inert alloplastic materials, which are available in many different forms, including porous polyethylene and metal alloys.

ORBITAL SURGERY

In addition to the decompression procedure for TAO and optic nerve sheath fenestration, orbitotomy is performed for biopsy and removal of mass lesions. The specific surgical approach is guided by the location of the lesion and broadly can be grouped as anterior, lateral, and superior.[273–276] A combination approach is occasionally used, requiring the cooperation of otolaryngologists, neurosurgeons, and reconstructive surgeons. The anterior approach is the most frequently employed and incisions may be made either transconjunctivally or through the skin. This technique may involve surgery through the orbital septum or can be extraperiosteal. This technique can be used to biopsy lesions anywhere in the orbit and to remove palpable mass lesions. The retrobulbar space may be accessed through a conjunctival incision with temporary displacement of the medial rectus muscle. This technique is particularly useful for optic nerve sheath fenestration. The anterior extraperiosteal approach is particularly useful for lesions that are based in or involve the bone or sinuses.

Lateral orbitotomy allows access to the retrobulbar space and involves a lateral and subbrow skin incision with removal of portions of the lateral wall of the orbit and zygomatic arch. In the superior approaches the orbit is accessed through a frontal or frontotemporal craniotomy. The superior procedures are usually necessary for removal of orbital apex lesions or lesions that involve the optic canal and intracranial contents. The procedure allows for en-bloc excision of the roof and lateral wall of the orbit and provides a wide view of the orbit and the adjacent intracranial structures. If removal of the optic nerve is planned, the canal must be unroofed and the annulus of Zinn incised.

Some malignant tumors of the orbit threaten to extend beyond the orbit and require exenteration. This definitive procedure involves removal of the entire orbital contents. When the eyelids are also removed, this is called *superexenteration.* With malignant lacrimal gland tumors that involve bone, exenteration may include removal of involved portions of bone. Exenteration is also used in the surgical management of malignant tumors of the paranasal sinus and nasopharynx that extend into the orbit.

REFERENCES

1. Beard C, Quickert MH: Anatomy of the Orbit (A Dissection Manual). Birmingham, AL, Aesculapius Publishing, 1969.
2. Doxanas MT, Anderson RL: Clinical Orbital Anatomy. Baltimore, Williams & Wilkins, 1984.
3. Jakobiec FA: Ocular Anatomy, Embryology and Teratology. Philadelphia, Harper & Row, 1982.
4. Jakobiec FA, Iwamoto T: Ocular adnexa: Introduction to the lids, conjunctiva and orbit. In: Jakobiec FA (ed): Ocular Anatomy, Embryology and Teratology, pp 677–732. Philadelphia, Harper & Row, 1982.
5. Liu GT: Anatomy and physiology of the trigeminal nerve. In: Miller NR, Newman NJ (eds): Walsh and Hoyt's Clinical Neuro-ophthalmology, 5th edition, pp 1595–1648. Baltimore, Williams & Wilkins, 1998.
6. Hayreh SS: Arteries of the orbit in the human being. Br J Surg 1963;50:948–953.
7. Bergen MP: Spatial aspects of the orbital vascular system. In: Jakobiec FA (ed): Ocular Anatomy, Embryology and Teratology, pp 859–868. Philadelphia, Harper & Row, 1982.
8. Eggers HM: Functional anatomy of the extraocular muscles. In: Jakobiec FA (ed): Ocular Anatomy, Embryology and Teratology, pp 783–834. Philadelphia, Harper & Row, 1982.
9. Greiner JV, Covington HI, Allansmith MR: The human limbus. A scanning electron microscopic study. Arch Ophthalmol. 1979;97:1159–1165.
10. Koornneef L: Orbital septa: anatomy and function. Ophthalmology 1979;86:876–880.
11. Bradbury PG, Levy IS, McDonald WI: Transient uniocular visual loss on deviation of the eye in association with intraorbital turnours. J Neurol Neurosurg Psychiatry 1987;50:615–619.

12. De-LaPaz; MA, Boniuk M: Fundus manifestations of orbital disease and treatment of orbital disease. Surv Ophthalmol 1995;40:3–21.
13. Newell FW: Choridal folds. Am J Ophthalmol 1973; 75:930–942.
14. Norton EWD: A characteristic fluorescein angiographic appearance in choroidal folds. Proc R Soc Med 1969;62:119–128.
15. Byrne SF: Standardized echography in the differentiation of orbital lesions. Surv Ophthalmol 1984;29: 226–228.
16. Byrne SF: Standardized echography of the eye and orbit. Neuroradiology 1986;28:618–640.
17. Dallow RL, Momose KJ, Weber AL, et al: Comparison of ultrasonography, computerized tomography (EMI scan), and radiographic techniques in evaluation of exophthalmos. Trans Am Acad Ophthalmol Otolaryngol 1976;81:305–322.
18. Byrne SF, Gendron EK, Glaser JS, et al: Diameter of normal extraocular recti muscles with echography. Am J Ophthalmol 1991;112:706–713.
19. Williamson TH, Harris A: Color Doppler ultrasound imaging of the eye and orbit. Surv Ophthalmol 1996;40:255–267.
20. Kodsi SR, Shetlar DJ, Campbell RJ, et al: A review of 340 orbital tumors in children during a 60-year period. Am J Ophthalmol 1994;117:177–182.
21. Haik BG, Ellsworth RM: Pediatric orbital tumors. Trans New Orleans Acad Ophthalmol 1986;109.
22. Gunalp I, Gunduz K: Pediatric orbital tumors in Turkey. Ophthal Plast Reconstr Surg 1995;11: 193–199.
23. Grossniklaus HE, Lass JH, Abrarnowsky CR, et al: Childhood orbital pseudotumor. Ann Ophthalmol 1985;17:372–377.
24. Bullock JD, Goldberg SH, Rakes SM: Orbital tumors in children. Ophthal Plast Reconstr Surg 1989;5: 13–16.
25. Volpe NJ, Jakobiec FA: Pediatric orbital tumors. Int Ophthalmol Clin 1992;32:201–221.
26. Margo CE, Mulla ZD: Malignant tumors of the orbit. Analysis of the Florida Cancer Registry. Ophthalmology 1998;105:185–190.
27. Dallow RL, Pratt SG: Approach to orbital disorders and frequency of disease occurence. In: Albert DM, Jakobiec FA (eds.): Principles and Practice of Ophthalmology, pp 1881–1890. Philadelphia,WB Saunders, 1994.
28. Rootman J: Frequency and differential diagnosis of orbital disease. In: Rootman J. (ed): Diseases of the Orbit: A Multidisciplinary Approach, pp 119–139 Philadelphia, JB Lippincott, 1988.
29. Shields JA, Bakewell B, Augsburger JJ, et al: Classification and incidence of space-occupying lesions of the orbit. A survey of 645 biopsies. Arch Ophthalmol 1984;102:1606–1611.
30. Kennedy RE: An evaluation of 820 orbital cases. Trans Am Ophthalmol Soc 1984;82:134–157.
31. Volpe R: Immunological aspects of autoimmune thyroid disease. Prog Clin Biol Res 1981;74:1–27.
32. Volpe R: Autoimmune thyroid disease—a perspective. Mol Biol Med 1986;3:25–51.
33. Volpe R: Immunoregulation in autoimmune thyroid disease [editorial]. N EngI J Med 1987;316:44–46.
34. Weetman AP, Yateman ME, Ealey PA, et al: Thyroid-stimulating antibody activity between different immunoglobulin G subclasses. J Clin Invest 1990;86: 723–727.
35. Char DH: Normal thyroid gland and mechanisms of hyperthyroidism. In: Throid Eye Disease, 3rd edition, pp 5–23. Boston, Butterworth–Heinemann, 1997.
36. Char DH: Systemic diagnostic tests for thyroid ophthalmopathy and euthyroid ophthalmopathy. In: Thyroid Eye Disease, 3rd edition, pp 23–37. Boston, Butterworth–Heinemann, 1997.
37. Spencer CA, Schwarzbein D, Guttler RB, et al: Thyrotropin (TSH)-releasing hormone stimulation test responses employing third and fourth generation TSH assays. J Clin Endocrinol Metab 1993;76:494–498.
38. Helfand M, Reffern CC: Clinical guideline, part 2. Screening for thyroid disease: an update. American College of Physicians. Ann Intern Med 1998;129: 144–158.
39. Bartley GB, Fatourechi V, Kadrmas EF, et al: The incidence of Graves' ophthalmopathy in Olmsted County, Minnesota. Am J Ophthalmol 1995;120: 511–517.
40. Marcocci C, Bartalena L, Bogazzi F, et al: Studies on the occurrence of ophthalmopathy in Graves' disease. Acta Endocrinol Copenh 1989;120:473–478.
41. Wiersinga WM, Smit T, van der Gaag R, et al: Temporal relationship between onset of Graves' ophthalmopathy and onset of thyroidal Graves' disease. J Endocrinol Invest 1988;11:615–619.
42. Bartley GB, Fatourechi V, Kadrmas EF, et al: Chronology of Graves' ophthalmopathy in an incidence cohort. Am J Ophthalmol 1996; 121:426–434.
43. Sridama V, DeGroot LJ: Treatment of Graves' disease and the course of ophthalmopathy. Am J Med 1989;87:70–73.
44. Tallstedt L, Lundell G, Taube A: Graves' ophthalmopathy and tobacco smoking. Acta Endocrinot Copenh 1993;129:147–150.
45. Prummel W, Wiersinga WM: Smoking and risk of Graves' disease. JAMA 1993;269:479–482.
46. Kung AW, Yau CC, Cheng A: The incidence of ophthalmopathy after radioiodine therapy for Graves' disease: prognostic factors and the role of methimazole. J Clin Endocrinol Metab 1994;79:542–546.
47. Bartalena L, Martino E, Marcocci C, et al: More on smoking habits and Graves' ophthalmopathy. J Endocrinol Invest 1989;12:733–737.
48. Perros P, Crombie AL, Matthews JN, et al: Age and gender influence the severity of thyroid-associated ophthalmopathy: a study of 101 patients attending a combined thyroid–eye clinic. Clin Endocrinol (Oxf) 1993;38:367–372.
49. Tallstedt L, Lundell G: Radioiodine treatment, ablation, and ophthalmopathy: a balanced perspective. Thyroid 1997;7:241–245.
50. Bartalena L, Marcocci C, Bogazzi F, et al: Relation between therapy for hyperthyroidism and the course of Graves' ophthalmopathy. N Engl J Med 1998; 338:73–78.
51. Prummel MF, Wiersinga. WM: Medical management of Graves' ophthalmopathy. Thyroid 1995;5:231–234.
52. Sergott RC, Felberg NT, Savinco PJ, et al: Association of HLA antigen BW35 with severe Graves' ophthalmopathy. Invest Ophthalmol Vis Sci 1983;24:124–127.
53. Mariotti S, Chiovato L, Vitti P, et al: Recent advances in the understanding of humoral and cellular mechanisms implicated in thyroid autoimmune disorders. Clin Immunol Immunopathol 1989;50:S73–84.
54. Ofosu MH, Dunston G, Henry L, et al: HLA-DQ3 is associated with Graves' disease in African-Americans. Immunol Invest 1996;25:103–110.

55. Barlow AB, Wheatcroft N, Watson P, et al: Association of HLA-DQA1*0501 with Graves' disease in English Caucasian men and women. Clin Endocrinol (Oxf) 1996;44:73–77.
56. Yanagawa T, DeGroot LJ: HLA class II associations in African-American female patients with Graves' disease. Thyroid 1996;6:37–39.
57. Donner H, Rau H, Walfish PG, et al: CTLA4 alanine-17 confers genetic susceptibility to Graves' disease and to type 1 diabetes mellitus. J Clin Endocrinol Metab 1997;82:143–146.
58. Tomer Y, Barbesino G, Keddache M, et al: Mapping of a major susceptibility locus for Graves' disease (GD-1) to chromosome 14q3l. J Clin Endocrinol Metab 1997;82:1645-1648.
59. Faure GC, Bensoussan Lejzerowicz D, Bene MC, et al: Coexpression of CD40 and class II antigen HLA-DR in Graves' disease thyroid epithelial cells. Clin Immunol Immunopathol 1997;84:212–215.
60. Sergott RC, Glaser JS: Graves' ophthalmopathy. A clinical and immunologic review. Surv Ophthalmol 1981;26:1–21.
61. Balazs C, Kiss E, Vamos A, et al: Beneficial effect of pentoxifylline on thyroid associated ophthalmopathy (TAO): a pilot study. J Clin Endocrinol Metab 1997;82:1999–2002.
62. Weetman AP, Fells P, Shine B: T and B cell reactivity to extraocular and skeletal muscle in Graves' ophthalmopathy. Br J Ophthalmol 1989;73:323–327.
63. Baker JR Jr: Autoimmune endocrine disease. JAMA 1997;278:1931–1937.
64. Perros P, Kendall Taylor P: The pathogenesis of thyroid-associated ophthalmopathy. J Endocrinol 1989;122:619–624.
65. Perros P, Kendall Taylor P: Antibodies to orbital tissues in thyroid-associated ophthalmopathy. Acta Endocrinol Copenh 1992;126:137–142.
66. Heufelder AE: Pathogenesis of Graves' ophthalmopathy: recent controversies and progress. Eur J Endocrinol 1995;132:532–541.
67. Kubota S, Gunji K, Stolarski C, et al: Reevaluation of the prevalences of serum autoantibodies reactive with "64-kd eye muscle proteins" in patients with thyroid-associated ophthalmopathy. Thyroid 1998;8: 175–179.
68. Gunji K, Kubota S, Swanson J, et al: Role of the eye muscles in thyroid eye disease: identification of the principal autoantigens. Thyroid 1998;8:553–556.
69. Wall J, Barsouk A, Stolarski C, et al: Serum antibodies reactive with eye muscle antigens and the TSH receptor in a euthyroid subject who developed ophthalmopathy and Graves' hyperthyroidism. Thyroid 1996;6:353–358.
70. Wall JR, Salvi M, Bernard NF, et al: Thyroid-associated ophthalmopathy—a model for the association of organ-specific autoimmune disorders. Immunol Today 1991;12:150–153.
71. Wall JR, Bernard N, Boucher A, et al: Pathogenesis of thyroid-associated ophthalmopathy: an autoimmune disorder of the eye muscle associated with Graves' hyperthyroidism and Hashimoto's thyroiditis. Clin Immunol Immunopathol 1993;68:1–8.
72. Wall J, Kennerdell JS: Progress in thyroid-associated ophthalmopathy. Autoimmunity 1995;22:191–195.
73. Bartley GB, Fatourechi V, Kadrmas EF, et al: Clinical features of Graves' ophthalmopathy in an incidence cohort. Am J Ophthalmol 1996; 121:284–290.
74. Feldon SE, Levin L: Graves' ophthalmopathy: V. Aetiology of upper eyelid retraction in Graves' ophthalmopathy. Br J Ophthalmol 1990;74:484–485.
75. Mourits MP, Prummel MF, Wiersinga WM, et al: Measuring eye movements in Graves ophthalmopathy. Ophthalmology 1994;101:1341–1346.
76. Trobe JD: Cyclodeviation in acquired vertical strabismus. Arch Ophthalmol 1984;102:717–720.
77. Garrity JA, Saggau DD, Gorman CA, et al: Torsional diplopia after transantral orbital decompression and extraocular muscle surgery associated with Graves' orbitopathy. Am J Ophthalmol 1992;113:363–373.
78. Scott WE, Thalacker JA: Diagnosis and treatment of thyroid myopathy. Ophthalmology 1981;88:493–498.
79. Spierer A, Eisenstein Z: The role of increased intraocular pressure on upgaze in the assessment of Graves ophthalmopathy. Ophthalmology 1991;98: 1491–1494.
80. Chung SM, Lee AG, Holds JB, et al: Ocular neuromyotonia in Graves dysthyroid orbitopathy. Arch Ophthalmol 1997;115:365–370.
81. Vargas ME, Warren FA, Kupersmith MJ: Exotropia as a sign of myasthenia gravis in dysthyroid ophthalmopathy. Br J Ophthalmol 1993;77:822–823.
82. Jacobson DM: Acetylcholine receptor antibodies in patients with Graves' ophthalmopathy. J Neuro-ophthalmol 1995;15:166–170.
83. Neigel JM, Rootman J, Belkin RI, et al: Dysthyroid optic neuropathy. The crowded orbital apex syndrome. Ophthalmology 1988;95:1515–1521.
84. Bartley GB, Fatourechi V, Kadrmas EF, et al: Long-term follow-up of Graves ophthalmopathy in an incidence cohort. Ophthalmology 1996;103:958–962.
85. Garrity JA, Fatourechi V, Bergstralh EJ, et al: Results of transantral orbital decompression in 428 patients with severe Graves' ophthahlmopathy. Am J Ophthalmol 1993;116:533–547.
86. Kennerdell JS, Rosenbaum AE, El-Hoshy MH: Apical optic nerve compression of dysthyroid optic neuropathy on computed tomography. Arch Ophthalmol 1981;99:807–809.
87. Trobe JD, Glaser JS, Laflamme P: Dysthyroid optic neuropathy: clinical profile and rationale for management. Arch Ophthalmol 1978;96:1199–1209.
88. Cockerham KP, Pal C, Jani B, et al: The prevalence and implications of ocular hypertension and glaucoma in thyroid-associated orbitopathy. Ophthalmology 1997;104:914–917.
89. Feldon SE, Lee CP, Muramatsu SK, et al: Quantitative computed tomography of Graves' ophthalmopathy. Extraocular muscle and orbital fat in development of optic neuropathy. Arch Ophthalmol 1985;103: 213–215.
90. Feldon SE, Muramatsu S, Weiner JM: Clinical classification of Graves' ophthalmopathy. Identification of risk factors for optic neuropathy. Arch Ophthalmol 1984;102:1469–1472.
91. Enzmann DR, Donaldson SS, Kriss JP: Appearance of Graves' disease on orbital computed tomography. J Comput Assist Tomogr 1979;3:815–819.
92. Nugent RA, Belkin RI, Neigel JM, et al: Graves orbitopathy: correlation of CT and clinical findings. Radiology 1990;177:675–682.
93. Rothfus WE, Curtin HD: Extraocular muscle enlargement: a CT review. Radiology 1984;151:677–681.
94. Trokel SL, Jakobiec FA: Correlation of CT scanning and pathologic features of ophthalmic Graves' disease. Ophthalmology 1981;88:553–564.
95. Bailey CC, Kabala J, Laitt R, et al: Magnetic resonance imaging in thyroid eye disease. Eye 1996;10:617–619.
96. Hiromatsu Y, Kojima K, Ishisaka N, et al: Role of magnetic resonance imaging in thyroid-associated

ophthalmopathy: its predictive value for therapeutic outcome of immunosuppressive therapy. Thyroid 1992;2:299–305.
97. Hoh HB, Laitt RD, Wakeley C, et al: The STIR sequence MRI in the assessment of extraocular muscles in thyroid eye disease. Eye 1994;8:506–510.
98. Holt JE, O'Connor PS, Douglas JP, et al: Extraocular muscle size comparison using standardized A-scan echography and computerized tomography scan measurements. Ophthalmology 1985;92:1351–1355.
99. Dallow RL: Evaluation of unilateral exophthalmos with ultrasonography: analysis of 258 consecutive cases. Laryngoscope 1975;85:1905–1919.
100. Delint PJ, Mourits MP, Kerlen CH, et al: B-scan ultrasonography in Graves' orbitopathy. Doc Ophthalmol 1993;85:1–4.
101. Shammas HJ, Minckler DS, Ogden C: Ultrasound in early thyroid orbitopathy. Arch Ophthalmol 1980; 98:277–279.
102. Werner SC: Modification of the classification of the eye changes of Graves' disease. Am J Ophthalmol 1977;83:725–727.
103. Werner SC: Modification of the classification of the eye changes of Graves' disease: recommendations of the Ad Hoc Committee of the American Thyroid Association [letter]. J Clin Endocrinol Metab 1977; 44:203–204.
104. Bartley GB: Evolution of classification systems for Graves' ophthalmopathy. Ophthal Plast Reconstr Surg 1995;11:229–237.
105. Frueh BR: Why the NOSPECS classification of Graves' eye disease should be abandoned, with suggestions for the characterization of this disease. Thyroid 1992;2:85–88.
106. Van Dyk HJ: Orbital Graves' disease. A modification of the "NO SPECS" classification. Ophthalmology 1981;88:479–483.
107. Bartley GB, Fatourechi V, Kadrmas EF, et al: The treatment of Graves' ophthalmopathy in an incidence cohort. Am J Ophthalmol 1996;121:200–206.
108. Perros P, Crombie AL, Kendall Taylor P: Natural history of thyroid associated ophthalmopathy. Clin Endocrinol (Oxf) 1995;42:45–50.
109. Rootman J: Graves' orbitopathy. In: Rootman J (ed): Disease of the Orbit: A Multidisciplinary Approach, pp 241–280. Philadelphia, JB. Lippincott, 1988.
110. Wiersinga WM, Smit T, Schuster Uittenhoeve AL, et al: Therapeutic outcome of prednisone medication and of orbital irradiation in patients with Graves' ophthalmopathy. Ophthalmologica 1988;197:75–84.
111. Kendall Taylor P, Crombie AL, Stephenson AM, et al: Intravenous methylprednisolone in the treatment of Graves' ophthalmopathy. BMJ 1988;297:1574–1578.
112. Tagami T, Tanaka Y, Sugawa H, et al: High-dose intravenous steroid pulse therapy in thyroid-associated ophthalmopathy. Endocr J 1996;43: 689–699.
113. Koshiyama H, Koh T, Fujiwara K, et al: Therapy of Graves' ophthalmopathy with intravenous high-dose steroid followed by orbital irradiation. Thyroid 1994;4:409–413.
114. Atabay C, Schrooyen M, Zhang ZG, et al: Use of eye muscle antibody measurements to monitor response to plasmapheresis in patients with thyroid-associated ophthalmopathy. J Endocrinol Invest 1993;16:669–674.
115. Antonelli A, Saracino A, Alberti B, et al: High-dose intravenous immunoglobulin treatment in Graves' ophthalmopathy. Acta Endocrinol Copenh 1992; 126:13–23.
116. Baschieri L, Antonelli A, Nardi S, et al: Intravenous immunoglobulin versus corticosteroid in treatment of Graves' ophthalmopathy. Thyroid 1997;7:579–585.
117. Kahaly G, Pitz S, Muller Forell W, et al: Randomized trial of intravenous immunoglobulins versus prednisolone in Graves' ophthalmopathy. Clin Exp Immunol 1996;106:197–202.
118. Kung AW, Michon J, Tai KS, et al: The effect of somatostatin versus corticosteroid in the treatment of Graves' ophthalmopathy. Thyroid 1996;6:381–384.
119. Prummel MF, Mourits MP, Berghout A, et al: Prednisone, and cyclosporine, in the treatment of severe Graves' ophthalmopathy. N Engl J Med 1989; 321:1353–1359.
120. Bartalena L, Marcocci C, Bogazzi F, et al: Use of corticosteroids to prevent progression of Graves' ophthalmopathy after radioiodine therapy for hyperthyroidism. N Engl J Med 1989;321:1349–1352.
121. Hurbli T, Char DH, Harris J, et al: Radiation therapy for thyroid eye diseases. Am J Ophthalmol 1985;99: 633–637.
122. Bartalena L, Marcocci C, Chiovato L, et al: Orbital cobalt irradiation combined with systemic corticosteroids for Graves' ophthalmopathy: comparison with systemic corticosteroids alone. J Clin Endocrinol Metab 1983;56:1139–1144.
123. Lloyd WCd, Leone CR, Jr: Supervoltage orbital radiotherapy in 36 cases of Graves' disease. Am J Ophthalmol 1992;113:374–380.
124. Marcocci C, Bartalena L, Panicucci M, et al: Orbital cobalt irradiation combined with retrobulbar or systemic corticosteroids for Graves' ophthalmopathy: a comparative study. Clin Endocrinol (Oxf) 1987; 27:33–42.
125. Nakahara H, Noguchi S, Murakarm N, et al: Graves ophthalmopathy: MR evaluation of 10-Gy versus 24-Gy irradiation combined with systemic corticosteroids. Radiology 1995;196:857–862.
126. Palmer D, Greenberg P, Cornell P, et al: Radiation therapy for Graves' ophthalmopathy: a retrospective analysis. Int J Radiat Oncol Biol Phys 1987;13:1815–1820.
127. Kazim M, Trokel S, Moore S: Treatment of acute Graves orbitopathy. Ophthalmology 1991;98:1443–1448.
128. Wilson WB, Prochoda M: Radiotherapy for thyroid orbitopathy. Effects on extraocular muscle balance. Arch Ophthalmol 1995;113:1420–1425.
129. Miller MI, Goldberg SH, Bullock JD: Radiation retinopathy after standard radiotherapy for thyroid-related ophthalmopathy [letter]. Am J Ophthalmol 1991;112:600–601.
130. Carter KD, Frueh BR, Hessburg TP, et al: Long-term efficacy of orbital decompression for compressive optic neuropathy of Graves' eye disease. Ophthalmology 1991;98:1435–1442.
131. Fatourechi V, Garrity JA, Bartley GB, et al: Graves ophthalmopathy. Results of transantral orbital decompression performed primarily for cosmetic indications. Ophthalmology 1994;101:938–942.
132. Fells P: Orbital decompression for severe dysthyroid eye disease. Br J Ophthalmol 1987;71:107–111.
133. Girod DA, Orcutt JC, Cummings CW: Orbital decompression for preservation of vision in Graves' ophthalmopathy. Arch Otolaryngol Head Neck Surg 1993;119:229–233.

134. Goldberg RA, Weinberg DA, Shorr N, et al. Maximal, three-wall, orbital decompression through a coronal approach. Ophthalmic Surg Lasers 1997;28:832–843.
135. Hutchison BM, Kyle PM. Long-term visual outcome following orbital decompression for dysthyroid eye disease. Eye 1995;9:578–581.
136. Kennerdell JS, Maroon JC: An orbital decompression for severe dysthyroid exophthalmos. Ophthalmology 1982;89:467–472.
137. Maroon JC, Kennerdell JS: Radical orbital decompression for severe dysthyroid exophthalmos. J Neurosurg 1982;56:260–266.
138. McNab AA: Orbital decompression for thyroid orbitopathy. Aust NZ J Ophthalmol 1997;25:55–61.
139. Neugebauer A, Nishino K, Neugebauer P, et al: Effects of bilateral orbital decompression by an endoscopic endonasal approach in dysthyroid orbitopathy. Br J Ophthalmol 1996;80:58–62.
140. Schaefer SD, Merritt JH, Close LG: Orbital decompression for optic neuropathy secondary to thyroid eye disease. Laryngoscope 1988;98:712–716.
141. McCord CD, Jr: Current trends in orbital decompression. Ophthalmology 1985;92:21–33.
142. Mourits MP, Koornneef L, Wiersinga WM, et al: Orbital decompression for Graves' ophthalmopathy by inferomedial, by inferomedial plus lateral, and by coronal approach. Ophthalmology 1990;97:636–641.
143. Metson R, Dallow RL, Shore JW: Endoscopic orbital decompression. Laryngoscope 1994;104:950–957.
144. Metson R, Shore JW, Gliklich RE, et al: Endosopic orbital decompression under local anesthesia. Otolaryngol Head Neck Surg 1995;113:661–667.
145. Khan JA, Wagner DV, Tiojanco JK, et al: Combined transconjunctival and external approach for endoscopic orbital apex decompression in Graves' disease. Laryngoscope 1995;105:203–206.
146. DeSanto LW: The total rehabilitation of Graves' ophthalmopathy. Laryngoscope 1980;90:1652–1678.
147. Shorr N, Neuhaus RW, Baylis HI: Ocular motility problems after orbital decompression for dysthyroid ophthalmopathy. Ophthalmology 1982;89:323–328.
148. Shorr N, Seiff SR: The four stages of surgical rehabilitation of the patient with dysthyroid ophthalmopathy. Ophthalmology 1986;93:476–483.
149. Lyons CJ, Rootman J: Orbital decompression for disfiguring exophthalmos in thyroid orbitopathy. Ophthalmology 1994;101:223–230.
150. Trokel S, Kazim M, Moore S: Orbital fat removal. Decompression for Graves orbitopathy. Ophthalmology 1993;100:674–682.
151. Fells P, Kousoulides L, Pappa, A, et al: Extraocular muscle problems in thyroid eye disease. Eye 1994; 8:497–505.
152. Sprunger DT, Helveston EM: Progressive overcorrection after inferior rectus recession. J Pediatr Ophthalmol Strabismus 1993;30:145–148.
153. Evans D, Kennerdell JS: Extraocular muscle surgery for dysthyroid myopathy. Am J Ophthalmol 1983; 95:767–771.
154. Young LA: Dysthyroid ophthalmopathy in children. J Pediatr Ophthalmol Strabismus 1979;16:105–107.
155. Liu GT, Heher KL, Katowitz JA, et al: Prominent proptosis in childhood thyroid eye disease. Ophthalmology 1996;103:779–784.
156. Jakobiec FA, Lefkowitch J, Knowles DM: B- and T-lymphocytes in ocular disease. Ophthalmology 1984; 91:635–654.
157. Mombaerts I, Goldschmeding R, Schlingemann RO, et al: What is orbital pseudotumor? Surv Ophthalmol 1996;41:66–78.
158. Atabay C, Tyutyunikov A, Scalise D, et al: Serum antibodies reactive with eye muscle membrane antigens are detected in patients with nonspecific orbital inflammation. Ophthalmology 1995;102:145–153.
159. Purcell JJ, Jr., Taulbee WA: Orbital myositis after upper respiratory tract infection. Arch Ophthalmol 1981;99:437–438.
160. Slavin ML, Glaser JS: Idiopathic orbital myositis: report of six cases. Arch Ophthalmol 1982;100:1261–1265.
161. Ludwig I, Tomsak RL: Acute recurrent orbital myositis. J Clin Neuro-ophthalmol 1983;3:41–47.
162. Eshaghian J, Anderson RL: Sinus involvement in inflammatory orbital pseudotumor. Arch Ophthalmol 1981;99:627–630.
163. Pillai P, Saini JS: Bilateral sino-orbital pseudotumour. Can J Ophthalmol 1988;23:177–180.
164. Fujii H, Fujisada H, Kondo T, et al: Orbital pseudotumor: histopathological classification and treatment. Ophthalmologica 1985;190:230–242.
165. Rootman J, Nugent R: The classification and management of acute orbital pseudotumors. Ophthalmology 1982;89:1040–1048.
166. Mottow Lippa L, Jakobiec FA, Smith M: Idiopathic inflammatory orbital pseudotumor in childhood. II. Results of diagnostic tests and biopsies. Ophthalmology 1981;88:565–574.
167. Kennerdell JS, Dresner SC: The nonspecific orbital inflammatory syndromes. Surv Ophthalmol 1984;29: 93–103.
168. Benson WE: Posterior scleritis. Surv Ophthalmol 1988;32:297–316.
169. Ohtsuka K, Hashimoto M, Miura M, et al: Posterior scleritis with optic perineuritis and interal ophthalmoplegia [letter]. Br J Ophthalmol 1997;81:514.
170. Rootman J, Robertson W, Lapointe JS: Inflammatory diseases. In: Rootman J (ed): Diseases of the Orbit: A Multidisciplinary Approach, pp 143–204, Philadelphia, JB Lippincott, 1988.
171. Tychsen L, Tse DT, Ossoinig K, et al: Trochleitis with superior oblique myositis. Ophthalmology 1984;91: 1075–1079.
172. Frohman L, Wolansky L: Magnetic resonance imaging of syphilitic optic neuritis/perineuritis. J Neuro-ophthalmol 1997;17:57–59.
173. Toshniwal P: Optic perineuritis with secondary syphilis. J Clin Neuro-ophthalmol 1987;7:6–10.
174. Rush JA, Ryan EJ: Syphilitic optic perineuritis. Am J Ophthalmol 1981;91:404–406.
175. Abramovitz JN, Kasdon DL, Sutula F, et al: Sclerosing orbital pseudotumor. Neurosurgery 1983;12: 463–468.
176. Cervellini P, Volpin L, Curri D, et al: Sclerosing orbital pseudotumor. Ophthalmologica 1986;193: 39–44.
177. Kennerdell JS: The management of sclerosing nonspecific orbital inflammation. Ophthalmic Surg 1991; 22:512–518.
178. McCarthy JM, White VA, Harris G, et al: Idiopathic sclerosing inflammation of the orbit: immunohistologic analysis and comparison with retroperitioneal fibrosis. Mod Pathol 1993;6:581–587.
179. Paris GL, Waltuch GF, Egbert PR: Treatment of refractory orbital pseudotumors with pulsed chemotherapy. Ophthal Plast Reconstr Surg 1990;6:96–101.
180. Rootman J, McCarthy M, White V, et al: Idiopathic sclerosing inflammation of the orbit. A distinct clinicopathologic entity. Ophthalmology 1994;101: 570–584.

181. Weissler MC, Miller E, Fortune MA: Sclerosing orbital pseudotumor: a unique clinicopathologic entity. Ann Otol Rhinol Laryngol 1989;98:496–501.
182. de Jesus O, Inserni JA, Gonzalez A, et al: Idiopathic orbital inflammation with intracranial extension. Case report. J Neurosurg 1996;85:510–513.
183. Frohman LP, Kupersmith MJ, Lang J, et al: Intracranial extension and bone destruction in orbital pseudotumor. Arch Ophthalmol 1986;104:380–384.
184. Kaye AH, Hahn JF, Craciun A, et al: Intracranial extension of inflammatory pseudotumor of the orbit. Case report. J Neurosurg 1984;60:625–629.
185. Nishi T, Saito Y, Watanabe K, et al: Intracranial extension of an orbital pseudotumor accompanied by internal carotid artery occlusion—case report. Neurol Med Chir Tokyo 1992;32:758–761.
186. Noble SC, Chandler WF, Lloyd RV: Intracranial extension of orbital pseudotumor: a case report. Neurosurgery 1986;18:798–801.
187. Richards AB, Shalka HW, Roberts FJ, et al: Psuedotumor of the orbit and retroperitoneal fibrosis. A form of multifocal fibrosclerosis. Arch Ophthalmol 1980; 98:1617–1620.
188. Berger JR, Snodgrass, S, Glaser J, et al: Multifocal fibrosclerosis with hypertrophic intracranial pachymeningitis. Neurology 1989;39:1345–1349.
189. Brazier DJ, Sanders MD: Multifocal fibrosclerosis associated with suprasellar and macular lesions. Br J Ophthalmol 1983;67:292–296.
190. Flanders AE, Mafee MF, Rao VM, et al: CT characteristics of orbital pseudotumors and other orbital inflammatory processes. J Comput Assist Tomogr 1989; 13:40–47.
191. Atlas SW, Grossman RI, Savino PJ, et al: Surface-coil MR of orbital pseudotumor. AJR Am J Roentgenol 1987;148:803–808.
192. Mombaerts I, Schlingemann RO, Goldschmeding R, et al: Are systemic corticosteroids useful in the management of orbital pseudotumors? Ophthalmology 1996;103:521–528.
193. Leone CR, Jr., Lloyd WC: Treatment protocol for orbital inflammatory disease. Ophthalmology 1985;92: 1325–1331.
194. Bielory L, Frohman LP: Low-dose cyclosporine therapy of granulomatous optic neuropathy and orbitopathy. Ophthalmology 1991;98:1732–1736.
195. Diaz Llopis M, Menezo JL: Idiopathic inflammatory orbital pseudotumor and low-dose cyclosporine. Am J Ophthalmol 1989;107:547–548.
196. Donaldson SS, McDougall IR, Egbert PR, et al: Treatment of orbital pseudotumor (idiopathic orbital inflammation) by radiation therapy. Int J Radiat Oncol Biol Phys 1980;6:79–86.
197. Lanciano R, Fowble B, Sergott RC, et al: The results of radiotherapy for orbital pseudotumor. Int J Radiat Oncol Biol Phys 1990;18:407–411.
198. Sergott RC, Glaser JS, Charyulu K: Radiotherapy for idiopathic inflammatory orbital pseudotumor. Indications and results. Arch Ophthalmol 1981;99: 853–856.
199. Nishino H, Rubino FA, DeRemee RA, et al: Neurological involvement in Wegener's granulomatosis: an analysis of 324 consecutive patients at the Mayo Clinic. Ann Neurol 1993;33:4–9.
200. Patrinely JR, Osborn AG, Anderson RL, et al: Computed tomographic features of nonthyroid extraocular muscle enlargement. Ophthalmology 1989;96: 1038–1047.
201. Slamovits TL, Burde RM: Bumpy muscles. Surv Ophthalmol 1988;33:189–199.
202. Capone A, Jr., Slamovits TL: Discrete metastasis of solid tumors to extraocular muscles. Arch Ophthalmol 1990;108:237–243.
203. Hornblass A, Jakobiec FA, Reifler DM, et al: Orbital lymphoid tumors located predominantly within extraocular muscles. Ophthalmology 1984;94:688–697.
204. Nicol JL, Massin M, Ullern M: [A case of bilateral exophthalmos disclosing trichinosis]. Bull Soc Ophtalmol Fr 1987;87:577–578, 581–573.
205. Pasco M: [Ocular manifestations of trichinosis. Considerations on an epidemic of trichinosis]. Bull Mem Soc Fr Ophthalmol 1986;97:74–76.
206. Behrens Baumann W, Freissler G: Computed tomographic appearance of extraocular muscle calcification in a patient with seropositive trichinosis [letter]. Am J Ophthalmol 1990;110:709–710.
207. Dal Pozzo G, Boschi MC: Extraocular muscle enlargement in acromegaly. J Comput Assist Tomogr 1982; 6:706–707.
208. Katz B, Leja S, Melles RB, et al: Amyloid ophthalmoplegia. Ophthalmoparesis secondary to primary systemic amyloidosis. J Clin Neuro-ophthalmol 1989; 9:39–42.
209. Patel AS, Kelman SE, Duncan GW, et al: Painless diplopia caused by extraocular muscle sarcoid [letter]. Arch Ophthalmol 1994;112:879–880.
210. Cornblath WT, Elner V, Rolfe M: Extraocular muscle involvement in sarcoidosis. Ophthalmology 1993;100: 501–505.
211. Simon EM, Zoarski GH, Rothman MI, et al: Systemic sarcoidosis with bilateral orbital involvement: MR findings. AJNR Am J Neuroradiol 1998;19:336–337.
212. Wende S, Aulich A, Nover A, et al: Computed tomography or orbital lesions. A cooperative study of 210 cases. Neuroradiology 1977;13:123–134.
213. Moshfeghi DM, Finger PT, Cohen RB, et al: Visual recovery after radiation therapy of orbital lymphoma [letter]. Am J Ophthalmol 1992;114:645–646.
214. Reddy EK, Bhatia P, Evans RG: Primary orbital lymphomas. 1988;15:1239–1241.
215. Rootman J, Goldberg C, Robertson W: Primary orbital schwannomas. Br J Ophthalmol 1982;66:194–204.
216. Gunalp I, Gunduz K, Duruk K, et al: Neurogenic tumors of the orbit. Jpn J Ophthalmol 1994;38: 185–190.
217. Konrad EA, Thiel HJ: Schwannoma of the orbit. Ophthalmologica 1984;188:118–127.
218. Cantore G, Ciappetta P, Raco A, et al: Orbital schwannomas: report of nine cases and review of the literature. Neurosurgery 1986;19:583–588.
219. Ni C, Cheng SC, Dryja TP, et al: Lacrimal gland tumors: a clinicopathological analysis of 160 cases. Int Ophthalmol Clin 1982;22:99–120.
220. Wright JE, Rose GE, Garner A: Primary malignant neoplasms of the lacrimal gland. Br J Ophthalmol 1992;76:401–407.
221. Wright JE, Stewart WB, Krohel GB: Clinical presentation and management of lacrimal gland tumours. Br J Ophthalmol 1979;63:600–606.
222. Stewart WB, Krohel GB, Wright JE: Lacrimal gland and fossa lesions: an approach to diagnosis and management. Ophthalmology 1979;86:886–895.
223. Gamel JW, Font RL: Adenoid cystic carcinoma of the lacrimal gland: the clinical significance of a basaloid histologic pattern. Hum Pathol 1982;13:219–225.
224. Tyl JW, Blank LE, Koornneef L: Brachytherapy in orbital tumors. Ophthalmology 1997;104:1475–1479.

225. Goldberg RA, Rootman J, Cline RA: Tumors metastatic to the orbit: a changing picture. Surv Ophthalmol 1990;35:1–24.
226. Goldberg RA, Rootman J: Clinical characteristics of metastatic orbital tumors. Ophthalmology 1990;97: 620–624.
227. Gunalp I, Gunduz K: Metastatic orbital tumors. Jpn J Ophthalmol 1995;39:65–70.
228. Cline RA, Rootman J: Enophthalmos: a clinical review. Ophthalmology 1984;91:229–237.
229. Healy JF: Computed tomographic evaluation of metatases to the orbit. Ann Ophthalmol 1983;15:1026–1029.
230. Johnson TE, Tabbara KF, Weatherhead RG, et al: Secondary squamous cell carcinoma of the orbit. Arch Ophthalmol 1997;115:75–78.
231. Weaver DT, Bartley GB: Malignant neoplasia of the paranasal sinuses associated with mucocele. Ophthalmology 1991;98:342–346.
232. Gunalp I, Gunduz K: Secondary orbital tumors. Ophthal Plast Reconstr Surg 1997;13:31–35.
233. Ferry AP, Haddad HM, Goldman JL: Orbital invasion by an intracranial chordoma. Am J Ophthalmol 1981; 92:7–12.
234. Yamasaki T, Handa H, Yamashita J, et al: Intracranial and orbital cavernous angiomas. A review of 30 cases. J Neurosurg 1986;64:197–208.
235. Ohtsuka K, Hashimoto M, Akiba H: Serial dynamic magnetic resonance imaging of orbital cavernous hemangioma. Am J Ophthalmol 1997;123:396–398.
236. In S, Miyagi J, Kojho N, et al: Intraorbital optic nerve hemangioblastoma with von Hippel–Lindau disease. Case report. J Neurosurg 1982;56:426–429.
237. Nerad JA, Kersten RC, Anderson RL: Hemangioblastoma of the optic nerve. Report of a case and review of literature. Ophthalmology 1988;95:398–402.
238. Kerr DJ, Scheithauer BW, Miller GM, et al: Hemangioblastoma of the optic nerve: case report. Neurosurgery 1995;36:573–580.
239. Karcioglu ZA, Nasr AM, Haik BG: Orbital hemangiopericytoma: clinical and morphologic features. Am J Ophthalmol 1997;124:661–672.
240. Kikuchi K, Kowada M, Sageshima M: Orbital hemangiopericytoma: CT, MR, and angiographic findings. Comput Med Imaging Graph 1994;18:217–222.
241. Musarella MA, Chan HS, DeBoer G, et al: Ocular involvement in neuroblastoma: prognostic implications. Ophthalmology 1984;91:936–940.
242. Katz BJ, Nerad JA: Ophthalmic manifestations of fibrous dysplasia. A disease of children and adults. Ophthalmology 1998;105:2207–2215.
243. Bibby K, McFadzean R: Fibrous dysplasia of the orbit. Br J Ophthalmol 1994;78:266–270.
244. Rootman J, Kemp E, Lapointe JS: Orbital tumors originating in bone. In: Rootman J (ed): Diseases of the Orbit. A Multidisciplinary approach, pp 354–379. Philadelphia, JB Lippincott, 1988.
245. Casselman JW, De Jonge I, Neyt L, et al: MRI in craniofacial fibrous dysplasia. Neuroradiology 1993; 35:234–237.
246. Moore AT, Buncic JR, Munro IR: Fibrous dysplasia of the orbit in childhood. Clinical features and management. Ophthalmology 1985;92:12–20.
247. Osguthorpe JD, Gudeman SK: Orbital complications of fibrous dysplasia. Otolaryngol Head Neck Surg 1987;97:403–405.
248. Arroyo JG, Lessell S, Montgomery WW: Steroid-induced visual recovery in fibrous dysplasia. J Clin Neuro-ophthalmol 1991;11:259–261.
249. Weisman JS, Hepler RS, Vinters HV: Reversible visual loss caused by fibrous dysplasia. Am J Ophthalmol 1990;110:244–249.
250. Chen YR, Breidahl A, Chang CN: Optic nerve decompression in fibrous dysplasia: indications, efficacy, and safety. Plast Reconstr Surg 1997;99:22–30.
251. Seiff SR: Optic nerve decompression in fibrous dysplasia: indications, efficacy, and safety [letter]. Plast Reconstr Surg 1997;100:1611–1612.
252. Edelstein C, Goldberg RA, Rubino G: Unilateral blindness after ipsilateral prophylactic transcranial optic canal decompression for fibrous dysplasia. Am J Ophthalmol 1998;126:469–471.
253. Rubin SE, Slavin ML, Rubin LG: Eyelid swelling and erythema as the only signs of subperiosteal abscess. Br J Ophthalmol 1989;73:576–578.
254. Hornblass A, Herschorn BJ, Stern K, et al: Orbital abscess. Surv Ophthalmol 1984;29:169–178.
255. Donahue SP, Schwartz G: Preseptal and orbital cellulitis in childhood. A changing microbiologic spectrum. Ophthalmology 1998;105:1902-1905.
256. Weiss A, Friendly D, Eglin K, et al: Bacterial periorbital and orbital cellulitis in childhood. Ophthalmology 1983;90:195–203.
257. Slavin ML, Glaser JS: Acute severe irreversible visual loss with sphenoethmoiditis-'posterior' orbital cellulitis. Arch Ophthalmol 1987;105:345–348.
258. Gutierrez Diaz A, del Palacio Hernanz A, Larregla S, et al: Orbital phycomycosis. Ophthalmologica 1981;182:165–170.
259. Schwartze GM, Kilgo GR, Ford CS: Internal ophthalmoplegia resulting from acute orbital phycomycosis. J Clin Neuro-ophthalmol 1984;4:105–108.
260. Kohn R, Hepler R: Management of limited rhino-orbital mucormycosis without exenteration. Ophthalmology 1985;92:1440–1444.
261. Bray WH, Giangiacomo J, Ide CH: Orbital apex syndrome. Surv Ophthalmol 1987;32:136–140.
262. Ferry AP, Abedi S: Diagnosis and management of rhino-orbitocerebral mucormycosis (phycomycosis). A report of 16 personally observed cases. Ophthalmology 1983;90:1096–1104.
263. Dortzbach RK, Segrest DR: Orbital aspergillosis. Ophthalmic Surg 1983;14:240–244.
264. Spoor TC, Hartel WC, Harding S, et al: Aspergillosis presenting as a corticosteroid-responsive optic neuropathy. J Clin Neuro-ophthalmol 1982;2:103–107.
265. Klapper SR, Lee AG, Patrinely JR, et al: Orbital involvement in allergic fungal sinusitis. Ophthalmology 1997;104:2094–2100.
266. Chang WJ, Shields CL, Shields JA, et al: Bilateral orbital involvement with massive allergic fungal sinusitis [letter]. Arch Ophthalmol 1996;114:767–768.
267. Brown P, Demaerel P, McNaught A, et al: Neuro-ophthalmological presentation of non-invasive *Aspergillus* sinus disease in the non-immunocompromised host. J Neurol Neurosurg Psychiatry 1994;57: 234–237.
268. Jacobson M, Galetta SL, Atlas SW, et al: Bipolaris-induced orbital cellulitis. J Clin Neuro-ophthalmol 1992;12:250–256.
269. Dunlop IS, Billson FA: Visual failure in allergic aspergillus sinusitis: case report. Br J Ophthalmol 1988; 72:127–130.
270. Brummund W, Kurup VP, Harris GJ, et al: Allergic sino-orbital mycosis. A clinical and immunologic study. JAMA 1986;256:3249–3253.
271. Adam RD, Paquin ML, Petersen EA, et al: Phaeohyphomycosis caused by the fungal genera *Bipolaris* and

Exserohilum. A report of 9 cases and review of the literature. Medicine Baltimore 1986;65:203–217.
272. Cody DTI, Neel HBI, Ferreiro JA, et al: Allergic fungal sinusitis: The Mayo Clinic experience. Laryngoscope 1994;104:1074–1079.
273. Kennerdell JS, Maroon JC: Microsurgical approach to intraorbital tumors. Technique and instrumentation. Arch Ophthalmol 1976;94:1333–1336.
274. Kennerdell JS, Maroon JC, Malton ML: Surgical approaches to orbital tumors. Clin Plast Surg 1988; 273–282.
275. Maroon JC, Kennerdell JS: Microsurgical approach to orbital tumors. Clin Neurosurg 1979;26:479–489.
276. Maroon JC, Kennerdell JS: Surgical approaches to the orbit. Indications and techniques. 1984;60:1226–1235.

PART IV

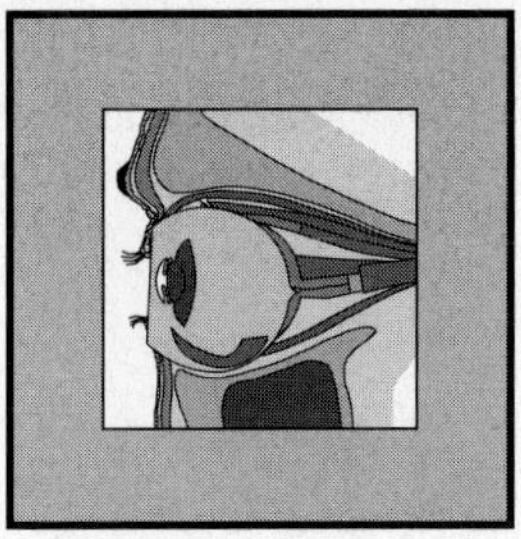

OTHER TOPICS

CHAPTER 19

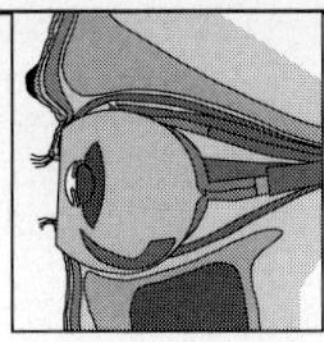

Headache, Facial Pain, and Disorders of Facial Sensation

Headache is nearly a universal experience as over 90% of individuals have noted at least one headache during their lifetime.[1] Since the eye receives a rich innervation from the trigeminal nerve, it is not surprising that many headache syndromes are associated with pain concentrated around the eye. Furthermore, many of the primary headaches syndromes such as migraine and cluster headaches have prominent visual signs and symptoms. As such, the reader should become familiar with the many types of headache, facial pains, and disorders of facial sensation.

HEADACHE

Approach

History. The cause of the patient's headache is usually established from the history. Important features include the frequency, location, mode of onset, duration, nature of the headache (throbbing, aching, pressure, dull or sharp), and the presence of prodromal symptoms, along with precipitating and alleviating factors. Naturally, the patient's medical and psychiatric history and medication list provide essential information.

Classification. It is useful to classify headaches into those that are primary or without specific cause and those with an organic cause. Migraine, cluster; and tension-type headaches are the most common forms of primary headache. In 1988, the International Headache Society (IHS) established diagnostic criteria for a variety of headache disorders to provide uniformity in classification (Tables 19–1, 19–2, and 19–3).[2, 3]

These guidelines were primarily created for the purpose of collecting epidemiologic and clinical trial data and may not always be practical for use in the clinical setting.[4] Diagnostic difficulty occurs in patients with multiple headache syndromes and from the fact that headache characteristics may change over time. Visual aura is highly suggestive of a migraine disturbance. Although nonspecific, photophobia, phonophobia, osmophobia, and gastrointestinal symptoms may also help to discriminate migraine from other causes of headache.

Headaches that suggest a more ominous cause include those with (1) abrupt onset; (2) onset after the 4th decade; (3) progressive symptoms; (4) focal neurologic signs; (5) change with position or exertion; and (6) those associated with fever, coughing, straining, or sexual activity. These types of headaches require more aggressive evaluation, including neuroimaging and possibly lumbar puncture.

MIGRAINE

Because it is such a common disorder, migraine will be discussed first. This section will review the epidemiology, genetic and clinical factors, pathophysiology, and treatment of migraine.

TABLE 19–1. International Headache Society (IHS) Criteria for Migraine Without Aura

A. Five attacks fulfilling criteria B–D
B. Headache lasting 4 to 72 hours (untreated or unsuccessfully treated)
C. Headache has two of the following characteristics:
   1. Unilateral location
   2. Pulsating quality
   3. Moderate to severe intensity
   4. Aggravation by walking stairs or similar routine physical activity
D. During headache at least one of the following:
   1. Nausea or vomiting
   2. Photophobia or phonophobia

Epidemiology

Approximately 18% of women and 6% of men endure recurrent headache classified as migraine.[5] Despite beliefs that migraine is a disorder associated with high socioeconomic status, studies show a progressive decline in migraine with rising income.[5] Approximately 80% of patients with migraine report some disability associated with their headache and one third have severe disability.[5] In fact, patients with migraine on average lose 4 to 8 days of work per year related to headache.[6] Despite the high frequency of disability associated with migraine, many patients do not seek medical attention for their headache. Physicians were never consulted by 85% of men and 72% of women who had one or more headaches over a 12-month period.[5] Most of these patients rely on over-the-counter medications and the majority are probably inadequately treated. Although the exact annual cost of migraine disability and treatment is unknown, estimates range from 1.4 to 17.2 billion dollars.[7]

The incidence of migraine actually peaks in early life[8] while the prevalence of migraine is highest between the ages of 25 and 55.[9] The prevalence of migraine also varies with race. Population-based studies show the prevalence to be highest for Caucasians and lowest for Asians.[10]

TABLE 19–2. International Headache Society (IHS) Criteria for Episodic Tension Headaches

A. At least 10 previous headaches episodes for filling criteria B–D listed below; number of days with such headaches: less than 180 per year or less than 15 per month
B. Headache lasting from 30 minutes to 7 days
C. At least two of the following pain characteristics:
   1. Pressure/tightening (nonpulsating) quality
   2. Mild or moderate intensity
   3. Bilateral location
   4. No aggravation with routine physical activity
D. Both of the following:
   1. No nausea or vomiting
   2. Photophobia and phonophobia are absent, or one but not the other is present

TABLE 19–3. International Headache Society (IHS) Criteria for Cluster Headaches

A. At least five attacks fulfilling criteria B–D
B. Severe unilateral orbital, supraorbital, and/or temporal pain lasting 15 to 180 minutes untreated
C. Headache associated with at least one of the following signs, which have to be present on the painful side:
   1. Conjunctival injection
   2. Lacrimation
   3. Nasal congestion
   4. Rhinorrhea
   5. Forehead and facial sweating
   6. Miosis
   7. Ptosis
   8. Eyelid edema
D. Frequency of attacks: from one to eight per day

A variety of neurologic and psychiatric disorders may also have an association with migraine. According to one study, epilepsy patients have twice the risk of developing migraine as those without seizures.[11] Stroke also appears to be related to migraine. The rate of stroke in migraine patients is approximately 1.44/100,000 per year if all other stroke factors are eliminated.[12] A variety of affective disorders are related to migraine, including depression, manic depressive illness, and panic disorder. The relationship of these neurologic and psychiatric conditions suggest a common genetic or environmental factor.[13]

Genetic Factors. A genetic basis for migraine has been long suggested by the observation that 70% to 90% of migraine patients have a positive family history.[14] Recently, Joutel et al[15] have linked familial hemiplegic migraine to chromosome 19. Evidence suggests that the defective gene encodes for a voltage-dependent P-type calcium channel.[16] A link to chromosome 19 has also been established for the entity known as CADASIL (cerebral autosomal dominant arteriopathy with subcortical infarcts and leukoencephalopathy). This is an autosomal dominant arteriopathy characterized by leukoencephalopathy and subcortical infarction. Other studies of familial hemiplegic migraine also suggest a link to chromosome 1 and a defect in calcium and potassium channels.[17, 18] Thus, accumulating data suggest that migraine in some instances may be a channelopathy, a condition that ultimately leads to neuronal hyperexcitability.

Pathophysiology

Pain-sensitive structures of the head and face include the skin and blood vessels of the scalp, the dura, the venous sinuses, the arteries, and the sensory fibers of the fifth, ninth, and tenth nerves (Fig. 19–1).

Although the precise mechanism of migraine remains uncertain, evidence suggests an important role for the trigeminal–vascular projections and the neurochemical serotonin.[19, 20] The trigeminal nerve has terminals on the pial and dural blood vessels that release a variety of vasoactive neuropeptides, including substance P, neurokinin A, and calcitonin gene-related peptide (CGRP) (Fig. 19–2). Release of these neuromediators produces sterile neurogenic inflammation by dilating meningeal blood vessels and increasing vascular permeability. Sumatriptan and dihydroergotamine (DHE) act on presynaptic 5-HT$_1$D receptors to block the release of these neuroactive peptides and 5HT$_1$B receptors to selectively constrict dilated meningeal vessels. In addition, 5HT$_1$B/D agonists such as zolmitriptan that cross the blood–brain barrier may also block neurons of the trigeminal nucleus caudalis within the medulla.[21]

Further evidence for the involvement of brain stem structures is supported by positron emission tomography studies that show increased blood flow in the reticular activating formation during the migraine episode.[22] The median raphe nucleus and the periaqueductal gray matter along with the locus ceruleus are regions thought to be activated during a migraine attack. In addition, activated parasympathetic projections from the superior salivatory nucleus may produce vasodilation of meningeal vessels. Projections from parasympathetic structures may also release nitric oxide and secondarily result in vasodilation and activation of perivascular and sensory nerves.[23]

The cause of the migraine aura is probably unrelated to a primary vasoconstrictive process. Blood flow studies have demonstrated reduced flow preceding the onset of the aura and continuing into the headache phase[24] (Fig. 19–3). One theory for the aura of migraine involves the concept of spreading depression.[25] This concept of cortical depression was promulgated by Leao,[26] who demonstrated that electrical depression moved over the cortex at a rate of 2 to 3mm per minute. The observation of Leao was supported by Lashley,[27] who calculated his own aura progressing over the visual cortex at the same rate of 2 to 3 mm per minute. Although blood flow reduction spreads over the cortex at this rate, it is believed to be a secondary event triggered by a primary neurogenic process. Lance[19] proposed that the neuroadrenergic locus ceruleus, which

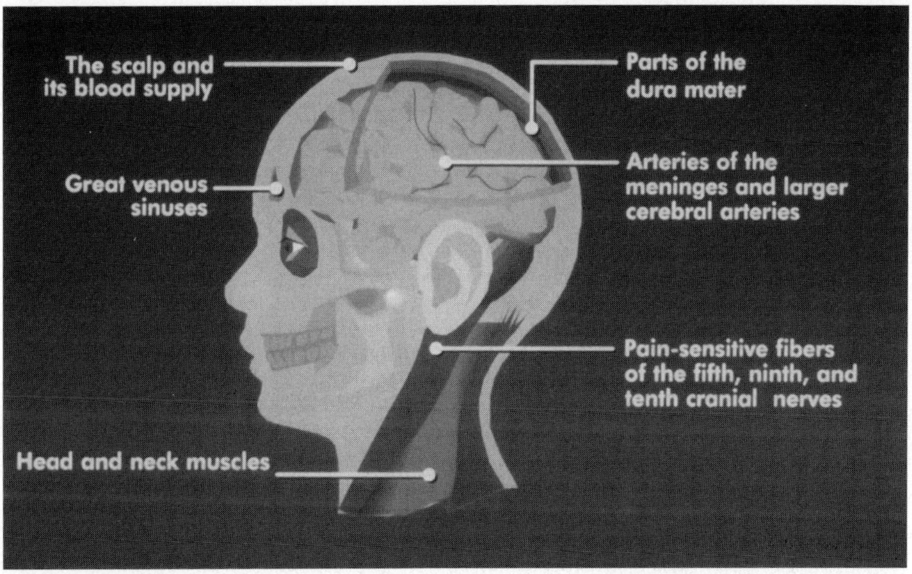

FIGURE 19–1. Pain-sensitive structures of the head and neck. The brain parenchyma itself does not sense pain. (From Novartis, with permission.)

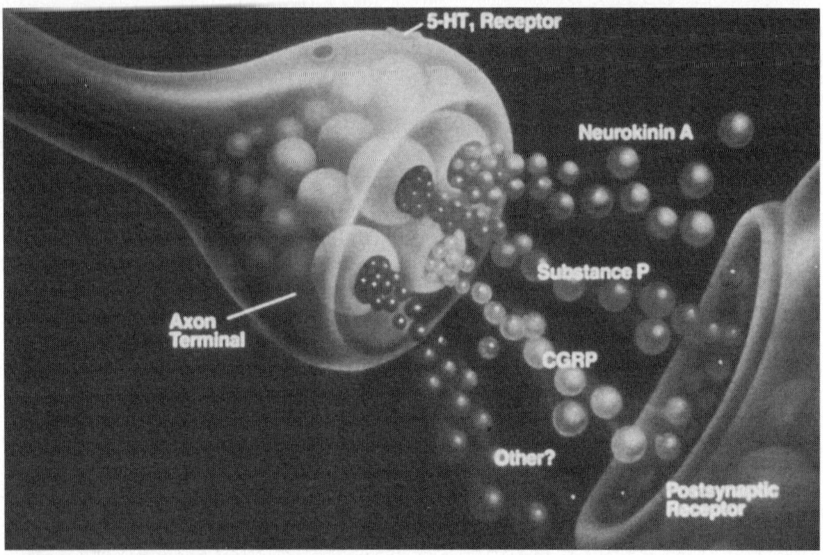

FIGURE 19–2. Trigeminal nerve terminal in close proximity to a pial blood vessel. Release of neurokinin A, substance P, and calcitonin gene-related peptide (CGRP) produces a sterile inflammation around the vessel. The $5HT_1$ receptor lies at the axon terminal. Binding of this receptor with a serotonin agonist such as sumatriptan blocks the release of the offending neuropeptides. (From Novartis, with permission.)

diffusely projects to the cerebral cortex, may be one neural network that triggers the migraine aura. Ultimately, the locus ceruleus and the spinal nucleus of the trigeminal nerve are influenced by the cortex and other higher structures.

Integrated Theory. At this time, the precise pathophysiology of migraine remains uncertain, but a cascade of events seems likely. In summary, migraine appears to be initiated by hyperexcitability of brain stem neurons (Fig. 19–4). The overactivation of these neurons may be the result of an underlying channelopathy seen in genetically predisposed individuals. Presumably, these hyperexcitable neurons are responsible for activating portions of the cortex (aura) and meningeal vessels (pain). The

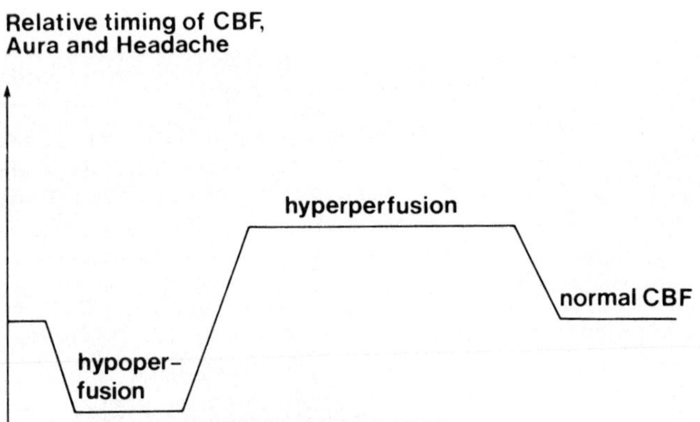

FIGURE 19–3. Schematic drawing illustrating the temporal relationship between angiography (time 1 hour) and provoked migraine. Hypoperfusion, aura, headache, hyperperfusion, disappearance of headache, and disappearance of hyperperfusion are diagrammed. The time axis is chosen to illustrate what is typical. It does not depict actually recorded times in a single patient or in a group of patients. (From Olesen J, et al: Ann Neurol 1990;28:794, with permission.)

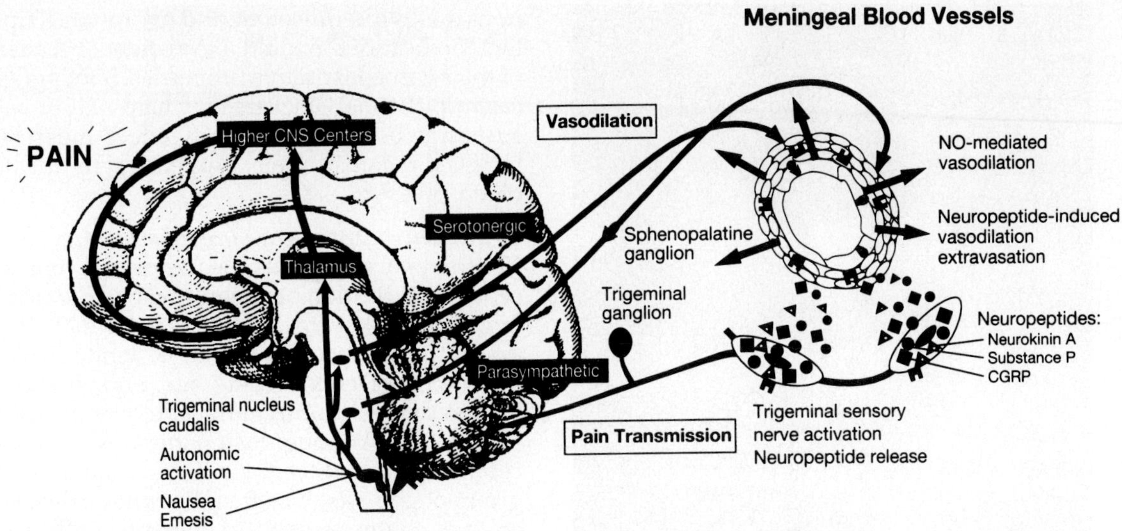

FIGURE 19–4. Migraine represented as a disorder of brain stem hyperexcitability. Overfiring of serotonin, parasympathetic, and trigeminal systems results in neuropeptide- and nitric oxide (NO)-mediated pial vessel inflammation and vasodilatation. (Courtesy of Merck & Co., Inc. U.S. Human Health Division, West Point, Pennsylvania, with permission.)

activation of these brain stem neurons may be influenced by internal and external factors such as hormonal balance, foodstuffs, stress, and sleep deprivation. The different symptoms observed in migraine probably reflect differential activation of cortical, brain stem; and vascular structures.

Symptoms and Signs

A variety of factors may provoke migraine, including menstruation, change in sleep patterns, hunger, stress, certain foods, odors, and even the type of lighting.[4] Hours to days before the onset of migraine, the patient may experience prodromal symptoms manifesting as mood swings, food cravings, anorexia, fluid retention, or urinary frequency.

Headache. The headache of migraine is usually unilateral, throbbing, and of moderate severity. It may start any time of the day or night, but has a tendency to start in the morning. The onset is usually gradual, and it is this feature that helps to distinguish migraine from a more ominous cause such as a subarachnoid hemorrhage. Migraine headaches usually last 4 to 72 hours, and may be exacerbated by physical exercise. A variety of symptoms may accompany the headache, including photophobia, phonophobia, osmophobia, nausea, vomiting, and autonomic symptoms (Table 19–1). Patients may become irritable, anxious, or depressed.

Aura. The aura of migraine usually begins before the headache phase but occasionally it will occur simultaneously or follow it. The most characteristic aura is visual, but sensory or motor dysfunction may also occur. The visual symptoms typically build up over several minutes and resolve by 20 to 40 minutes. Occasionally, the aura will extend to 60 minutes. Some patients will have recurrent auras during the day. Most patients are unable to determine whether the phenomenon occurred in one or both eyes. In fact, the vast majority of patients believe the hemifield disturbance occurred in one eye. Although fortification scotomas are the most characteristic visual disturbance, the patient may also complain of bright flashing lights or distorted vision. Some described the sensation as if they were looking through clouded or prismatic glass. Classically, an arc of flashing zigzag light starts in the paracentral area of one hemifield and expands peripherally. As the wave of visual disturbance travels across the visual field it may rotate or undulate. Other patients will experience tunnel vision or a disturbance in both hemifields. Unusual disturbances of vision may occur, such as palinopsia (perseveration of visual image) or the Alice in Wonderland syndrome. In the latter, the patient may appreciate objects as overly large, small, or distorted. Rare patients

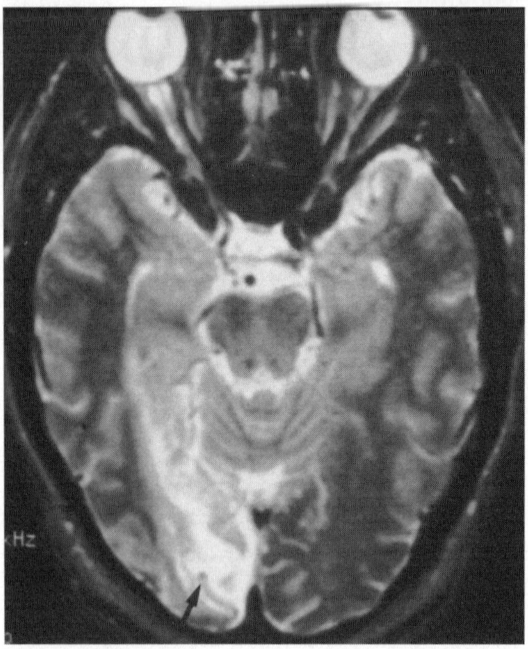

FIGURE 19–5. T_2-weighted image of patient with migrainous infarction, demonstrating high signal abnormality (*arrow*) in the right occipital lobe.

may experience persistent positive visual phenomena.[28] The various types of positive migraine visual aura are discussed in more detail and with figures in Chapter 12, and the negative visual auras (vision loss) in Chapter 10.

Sensory disturbance may include paresthesias, dysesthesias, or hyperesthesia. It is not unusual for the sensory symptoms to follow the headache. Classically, the sensory symptoms[19] begin in the fingertips and march up the arm and into the perioral area. Sensory auras are most convincingly migraine when they have been preceded by a classic visual aura. Most worrisome are aphasic and motor auras. Fortunately, these auras are uncommon.

Complicated Migraine

The term *complicated migraine* refers to a permanent neurologic deficit whether it be visual, motor, or sensory in origin. In these patients, magnetic resonance imaging (MRI) may demonstrate the cerebral ischemic changes that typically occur in the occipital–parietal regions (Fig. 19–5).

There is no effective therapy for evolving complicated migraine. We treat suspected complicated migraine with high-dose intravenous methylprednisolone and hydration. Triptan medications should be avoided because of their vasoconstrictive properties. Sublingual calcium channel blockers may help reduce vasospasm, but this beneficial effect must be weighed against their propensity to lower blood pressure.

Oral Contraceptives and Stroke in Migraine. Controversy surrounds the use of oral contraceptive medication in patients who suffer from migraine with aura. Migraine itself may significantly increase the risk of ischemic stroke in women of childbearing age, and in some studies the use of oral contraceptives enhanced this risk.[29–33] Although using low-dose contraceptives may reduce the risk of stroke in this group of patients, we often discourage the use of oral contraceptives in patients with migraine. The risk of stroke may be most significant in female migraineurs who are over the age of 35, use contraceptives, and smoke cigarettes.

Retinal Migraine

These events typically occur in one eye. Unlike the patient with occipital auras, the patient frequently experiences a negative visual phenomenon that is described as graying or a blackout of vision. The pattern of visual loss is often described as a tunnel, but may be altitudinal or quandrantic in nature.[34] As such, the diagnosis of retinal migraine is often one of exclusion, and a noninvasive evaluation in most patients is necessary. This usually consists of noninvasive studies of the neck, and checking for antiphospholipid antibodies. In some patients, echocardiography and a hypercoagulation workup will prove helpful to exclude a nonmigranous cause. Rarely, patients have permanent visual loss as the result of retinal or optic nerve damage (Table 19–4).[35,36] Observers have occasionally noted constriction of the retinal arterioles and venules during

TABLE 19–4. Ocular Complications of Migraine

Anterior ischemic optic neuropathy
Central retinal artery occlusion
Branch retinal artery occlusion
Central retinal vein occlusion
Retinal hemorrhage
Vitreous hemorrhage
Retinal pigment changes
Central serous chorioretinopathy

an attack (Fig. 19–6).[37] During these episodes, the retina will transiently lose its orange color. It seems likely that retinal changes are primarily induced by local vascular changes.[38] Calcium blockers have been particularly effective for these patients.[39] Occasionally, one aspirin a day will also reduce the frequency of retinal migraine.

This entity, and other types of transient visual loss in migraine, are also discussed in Chapter 10.

Ophthalmoplegic Migraine

This rare disorder usually begins before the age of 10 in the patient with an otherwise typical migraine pattern.[40] The ophthalmoplegia usually follows the headache by several days but occasionally it will occur simultaneously or precede it. The most common motility disturbance is a third nerve palsy, and the pupil is often involved.[41] Rarely, fourth and sixth nerve palsies or a combination of ocular motor palsies may be a manifestation of migraine. Clearly, other causes of a cavernous sinus syndrome need to be excluded fully in such situations. It usually takes 1 to 4 weeks for the ophthalmoparesis to resolve. After several episodes, a partial palsy may persist.

In patients under the age of 10, MRI should suffice to exclude most serious conditions when a pupil involving third nerve palsy is present. However, above age 10, an aneurysm is an increasing concern and arteriography is recommended. The differential diagnosis of ophthalmoplegic migraine includes an inflammatory or a neoplastic process involving the cavernous sinus, a posterior communicating artery aneurysm, herpes zoster ophthalmicus, and vasculopathic palsies.

The cause of the ophthalmoparesis in migraine is uncertain; the two leading possibilities are microvascular occlusion and swelling of the intracavernous carotid. In patients with recurrent attacks, prophylactic therapy has been tried with variable success. Because of the age of the patient, a beta blocker or calcium channel blocker is usually started.

This entity is also discussed in further detail in Chapter 15.

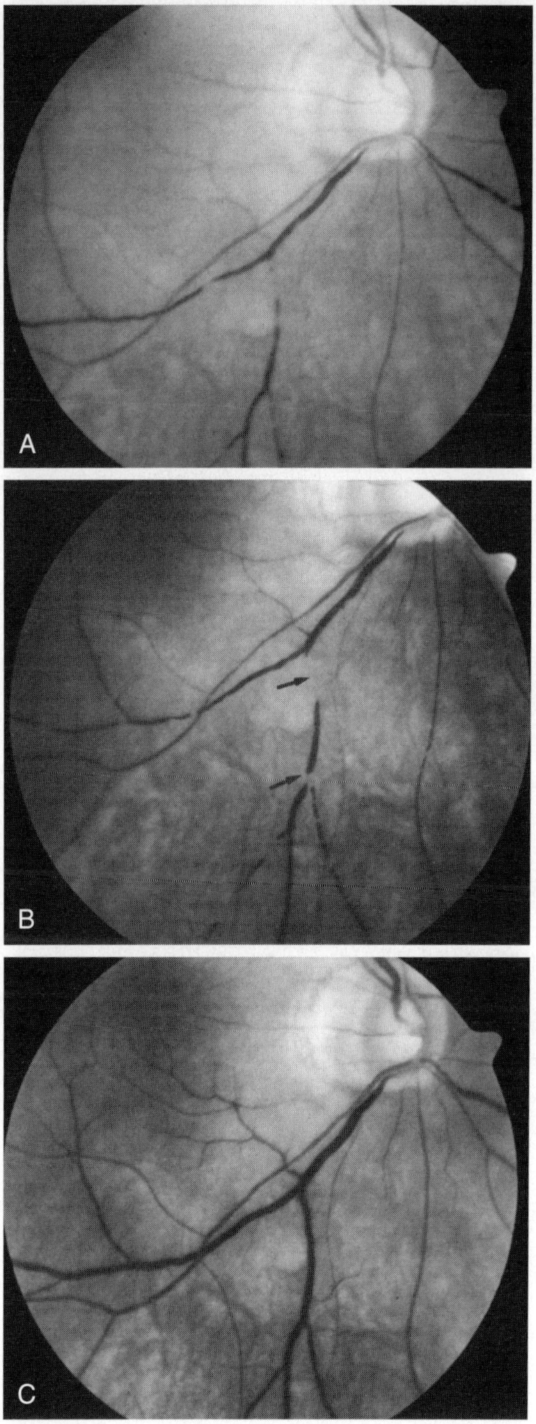

FIGURE 19–6. Patient with retinal migraine. **A.** Early in the attack, the retinal arteries and veins narrow and flow becomes segmented. The retina is pale in appearance. **B.** Later in the attack, gaps in retinal vein flow (*arrows*) become more obvious. **C.** After the attack, there is resumption of normal flow. (Photos courtesy of Dr. Jeffrey Bennett.)

Benign Episodic Mydriasis

Rarely, a dilated pupil may be a manifestation of migraine, and other signs of a third nerve palsy such as ptosis or ophthalmoparesis are absent. Angle-closure glaucoma should be excluded. This entity is discussed in more detail in Chapter 13.

Basilar (Bickerstaff) Migraine

These patients may experience transient symptoms of posterior circulation insufficiency, including visual field defects, vertigo, nystagmus, ataxia, impaired hearing, dysarthria, and motor and sensory symptoms.[42] Some patients may have an alteration of consciousness, presumably from involvement of the reticular activating system.[41] This disorder usually occurs in young women. This form of migraine may be the cause of episodic vertigo seen in young children. These patients may be more sensitive to the vasoconstrictive effects of triptan medication. As such, the triptan compounds are contraindicated in these groups of patients. Unfortunately, solid data regarding this important issue are lacking.

Hemiplegic Migraine

This disorder usually occurs early in life as a prelude to headache. This disorder has a male predominance and may be familial. The hemiplegia usually lasts less than 1 hour, but it may persist for several days. Like the sensory aura, the headache may precede the hemiplegia. Recently familial hemiplegic migraine has been linked to chromosome 19 and less frequently to chromosome 1. The gene defect in familial hemiplegia appears to result from a defect in the calcium channel.[16] Likewise, these patients may be overly sensitive to the triptan compounds and their use in this subgroup of patients should be avoided until further data are available.

Migraine and Vertigo

Patients with migraine commonly have vertigo as an associated symptom. In some patients, episodic vertigo may be the only complaint and confusion may exist with Meniere's disease. Although phonophobia is another common symptom in migraine, a small percentage of patients may experience acute permanent hearing loss. The episodes of vertigo may begin abruptly and last minutes to days.[132] It is quite common for them to occur without headache. These patients may also experience a variety of abnormalities on vestibular testing, including caloric paresis, spontaneous nystagmus, positional nystagmus, and abnormal rotary-chair testing.[43, 44] Baloh[45] has proposed that such patients may have a defective calcium channel manifesting within the inner ear and brain. The treatment is similar to that for other forms of migraine.

Diagnostic Testing in a Patient With Suspected Migraine

Visual fields should be assessed in all new patients with suspected migraine visual aura to exclude field defects. A homonymous defect, for instance, would suggest alternative diagnoses such as release hallucinations or seizures due to a neoplasm.

If the patient has a long history of typical migraine and a normal examination, it may be reasonable to defer neuroimaging. However, we have a low threshold for performing MRI in most patients because there are many causes of headache, and several organic disorders may mimic or even trigger migraine.[4] This is particularly true in patients with new onset of symptoms in middle age, atypical features, or marked increase in frequency of headache. Routine blood work is often unhelpful in young patients, but a sedimentation rate is extremely important in the elderly patients with transient loss of vision or headache to help exclude temporal arteritis. Lumbar puncture, almost always following neuroimaging, is an important test when suspecting a diagnosis of subarachnoid hemorrhage, meningitis, or pseudotumor cerebri.

Treatment

Migraine treatment depends on the frequency, duration, and intensity of the pain. Symptomatic or abortive treatment is most helpful when the attacks occur less than twice a week and are short lived (Table 19–5). Prophylactic or preventative therapy should be added when the headaches are more frequent.

Abortive Therapy

Mild to Moderate Headaches. There are many patients who find relief with acetaminophen, nonsteroidal anti-inflammatory drugs (NSAIDs), or aspirin. Many of these patients do not seek medical attention. In fact, the non-

TABLE 19–5. Pharmacologic Abortive Therapy in Migraine, Including Initial Dosages and Route of Administration

Triptan Medications	Dose	Route
Sumatriptan	50 mg	PO
Sumatriptan	20 mg	IN
Sumatriptan	6 mg	SQ
Naratriptan	2.5 mg	PO
Rizatriptan	5 mg, 10 mg	PO
Zolmitriptan	2.5 mg, 5.0 mg	PO
Nonsteroidal Anti-inflammatory Drugs (NSAIDs)		
Naproxyn	375 mg, 500 mg	PO
Indomethacin	75 mg	SR
Ketoralac	10 mg	PO
Antiemetics		
Droperidol	2.5 mg	IV
Prochlorperazine	2 mg to 10 mg	IV
Metoclopramide	10 mg	PO, IV
Corticosteroids		
Prednisone	60 mg	IV, PO
Methylprednisolone	60 mg	IV, PO
Miscellaneous		
Butorphanol	1 spray	IN
Butalbital, caffeine, and acetaminophen preparation	1–2 pills	PO
Isometheptene mucate	1–2 capsules	PO
Dihydroergotamine	0.5–1 mg	IV
	2 mg	IN
Ergotamine	2 mg	SL

IN = intranasal, IV = intravenous, PO = oral, SQ = subcutaneous, SR = sustained release, SL = sublinqual.

prescription combination of acetaminophen, aspirin, and caffeine may be quite effective. In one study, pain intensity was reduced to mild or none in 59.3% of treated patients compared to 32.8% of placebo patients, 2 hours after the dose.[46] NSAIDs are very helpful in patients with occasional headaches and may be used prophylactically in menstrual or orgasmic migraine.[4] NSAIDs are also very helpful for the brief lancinating pain that lasts seconds that plague certain migraine patients. These pains are referred to as ice-pick-like (idiopathic stabbing pain) and may occur over the scalp, particularly over the temporal regions.

Other options for abortive therapy in patients with mild to moderate headache include butorphanol nasal spray, a isometheptene–dichloralphenazone–acetaminophen combination, a butalbital–caffeine–acetaminophen combination, and oral ergotamine. We use the butalbital–caffeine–acetaminophen combination sparingly because of its high abuse potential and its tendency to produce rebound headaches when it is used frequently. Butorphanol nasal spray is a mixed opiate agonist–antagonist. It is effective in aborting 50% to 60% of migraine headaches. The dose is one spray in one nostril, which may be repeated in 1 hour if pain relief is inadequate. However, the abuse potential of butorphanol is high, which limits its routine use. Intranasal lidocaine (4% soln, 0.5-mL dose) may also abort migraine headaches. In one study, 55% of patients responded to intranasal lidocaine compared to 21% of placebo patients. However, 42% of the responders had a recurrence of their headache, usually within 30 to 60 minutes.[47]

Moderate to Severe Headache. For patients with moderate to severe pain, the options for therapy are also numerous. If the patient is not suffering from nausea, oral sumatriptan or one of the other triptans is an excellent option. The usual dose of sumatriptan is 50 mg, but a small number of patients benefit from a slightly higher dose.[48] The maximum single dose is 100 mg per day and the dosage taken over 24 hours should not exceed 200 mg. Patients with ischemic heart disease, poorly controlled hypertension, or Prinzmetal's angina should not receive sumatriptan or any other triptan. Sumatriptan should not be used within 24 hours of the patient taking an ergot-containing compound or with monoamine oxidase inhibitors (Physicians' Desk Reference, 2000). Sumatriptan should not be administered to patients with possible cerebral vasospasm such as those with hemiplegic or basilar migraine. The drug should be used with caution in menopausal women, males over 40, and patients with other cardiovascular risk factors. In these patients, a cardiovascular evaluation is warranted first before administering sumatriptan. Fortunately, serious cardiovascular events are rare and occur in less than one in a million treatments. Both electrocardiography and positron emission tomography perfusion studies suggest that most cases of chest pain associated with sumatriptan are not cardiac related.[49, 50] The main side effects of oral sumatriptan are paresthesias and nasal discomfort.[48] Subcutaneous and intranasal sumatriptan are important alternative routes of triptan administration. Since both of these routes of administration are quick, they may not be effective during the aura phase. Patients should be advised to take subcutaneous or intranasal sumatriptan at the headache onset. However oral sumatriptan may be taken at the onset of the aura, because of its slower onset.

Intranasal sumatriptan provides an alternative to injection for migraine patients needing quick onset or suffering from nausea.[51] The onset of action of intranasal sumatriptan may be as quick as 15 minutes, and at 2 hours approximately 62% of patients taking the 20-mg dose have responded.[51] This compares to the 81% response rate to subcutaneous sumatriptan and the 50% to 60% efficacy of oral sumatriptan at 2 hours. The major adverse effect of intranasal sumatriptan is a bitter taste that occurs in 25% to 30% of patients. Intranasal dihydroergotamine (DHE) may also be used, but it may be slightly less efficacious when compared to sumatriptan.[52] However, the recurrence rate is less frequent with intranasal DHE. Patients using the nasal form of sumatriptan should instructed to tilt their head forward during administration. This technique reduces the amount of the drug delivered to the gastrointestinal tract and helps eliminate some of the bitter taste.

Zolmitriptan is structurally similar to the serotonin agonist sumatriptan and has a high affinity for the $5HT_1D$ and $5HT_1B$ receptors.[53, 54] It was designed to enhance oral availability and, because of its greater lipid solubility, better penetrate the blood–brain barrier. Zolmitriptan at a dose of 2.5 mg improves headache pain in 65% to 67% of patients at 2 hours. At 4 hours 70% to 75% of patients have responded.[53, 54]

Naratriptan (2.5 mg) is also effective in the acute treatment of migraine.[55] It is well tolerated and its major advantage is its relatively long half-life of 6 hours. Therefore, it has its greatest utility in patients prone to recurrence of their migraine after an initial therapeutic response. As such it seems well suited for many patients who suffer from prolonged menstrual migraine. New $5HT_1B/D$ oral serotonin agonists such as eletriptan and rizatriptan are other alternatives.[56, 57, 133, 137] Rizatriptan (5 to 10 mg) comes in a wafer form, providing an alternative route of oral administration, even though its absorption is primarily in the gastrointestinal tract.[58] The wafer contains aspartame, so it may have limited use in patients who have their headache triggered by this artificial substance. Rizatriptan also interacts with propranolol, requiring the physician to half the dose of rizatriptan with concurrent use.[57, 59] Rizatriptan has efficacy rates similar to those of sumatriptan and zolmitriptan.

The decision of which triptan to use largely depends on the rapidity and the length of the migraine headache (Table 19–6). The presence of nausea and vomiting are other important considerations. For patients with rapid onset of headache and prominent gastrointestinal complaints, subcutaneous and intranasal sumatriptan tend to be most efficacious. Headaches of slower onset may be effectively treated with one of the oral triptans. For patients with prolonged or recurrent migraine, naratriptan may be most beneficial. Oral sumatriptan may not be as effective in children as in adults, however, the studies to date have been relatively small.[60] Intranasal sumatriptan may provide a better route of administration for children with acute migraine.[61]

Recent attention has been turned to the role of dopamine in migraine.[62, 63] Dopamine stimulation may induce the symptoms of migraine, including yawning, irritability, nausea, vomiting, and hypotension. In addition, dopamine receptor antagonists are effective in terminating acute migraine symptoms. Haloperidol, droperidol, prochlorperazine, chlorpromazine, and metoclopramide have been shown in small studies to be quite effective in treating acute migraine, with success rates in the 70% to 90% range.[62, 64, 65] Furthermore, metoclopramide may also have a beneficial effect in migraine prophylaxis. This effect correlates well with the agent's ability to block the D_2 dopamine receptor.[62, 66]

Currently there is no effective treatment for aborting the visual aura of migraine. Observation is usually the safest approach. In cases where it is suspected that migrainous infarction is about to evolve, one may try 10 mg of nifedipine sublingually, keeping in mind that hypotension is a possible side effect. Inhaled amyl nitrate and isoproterenol are alternatives but the efficacy of all these regimens are unproven.

Severe Migraine Headache in the Emergency Department. For the patient with severe pain and nausea, the following regimens may be tried:

1. Subcutaneous sumatriptan.[67, 68]
2. Intramuscular ketorolac 30 to 60 mg. Prochlorperazine 10 mg could also be given before the ketorolac to lessen nausea.
3. Intravenous dihydroergotamine. Prochlorperazine 10 mg is combined with 1 mg of dihydroergotamine. One half of the solution is given intravenously over 1 to 2 minutes. If chest pain ensues, the drug is discontinued. If there is no response, the remaining solution is administered in 15 to

TABLE 19–6. Comparison of Triptan Drugs

	Sumatriptan Injection	**Sumatriptan Oral**	**Sumatriptan Intranasal**	**Naratriptan Oral**	**Rizatriptan Oral**	**Zolmatriptan Oral**
Optimal dose	6 mg	50 mg	20 mg	2.5 mg	10 mg	2.5 mg
Efficacy						
% getting headache relief						
At 2 hours:	82%	50–61%	62%	40–50%	67–77%	62–65%
At 4 hours:	N/A	68–78%	62%	60–66%	84%[b]	78%
% experiencing recurrence[a]	36%	25–42%	30–41%	19–28%	33–47%	25–40%
Most common side effects	Injection site reactions: 59% Atypical sensations: 42% Dizziness: 12%	Tingling: 6% Fatigue: 2% Dizziness: 1%	Disturbance of taste: 24% Nausea &/or vomiting: 14% Nasal discomfort: 4%	Malaise/ fatigue: 2% Dizziness: 2% Drowsiness: 2%	Malaise/ fatigue: 7% Dizziness: 9% Drowsiness: 8%	Dizziness: 8% Drowsiness: 6%
Half-life ($t_{1/2}$)	2 hours	2 hours	2 hours	6 hours	2 hours	3 hours

[a] *Recurrence* is defined as headache relief followed by return of head pain within 24 hours, not due to rebound.
[b] Placebo response rate was high at 60%.

20 minutes. In rare cases of refractory migraine, dihydroergotamine 0.5 to 1 mg may be given every 8 hours for 3 days.
4. Intravenous prochlorperazine 10 mg. Boluses of 2 mg are given every 5 minutes until the headache abates or a total of 10 mg is given. When one administers prochlorperazine, it is important that the patient not drive home alone because of its sedative effect. Intravenous hydration is also a very effective adjunct as most patients with severe acute migraine have become dehydrated. Droperidol 2.5 mg IV every hour to a maximum of 10 mg can also be tried.[65, 69] Premedication with 1 mg of benztropine mesylate may help eliminate some of the side effects of this regimen.
5. A combination of 50% nitrous oxide (N_2O) and 50% oxygen, which was effective in one emergency room study of acute migraine.[70]
6. Intravenous valproic acid 10 mg/kg over 60 minutes.

TABLE 19–7. Pharmacologic Preventative Therapy in Migraine, Including Oral Daily Dosages

Beta Blockers	**Dose**
Propranolol	60–320 mg LA
Nadolol	40–160 mg
Metoprolol	50–200 mg
Atenolol	50–200 mg
Timolol	20–30 mg
Calcium Channel Blockers	
Verapamil	120–480 mg SR
Nifedipine	30–90 mg
Amlodipine	2.5–10 mg
Antidepressants	
Nortriptyline	50–150 mg
Amitriptyline	50–150 mg
Doxepin	75–300 mg
Fluoxetine	20–80 mg
Sertraline	50–100 mg
Anticonvulsants	
Valproic acid	500–2000 mg
Gabapentin	900–3600 mg
Topiramate	50–300 mg (slow titration)
Lamotrigine	50–300 mg (slow titration)
Other	
Lithium	600–1800 mg
Methysergide	2 mg three times per day

SR = sustained release.

Preventive Therapy

Preventive (prophylactic) therapy is indicated when headaches occur more than twice a week or produce significant disability, or when symptomatic therapy fails (Table 19–7). The goal of prophylaxis is to reduce or eliminate the need for acute therapy. Even if preventive therapy is not completely effective, it may render acute therapy more efficacious and lessen the risk of rebound headaches. Elimination of triggering factors such as certain foodstuffs, smoking, or alcohol (red wine, particularly) may also contribute to the effect of preventive therapy. Culprit foods include chocolate, cheeses, and nuts. We usually try to tailor preventive therapy to meet the individual needs of the patient. For instance, patients who are depressed may fare better with an antidepressant like nortriptyline, while other patients with mood swings might benefit from valproic acid. The medications most frequently used to prevent migraine headaches include (1) beta blockers, (2) calcium channel blockers, (3) antidepressants, and (4) anticonvulsants.

Beta Blockers. Most of these drugs have to be administered for at least a month to assess their efficacy. Beta blockers are often used as first-line agents and have an efficacy in the range of 60% to 80%.[71] Propranolol 60 mg LA (long-acting) is the usual starting dose, and patients are instructed to increase the dose to 120 mg LA after 5 days if the initial 60-mg dose is well tolerated. Thereafter, the dosage can be raised in 60-mg increments up to 320 mg a day. Occasionally, patients will not respond to propranolol but will to other beta blockers such as metroprolol or atenolol. Side effects of beta blockers include congestive heart failure, asthma, hypotension, bradycardia, and depression. Men may suffer reversible impotence. If the patient is headache free for 2 to 3 months, a taper of the beta blocker over several weeks can be attempted.

Calcium Channel Blockers. Calcium channel blockers are also an excellent choice for prophylactic therapy.[72] One of their main advantages is their limited side effects in most patients. Constipation, arrhythmias, heart failure, and hypotension are among the most common side effects. Verapamil is an excellent choice in this category. The initial dose is usually 120 mg SR (sustained release), which can be increased by 120-mg SR increments as necessary. Most patients respond by 360 mg, but occasionally 480 mg a day is necessary. Verapamil works in 60% to 70% of patients with migraine. Amlodipine is another good alternative. Doses of 2.5 to 5.0 mg are usually sufficient.

Antidepressants. Antidepressants are also highly effective, particularly when patients have sleeping problems, depressive symptoms, or a combination of migraine and tension-type headaches. Amitriptyline and nortriptyline seem to be the most effective in this category although some patients may respond to fluoxetine, nefazodone hydrochloride, sertraline hydrochloride, venlafaxine hydrochloride, and desipramine.[73] It is those compounds that block norepinephrine uptake that seem to be the most effective. Nortriptyline is typically chosen over amitriptyline because the latter has more anticholinergic side effects. In addition, these compounds produce dry mouth, constipation, urinary retention, tachycardia, and weight gain. Nortriptyline is started at either 10 or 25 mg depending on the size and age of the patient. From there, the dosage can be increased as necessary. If symptoms have not improved by 75 mg at bedtime, it is often useful to check a drug level before proceeding to higher doses. Most patients, if they are going to respond to nortriptyline, will do so by 100 mg a day.

Anticonvulsant Drugs. Recently anticonvulsant drugs, in particular valproic acid, have proven to be very effective in the prevention of migraine.[74,75] Carbamazepine and phenytoin may be used with more variable success. Gabapentin also shows significant promise in the treatment of both migraine and chronic daily headaches.[76] High doses of gabapentin in the 2400 to 3600 mg per day range may be necessary to achieve a beneficial effect. Valproic acid may be started at 125 mg twice a day and slowly increased to 500 to 1000 mg per day in divided doses. Patients often do not require large doses for a therapeutic effect. The side effects of valproate are nausea, alopecia, tremor, and weight gain. Hepatoxicity is a concern, particularly in young children on multiple medications. Since valproic acid is teratogenic and associated with a 1% risk of neural tube defects, this drug needs to be used with caution in women of childbearing age. They should be advised of the risk and use appropriate contraception. The anticonvulsant drugs may be best utilized in patients with cardiac disease or mood disorders, or in those with concerns regarding exercise intolerance. Newer anticonvulsants such as topiramate and lamotrigine have also been successful in the treatment of vascular headache.[77]

Miscellaneous Drugs. Riboflavin in high doses (400 mg per day) may be effective in migraine prevention. Riboflavin may enhance a deficient mitochondrial energy reserve, a potential factor in the genesis of migraine.[78] Magnesium deficiency in the brain has also been suggested as a potential mechanism of migraine. Unfortunately, magnesium supplementation has not been convincingly effective.[79] Intermittent use of oral sumatriptan or naratriptan may be effective in treating menstrual migraine. One regiment used 25 mg of sumatriptan three times per day for a total of 5 days.[80] Transdermal estrogen, ergotamine tartrate, and NSAIDS may be used as prophylaxis for menstrual-related migraine.[134] Cyproheptadine is frequently used as migraine prophylaxis in children.

Acephalgic Migraine

Patients with migraine may have transient neurologic events without headache. When these events occur in patients over the age of 40, concern over the possibility of a transient ischemic attack (TIA) is raised. In any age group, seizures may also be considered. Fortunately, there are some features that may differentiate these disorders. The migraine aura has a characteristic buildup of scintillations. The episodes may occur in a flurry and tend to last longer than a typical TIA. Patients often have a remote history of migraine headaches. Some even have mild accompanying discomfort but do not think it is important to report it. The intensity of their headache is often not as severe as it was previously.

In a relatively young patient with visual aura without headache, but with a previous history of migraine, further testing may not be necessary. However, in patients over age 40, the new onset of acephalgic migraine is a diagnosis of exclusion. Workup would include neuroimaging to exclude a structural lesion of the occipital cortex such as an arteriovenous malformation or meningioma and to check for ischemic changes. In some instances electroencephalography can be performed to rule out an irritative lesion. When the aura is characterized by visual loss, cardiac emboli, carotid insufficiency, and hypercoagulable states should also be considered.

Treatment of Acephalgic Migraine. If tolerated, 325 mg of aspirin per day may be given, particularly in elderly individuals in whom the diagnosis may not be certain. It may lessen acephalgic migraine episodes and help prevent stroke in case the events were in fact TIAs. In patients in whom aspirin is ineffective or not tolerated, calcium channel blockers such as verapamil, 120 to 360 mg (SR) per day, can be considered for those with recurrent disabling episodes. In many instances, patients are reassured knowing that their visual episodes are migrainous and benign, and choose to eschew pharmacologic treatment.

OTHER HEADACHE TYPES

Tension Type Headaches

Tension headaches are probably a continuum of migraine headaches (Fig. 19–7). The pain is mild to moderate in intensity and is often described as pressure or tightness. There is no aura, nausea, or vomiting, and the headaches are usually not aggravated by exercise. Photophobia and phonophobia are rarely present. The location of the headache is often bilateral. Common locations for tension headaches are over the eyes, on top of the head, over the temples, and over the occipital region. These patients often have tender spots over the shoulder girdle muscles. Most tension headaches are episodic. However, some patients have chronic tension-type headaches and are without pain-free intervals.[81] The International Headache Society has compiled a set of criteria for episodic tension headache similar to those of migraine (Table 19–2).

Many patients with chronic daily tension headaches have a history of migraine. In fact, migraine episodes may periodically occur in such patients. A significant proportion of this patient population has concurrent depression. In patients with tension headache, one also has to be aware of the possibility of secondary headache disorders or rebound headaches from over-the-counter analgesic abuse (see below).

Treatment. Patients with tension headaches, particularly those with chronic daily headaches, pose a therapeutic challenge. The abortive and prophylactic medications used to treat migraine may be tried in patients with tension headaches. The antidepressants nortriptyline and amitriptyline may be the first-line agents for these patients. It is important to make sure that patients with tension headaches do not have temporomandibular joint dysfunction or sinus disease before committing them to preventive therapy. Some tension headache patients do not respond to medication and may benefit from alternative therapies, including stretching exercises, meditation, and acupuncture. Botulinum toxin injected into the frontal and occipital muscles has been tried in refractory tension headache.[82]

Rebound Headache

These type of headaches share similar clinical characteristics with tension headaches as described above. However, there is the complicating history of long-standing misuse of headache medications. Although rebound headache is classically associated with overuse of narcotics or other over-the-counter analge-

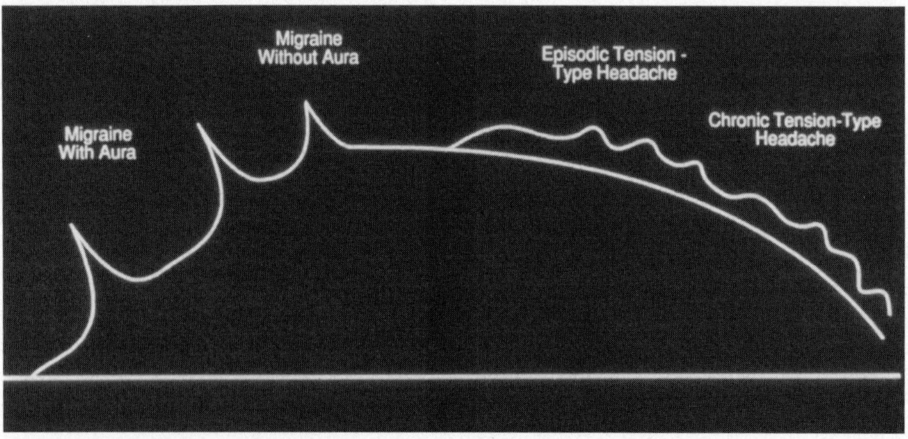

FIGURE 19–7. Tension and migraine headaches may represent a continuum of severity, frequency, and associated findings. (Modified from Raskin NH. In: Headache, 2nd edition, New York, Churchill Livingstone, 1988; Ch. 5, with permission.)

sics, this phenomenon also may be observed to a lesser degree with triptan and ergot overuse.

Treatment. In this condition, it is important to taper the overused medication. If not already contributing to the problem, NSAIDs or a short course of corticosteroids may help ameliorate some of the patient's symptoms. If outpatient detoxification fails, inpatient management may be necessary. Intravenous dihydroergotamine 1 mg combined with 10 mg of intravenous metoclopramide every 8 hours for 3 to 5 days is one effective regimen to treat analgesic overuse.

Cluster Headache

Cluster headache is a severe unilateral headache disorder that predominantly occurs in middle-aged men (Table 19–3). The ratio of men to women with this disorder ranges from 5 to 7:1.[83] These headaches occur in clusters or on a daily basis for weeks to months. Although most cluster headaches are usually episodic, in 10% of patients they are chronic and without remission.[83] Cluster headaches are often severe and may awaken a patient from sleep. They typically occur over the periorbital region and are often associated with rhinorrhea and tearing. Alcohol is a common trigger. The attacks are much shorter than migraine, lasting 1/2 hour to 3 hours. There is often no nausea or vomiting; aura is rare but can occur.[138] About 30% to 50% of patients will develop signs of a Horner syndrome (Fig. 19–8). Occasionally, only ptosis or miosis will be present. After several attacks, a permanent Horner syndrome may ensue. In contrast to the migraine patient who desires sleep, the cluster headache patient cannot stand still. The headache is so severe that some patients literally run around the room screaming, and some patients even contemplate suicide. In between the attacks, some patients will suffer typical migraine headaches.

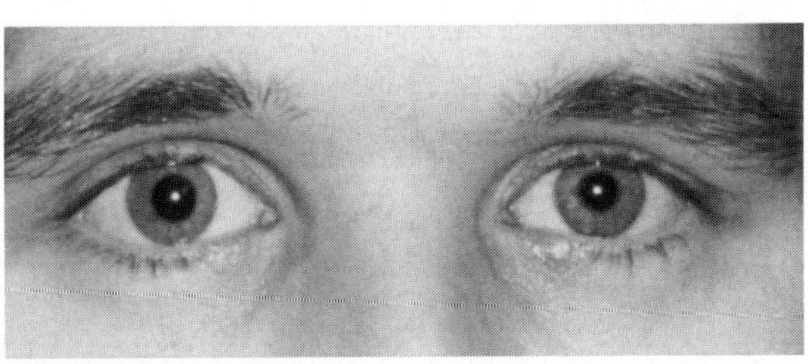

FIGURE 19–8. Patient with left Horner syndrome during cluster attack.

The major entity to exclude in a patient with a painful Horner syndrome is a carotid dissection (see Chapter 13 for further discussion). Other entities that may mimic cluster headaches include (1) arteriovenous malformation,[84] (2) brain stem compression by tumor,[85] (3) vertebral artery aneurysm,[86] (4) cavernous carotid artery aneurysms,[87] (5) sinusitis, (6) temporal arteritis, and (7) the Tolosa–Hunt syndrome. In patients presenting with a painful Horner syndrome, MRI of the neck, including axial T_1-weighted images and angiographic sequences, is recommended to exclude carotid dissection.

Treatment. The treatment of acute cluster attack may be difficult. In the emergency department, the following regimens may be tried:

1. 100% oxygen therapy via a face mask for 10 minutes.
2. Subcutaneous or intranasal sumatriptan.
3. Intranasal or intravenous dihydroergotamine.
4. Intranasal lidocaine 4%.
5. Corticosteroids (2-week prednisone taper).

Corticosteroids often take hours to begin to work. However, they may be useful in transition to other preventive therapies in cluster headache patients. The two most effective preventive therapies are lithium and verapamil.[135] Other options include methylsergide and twice-daily ergotamine therapy. Methylsergide should not be used for more than 3 months at a time because of the rare complication of retroperitoneal fibrosis. Indomethacin may provide benefit to certain patients, and valproic acid may also provide effective prophylaxis.

Occasionally, patients are refractory to monotherapy, and combination therapy may be necessary. Verapamil and lithium are usually tried together first. Valproate and verapamil is another effective combination.

Rare patients may require intravenous dihydroergotamine every 8 hours to break the cluster bout. If all medical therapy fails and headaches are strictly unilateral, then radiofrequency thermocoagulation of the gasserian ganglia may be tried.[88] However, the resultant corneal and trigeminal anesthesia may lead to their own set of complications.

Paroxysmal Hemicrania

Paroxysmal hemicrania refers to a headache syndrome characterized by brief episodes of unilateral pain lasting 2 to 45 minutes. The pain tends to occur over the orbital and temporal regions. Patients often experience multiple attacks a day and some have 40 to 50 attacks in a 24-hour period.[89] The pain is typically associated with autonomic dysfunction such as conjunctival injection, lacrimation, nasal congestion, ptosis, and eyelid edema. There are many similarities between paroxysmal hemicrania and cluster headache. Paroxysmal hemicrania is distinguished by its female predominance, shorter duration, and response to indomethacin.[83] Although indomethacin is a treatment of choice for paroxysmal hemicrania, other patients may respond to verapamil, acetazolamide, or other NSAIDs.[83] Some patients with paroxysmal hemicrania will have superimposed mild and dull hemicranial discomfort between episodes.

SUNCT Syndrome

The acronym for this syndrome stands for "*s*hort-lasting, *u*nilateral, *n*euralgiform headache with *c*onjunctival injection, and *t*earing." This rare condition is similar to the paroxysmal hemicranias, but is distinguished by less severe pain, more marked autonomic activation, and unresponsiveness to indomethacin.[89]

Ice Pick Headache (Idiopathic Stabbing Headache)

Some patients experience sudden stabbing pain that may be described as like being stabbed with an ice pick (Fig. 19–9).[89] The pain is often located in the temple region but the occipital area may also be involved. The pain often lasts seconds, but may persist for minutes. Many patients have underlying migraine or tension headaches. The pain may occur several times a day and may awaken the patient from sleep. Occasionally, the examiner can palpate the area and elicit the pain. The pain of a corneal erosion may be brief and present upon awakening and should be carefully considered in the patient with stabbing pain concentrated around the eye. Patients with stabbing pain respond best to indomethacin or other NSAIDs.

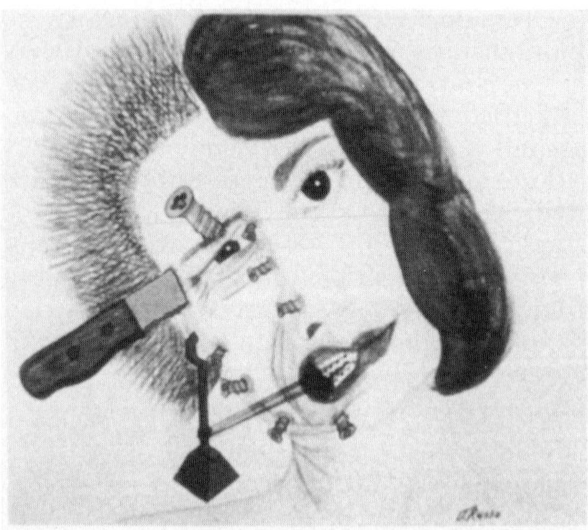

FIGURE 19–9. Artist's rendition of the pain of idiopathic stabbing headache. (From Novartis, with permission.)

Cough Headache

Patients with cough headache may be divided into two broad groups. First, cough-induced headaches may be associated with an intracranial lesion. The posterior fossa is the most frequent location for a lesion producing cough headache. An Arnold–Chiari malformation is a relatively common cause, but tumors and subdural hematomas are other reported causes.

Patients in the second group with cough-induced headache have no detectable intracranial lesions despite extensive investigation. These patients often respond to a course of indomethacin or other NSAID.

Thunderclap Headache

Thunderclap headache is a term used to describe a sudden and severe headache. Although controversy exists regarding the significance of such a headache, we believe an intracerebral hemorrhage or even an unruptured aneurysm has to be strongly considered. Raps et al[90] concluded that thunderclap headache may be induced by a variety of mechanisms, including thrombosis of the aneurysm, expansion of the aneurysm, or intramural hemorrhage. Some patients with thunderclap headache have no identifiable cause. Patients with thunderclap headache should be evaluated with emergent computed tomography (CT) and lumbar puncture. If both are negative, and the suspicion remains high for an unruptured aneurysm, MRI-angiography should be performed.

Greater Occipital Neuralgia

Some patients experience episodic pain in the greater occipital region. Occasionally the pain will radiate forward toward the ipsilateral eye. The pain usually only lasts seconds, but may recur frequently during the day. The patient typically has pain at the point where the greater occipital nerve pierces the tendinous insertion of the splenius capitus muscle at the skull base. Many patients have superimposed tension and migraine headaches.

Treatment with local injection of lidocaine has a high success rate. Occasionally repeated injections are necessary to break the cycle. If patients do not respond or are reluctant to have a local lidocaine injection, NSAIDS, carbamazepine, gabapentin, or a short course of corticosteroids may be tried.

Hypnic Headache

Elderly patients may experience headaches shortly after falling asleep.[91] The headache is throbbing and global in location. These headaches are short lived and usually resolve within an hour. This disorder is also recognized in the young patient and may be unilateral. Lithium may prevent the headaches, but the side effects of this medication in the elderly population may limit its use.

Carotid Dissection

Patients with acute carotid dissection may develop throbbing pain over the periorbital area.[41] Most patients will have accompanying neurologic signs such as a Horner syndrome or ipsilateral visual loss. A patient with an isolated painful Horner syndrome should be considered to have a carotid dissection until proven otherwise. Other clinical manifestations, radiographic features, and management of this condition are discussed in detail in Chapter 13.

Temporal Arteritis

The headache of temporal arteritis is often described as an ache concentrated over the temporal arteries. The pain can be severe and the area exquisitely sensitive to touch. Although the pain is often concentrated over the temporal region, it may occur over any portion of the head. The pain of giant cell arteritis typically abates within days of starting corticosteroids. This condition, particularly with regard to visual loss, pathophysiology, and management, is reviewed in Chapter 5.

Posttraumatic Headache

Mild to moderate headaches are common after head injury. Patients may or may not have experienced a loss of consciousness. Typically, the headache is one of many symptoms that accompany the posttraumatic syndrome. Vertigo, irritability, concentration difficulty, and short-term memory loss are other frequent complaints. The posttraumatic headache may simulate tension headaches or migraine headaches. The headache may improve spontaneously or persist indefinitely. The International Headache Society criteria require the onset of the headache within 2 weeks after the injury or upon return of consciousness.[2, 3] Migraine, common daily headache, and cluster may follow mild head trauma. Posttraumatic headaches may last for several years, regardless of financial compensation issues. If tolerated, antidepressant compounds may reduce some of the symptoms. Other prophylactic headache medications such as propranolol, verapamil, and valproic acid may also be tried with variable success.

Glossopharyngeal Neuralgia

Patients with glossopharyngeal neuralgia experience pain in the pharynx and base of the tongue. The pain may be triggered by swallowing, coughing, or talking. Like trigeminal neuralgia, the pain is usually sharp, stabbing, or lacinating. The condition is usually idiopathic but mass lesions should be carefully considered. Most cases result from compression by a dolichoectatic artery or venous structure. Treatment of glossopharyngeal neuralgia is similar to trigeminal neuralgia and includes anticonvulsants, antidepressants, and baclofen therapy. If medical therapy fails, the glossopharyngeal nerve may be thermocoagulated. Other patients may benefit from microvascular decompression.

Intracranial Hypotension

Headache is a prominent symptom of the patient suffering from intracranial hypotension. Patients may have associated nausea, vomiting, tinnitus, and photophobia. The hallmark feature of this disorder is pain aggravated by an upright posture.[92] Some patients will develop unilateral or bilateral sixth nerve palsies resulting from the traction on these nerves as the brain sinks downward from the intracranial hypotension.[93] Rarely, patients may complain of transient visual obscurations or blurred vision, and binasal field defects have been documented.[94] The downward displacement of the brain is frequently evident on sagittal MRI, and diffuse meningeal enhancement is often present.[95, 96, 136] If severe, bilateral subdural hematomas or organized hygromas may evolve.

Of course, most commonly the cause intracranial hypotension is iatrogenic, induced by lumbar puncture, spinal anesthesia, or shunting.[97, 98] Other causes of intracranial hypotension include traumatic injury, particularly those that lead to cerebrospinal fluid (CSF) rhinorrhea. Spontaneous intracranial hypotension may also occur when there is a spontaneous tear of the dura, especially along a spinal nerve root sleeve.[92] The source of the cerebrospinal fluid leak may be established with radionuclide cisternography or metrizamide myelography. In our experience, these tests have a low diagnostic yield.

Even, if no source of CSF leak is found, patients may still respond to blood patching.[92] If the source of the CSF leak is found, it should be repaired, if possible. Other nonspecific treatment measures include bedrest, caffeine, volume expansion, corticosteroids, and the use of an abdominal binder. In refractory cases, intrathecal saline solution may be tried. Some antecdotal success using theophylline has been reported in refractory cases.[92]

Intracranial Hypertension Without Papilledema

A small group of patients with chronic daily headaches may have raised intracranial pressure without evidence of papilledema.[99] These patients may be distinguished from other patients with chronic daily headaches by a high frequency of pulsatile tinnitus and obesity. Unfortunately, therapies aimed at lowering the increased intracranial pressure may not reduce the headaches. Intracranial hypertension without and with papilledema is also discussed in Chapter 6.

HEADACHES AND OCULAR DISEASES

A variety of ocular conditions may be associated with eye or periorbital pain. Headaches of ocular origin are often accompanied by other eye signs such as conjunctival or sclera injection. The frequency and intensity of the pain is often dependent on the ocular structure affected.

Corneal Diseases

Among the most common causes of periorbital discomfort is dry eyes. These patients complain of a gritty, achy, or burning sensation. These patients may have associated dry mouth and Sjögren syndrome. The diagnosis of dry eyes is established by checking the slit-lamp examination for a quick breakup of the tear film or punctate corneal epithelial defect or by performing the Schirmer test. An abnormal Schirmer test occurs when there is less than 15 mm of strip wetting at 5 minutes. The dry eye syndrome may be treated with lubricants or artificial tears. Dry eye as a cause of transient visual loss is discussed in Chapter 10.

Severe pain and foreign body sensation in one eye upon awakening suggests the possibility of recurrent corneal erosion. Slit-lamp examination can confirm a corneal epithelial defect. Corneal erosion may occur on an idiopathic basis, after previous corneal abrasion, or in association with a corneal dystrophy.

Intraocular Causes

Scleritis, iritis, and uveitis may be associated with severe eye pain. The pain may be referred to other regions of the face, but most often is concentrated over the eye. The eye may be exquisitely tender to palpation in this situation and photophobia is universal.

Angle closure glaucoma may be associated with variable pain, ranging from virtually none to severe. The patient's pain may be triggered by walking into a dark room or from pupillary dilation. The pain may be throbbing and associated with nausea and vomiting. As such, patients with angle-closure glaucoma may be thought to have migraine. Since the patients may have associated visual loss, temporal arteritis may also be confused with angle-closure glaucoma. The patient with angle-closure glaucoma often has a red eye and a cloudy cornea during the episode. The diagnosis of angle-closure glaucoma is established by slit-lamp examination, tonometry, and gonioscopy to evaluate the angle of the eye.

Optic Nerve Diseases

Nearly 90% of patients with optic neuritis have periocular pain. In fact, the absence of pain in such a situation raises the possibility of an alternative cause. The pain of optic neuritis usually occurs upon eye movements and the eye may be tender, but in some patients it manifests as a dull periocular ache. Pain may also rarely accompany anterior ischemic optic neuropathy (AION). Although pain has been described with nonarteritic AION, an arteritic process always needs to be strongly considered until proven otherwise.[100] Pain on eye movement may also accompany orbital myositis or idiopathic inflammatory orbital pseudotumor.

Eye Strain

Many patients attribute their headaches to eye strain. However, eye strain is a relatively uncommon cause of headaches presenting to a physician. Pain is often described as aching and is relieved by resting or not reading. The pain often begins over the brow and may spread to other scalp muscles. Often, an uncorrected hyperopic refractive error or an ocular motility problem such as convergence insufficiency is found in patients with headaches related to eye strain. Some patients will have eye strain while getting adjusted to a new pair of glasses.

Photophobia

Pain produced by a bright light is known as photophobia. The pain is transmitted to the brain stem from the ophthalmic division of the trigeminal nerve. As discussed above, migraine may be associated with photophobia. Even between episodes of headache, migraine patients may have a heightened sensitivity to glare. Migraine patients may have impaired inhibitory subcortical function that normally suppresses glare-induced pain.[101] Photophobia may also be symptom of meningeal irritation, and such a possibility should always be carefully considered in patients with light sensitivity. A variety of ocular inflammatory disorders may also be associated with photophobia. However, many patients have no clear cause for their photophobia. Tinted glasses or lenses that block ultraviolet ray transmission may help relief the discomfort of photophobia.

Miscellaneous

Table 19–8 outlines some other causes of headache not reviewed in the text.

TABLE 19–8. The Differential Diagnosis of Other Miscellaneous Headache Disorders and Their Clinical Features

Entity	Onset	Location	Pain Characteristics	Duration	Associated Symptoms	Diagnostic Evaluation
Subarachnoid hemorrhage	Acute	Global, occipital	Worst ever	Brief or prolonged	Meningismus	CT, LP
Brain tumor	Subacute	Focal	Dull pressure	Prolonged	Focal signs	Brain MRI
Painful eye movements	Acute	Retrobulbar	Sharp	Days	Optic neuritis—reduced vision myositis—ptosis, diplopia	Orbit MRI
Hypertension	Acute	Frontal, occipital	Throbbing	Brief	Focal signs suggest hemorrhage	Consider CT
Pseudotumor cerebri	Subacute	Bifrontal	Dull or throbbing	Prolonged	Pulsatile tinnitus, papilledema, transient visual obscuration	Neuroimaging, then LP
Meningitis	Acute or chronic	Neck	Throbbing severe	Brief or prolonged	Fever, meningismus	LP

CT = computed tomography; MRI = magnetic resonance imaging; LP = lumbar puncture.

FACIAL PAIN AND DISORDERS OF FACIAL SENSATION

Approach

Many patients with facial pain will suffer from migraine or local conditions such as sinusitis or dental disease. However, a group of patients with facial pain will have sensory or motor dysfunction within the trigeminal nerve distribution. Trigeminal nerve dysfunction commonly manifests with sensory changes such as paresthesias, dysethesias, or anesthesia. Other patients complain of paroxysmal or chronic facial pain.

Understanding the nature of the patient's complaint is often critical in establishing a proper diagnosis. For example, the lancinating, excruciating pain of trigeminal neuralgia must be distinguished from the more tolerable yet disturbing paresthesias of trigeminal sensory neuropathy. The temporal profile of symptom onset often provides invaluable diagnostic clues. For instance, sudden complaints of sensory loss, paresthesias, or motor dysfunction in the face are consistent with vascular, traumatic, or demyelinating processes, whereas similar complaints developing over weeks to months are more suggestive of neoplastic or infiltrative processes.

Neuroanatomy

The trigeminal nerve is a mixed nerve conveying both sensory input from and motor information to the face. Sensory neurons of the trigeminal fibers V_1 to V_3 lie in the gasserian ganglion, which is embedded in the temporal bone within the middle cranial fossa.[102, 103] The dura-lined cavity in the middle cranial fossa that surrounds the gasserian ganglion and its branches as they exit into the petrous temporal bone is known as Meckel's cave. From the gasserian ganglion, three trigeminal divisions proceed forward and exit from distinct skull-base foramina: V_1 exits the superior orbital fissure, V_2 via foramen rotundum, and V_3 via the foramen ovale (Fig. 19–10).

The *ophthalmic division* (V_1) is entirely sensory, and its branches innervate the orbit and the eye (lacrimal and nasociliary branches), upper eyelid, forehead and nose (frontal branches), nasal cavity, and nasal sinus (nasociliary branches) (Fig. 19–11). V_1 passes within the cavernous sinus, where it lies inferolateral to the oculomotor, trochlear, and abducens nerves. From the cavernous sinus, V_1 extends through the superior orbital fissure in association with the ocular motor nerves before dividing into lacrimal, frontal, and nasociliary nerves. Cutaneous fibers reach the skin via the supraorbital foramen along the ridge of the brow (Fig. 19–11). V_1 sensory fibers provide afferents for the corneal reflex. Smaller tentorial and dural branches innervate the tentorium and dura mater.[104] The trigeminal system also provides inputs to the intracranial vessels (trigeminovascular system) that are considered important in the pathogenesis of migraine (see earlier discussion of migraine pathophysiology). Autonomic fibers that originate from the facial nerve run with the lacrimal nerve of V_1 to innervate the lacrimal gland.

The *maxillary division* (V_2) is also completely sensory and innervates the skin of the cheek, upper lip, maxillary sinus, nasopharynx, soft and hard palate, and upper teeth. A small meningeal branch follows the middle meningeal artery and supplies dura.[104] These fibers leave the gasserian ganglion and run inferior within the cavernous sinus before exiting the foramen rotundum. V_2 axons pass through the pterygopalatine fossa to exit the infraorbital foramen. The cutaneous branches of V_2 include the zygomaticotemporal, zygomaticofacial, and infraorbital nerves (Fig. 19–11). Branches innervating the nasopharynx and maxillary sinus include the greater lesser palatine nerves, the nasopalatine nerves, and pharyngeal nerve. V_2 also supplies innervation to the upper teeth, maxillary sinus, and palate via the anterior, middle, and posterior superior alveolar nerves, respectively. Autonomic fibers that originate in the facial nerve (superior salivatory) nuclei accompany V_2 branches and comprise the superficial petrosal nerve. Superficial petrosal nerve fibers synapse within the pterygopalatine ganglion and provide parasympathetic input to the lacrimal, nasal, and palatine glands. Fibers of the superficial petrosal nerve join the deep petrosal nerve to form the nerve of the pterygoid canal. The deep petrosal nerve is a branch of the internal carotid plexus and carries postganglionic sympathetic fibers from the superior cervical ganglion to the lacrimal glands.

The *mandibular division* (V_3) carries both sensory fibers from and motor axons to the lower face. V_3 axons leave the gasserian gan-

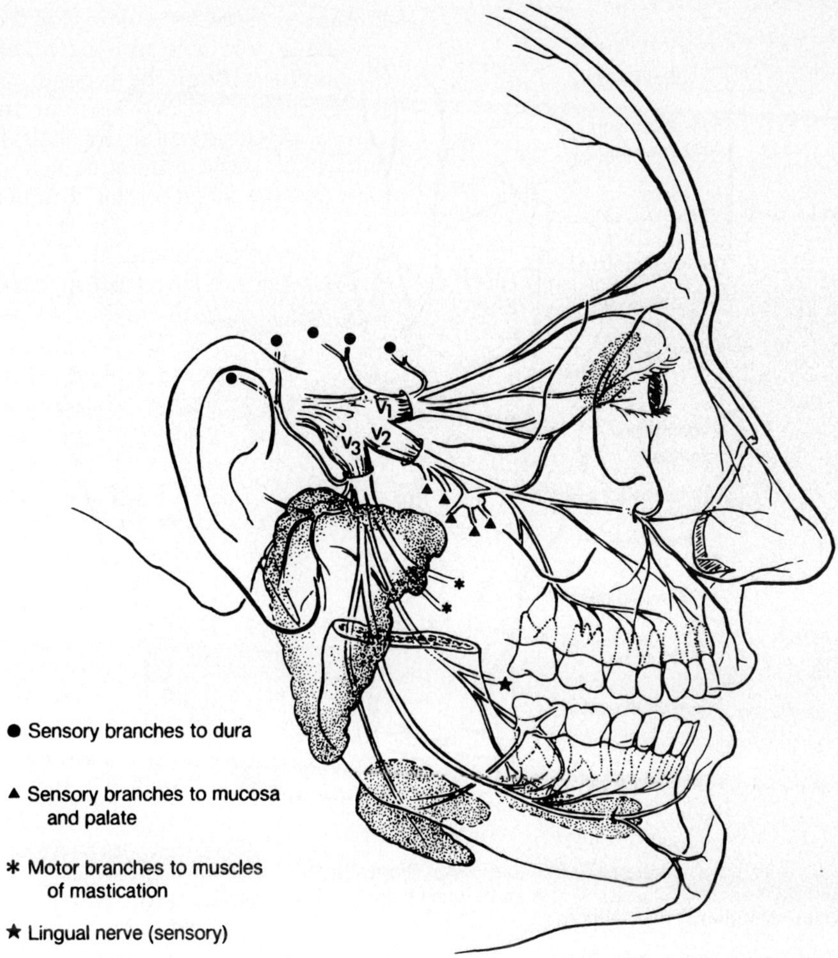

FIGURE 19–10. The peripheral sensory and motor branches of the trigeminal nerve. (From Liu GT: Anatomy and physiology of the trigeminal nerve. In: Miller NR, Newman NJ (eds): Walsh and Hoyt's Clinical Neuro-ophthalmology, 4th edition, pp 1595–1648. Baltimore, Williams & Wilkins, 1998, with permission.)

glion posterior to the cavernous sinus and exit the skull base via the foramen ovale. The fibers ramify through the deep face lateral to the middle pterygoid muscles then divide into branches that provide sensation to the skin around the mandible, chin, and ear (lingual, auriculotemporal, and mental branches), mucosa around the inner cheek (buccal branch), lower teeth (inferior alveolar nerve), and dura (meningeal branch) (Fig. 19–11). Parasympathetic fibers synapse within the otic and submandibular ganglia and project to the submandibular and parotid glands, respectively.

Central Projections. Proximal connections of the primary sensory neurons travel within the trigeminal root before synapsing in the brain stem in three sensory subnuclei that extend from the cervical spine to the pontomesencephalic junction. These include (1) the spinal (descending) trigeminal tract and nucleus, which is organized rostrally–caudally to receive fibers responsible for pain perception on the face from the inside out in an "onion-skin" fashion; (2) the principal sensory nucleus, which governs tactile sensation on the face; and (3) the mesencephalic nucleus, which mediates proprioception for V_3-innervated muscles. Neurons from these nuclei primarily cross and head rostrally within the ventral trigeminothalmic tract before reaching the ventral posteromedial nucleus of the thalamus. From there, thalamic neurons project to the facial portion of the somatosensory cortex.[105, 106]

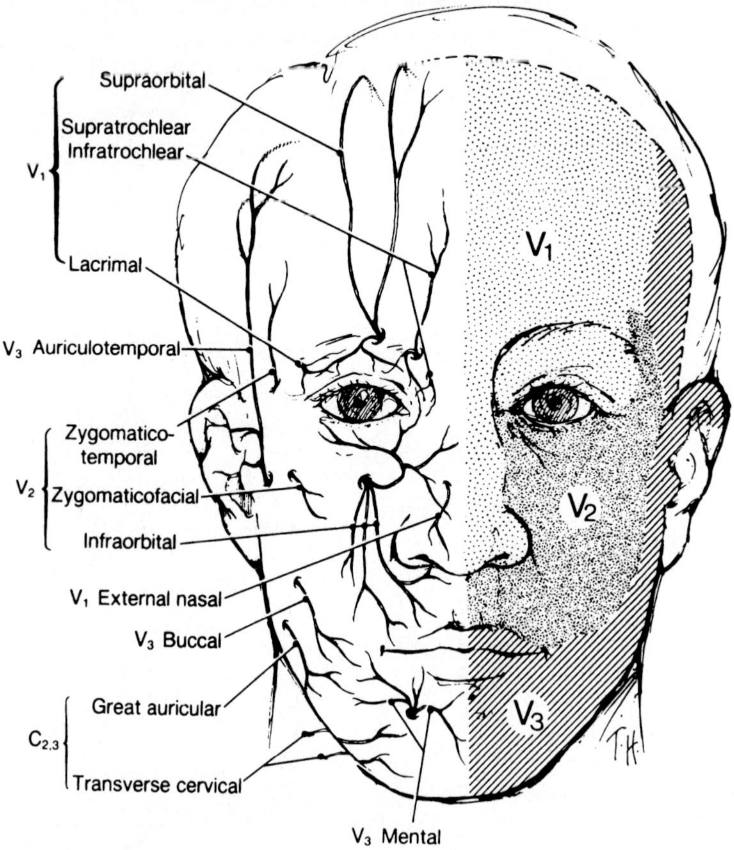

FIGURE 19–11. Sensory innervation of the face and scalp. (From Liu GT: Anatomy and physiology of the trigeminal nerve. In: Miller NR, Newman NJ (eds): Walsh and Hoyt's Clinical Neuro-ophthalmology, 4th edition, pp 1595–1648. Baltimore, Williams & Wilkins, 1998, with permission.)

Clinical Syndromes Causing Face Pain and Sensory Loss

Lesions involving the proximal portion of the trigeminal nerve usually present no diagnostic problem as concomitant neurologic features usually help in localization. For instance, thalamic lesions usually cause facial and ipsilateral hemibody numbness together. In Wallenberg's lateral medullary syndrome, the facial anesthesia is contralateral to the hemibody sensory loss. Syringobulbia, which can affect the nucleus of the spinal tract in the medulla, might cause ipsilateral facial anesthesia, tongue fasciculations, and weakness and atrophy of upper extremity muscles. Cavernous sinus and superior orbital fissure disturbances (see Chapter 15) and orbital apex lesions (see Chapter 18) will be characterized by concomitant ocular motor palsies or Horner syndrome.

The rest of this section will focus on the more diagnostically challenging conditions that might present with isolated facial pain or sensory loss in the trigeminal distribution.

Isolated Trigeminal Neuropathy

A benign, self-limited trigeminal neuropathy may be seen 7 to 21 days after a nonspecific viral illness or upper respiratory infection, similar to the postinfectious cranial neuropathy affecting the abducens, facial, or hypoglossal nerves. Diagnostic evaluations are unremarkable or demonstrate a mild CSF pleocytosis.[107] Symptoms usually resolve within 3 months. It is unclear whether these postinfectious neuropathies result from brain stem, gasserian ganglion, or peripheral nerve dysfunction.

Trigeminal sensory neuropathy may also occur in association with connective tissue disorders such as Sjögren syndrome, systemic sclerosis, and systemic lupus erythematosus.[108, 109]

On the basis of radiographic and electrophysiologic studies, the gasserian ganglion has been suggested as the site of injury in such cases.[110] A variety of other conditions may also produce a trigeminal sensory neuropathy, such as tuberculosis, syphilis, and Lyme disease. Likewise, neoplasms of the middle cranial fossa, such as schwannomas and meningiomas, may produce trigeminal sensory dysfunction. In young patients with facial sensory loss and lancinating pain, a central demyelinating process should be considered. Occasionally, such a symptom may be an initial manifestation of multiple sclerosis.

Facial parenthesis in the V_1 to V_3 distributions may occur in patients with peripheral nerve disorders such as the Guillain–Barré syndrome, diabetes, hereditary sensory-motor neuropathy,[111] and chronic inflammatory demyelinating polyneuropathy. Compressive or infiltrative conditions affecting the peripheral nerve branches may also produce circumscribed sensory loss.

Numb Chin Syndrome (Mental Neuropathy)

The numb chin syndrome typically results from a bony lesion affecting the mental foramen through which V_3 passes to innervate the chin and mandible.[112, 113] Patients often complain of numbness of chin that spreads to the lower lip but respects the midline. The numb chin syndrome is an ominous sign that may be produced by a variety of mass lesions, including metastatic lung, breast, and prostate carcinoma.[114] Lymphoma, particularly of the non-Hodgkin's type, may also be responsible for this syndrome. Primary bony malignancies such as osteosarcoma, fibrosarcoma, and plasmacytoma are other considerations. Development of the numb chin syndrome in a patient previously treated for cancer may signal a recurrence. Nonmalignant causes include granulomatous processes, collagen vascular disorders, trauma, periodontal disease, bony cysts, focal idiopathic osteolysis (Gorham's disease),[115] and sickle cell disease.

The numb cheek syndrome is a variant of the numb chin syndrome and results from a bony lesion involving the infraorbital foramen and the trigeminal branch V_2.[116] Patients with the numb chin or cheek syndrome require an aggressive evaluation. Careful examination of the oropharynx, dentition, and skin of the face should be performed. CT through the mandible with bone windows is the test of choice. Bone scans can occasionally be helpful when the CT scan is negative. A search for occult malignancy may be necessary to include CT of the chest and abdomen, prostate-specific antigen, and even bone marrow biopsy. Since brain stem lesions or carcinomatous meningitis may also cause focal trigeminal dysfunction, brain MRI and a lumbar puncture for cytology may be necessary.

Trigeminal Neuralgia

Trigeminal neuralgia (tic douloureux) describes a brief lancinating pain that occurs in the distribution of the trigeminal nerve. The pain is often triggered by chewing, speaking, or simply touching the affected area.[117] Most cases are idiopathic with a tendency to occur in the middle-aged or elderly population. The pain typically occurs in the second and third trigeminal divisions, lasts seconds, and may recur several times a day. Most cases are believed to result from irritation of the trigeminal nerve by a dolichoectatic superior cerebellar artery or an adjacent venous structure. Other causes include posterior fossa mass lesions,[118] pontine demyelination in multiple sclerosis,[119] and dental disease. In cases with a structural cause, one can usually detect an area of numbness in the trigeminal territory to distinguish them from idiopathic cases. Patients with multiple sclerosis also have an increased frequency of bilateral trigeminal neuralgia.[120]

Treatment. Many patients respond to carbamazepine, phenytoin, gabapentin, baclofen, or tricyclic antidepressants.[121, 122] Sometimes trigeminal neuralgia may spontaneously remit. Acupuncture may help in others. Patients who do not respond to medical therapy may require trigeminal nerve root or ganglion destruction. Glycerol injection,[123] radiofrequency thermocoagulation, and balloon occlusion are commonly used percutaneous methods.

In certain centers, microvascular decompression of the trigeminal nerve is the preferred surgical method because it tends to spare facial sensation and has an 80% to 90% chance of producing immediate relief.[117] Long-term outcome is also excellent as approximately 70% of patients will remain pain free 10 years later.[124] Major complications of microvascular surgery are low, but in one series included brain stem stroke (0.1%), hearing loss (1%), and abducens or trochlear nerve palsies (1%).[124]

Gamma knife radiosurgery is also being used in some centers.[125, 126] Early studies show excellent short-term results, with 70% to 80% of patients experiencing improvement or complete resolution of their pain.[126, 127] The mechanism of action of radiosurgery in trigeminal neuralgia is unclear, but it may reduce ephaptic transmission.[128] Complications are low, but 5% to 10% of patients may experience increased facial numbness or paresthesias.[126]

Herpes Zoster Ophthalmicus

Herpes zoster ophthalmicus results when the herpes virus lying dormant in the gasserian ganglion reactivates and spreads to the face along the V_1 dermatome. The infection is primarily observed in older patients, but young patients, particularly those who are immunocompromised, may also experience this unpleasant condition. The pain of herpes zoster ophthalmicus may begin a week before the onset of the rash.[129] In some cases the rash never appears. The pain, which is often described as aching or burning, may be quite severe but usually resolves in several weeks. Acutely, associated uveitis and keratitis should be excluded as alternative causes of pain.

Postherpetic Neuralgia. The pain of herpes zoster ophthalmicus may evolve directly into postherpetic neuralgia, but some patients have a grace period of several weeks. Postherpetic pain can be unrelenting and is often described as aching, burning, or boring in nature. In the affected dermatome, the patient may have an area of increased or decreased sensation. Postherpetic neuralgia may improve over months.[130] Unfortunately, the pain may persist indefinitely.

Treatment of postherpetic neuralgia can be extremely difficult. It is always reasonable to give the patient a trial of antiviral therapy for either the acute infection or the postherpetic phase.[129] Early in the infection, corticosteroids may be helpful to reduce the acute pain and possibly abort the delayed neuralgia. Topical capsaicin can be tried, but the patient has to be meticulous about avoiding cream in the eye. In one third of patients, the ointment intensifies the burning pain and cannot be tolerated.[130] Anticonvulsants (carbamazepine, gabapentin, phenytoin) and antidepressant compounds (eg, nortriptyline) may be effective in reducing postherpetic neuralgia.[130, 131] Acupuncture and biofeedback are some alternative approaches that occasionally work. Narcotics have be required for both the acute and chronic pain that complicates this disorder.

Atypical Facial Pain

There is a group of patients who have facial pain that defies classification. The pain tends to be deep and boring. It is separated from trigeminal neuralgia by its persistent nature and its tendency not to respect a single dermatome. Many patients relate their pain to prior surgery whether it be dental, sinus, or cosmetic in nature. Again, an underlying structural lesion needs to be carefully considered.

Treatment of atypical facial pain may be difficult. A variety of measures can be taken, with variable success. Trials of anticonvulsants and antidepressant compounds may be tried. Local nerve blocks usually only provide short-term relief. Again, alternative treatments, such as acupuncture, occasionally benefits the refractory patient. The pain may persist for years, but some patients have a spontaneous remission.

REFERENCES

1. Linet MS, Stewart WF, Celentano DD: An epidemiologic study of headache among adolescents and young adults. JAMA 1989;261:2211–2216.
2. Headache classification committee of the International Headache Society: Classification and diagnostic criteria for headache disorders, cranial neuralgias and facial pain. Cephalalgia 1988;8 (Suppl 7):1–96.
3. ICD-10 guide for headaches: Cephalalgia 1997;17 (Suppl 19):1–82.
4. Saper JR, Silberstein S, Gordon CD, et al: Handbook of Headache Management. Baltimore, Williams & Wilkins, 1993.
5. Lipton RB, Stewart WF: Migraine in the United States: A review of epidemiology and health care use. Neurology 1993;43(Suppl 1):S6–S10.
6. Stewart WF, Lipton RB, Simon D: Work-related disability. Results from the American migraine study. Cephalalgia 1996;16:231–238.
7. Lissovoy G, Lazarus SS: The economic cost of migraine: present state of knowledge. Neurology 1994;44(Suppl 4):S56–S62.
8. Stewart WF, Linet MS, Celentano DO: Age and sex-specific incidence rates of migraine with and without aura. Am J Epidemiol 1993;34:1111–1120.
9. Lipton RB, Stewart WF: Migraine headaches: epidemiology and comorbidity. Clin Neurosci 1998;5:2–9.
10. Stewart WF, Lipton RB, Lieberman J: Variation in migraine prevalence by race. Neurology 1996;47: 52–59.
11. Ottman R, Lipton RB: Cormorbidity of migraine and epilepsy. Neurology 1994;44:2105–2110.
12. Welch KMA: Relationship of stroke and migraine. Neurology 1994;44(Suppl 7):S33-S36.

13. Breslau N, Davis GC: Migraine, physical health and psychiatric disorders. A prospective epidemiologic study of young adults. J Psychiatr Res 1993;27: 211–221.
14. Peroutka SJ, Howell TA: The genetic evaluation of migraine: clinical database requirements. In: Rose FC (ed): Towards Migraine 2000, pp 34-48. Amsterdam, Elsevier Science, 1996.
15. Joutel A, Bousser MG, Biousse V, et al: A gene for familial hemiplegic migraine maps to chromosome 19. Nature Genet 1993;5:40–45.
16. Ophoff RA, Terwindt GM, Vergouwe MN, et al: Familial hemiplegic migraine and episodic ataxia type 2 are caused by mutation in the calcium channel gene CACNLA4. Cell 1996;87:543–552.
17. Ducros A, Joutel A, Vahedi K, et al: Mapping of a second locus for familial hemiplegic migraine to 1q21–q23 and evidence of further heterogeneity. Ann Neurol 1997;42:885–890.
18. Gardner K, Barmada MM, Ptacek LJ, et al: A new locus for hemiplegic migraine maps to chromosome 1q31. Neurology 1997;49:1231–1238.
19. Lance JW: Current concepts of migraine pathogenesis. Neurology 1993;43(Suppl 1):S11-S15.
20. Moskowitz MA: Neurogenic inflammation in the pathophysiology and treatment of migraine. Neurology 1993;43(Suppl 1):S16–S20.
21. Goadsby PJ, Knight YE: Direct evidence for central sites of action of zolmitriptan (311C90): An autoradiographic study in cat. Cephalalgia 1997;17:153–158.
22. Weiller C, May A, Limmroth V, et al: Brainstem activation in spontaneous human migraine attacks. Nature Med 1995;1:658–660.
23. Goadsby PJ, Uddmann R, Edvinsson L: Cerebral vasodilation in the cat appears to result from nitric oxide released from parasympathetic nerves. Brain Res 1996 1996;707:110–118.
24. Olesen J: Understanding the biologic basis of migraine (editorial). N Engl J Med 1994;331:1713–1714.
25. Welch KMA, Barkley GL, Tepley N, et al: Central neurogenic mechanisms of migraine. Neurology 1993;43(Suppl 1):S21–S25.
26. Leao AAP: Spreading depression of activity in the cerebral cortex. J Neurophysiol 1944;7:359–390.
27. Lashley KS: Patterns of cerebral integration indicated by the scotomas of migraine. Arch Neurol Psychiatry 1941;46:331–339.
28. Liu GT, Schatz NJ, Galetta SL, et al: Persistent positive visual phenomena in migraine. Neurology 1995; 45:664–668.
29. Carolei A, Marini C, De Matteis G: History of migraine and risk of cerebral ischaemia in young adults. The Italian National Research Council Study Group on stroke in the young. Lancet 1996;347:1503–1506.
30. Pettiti DB, Sidney S, Bernstein A: Stroke in users of low dose oral contraceptives. N Engl J Med 1996; 335:8–15.
31. Tzourio C, Tehindrazanarivielo A, Iglesias S, et al: Case control study of migraine and risk of ischaemia stroke in young women. Br Med J 1995;310:830–833.
32. Collaborative group for the study of stroke in young women: JAMA 1975;231:718–720.
33. Chang CL, Donaghy M, Poulter N, et al: Migraine and stroke in young women: case-control study. BMJ 1999;318:13–18.
34. Hupp SL, Kline LB, Corbett JJ: Visual disturbances of migraine. Surv Ophthalmol 1989;33:221–236.
35. Krapin D: Occlusion of the central retinal artery in migraine. N Engl J Med 1964;270:359.
36. Lewis RA, Vijayan N, Watson C, et al: Visual field loss in migraine. Ophthalmology 1989;96:321–326.
37. Burger SK, Saul RF, Selhorst JB, et al: Transient monocular blindness caused by vasospasm. N Engl J Med 1991;12:870–873.
38. Tomsak RL, Jergens PB: Benign recurrent transient monocular blindness: a possible variant of acephalgic migraine. Headache 1987;27:66–69.
39. Winterkorn JMS, Kupersmith MJ, Wirtschafter JD, et al: Treatment of vasospastic amaurosis fugax with calcium channel blockers. N Engl J Med 1993;329: 396–398.
40. Friedman AP, Harter DH, Merritt HH: Ophthalmoplegic migraine. Arch Neurol 1962;7:320–327.
41. Troost BT: Migraine and other headaches. In: Glaser JS (ed): Neuro-ophthalmology, 2nd edition, pp 487–518. Philadelphia, JB Lippincott, 1990.
42. Bickerstaff ER: Basilar artery migraine. Lancet 1961;1:15–17.
43. Johnson GD: Medical management of migraine-related dizziness and vertigo. Laryngoscope 1998;108 (Jan. suppl):1–28.
44. Cutrer FM, Baloh RW: Migraine-associated dizziness. Headache 1992;32:300–304.
45. Baloh RW: Neurotology of migraine. Headache 1997;37:615–621.
46. Lipton RB, Stewart WF, Ryan RE, Jr, et al: Efficacy and safety of acetaminophen, aspirin, and caffeine in alleviating migraine headache pain: three double-blind, randomized, placebo-controlled trials. Arch Neurol 1998;55:210–217.
47. Maizels M, Scott B, Cohen W, et al: Intranasal lidocaine for treatment of migraine: a randomized, double-blind, controlled trial. JAMA 1996;276:319-321.
48. Pfaffenrath V, Cunin G, Sjonell G, et al: Efficacy and safety of sumatriptan tablets (25 mg, 50 mg, and 100 mg) in the acute treatment of migraine: defining the optimum doses of oral sumatriptan. Headache 1998;38:184–190.
49. MaassenVanDenBrink A, Reekers M, Bax WA, et al: Coronary side-effect potential of current and prospective antimigraine drugs. Circulation 1998;98: 25–30.
50. Lewis PJ, Barrington SF, Marsden PK, et al: A study of the effects of sumatriptan on myocardial perfusion in healthy female migraineurs using 13NH3 positron emission tomography. Neurology 1997;48:1542–1550.
51. Ryan R, Elkind A, Baker CC, et al: Sumatriptan nasal spray for the acute treatment of migraine. Results of two clinical studies. Neurology 1997;49:1225–1230.
52. Massiou H, on behalf of study groups: A comparison of sumatriptan nasal spray 20 mg and intranasal dihydroergotamine in the acute treatment of migraine. Poster presentation at the 3rd European Headache Conference, Sardinia, 1996; June 5–8.
53. Rapoport AM, Ramadan NM, Adelman JU, et al: Optimizing the dose of zolmitriptan (Zomig, 311C90) for the acute treatment of migraine. A multicenter, double-blind, placebo-controlled, dose range-finding study. The 017 Clinical Trial Study Group. Neurology 1997;49:1210–1218.
54. Solomon GD, Cady RK, Klapper JA, et al: Clinical efficacy and tolerability of 2.5 mg zolmitriptan for the acute treatment of migraine. The 042 Clinical Trial Study Group. Neurology 1997;49:1219–1225.
55. Mathew NT, Asgharnejad M, Peykamian M, et al: Naratriptan is effective and well tolerated in the acute

treatment of migraine. Results of a double-blind, placebo-controlled, crossover study. The Naratriptan S2WA3003 Study Group. Neurology 1997;49:1485–1490.

56. Jackson NC: A comparison of oral eletriptan (vk-116,044)(20–80 mg) and oral sumatriptan (100 mg) in the acute treatment of migraine (for the eletriptan steering committee). Cephalalgia 1996;16:368.
57. Kramer MS, Matzura-Wolfe D, Polis A, et al: A placebo-controlled crossover study of rizatriptan in the treatment of multiple migraine attacks. Rizatriptan Multiple Attack Study Group. Neurology 1998; 51:773–781.
58. Ahrens SP, Farmer MV, Williams DL, et al: Efficacy and safety of rizatriptan wafer for the acute treatment of migraine. Rizatriptan Wafer Protocol 049 Study Group. Cephalalgia 1999;19:525–530.
59. Moskowitz MA, Cutrer FM: Attacking migraine headache from beginning to end (editorial). Neurology 1997;49:1193–1195.
60. Hamalainen ML, Hoppu K, Santavuori P: Sumatriptan for migraine attacks in children: a randomized placebo-controlled study. Do children with migraine respond to oral sumatriptan differently from adults? Neurology 1997;48:1100–1103.
61. Ueberall MA, Wenzel D: Intranasal sumatriptan for the acute treatment of migraine in children. Neurology 1999;52:1507–1510.
62. Peroutka SJ: Dopamine and migraine. Neurology 1997;49:650–656.
63. Welch KMA: Drug therapy of migraine. N Engl J Med 1993;329:1476–1483.
64. Matts SG: Metoclopramide in the treatment of migraine. Practitioner 1974;212:887–890.
65. Richman PB, Reischel U, Ostrow A, et al: Droperidol for acute migraine headache. Am J Emer Med 1999;17:398–400.
66. Ison PJ, Peroutka SJ: Neurotransmitter receptor binding studies predict antiemetic efficacy and side-effects. Cancer Treat Rep 1986;70:637–641.
67. The subcutaneous sumatriptan international study group: Treatment of migraine attacks with sumatriptan. N Engl J Med 1991;325:316–326.
68. Cady RK, Wendt JK, Kirchner JR, et al: Treatment of acute migraine with subcutaneous sumatriptan. JAMA 1991;265:2831–2835.
69. Wang SJ, Silberstein SD, Young WB: Droperidol treatment of status migrainosus and refractory migraine. Headache 1997;37:377–382.
70. Triner WR, Bartfield JM, Birdwell M, et al: Nitrous oxide for the treatment of acute migraine headache. Am J Emerg Med 1999;17:252–254.
71. Diamond S, Kudrow L, Stevens J, et al: Long term study of propranolol in the treatment of migraine. Headache 1982;22:268–271.
72. Jonsdottir M, Meyer JS, Rogers RL: Efficacy, side effects and tolerance compared during headache treatment with three different calcium blockers. Headache 1987;27:364–369.
73. Couch JR, Hassanein RS: Amitriptyline in migraine prophylaxis. Arch Neurol 1979;36:695–699.
74. Raskin NH: Acute and prophylactic treatment of migraine: Practical approaches and pharmacologic rationale. Neurology 1996;43:93–96, 101–104.
75. Mathew NT, Saper JR, Silberstein SD, et al: Migraine prophylaxis with divalproex. Arch Neurol 1995; 52:281–286.
76. Mathew N: Gabapentin in migraine prophylaxis. Cephalalgia 1996;16:397.
77. Wheeler SD, Carrazana EJ: Topiramate-treated cluster headache. Neurology 1999;53:234–236.
78. Schoenen J, Jacquy J, Lenaerts M: Effectiveness of high-dose riboflavin in migraine prophylaxis: a randomized controlled trial. Neurology 1998;50:466–469.
79. Pfaffenrath V, Wessely P, Meyer C, et al: Magnesium in the prophylaxis of migraine. A double blind placebo controlled study. Cephalalgia 1996;16:436–440.
80. Newman LC, Lipton RB, Lay CL, et al: A pilot study of oral sumatriptan as intermittent prophylaxis of menstruation-related migraine. Neurology 1998;51: 307–308.
81. Silberstein SD, Lipton RB, Sliwinski M: Classification of daily and near-daily headaches: field trial and revised IHS criteria. Neurology 1996;47:871–875.
82. Schulte-Mattler WJ, Wieser T, Zierz S: Treatment of tension-type headache with botulinum toxin: a pilot study. Eur J Med Res 1999;4:183–186.
83. Silberstein SD, Lipton RB, Goadsby PJ: Headache in Clinical Practice. Oxford, ISIS Medical Media, 1998.
84. Mani S, Deeter J: Arteriovenous malformation of the brain presenting as a cluster headache—a case report. Headache 1982;22:184–185.
85. Kuritzky A: Cluster headache-like pain caused by an upper cervical meningioma. Cephalalgia 1984;4:185–186.
86. West P, Todman D: Chronic cluster associated with a vertebral artery aneurysm. Headache 1991;31: 210–212.
87. Koenigsberg AD, Solomon GD, Kosmorsky GO: Pseudoaneurysm within the cavernous sinus presenting as cluster headache. Headache 1994;34: 111–113.
88. Mathew NT, Hurt W: Percutaneous radiofrequency trigeminal gangliorhizolysis in intractable cluster headache. Headache 1988;28:328–331.
89. Goadsby PJ, Lipton RB: A review of paroxysmal hemicranias, SUNCT syndrome and other short lasting headaches with autonomic feature, including new cases. Brain 1997;120:193–209.
90. Raps EC, Rogers JD, Galetta SL, et al: The clinical spectrum of unruptured intracranial aneurysms. Arch Neurol 1993;50:265–268.
91. Gould JD, Silberstein SD: Unilateral hypnic headache: a case study. Neurology 1997;49:1749–1751.
92. Rando TA, Fishman RA: Spontaneous intracranial hypotension: report of two cases and review of literature. Neurology 1992;42:481–487.
93. Case records of the Massachusetts General Hospital: Case 2-1998. N Engl J Med 1998;338:180–188.
94. Horton JC, Fishman RA: Neurovisual findings in the syndrome of spontaneous intracranial hyptension from dural cerebrospinal fluid leak. Ophthalmology 1994;101:244–251.
95. Pannullo SC, Reich JB, Krol G, et al: MRI changes in intracranial hypotension. Neurology 1993;43:919–926.
96. Krause I, Kornreich L, Waldman D, et al: MRI meningeal enhancement with intracranial hypotension caused by lumbar puncture. Pediatr Neurol 1997;16:163–165.
97. Kosmorsky G: Spontaneous intracranial hypotension. A review. J Neuro-ophthalmol 1995;15:79–83.
98. Hochman MS, Naidich TP: Diffuse meningeal enhancement in patients with overdraining, longstanding ventricular shunts. Neurology 1999;52: 406–409.

99. Wang SJ, Silberstein SD, Patterson S, et al: Idiopathic intracranial hypertension without papilledema: a case control study in a headache center. Neurology 1998;51:245–249.
100. Swartz NG, Beck RW, Savino PJ, et al: Pain in anterior ischemic optic neuropathy. J Neuro-ophthalmol 1995;15:9–10.
101. Drummond P: Photophobia and autonomic responses to facial pain in migraine. Brain 1997;120: 1857–1864.
102. Burr HS, Robinson GB: An anatomical study of the gasserian ganglion, with particular reference to the nature and extent of Meckel's cave. Anat Rec 1925;29:269–282.
103. Gudmundsson K, Rhoton AL, Rushton JG: Detailed anatomy of the intracranial portion of the trigeminal nerve. J Neurosurg 1971;35:592–600.
104. Feindel W, Penfield W, McNaughton F: The tentorial nerves and localization of intracranial pain in man. Neurology 1960;10:555–563.
105. Liu GT: Anatomy and physiology of the trigeminal nerve. In: Miller NR, Newman NJ (eds): Walsh and Hoyt's Clinical Neuro-ophthalmology, 4th edition, pp 1595–1648. Baltimore, Williams & Wilkins, 1998.
106. Crino PB, Galetta SL: CN V: The trigeminal nerve. In: Goetz GC, Pappert EJ (eds): Textbook of Clinical Neurology, pp 155–170. Philadelphia, WB Saunders, 1998.
107. Blau JN, Harris M, Kennett S: Trigeminal sensory neuropathy. N Engl J Med 1969;281:873–877.
108. Leck BRF, Hughes RAC, Murray NMF: Trigeminal sensory neuropathy. Brain 1987;110:1463–1485.
109. Olney RK: AAEM minimonograph #38: neuropathies in connective tissue disease. Muscle Nerve 1992; 15:531–542.
110. Forster C, Brandt T, Hund E, et al: Trigeminal sensory neuropathy in connective tissue disease; evidence for the site of the lesion. Neurology 1996;46:270–271.
111. Coffey RJ, Fromm GH: Familial trigeminal neuralgia and Charcot–Marie–Tooth neuropathy. Report of two families and review. Surg Neurol 1991;35:49–53.
112. Massey EW, Moore J, Schold SC: Mental neuropathy. Neurology 1981;31:1277–1281.
113. Brazis PW, Vogler JB, Shaw KE: The "numb cheek–lip–lower lid" syndrome. Neurology 1991;41:327–328.
114. Lossos A, Siegal T: Numb chin syndrome in cancer patients: etiology, response to treatment, and prognostic significance. Neurology 1992;42:1181–1184.
115. Malter IM: Massive osteolysis of the mandible: report of a case. J Am Dental Assoc 1972;85:148–150.
116. Campbell WW: The numb cheek syndrome: a sign of infraorbital neuropathy. Neurology 1986;36:421–423.
117. Walchenbach R, Voormolen JHC: Surgical treatment for trigeminal neuralgia: We must have a direct, randomized comparison between decompression and thermocoagulation. Br Med J 1996;313:1027–1028.
118. Cheng TMW, Cascino TL, Onofrio BM: Comprehensive study of diagnosis and treatment of trigeminal neuralgia secondary to tumors. Neurology 1993;43:2298–2302.
119. Gass A, Kitchen N, MacManus DG, et al: Trigeminal neuralgia in patients with multiple sclerosis: lesion localization with magnetic resonance imaging. Neurology 1997;49:1142–1144.
120. Hooge JP, Redekop WK: Trigeminal neuralgia in multiple sclerosis. Neurology 1995;45:1294–1296.
121. Sist T, Filadora V, Miner M, et al: Gabapentin for idiopathic trigeminal neuralgia: report of two cases. Neurology 1997;48:1467–1471.
122. Khan OA: Gabapentin relieves trigeminal neuralgia in multiple sclerosis patients. Neurology 1998; 51:611–614.
123. Cappabianca P, Spaziante R, Graziussi G, et al: Percutaneous retrogasserian glycerol rhizolysis for treatment of trigeminal neuralgia. Technique and results in 191 patients. J Neurosci 1995;39:37–45.
124. Barker FG, Jannetta PJ, Bissonette DJ, et al: The long-term outcome of microvascular decompression for trigeminal neuralgia. N Engl J Med 1996;334:1077–1083.
125. Maciewicz R, Scrivani S: Trigeminal neuralgia: gamma radiosurgery may provide new options for treatment (editorial). Neurology 1997;48:565–566.
126. Kondziolka D, Perez B, Flickinger JC, et al: Gamma knife radiosurgery for trigeminal neuralgia. Results and expectations. Arch Neurol 1998;55:1524–1529.
127. Young RF, Vermeulen SS, Grimm P, et al: Gamma knife radiosurgery for treatment of trigeminal neuralgia. Idiopathic and tumor related. Neurology 1997; 48:608–614.
128. Tenser RB: Trigeminal neuralgia. Mechanisms of treatment. Neurology 1998;51:17–19.
129. Straus SE: Shingles: sorrows, salves, and solutions. JAMA 1993;269:1836–1839.
130. Robertson DR, George CF: Treatment of post herpetic neuralgia in the elderly. Br Med Bull 1990;46:113–123.
131. Rowbotham M, Harden N, Stacey B, et al: Gabapentin for the treatment of postherpetic neuralgia. A randomized controlled trial. JAMA 1998;280:1837–1842.
132. Dieterich M, Brandt T: Episodic vertigo related to migraine (90 cases): vestibular migraine? Journal of Neurology 1999;246:883–892.
133. Dooley M, Faulds D: Rizatriptan: a review of its efficacy in the management of migraine. Drugs 1999; 58:699–723.
134. Boyle CA: Management of menstrual migraine. Neurology 1999;53 (Suppl 1):S14–18.
135. Leone M, D'Amico D, Frediani F, et al: Verapamil in the prophylaxis of episodic cluster headache: a double-blind study versus placebo. Neurology 2000;54:1382–1385.
136. Mokri B: Spontaneous cerebrospinal fluid leaks; from intracranial hypotension to cerebrospinal fluid hypovolemia—evolution of a concept. Mayo Clin Proc 1999;74:1113–1123.
137. Goadsby PJ, Ferrari MD, Olesen J, et al: Eletriptan in acute migraine: a double-blind, placebo-controlled comparison to sumatriptan. Neurology 2000;54: 156–163.
138. Silberstein SD, Niknam R, Rozen TD, et al: Cluster headache with aura. Neurology 2000;54:219–221.

Index

Page numbers in *italics* refer to figures; page numbers followed by t refer to tables; page numbers followed by cp refer to color plates.

ISBN 0-7216-6533-0

90038

9 780721 665337